Chronic obstructive pulmonary disease

Second edition

Edited by

Peter MA Calverley MB FRCP FRCPE
Professor of Medicine, Pulmonary and
Rehabilitation Research Group, University of
Liverpool, UK

William MacNee MB ChB MD FRCP FRCPE
Professor of Respiratory and Environmental
Medicine, University of Edinburgh, UK

Neil B Pride MD FRCP
Emeritus Professor of Respiratory Medicine
National Heart and Lung Institute, Imperial College,
London, UK

and

Stephen I Rennard MD
Larson Professor, Pulmonary and Critical Care
Medicine Section, University of Nebraska Medical
Center, Omaha, NE, USA

ARNOLD

A member of the Hodder Headline Group

LONDON

First published in Great Britain in 1995 by Chapman & Hall
Reprinted in 1999 by Arnold
This second edition published in 2003 by Arnold,
a member of the Hodder Headline Group,
338 Euston Road, London NW1 3BH

http://www.arnoldpublishers.com

Distributed in the United States of America by
Oxford University Press Inc.,
198 Madison Avenue, New York, NY10016
Oxford is a registered trademark of Oxford University Press

Whilst the advice and information in this book are believed to be
true and accurate at the date of going to press, neither the
author[s] nor the publisher can accept any legal responsibility
or liability for any errors or omissions that may be made.
In particular (but without limiting the generality of the preceding
disclaimer) every effort has been made to check drug dosages;
however it is still possible that errors have been missed.
Furthermore, dosage schedules are constantly being revised and
new side-effects recognized. For these reasons the reader is
strongly urged to consult the drug companies' printed
instructions before administering any of the drugs recommended
in this book.

British Library Cataloguing in Publication Data
A catalogue record for this book is available from the British Library

Library of Congress Cataloging-in-Publication Data
A catalog record for this book is available from the Library of Congress

ISBN 0 340 80718 0

1 2 3 4 5 6 7 8 9 10

Commissioning Editor: Joanna Koster
Development Editor: Sarah Burrows
Project Management: Nora Naughton, Samantha Gear
Production Controller: Deborah Smith
Cover Design: Lee-May Lim

Typeset in 10/12 Minion by Charon Tec Pvt Ltd., Chennai, India
Printed and bound in the UK by Butler & Tanner

What do you think about this book? Or any other Arnold title?
Please send your comments to feedback.arnold@hodder.co.uk

This book is dedicated to George William Tatam,
who faced this terrible disease with such dignity and courage.

Contents

Contributors

JA Barberà MD
Servei de Pneumologia, Hospital Clinic, Villarroel, Barcelona, Spain

Peter J Barnes DM
Professor, Department of Thoracic Medicine, National Heart and Lung Institute, Imperial College, London, UK

A Sonia Buist MD
Professor of Medicine, Department of Pulmonary and Critical Care Medicine, Oregon Health and Science University, Portland, OR, USA

P Sherwood Burge MSc MD FFOM FRCP FRCPE
Director of the Occupational Lung Disease Unit, Birmingham Heartlands Hospital, Birmingham, UK

Peter MA Calverley MB FRCP FRCPE
Professor of Medicine, Pulmonary and Rehabilitation Research Group, University of Liverpool; and University Clinical Departments, University Hospital Aintree, Liverpool, UK

Bartolome R Celli MD
Chief Pulmonary and Critical Care Medicine, St Elizabeth's Medical Center, Professor of Medicine, Tufts University; and Pulmonary and Critical Care Division, St Elizabeth's Medical Center, Boston, MA, USA

Paul A Corris MB, FRCP (LOND & EDIN)
Professor of Thoracic Medicine, University of Newcastle-upon-Tyne and Freeman Hospital, Newcastle-upon-Tyne, UK

Richard Costello MB MD FRCPI
Consultant Chest Physician and Senior Lecturer, Department of Medicine, Royal College of Surgeons in Ireland, Beaumont Hospital, Dublin, Ireland

David M Daughton MS
Pulmonary and Critical Care Medicine Section, Department of Internal Medicine, University of Nebraska Medical Center, Omaha, NE, USA

Asger Dirksen MD DMSc
Professor of Respiratory Medicine, Department of Respiratory Medicine, Gentofte University Hospital, Hellerup, Denmark

Karen-Lisbeth Dirksen MD
Chief Radiologist, Department of Radiology, Gentofte University Hospital, Hellerup, Denmark

Kenneth Donaldson BSC PhD DSC FIBiol FRCPath FFOM
Professor, ELEGI Colt Research Laboratories, Napier University, Edinburgh, UK

Neil J Douglas MD FRCP FRCPE
Professor of Respiratory and Sleep Medicine, The University of Edinburgh; and Respiratory Medicine Unit, Department of Medicine, Royal Infirmary, Edinburgh, UK

Mark W Elliott MD FRCP
Consultant Respiratory Physician, St James University Hospital, Leeds, UK

William J Gibbons MD
Assistant Professor of Medicine, Division of Pulmonary, Critical Care and Sleep Medicine, State University of New York at Buffalo, Kaleida Health, Buffalo General Hospital, Buffalo, NY, USA

Adam Hill MD MRCP
Consultant Physician, Department of Respiratory Medicine, Royal Infirmary Edinburgh, UK

James C Hogg MD
UBC McDonald Research Laboratory/iCAPTURE Centre, St Paul's Hospital, Vancouver, BC, Canada

Paul W Jones
Professor of Medicine, Department of Physiological Medicine, St George's Hospital Medical School, London, UK

Peter Lange MD PhD
Clinical Head, Department of Respiratory Medicine, Hvidovre University Hospital, Denmark

David A Lomas PhD FRCP FMedsci
Professor of Respiratory Biology/Honorary Consultant Physician, Respiratory Medicine Unit, Department of Medicine, University of Cambridge; and Cambridge Institute for Medical Research, Wellcome Trust, Cambridge, UK

William MacNee MB ChB MD FRCP FRCPE
Professor of Respiratory and Environmental Medicine,
ELEGI, Colt Research Laboratories, University of Edinburgh
Medical School, Edinburgh, UK

M Jeffery Mador MD
Associate Professor of Medicine, Division of Pulmonary,
Critical Care and Sleep Medicine, State University of
New York at Buffalo, Veterans Administration Medical
Center, Buffalo, NY, USA

Joseph Milic-Emili CM MD FRSC
Professor, Departments of Physiology and Medicine,
Meakins-Christie Laboratories, McGill University, Montreal,
Quebec, Canada

John Moxham MD FRCP
Department of Respiratory Medicine,
Kings College Hospital, London

Robert Naeije MD
Professor, Dept des Soins Intensifs, Hopital Universitaire
Erasme, Brussels, Belgium

Denis E O'Donnell MD FRCP(I) FRCP(C)
Professor (Medicine and Physiology), Head, Division of
Respiratory and Critical Care Medicine, Department of
Medicine, Queen's University, Kingston, ON, Canada

Michael G Pearson
Aintree Chest Centre, University Hospital Aintree,
Liverpool, UK

Michael I Polkey PhD MRCP
Consultant Physician and Reader in Respiratory Medicine,
Royal Brompton Hospital/National Heart and Lung Institute,
London, UK

Dirkje Postma MD
Professor, Department of Pulmonary Diseases,
University Hospital, Groningen, The Netherlands

Neil B Pride MD FRCP
Emeritus Professor of Respiratory Medicine, National
Heart and Lung Institute, Imperial College, London, UK

Irfan Rahman
ELEGI, Colt Research Laboratories,
MRC Centre for Inflammation Research,
Respiratory Medicine Unit,
University of Edinburgh Medical School, Edinburgh, UK

Stephen I Rennard MD
Larson Professor, Pulmonary and Critical Care Medicine
Section, Department of Internal Medicine, University of
Nebraska Medical Center, Omaha, NE, USA

Josep Roca
Servei de Preumologia, Hospital Clinic,
Villarroel, Barcelona, Spain

Roberto Rodriguez-Roisin
Professor, Servei de Pneumologia, Hospital Clinic,
Villarroel, Barcelona, Spain

Marina Saetta MD
Instituto di Medicina del Lavoro, Servizio di Fisiopatologia
Respiratoria, Universita di Padova, Italy

Edwin K Silverman MD PhD
Assistant Professor of Medicine, Channing Laboratory and
Pulmonary and Critical Care Division,
Brigham and Womens Hospital, Boston, USA

Gordon L Snider MD
Maurice B Strauss Professor of Medicine, Boston University
School of Medicine, Boston, USA

Robert A Stockley MD DSc FRCP
Professor, Department of Respiratory Medicine, Lung
Resource Centre, Queen Elizabeth Hospital, Birmingham

Jørgen Vestbo MD PhD
Professor, North West Lung Centre,
Wythenshawe Hospital, Manchester, UK

Katherine A Webb MSC
Senior Research Associate, Respiratory Investigation Unit,
Department of Medicine, Queen's University, Kingston,
Ontario, Canada

Jadwiga A Wedzicha MA MD FRCP
Professor of Respiratory Medicine, St Bartholomew's and
Royal London School of Medicine,
St Bartholomew's Hospital, London, UK

Emiel FM Wouters MD
Department of Pulmonology, University of Maastricht,
Maastricht, The Netherlands

Jan Zieliski MD PhD
Professor of Medicine, Department of Respiratory
Medicine, National Research Institute of Tuberculosis and
Lung Disease, Warsaw, Poland

Foreword to first edition

Historically, the recognition of pulmonary emphysema and, less certainly, of chronic bronchitis can probably be attributed to Laennec. The two conditions became coupled and the relationship confused throughout the latter part of the last century and the first part of this. In the 1940s, the common story was as follows. Acute bronchitis is a bacterial infection, usually following viral upper respiratory infection. In some people, this acute bronchitis invariably followed such upper respiratory infections and persisted for increasingly long periods until, for most of the winter, they had cough and sputum. They were then said to have chronic bronchitis. This went on for years until they began to have troublesome breathlessness. At which time, it was thought that their lungs were destroyed by emphysema. This put a strain on the right heart and they became edematous and were said to have cor pulmonale. Usually, they died during an acute infection, and probably in respiratory failure but blood gases were not, of course, measurable until the 1960s. Throughout the 1930s, 1940s and 1950s, the situation was complicated by a difference in verbal habits on the two sides of the Atlantic. In Britain, many patients were said to have chronic bronchitis who, in the United States, were said to have emphysema. The situation was greatly clarified by the CIBA Symposium in 1958 which gave a sound basis for the discrimination of chronic bronchitis, emphysema and asthma, and led to the adoption of terms such as chronic airflow obstruction or chronic obstructive lung disease. Recognition of the common factor of chronic airflow obstruction or limitation can fairly be attributed to the Bellevue group in the late 1930s, and of emphysema and its subtypes to Gough.

In the late 1950s, it was recognized that bronchitis and emphysema did not necessarily follow each other in the order outlined above. Some patients died with little evidence of emphysema; some patients with emphysema had little bronchitis. With the advent of methods for measuring blood gases, it also became recognized that the hypoxemia which was quite profound during acute infections required careful management; otherwise the patient died in CO_2 narcosis. It is to be wondered that until the 1950s cigarette smoking was not linked as an important factor in either chronic bronchitis or emphysema.

The chapters in this book fill out this sketch, give authoritative accounts of recent developments, point out the areas of ignorance and thus indicate the likely paths of future research.

When I was a student and houseman, chronic bronchitis and emphysema were unfashionable diseases, and not generally seen in teaching hospitals and the vestige of this neglect is perhaps the fact that this is one of the few books devoted to the subject of chronic airflow obstruction.

E.J.M. Campbell

Preface to first edition

Chronic obstructive pulmonary disease (COPD) is one of the commonest respiratory diseases of the developed world. It kills many more people each year than does bronchial asthma and has a similar prevalence in adults but has not attracted an equivalent amount of attention from either research funding agencies or textbook writers. This surprising state of affairs is likely to have several causes COPD is perceived as being a 'dull' chronic illness with undramatic physical signs which result from largely irreversible lung damage. As a result prognosis cannot usually be radically altered and is often the patient's own fault for having smoked. We reject this view and this book is an attempt to redress this unduly pessimistic perception. It cannot hope to be comprehensive given the wide range of disciplines needed to understand all aspects of COPD but we hope that the reader will find insights into scientific basis of this illness and some guidance on the practical care of these patients.

Much of the scientific basis of COPD which is the subject of the first chapters is far from settled. Even the definition, particularly the borderlands between COPD and persistent asthma, remains controversial (indeed the remaining chapters diverge from Chapter 1 in *not* following the recommendation to include incompletely reversible asthma as a sub-category of COPD). Readers coming fresh to the field may be surprised that it is still unclear whether airway disease (Chapter 3) or emphysema (Chapter 2) is the more important factor determining obstruction; perhaps we are on the edge of some quantitative morphology of airways and airspace with increasing concentration on the microscopic rather than macroscopic changes in lung structure ("the doughnut, not the hole"). Epidemiologic studies not only perform their traditional role of defining the scale of the problem, but have been important in defining the "preclinical" course of the disease. The proteolytic theory of emphysema has provided a rational biochemical basis for the disease but remains a reasonable theory rather than an established fact, a point stressed in Chapter 6. Apart from their intellectual value these differing pathologic, etiologic and biochemical approaches have identified areas where intervention may modify the natural history. The most familiar is smoking cessation but modifications of small airways "inflammation" by corticosteroids or even

enhancement of antiprotease activity by appropriate supplementations are all under active investigation.

Physiologic abnormalities in lung mechanics gas exchange and ventilatory control have been exhaustively studied and explain most of the clinical features with which the COPD patient presents. Even here new data are still emerging to challenge previous orthodoxy. The role of pulmonary hyperinflation especially in acute and chronic respiratory failure in COPD, the new understanding of ventilation-perfusion abnormalities using the multiple inert gas elimination technique and the importance of behavioral influences on the control of breathing are all relatively recent themes under-represented in most textbooks. The activities of the respiratory muscles and how they cope with the altered geometry of advanced COPD now merits separate consideration. Much of the research which led to long-term domiciliary oxygen treatment was based on studies of pulmonary circulation and its effects on cardiac function and fluid retention. This is reviewed in detail in Chapter 11 where some of the contradictions and misconceptions of the terms cor pulmonale and right heart failure are highlighted with the aid of more current investigational methods. Finally, the role of sleep and sleep-disordered breathing in the genesis of the daytime complications of COPD are authoritatively addressed in Chapter 12.

The remaining chapters look at the diagnosis, investigation and management of the COPD patient, hopefully in an equally critical fashion. They stress the importance of physiologic assessment for both the diagnosis and treatment selection and the range of imaging techniques available as well as their limitations. In considering management a graded approach seems reasonable. Thus all continuing smokers will need advice about nicotine withdrawal (Chapter 15) whilst many will benefit from symptomatic bronchodilator therapy although the exact choice of dose and type of drug may vary with the circumstance as indicated in Chapter 17. At present, guidelines for routine corticosteroid prescription are lacking and the evidence of the benefits of this treatment are reviewed in Chapter 18. Many patients will present for the first time to hospital in an acute exacerbation and the modern approach to diagnosis and management is comprehensively addressed in Chapter 19. The more severe patient will need more specialized rehabilitation which will certainly include assessment for domiciliary oxygen (Chapters 20 and 21) as well as exclusion of surgically resectable bullous disease (Chapter 22). For the younger patient single or double lung transplantation may offer an escape from otherwise inevitable early death. Whether this treatment will be widely used is as likely to depend on the availability of donor organs as on technical considerations as pointed out in Chapter 23.

Although this book considers many aspects of COPD we have not specifically addressed the politics of its principal cause, tobacco smoking. Others, better qualified than ourselves, have already done so and we feel that to do so here would merely be to preach to the converted. Yet the global impact of tobacco is enormous and as the pressures increase within the developed world to restrict its consumption so the commercial energies of the relevant multinationals have switches their merchandising to the easier markets of the developing world and, in particular, the rapidly expanding economies of the Pacific rim. Given this depressing development, it is likely that COPD will continue to be an important component of the work of all respiratory physicians. Moreover, since many patients who stop smoking in their fifties may still have done sufficient damage to develop physiologically important COPD in their seventies all responsible for the care of older patients are likely to be seeing new cases of this widespread illness.

This book would not have been completed without a great deal of effort by many people. We are especially grateful to our distinguished contributors who have borne the vagaries of our extended editing, resultant faxes and rewriting with great patience and understanding. It is a particular pleasure for us to have a foreword by Professor Moran Campbell whose contributions to COPD, through his insights into respiratory mechanics and breathlessness, and his impact on patient care with the development of controlled oxygen therapy, made him our obvious choice. Our secretaries have coped stoically with the further burden this project has produced in an already busy schedule whilst Ms Annalisa Page, the Commissioning Editor from Chapman & Hall, has shepherded us with patience and perseverance to the end of this project which has proven to be a greater task than either the Editors or she initially envisaged. The publishers hope the use of American spelling will make this book accessible to a wider market.

Finally, our wives and families have, as ever, had to put up with even more disruption than are their usual lot and, for their sakes as well as that of our present and future patients, we hope that you feel that the effort has been worthwhile.

Peter Calverley
Neil Pride

Preface

In the eight years since this book was first published there has been a remarkable resurgence of interest in the science and clinical care of patients suffering from chronic obstructive pulmonary disease (COPD). While the first edition of the book can lay no claims to have stimulated this overdue process, we hope that it helped those who were seeking an up-to-date overview of this important clinical problem. Interest in COPD has certainly blossomed at specialist and general medical congresses with several stand-alone international meetings now devoted to this topic. Sadly, public awareness of the hazard that COPD poses and the need to identify the disease early has been slower to develop. Nonetheless, the advent of a specific international agency, the Global initiative for chronic Obstructive Lung Disease (GOLD), charged with providing up-to-date information about clinical practice and the risks of COPD, is to be welcomed. The GOLD initiative was sponsored by the World Health Organisation (WHO) and the National Heart, Lung and Blood Institute in the USA and is specifically responsible for raising awareness among patients and doctors of the importance of COPD and of how it can best be managed. Its guidance is regularly updated on the Internet and provides an accurate and accessible resource to help the practicing doctor.

Why then bother with another edition of this textbook? Several answers suggest themselves. Although data in the background documents of initiatives like GOLD (and in the national and international societies who produce treatment guidelines) is valuable in terms of current management, it tends to be didactic and does not permit the reader to understand how the ideas described have been developed and are developing. We hope that the latest edition of this book will allow the reader more time to understand what are the key ideas that underpin our knowledge of this disease and to bring themselves up-to-date with how these are changing. Secondly, guidance from expert committees inevitably tends to simplify complex issues and the space available in a textbook allows this to be discussed in more detail than is normally possible in brief executive summaries or action plans. Finally, the level of referencing to the literature available for citation by our contributors is much greater than that which can be practicably housed in even the rather encyclopedic guidelines currently offered. Thus we believe that a textbook of this type is complementary to information available from other sources and can help in the understanding of the complex problems presented by chronic obstructive pulmonary disease.

The current edition contains many significant changes from its predecessor, not least, the inclusion of two new editors whose energy and enthusiasm has been greatly appreciated. We feel there is now more to say about the science of COPD than was the case previously and new chapters devoted to genetics, alpha-1-anti-trypsin deficiency, inflammatory processes and repair reflect this emphasis. Important areas with a more direct clinical relevance have demanded more detailed coverage. Thus, there are new chapters about occupational aspects of COPD, bronchial hyper-responsiveness, infection, exercise performance and surgery for COPD as well as a review of the rapidly growing area of health status assessment in COPD patients. Extensive changing and updating can be seen in chapters published previously and we believe that the book is as current as our publication deadlines could make it.

COPD is an international disease that knows no boundaries and seems set to increase disastrously in areas of the world where economic progress is being made, especially in South-east Asia. Our contributors reflect the international efforts made to combat this illness and we are deeply grateful to them for the time and energy they have put into writing and/or revising their contributions. Likewise, we now have a new publisher and, we feel, a more attractive format in which to present the contents of this book. We are grateful for all in the publication process at Edward Arnold for their patience and courtesy and especially to Jo Koster for her unfailing optimism and enthusiasm, which has ensured that her recalcitrant editors finally produced a book in something approaching an acceptable timescale.

We remain deeply indebted to our secretaries for their efforts in deciphering what we have written, to our families for their patience and tolerance of our continued absences and to our patients for whom we still hope to do good and persuade others to do better. Hopefully, all of these people will feel that the effort involved in revising this book has been worthwhile.

Peter Calverley
William MacNee
Neil Pride
Stephen Rennard

Glossary

RESPIRATORY MECHANICS

STATIC LUNG VOLUMES

TLC	Total lung capacity
VC	(Slow) vital capacity
RV	Residual volume
FRC	Functional residual capacity (=end-expiratory volume at rest)
Vr	Relaxation volume of the respiratory system
ERV	Expiratory reserve volume (FRC − RV)
EELV	End expired lung volume (often used on exercise when usually does not equal FRC)
IC	Inspiratory capacity (TLC − FRC at rest, TLC − EELV during exercise)
EILV	End inspired lung volume
IRV	Inspiratory reserve volume (TLC − EILV)

SINGLE BREATH N_2 TEST

SBN_2	Single breath nitrogen text
CV	Closing volume
CC	Closing capacity (sum of residual volume and closing volume)

CONTROL OF BREATHING

V_T	Tidal volume
T_I	Inspiratory time
T_E	Expiratory time
T_{TOT}	Total respiratory cycle time
V_E	Expired minute ventilation
$P_{0.1}$	Mouth occlusion pressure 0.1 s after onset of inspiration
F	Frequency of breathing

FORCED VITAL CAPACITY MANEUVERS

FEV_1	Forced expiratory volume in one second
FVC	Forced vital capacity
MEFV	Maximum expiratory flow-volume
MIFV	Maximum inspiratory flow-volume
MBC	Maximum breathing capacity (syn. Maximum ventilatory capacity, MVC)
PEF	Peak expiratory flow
PIF	Peak inspiratory flow
$\dot{V}_E$ max	Maximum expiratory flow

$\Delta\dot{V}max_{50}$	Difference between maximum expiratory flow at 50% vital capacity breathing air and breathing a helium-oxygen mixture
Viso$\dot{V}$	Volume at which maximum expiratory flow is same breathing air and a helium-oxygen mixture

MECHANICS OF BREATHING

Pressure measurements

P_L	Static transpulmonary pressure (syn. Lung recoil pressure)
P_L max	P_L at TLC
Palv	Alveolar pressure
Ppl, Poes	Pleural pressure, usually estimated from esophageal pressure)
Ppl min	Lowest Ppl during a maximum inspiratory effort
P_I max	Lowest mouth pressure during a maximum inspiratory effort
P_E max	Highest mouth pressure during a maximum expiratory effort
Pab (ga)	Abdominal (gastric) pressure
Pdi	Transdiaphragmatic pressure (= Pab − Ppl), estimated as Pga − Poes
Pdi max	Pdi during a maximum inspiratory effort
Pao	Pressure at airway opening (mouth, nose or tracheotomy)
PEEPi	Intrinsic positive end-expiratory pressure (syn. Auto-PEEP)
TTdi	Tension-time index of diaphragm

Resistance and compliance

Raw	Airways resistance
SGaw	Specific airway conductance
Rrs	Total respiratory resistance
ΔRrs	Additional total respiratory resistance
Est,rs	Static elastance of respiratory system
Edyn,L	Dynamic elastance of lungs
Cdyn,L	Dynamic compliance of lungs
VP	Static volume-pressure curve of the lungs (often pressure-volume, PV curve)
k	Shape factor of VP curve
Gus	Upstream conductance (ratio of maximum expiratory flow/P_L)

IVPF	iso-volume pressure-flow curve
MFSR	maximum flow-static recoil curve

Work of breathing

$W_{I,rs}$	Total inspiratory work (static and dynamic) on the respiratory system
$W_{Ist,rs}$	Static component of total inspiratory work
$W_{I,PEEPi}$	Static work required to overcome PEEPi
$W_{Idyn,rs}$	Dynamic component of total inspiratory work
$W_{I,aw}$	Dynamic work to overcome subject's airway resistance
$W_{I,L}$	Dynamic work due to time constant inequality and viscoelastic pressure dissipation
$W_{I,w}$	Dynamic work to overcome chest wall tissue resistance

Assisted ventilation

NIV	Non-invasive ventilation, applied at nose and/or mouth
NIPPV	Nasal intermittent positive pressure ventilation
CPAP	Continuous positive airway pressure
PEEPe	Externally applied positive end-expired pressure
IMV	Intermittent mandatory ventilation
PAV	Proportional assisted ventilation

BLOOD AND ALVEOLAR GAS EXCHANGE AND PULMONARY CIRCULATION

Blood and Alveolar O_2 and CO_2

SaO_2	arterial O_2 saturation
CaO_2	arterial O_2 content
DO_2	O_2 delivery
Pa_{O_2}	Arterial O_2 tension
$PaCO_2$	Arterial CO_2 tension
PAO_2	Alveolar O_2 tension
PAO_2-Pao_2	Alveolar-arterial PO_2 difference
PvO_2	Mixed venous O_2 tension
$PtcO_2$	Transcutaneous O_2 tension
$PACO_2$	Alveolar CO_2 tension
Pet_{CO_2}	End tidal CO_2 tension
$\dot{V}O_2$	O_2 consumption

$\dot{V}O_2$ max	maximum O_2 consumption
$\dot{V}CO_2$	CO_2 production
RQ	Respiratory quotient
RE	Respiratory exchange ratio
FIO_2	Fractional concentration of O_2 in inspired air
Q	Cardiac output
$\dot{V}A$	Alveolar ventilation
$\dot{V}A/\dot{Q}$	Ventilation-perfusion ratio
VD	Deadspace
VD/VT	Deadspace as a proportion of tidal volume
Qs/Qt	Proportion of shunt to total cardiac output

CARBON MONOXIDE TRANSFER

$TLCO$	Carbon monoxide transfer factor (syn. Diffusing capacity for CO, $DLCO$)
$TLco/Va$	$TLCO$ per unit alveolar volume (Va) (syn. Carbon monoxide transfer coefficient)
KCO	Krogh constant for CO, analogous to $TLCO/VA$

PULMONARY CIRCULATION

Ppa	Pulmonary artery pressure
Ppw	Pulmonary artery wedge pressure
Ppv	Pulmonary venous pressure

MISCELLANEOUS

BMI	Body mass index (wt/height^2)
CT (HRCT)	Computerised tomography (high resolution CT)
DH	Dynamic hyperinflation
EFL	Expiratory flow limitation (during tidal breathing)
EXT	Exercise training
FFM	Fat free mass
LTOT	Long term oxygen treatment
LVRS	Lung volume reduction surgery
MRC	Medical research council
NEP	Negative expiratory pressure (used to detect EFL)
SGRQ	St George's respiratory questionnaire
TDI	Transitional dyspnea index

Definition of chronic obstructive pulmonary disease

GORDON L SNIDER

'Then you should say what you mean', the March Hare went on.

'I do', Alice hastily replied; 'at least I mean what I say– that's the same thing, you know'.

'Not the same thing a bit!' said the Hatter. 'Why, you might just as well say that "I see what I eat" is the same thing as "I eat what I see"!'

Alice's Adventures in Wonderland,
Lewis Carroll.[1]

The opening sentence of my chapter in the first edition of this book reads as follows: That the initial chapter of this book is on the definition of chronic obstructive pulmonary disease (COPD) reflects not only the confusion that exists in the field of the obstructive airflow diseases, but also the confusion in nosology and definitions that has historically pervaded all of medicine. There is not even a generally accepted definition of the widely used term 'disease'.

In my view, the situation has not changed much since the first edition of this book was published. There is still confusion in the periodical medical literature on how to define a disease. The definition and the diagnostic criteria of a particular disease or syndrome are often conflated. Since 1995, four different expert panels have approached the definition, diagnostic criteria and staging systems for COPD in quite different ways.[2–5] The recently published Global Initiative for Chronic Obstructive Lung Disease (GOLD) guidelines have been reviewed by many experts worldwide and have been sponsored or accepted by many national and international respiratory societies. The definition established by GOLD, therefore, is likely to be in common use for some time. All definitions offer some advantages and have some limitations and these will be reviewed for the four published definitions of COPD.

NOSOLOGY

Nosology is the discipline of classification and terminology of diseases. In this chapter I shall define the general term 'disease' and how it is used in modern medical discourse. The features that govern the terminology of a particular disease will be elucidated, using COPD as an illustration. J.G. Scadding has written extensively on this topic in recent years[6–11] and he suggested some simple rules to govern the nosology of COPD.

Background

In the era of Hippocrates, disease was considered to be a morbid phenomenon *sui generis*; disease manifestations such as *fever, dropsy, diarrhoea* or *cyanosis* were used as names of diseases.[12] During the 17th century, Thomas Sydenham founded the discipline of nosology by insisting that diseases had their own natural history and could be described and classified on the basis of their specific characteristics.[13] This concept did not have a major impact until the latter part of the 19th century, when the observational techniques of physical examination – percussion, auscultation, sphygmomanometry and thermometry – had been developed.[14] The correlation of first the gross and later the microscopic findings at necropsy with the clinical history and physical examination completely changed the concepts and names of diseases. This process accelerated in the 20th century as the result of a torrent of new information coming from radiography, ultrasonography and other biophysical techniques of imaging, and from epidemiology, microbiology, immunology, biochemistry, electron microscopy and genetics.

In the modern era, we do not use the names of diseases as if they were independent morbid entities with external existences that are causing the patient's illness. In the terms of philosophy, this approach represents a *realist or essentialist* definition.[15,16] As Popper has pointed out,[16] *methodological essentialism*, the method of our Greek forbears, posits that we can know the unchanging reality or essence of a thing simply by intellectual consideration; we can know the definition of the essence; and we can give it a name. An example of such usage would be to say that a patient was ill *because* of COPD. Such usage implies a finite number of diseases in the universe.

THE GENERAL CONCEPT OF DISEASE

Current belief is that diseases are due to interactions between the host and one or more causes of disease, thus permitting an infinite number of interactions. Every patient's illness is unique. However, there *are* groups of patients who have some common features to their illness. We have developed names for the diseases these groups of patients represent, which is an arbitrary way of referring to them, and which permits making a diagnosis on a particular patient within the group. The names are verbal symbols designed to refer to an area of interest. A diagnosis provides an abbreviated way of referring to a particular illness and is an important tool for effective communication. In the terms of philosophy, this approach represents a *nominalist* definition.[15,16]

Given that nosology attempts to lump together a large group of unique patients who have some common feature of a disease (but many unique features), it is not surprising that success is far from complete. It is inevitable that, no matter what system we devise, some patients will not fit.

Popper[16] makes the point that scientists do not depend on definitions; all definitions can be omitted without loss to the information imparted. They take care that the statements made should never *depend* on the meaning of their terms. Terms are always a little vague (since they are used only in practical applications). Precision is attained not by reducing vagueness, but rather by keeping well within it; by carefully phrasing sentences in such a way that the possible shades of meaning do not matter.

Definition of the general term 'disease'

I have modified Scadding's definition of the term 'disease':[11]

> The term *disease* is defined as a condition or state in a group of persons who have specified characteristics by which they differ from the norm in a way that is biologically disadvantageous. The name of the disease should refer succinctly to the etiology of the disease or the abnormal phenomena displayed by the affected group of persons.

The name of a disease should be as brief and descriptive as possible and need give no indication of its cause. Even when a disease is defined in terms of etiology, using the name of the disease as the patient's diagnosis gives only limited information as to the disease manifestations in the sick person. The diagnosis of tuberculosis reveals that a disease caused by *Mycobacterium tuberculosis* is present, but gives little indication of the exact nature of the patient's illness or even whether an illness is overtly manifest.

TERMINOLOGY OF PARTICULAR DISEASES

The need to pay attention to defining and naming a particular disease arises when preliminary descriptions have identified a group of persons with similar clinical, pathologic or physiological features who fit the definition of having a 'disease'.

There are three main features of terminology of particular diseases, the definition, diagnostic criteria and a system for staging severity. As new knowledge accumulates, the definition, diagnostic criteria and staging may all need to change.

Defining characteristics of a particular disease

The *defining characteristics* of a disease are the common properties specifying the group of abnormal persons upon whom the description of the disease is based,[11] although the current definition should leave no doubt about the field of study from which the defining characteristics are drawn.

The characteristics specifying the population of interest may have different origins. They may be the effects in a particular group of persons of a particular etiological agent. They may be a specified disorder of structure or function of unknown etiology. Or, they may be a consistent syndrome (a set of clinical findings) whose etiology is unknown. These three levels indicate progressively decreasing knowledge of the disease and therefore decreasing priority as defining characteristics:

- Etiology has the highest priority.
- Altered structure or function have intermediate priority.
- The clinical features of a disease have the lowest priority.

Etiology has highest priority in this scheme but is the most difficult to use; etiology-based definitions are most easily written for diseases caused by infectious agents. It is difficult to use etiology as a defining characteristic for chronic diseases that have multiple risk factors as well as genetically based susceptibility factors. For chronic diseases, the pathologic, physiologic and clinical features of the disease will be most often used as defining characteristics; such definitions often provide a useful basis for discussing the conditions that are included or excluded from the chronic disease.

Compound definitions

A group of patients selected because they have a common characteristic in one field of study will not necessarily share common characteristics in another field. Compound definitions, which utilize defining characteristics from two or more fields of study, define subsets of patients with overlapping characteristics.[11] For example, pneumococcal pneumonia represents an overlapping subset of patients with pneumonia (defined in pathologic terms) and infection with *S. pneumoniae* (defined in etiological terms). Etiological factors may be included in compound definitions.

Diagnostic criteria

Diagnostic criteria are features of the disease, chosen from the description of the disease, which are found by empirical research to best distinguish the disease from other diseases that resemble it. The diagnostic criteria may or may not include features of the defining criteria and diagnostic criteria frequently contain disease features that do not appear in the definition. When the defining characteristic is clinically based, the diagnostic criteria must perforce include them. However, when the diagnostic criteria are based on etiology, the diagnostic

criteria may not include the defining characteristics. For example, the diagnosis of viral diseases is regularly made without directly demonstrating the presence of the virus in the patient.

Another illustration of the dichotomy between definition and diagnostic criteria is found in mitral stenosis. This disease is defined using pathology as the defining characteristic. Although rheumatic fever is responsible for 99% of instances of mitral stenosis, a variety of causes account for the remaining 1%. The diagnostic criteria of mitral stenosis include the characteristic heart murmur, an image of the valve and other findings in two-dimensional transthoracic or transesophageal echocardiography and, to decreasing extent, an estimation of valve orifice diameter from physiologic data obtained during left heart catheterization. None of these methods actually demonstrate the pathology that is the major defining characteristic of mitral stenosis. The diagnostic criteria come from empirical studies correlating pathological anatomy and the diagnostic criterion.[17]

Staging severity of a disease

Staging systems may be based on clinical features, physiological alterations, the pattern of the pathology or a combination of features. The features of a disease that are used in staging, whether of clinical or laboratory origin, should be validated by comparison with independent outcome variables of disease such as mortality, morbidity or quality of life. Staging can be useful in planning and gauging the effectiveness of therapy, in stratifying groups of patients in clinical trials, in making a prognosis, in predicting effects on health-related quality of life or in predicting medical resource utilization.

Description of a disease – a continuing process

Once a disease has been defined, the process of description of the disease should resume. Subjects with the defining characteristics should be studied by all available means, thereby determining all ascertainable features. In this way the description of the disease is extended, including features that are of frequent as well as of infrequent occurrence. Nosology is a dynamic process and as more information becomes available, the description, definition and diagnostic criteria may undergo revision. If the population studied is large enough, the frequency of inconstant features can be estimated, although we do not usually redefine the disease in order to include the inconstant features; there will inevitably be rare patients who do not fit the defining characteristics or diagnostic criteria.

OBSTRUCTIVE AIRWAY DISEASES

In the mid 20th century, as tuberculosis came under control in developed countries, attention was turned to the high morbidity and mortality from chronic obstructive respiratory diseases and studies were undertaken to determine the nature, frequency and causes of these disorders.[18–20] In 1958, a Ciba Guest Symposium was convened and subsequently published the first attempt to achieve a consensus on definitions of disorders associated with chronic airflow obstruction.[21] In 1962, definitions that were similar to those of the Ciba Symposium were published by the American Thoracic Society.[22] The subsequent history of definitions of these diseases has been reviewed by Samet.[23]

CHRONIC OBSTRUCTIVE PULMONARY DISEASE

Description

Chronic obstructive pulmonary disease most commonly afflicts a group of persons with longstanding exposure to cigarette smoke and other toxic inhalants. These persons have non-remitting airflow obstruction of variable severity, which is associated with airway hyperreactivity, chronic productive cough and decreased tolerance for exercise. As the disease progresses, hypoxemia followed by hypercapnia and worsening hypoxemia supervene. Cor pulmonale may be manifest. Altered oxidant/antioxidant balance, circulating levels of inflammatory mediators and acute-phase proteins, weight loss, loss of muscle mass and muscle dysfunction, which may be due to abnormal levels of circulating cytokines, are evidence of a systemic component to the disease.[24–26]

COPD definitions

While the writings of a single author have sometimes been highly influential in establishing a definition,[27] given the important communication systems that depend on these definitions, such as morbidity and mortality statistics, statements by expert groups are most commonly used. Definitions of COPD have recently been prepared by expert panels of the American Thoracic Society (ATS) in 1995,[3] The European Respiratory Society (ERS) in 1995,[2] The British Thoracic Society (BTS) in 1997[4] and the Global Initiative for Chronic Obstructive Lung Disease (GOLD) in 2001.[5] The definitions by these four expert groups will be presented and briefly discussed.

American Thoracic Society (ATS 1995)[3] definition

> Chronic obstructive pulmonary disease is defined as a disease state characterized by the presence of airflow obstruction due to chronic bronchitis or emphysema; the airflow obstruction is generally progressive, may be accompanied by airway hyperreactivity and may be partially reversible.

This compound definition uses the combination of chronic bronchitis defined in clinical terms, emphysema in anatomic terms, and airflow obstruction representing a physiologic state (Figure 1.1).

- Patients with chronic airflow obstruction that is not due to chronic bronchitis, emphysema or persistent asthma are not considered to have COPD, for example patients with cystic fibrosis or obliterative bronchiolitis. Readers are referred to two excellent

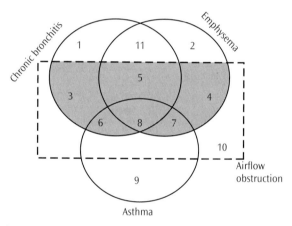

Figure 1.1 *Schema of COPD. A non-proportional Venn diagram shows subsets of patients with chronic bronchitis, emphysema and asthma in three overlapping circles; the subsets comprising COPD are shaded. The areas of the subsets are not proportional to the size of the subset. Most patients with severe disease have features of both chronic bronchitis and emphysema and fall into subset 5; some patients have features of asthma as well and fall into subset 8. Patients with features of asthma and chronic bronchitis (asthmatic bronchitis or the asthmatic form of COPD) fall into subset 6. Patients with asthma whose airflow obstruction is completely reversible (subset 9) are classified as asthma; these, and patients with chronic bronchitis or emphysema without airflow obstruction (subsets 1, 2 and 11), are not classed as COPD. With permission from ATS, 1995. Standards for the diagnosis and care of patients with chronic obstructive pulmonary disease. Official statement Am J Respir Crit Care Med **152** S77–121. Official Journal of American Thoracic Society © American Lung Association.*

recent reviews that discuss other causes of chronic airflow limitation;[28,29] Table 1.1 lists many of these other causes.

- Patients with airflow obstruction and either chronic bronchitis or emphysema are diagnosed COPD. Most COPD patients have both chronic bronchitis and emphysema.
- Although the lack of specificity of the airways pathology in chronic bronchitis precludes its use as a defining characteristic, the pathology *is* well defined and we know that bronchiolitis is a cause of airflow obstruction in COPD, in addition to the loss of elastic recoil and rupture of alveolar attachments to small airways caused by emphysema.
- Patients with asthma who have completely reversible airways obstruction are diagnosed asthma and not COPD. It is difficult to distinguish patients with non-remitting asthma from patients with chronic bronchitis or emphysema who have airway hyperreactivity, and such patients are included within the rubric COPD.

Table 1.1 *Some conditions other than COPD that cause chronic airflow limitation. (Adapted from refs 28, 29)*

Site of airflow obstruction	Disease
Upper airway	Bilateral vocal cord paralysis
	Laryngeal tumors
Trachea	Neoplasm
	Stenosis
	Amyloidosis
	Tracheobronchomegaly
	Polychondritis
Central airways*	Bronchial tumors
	Stenosis
	Bronchiectasis
	Cystic fibrosis
	Amyloidosis
	Sarcoidosis
	Polychondritis
Peripheral airways*	Sarcoidosis
	Bronchiectasis
	Cystic fibrosis
	Infectious granulomas
	Hypersensitivity pneumonia
	Pneumoconioses
	Bronchiolitis obliterans
	Lymphangiomyomatosis
	Eosinophilic granuloma
	Diffuse panbronchiolitis
	Lymphocytic bronchiolitis
	Obliterative bronchiolitis

*The separation between central and peripheral airways is somewhat artificial; many disorders involve both.

European Respiratory Society (ERS 1995)[2] definition

COPD is defined as a disorder characterized by reduced maximum expiratory flow and slow forced emptying of the lungs, features which do not change markedly over several months. Most of the airflow limitation is slowly progressive and irreversible. The airflow limitation is due to varying combinations of airway disease and emphysema; the relative contribution of the two processes is difficult to define *in vivo*.

- The report reviews the mechanisms of production of airflow obstruction by small airway disease and by emphysema, which were discussed earlier.
- It is pointed out that patients with COPD often exhibit minimal reversibility of airflow obstruction with bronchodilators and that airway hyperresponsiveness and recurrent or persistent cough is common. It is usually, but not always, possible to distinguish between asthma and COPD.
- By convention, a number of specific causes of chronic airflow obstruction, including cystic fibrosis, bronchiectasis and bronchiolitis obliterans, have been excluded from COPD.

British Thoracic Society (BTS 1997)[4] definition

COPD is defined as a chronic, slowly progressive disorder characterized by airways obstruction ($FEV_1 < 80\%$ predicted and $FEV_1/FVC < 70\%$) which does not change markedly over several months. The impairment of lung function is largely fixed but is partially reversible by bronchodilator (or other) therapy.

Comments following the definition state:

- COPD arises from varying combinations of airway disease and pulmonary emphysema; it is difficult to define the relative importance of each in an individual patient.
- Chronic bronchitis, defined as chronic productive cough for at least 3 months in each of two successive years, does not necessarily signify the presence of airway obstruction.
- The differentiation of severe COPD from chronic severe asthma is difficult, since some improvement in FEV_1 (reversibility) can often be produced by bronchodilator therapy. Unlike asthma, airflow limitation in COPD as measured by the FEV_1 can never be returned to normal values.
- Most (but not all) cases of COPD are caused by tobacco smoking.

- The term COPD is not conventionally used to include other specific conditions that can cause airways obstruction such as cystic fibrosis, bronchiectasis or bronchiolitis obliterans.

Global Initiative for Chronic Obstructive Lung Disease (GOLD 2001)[5] definition

Most recently, an international workshop on COPD, GOLD[5], based their definition on physiology, etiology and pathology:

COPD is a disease state characterized by airflow limitation that is not fully reversible. The airflow obstruction is usually both progressive and associated with an abnormal inflammatory response of the lungs to noxious particles or gases.

In discussion in the Workshop Report, it is stated:

- Chronic airflow limitation is caused by a mixture of small airway disease (obstructive bronchiolitis) and parenchymal destruction (emphysema), the relative contributions of which vary from person to person. Chronic inflammation produces remodeling and narrowing of the small airways. Destruction of the lung parenchyma, also by inflammatory processes, leads to the loss of alveolar attachments to the small airways and decreases lung elastic recoil; in turn these changes diminish the ability of airways to remain open during expiration.
- Airflow limitation is measured by spirometry, as this is the most widely available, reproducible test of lung function.
- The authors state that the terms emphysema and chronic bronchitis were not used in the GOLD report because the term emphysema is often incorrectly used clinically; emphysema is only one of several structural abnormalities present in the lungs of persons with COPD. Chronic bronchitis, essentially chronic productive cough for at least two months in each of two successive years, remains a clinically and epidemiologically useful term. However, it does not reflect the major impact of airflow limitation on morbidity and mortality of COPD patients. Also, productive cough may precede the development of airflow limitation; conversely some patients develop significant airflow limitation without chronic cough and sputum production.
- Asthma and COPD are both characterized by airflow obstruction, although the airway inflammation underlying them has important differences.
- Airflow limitation in asthma is often completely reversible, either spontaneously or with treatment, while in COPD it is never completely reversible.

Some patients have features of both diseases, with asthma-like and COPD-like inflammation. While asthma can usually be differentiated from COPD, this is not possible in some patients.
- Poorly reversible airflow limitation associated with bronchiectasis, cystic fibrosis, tuberculosis or asthma is not included except insofar as these conditions overlap with COPD.

DISCUSSION: THE FOUR DIAGNOSTIC SYSTEMS

There is much conflation of definitions and diagnostic criteria in these reports, a condition that pervades the medical literature generally. However, in the combination of their definitions, discussions and diagnostic criteria, which will here be called 'diagnostic systems', all four expert panels make essentially the same key points:

- Irreversible airflow obstruction is a cardinal feature of COPD.
- Limited reversibility of airflow obstruction in response to bronchodilator drugs is common; the absence of such reversibility does not preclude bronchodilator treatment.
- Asthma with complete reversibility is not included within the rubric COPD.
- Chronic airflow obstruction due to other diagnosable conditions such as cystic fibrosis, obliterative bronchiolitis or panbronchiolitis is not included in COPD.
- Tobacco smoking is the major but not the only risk factor for COPD.
- The cause of the irreversible airflow obstruction in COPD is the presence in the lungs of bronchiolitis or small airway disease, and emphysema, which is present in a variable mix among patients.

There are some differences among the four systems. All four systems exclude from the diagnosis COPD patients with emphysema or chronic bronchitis who do not have airflow obstruction. The GOLD staging system classifies patients with normal spirometry but chronic cough or sputum production as 'at risk'; with a severity grade of '0'. The ATS 1995 system does not mention the use of a decreased FEV_1/FVC ratio as an indicator of airflow obstruction; the ERS 1995 system does so and makes the point that the ratio is a relatively sensitive index of mild airflow limitation. The BTS 1997 and the GOLD systems both stress that the spirometric diagnosis of airflow obstruction require both an FEV_1/FVC ratio less than 70% and an FEV_1 less than 80% predicted. GOLD specifies that the spirometric measurements should be made post-bronchodilator treatment.

A major strength of the GOLD definition is its widespread acceptance, simplicity and emphasis on spirometry as the standard for the diagnosis of airflow obstruction. This approach should permit reasonable comparisons among various populations in different countries. Inflammation may be simply defined as the response of tissues to injury; accordingly, the meaning of the term '... abnormal inflammatory response of the lungs...' is not clear.

The literature on COPD often uses the terms airflow limitation and airflow obstruction as synonyms. Expiratory airflow can be limited by severe restrictive disease or impaired muscle function, although the use of the FEV_1/FVC ratio in the staging system should exclude these conditions. Airflow obstruction means that something is blocking the expiratory flow of air. As pointed out earlier, in COPD the airflow obstruction is due either to small airway disease or, with emphysema, collapse of small airways due to loss of elastic recoil and small airway tethering; the latter causes closure of small airways at abnormally large lung volumes during exhalation. The term 'airflow obstruction' seems preferable to 'airflow limitation'.

I suggest that the next iteration of the GOLD definition might read:

> COPD is a disease state characterized by incompletely reversible, progressive airflow obstruction that is associated with inflammation in the lungs due to prolonged exposure to tobacco smoke and other noxious particles and gases.

Definitions of diseases encompassed in COPD

CHRONIC BRONCHITIS

Chronic bronchitis is defined as the presence of chronic productive cough for three months in each of two successive years in a patient in whom other causes of chronic cough have been excluded.[3]

EMPHYSEMA

Emphysema has been defined in morphologic terms since the Ciba symposium.[21] There have been clarifications from time to time.[30,31] In the latest of these, emphysema was defined as follows:

> Emphysema is defined as a condition of the lung characterized by abnormal permanent enlargement of the airspaces distal to the terminal bronchioles accompanied by destruction of their walls and without obvious fibrosis. Destruction is defined as non-uniformity in the pattern of respiratory airspace enlargement; the orderly appearance of the acinus and its components is disturbed and may be lost. Emphysema may occur with or without airflow obstruction.

FIBROSIS AND EMPHYSEMA

In 1985[30] the expert panel also defined a condition termed airspace enlargement with fibrosis:

> Air space enlargement with fibrosis occurs with obvious fibrosis, associated with infectious granulomatous disease such as tuberculosis, noninfectious granulomatous disease such as sarcoidosis, or fibrosis of undetermined etiology. The scarring is readily evident in the chest radiograph, or in the inflation-fixed lung specimen, and is apparent to the naked eye. This form of airspace enlargement with fibrosis was formerly termed irregular or paracicatricial emphysema. It is not included under the umbrella of COPD, although it may occur with or without airflow obstruction.

The separation of airspace enlargement with fibrosis and emphysema is not as clean as was formerly thought. A recent review[32] presents evidence suggesting that emphysema is multifactorial in its pathogenesis and respiratory airspace enlargement is a stereotyped response of the lungs to a variety of injuries. Fibrosis may be part of the healing process after some injuries. Microscopic fibrosis is observed in the mild airspace enlargement of centriacinar emphysema;[33] biochemically, collagen concentration is increased in these lesions.[34–36] These lesions may represent a form of focal airspace enlargement with fibrosis. It may be time to remove the phrase 'without obvious fibrosis' from the 1985 ATS definition of emphysema. Also, it seems preferable to use the term 'scar emphysema', for this lesion.

> Scar emphysema is defined as respiratory air space enlargement occurring with obvious fibrosis that is associated with infectious or non-infectious granulomatous disease, pneumoconiosis or fibrosis of undetermined etiology. The scarring is readily evident in the chest radiograph and is apparent to the naked eye in the inflation-fixed lung specimen. Scar emphysema may occur with or without airflow obstruction.

The airspace enlargement of sarcoidosis, tuberculosis or silicosis and the honeycombing of interstitial pulmonary fibrosis would be called scar emphysema. I suggest that a patient with a fibrosing condition of the lungs who has scar emphysema with chronic airflow obstruction, should be diagnosed as having the primary diagnosis causing the scarring, for example tuberculosis, with COPD as a secondary diagnosis.

Etiology in definition of COPD

Tobacco smoking has been identified as the major risk factor for the development of COPD, accounting for 80–90% of the risk for developing the disease in the

United States.[36] The smoking-attributable fraction of United States COPD mortality in 1984 was 0.850 for men and 0.694 for women;[37] however, the proportion of individuals exposed to tobacco smoke who develop chronic bronchitis and emphysema has been stated to be relatively small – about 15%.[38,39] Nevertheless, the percentage who develop disease depends entirely on the diagnostic criteria. Those which recognize milder conditions will result in increased prevalence of disease (see below). It is evident that host factors, most likely genetic in origin, must play an important role in pathogenesis, suggesting strong gene/environment interactions. The only genetic factor unequivocally predisposing to COPD in meaningful numbers of patients with COPD is severe alpha$_1$ antitrypsin deficiency, which accounts for 1–2% of COPD.[25]

Since 1990, experimental exposure of rodents to cigarette smoke has been shown to consistently produce emphysema.[40,41] The emphysema is mild, requiring about 6 months of smoke exposure for its induction. The strong epidemiologic evidence indicting cigarette smoke as a risk factor for COPD proves an *association* between cigarette smoke exposure and COPD. The evidence that prolonged cigarette smoke induces emphysema in rodents establishes an *etiological* role for cigarette smoke exposure in COPD.

New information has added greatly to understanding the etiology of COPD. However, there are multiple risk factors and large gaps in knowledge are evident. For example recent studies indicate that inhalation of smoke from burning biomass fuels in unventilated indoor spaces accounts for more than 400 000 persons with COPD in the developing world.[42] Other, minor risk factors include exposure to siliceous dusts and irritant gases and particulate urban air pollutants $<10\,\mu$m in diameter. There are also possible roles for infection and atopic disease.[41,43] It is thus inappropriate to attempt to write a purely etiology-based definition for COPD at this time.

Diagnostic criteria for COPD

Diagnostic criteria are much more important than definitions in either clinical practice or research. As long as diagnostic criteria are clearly stated, the definition does not matter. It is the diagnostic criteria and not the definition that determine the diagnosis of a particular patient's disease. It is the diagnostic criteria and the specific inclusion and exclusion criteria that determine the precise makeup of a population of research participants.

A diagnosis of COPD requires a history of chronic progressive symptoms (cough, sputum production, wheeze or dyspnea). Physical examination may reveal evidence of airflow obstruction in the form of wheezes on auscultation during quiet or forced expiration; the forced expiratory time may be found to be prolonged.[44]

However the objective evidence of airway obstruction determined by forced expiratory spirometry is the standard for demonstrating and quantifying airflow obstruction. Indices such as the FEV$_1$ and FEV$_1$/FVC ratio should be measured after bronchodilator drug inhalation. It may also be necessary in some instances to show that spirometric values do not return to normal with treatment over an extended period of time. There will usually but not always be a history of prolonged cigarette smoking; other risk factors, particularly the inhalation of toxic gases and particles, should be sought. Other diseases causing airflow obstruction should be excluded by chest X-ray and other appropriate studies.

Staging severity of COPD

Staging the severity of a disease can be helpful in establishing a prognosis, in setting standards for appropriate investigation of patients, in making recommendations for treatment and for allocating healthcare resources. Staging should ideally be based on a composite of factors including symptoms, severity of airflow obstruction, degree of blood gas abnormality and a measure of the systemic effects of the illness such as body mass index. Obviously, one would like the predictive power of a staging system to be as great as possible. The staging of a disease should be based on correlative studies; for example, there should be a strong correlation between stage of the disease and morbidity and mortality data. Such a correlation exists between FEV$_1$ and mortality[45] and between body mass index and mortality.[46] Interestingly, FEV$_1$ correlates with health status, but weakly,[47] suggesting that a multidimensional staging system might be needed for COPD. The four expert panels have recommended different cut points for staging severity of COPD. These are compared in Table 1.2. In all four of these guidelines, the intensity of therapy was staged to disease severity.

Table 1.2 *FEV$_1$ standards for staging severity of COPD*

Staging system	At risk	Mild (%)	Moderate (%)	Severe (%)
ATS[3]		≥50	35–49	<35
ERS[2]		≥70	50–69	<50
BTS[4]		60–79	40–59	<40
GOLD[5]	Normal*	≥80	30–79	<30[†]
			Mod A: 50–79 % predicted**	
			Mod B: 30–49 % predicted	

*Chronic symptoms (cough, sputum production) are present.
[†]Classified as severe regardless of FEV$_1$ in presence of right heart failure or respiratory failure (Pao_2 < 60 mmHg with or without Paco_2 > 50 mmHg breathing air at sea level).
**Moderate is divided into two subcategories, A and B.

CONCLUSIONS

This chapter reviews currently used nominalist methodology in defining diseases. It provides a definition of the general term 'disease'. For specific diseases, it recommends that in choosing defining characteristics, highest priority should be assigned to etiology, intermediate priority to pathology and lowest priority to clinical features of disease. However, etiology is incompletely known for many chronic diseases and is the most difficult defining characteristic to use. Although definitions are useful in communication they are not critical to doing good clinical or scientific work. However, diagnostic criteria, which will vary depending on how they are to be used, are critically important for both sound clinical and research work. They should be specified as precisely as possible.

Staging of disease is useful for establishing a prognosis, setting standards for appropriate investigation of patients, planning treatment and for allocating healthcare resources. The variables used in a staging system should be based on the empirical demonstration that the variables, whether clinical, physiologic or pathologic, bear a relation to outcome variables such as morbidity, mortality or health status. The cut points separating particular stages will generally be arbitrary.

No doubt, definitions will change as understanding of the disorders which comprise COPD increase. Hopefully the rapid advances in the biological sciences will bring many benefits to COPD patients. If so, it seems certain that current definitions, and the generalized statements made about COPD which are based on those definitions, will be rapidly outdated.

REFERENCES

1. Carroll Lewis; pseudonym of C.L. Dodgson. *Alice's Adventures in Wonderland*. R Clay, Son, and Taylor, London, 1865.
2. Siafakas NM, Vermeire P, Pride NB, *et al.* Optimal assessment and management of chronic obstructive pulmonary disease (COPD). The European Respiratory Society Task Force. *Eur Respir J* 1995;**8**:1398–420.
3. American Thoracic Society. Standards for the diagnosis and care of patients with chronic obstructive pulmonary disease. Official Statement. *Am J Respir Crit Care Med* 1995;**152**: S77–121.
4. British Thoracic Society Group of the Standards of Care Committee. BTS guidelines for the management of chronic obstructive pulmonary disease. The COPD Guidelines Group of the Standards of Care Committee of the BTS. *Thorax* 1997; **52**:S1–28.
5. Pauwels RA, Buist AS, Calverley PM, Jenkins CR, Hurd SS. Global strategy for the diagnosis, management, and prevention of chronic obstructive pulmonary disease. NHLBI/WHO Global Initiative for Chronic Obstructive Lung Disease (GOLD) Workshop summary. *Am J Respir Crit Care Med* 2001;**163**:1256–76.
6. Scadding JG. Principles of definition in medicine. *Lancet* 1959;**1**:323–5.
7. Scadding JG. Meaning of diagnostic terms in bronchopulmonary disease. *Br Med J* 1963;**2**:1425–30.
8. Scadding JG. The semantics of medical diagnosis. *Biomed Comput* 1972;**3**:83–90.
9. Scadding JG. Talking clearly about bronchopulmonary diseases. In: JG Scadding, G Cumming, eds. *Scientific Foundations of Respiratory Medicine*. WB Saunders, Philadelphia, 1981, Ch 2.
10. Scadding JG. Health and disease: what can medicine do for philosophy? *J Med Ethics* 1988;**14**:118–24.
11. Scadding JG. Definition of asthma. In: EB Weiss, M Stein, eds. *Bronchial Asthma, Mechanisms and Therapeutics*, 3rd edn. Little Brown and Co, Boston, 1993, pp. 1–13.
12. Adams F. *The Genuine Works of Hippocrates, Translated from the Greek, With a Preliminary Discourse and Annotations*, Vol II, *Aphorisms iii – 12 and 31*. Sydenham Society, London.
13. Garrison FH. *An Introduction to the History of Medicine*. WB Saunders, Philadelphia.
14. Feinstein AR. An analysis of diagnostic reasoning; 1. The domains and disorders of clinical macrobiology. *Yale J Biol Med* 1973;**46**:212–32.
15. Crookshank FG. The importance of a theory of signs and a critique of language in the study of medicine. In: CK Ogden, IA Richards, eds. *The Meaning of Meaning*, first published in 1923. Harcourt Brace Jovanovich, New York, 1956, pp. 327–55.
16. Popper KR. *The Open Society and Its Enemies*. Princeton University Press, Princeton, 1963.
17. Braunwald E. Valvular heart disease. In: E Braunwald, DP Zipes, P Libby, eds. *Heart Disease*, 6th edn. WB Saunders, Philadelphia, 2001, pp. 1643–722.
18. Stuart-Harris CH, Hanley T, Clifton M, Platts MM, Hammond JDS, Whitaker W. *Chronic Bronchitis, Emphysema and Cor Pulmonale*. John Wright and Sons, Bristol, 1957.
19. Oswald NC, Medvei VC. Chronic bronchitis; the effect of cigarette smoking. *Lancet* 1955;**2**:843–4.
20. Reid LM. Pathology of chronic bronchitis. *Lancet* 1954;**1**:275–9.
21. Ciba Foundation Guest Symposium. Terminology, definitions and classification of chronic pulmonary emphysema and related conditions. *Thorax* 1959;**14**:286–99.
22. American Thoracic Society. Chronic bronchitis, asthma and pulmonary emphysema. A statement by the Committee on Diagnostic Standards for Nontuberculous Respiratory Diseases. *Am Rev Respir Dis* 1962;**85**:762–8.
23. Samet JM. Definitions and methodology in COPD research. In: MJ Hensley, NA Saunders, eds. *Clinical Epidemiology of Chronic Obstructive Pulmonary Disease*. Marcel Dekker, New York, 1989, pp. 1–22.
24. Wouters EFM, Creutzberg EC, Schols AMJW. Systemic effects of COPD. *Chest* 2002;**121**:127S–30S.
25. Piquette CA, Rennard SI, Snider GL. Chronic bronchitis and emphysema. In: JF Murray, JA Nadel, RJ Mason, HA Boushey Jr, eds. *Textbook of Respiratory Medicine*, 3rd edn. WB Saunders, Philadelphia, 2000, pp. 1187–246.
26. Maltais F, LeBlanc P, Jobin J, Casaburi R. Peripheral muscle dysfunction in chronic obstructive pulmonary disease. *Clin Chest Med* 2000;**21**:665–77.
27. Anthonisen NR, Manfreda J, Warren CPW, Hershfield ES, Harding GKM, Nelson NA. Antibiotic therapy in exacerbations of chronic obstructive pulmonary disease. *Ann Intern Med* 1987;**106**:196–204.

28. Girod CE, Schwartz MI. Other large-airway diseases that limit airflow. In: NF Voelkel, W MacNee, eds. *Chronic Obstructive Lung Diseases*. BC Decker, Hamilton, 2002, pp. 184–98.

29. Girod CE, Schwartz MI. Diffuse interstitial lung diseases resulting in airflow limitation. In: NF Voelkel, W MacNee, ed. *Chronic Obstructive Lung Diseases*. BC Decker, Hamilton, 2002, pp. 199–213.

30. National Heart Lung and Blood Institute. The definition of emphysema. Report of a Division of Lung Diseases workshop. *Am Rev Respir Dis* 1985;**132**:182–5.

31. World Health Organization. Epidemiology of chronic non-specific lung diseases. *Bull World Health Org* 1975;**52**:251–60.

32. Snider GL. Emphysema: the first two centuries – and beyond. A historical overview, with suggestions for future research: part 2. *Am Rev Respir Dis* 1992;**146**:1615–22.

33. Leopold JG, Gough J. The centrilobular form of hypertrophic emphysema and its relation to chronic bronchitis. *Thorax* 1957;**12**:219–35.

34. Cardoso WV, Sekhon HS, Hyde DM, Thurlbeck WM. Collagen and elastin in human pulmonary emphysema. *Am Rev Respir Dis* 1993;**147**:975–81.

35. Lang MR, Fiaux GW, Gillooly M, Stewart JA, Hulmes DJ, Lamb D. Collagen content of alveolar wall tissue in emphysematous and non-emphysematous lungs. *Thorax* 1994;**49**:319–26.

36. US Surgeon General, ed. *The Health Consequences of Smoking: Chronic Obstructive Lung Disease*. USDHHS Publ No 84–50205. Washington DC, 1984, p. 135.

37. Davis RM, Novotny TE. The epidemiology of cigarette smoking and its impact on chronic obstructive pulmonary disease. *Am Rev Respir Dis* 1989;**140**:S82–4.

38. Burrows B, Knudson RJ, Cline MG, Lebowitz MD. Quantitative relationships between cigarette smoking and ventilatory function. *Am Rev Respir Dis* 1977;**115**:195–205.

39. Silverman EK, Speizer FE. Risk factors for the development of chronic obstructive pulmonary disease. *Med Clin North Am* 1996;**80**:501–22.

40. Wright JL, Churg A. Cigarette smoke causes physiologic and morphologic changes of emphysema in the guinea pig. *Am Rev Respir Dis* 1990;**142**:1422–8.

41. Hautamaki RD, Kobayashi DK, Senior RM, Shapiro SD. Requirement for macrophage elastase for cigarette smoke-induced emphysema in mice. *Science* 1997;**277**:2002–4.

42. Smith KR. Inaugural article: national burden of disease in India from indoor air pollution. *Proc Natl Acad Sci USA* 2000;**97**:13286–93.

43. Garshick E, Schenker MB, Dosman JA. Occupationally induced airways obstruction. *Med Clin North Am* 1996;**80**:851–78.

44. Straus SE, McAlister FA, Sackett DL, Deeks JJ. Accuracy of history, wheezing, and forced expiratory time in the diagnosis of chronic obstructive pulmonary disease. *J Gen Intern Med* 2002;**17**:684–8.

45. Hodgkin JE. Prognosis in chronic obstructive pulmonary disease. *Clin Chest Med* 1990;**11**:555–69.

46. Landbo C, Prescott E, Lange P, Vestbo J, Almdal TP. Prognostic value of nutritional status in chronic obstructive pulmonary disease. *Am J Respir Crit Care Med* 1999;**160**:1856–61.

47. Harper R, Brazier JE, Waterhouse JC, Walters SJ, Jones NM, Howard P. Comparison of outcome measures for patients with chronic obstructive pulmonary disease (COPD) in an outpatient setting. *Thorax* 1997;**52**:879–87.

2

Pathology

JAMES C HOGG AND MARINA SAETTA

INTRODUCTION

Chronic obstructive pulmonary disease (COPD) is the result of pathologic changes in the central airways that are responsible for chronic cough and sputum production,[1–3] lesions in the smaller conducting airways that cause airway obstruction[4,5] and emphysematous destruction of the lung surface.[6–8] These abnormalities are also accompanied by pulmonary vascular changes that contribute to right heart failure,[9,10] and less well defined lesions[11] that are associated with the acute exacerbations of COPD.[12] Although their location and appearance differ, their pathogenesis is determined by the inflammatory process, and the purpose of this chapter is to provide an overview of their structural features.

The tobacco smoking habit causes lung inflammation in everyone that smokes[13,14] and is the major risk factor for developing COPD. However, the linkage between cigarette smoke-induced lung inflammation and COPD is not simple and does not explain why only a minority of heavy smokers develop clinically significant disease.[15,16] Recent evidence suggests that cigarette smoke-induced lung inflammation is amplified in those who develop advanced disease.[17] Data obtained using quantitative methods suggest that approximately 20×10^{12} polymorphonuclear cells (PMN) are present in the parenchyma and airspaces of the lungs of cigarette smokers with preserved lung function compared to approximately 300×10^{12} in the lungs of patients with similar smoking histories who have advanced emphysema. As there are

only 5×10^9 PMN/liter of blood, a cardiac output of 6 liters/min delivers approximately 43×10^{12} PMN cells to the lungs over 24 hours. Therefore, the airspaces of heavy smokers with preserved lung function contain approximately 50% of the PMN delivered to the lungs in a 24-hour period and the lungs of patients with advanced emphysema contain the equivalent of several days' delivery of PMN. This is very different to the 2% of delivered PMN that migrate into the airspaces in experimental pneumonia[18] and suggests a very marked accumulation of PMN in the lungs of smokers that is further enhanced in severe COPD. Unfortunately we know very little about the nature and causes of this remarkable accumulation of PMN, and it probably involves both increased migration into the airspaces and a prolonged life span after they arrive. The kinetics of the other inflammatory cells are more difficult to understand because macrophages and lymphocytes can divide after they leave the vascular space and the PMN cannot.

CENTRAL AIRWAYS

The central airways are the site of the mucus hypersecretion that is expressed clinically as chronic bronchitis.[1,16,23] Mucous gland enlargement was considered a histologic hallmark of the disease, and Reid[19] used the size of the mucus glands as a yardstick for measuring chronic bronchitis. In a re-evaluation of this problem some years later, Mullen and coworkers[1] found that airway inflammation provided a better morphological indicator of chronic bronchitis than did mucous gland hypertrophy. They found that inflammation was present in the airway wall, mucous glands and ducts particularly in cartilaginous bronchi between 2 and 4 mm diameter in patients with chronic bronchitis.[1] Saetta and colleagues extended these observations and characterized the inflammatory response.[2,20]

The morphologic and cellular changes in central airways have been the focus of several biopsy studies conducted in smokers with symptoms of chronic bronchitis.[2,3,20–24] The epithelium is normally intact and shows squamous metaplastic change as well as increase in the number of goblet cells. Differently from asthma, the thickness of the reticular basement membrane is within the normal range, in the majority of subjects. Mononuclear cells predominate in the subepithelium and this population contains an increased number of CD3 (T-lymphocytes), CD25+ cells (early activation), VLA-1 positive cells (late activation) and macrophages.[20] There have also been reports of tissue eosinophilia in chronic bronchitis,[21] particularly during exacerbations of the disease.[22] Interestingly, the high numbers of neutrophils found in lavage fluid from subjects with chronic bronchitis[23] is not reflected in their numbers in the bronchial subepithelium. This discrepancy could result from rapid migration of neutrophils through the tissue, across the epithelium into the airway lumen, with accumulation of these cells on the surface where they might be undetectable by tissue analysis but present in lavage fluid. However, lavage findings may reflect the pathology of alveolar surface more than the airway mucosa.[24] Although the mechanism of neutrophil accumulation into the airway lumen in smokers with chronic bronchitis is not entirely clear, an imbalance between pro- and anti-inflammatory cytokines could be important. Interleukin 10 (IL-10), a cytokine that reduces inflammatory responses, is decreased in sputum of smokers with COPD,[25] whereas IL-8, a cytokine that promotes neutrophil chemotaxis, and tumor necrosis factor alpha (TNF-α), a cytokine that activates adhesion molecules, are increased.[26] The observation of an upregulation of the adhesion molecules E-selectin and ICAM-1 (intercellular adhesion molecule 1) on subepithelial vessels and on bronchial epithelium of smokers with chronic bronchitis[27] is consistent with active neutrophil migration into the bronchial epithelium.

The mucous glands are inflamed in chronic bronchitis[1] and this response contains an increased number of mast cells,[28] macrophages, CD8 T-lymphocytes and neutrophils.[2] Neutrophil elastase is a potent secretagogue for mucus secretion in cultured gland cells[29] and it is possible that the location of neutrophils within the bronchial glands is crucial for the activation of mucus secretion and sputum production in subjects with chronic bronchitis. This mucus hypersecretion was not considered important

to the development of chronic airflow limitation in smokers,[30] but a recent study suggests there is an association between chronic bronchitis and decline in FEV_1 and an increased risk of subsequent hospitalization because of COPD.[31]

Chronic bronchitis may or may not be associated with airflow limitation.[1] When airflow obstruction is present, a further increase in macrophages and T-lymphocytes has been reported in the subepithelium of the bronchial mucosa.[32] The association between CD8+ T-lymphocytes in central airway biopsies and a decline in FEV_1[33] suggests that the inflammatory process extends beyond the reach of the biopsy forceps to the site of obstruction in the small airways. A major function of CD8+ T-lymphocytes is the removal of host cells that are infected with a virus, and their excessive recruitment to the parenchymal tissue in patients with COPD has been correlated with latent adenoviral infection.[17] The upregulation of ICAM-1 expression in the epithelium of smokers with COPD[27,34] suggests a mechanism for the increased incidence of rhinovirus infection in patients with COPD as ICAM-1 serves as the receptor for this virus.[35]

In smokers with COPD the increase in the number of CD8 T-lymphocytes results in a shift in the balance of the CD4/CD8 cell ratio in favor of a CD8 predominance.[33,36] This contrasts with the predominance and activation of the CD4 T-cell subset in asthma.[36] A current paradigm in immunology is that the nature of an immune response to an antigenic stimulus is determined largely by the pattern of cytokines produced by activated CD4+ and CD8+ T cells. Both CD4 and CD8 T-lymphocytes include subsets that make interferon gamma (IFN-γ) but not IL-4 (Th1 or Tc1) as well as IL-4 but not IFN-γ (Th2 or Tc2). Differently from asthma, where several studies have shown a prevalent infiltration of Th2 lymphocytes, little is known about CD8 T-lymphocytes subsets in COPD.[37]

As airflow limitation progressively worsens in subjects with COPD, neutrophils increase in the subepithelium and this increase is correlated with the degree of airflow limitation.[38] Interestingly, an association between neutrophilia and severity of disease has been recently reported in asthma,[39] suggesting a role for these cells in the progression of both asthma and COPD.

There are very few observations of airway pathology in longitudinal studies of COPD. In one pioneer study involving a 15-year follow-up, Stanescu and colleagues found that an accelerated decline in lung function was associated with an increased number of neutrophils in the airway lumen.[40] In addition, in subjects with a more rapid decline in FEV_1, neutrophils exhibited an increased expression of the adhesion molecule CD11b/CD18, the ligand for ICAM-1. The correlation that is observed between increased expression of CD11b/CD18 and reduced expiratory flow in these subjects[41] shows that the adhesion molecules responsible for PMN migration are upregulated in COPD.

Although smoking cessation has beneficial effects on pulmonary function, there is relatively little information about the effect of smoking cessation on the airway inflammatory process. The few studies that have made a direct assessment of airway inflammation after smoking cessation suggest that an airway inflammatory response is present, even in the absence of cigarette smoking.[17,42–45] Although the inflammatory process in the central airways consists predominantly of mononuclear cells, there is a subgroup of patients with COPD that shows increased numbers of eosinophils in the inflammatory exudate. A prominent eosinophilia has recently been reported in bronchial biopsies of subjects with chronic bronchitis examined during an acute exacerbation of the disease,[22] as well as in sputum and bronchial lavage fluid of patients who improved their pulmonary function in response to a short course of oral corticosteroids.[46,47] These findings suggest that COPD represents a heterogeneous disease that includes a subgroup of patients with features of asthma such as airway eosinophilia and reversibility of airway obstruction in response to corticosteroids.

PERIPHERAL AIRWAYS

The smaller bronchi and bronchioles less than 2 mm in diameter are the major site of airway obstruction in COPD,[4] but the proportion of the total resistance that these small airways contribute to in normal subjects is controversial.[4,48,49] The reasons for the difference of opinion are too technical to be debated here but there are compelling reasons to believe that the small airways represent the lungs 'quiet zone' where disease can accumulate for many years before symptoms of airway obstruction appear.[50]

Some authors have suggested that small airway resistance is increased because of a reduction in the support they receive from the surrounding parenchyma.[51,52] Dayman[51] postulated that the destruction of the alveolar walls attached to the outer surface of the small airways caused them to behave like check valves. However, direct measurements of small airway pressure and flow established that the inspiratory and expiratory resistance of the small airways was the same over a wide range of lung volume.[4] Butler et al.[52] suggested the alternate hypothesis that the overall loss in lung elastic recoil produced by emphysema caused the small airways to narrow by reducing the stretch on the outer airway wall. If this were true then the increased lung elastic recoil generated by inflating the lung should have caused the small airway resistance to decrease toward normal in diseased lungs but it did not.[4] Mead et al.[53] subsequently showed that lung elastic recoil provides the driving pressure for flow out of the lungs during forced expiration and suggested that reduced lung recoil caused airflow limitation in COPD by decreasing

the pressure available to drive air out of the lung during maximum expiration. These data suggest that the increase in small airway resistance in COPD is related to the inflammatory disease in the wall and lumen of the airway that are independent of the changes in elastic recoil in the surrounding lung parenchyma.

Dunnill recognized that the inflammatory process that involves the small airways in emphysematous lungs is peribronchiolar in nature and consists of a mixture of mononuclear and polymorphonuclear leucocytes.[54] Matsuba and Thurlbeck[55] showed that this process progressed with connective tissue deposition and fixed airway narrowing due to peribronchial fibrosis. The types of inflammatory cells in the peripheral lung in COPD[17] are similar to those found in the central airways,[20,33,38] although it is clear that the disease responsible for both chronic bronchitis and small airway obstruction can occur independently and need not be found together.

EMPHYSEMA

Pulmonary emphysema

Laennec first described pulmonary emphysema in 1834 from observations of the cut surface of post-mortem human lungs that had been air dried in inflation.[56] He postulated that the lesions were due to overinflation of the lung, which compressed capillaries and led to atrophy of lung tissue. This hypothesis appeared in a major textbook of pathology as late as 1940[57] when reports implicating infection and inflammation in the pathogenesis of emphysema began to appear. Both McLean[6] and Leopold and Gough[58] implicated the inflammatory response in their early description of centrilobular emphysema, but it was difficult to be sure of its importance because their post-mortem observations might have been influenced by pre terminal pneumonia. The subsequent observations that emphysema could be produced experimentally by depositing the enzyme papain in the lung,[59] and was expressed as part of the phenotype of α_1 antitrypsin deficiency,[60] led naturally to the current hypothesis that emphysema results from a proteolytic imbalance within the cigarette smoke-induced inflammatory response.[7,28] The source of the proteolytic enzymes that might contribute to lung destruction and their inhibitors is discussed elsewhere in this book (Chapter 9).

The definition of pulmonary emphysema is 'abnormal permanent enlargement of airspaces distal to terminal bronchioles, accompanied by destruction of their walls without obvious fibrosis'.[61,62] The terms used to describe the emphysematous lesions (i.e. centrilobular or centriacinar vs. panlobular or panacinar) are based on the anatomy of the normal lung where the acinus is defined as the portion of the lung parenchyma supplied by a single terminal bronchiole (Figure 2.1(b)) whereas the 'secondary lobule' is that part of the lung surrounded by connective tissue septa which contains several terminal bronchioles and therefore several acini (Figure 2.1(a)).

Centrilobular/centriacinar emphysema

Centrilobular emphysema was briefly described by Gough in 1952,[63] by McLean in Australia in 1956[64] and in a more detailed report by Leopold and Gough in 1957.[58] Figure 2.1(c) shows a line drawing from Leopold and Gough's description as well as a post-mortem radiograph illustrating the effect of dilatation and destruction of the respiratory bronchioles. These lesions affect the upper regions of the lung more commonly than the lower and are also larger and more numerous in the upper lung.[65,66] Heppleston and Leopold[67] used the term 'focal

emphysema' to describe a less severe form of the disease. But Dunnill concluded that this separation is based largely on semantic arguments.[54] His review suggests that the two conditions have a similar origin with focal emphysema being more widely distributed in the lung and less severe than the classic centrilobular form.[58] Dunnill also preferred the term centriacinar to centrilobular, which is logical, based on the fact that each secondary lobule contains several acini (Figure 2.1) and not all of them need be involved in emphysematous destruction.

Panacinar/panlobular emphysema

In panacinar emphysema, there is more uniform destruction of the acinus and all of the acini within the secondary lobule are involved. Wyatt et al.[68] provided a detailed account of this lesion in 1962 and Thurlbeck[66] pointed out that in its mildest forms, it is difficult to discern from

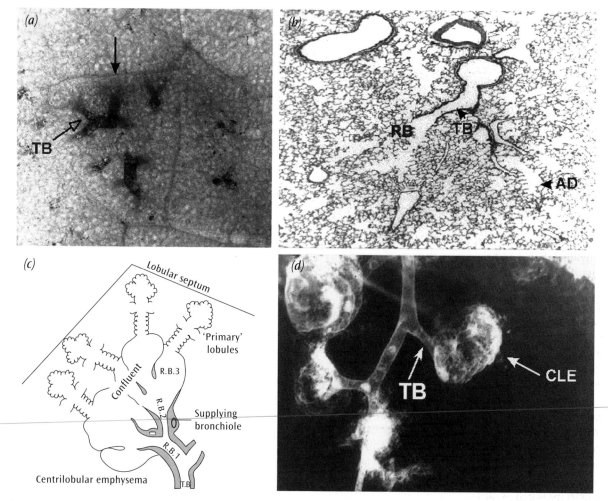

Figure 2.1 *Normal anatomy of the secondary lobule (a) and the acinus (b). The solid arrow indicates the lobular septae and TB indicates the terminal bronchiole supplying the acinus in both (a) and (b). (c) Diagram of a lobule containing the centrilobular emphysematous lesion. (From ref. 34 with permission.) (d) Post-mortem bronchogram illustrating a terminal bronchiole (TB) supplying a centrilobular space (CLE). RB = Respiratory bronchial; AD = Alveolar duct.*

normal lung unless fixed inflated lung slices are impregnated with barium sulfate and examined under water using low power magnification. In contrast to centrilobular emphysema, the panacinar form tends to be more severe in the lower compared to the upper lobe but this difference only becomes statistically significant in severe disease.[66] Panacinar emphysema is the type of lesion commonly associated with α_1 antitrypsin deficiency but is also found in cases where no genetic abnormality has been identified.[69]

Other forms of emphysema

Distal acinar, mantle or paraseptal emphysema are terms used to describe lesions that occur in the periphery of the lobule. This type of lesion can be commonly found along the lobular septae particularly in the subpleural region. It can also occur in isolation and it has been associated with spontaneous pneumothorax in young adults[70] and bullous lung disease in older individuals where individual cysts may become large enough to interfere with lung function.[71] Unilateral emphysema or McLeod's syndrome is a complication of severe childhood infections caused by rubella or adenovirus and congenital lobar emphysema is a developmental abnormality affecting newborn children. The emphysema that forms around scars lacks any special distribution within the acinus or lobule and is referred to as irregular or paracicatricial emphysema.[54,69]

DIAGNOSIS OF EMPHYSEMA

The definition of emphysema presupposes knowledge of normal airspace size. This varies considerably between individuals based on height, weight and sex and within a single individual based on the level of lung inflation. The problem of separating fully inflated normal lung from mild emphysema restricted the diagnosis of emphysema to pathologists who were willing to examine post-mortem specimens that were fixed in inflation.[61–69] The Edinburgh group[72] were the first to provide a quantitative diagnosis of emphysema in living patients using the frequency distribution of computed tomographic EMI units to separate normal lung from permanent distal airspace enlargement. The Hounsfield unit has subsequently replaced the EMI unit; it measures the degree to which X-rays are attenuated by tissue and can be calibrated between −1000 (air) to 0 (water) and +1000 (bone). The Hounsfield unit can be converted to density by adding 1000 to the number of units measured in each three-dimensional unit (voxels) of the CT scan and dividing that sum by 1000. Muller and colleagues[73] developed a density mask to separate the CT voxels below a fixed density (0.910 HU) and used it to separate normal from emphysematous lung. The same

group subsequently showed that this method identified emphysematous lesions down to those that were approximately 5 mm in diameter but did not identify the milder forms of the disease.[74]

Measurements of density have the units of weight/volume and can be converted to specific volume (volume/weight) and used to calculate regional lung volumes in ml/gram of lung.[75] This approach was first used to calculate the regional lung volume in dogs where the thorax had been frozen intact and the density determined directly from measurements of weight and volume of frozen lung samples.[75] Similar measurements obtained using CT provided measurements of regional lung volume and estimates of the pleural pressure gradient in humans.[76] These results also showed that the summed weight of each voxel (density × volume) measured from the preoperative CT scan of a lung or lobe compared favorably with the weight of the resected specimen.[76] These measurements of regional lung expansion allow emphysema to be identified by its definition, which is expansion beyond normal[61,62] where the normal value for maximum lung expansion ranges from 5.7 to 6.8 ml/gram depending on the age, height and sex of the subject.[77]

Analysis of the frequency distribution of the volume of gas/gram tissue of all of the voxels in the CT scan of lungs from patients with normal lung function show that they are normally distributed in patients with preserved lung function.[78] This distribution shifts to the right in mild emphysema and further to the right with severe disease (Figure 2.2). The value added by analyzing the CT scan in terms of volume[75–78] rather than density[72–74] is that

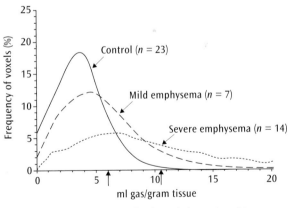

Figure 2.2 *Frequency distribution of the regional lung volume of all of the lung voxels in CT scans from 23 control cases with normal lung function, 7 cases with mild emphysema and 14 cases with severe emphysema. The arrows indicate the upper limits of normal lung volume (6.0 ± 1.1 ml gas/gram tissue) and the lung volume determined by the cutoff defined by the density mask used in ref. 48 (10.2 ml/gram). Lesions less than 0.5 mm in diameter are not found using the density mask but are identified between 6 and 10 ml/gram. (Data from ref. 78.)*

it can separate fully inflated normal lung from the mild emphysema based on the definition of emphysema as expansion of the lung beyond the normal range.[61,62]

Combining CT measurements with quantitative histology

Cruz-Orive and Weibel[79] introduced a robust cascade sampling design that used the fixed inflated lung as a reference volume and random samples of the lung examined at increasing levels of magnification to quantitate lung structure from the gross to the electron microscopic level. Coxson and associates[80] modified this technique for use with lung biopsy in living patients by substituting the CT-determined lung volume as the reference in the cascade. This approach was subsequently applied to tissue from resected lobes[76] and more recently from lung volume reduction surgery[78] where an equation (surface area/volume $= e^{6.84 - 0.32 \text{ ml gas/gram tissue}}$) was used to link the CT-determined volume to histologically measured surface area/volume ratio. This approach provides a method of estimating the surface area to volume ratio and total surface area of the lung from the CT scan which show good correlation with measurements of diffusing capacity made in the same subjects.[78] This type of analysis provides a quantitative estimate of the extent and severity of lung destruction, as well as its location within the lung. It could be helpful in following the natural history of the emphysema and as an outcome measure for trials of surgical and medical treatment.

PULMONARY VASCULAR CHANGES IN COPD

The resistance to airflow ($cmH_2O/L/s$) and the compliance (L/cmH_2O) of the lung both increase as COPD develops. The combined effect of these two mechanical changes has the units of time and is referred to as the time constant of the lung. When the time constant for lung emptying exceeds that of the chest wall, intrathoracic pressure increases and is transmitted to the pulmonary vasculature and the alveolar gas. This increases intravascular pressure relative to the atmosphere but has no effect on the transmural pressure of the vessels within the thorax because transmural pressure (the difference between intravascular and intrathoracic pressure) remains the same. However, in regions of diseased lung where the time constant is abnormally prolonged, the alveolar gas is compressed and when its pressure rises above intrathoracic pressure the lung capillaries are compressed and alveolar vascular resistance increases. Wright et al.[9] studied cardiac output and pulmonary vascular pressures in patients with mild to moderate COPD that required lung

resection for a peripheral tumor and correlated these physiologic measurements to the histologic changes in the pulmonary vessels in the resected specimens. These hemodynamic measurements were made in the supine position with the majority of the lung under zone 3 conditions and normal pulmonary vascular pressures and cardiac output at rest. Mild exercise performed in this position increased cardiac output, pulmonary arterial and pulmonary venous pressures without changing the driving pressure (i.e. the difference between pulmonary arterial and pulmonary venous pressure) because the rise in both pulmonary arterial and venous pressure was due to the rise in intrathoracic pressure. Switching from air to oxygen breathing reduced both pulmonary artery and venous pressures, suggesting that intrathoracic pressure fell because of a reduction in the lung time constant. Just how an increase in oxygen tension decreased either the lung compliance or airway resistance was not clear from these experiments.

Wright et al. found that even the modest changes in pulmonary vascular physiology found in these patients with mild COPD were associated with structural changes in the peripheral lung vessels. These included a thickening of the intima, media and adventitial layers in the peripheral lung vessel walls. Peinado et al.[10] have subsequently studied resected lung tissue from a similar group of patients and shown that there is also an inflammatory reaction in the wall of the muscular arteries that contain large numbers of CD8+ lymphocytes. Just how much of the structural change seen in the vascular wall is due to changes in hemodynamics and how much is due to the inflammatory response remains to be determined. Both probably contribute to the progression to the more severe arterial lesions that have been associated with right heart failure in COPD.

ACUTE EXACERBATION OF COPD

Acute exacerbations of cough, sputum production and dyspnea are an important feature of the natural history of COPD.[11,12,15,16] These symptoms may go unreported, be treated on an ambulatory basis or require hospital admission to an ICU for acute respiratory failure.[81] Although an exacerbation is one of the principal reasons that patients with COPD seek medical attention, they are not included in the definition of COPD and their pathology is very poorly understood.[82] A proportion responds to antibiotics in a way that suggests they are initiated by bacteria.[12] But the pathologic basis of the lesions that are responsible for the wide range of presenting symptoms has not been adequately determined during life.

The reason for the inadequate state of our understanding of the pathology of an acute exacerbation is that invasive procedures cannot be performed on these severely ill patients. Studies of an exacerbation in patients with mild COPD show a prominent inflammatory response with numbers of eosinophils similar to those reported in stable asthma.[83] However in contrast to asthma, the tissue eosinophils found in COPD do not degranulate as they do in asthma and were not associated with an increased expression of IL-5.[84] Viral infections may have a role in producing this eosinophilia because certain respiratory viruses are able to stimulate the production of eotaxin, a potent eosinophil chemoattractant.[85] In exacerbations of bacterial origin, myeloperoxidase, a marker of neutrophil activation, and IL-8, a potent neutrophil chemoattractant, were increased in the airway lumen, suggesting a neutrophilic inflammatory reaction.[86] A recent study of a large cohort of severe COPD patients failed to demonstrate any change in the total number of cells in the sputum of the differential counts between exacerbated and stable disease. The only difference in the exacerbated group was a higher level of the proinflammatory cytokine IL-6.[87]

Several early studies suggested that these exacerbations had no effect on the decline in lung function,[15,88,89] but a recent report from the National Institute of Health sponsored Lung Health Study suggests that they do increase the decline in lung function in patients who continue to smoke.[90] Interestingly long-term treatment with high doses of inhaled corticosteroids apparently reduces the incidence of acute exacerbations of COPD[91] without reducing the progressive fall in FEV$_1$.[91–93] In a mild exacerbation the effectiveness of corticosteroids could be related to the presence of airway eosinophilia.[83] Long-term treatment with inhaled corticosteroids might also reduce the frequency of exacerbations in patients that have either asthmatic features[46] or sputum eosinophilia[47] and show improvement in pulmonary function in response to a short course of steroids. The structural changes that are responsible for the long-term decline in lung function appear to progress following an exacerbation when the patient continues to smoke[90] and are apparently unchanged by long-term inhaled corticosteroid treatment.[91–93]

SUMMARY

The lung inflammatory response that is present in all cigarette smokers is amplified in the minority that develop COPD and persists even after smoking has stopped. In chronic bronchitis, this process is located in the mucosa, gland ducts and glands of intermediate sized bronchi between 2–4 mm internal diameter. Airway obstruction is caused by a similar inflammatory process in the smaller bronchi and bronchioles less than 2 mm in internal diameter that may be present with or without chronic bronchitis. The inflammatory response in the alveolar

tissue and airspaces of the subgroup of smokers with severe emphysema provides several opportunities for the proteolytic imbalance that underlies the emphysematous destruction of the lung surface. Both the increase in small airway resistance and the loss of lung elastic recoil caused by emphysema contribute to the decline in FEV$_1$ and FEV$_1$/FVC ratio, whereas the reduction in lung surface area/volume ratio and total surface area of the lung contribute to the reduction in diffusing capacity.

The behavior of the pulmonary circulation is influenced by the changes in lung mechanics that occur in patients with COPD. The increase in airway resistance and in lung compliance lengthens the time constant (i.e. the product of resistance and compliance) of the lung and when the time constant of the lung exceeds that of the chest wall intrathoracic pressure begins to rise. In regions of the lung where the rise in alveolar pressure exceeds that in intrathoracic pressure the alveolar vessels are compressed and alveolar vascular resistance is increased. An inflammatory process that has been demonstrated in the wall of the small blood vessels contributes to the vascular changes that are associated with pulmonary hypertension in COPD.

The pathology of the acute exacerbations that punctuate the progressive decline in lung function in COPD is only beginning to be understood. Some of these attacks are caused by bacterial infection, others by atmospheric pollution, but recent evidence suggests that viral infection may have an important role in precipitating these episodes. Viral infection has been implicated in the tissue and sputum eosinophilia as well as the response to steroids observed in patients with relatively mild COPD who have exacerbations. Unfortunately very little is known about the pathology of exacerbations in patients with more severe COPD because they are generally too sick to be studied using the invasive methods that have become common in less severe disease.

REFERENCES

1. Mullen JBM, Wright JL, Wiggs B, Pare PD, Hogg JC. Reassessment of inflammation in the airways of chronic bronchitis. *Br Med J* 1985;**291**:1235–9.
2. Saetta M, Turato G, Facchini FM, *et al*. Inflammatory cells in the bronchial glands of smokers with chronic bronchitis. *Am J Respir Crit Care Med* 1997;**156**:1633–9.
3. Jeffery PK. Comparison of the structural and inflammatory features of COPD and asthma. *Chest* 2000;**117**:251S–60S.
4. Hogg JC, Macklem PT, Thurlbeck WM. Site and nature of airways obstruction in chronic obstructive lung disease. *N Engl J Med* 1968;**278**:1355–60.
5. Cosio M, Ghezzo M, Hogg JC, *et al*. The relation between structural changes in small airways and pulmonary function tests. *New Engl J Med* 1978;**298**:1277–81.
6. McLean KA. Pathogenesis of pulmonary emphysema. *Am J Med* 1958;**25**:62–74.

7. Gadek JE, Fells JA, Crystal RG. Cigarette smoke induces a functional anti-protease deficiency in the lower respiratory tract. *Science* 1979;**206**:315–16.

8. Janoff A. Biochemical links between cigarette smoking and pulmonary emphysema. *J Appl Physiol* 1983;**55**:285–93.

9. Wright JL, Lawson L, Pare PD, *et al.* The structure and function of the pulmonary vasculature in mild chronic obstructive pulmonary disease. *Am Rev Respir Dis* 1983;**128**:702–7.

10. Peinado VI, Barbera JA, Abate P, Ramirez J, Roca J, Santos S, Rodriguez-Roisin R. Inflammatory reaction in pulmonary muscular arteries of patients with mild chronic obstructive pulmonary disease. *Am J Respir Crit Care Med* 1999;**159**:1605–11.

11. Saetta M, Di Stefano A, Maestrelli P, *et al.* Airway eosinophilia in chronic bronchitis during exacerbations. *Am J Respir Crit Care Med* 1994;**150**:1646–52.

12. Anthonisen NR, Manfreda J, Warren CP, Hershfield ES, Harding GK, Nelson NA. Antibiotic therapy in exacerbations of chronic obstructive pulmonary disease. *Ann Intern Med* 1987;**106**:196–204.

13. Niewoehner DE, Kleinerman J, Reisst DB. Pathologic changes in the peripheral airways of young cigarette smokers. *N Engl J Med* 1974;**291**:755–8.

14. Hunninghake BW, Crystal RG. Cigarette smoking and lung destruction: accumulation of neutrophils in the lung. *Am Rev Respir Dis* 1983;**128**:833–8.

15. Fletcher C, Peto R, Tinker C, Speizer FE. *The Natural History of Chronic Bronchitis and Emphysema*. Oxford University Press, Oxford, 1976.

16. Speizer FE, Tager IB. Epidemiology of chronic mucus hypersecretion and obstructive airways disease. *Epidemiol Rev* 1970;**1**:124–42.

17. Ratemales I, Elliott WM, Meshi B, *et al.* The amplification of inflammation in emphysema and its association with latent adenoviral infection. *Am J Respir Crit Care Med* 2001;**164**:469–73.

18. Doerschuk CM, Markos J, Coxson HO, English D, Hogg JC. Quantitation of neutrophil migration into acute bacterial pneumonia in rabbits. *J Appl Physiol* 1994;**77**:2593–9.

19. Reid L. Measurement of the bronchial mucous gland layer: a diagnostic yardstick in chronic bronchitis. *Thorax* 1960;**15**:132–41.

20. Saetta M, Di Stefano A, Maestrelli P, *et al.* Activated T-lymphocytes and macrophages in bronchial mucosa of subjects with chronic bronchitis. *Am Rev Respir Dis* 1993;**147**:301–6.

21. Lacoste JY, Bousquet J, Chanez P, *et al.* Eosinophilic and neutrophilic inflammation in asthma, chronic bronchitis, and chronic obstructive pulmonary disease. *J Allerg Clin Immunol* 1993;**92**:537–48.

22. Saetta M, Di Stefano A, Maestrelli P, *et al.* Airway eosinophilia in chronic bronchitis during exacerbations. *Am J Respir Crit Care Med* 1994;**150**:1646–52.

23. Thompson AB, Daughton D, Robbins GA, Ghafouri MA, Oehlerking M, Rennard MI. Intraluminal airway inflammation in chronic bronchitis. Characterization and correlation with clinical parameters. *Am Rev Respir Dis* 1989;**140**:1527–37.

24. Maestrelli P, Saetta M, Di Stefano A, *et al.* Comparison of leukocyte counts in sputum, bronchial biopsies and bronchoalveolar lavage. *Am J Respir Crit Care Med* 1995;**152**:1926–31.

25. Takanashi S, Hasegawa Y, Kanehira Y, *et al.* Interleukin-10 level in sputum is reduced in bronchial asthma, COPD and in smokers. *Eur Respir J* 1999;**14**:309–14.

26. Keatings VM, Collins PD, Scott DM, Barnes PJ. Differences in interleukin-8 and tumour necrosis factor-alpha in induced sputum from patients with chronic obstructive pulmonary disease or asthma. *Am J Respir Crit Care Med* 1996;**153**:530–4.

27. Di Stefano A, Maestrelli P, Roggeri A, *et al.* Upregulation of adhesion molecules in the bronchial mucosa of subjects with chronic obstructive bronchitis. *Am J Respir Crit Care Med* 1994;**149**:803–10.

28. Pesci A, Rossi GA, Bertorelli G, Aufiero A, Zanon P, Olivieri D. Mast cells in the airway lumen and bronchial mucosa of patients with chronic bronchitis. *Am J Respir Crit Care Med* 1994;**152**:260–6.

29. Nadel JA. Role of mast cell and neutrophil proteases in airway secretion. *Am Rev Respir Dis* 1991;**144**:S48–51.

30. Peto R, Speizer FE, Cochrane AL, *et al.* The relevance in adults of airflow obstruction, but not of mucous hypersecretion, to mortality from chronic lung disease. *Am Rev Respir Dis* 1983;**128**:491–500.

31. Vestbo J, Prescott E, Lange P, and the Copenhagen City Heart Study Group. Association of chronic mucus hypersecretion with FEV_1 decline and chronic obstructive pulmonary disease morbidity. *Am J Respir Crit Care Med* 1996;**153**:1530–5.

32. Di Stefano A, Turato G, Maestrelli P, *et al.* Airflow limitation in chronic bronchitis is associated with T-lymphocyte and macrophage infiltration in the bronchial mucosa. *Am J Respir Crit Care Med* 1996;**153**:629–32.

33. O'Shaughnessy TC, Ansari TW, Barnes NC, Jeffery PK. Inflammation in bronchial biopsies of subjects with chronic bronchitis: inverse relationship of CD8+ T-lymphocytes with FEV_1. *Am J Respir Crit Care Med* 1997;**155**:852–7.

34. Vignola AM, Campbell AM, Chanez P, Bousquet J, Paul-Lacoste P, Michel F-B, Godard P. HLA-DR and ICAM-1 expression on bronchial epithelial cells in asthma and chronic bronchitis. *Am Rev Respir Dis* 1993;**148**:689–94.

35. Papi A, Johnston SL. Rhinovirus infection induces expression of its own Receptor Intercellular Adhesion Molecule 1 (ICAM-1) via increased NF-kB-mediated transcription. *J Biol Chem* 1999;**274**:9707–20.

36. Jeffery PK. Differences and similarities between chronic obstructive pulmonary disease and asthma. *Clin Exp Allergy* 1999;**29**:14–26.

37. Kemeny DM, Vyas B, Vukmanovic-Stejic M, Thomas MJ, Noble A, Loh LC, O'Connor BJ. CD8+ T cell subsets and chronic obstructive pulmonary disease. *Am J Respir Crit Care Med* 1999;**160**:S33–7.

38. Di Stefano A, Capelli A, Lusuardi M, *et al.* Severity of airflow limitation is associated with severity of airway inflammation in smokers. *Am J Respir Crit Care Med* 1998;**158**:1277–85.

39. Wenzel SE, Szefler SJ, Leung DYM, Sloan SI, Rex MD, Martin RJ. Broncoscopic evaluation of severe asthma: persistent inflammation associated with high dose glucocorticoids. *Am J Respir Crit Care Med* 1997;**156**:737–43.

40. Stanescu D, Sanna A, Veriter C, *et al.* Airways obstruction, chronic expectoration, and rapid decline of FEV_1 in smokers are associated with increased levels of sputum neutrophils. *Thorax* 1996;**51**:267–71.

41. Maestrelli P, Calcagni PG, Saetta M, *et al.* Integrin upregulation on sputum neutrophils in smokers with chronic airway obstruction. *Am J Respir Crit Care Med* 1996;**154**:1296–300.

42. Turato G, Di Stefano A, Maestrelli P, *et al.* Effect of smoking cessation on airway inflammation in chronic bronchitis. *Am J Respir Crit Care Med* 1995;**152**:1262–7.

43. Rutgers SR, Postma DS, ten Hacken NHT, *et al.* Ongoing inflammation in patients with COPD who do not currently smoke. *Thorax* 2000;**55**:12–18.

44. Wright GL, Lawson LM, Parè PD, Wiggs BJ, Kennedy S, Hogg JC. Morphology of peripheral airways in current smokers and ex smokers. *Am Rev Respir Dis* 1983;**127**:474–7.

45. Shapiro S. End stage chronic obstructive pulmonary disease: the cigarette is burned out but the inflammation rages on. *Am J Respir Crit Care Med* 2001;**164**:339–40.

46. Chanez P, Vignola AM, O'Shaugnessy M, *et al.* Corticosteroid reversibility in COPD is related to features of asthma. *Am J Respir Crit Care Med* 1997;**155**:1529–34.

47. Pizzichini E, Pizzichini MMM, Gibson P, *et al.* Sputum eosinophilia predicts benefit from prednisone in smokers with chronic obstructive bronchitis. *Am J Respir Crit Care Med* 1998;**158**:1511–17.

48. Macklem PT, Mead J. Resistance of central and peripheral airways measured by the retrograde catheter. *J Appl Physiol* 1967;**22**:395–401.

49. van Brabant T, Cauberghs M, Verbeken E, Moerman P, Lauweryns JM, van de Woestijne KP. Partitioning of pulmonary impedance in excised human and canine lungs. *J Appl Physiol: Respir Environ Exercise Physiol* 1983;**55**:1733–42.

50. Mead J. The lung's 'quiet zone'. *N Engl J Med* 1970;**282**:1318–19.

51. Dayman H. Mechanics of airflow in health and emphysema. *J Clin Invest* 1951;**3031**:1175–90.

52. Butler J, Caro C, Alkaler R, Dubois AB. Physiological factors affecting airway resistance in normal subjects and in patients with obstructive airways disease. *J Clin Invest* 1960;**39**:584–91.

53. Mead J, Turner JM, Macklem PT, Little J. Significance of the relationship between lung recoil and maximum expiratory flow. *J Appl Physiol* 1967;**22**:95–108.

54. Dunnill MS. Emphysema. In: *Pulmonary Pathology*. Churchill Livingstone, Edinburgh, 1982, pp 81–112.

55. Matsuba K, Thurlbeck WM. The number and dimensions of small airways in emphysematous lungs. *Am J Pathol* 1972;**67**:265–75.

56. Laennec RTH, translated Forbes J. *A Treatise on Diseases of the Chest and on Mediate Auscultations*, 4th edn. Longmans, London.

57. McCallum WG. A Textbook of Pathology. WB Saunders, 1940. 7th edition. Chapter 21 Types of Injury – Destruction of the Respiratory Tract. pp 419–28.

58. Leopold JG, Gough J. Centrilobular form of hypertrophic emphysema and its relation to chronic bronchitis. *Thorax* 1957;**12**:219–35.

59. Gross P, Babyuk MA, Toller E, Kashak M. Enzymatically produced pulmonary emphysema. *J Occup Med* 1964;**6**:481–4.

60. Laurell CB, Erickson S. The electrophoretic alpha-1 globulin pattern of serum alpha-1 anti-trypsin deficiency. *Scand J Clin Lab Invest* 1963;**15**:132–40.

61. Ciba Guest Symposium Report: terminology, definitions and classifications of chronic pulmonary emphysema and related conditions. *Thorax* 1959;**14**:286–99.

62. Snider GL, Kleinerman JL, Thurlbeck WM, Bengally ZH. Definition of emphysema. Report of a National Heart, Lung and Blood Institute, Division of Lung Diseases. *Am Rev Respir Dis* 1985;**132**:182–5.

63. Gough J. Discussion of diagnosis of pulmonary emphysema. *Proc R Soc Med* 1952;**45**:576–7.

64. McLean KH. Microscopic anatomy of pulmonary emphysema. *Aust Ann Intern Med* 1956;**5**:73–88.

65. Heard BE. Further observations on the pathology of pulmonary emphysema in chronic bronchitis. *Thorax* 1958;**14**:58–90.

66. Thurlbeck WM. The incidence of pulmonary emphysema with observations on the relative incidence and spatial distribution of various types of emphysema. *Am Rev Respir Dis* 1963;**87**:207–15.

67. Heppleston AG, Leopold JG. Chronic pulmonary emphysema: anatomy and pathogenesis. *Am J Med* 1961;**31**:279–91.

68. Wyatt JP, Fischer VW, Sweet AC. Panlobular emphysema: anatomy and pathogenesis. *Dis Chest* 1962;**41**:239–59.

69. Thurlbeck WM. Chronic airflow obstruction. In: WM Thurlbeck, AM Churg, eds. *Pathology of the Lung*. Theime Medical, Stuttgart, 1995, pp 739–825.

70. Ohtaka M, Suzuki H. Pathogenesis of spontaneous pneumothorax with special reference to the ultrastructure of emphysematous bullae. *Chest* 1980;**77**:771–6.

71. Morgan MDL. Bullous lung disease. In: P Calverley, N Pride, eds. *Chronic Obstructive Pulmonary Disease*. Chapman and Hall, London, 1995, pp 548–60.

72. Hayhurst MD, MacNee W, Flenley DC, *et al.* Diagnosis of pulmonary emphysema by computerized tomography. *Lancet* 1984;**2**:32–322.

73. Muller NL, Staples CA, Miller RR, Alboud RT. Density mask. An objective method to quantitate emphysema using computed tomography. *Chest* 1988;**94**:782–7.

74. Miller RR, Muller NL, Vedal S, *et al.* Limitations of computed tomography in the assessment of emphysema. *Am Rev Resp Dis* 1989;**139**:980–3.

75. Hogg JC, Nepszy S. Regional lung volume and pleural pressure gradient estimated from lung density in dogs. *J Appl Physiol* 1969;**27**:198–203.

76. Coxson HO, Mayo JR, Behzad H, *et al.* The measurement of lung expansion with computed tomography and comparison with quantitative histology. *J Appl Physiol* 1995;**79**:1525–30.

77. Nakano Y, Coxson HO, Moore BR, van Eeden SF, Hogg JC. *Am J Resp Crit Care Med* 2001;**163**:907 (abstract).

78. Coxson HO, Rogers RM, Whittall P, *et al.* Quantification of the lung surface area in emphysema using computed tomography. *Am J Respir Crit Care Med* 1999;**159**:851–6.

79. Cruz-Orive LM, Weibel ER. Sampling designs for stereology. *J Microsc* 1981;**122**:235–57.

80. Coxson HO, Hogg JC, Mayo JR, *et al.* Quantification of idiopathic pulmonary fibrosis using computed tomography and histology. *Am J Respir Crit Care Med* 1997;**155**:1649–56.

81. Barnes PJ. Chronic obstructive pulmonary disease. *N Engl J Med* 2000;**343**:269–80.

82. Fabbri LM, Beghè B, Caramori G, Papi A, Saetta M. Similarities and discrepancies between exacerbations of asthma and chronic obstructive pulmonary disease. *Thorax* 1998;**53**:803–8.

83. Saetta M, Di Stefano A, Maestrelli P, *et al.* Airway eosinophilia in chronic bronchitis during exacerbations. *Am J Respir Crit Care Med* 1994;**150**:1646–52.

84. Saetta M, Di Stefano A, Maestrelli P, *et al.* Airway eosinophilia and expression of IL-5 in asthma and in exacerbations of chronic bronchitis. *Clin Exp Allergy* 1996;**26**:766–74.

85. Scheerens J, Folkerts G, van der Linde H, *et al.* Eotaxin levels and eosinophils in guinea pig bronchoalveolar lavage fluid are increased at the onset of a viral respiratory infection. *Clin Exp Allergy* 1999;**29**(suppl)2:74–7.

86. Crooks SW, Bayley DL, Hill SL, Stockley RA. Bronchial inflammation in acute bacterial exacerbations of chronic bronchitis: the role of leukotriene B4. *Eur Respir J* 2000;**15**:274–80.

87. Bhowmik A, Seemungal TAR, Sapsford RJ, Wedzicha JA. Relation of sputum inflammatory markers to symptoms and lung function changes in COPD exacerbations. *Thorax* 2000;**55**:114–20.

88. Howard P. Long term follow up of respiratory symptoms and ventilatory function in a group of working men. *Br J Industr Med* 1970;**27**:326–33.

89. Bates D. The fate of the chronic bronchitic: a report of the 10 year follow up in the Canadian Department of Veterans Affairs co-ordinated study on chronic bronchitis. *Am Rev Respir Dis* 1973;**108**:1043–65.

90. Kanner RE, Anthonisen NR, Connett JE, *et al.* Lower respiratory illnesses promote FEV_1 decline in current smokers but not ex smokers with mild COPD. *Am J Respir Crit Care Med* 2001;**164**:358–64.

91. Burge PS, Calverley PMA, Jones PW, Spencer S, Anderson JA, Maslen TK. Randomised, double blind, placebo controlled study of fluticasone proportionate in patients with moderate to severe chronic obstructive pulmonary disease: the ISOLDE trial. *Br Med J* 2000;**320**:1297–303.

92. Pauwels RA, Lofdahl CG, Laitinen LA, *et al.* for the European Respiratory Society Study on Chronic Obstructive Pulmonary Disease. Long-term treatment with inhaled budesonide in patients with mild chronic obstructive pulmonary disease who continue smoking. *N Engl J Med* 1999;**340**:1948–53.

93. Vestbo J, Sorensen T, Lange P, Brix A, Torre P, Viskum K. Long-term effect of inhaled budesonide in mild and moderate chronic obstructive pulmonary disease: a randomised controlled trial. *Lancet* 1999;**353**:1819–23.

3

Epidemiology

JØRGEN VESTBO AND PETER LANGE

INTRODUCTION

As a consequence of the declining incidence of tuberculosis in Western countries that took place at the beginning of the last century, increasing attention was paid to other causes of chronic lung diseases. Interest in the epidemiology of chronic respiratory disease was further enforced by the air pollution disasters like that in the Meuse Valley in 1930 and in London in 1952, and in particular in response to the universal spread of the smoking epidemic that took place after the second world war. In this introduction we will give a short overview of the epidemiologic definitions of bronchitis and COPD and the tools and limitations for studying COPD in an epidemiologic setting.

Definitions of diseases frequently vary between clinical and epidemiologic settings. Often, more simple diagnostic tools are used in epidemiology, where for practical reasons the use of the sophisticated investigation methods available in clinical practice is impossible. For this reason it may be difficult to compare rates of disease in the population with the number of patients in the clinical situation in a way which makes sense to both the clinician and the epidemiologist. Fortunately, this is only true to some extent for COPD and has mainly been a problem for the study of subtypes of COPD, especially emphysema, where little can be accomplished with the usual epidemiologic tools, which often only comprise standardized questionnaires of respiratory symptoms and spirometry.

Since the study by Fletcher *et al.* published 25 years ago,[1] the FEV_1 has been established as the key measurement in the epidemiology of COPD. The increasing attention paid to measurement of lung function has been adopted very early by respiratory epidemiologists since measurement of the FEV_1 and FVC is easy to perform in the epidemiological setting, where large sources of data based on samples of the general population and occupational cohorts have been available for many decades. Spirometric measurements have among others the advantage of being described on a continuous scale, allowing reanalyses if new criteria for assessing the presence of significant COPD are introduced, resulting in new cut-off values between normal lung function and significant airway obstruction. Therefore, it has been easy to adjust the epidemiologic definition of COPD to the clinical definition, based on the presence of airway obstruction. As in the clinical setting, COPD in epidemiology is defined as the presence of reduced maximal expiratory flow not caused by a specific airway disease, which in practice means a FEV_1/FVC ratio of less than 88% predicted in males and less than 89% predicted in women according to the European Respiratory Society (ERS) statement[2] or FEV_1/FVC less than 70% according to the recently published GOLD guidelines.[3] However, compared with the clinical situation, it is much more difficult in population studies to exclude specific causes of airway obstruction like cystic fibrosis, bronchiectases, obliterative broncholitis and, in particular, bronchial asthma. With regard to the latter condition one may rely on the presence of reversibility of airway obstruction or hyperresponsiveness, data which are now available in some epidemiologic studies. However, both a degree of reversibility and hyperresponsiveness may be present in COPD – and absent in asthma – and underline the need for better diagnostic markers. Although spirometry ought to be an essential measurement in epidemiologic studies of COPD, it is unfortunately not always available and in many circumstances we still have to rely on reported diagnoses from death certificates, hospital discharge forms and patients' own perception of disease with all the expected limitations and potential sources of bias. In order to minimize this latter bias, respiratory epidemiologists have over the years developed and validated several standardized questionnaires on respiratory symptoms, beginning with the British Medical Research Council (BMRC) questionnaire in 1960[4,5] and followed by the European Community of Coal and Steel (ECCS) questionnaire,[6] the National Heart and Lung Institute (NHLI) questionnaire and the American Thoracic Society (ATS-DLD) questionnaire.[7] Initially, these questionnaires focused mainly on cough, sputum production, breathlessness and chest infections but more recently, the focus has been expanded to include questions on asthma and asthma symptoms like wheezing, nocturnal coughing and nasal allergies, making attempts to differentiate between COPD and asthma more easily. The recognition of cultural and language barriers has within the last years resulted in the development of video questionnaires especially suited for investigating school children.

In addition to measurement techniques, tools in epidemiology include both study design and methodology. Health statistics providing large-scale data enable us to study the impact of the disease in society, make crude comparisons between countries and continents, detect major changes in disease distribution over time, and make qualified predictions for the future. Such data have limited use in establishing anything close to a causal relationship and are often affected by universal and time-dependent biases which can be difficult and sometimes impossible to adjust properly for. An important problem with the use of health statistics to measure the burden of COPD has been the lack of a specific diagnostic category in the International Classification of Diseases (ICD) describing COPD. Therefore, data are often generated, on the one hand, by combining diagnoses of chronic bronchitis, emphysema, chronic airway obstruction and sometimes even asthma. Population surveys on the other hand provide data on a limited number of individuals, but the loss of quantity is made up for by the possibility of information gathered in a standardized way, including questionnaire-derived information such as symptoms, smoking habits, etc., as well as measurement of lung function and airway responsiveness, blood tests and genetic information. Finally, databases from population surveys, including data on repeated screenings, can be merged with locally existing health registers, combining the advantages of the two strategies.

IMPACT OF COPD: PREVALENCE, MORTALITY, MORBIDITY AND COSTS

The estimates of the distribution of COPD are incomplete for several reasons. As for asthma there has for decades been an ongoing debate on the definition, and although spirometry is now considered a gold standard, there is still much discussion on how to discriminate between COPD and other diseases causing cough and airway obstruction. Most importantly, however, is the fact that large-scale estimates of morbidity and mortality based on health statistics do not contain any information on the presence of airway obstruction and must therefore rely on the diagnosis made by doctors reporting the case (e.g. mortality statistics, statistics on consultation in general practice, hospital discharges, etc.). As diagnostic habits differ greatly between different geographical regions, the comparison of health statistics data between countries may be difficult or even impossible. In addition it seems that misclassification may underestimate the impact of COPD more than for conditions such as cancer or ischemic heart disease. COPD is often not included in the vital statistics as it is mentioned on death certificates more often as a contributory and not as an underlying cause of death.[8] It is also a clinical impression that the fact that COPD develops slowly and without dramatic manifestations results in underdiagnosis and that dyspnea caused by COPD is interpreted as being caused by other conditions like heart disease or simply old age.

Despite these methodologic problems there is no doubt that COPD is a very prevalent disease worldwide. Although it may already be detectable in young adults, where FEV_1 may be within the normal range whereas FEV_1/FVC has already started to decrease below normal limits, its greatest impact is in the middle aged and elderly population. Data from random samples of the population show that prevalences of COPD, defined as irreversible obstructive lung function impairment, vary from 4% to 10% in the adult population.[9,10] The prevalence is approximately twice as high in subjects older than 65 years compared with the 45–65-year age group. Generally, it is higher in men than in women although in countries where smoking is more prevalent in younger women than in men, the prevalence in young adults is also highest in women. The prevalence is three to four times higher in smokers compared to non-smokers, although this gradient is less prominent among women in the developing countries.[9,10] Even in developed countries there is still a clearly detectable and poorly understood social gradient, which cannot be explained by differences in smoking habits or occupational exposures.[11] As international comparisons of COPD prevalence rates are difficult and as data on prevalence in many countries are non-existent, attempts have been made to estimate the prevalence using data on smoking habits. This approach seems reasonable for industrialized countries where smoking is responsible for between 85% and 90% of all cases. Such estimates suggest that the total prevalence of COPD in adults older than 40 years of age is 17.1 million people in the USA, 3 million people in the UK, 2.7 million in Germany, and 2.6 million in Italy as well as in France.[12]

The investigation of time trends in prevalence is difficult because of the changes in diagnostic coding that took place with the implementation of new codes on revision of the International Classification of Diseases (ICD-8 to ICD-10). In addition, older population studies require a reduction of FEV_1/FVC below 60% and FEV_1 in per cent predicted below 60% to include a participant as having COPD, whereas the newer studies require less impaired values. The prevalence of irritative bronchial symptoms like chronic cough or phlegm production is usually higher than that of airway obstruction: chronic cough and phlegm is present in about 5% of non-smokers in the general population, whereas it is observed in 15–25% of smokers.[9] These symptoms are usually more prevalent in men, possibly due to under-reporting among women.

Analyses by Murray and Lopez have shown that COPD ranked sixth among causes of death globally in 1990 and is expected to be the third most important cause of death in 2020.[13] This development is illustrated in Figure 3.1, where for comparison numbers of deaths from COPD are shown together with the estimated deaths from HIV infection. Furthermore, disability from COPD is believed to be increasing and will be the fifth leading cause of disability-adjusted life years (DALYs) lost in 2020. The dramatic increase is mainly due to a steep rise in COPD in the third world, a result of the spread of the tobacco epidemic. As the tobacco industry is unable to maintain profit in the industrialized countries, new markets are eagerly being sought in less developed countries. An increase will, however, also be seen in industrialized countries as the burden of COPD in women is rising and in many countries outweighs the effect of smoking cessation. To many health administrators this seems like a paradox as the immediate beneficial effects of smoking cessation are less apparent in COPD than in, for example, ischemic heart disease and maybe even lung cancer. This of course only illustrates the course of COPD where effects of smoking

cessation on COPD mortality may take decades before having the true expected effect.[14] In the Global Burden of Disease Study from WHO, the worldwide prevalence of COPD in 1990 was estimated at 9.34/1000 in men and 7.33/1000 in women.[3] These estimates, however, make little sense as they include all ages and therefore underestimate the true prevalence of COPD in older adults.

In the USA age-adjusted COPD mortality rates increased 17.1% among men from 1979 to 1993, from 96.3/100 000 to 112.8/100 000;[15] among women, rates increased 126.1% from 24.5/100 000 in 1979 to 55.4/100 000 in 1993. In Canada the total number of deaths from COPD almost doubled from 1980 to 1995 and this increase was not merely due to the change from ICD-9 to ICD-10. The increase was mainly a result of the population living longer, although a real increase was seen in women, where the age-standardized mortality rate rose from 8.3 to 17.3 per 100 000.[16] The effect of aging of the population is indeed very important for the prevalence of COPD. As shown in Holland by Feenstra et al.,[17] the effects of aging are more prominent than the effects of the expected changes in smoking habits over a 30-year period. In line with the high prevalence of COPD in middle-aged women in areas of the world where smoking has been prevalent for decades, such as Denmark, mortality rates are now higher among women than among men in certain age groups. With the expected increase in female COPD mortality globally, equal mortality rates are also estimated to occur within a decade elsewhere.[18]

Significant variations exist in mortality rates between countries as shown for both men and women in Figure 3.2. Differences in smoking habits also exist and patterns of smoking may vary from one country to another. This may partly explain why differences in COPD mortality cannot be completely explained by differences in crude measures of smoking between countries.[19] Also, it is difficult to adjust for changes in smoking as the lag time between changes in smoking habits and the impact in society may be very long. Finally, it may also be worthwhile taking into account that although trends in COPD mortality over decades may have value within a country, differences between countries may exist because of different diagnostic traditions alone.[20] Trends in subtypes of COPD cannot be ascertained from mortality statistics. There are clear variations in labeling geographically, over time, and independent of time.

Morbidity data are often regarded as superior to mortality data, due to the chronicity of COPD, and to the fact that many patients with mild or moderate COPD die from other smoking-related diseases, such as cancer or cardiovascular disease, rather than from COPD. Analyses of hospitalizations suggest that up to 25% of medical admissions in the UK are due to respiratory diseases and that half of these are COPD.[21] The high prevalence of COPD is reflected in the number of general practice consultations. In Copenhagen, general practice annual consultation

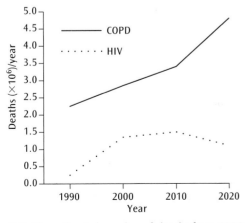

Figure 3.1 *The estimated number of deaths from COPD and HIV infection: 1990–2020. (Based on calculations in ref. 13.)*

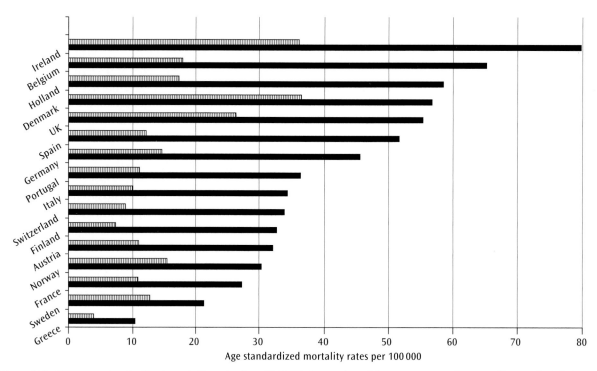

Figure 3.2 *COPD age-standardized mortality rates (per 100 000) from selected European countries according to the WHO Health For All database. Rates for men are shown in solid bars and for women in striped bars.*

rates for chronic bronchitis and COPD are 1000–1500 per 100 000. In the UK annual consultation rates increase from 4170 per 100 000 at age 45–64 to 8860 at age 65–74 and 10 320 per 100 000 at age 75–84.[22] There are, however, as least as many sources of diagnostic biases in data available on morbidity as on mortality. As an example, hospital admissions among US men decreased in 1980–85 in parallel with an increase in outpatient visits,[23] and contacts with general practitioners in the UK have remained almost constant over 20 years in spite of obvious changes in distribution of disease.[24]

The costs of COPD are considerable,[3,25] particularly for patients with severe COPD, and hospitalization-related costs in this group are large.[26] In a US study approximately 70% of the direct medical costs were for inpatient hospitalization,[27] and since exacerbations of COPD represent a large proportion of the total cost of the disease, Price *et al.*[28] have recently suggested that expensive medication such as inhaled corticosteroids, although having only a modest impact on the natural history of COPD, by slightly reducing the number of severe exacerbations may be cost-effective in the long run.

NATURAL HISTORY OF COPD

Development of COPD

Epidemiologic studies of the natural history of chronic respiratory symptoms and of obstructive lung function

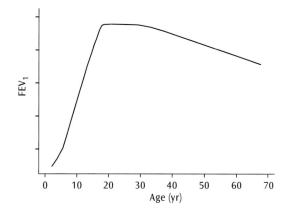

Figure 3.3 *The course of FEV_1 based on cumulated data from population studies.*

impairment have had a profound impact on the clinical definition and comprehension of COPD. Since the introduction and acceptance of spirometric measurements of airflow obstruction as the key physiologic findings and the hallmark of COPD, many longitudinal epidemiologic studies have been conducted to describe the course of lung function in different stages of life in healthy and affected individuals. Although no single study has followed its participants with lung function measurements from birth to old age, by juxtaposing the results of different studies a clear picture of the natural history of FEV_1 (and FVC) in healthy non-smokers has gradually emerged (Figure 3.3). The growth phase of FEV_1 continues until approximately the age of 20–25 years, when the maximum

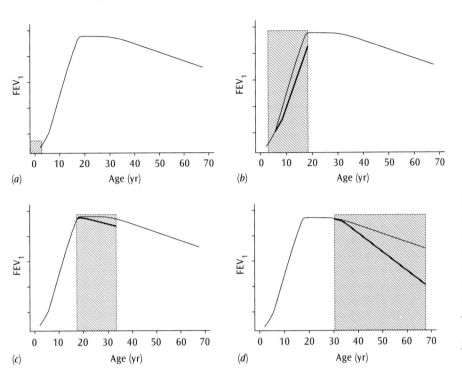

Figure 3.4 *Theoretical model of risk factors in COPD showing effect of risk factors during pregnancy (a), during growth of lung function (b), during plateau phase (c) and during phase of decline (d). (Modified from ref. 29.) Hatched areas indicate where in time risk factors act during the natural history of the disease.*

values are reached. This is followed by a phase of relatively stable lung function, the so-called 'plateau phase' which may last until approximately 35 years of age. Thereafter as part of the aging process the FEV_1 starts to decline in an accelerating fashion. This is the best described part of the lung function curve and the decline in FEV_1 is often reported in ml/yr rather than as percentage change of FEV_1/year. The mean values of FEV_1 decline in healthy men and women are around 30 ml/yr and 25 ml/yr respectively.[9,10] This means that an average reduction in FEV_1 for a healthy non-smoking man is around 1.2 liter from the 40th to the 80th year of life. This concept of the changes in FEV_1 implies that reduced lung function may be caused by inadequate growth of the lungs during childhood (or even in utero) and adolescence, premature start of decline in FEV_1 in early adulthood, accelerated decline after the age of 30 throughout middle and old age or even a combination of all these factors. Another interesting observation from longitudinal studies is the phenomenon called tracking, which means that a measurement of FEV_1 before the age of 10 years is a strong predictor of the level of FEV_1 in early adulthood, midlife and probably even in old age, a finding similar to the course of body height throughout life.

The lung function impairment which defines COPD is generally believed to be the result of changes which take place over decades. The most important and also best investigated deviation from the normal course of changes in lung function is the accelerated decline of FEV_1, in the middle-aged or elderly smoker. Adult smokers experience on average an FEV_1 decline of 40–50 ml/yr, an excess of

the normal annual decline of 15–20 ml/yr. Yet, the FEV_1 of some smokers may decline by 80–100 ml/yr. Thus, although the rate of decline in FEV_1 shows considerable interindividual variation in the literature, the notion of rapid decliners seems justified. These smokers who are susceptible to the deleterious effects of tobacco may lose 3–4 liters of FEV_1 during four decades, a process with devastating clinical consequences. Besides smoking, other intrinsic and extrinsic risk factors like an asthmatic predisposition, occupational exposures and air pollution may operate, resulting in an accelerated decline in FEV_1, as described later. This is illustrated in Figure 3.4 from the recent review by Rijcken and Britton.[29] In addition to being faster than normal, the decline of FEV_1 may start earlier than usual and although the evidence in this field is sparse,[30] it seems that in smokers and subjects with respiratory symptoms the plateau phase may be shorter – or even missing – resulting in an earlier onset of decline in lung function which may contribute to the development of COPD (Figure 3.4).

It has, however, become apparent that the maximally attained FEV_1 prior to the normal decline from adulthood may be important.[31] Even a normal decline in FEV_1 may result in reduced lung function in old age if the starting point at age 25 years is very low. As with other chronic diseases, such as ischemic heart disease, genetic and non-genetic prenatal factors, as well as perinatal factors may be of importance. So far, good research in this area is sparse, but perinatal factors may contribute by determining the level of lung function at birth and the rate of growth of lung function in childhood and adolescence. An altered growth of lung function, either due to genetics, perinatal factors or exposures during childhood and adolescence, such as recurrent infections or smoking, will result in a suboptimal level of lung function in early adulthood. Depending on subsequent lifestyle, this may increase the risk of developing COPD.

Hypotheses on the development of COPD

Historically, attempts at understanding the natural history of COPD have been influenced by the anatomic, pathophysiologic and clinical descriptions of the disease, which have varied over the last decades. In addition, the heterogeneity of COPD, which sometimes manifests primarily as a disease of the airways and therefore resembles asthma and sometimes mainly as the disease of the pulmonary parenchyma (emphysema), made it difficult to provide a single hypothesis describing the development and progression of the disease.

Initially, COPD was not defined, but described as 'obstructive bronchitis' in contrast to 'simple bronchitis'. This was the basis for the 'The British hypothesis' which claimed that chronic mucus hypersecretion (CMH), by setting the stage for recurrent airway infection, was causative in the development of airway obstruction. Fletcher and coworkers in the 1960s performed a 7-year longitudinal study of 30–60-year-old working males, most of whom were heavy smokers and all of whom had lived in London during a period of heavy air pollution. Men with asthmatic features were excluded from the analyses. The seminal work by Fletcher et al.,[1] clearly rejected the British hypothesis by showing that in middle-aged men CMH and progressive airway obstruction were two separate entities, although often occurring concomitantly, because of a common risk factor – smoking. Whereas progressive airway obstruction was the most important disease process resulting in progressive dyspnea, which is the main cause of disability in COPD patients, the presence of mucus hypersecretion clearly predisposed to recurrent bronchopulmonary infections causing increased morbidity and absence from work. Although bronchial infections are very unlikely to affect the FEV_1 decline in the long term in most patients, they may play a significant role with regard to the course of disease once significant obstruction has developed, as described later in the chapter. One of the most important findings from the London study was the observation that quitting smoking resulted in normalization of the FEV_1 decline and reduction of the irritative bronchial symptoms like cough and phlegm. This finding has been reproduced in several observational studies and in a major intervention study, the Lung Health Study.[32] Yet, after stopping smoking subjects with reduced FEV_1 do not normalize their FEV_1, although a small increase around 50 ml is observed, probably due to disappearance of acute inflammatory changes caused by tobacco smoke.

With the rejection of the British hypothesis a new approach to the understanding of factors related to the development of chronic bronchitis and emphysema was both needed and possible. Already in 1961 a group of Dutch investigators put forward the hypothesis that various forms of airway obstruction such as asthma, chronic bronchitis and even emphysema should be considered as different expressions of the same underlying abnormality and introduced the term 'chronic non-specific lung disease'. They suggested that host factors, airway hyperresponsiveness and allergy define susceptibility to the development of airway obstruction by interacting with environmental factors like smoking and air pollution. This was subsequently named 'the Dutch hypothesis'.[33,34] Although the idea of combining asthma together with bronchitis and emphysema into a single disease category has not gained wide acceptance outside The Netherlands, several prospective studies have until now shown that airway hyperresponsiveness is a significant predictor of FEV_1 decline, development of respiratory symptoms and even mortality from COPD.[35,36] One of the problems of interpreting the role of airway hyperresponsiveness as a host susceptibility factor for the development of COPD is the fact that it may develop secondary to development of airway obstruction due to changes in airway geometry. Yet, it seems that airway hyperresponsiveness is a significant predictor of both the preclinical and clinical course of COPD and asthma, even after some adjustment for the impact of airway geometry. With regard to allergy, which in epidemiologic studies is usually measured as skin prick test positivity or elevated levels of IgE, it has been shown that these allergy markers may interact with smoking in predicting FEV_1 decline and survival.

Based on the analyses of survival and the course of lung function of the participants in the longitudinal Tucson respiratory study, Burrows et al. suggested that the Dutch hypothesis is valid for the subgroup of COPD patients with obstructive lung function impairment mainly caused by airway disease – patients who clinically share some common characteristics with asthma – and that the term asthmatic bronchitis is a relevant description of this group.[37] However, the Dutch hypothesis is probably less relevant to COPD patients with a more 'malignant type of disease', where emphysema is the main cause of airway obstruction. An important consequence of the Dutch hypothesis is that asthma could be regarded as a risk factor for COPD (at least the subtype with predominant airway disease). This latter notion is in line with epidemiologic observations that some asthmatic patients have a very rapid FEV_1 decline (already observed by Fletcher) and high mortality[38,39] and clinical studies showing irreversible airway obstruction as a consequence of longstanding and severe asthma.[40] Whether the latter type of obstructive disease should be named progressive irreversible asthma or COPD is a matter of semantics. As longstanding asthma does not result in emphysema in the absence of smoking, it may well be that the risk factors of the emphysematous type of COPD are different. In general much more research is needed about the natural history of different subtypes of COPD.[41] This may, however, prove to be difficult to disentangle as most patients cannot be clearly sub-typed into bronchitic and emphysematous, and most patients in fact have features of both *and* small airways disease.

Prognosis in established COPD

Once airway obstruction has developed the further course of disease is characterized by accelerated decline of lung function and the development of dyspnea. In addition, patients with chronic mucus hypersecretion are particularly prone to recurrent lower airway infections, resulting in acute exacerbations with a frequency up to several exacerbations each year. In the latter group, recurrent infections may further accelerate the decline of lung function.[42] Along with the decline of FEV_1 and recurrent exacerbations, patients experience the gradual loss of health status or health-related quality of life.[43,44] Late in the course of the disease disability is present as a result of the severely reduced lung function. The progressive loss of FEV_1 may be accompanied by a decrease in the volume-adjusted diffusion capacity (diffusion constant) due to emphysema. Stopping smoking is the only established measure that reduces the excessive FEV_1 decline, whereas treatment with inhaled bronchodilators and inhaled steroids does not affect the decline.[32,45]

With a more severe decrease in lung function hypoxemia develops and secondary to this elevation of the pulmonary arterial pressure. In severe COPD the mean pulmonary artery pressure increases by approximately 0.5–3 mmHg/yr.[46] As a consequence of the high pressure in the pulmonary vascular bed, right ventricular hypertrophy, or 'cor pulmonale', develops. Since severe COPD is a disease of current and former elderly smokers, comorbidity caused by other smoking-related diseases, such as ischemic heart disease, general artheriosclerosis and cancer, are important features of COPD. Although many COPD patients may die from cardiovascular diseases, the risk of dying from respiratory failure or respiratory infections is high, especially in patients with chronic hypoxemia.[47,48]

Reduced FEV_1 is a strong predictor of morbidity and mortality in established COPD. Survival is more closely related to post-bronchodilator FEV_1 than to the pre-bronchodilator value,[49] whereas it is unclear whether bronchodilator reversibility as such is a significant predictor of prognosis.[50] As a rule of thumb the median survival in patients with an FEV_1 of approximately 1 liter is around 5 years, strongly depending on age, the presence of hypoxemia and comorbidity.[51] COPD patients with peripheral edema due to cor pulmonale have a 5-year survival of 30–40%.[52] Long-term oxygen therapy in severe hypoxemia ($PaO_2 < 7.3$ kPa) prolongs survival, whereas there is no significant effect on survival of oxygen therapy in patients with moderate hypoxemia.[53] Other predictors of survival in established COPD include smoking, low body weight for height, chronic mucus hypersecretion, signs of ischemic heart disease and male gender. Low body weight, expressed as low body mass index (BMI), is an indicator of malnutrition and probably systemic disease in patients with COPD causing weakness of respiratory muscles, impaired immune response and gas exchange. Low BMI (< 20 kg/m^2) interacts with the level of FEV_1 with regard to mortality, being a much stronger predictor of death in severe COPD, with a relative risk of death of 4.3, than in mild and moderate COPD, where the relative risk is 1.8.[54] The importance of CMH for mortality has been a subject of dispute, yet in severe COPD, the presence of CMH indicated a 4.2 times higher risk of death from COPD, mainly due to infective exacerbations, whereas the increase in relative risk connected with CMH was only 1.2 if lung function was preserved.[55]

Possibilities of early detection of COPD

In population studies and in studies of patients with COPD a reduced FEV_1 is a powerful predictor of morbidity and mortality from COPD. As it usually takes 20–30 years to develop clinically significant COPD and as FEV_1 shows a very strong tracking effect, it has been advocated that one – or at least a few – measurements of FEV_1 would be sufficient to identify a subject who is susceptible to, for example, tobacco smoking. This assumes that a low value at any time predicts a subject would have a subsequent fast decline, thereby staying in his or her own 'track'.[29] This notion was introduced after the study of Fletcher and colleagues and has been named the 'horse-racing effect'.[1,56] It indicates that a minor impairment would lead to increasingly lower lung function, disability, and perhaps death from COPD. Although this phenomenon is seen in population studies and is even stronger for FEV_1/FVC than for FEV_1, it may, however, not be entirely true in individual smokers. Firstly, the initial changes in COPD take place in the small airways and may not be reflected initially in FEV_1, which is mainly a measurement of large airway function. Because of this, the full effects of these changes may not be reflected in the FEV_1 and respiratory symptoms until late middle age. Secondly, rates of decline may change over time, which could change the course considerably. Also, the variation in a single FEV_1 measurement is 175–200 ml, which is 3–8 years of excess decline in the susceptible smoker. Thus, it is apparent that several measurements years apart are necessary to determine the rate of decline in a single individual. As an approximation, annual measurements will have to be undertaken for at least 3–5 years for an excess decline in FEV_1 to become apparent. For many years there has been an ongoing search for an alternative test that would predict subsequent FEV_1 decline with enough precision to be feasible in the clinical practice. However, inclusion of more sophisticated measurements of airway function like end- or mid-expiratory flow rates, closing volume and nitrogen slope of alveolar plateau have not improved prediction equations substantially.[57–59] (See Chapter 13) Although the prediction for the individual patients may be quite imprecise, it is still reasonable to recommend spirometry in primary health care for all smokers older than 45 years of age and patients with respiratory symptoms such as coughing and/or episodic wheezing. These measurements will hopefully increase the success of antismoking advice.[60]

RISK FACTORS

Epidemiology has been crucial in the investigation of risk factors and the determination of their importance and relevance in different populations. However, this task has often been looked at with some condescension by basic scientists and some clinicians, as it has been regarded as merely determining associations without much evidence of causation. From an epidemiologic point of view it is not necessary to completely understand a complex chain of causation if the ability to pick up a prevalent cause can produce an effective target for intervention or even prevention. Often, increasingly advanced epidemiology or simply the consistency of several studies can be so impressive that risk factor epidemiology can actually contribute to knowledge enabling the establishment of causation through observational studies.[61] The best example is of course the relationship between smoking and COPD where the major breakthrough occurred in 1964 when the Report of The Surgeon General in the USA recognized smoking as the most important cause of non-neoplastic chronic respiratory disease in the USA.[62]

Risk factors for COPD in epidemiology are most convincingly determined from studies showing an association between the risk factor under study and change in FEV_1 (longitudinal assessment). However, as mentioned previously 'change in FEV_1' often refers to decline in FEV_1 as most studies so far have looked at decline in FEV_1 only. The ideal is still to consider both growth and decline of lung function and there is still an obvious lack of studies assessing changes in growth of lung function associated with well-defined factors. Often longitudinal assessment is not possible and cross-sectional findings have to be relied on. This may cause bias[63] but will not necessarily do so. The introduction of statistical models which can

Table 3.1 *Risk factors for COPD in an attempted descending order; external and internal factors presumably have similar impact*

External factors	Internal factors
Smoking	Genetic factors
Socioeconomic status	Gender
Occupation	Chronic mucus
Environmental	hypersecretion
pollution	Airway hyperresponsiveness,
Perinatal events and	↑ IgE and asthma
childhood respiratory	
illness	
Recurrent	
bronchopulmonary	
infections	
Diet	

handle cross-sectional data and longitudinal data on the same population simultaneously will further increase our ability to properly assess risk factors.[64]

Although smoking is by far the strongest risk factor for COPD, it is worthwhile remembering that our detailed knowledge of this particular risk factor is mainly the result of the ease with which large population surveys have been able to collect information on smoking and relate this to change in lung function. However, other factors definitely play a role and deserve attention, both because of their impact, but also because several of them can be affected by preventive measures just as with smoking.

Risk factors cannot be studied independent of the time. In this respect, 'time' refers to both calendar time and time in the individual's life. Whereas smoking presumably has a profound effect on both growth and decline in FEV_1, other features or exposures may only have an effect at limited time intervals and can more easily be overlooked. In the subsequent sections each factor believed to be of relevance is discussed. In Table 3.1 risk factors for COPD have been listed in an approximated descending order of importance.

Genetic determinants

The term genetic determinants mainly includes genetic products that may affect the individual's susceptibility to smoking and presumably a wide variety of other environmental factors. Both family and twin studies have confirmed a significant genetic contribution to the variance in pulmonary function.[65–68] In spite of this, few other specific genetic factors than alpha-1-antitrypsin are known. The genetic determinants of COPD are likely to be complex and only recently have started to receive attention. Genes coding for a number of proteins and proteases likely to be associated with increased susceptibility have been identified, but seem to explain little of the variation in susceptibility.[69]

Thus, so far only the gene for alpha-1-antitrypsin (α_1-AT) has proven relevance. The gene is highly polymorphic with more than 75 different alleles described, although only a minority convey a true risk of low serum levels of α_1-AT likely to give rise to emphysema. The more common variants are the alleles M, S and Z with population frequencies of about 0.93, 0.05 and 0.02, respectively. Usually α_1-AT deficiency denotes those homozygous for the Z allele (PiZZ) who have very low levels of α_1-AT in the blood. Because of the low prevalence of this variant the proportion of COPD attributable to this gene is about 1%. A few studies assessing the association between different genotypes and the development of COPD suggested that those with a MZ genotype could be at higher risk of COPD than those with a MM genotype.[70,71] Several large registers containing both patients with α_1-AT deficiency and their relatives have been established for the purpose of providing a better understanding of the development of emphysema in this subset of COPD patients. Some important points have already emerged. Whereas prognosis is generally poor, due to an abnormally rapid decline in FEV_1 in patients with α_1-AT deficiency identified as COPD patients,[72] subjects identified as non-index cases, through a Danish register based on family studies, had a much more favorable prognosis.[73,74] Lung function decline seems well characterized from cohorts of PiZZ subjects,[75,76] whereas the importance of PiMZ for decline in FEV_1 is more questionable.[77]

Gender

Until recently, little research has taken place concerning the effect of gender on COPD. The reason for this is obvious as COPD has for years been a disease of men, merely reflecting that men for decades have had higher smoking rates and more occupational exposures than women. This, however, has nothing to do with the influence of gender on susceptibility as this requires careful studies of risk of COPD for the same environmental exposure. As smoking in women has been rare until after the second world war, such studies have not been performed; this is presumably also because of a lack of obvious reasons to suspect an impact of sex hormones on the susceptibility to tobacco smoking. This is not an easy issue to study. A direct comparison of lung function in men and women makes little sense for obvious physical/geometric reasons. More importantly, it is a difficult task to compare the typical male smoker with the typical female smoker. Such a comparison will invariably be biased by the fact that proper controlling for smoking in terms of gender differences is very difficult, if not impossible. In addition to smoking more

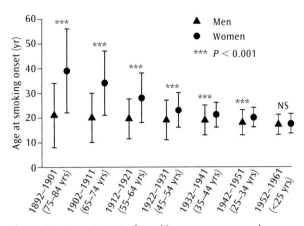

Figure 3.5 *Age at onset of smoking among men and women from different birth cohorts. (Data from Danish population studies. Modified from ref. 78.)*

than women (which is the measurement most often controlled for), men inhale more often, and they start smoking at an earlier age as illustrated in Figure 3.5.[78] Thus, most biases at work in this area will tend to underestimate the true effect of smoking in women compared to men. Recent studies indicate that when controlling correctly for differences in smoking patterns women have a higher risk of loss in FEV_1 and subsequent hospitalization for COPD.[79,80] In two populations from Copenhagen, women tended to show a larger effect of smoking on FEV_1 assessed cross-sectionally and their risk of hospitalization due to COPD was increased by a factor of 1.5–3.5. Further studies on different aspects of gender differences are needed,[81] especially longitudinal studies, although this may prove difficult due to the relatively rapid gender-specific changes in smoking habits.

As more women in many countries started smoking after the second world war, more reliable data on the effects of heavy smoking in women become available from national health statistics. In Denmark, where women had taken up smoking on a broad scale already in the 1950s, death rates for COPD among women aged 65–74 years have now exceeded those of men as shown previously in Figure 3.6. This clearly serves as a warning to countries still in an earlier phase of what has been termed the female smoking epidemic. In a recent study by Gold *et al.* on growth of lung function in adolescents, it also seemed that girls were more vulnerable to the harmful effects of smoking than boys.[82] We are currently awaiting more studies in this area. We also need more knowledge about the basis for an increased susceptibility in women. Whereas an excess risk of cardiovascular disease in smoking women has been suggested to be due to the anti-estrogenic properties of tobacco smoke,[83,84] it is not apparent that this effect of tobacco plays any role in the development of COPD.

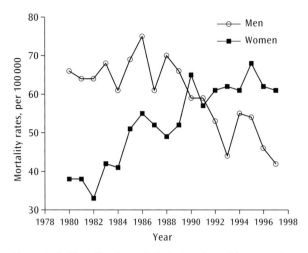

Figure 3.6 *Mortality from COPD in Danish subjects aged 65–74 years.*

Perinatal events and childhood respiratory illness

Low birth weight has in some studies been shown to predict low lung function in adult life.[85,86] Although exposures early in life have been considered important for subsequent development of COPD for almost 40 years,[87,88] the theory connecting pre- and perinatal events with many chronic diseases is generally termed the 'Barker theory'. It may, however, be difficult to disentangle the effects of pure perinatal events from those of other strong risk factors, especially socioeconomic status and subsequent smoking habits, but also maternal smoking has to be considered as it is associated with lower lung function at birth.[89,90] In the Barker study[85] the effect of birth weight was not limited to lung function in adult life, but was also related to subsequent death from COPD. The effect of birth weight on FEV_1 was statistically significant, but the difference in FEV_1 between those who were small or large at birth was only 250 ml, of which 100–150 ml were due to differences in childhood infections, bronchitis, pneumonia and whooping cough. The effect of childhood infections is in accordance with other cohort studies linking chronic childhood disease to reduced lung function in both early[91] and late adult life.[92] The mechanism is generally believed to be related to impaired growth of lung function.

Airway hyperresponsiveness and asthma

For years it has been hypothesized that susceptibility to COPD is determined by an allergic constitution manifest as airway hyperresponsiveness (AHR). Dutch researchers especially have favored this hypothesis which has been generally known as 'the Dutch hypothesis'.[33,34] Unfortunately for the hypothesis it seems that the distinction between asthma and COPD has turned out to be the key in discussions of the Dutch hypothesis. However, the principal question seems to be if AHR has a prominent role in the natural history in COPD; i.e. if the presence of AHR in smokers predicts subsequent accelerated decline in FEV_1?

This question is, however, not easy to answer. AHR is present in patients with COPD[93] most likely because of geometrical relations. For this reason longitudinal assessments are crucial. AHR has been shown to be an independent risk factor for an accelerated FEV_1 decline in a number of large cohort studies, including a study from the Groningen group,[94] a study by Villar *et al.* in the elderly,[95] the Normative Aging study[96,97] and the Lung Health Study.[98] The impact of AHR on FEV_1 decline has varied between studies, but on average AHR adds approximately 10 ml/yr to the decline in FEV_1. There is also no clear-cut interaction between AHR and smoking – indicating that AHR could be a determinator of susceptibility. A review of the epidemiologic literature on AHR and FEV_1 decline has been given by Rijcken and Weiss.[93]

Recently, Xu *et al.* have assessed the association between bronchial responsiveness in both incidence and remission of chronic cough and phlegm in a 24-year follow-up of 2684 subjects from the two towns Vlagtwedde and Vlaardingen in The Netherlands.[99] After adjusting for age, sex, area and smoking, incident cases of chronic cough and chronic phlegm were twice as likely to have AHR as those who persistently were without these symptoms. A similar association was seen for the remission of these symptoms. The same results were obtained after excluding subjects with asthma from the analysis, but no details on this are given. In the same population AHR was a significant predictor of COPD mortality.[35,36]

Generally, asthma should be separated from COPD as the two diseases differ in a number of ways and each have specific features enabling us to distinguish the two disease entities. It may thus seem confusing to add asthma to the risk factors for COPD. There is, however, increasing evidence from longitudinal population studies that asthmatics have a more rapid decline in FEV_1 than non-asthmatics.[38,100] This is likely to be seen in only a proportion of asthmatics and could possibly be related to degree of asthma control as discussed previously. Asthmatics also experience an increased mortality, primarily due to an increased COPD mortality.[39]

Recurrent bronchopulmonary infections and chronic mucus hypersecretion

In the 1950s recurrent bronchopulmonary infections in adulthood were believed to play a major role in the development of chronic bronchitis and emphysema, forming the basis for 'the British hypothesis' as described earlier in this chapter. The hypothesis was rejected by Fletcher *et al.*,[1] but the debate about the impact of chronic mucus hyper-secretion and recurrent bronchopulmonary infections continues. In this regard the role of childhood infections is not quite clear. In some studies, the presence of lower respiratory infection during childhood has been found to increase the risk of respiratory symptoms[101] and of functional impairment.[102] In the study reported by Barker et al.,[85] childhood infections such as bronchitis, pneumonia and whooping cough had an effect on both lung function and mortality, and other cohort studies have also linked chronic childhood disease to lowered lung function in both early[91] and late adult life.[92] The mechanism is generally believed to be related to impaired growth of lung function. A major drawback is the uncertainty associated with research in this area. Most studies rely on combining lung function measurements with information on childhood respiratory infections often collected in ways which are unable to preclude significant recall bias and other sources of bias.[103] With increasing severity of airflow obstruction it is both an epidemiologic and a clinical observation that recurrent bronchopulmonary infections occur with increasing frequency. Several epidemiologic studies have shown that bronchopulmonary infections lead to a temporary decrease in lung function and one could speculate that recurrent bronchopulmonary infections could, in selected individuals, play a role in the course of the disease as suggested by Kanner et al., when analyzing data from the Lung Health Study.[42]

Independent of the actual mechanism, the presence of chronic mucus hypersecretion (CMH) influences the course of COPD. As stated earlier in this chapter, initial epidemiologic studies ruled out CMH as an important risk factor for subsequent FEV_1 decline[1] and COPD mortality.[104] Nevertheless, recent findings have revived interest in CMH. Longitudinal population-based studies have demonstrated an independent association between CMH and FEV_1 decline,[105,106] COPD morbidity[106,107] and COPD mortality.[55] In the Copenhagen study the effect of CMH on FEV_1 decline was of considerable size; i.e. 10–25 ml/yr after adjusting for smoking.[106] The discrepancy between these results and earlier findings cannot easily be explained, but the change over time may reflect the fact that whereas CMH previously was frequent in working males as a response to irritation from widespread particulate pollution, CMH could today serve as a marker of ongoing inflammation. The possible effect of CMH on COPD mortality may of course be mediated by FEV_1 alone, but it is also plausible that subjects with CMH are simply more prone to terminal respiratory infection.[108]

Smoking

By far the most important cause of COPD is tobacco smoking,[109] which is believed to be the cause of 85–90%

of all COPD in men in the industrialized world.[110] Epidemiologic studies have been crucial in determining this association.[1,9,111,112] The association has been demonstrated in both cross-sectional and longitudinal studies and the effect of smoking seems to be present from the cradle to the grave.

In a recent review Le Souëf clearly pointed out how a disease like COPD, which is generally considered a disease secondary to adult smoking, indeed has its roots in childhood.[113] Smoking during pregnancy affects growth in utero and presumably also lung growth, as it leads to decreased lung function at birth.[89,90,114] The significance of this for the subsequent risk of the development of COPD is of course difficult to determine. It seems highly plausible, however, that decreased lung function at birth may lead to a decreased level of lung function in early adulthood, which would increase the risk of COPD pending subsequent lifestyle, especially the subject's own smoking career.[31]

Evidence of mild airway obstruction and slowed growth of lung function was recently found in smoking American adolescents,[82] and this is in accordance with a previous study showing a slowing of growth of FEV_1 in smoking adolescents with respiratory symptoms.[115] Although the growth of lung function was only slowed by 1–2% on average, the variation was large, and this indicates that the susceptible adolescents may suffer substantial growth impairment due to smoking.

In adulthood the effect of smoking on FEV_1 decline is well documented. Just as in never smokers, FEV_1 decline varies considerably among smokers. Most longitudinal studies have included men and FEV_1 decline ranges from 45 to 90 ml/yr, in contrast to the normal 30 ml/yr. As described earlier in this chapter, these values are mean values from population studies; a single individual may experience a decline significantly larger, at least temporarily, explaining why COPD may seem to surface within a few years during the fifth or sixth decade. Most studies link COPD to cigarette smoking, mainly because cigarettes are smoked much more often than cigars, cheroots or pipes. From studies including all types of smokers it seems that the type of tobacco smoked plays a minor role, if any.[9] The crucial factor seems to be the amount smoked and the extent of inhalation.[116] Filter cigarettes do not differ significantly from non-filter cigarettes, presumably because the substances causing lung function impairment originate from the volatile part of cigarettes which is not reduced by filters.

The role of environmental tobacco smoking (ETS), or passive smoking as it is often called, has for years been difficult to comprehend. In a recent review on the effect of passive smoking on children,[117] it was concluded that maternal smoking is associated with small but statistically significant deficits in FEV_1 and other spirometric indices and that the association was almost certainly causal.

In adults the role of ETS is less clear. The effect of ETS on lung function and COPD seems to depend strongly on the setting in which it is studied and in particular in which country it is studied. Even if studies from China, which show the largest effects, are excluded, a possible effect of ETS seems to be present. A very thorough review on this topic has recently been published.[118]

Smoking cessation has, in several surveys, been shown to be favorably associated with both prevalence of respiratory symptoms and the decline in FEV_1.[116,119,120] The first change in lung function seen after smoking cessation is a small increase, usually in the region of 50–100 ml for FEV_1. This is presumably due to the disappearance of the acute inflammatory edema in the smoker's airways. The favorable change in subsequent decline in lung function is seen in younger subjects and in those without apparent COPD, whereas the beneficial changes are less apparent in older subjects with overt COPD.[116,120] In young and middle-aged subjects, it is a matter of debate whether the decline in FEV_1 after smoking cessation normalizes completely and at present it seems that in general quitters continue to have an FEV_1 decline which is slightly larger than that seen in never-smokers.[32,120] Whether this is due to a small number of the quitters having continuous respiratory symptoms indicating an ongoing inflammation in the airways remains to be seen.

Until recently 'a smoker' used to be a person who smoked practically from adolescense to the grave. This has changed considerably within recent decades, as a large number of smokers have quit. As smokers are highly addicted to nicotine, a number of ex-smokers may restart smoking and at present our knowledge on restarting is sparse. Recent findings from the Tucson population study indicate that quitting and restarting smoking may be even more harmful than continued smoking. In a subset of smokers who quit and subsequently restarted smoking, it was estimated that the decline in FEV_1 after restarting was even greater than that seen in the initial smoking phase before quitting.[121]

The most interesting issue concerning smoking is susceptibility. Research in COPD is indeed challenged by the fact that only 15–20% of smokers are susceptible to the harmful effects of smoking on FEV_1 decline. Genetic factors are likely to play a major role. However, it is also important to realize that the 15–20% refer to smokers with a significant reduction in FEV_1. More detailed studies have shown that many more elderly smokers have abnormalities in their lung function because of their smoking.

Air pollution

The effect of air pollution on COPD has been reviewed recently.[122,129] It is important to distinguish the acute effects of air pollution on aggravating already established COPD (see Chapter 6) and its effect on the natural history of the disease. The acute effects of air pollution seem firmly established, not least from the effects of specific air pollution episodes; for example the London smog of 1952. Also less pronounced variations in air pollution play a role in temporary worsening of COPD. Studies from both Europe and the USA have shown that day-to-day variations in environmental pollution are associated with variations in admissions to hospital[124–126] and mortality.[126–129] Whether long-term exposure to outdoor air pollution is a predictor for the development of COPD is more dubious. Air pollution is a risk factor for increased phlegm – and thus chronic bronchitis – but less so for the development of airway obstruction or an accelerated decline in FEV_1.[122] Previous studies showing lower FEV_1 in urban areas than in rural areas may not have adjusted appropriately for socioeconomic factors. However, air pollution may affect growth of lung function as shown recently by Gauderman et al.,[130] and this mechanism may increase the risk of COPD in adulthood. Also, a number of components of air pollution have been linked to an increase in bronchial responsiveness and an effect of air pollution in causing COPD cannot be excluded.

In recent decades it has been documented that indoor air pollution derived from combustion of biomass fuel in fires and stoves may be an important source of COPD in developing countries. It has been estimated that up to 75% of the population of the developing countries cooks daily using unprocessed biomass fuels, which often consist of wood, corn husks, straw or animal dung.[131] Therefore, women and small children living in houses with indoor cooking are at particularly risk. Numerous studies have shown high prevalences of cough and CMH in non-smoking women exposed to smoke and fumes from stoves using wood and cow dung as fuel. In some cases the irritative symptoms are accompanied by irreversible obstructive lung function impairment,[123,132] whereas in other cases restrictive impairment is observed in which case the lung disease resembles pulmonary fibrosis more than COPD.[133] In some areas it has been estimated that exposure to smoke due to indoor cooking may explain up to 50% of COPD cases.[132]

Occupation (see also Chapter 5)

For decades it has been generally accepted that occupational dust exposure could lead to cough and sputum production; this association has been shown in several occupational cohorts. An association between occupational exposures and excess decline in lung function has been the topic of heated debate, not least because of the implications regarding health and safety at work and discussions on workers compensation. Recently, Hendrick pointed out that difficulties and weaknesses in study design have seriously influenced our understanding of the role of occupational exposures in COPD.[134]

The most important study leading to a change in opinion about the role of occupational exposures investigated a group of Paris area workers, in which working men with exposure to gases, dust or heat had an accelerated decline in FEV_1.[135] In this study the effect of different exposures on FEV_1 decline was examined and on average the exposed men had 5–15 ml/yr excess decline in FEV_1 due to the exposure. These and other findings from occupational cohorts have led to a general acceptance of a causal relationship between occupational exposure to dust and development of COPD; the effect is likely to be less potent than the smoking effect, but with probable interactions between smoking and occupation.[136,137] Important information has also been gathered from studies of the general population, including data on occupational exposures. Although the quality of information on occupation in population surveys can be questioned, these study populations are generally less affected by selection biases, especially the 'healthy worker effect'. Findings from cross-sectional surveys have been reported,[138–140] and in these studies subjects who in a questionnaire described themselves as being exposed to inorganic dusts, for example, experienced an FEV_1 decline comparable to that seen in moderate smokers. Findings from very thorough analyses of 1933 randomly sampled men from Bergen in Norway have convincingly demonstrated a significant dose-effect relationship between the number of occupational agents exposed to and decline in FEV_1,[141] as shown in Figure 3.7. An important contribution of population-based studies is that they provide an estimate of the attributable risk of occupational exposure on COPD. In the Zutphen Study

almost 40% of men were occupationally exposed to dust and had a risk ratio of 1.46.[142] These results suggest that, although the effect is smaller than that of smoking, they do affect a large proportion of the population and could therefore contribute considerably to the overall incidence and prevalence of COPD.

Nutrition

In recent years the role of nutrition in the development of COPD has been the subject of several studies. As a consequence of the potential role of oxidative stress in the pathogenesis of emphysema, it has been suggested that dietary antioxidants such as vitamins A, C and E could have a protective effect in smokers. An ecological analysis using information on baseline diet and 25-year COPD mortality rates in the Seven Countries Study revealed an inverse relationship between baseline intake of fruit and fish and subsequent COPD mortality.[143] Further support for a beneficial effect of vitamin C came from a Dutch study[144] and the American NHANES study,[145] but the value of both studies is somewhat limited by the unclear differentiation between asthma and COPD. More convincing data came from two British studies[146–148] in which COPD was more clearly defined.

Regarding other nutrients, data have been published suggesting a protective role of fish oil due to the presence of marine n-3 fatty acids. Shahar *et al.*[148] found a decreased risk of COPD in subjects with a high intake of n-3 fatty acids, and at least three other studies have suggested a similar mechanism.[149–151] However, the only longitudinal study to date could not support the hypothesis of a beneficial effect of these nutritional contents.[144] The whole area is not clear and awaits further studies.[152]

Socioeconomic status

For a considerable time it has been clear that COPD was strongly associated with socioeconomic status, 'social class'.[11] The association between socioeconomic status and general health has been consistently shown over decades in British studies of social class variations in both doctor consultations and mortality.[153,154] This is not limited to the socioeconomic status of the individual, but is probably also an effect of social deprivation in general.[155] However, in a cross-sectional study carried out in Pelotas, Brasil, Menezes *et al.* found an association between chronic bronchitis and a low socioeconomic status after multivariate adjustment including smoking.[156] Likewise, Bakke *et al.* found an association between educational level and lung function after adjusting for age, sex, smoking, and occupation.[157] In the paper on occupation and FEV_1 decline from Paris, unskilled workers also had a significantly steeper FEV_1 decline than skilled workers, after

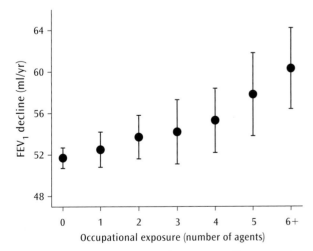

Figure 3.7 *Excess FEV_1 declines in men according to number of occupational exposures. Error bars show 95% confidence intervals for the estimated declines. Compare the effects of occupation with the baseline decline of 52 ml/yr most likely reflecting the effect of smoking. (Modified from ref. 140.)*

adjustment for smoking and occupational exposures.[135] The effects of socioeconomic status on lung function are not trivial. A recent Danish cohort study, which in spite of relatively small differences between social classes, revealed marked associations between both education and level of income and lung function and COPD hospitalizations.[158] Concerning FEV_1, the differences between men with long education and high income and those with short education and low income was 400 ml and the risk of subsequent COPD hospitalization varied by a factor of 3; in both instances smoking was adjusted for in the analyses. The difference was profound in both men and women, suggesting that occupational exposures alone were not to blame. As the effect was more or less constant over all age groups, the possibility that socioeconomic status in early life could be a relevant risk factor for COPD is worth considering. In a longitudinal analysis of the Medical Research Council's national survey of health and development of the 1946 birth cohort, Britten and coworkers assessed the presence of respiratory symptoms and peak expiratory flow when the subjects included in the study were 36 years old. They found that these respiratory events were indeed associated with both current indices of poor socioeconomic status and poor home environment at age 2.[159]

It is unlikely that just a few factors taken together make up the risk factor socioeconomic status. Most likely, socioeconomic risk factors are multifactorial and may cover the entire range from intrauterine exposure[85,160] to childhood infections[85,161] and childhood environment,[162] diet,[163–165] housing conditions[166–168] and occupational factors.[135,141]

REFERENCES

1. Fletcher CM, Peto R, Tinker CM, Speizer FE. *The Natural History of Chronic Bronchitis and Emphysema.* University Press, Oxford, 1976.
2. Siafakas NM, Vermeire P, Pride NB, *et al.*, on behalf of the European Respiratory Society Task Force. Optimal assessment and management of chronic obstructive pulmonary disease (COPD). *Eur Respir J* 1995;**8**:1398–420.
3. Pauwels R, Buist A, Calverley P, Jenkins C, Hurd S. Global strategy for the diagnosis, management and prevention of chronic obstructive pulmonary disease. NHLBI/WHO global initiative for chronic obstructive lung disease (GOLD) workshop summary. *Am J Respir Crit Care Med* 2001;**163**:1256–76.
4. Medical Research Council committee on the aetiology of chronic bronchitis. Standardized questionnaires on respiratory symptoms. *Br Med J* 1960;**2**:1665.
5. Medical Research Council. *Instructions for the use of the questionnaire on respiratory symptoms.* WJ Holman, Devon, 1966.
6. Minette A. Questionnaire of the European Community for Coal and Steel (ECCS) on respiratory symptoms. 1987-updating of the 1962 and 1967 questionnaires for studying chronic bronchitis and emphysema. *Eur Respir J* 1989;**2**:165–77.
7. Ferris BG. Epidemiology standardization project. *Am Rev Respir Dis* 1978;**118**:1–53.
8. Mannino DM, Gangnon RC, Petty TL, Lydick E. Obstructive lung disease and low lung function in adults in the United States. *Arch Intern Med* 2000;**160**:1683–9.
9. Lange P. Development and prognosis of chronic obstructive pulmonary disease with special reference to the role of tobacco smoking. *Dan Med Bull* 1992;**39**:30–48.
10. Anto JM, Vermeire P, Vestbo J, Sunyer J. Epidemiology of chronic obstructive pulmonary disease. *Eur Respir J* 2001;**17**:982–94.
11. Prescott E, Vestbo J. Socioeconomic status and chronic obstructive pulmonary disease. *Thorax* 1999;**54**:737–41.
12. Stang P, Lydick E, Silberman C, Kempel A, Keating ET. The prevalence of COPD. Using smoking rates to estimate disease frequency in the general population. *Chest* 2000;**117**:354–9s.
13. Murray CJL, Lopez AD. Alternative projections of mortality and disability by cause 1990–2020: Global Burden of Disease Study. *Lancet* 1997;**349**:1498–504.
14. Wise RA. Changing smoking patterns and mortality from chronic obstructive pulmonary disease. *Prev Med* 1997;**26**: 418–21.
15. Mannino DM, Brown C, Giovino GA. Obstructive lung disease deaths in the United States from 1979 through 1993. An analysis using multiple-cause mortality data. *Am J Respir Crit Care Med* 1997;**156**:814–18.
16. Lacasse Y, Brooks D, Goldstein RS. Trends in the epidemiology of COPD in Canada, 1980 to 1995. *Chest* 1999;**116**:306–13.
17. Feenstra TL, van Genugten MLL, Hoogenveen RT, Wouters EF, Rutten-van Mölken MPMH. The impact of aging and smoking on the future burden of chronic obstructive pulmonary disease. *Am J Respir Crit Care Med* 2001;**164**:590–6.
18. Crockett AJ, Cranston JM, Moss JR, Alpers JH. Trends in chronic obstructive pulmonary disease in Australia. *Med J Aust* 1994;**161**:600–3.
19. Brown CA, Crombie IK, Tunstall-Pedoe H. Failure of cigarette smoking to explain international differences in mortality from chronic obstructive pulmonary disease. *J Epidemiol Community Health* 1994;**48**:134–9.
20. Farebrother MJB, Kelson MC, Heller RF. Death certification of farmer's lung and chronic airway diseases in different countries of the EEC. *Br J Dis Chest* 1985;**79**:352–60.
21. Pearson MG, Littler J, Davies PDO. An analysis of medical workload by specialty and diagnosis in Mersey: evidence of a specialist to patient mismatch. *J R Coll Phys* 1994;**28**: 230–4.
22. British Thoracic Society guidelines for the management of chronic obstructive pulmonary disease. *Thorax* 1997;**52**:S1–28.
23. Feinleib M, Rosenberg HM, Cillons JG, Delozier JE, Pokras R, Chevarley FM. Trends in COPD morbidity and mortality in the United States. *Am Rev Respir Dis* 1989;**140**:S9–18.
24. Lung and Asthma Information Agency. *Respiratory Morbidity In General Practice, 1971–1991.* London. 1996; 92/4.
25. Sullivan SD, Ramsey SD, Lee TA. The economic burden of COPD. *Chest* 2000;**117**:5–9S.
26. Crisostomo MIL, Rubinstein I. Socioeconomic effects and health economics. *Eur Respir Mon* 1998;**7**:297–8.
27. Strassels SA, Smith DH, Sullivan SD, Mahajan PS. The costs of treating COPD in the United States. *Chest* 2001;**119**:344–52.
28. Price MJ, Hurrell C, Medley HV, Efthimiou J. Cost-effectiveness of fluticasone propionate in the management of symptomatic COPD patients. *Eur Respir J* 1999;**14**(suppl 30):379s.
29. Rijcken B, Britton J. Epidemiology of chronic obstructive pulmonary disease. *Eur Respir Mon* 1998;**7**:74–83.
30. Robbins DR, Enright PL, Sherrill DL. Lung function development in young adults: is there a plateau phase? *Eur Respir J* 1995;**8**:768–72.

31. Kerstjens HAM, Rijcken B, Schouten JP, Postma DS. Decline of FEV$_1$ by age and smoking status: facts, figures, and fallacies. *Thorax* 1997;**52**:820–7.

32. Anthonisen NR, Connett JE, Kiley JP, *et al.* Effects of smoking intervention and the use of an inhaled anticholinergic bronchodilator on the rate of decline of FEV$_1$: the Lung Health Study. *JAMA* 1994;**272**:1497–505.

33. Orie NGM, Sluiter HJ, de Vries K, Tammeling GJ, Witkop J. The host factor in bronchitis. In: NGM Orie, HJ Sluiter, eds. *Bronchitis: An International Symposium*. Royal van Gorcum, Assen, Netherlands, 1961.

34. Vestbo J, Prescott E. An update on the Dutch hypothesis and chronic respiratory disease. *Thorax* 1998;**53**(suppl 2):S15–19.

35. Hospers JJ, Postma DS, Rijcken B, Weiss ST, Schouten JP. Histamine airway hyper-responsiveness and mortality from chronic obstructive pulmonary disease: a cohort study. *Lancet* 2000;**356**:1313–17.

36. Vestbo J, Hansen EF. Airway hyper-responsiveness and COPD mortality. *Thorax* 2001;**56**(suppl 2):11–14.

37. Burrows B, Bloom JW, Traver GA, Cline MG. The course and prognosis of different forms of chronic airways obstruction in a sample of the general population. *N Engl J Med* 1987;**317**:1309–14.

38. Lange P, Parner J, Vestbo J, Jensen G, Schnohr P. A 15-year follow-up of ventilatory function in adults with asthma. *N Engl J Med* 1998;**339**:1194–200.

39. Lange P, Ulrik CS, Vestbo J, for The Copenhagen City Heart Study Group. Mortality in adults with self-reported bronchial asthma. A study of the general population. *Lancet* 1996;**347**:1285–9.

40. Hudon C, Trucotte H, Laviolette M, Carrier G, Boulet LP. Characteristics of bronchial asthma with incomplete reversibilitry to airflow obstruction. *Ann Allergy Asthma Immunol* 1997;**78**:195–202.

41. Kondoh Y, Taniguchi H, Yokoyama S, Taki F, Takagi K, Satake T. Emphysematous change in chronic asthma in relation to cigarette smoking. Assessment by computed tomography. *Chest* 1990;**97**:845–9.

42. Kanner RE, Anthonisen NR, Connett JE for the Lung Health Study Research Group. Lower respiratory illnesses promote FEV$_1$ decline in current smokers but not ex-smokers with mild chronic obstructive pulmonary disease. *Am J Respir Crit Care Med* 2001;**164**:358–64.

43. Burge PS, Calverley PM, Jones PW, Spencer S, Anderson JA, Maslen TK. Randomised, double blind, placebo controlled study of fluticasone propionate in patients with moderate to severe chronic obstructive pulmonary disease: the ISOLDE trial. *Br Med J* 2000;**320**:1297–303.

44. Spencer S, Calverley PM, Burge PS, Jones PW, on behalf of the ISOLDE Study Group. Health status deterioration in patients with chronic obstructive pulmonary disease. *Am J Respir Crit Care Med* 2001;**163**:122–8.

45. Mapp CE. Inhaled glucocorticoids in chronic obstructive pulmonary disease. *New Engl J Med* 2000;**343**:1960–1.

46. Weitzenblum E, Sautegeau A, Ehrhardt M, *et al.* Long-term course of pulmonary artery pressure in chronic obstructive pulmonary disease. *Am Rev Respir Dis* 1984;**130**:993–8.

47. Zielinski J, MacNee W, Wedzicha W, *et al.* Causes of death in patients with COPD and chronic respiratory failure. *Monaldi Arch Chest Dis* 1997;**52**:43–7.

48. Incalzi RA, Fuso L, De Rosa M, *et al.* Comorbidity contributors to predict mortality of patients with chronic obstructive pulmonary disease. *Eur Respir J* 1997;**10**:2794–800.

49. Anthonisen NR, Wright EC, Hodking JE. Prognosis in chronic obstructive pulmonary disease. *Am Rev Respir Dis* 1986;**133**:14–20.

50. Hansen EF, Phanareth K, Laursen LC, Kok-Jensen A, Dirksen A. Reversible and irreversible airflow obstruction as predictors of overall mortality in asthma and chronic obstructive pulmonary disease. *Am J Respir Crit Care Med* 1999;**159**:1267–71.

51. Burrows B, Earle RH. Prediction of survival in patients with chronic airway obstruction. *Am Rev Respir Dis* 1969;**99**:865–71.

52. Weitzenblum E, Hirth C, Ducolone A, *et al.* Prognostic value of pulmonary artery pressure in chronic obstructive pulmonary disease. *Thorax* 1981;**36**:752–8.

53. Gorecka D, Gorzelak K, Sliwinski P, Tobiasz M, Zielinski J. Effect of long-term oxygen therapy on survival in patients with chronic obstructive pulmonary disease with moderate hypoxaemia. *Thorax* 1997;**52**:674–9.

54. Landbo C, Prescott E, Lange P, Vestbo J, Almdal TP. Prognostic value of nutritional status in chronic obstructive pulmonary disease. *Am J Respir Crit Care Med* 1999;**160**:1856–61.

55. Lange P, Nyboe J, Appleyard M, Jensen G, Schnohr P. The relation of ventilatory impairment and of chronic mucus hypersecretion to mortality from obstructive lung disease and from all causes. *Thorax* 1990;**45**:579–85.

56. Burrows B, Knudson RJ, Camilli AE, Lyle SK, Lebowitz MD. The 'Horse-Racing Effect' and predicting decline in forced expiratory volume in one second from screening spirometry. *Am Rev Respir Dis* 1987;**135**:788–93.

57. Olofsson J, Bake B, Svärdsudd K, Skoogh B-E. The single breath N2-test predicts the rate of decline in FEV$_1$. The study of men born in 1913 and 1923. *Eur J Respir Dis* 1986;**69**:46–56.

58. Buist AS, Vollmer WM, Johnson LR, Mccamant LE. Does the single-breath N2 test identify the smoker who will develop chronic airflow limitation? *Am Rev Respir Dis* 1988;**137**:293–301.

59. Stanescu D, Sanna A, Veriter C, Robert A. Identification of smokers susceptible to development of chronic airflow limitation. A 13-year follow-up. *Chest* 1998;**114**:416–25.

60. Ferguson GT, Enright PL, Buist S, Higgins MW. Office spirometry for lung health assessment in adults. *Chest* 2000;**117**:1146–61.

61. Susser M. What is a cause and how do we know one? A grammaer for pragmatic epidemiology. *Am J Epidemiol* 1991;**133**:635–48.

62. United States Department of Health, Education and Welfare. *Smoking and Health: Report of the Advisory Committee of the Surgeon General of the Public Health Service*. PHS No 1103. Government Printing Office, Washington, DC, 1964.

63. Glindmeyer HW, Diem JE, Jones RN, Weill H. Non-comparability of longitudinally and cross-sectionally determined annual change in spirometry. *Am Rev Respir Dis* 1982;**125**:544–8.

64. American Thoracic Society – European Respiratory Society longitudinal data analysis workshop. *Am J Respir Crit Care Med* 1996;**154**:S207–84.

65. Larson RK, Barman ML, Kueppers F, Fudenberg HH. Genetic and environmental determinants of chronic obstructive pulmonary disease. *Ann Intern Med* 1970;**72**:627–32.

66. Kueppers F, Miller RD, Gordon H, Hepper NG, Offord K. Familial prevalence of chronic obstructive pulmonary disease in a matched pair study. *Am J Med* 1977;**63**:336–42.

67. Cohen BH, Ball WC, Jr, Brashears S, *et al.* Risk factors in chronic obstructive pulmonary disease (COPD). *Am J Epidemiol* 1977;**105**:223–32.

68. Silverman EK, Chapman HA, Drazen JM, *et al.* Genetic epidemiology of severe, early-onset chronic obstructive

pulmonary disease. Risk to relatives for airflow obstruction and chronic bronchitis. *Am J Respir Crit Care Med* 1998;**157**:1770–8.

69. Sandford AJ, Weir TD, Pare P. Genetic risk factors for chronic obstructive pulmonary disease. *Eur Respir J* 1997;**10**: 1380–91.

70. Tarjan E, Magyar P, Vaczi Z, Vaszar L. Longitudinal lung function study in heterozygous PiMZ phenotype subjects. *Eur Respir J* 1994;**7**:2199–204.

71. Seersholm N, Wilcke JTR, Kok-Jensen A, Dirksen A. Risk of hospital admission for obstructive pulmonary disease in alpha$_1$-antitrypsin heterozygotes of phenotype PiMZ. *Am J Respir Crit Care Med* 2000;**161**:81–4.

72. Janus ED, Phillips NT, Carrell RW. Smoking, lung function, and alpha-1-antitrypsin deficiency. *Lancet* 1985;**i**:152–4.

73. Seersholm N, Wilcke JT, Kok-Jensen A, Dirksen A. Risk of hospital admission for obstructive pulmonary disease in alpha$_1$-antitrypsin heterozygotes of phenotype PiMZ. *Am J Respir Crit Care Med* 2000;**161**:81–4.

74. Seersholm N, Kok-Jensen A, Dirksen A. Survival of patients with severe alpha-1-antitrypsin deficiency with special reference to non-index cases. *Thorax* 1994;**49**:695–8.

75. Seersholm N, Kok-Jensen A, Dirksen A. Decline in FEV_1 among patients with severe hereditary alpha-1-antitrypsin deficiency type PiZZ. *Am J Respir Crit Care Med* 1995;**152**: 1922–5.

76. Piitulainen E, Eriksson S. Decline in FEV_1 related to smoking status in individuals with severe alpha-1-antitrypsin deficiency (PiZZ). *Eur Respir J* 1999;**13**:247–51.

77. Dahl M, Nordestgaard BG, Lange P, Vestbo J, Tybjærg-Hansen A. Molecular diagnosis of severe and intermediate alpha-1-antitrypsin deficiency: MZ individuals with chronic obstructive pulmonary disease may have lower lung function than MM individuals. *Clin Chem* 2001;**47**:52–62.

78. Prescott E. Tobacco-related diseases: the role of gender. An epidemiologic study based on data from the Copenhagen Centre for Prospective Population Studies. *Dan Med Bull* 2000;**47**:115–31.

79. Prescott E, Bjerg AM, Andersen PK, Lange P, Vestbo J. Gender differences in smoking effects on lung function and risk of hospitalization for COPD: results from a Danish longitudinal population study. *Eur Respir J* 1997;**10**:822–7.

80. Prescott E, Osler M, Vestbo J. Importance of detailed adjustment for smoking when comparing morbidity and mortality in men and women in a Danish population study. *Eur J Publ Hlth* 1998;**8**:166–9.

81. Silverman EK, Weiss ST, Drazen JM, *et al.* Gender-related differences in severe, early-onset chronic obstructive pulmonary disease. *Am J Respir Crit Care Med* 2000;**162**: 2152–8.

82. Gold DR, Wang X, Wypij D, Spizer FE, Ware JH, Dockery DW. Effects of cigarette smoking on the pulmonary function in adolescent boys and girls. *N Engl J Med* 1996;**335**:931–7.

83. Prescott E, Hippe M, Schnohr P, Hein HO, Vestbo J. Comparison of smoking and risk of myocardial infarction in women and men. *Br Med J* 1998;**316**:1043–7.

84. Lindenström E, Boysen G, Nyboe J. Lifestyle factors and risk of cerebrovascular disease in women. *Stroke* 1993; **24**:1468–7.

85. Barker DJ, Godfrey KM, Fall C, Osmond C, Winter PD, Shaheen SO. Relation of birth weight and childhood respiratory infection to adult lung function and death from chronic obstructive airways disease. *Br Med J* 1991;**303**:671–5.

86. Stein CE, Kumaran K, Fall CH, Shaheen SO, Osmond C, Barker DJ. Relation of fetal growth to adult lung function in south India. *Thorax* 1997;**52**:895–9.

87. Reid DD, Fairburn AS. The natural history of chronic bronchitis. *Lancet* 1958;**i**:1147–52.

88. Rosenbaum S. Home localities of national servicemen with respiratory disease. *Br J Prev Soc Med* 1961;**15**:61–7.

89. Hanrahan JP, Tager IB, Segal MR, *et al.* The effect of maternal smoking during pregnancy on early infant lung function. *Am Rev Respir Dis* 1992;**145**:1129–35.

90. Carlsen HCL, Jaakkola JJK, Nafstad P, Carlsen K-H. In utero exposure to cigarette smoking influences lung function at birth. *Eur Respir J* 1997;**10**:1774–9.

91. Gold DR, Tager IB, Weiss ST, Tosteson TD, Speizer FE. Acute lower respiratory illness in childhood as a predictor of lung function and chronic respiratory symptoms. *Am Rev Respir Dis* 1989;**140**:877–84.

92. Shaheen SO, Barker DJ, Shiell AW, Crocker FJ, Wield GA, Holgate ST. The relationship between pneumonia in early childhood and impaired lung function in late adult life. *Am J Respir Crit Care Med* 1994;**149**:616–19.

93. Rijcken B, Weiss ST. Longitudinal analyses of airway responsiveness and pulmonary function decline. *Am J Respir Crit Care Med* 1996;**154**:S246–9.

94. Rijcken B, Scouten JP, Xu X, Rosner B, Weiss ST. Bronchial hyper-responsiveness to histamine is associated with accelerated decline of FEV_1. *Am J Respir Crit Care Med* 1995;**151**:1377–82.

95. Villar MT, Dow L, Coggon D, Lampe FC, Holgate ST. The influence of increased bronchial responsiveness, atopy, and serum IgE on decline in FEV_1: a longitudinal study in the elderly. *Am J Respir Crit Care Med* 1995;**151**:656–62.

96. Parker DR, O'Connor GT, Sparrow D, Segal MR, Weiss ST. The relationship of nonspecific airway responsiveness and atopy to the rate of decline of lung function. The Normative Aging Study. *Am Rev Respir Dis* 1990;**141**:589–94.

97. O'Connor GT, Sparrow D, Weiss ST. A prospective study of methacholine airway responsiveness as a predictor of pulmonary function decline: the Normative Aging Study. *Am J Respir Crit Care Med* 1995;**152**:87–92.

98. Tashkin DP, Altose MD, Connett JE, Kanner RE, Lee WW, Wise RA, for the Lung Health Study Research Group. Methacholine reactivity predicts changes in lung function over time in smokers with early chronic obstructive pulmonary disease. *Am J Respir Crit Care Med* 1996;**153**:1802–11.

99. Xu X, Rijcken B, Schouten JP, Weiss ST. Airways responsiveness and development and remission of chronic respiratory symptoms in adults. *Lancet* 1997;**350**:1431–4.

100. Peat JK, Woolcock AJ, Cullen K. Rate of decline of lung function in subjects with asthma. *Eur J Respir Dis* 1987; **70**:171–9.

101. Paoletti P, Prediletto R, Carrozzi L, *et al.* Effects of childhood and adolescence–adulthood respiratory infections in a general population. *Eur Respir J* 1989;**2**:428–36.

102. Burrows B, Knudson RJ, Cline MG, Lebowitz MD. A reexamination of risk factors for ventilatory impairment. *Am Rev Respir Dis* 1988;**138**:829–36.

103. Britton J, Martinez FD. The relationship of childhood respiratory infection to growth and decline in lung function. *Am J Respir Crit Care Med* 1996;**154**:S240–5.

104. Peto R, Speizer FE, Cochrane AL, *et al.* The relevance in adults of air-flow obstruction, but not of mucus hypersecretion, to mortality from chronic lung disease. *Am Rev Respir Dis* 1983;**128**:491–500.

105. Sherman CB, Xu X, Speizer FE, Ferris BG Jr, Weiss ST, Dockery DW. Longitudinal lung function decline in subjects with respiratory symptoms. *Am Rev Respir Dis* 1992;**146**: 855–9.

106. Vestbo J, Prescott E, Lange P, and The Copenhagen City Heart Study Group. Association of chronic mucus hypersecretion with FEV_1 decline and COPD morbidity. *Am J Respir Crit Care Med* 1996;**153**:1530–5.

107. Vestbo J, Rasmussen FV. Respiratory symptoms and FEV_1 as predictors of hospitalization and medication in the following 12 years due to respiratory disease. *Eur Respir J* 1989;**2**:710–15.

108. Prescott E, Lange P, Vestbo J. Chronic mucus hypersecretion in COPD and death from pulmonary infection. *Eur Respir J* 1995;**8**:1333–8.

109. US Surgeon General. *The Health Consequences of Smoking: Chronic Obstructive Lung Disease.* DHHS Publication No. 84–50205. US Department of Health and Human Services. Washington DC, 1984.

110. Davis RM, Novotny TE. The epidemiology of cigarette smoking and its impact on chronic obstructive pulmonary disease. *Am Rev Respir Dis* 1989;**140**:S82–4.

111. Tager IB, Segal MR, Speizer FE, Weiss ST. The natural history of forced expiratory volumes. Effect of cigarette smoking and respiratory symptoms. *Am Rev Respir Dis* 1988;**138**:837–49.

112. Xu X, Dockery DW, Ware JH, Speizer FE, Ferris BG Jr. Effects of cigarette smoking on rate of loss of pulmonary function in adults: a longitudinal assessment. *Am Rev Respir Dis* 1992;**146**:1345–8.

113. Le Souëf PN. Tobacco related lung diseases begin in childhood. *Thorax* 2000;**55**:1063–7.

114. Tager IB, Ngo L, Hanrahan JP. Maternal smoking during pregnancy. Effects on lung function during the first 18 months of life. *Am J Respir Crit Care Med* 1995;**152**:977–83.

115. Sherrill DL, Lebowitz MD, Knudson RJ, Burrows B. Smoking and symptom effects on the curves of lung function growth and decline. *Am Rev Respir Dis* 1991;**144**:17–22.

116. Lange P, Groth S, Nyboe J, *et al.* Effects of smoking and changes in smoking habits on the decline of FEV_1. *Eur Respir J* 1989;**2**:811–16.

117. Cook DG, Strachan DP. Summary of parental smoking on the effects of parental smoking on the respiratory health of children and implications for research. *Thorax* 1999;**54**:357–66.

118. Jaakkola MS. Environmental tobacco smoke and respiratory diseases. *Eur Respir Mon* 2000;**15**:322–83.

119. Royal College of Physicians of London. *Health or Smoking? Follow-up Report of the Royal College of Physicians.* Pitman, London, 1983.

120. Camilli AE, Burrows B, Knudson RJ, Lyle SK, Lebowitz MD. Longitudinal changes in forced expiratory volume in one second in adults. *Am Rev Respir Dis* 1987;**135**:794–9.

121. Sherrill DL, Enright P, Cline M, Burrows B, Lebowitz MD. Rates of decline in lung function among subjects who restart cigarette smoking. *Chest* 1996;**109**:1001–5.

122. Lebowitz MD. Epidemiological studies of the respiratory effects of air pollution. *Eur Respir J* 1996;**9**:1029–54.

123. Dennis RJ, Maldonado D, Norman S, Baena E, Martinez G. Woodsmoke exposure and risk for obstructive airways disease among women. *Chest* 1996;**109**:115–19.

124. Sunyer J, Antó JM, Murillo C, Sáez M. Effects of urban air pollution on emergency room admissions for chronic obstructive pulmonary disease. *Am J Epidemiol* 1991;**134**:277–88.

125. Sunyer J, Sáez M, Murillo C, Castellsague J, Martinez F, Anto JM. Air pollution and emergency room admissions for COPD: a five year study. *Am J Epidemiol* 1993;**137**:701–5.

126. Burnett RT, Dales R, Krewski D, Vincent R, Dann T, Brook JR. Associations between ambient particulate sulfate and admissions to Ontario hospitals for cardiac and respiratory diseases. *Am J Epidemiol* 1995;**142**:15–22.

127. Schwartz J, Dockery DW. Increased mortality in Philadelphia associated with daily air pollution concentrations. *Am Rev Respir Dis* 1992;**145**:600–4.

128. Dockery DW, Schwartz J, Spengler JD. Air pollution and daily mortality: associations with particulates and acid aerosols. *Environ Res* 1992;**59**:362–73.

129. Sunyer J, Schwartz J, Tobias A, Macfarlane D, Garcia J, Anto JM. Patients with chronic obstructive pulmonary disease are at increased risk of death associated with urban particle air pollution: a case-crossover analysis. *Am J Epidemiol* 2000;**151**:50–6.

130. Gauderman WJ, McConnell R, Gilliland F, *et al.* Association between air pollution and lung function growth in Southern California children. *Am J Respir Crit Care Med* 2000;**162**:1383–90.

131. Smith K. Fuel combustion, air pollution exposure, and health: the situation in the developing countries. *Ann Rev Environ Energy* 1993;**18**:529–66.

132. Dennis RJ, Maldonado D, Norman S, *et al.* Woodsmoke exposure and risk of obstructive airways disease among women. *Chest* 1996;**109**:115–19.

133. Gold JA, Jaishree J, Hay JG, *et al.* Hut lung. *Medicine* 2000;**79**:310–17.

134. Hendrick DJ. Occupation and chronic obstructive pulmonary disease. *Thorax* 1996;**51**:947–55.

135. Kauffmann F, Drouet D, Lellouch J, Brille D. Occupational exposure and 12-year spirometric changes among Paris area workers. *Br J Ind Med* 1982;**39**:221–32.

136. Becklake MR. Occupational exposures: evidence for a causal association with chronic obstructive pulmonary disease. *Am Rev Respir Dis* 1989;**140**:S85–91.

137. Heederik D. Epidemiology of occupational respiratory diseases and risk factors. *Eur Respir Mon* 2000;**15**:429–47.

138. Krzyzanowski M, Jedrychowski W, Wysocki M. Factors associated with the change in ventilatory function and the development of chronic obstructive pulmonary disease in a 13-year follow-up of the Cracow study. *Am Rev Respir Dis* 1986;**134**:1011–19.

139. Korn RJ, Dockery DW, Speizer FE, Ware JH, Ferris BG Jr. Occupational exposures and chronic respiratory symptoms. A population-based study. *Am Rev Respir Dis* 1987;**136**:298–304.

140. Heederik D, Pouwels H, Kromhout H, Kromhout D. Chronic non-specific lung disease and occupational exposures estimated by means of a job exposure matrix: the Zutphen Study. *Int J Epidemiol* 1989;**18**:382–9.

141. Humerfelt S, Gulsvik A, Skjærven R, *et al.* Decline in FEV_1 and airflow limitation related to occupational exposures in men of an urban community. *Eur Respir J* 1993;**6**:1095–103.

142. Post WK, Heederik D, Kromhout H, Kromhout D. Occupational exposures estimated by a population specific job exposure matrix and 25 year incidence rate of chronic non-specific lung disease (CNSLD): the Zutphen Study. *Eur Respir J* 1994;**7**:1048–55.

143. Tabak C, Feskens EJ, Heederik D, Kromhout D, Menotti A, Blackburn HW. Fruit and fish consumption: a possible explanation for population differences in COPD mortality (The Seven Countries Study). *Eur J Clin Nutr* 1998;**52**:819–25.

144. Miedema I, Feskens EJM, Heederik D, Kromhout D. Dietary determinants of long-term incidence of chronic nonspecific lung disease. The Zutphen study. *Am J Epidemiol* 1993;**138**:37–45.

145. Schwartz J, Weiss ST. Dietary factors and their relation to respiratory symptoms. *Am J Epidemiol* 1990;**132**:7–76.

146. Strachan DP, Cox BD, Erzinclioglu SW, Walters DE, Whichelow MJ. Ventilatory function and winter fresh fruit consumption in a random sample of British adults. *Thorax* 1991;**46**:624–9.

147. Dow L, Tracey M, Villar A, *et al*. Does dietary intake of vitamin C and E influence lung function in older people? *Am J Respir Crit Care Med* 1996;**154**:1401–4.

148. Shahar E, Folsom AR, Milnick SL, *et al*. Dietary n-3 polyunsaturated fatty acids and smoking-related chronic obstructive pulmonary disease. *N Engl J Med* 1994;**331**:228–33.

149. Sharp DS, Rodriguez BL, Shahar E, Hwang L, Burchfield CM. Fish consumption may limit the damage of smoking on the lung. *Am J Respir Crit Care Med* 1994;**150**:983–7.

150. Schwartz J, Weiss ST. The relationship of dietary fish intake to level of pulmonary function in the first national health and nutrition survey (NHANES I). *Eur Respir J* 1994;**7**:1821–4.

151. Tabak C, Smit HA, Rasanen L, *et al*. Dietary factors and pulmonary function: a cross sectional study in middle aged men from three European countries. *Thorax* 1999;**54**:1021–6.

152. Smit HA, Grievink L, Tabak C. Dietary influences on chronic obstructive lung disease and asthma: a review of the epidemiological evidence. *Proc Nutr Soc* 1999;**58**:309–19.

153. Marmot MG, Shipley MJ, Rose G. Inequalities in death – specific explanations of a general pattern? *Lancet* 1984;**i**:1003–6.

154. Marmot MG, McDowall ME. Mortality decline and widening in social inequalities. *Lancet* 1986;**i**:274–6.

155. Smith GD, Hart C, Blane D, Hole D. Adverse socioeconomic conditions in childhood cause specific adult mortality: prospective observational study. *Br Med J* 1998;**316**:1631–5.

156. Menezes AMB, Victora CG, Rigatto M. Prevalence and risk factors for chronic bronchitis in Pelotas, Brazil: a population-based study. *Thorax* 1994;**49**:1217–21.

157. Bakke PS, Hanoa R, Gulsvik A. Educational level and obstructive lung disease given smoking habits and occupational airborne exposure: a Norwegian community study. *Am J Epidemiol* 1995;**141**:1080–8.

158. Prescott E, Lange P, Vestbo J and the Copenhagen City Heart Study Group. Socioeconomic status, lung function, and admission to hospital for COPD. Results from the Copenhagen City Heart Study. *Eur Respir J* 1999;**13**:1109–14.

159. Britten N, Davies JMC, Colley JRT. Early respiratory experience and subsequent cough and peak expiratory flow rate in 36 year old men and women. *Br Med J* 1987;**294**:1317–20.

160. McCormick MC. The contribution of low birth weight to infant mortality and childhood morbidity. *N Engl J Med* 1985;**312**:82–90.

161. Shaheen SO, Barker DJ, Holgate ST. Do lower respiratory tract infections in early childhood cause chronic obstructive pulmonary disease? *Am J Respir Crit Care Med* 1995;**151**:1649–51.

162. Coggon D, Barker DJ, Inskip H, *et al*. Housing in early life and later mortality. *J Epidemiol Comm Health* 1993;**47**:345–8.

163. Schwartz J, Weiss ST. Relationship between dietary vitamin C intake and pulmonary function in the first national health and nutrition examination survey (NHANES). *Am J Clin Nutr* 1994;**59**:110–14.

164. Sharp DS, Rodriguez BL, Shahar E, *et al*. Fish consumption may limit the damage of smoking on the lung. *Am J Respir Crit Care Med* 1994;**150**:983–7.

165. Sridhar MK. Nutrition and lung health. *Br Med J* 1995;**3**:1075–6.

166. Rasmussen FV, Borcsenius L, Winsløw JB, Østergaard ER. Associations between housing conditions, smoking habits and ventilatory lung function in men with clean jobs. *Scand J Resp Dis* 1978;**59**:264–76.

167. Comstock GW, Meyer MB, Helsing KJ. Respiratory effects of household exposures to tobacco smoke and gas cooking. *Am Rev Respir Dis* 1981;**124**:143–8.

168. Viegi G, Paoletti P, Carozzi L, *et al*. Effects of home environment on respiratory symptoms and lung function in a general population sample in north Italy. *Eur Respir J* 1991;**4**:580–6.

4

Genetics

EDWIN K SILVERMAN

INTRODUCTION

Case reports of familial COPD were published in the 1950s,[1] but interest in the role of genetic factors in COPD largely began with the discovery of severe alpha-1-antitrypsin deficiency in 1963.[2] Severe alpha-1-antitrypsin deficiency is the most important known genetic determinant of COPD; therefore, we will discuss the molecular and population genetics of alpha-1-antitrypsin deficiency in detail. In addition, we will review the evidence for genetic factors in non-alpha-1-antitrypsin deficiency COPD, including assessment of risk to relatives for COPD-related phenotypes and association studies with candidate gene polymorphisms. We will also discuss the application of animal models to identify potential genetic determinants of COPD.

Although cigarette smoking is the major environmental risk factor for the development of COPD, the development of airflow obstruction in smokers is quite variable. In 1977, Burrows and colleagues demonstrated a dose–response relationship between FEV_1 (% predicted) and pack-years of cigarette smoking; heavier smokers were more likely to develop airflow obstruction, indicated by reduced FEV_1.[3] However, many smokers had pulmonary function within the normal range. In the Burrows study, pack-years, defined as the average number of packs of cigarettes smoked per day multiplied by the number of years of smoking, was the smoking-related variable which correlated most closely with FEV_1. However, pack-years of smoking only accounted for 15% of the variability in FEV_1.

Pathologic studies of emphysema have also demonstrated variability in the development of emphysema.[4] For example, Petty and colleagues demonstrated marked variability in the development of emphysema among smokers.[5] More recently, a study of lung pathology in smokers demonstrated that microscopic emphysema, assessed by quantitative measurements of airspace wall surface area per unit volume of lung tissue, was present in only 26% of smokers.[6]

In part, the variable relationship between cigarette smoking and COPD relates to competing risks; cigarette smokers may die from other smoking-related illnesses, such as lung cancer, prior to the development of COPD. However, genetic factors are also likely to influence the variable susceptibility to develop COPD. Because cigarette smoking is a proven major environmental risk factor for COPD that can be readily assessed by questionnaire, COPD offers unique opportunities and challenges to incorporate environmental influences in the study of genetics of complex diseases. Genetic determinants of COPD may well represent a genotype-by-environment interaction between cigarette smoking and susceptibility genes.

SEVERE ALPHA-1-ANTITRYPSIN DEFICIENCY

Only 1–2% of COPD patients inherit severe alpha-1-antitrypsin deficiency.[7] However, severe alpha-1-antitrypsin deficiency serves as a model of the manner in which genetic and environmental factors can interact to lead to COPD. Detailed discussion of the pathogenesis of emphysema in alpha-1-antitrypsin deficiency and treatment for severe alpha-1-antitrypsin deficiency is provided in Chapter 9.

Description of the PI locus and PI alleles

Alpha-1-antitrypsin is encoded by the PI (Protease Inhibitor) locus on chromosome 14q32.1.[8,9] The PI gene, which is 12.2 kb in length, has seven exons and six introns; the structure of the PI locus is shown in Figure 4.1. The first two exons and a short sequence of the third exon are encoded in the transcript for macrophages, but not for hepatocytes. Most of the fourth exon, and all of the remaining three exons, encode the protein sequence. The active inhibitor site PI amino acid residue, methionine 358, is encoded by exon V.

The dominant site of synthesis of alpha-1-antitrypsin is the liver, but alpha-1-antitrypsin is also synthesized in monocytes, macrophages and neutrophils.[10,11] Alpha-1-antitrypsin is a 394 amino acid protein (52 kDa); salt bridges within the molecule include glutamic acid 342 to lysine 290 and glutamic acid 264 to lysine 387.

The discovery of alpha-1-antitrypsin deficiency was made by observing the absence of an alpha-1-globulin band in serum protein electrophoresis.[2] Subsequently, differences in electrophoretic mobility of various alpha-1-antitrypsin forms, related to differences in molecular surface charge, were demonstrated.[12] The most common variant was designated M, for medium rate of migration. Variants that migrated faster and slower than M were called F and S, for faster and slower migration, respectively. The Z form of the protein migrated much slower than the S form.

More than 75 different PI alleles have been identified, a few of which result in decreased serum levels of alpha-1-antitrypsin.[13] The common M allele, with an allele frequency greater than 95% in Caucasian populations, is associated with normal alpha-1-antitrypsin levels. The S allele, which is associated with slightly reduced alpha-1-antitrypsin levels, and the Z allele, which is associated with markedly reduced alpha-1-antitrypsin levels, also occur in most Caucasian populations. A small percentage of subjects inherit null alleles, which lead to the absence of any alpha-1-antitrypsin production through a heterogeneous collection of mutations.[13] Individuals with two Z alleles or one Z and one null allele are referred to as PI Z, because they cannot be distinguished by the isoelectric focusing technique that is commonly used to assess PI type. PI Z individuals have approximately 15% of normal plasma antitrypsin levels.

Null alleles (also referred to as QO alleles) lead to the absence of alpha-1-antitrypsin protein production through a variety of mechanisms. Single base substitutions, insertions and deletions resulting in a premature stop codon have been reported; the consequences of premature termination of mRNA synthesis include the absence of mRNA production (as seen in QOgranite falls), intracellular accumulation of a truncated protein (as seen in QOhongkong) and intracellular degradation of a truncated protein (as seen in QOclayton).[14–16] Mechanisms other than premature stop codon formation that have resulted in null alleles include gene deletion (PI*QOisola di procida) and critical amino acid substitutions (PI*QOludwigshafen).[17,18] Brantly and colleagues noted that several different null alleles have been described which result from mutations in a series of seven cytosine nucleotides from codons 360 to 362.[16]

A small number of null-null individuals have been identified; these subjects have no detectable serum alpha-1-antitrypsin.[19] For example, Cox and Levison described three null-null siblings with COPD.[20] Null-null individuals

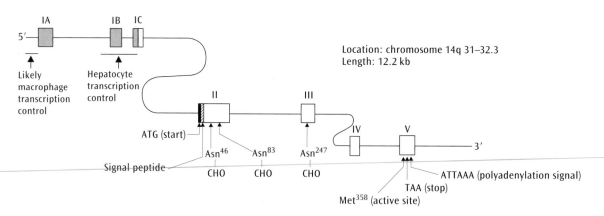

Figure 4.1 *Structure of PI Locus. The gene includes seven exons (IA, IB, IC, II, III, IV and V); the coding sequence is contained in exons II to V. A signal peptide is encoded by exon II, following the translation start site (ATG). Hepatocyte transcription begins within exon IC and is controlled by the region denoted by the solid line. Transcription in monocytes and macrophages begins with exon IA. The three carbohydrate attachment sites are noted at amino acid residues 46, 83 and 247. The site of the critical active site methionine (amino acid residue 358) is also indicated. (From ref. 13.) Reprinted from AJM, Vol 84; 16: Figure 2, with permission from Elsevier Science.*

seem to have an extremely high predisposition to develop COPD, but the number of subjects that have been identified is too small to quantitate the risk of null-null compared to PI Z individuals with certainty.

In addition to null alleles, a variety of very rare PI alleles with electrophoretic mobility similar to the M protein have been described, which are associated with very low serum levels of alpha-1-antitrypsin. Some of these rare variants, such as Mheerlen and Mprocida, are associated with reduced alpha-1-antitrypsin levels due to intracellular degradation of antitrypsin; other rare variants, such as Mmalton and Mnichinan are associated with reduced alpha-1-antitrypsin levels due to intracellular accumulation of protein.

Diagnosis of alpha-1-antitrypsin deficiency

The clinical laboratory test used most frequently to screen for alpha-1-antitrypsin deficiency is measurement of the immunologic level of alpha-1-antitrypsin in serum. The definitive diagnosis of alpha-1-antitrypsin deficiency requires PI type determination, but measurement of serum immunologic or functional levels can be used for screening, as long as appropriate methods to quantitate alpha-1-antitrypsin levels are used. Available assays for measurement of immunologic alpha-1-antitrypsin levels include immunoelectrophoresis, turbidometric assays, enzyme-linked immunoassays and radial immunodiffusion plates. Methods which are based on quantitation of the alpha-1-globulin peak (which is largely alpha-1-antitrypsin) from serum protein electrophoresis (SPEP) are unreliable, because the large albumin peak in SPEP analysis can provide falsely elevated estimates of alpha-1-globulin levels.

Isoelectric focusing of serum in polyacrylamide gels in the pH range of 4.0–5.0 remains the most common method for the determination of PI type. Alpha-1-antitrypsin is a negatively charged glycoprotein that resolves into eight bands when subjected to electrophoresis near its isoelectric point. Isoelectric focusing of serum can accurately determine PI type, which reflects the genotype at the PI locus for the common alleles. Molecular genotyping can be performed for the common PI alleles (M, S and Z) using oligonucleotide hybridization, denaturing gradient gel electrophoresis, or a variety of other molecular genotyping approaches, but molecular genetic tests for rare deficiency alleles are not widely available.[21]

The PI locus demonstrates autosomal codominant expression of protein variants, because individuals with, for example, PI MZ, will produce both M and Z protein. However, the development of COPD and liver disease are expressed in an autosomal recessive mode, because two deficiency alleles are required to cause a significant increase in risk for these diseases (see discussion of controversy

regarding the risk for COPD in PI MZ heterozygotes below).

The genotype at the PI locus is the primary genetic determinant of the serum alpha-1-antitrypsin level. Alpha-1-antitrypsin is an acute-phase reactant protein which increases with systemic infection or other stressors; therefore, environmental factors can influence alpha-1-antitrypsin serum levels. Martin and colleagues studied immunologic and functional levels of serum alpha-1-antitrypsin in 583 individuals from 114 pedigrees.[22] They noted that the PI locus appeared to be the only important genetic determinant of serum alpha-1-antitrypsin level, because adding polygenic determinants to quantitative genetic models which included PI type effects did not improve the fit of their models. Using measured genotype analysis in families of PI Z subjects, Silverman and colleagues estimated that, depending on adjustment for covariates, PI type explained between 72% and 92% of variation in immunologic serum alpha-1-antitrypsin levels.[23] Thus, most, if not all, of the genetic variation in serum alpha-1-antitrypsin levels appears to be controlled by the genotype at the PI locus.

Prevalence of severe alpha-1-antitrypsin deficiency

The prevalence of alpha-1-antitrypsin deficiency is elevated in populations of Scandinavian descent. Analysis of the haplotypes of polymorphic loci adjacent to the alpha-1-antitrypsin Z allele suggested that a common mutational origin for the majority of Z alleles may have occurred in southern Scandinavia.[24]

A variety of population screening studies for alpha-1-antitrypsin deficiency have been performed. Hutchison reviewed the European screening studies, and he noted that the highest Z allele frequencies were found in the northwestern section of Europe (including Southern Sweden, Norway, Denmark and the UK).[25] Prevalence surveys have typically found low Z allele frequencies in populations of African and Asian descent.[26] The largest screening study was a survey of 200 000 newborns in Sweden from 1972 to 1974; a prevalence estimate of 1/1639 for PI Z individuals was determined from this screening effort.[27] Early screening studies in the USA included only modest population samples, so that the prevalence of PI Z individuals (assumed to be PI ZZ homozygotes) was estimated from the Z allele frequency – which ranged from 0.0059 to 0.0229.[28]

A large newborn screening program in Oregon identified 21 PI Z infants in a population of 107 038, for a prevalence estimate of 1 in 5097.[29] However, confirmation of PI Z in the Oregon study required a follow-up test, so some PI Z infants may have been missed, resulting in an underestimate of PI Z prevalence. In a population of 20 000 blood donors in the USA, Silverman *et al.* found seven PI Z subjects, for a prevalence of approximately 1 in 2857.[28] Pooled data from 26 other screening studies of populations which included Z alleles (excluding Sweden and the USA) revealed a prevalence of eight subjects in 19 768 screened (1 in 2471).[28] Thus, although the highest prevalence rates of PI Z subjects have been noted in Sweden, the differences between the prevalence of PI Z subjects in Sweden compared to other Caucasian populations may not be as great as previously assumed.

Natural history of PI Z

PI Z individuals often develop early-onset COPD. Among PI Z subjects with COPD, panacinar emphysema with predominant involvement of the lung bases has been classically described. However, recent data based on chest CT scans indicate that PI Z subjects with COPD frequently have diffuse emphysema, without a basal predominance.[30]

Published series of PI Z individuals have usually included many PI Z subjects with COPD; however, these studies have largely included PI Z individuals who were tested for alpha-1-antitrypsin deficiency because they already had chronic obstructive lung disease.[31–34] Thus, the fraction of PI Z individuals who will develop COPD and the age-of-onset distribution for the development of COPD in PI Z subjects remain unknown. PI Z subjects are also at increased risk for liver diseases, including hepatic cirrhosis; however, discussion of liver disease is beyond the scope of this chapter.

Several large series of alpha-1-antitrypsin-deficient individuals reported in the 1970s and 1980s clearly demonstrated that PI Z subjects who smoke cigarettes tend to develop more severe pulmonary impairment at an earlier age than non-smoking PI Z individuals.[31–33] Larsson estimated survival probabilities in PI Z subjects using a life table approach.[32] He estimated that the median survival of PI Z smokers would be 23 years less than PI Z non-smokers.

Few studies have considered whether factors other than smoking influence the development of lung disease. Black and Kueppers compared 18 non-smoking PI Z individuals with 36 PI Z subjects who were current or ex-smokers.[35] They found significant variability in pulmonary function and clinical symptoms, especially among non-smoking PI Z individuals. They speculated that unidentified host factors contribute to this variability.

A significant fraction of the variability in pulmonary function among PI Z individuals is certainly explained by cigarette smoking; however, the development of COPD in PI Z subjects, even among current or ex-smokers, is not absolute. In a study performed at Washington University in St Louis, Silverman and colleagues enroled 52 PI Z

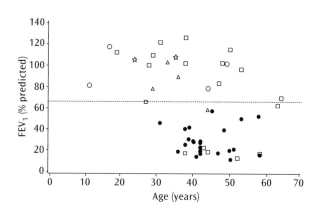

Figure 4.2 *Effect of ascertainment bias on per cent predicted FEV₁ among 52 severely alpha-1-antitrypsin-deficient subjects (PI Z) in the study by Silverman* et al.*[36] Closed circles represent index PI Z subjects (individuals diagnosed with severe alpha-1-antitrypsin deficiency because they had COPD, and who were the first PI Z subject identified in their family); open symbols represent non-index subjects. Non-index subjects were ascertained by liver disease (open circles), family studies (squares), population screening (triangles) and other pulmonary problems (stars). Marked variability in FEV₁ values is evident for the non-index PI Z subjects. (From ref. 36.) Reproduced from* Ann Intern Med *1989;**111**:982–991, Figure 2, with permission from ACP-ASIM.*

subjects;[36] significant variability in pulmonary function was found (Figure 4.2). In Figure 4.2, index PI Z subjects, who were tested for alpha-1-deficiency because they had COPD and who were the first PI Z identified in their family, all had significantly reduced FEV₁ values. Non-index PI Z subjects, who were ascertained by a variety of other means, including family studies, population screening and liver disease, suggest a much different natural history for severe alpha-1-antitrypsin deficiency than index PI Z subjects. Many non-index PI Z subjects have preserved pulmonary function. With subjects identified from the Danish Alpha-1-antitrypsin Register, Seersolm and colleagues also found significantly higher FEV₁ values in non-index PI Z subjects (not identified because they had COPD) compared to index PI Z subjects (identified because they had COPD) despite similar ages and smoking histories.[37] Moreover, Seersholm and colleagues demonstrated that index PI Z subjects had markedly reduced survival compared to non-index PI Z subjects (Figure 4.3).

Mayer and colleagues recently assessed occupational exposures as a potential contributor to variable expression of lung disease in severe alpha-1-antitrypsin deficiency.[38] They assessed 128 PI Z subjects with spirometry and a questionnaire that included detailed information regarding occupational exposures to dust and fumes. They found that cigarette smoking was a critical risk factor for the development of airflow obstruction and dyspnea. Of interest, they found that high mineral dust exposure

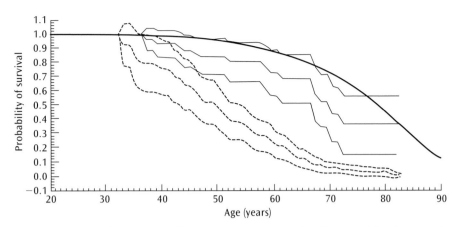

Figure 4.3 *Projected survival of 252 index (dashed lines) and 145 non-index (medium black lines) PI Z subjects in the Danish Alpha-1-antitrypsin Register. Estimated survival curves with 95% confidence intervals are provided; survival within the general Danish population (thick black line) is also presented. Survival among index PI Z subjects is significantly lower than non-index PI Z subjects; both groups have reduced survival compared to the general Danish population. (From ref. 97.) Taken from Chronic Obstructive Pulmonary Disease. 2nd ed. Chapter 4; eds: Calverely et al. with permission from BMJ Publishing Group.*

was associated with reduced FEV_1 and chronic cough, independent of smoking history. Thus, occupational exposures may also be important determinants of the development of lung disease in PI Z subjects.

The natural history of PI Z subjects in the general population remains uncertain. There are likely three groups of unidentified PI Z subjects in the general population:

1 PI Z subjects with diagnosed COPD who have not been tested for alpha-1-antitrypsin deficiency (possibly because they were not diagnosed with early-onset COPD).
2 PI Z subjects who have significant airflow obstruction but who have not been diagnosed with COPD.
3 PI Z subjects with normal pulmonary function.

However, the relative proportions of these groups are unknown.

Genetics of variable expression of severe alpha-1-antitrypsin deficiency

The primary focus of the St Louis Alpha-1-antitrypsin Study was to determine if genetic factors other than PI type influenced the variable development of lung disease among PI Z subjects. Therefore, first-degree relatives of the 52 PI Z subjects were enroled. Despite comparable smoking history, parents of PI Z subjects with reduced FEV_1 tended to have lower FEV_1 values themselves compared to parents of PI Z subjects with preserved FEV_1.[39] This difference in FEV_1 (% predicted) among parents of PI Z subjects, 95% vs. 75.3%, was of borderline statistical significance, with $P = 0.05$. These results, as well as the findings with segregation analysis from the St Louis study, suggested that additional genetic factors influence the development of airflow obstruction in alpha-1-antitrypsin

deficiency. Moreover, Silverman and colleagues demonstrated that significant genotype-by-environment interaction between PI type and pack-years of smoking was present.[23]

More recently, Novoradovsky and colleagues published a study in which they assessed whether variation in the endothelial nitric oxide synthase (NOS3) gene could be one of the genetic factors which influences the variable development of airflow obstruction in PI Z subjects.[40] They identified polymorphisms in the NOS3 gene, and they tested for genetic association of these variants with airflow obstruction in 55 PI Z subjects with FEV_1 less than 35% predicted, 122 PI Z subjects with FEV_1 greater than 35% predicted and 93 control subjects. Two polymorphisms in the coding region, which probably do not lead to functionally important changes in the NOS3 protein, were associated with severe airflow obstruction in PI Z subjects. Further work to replicate this finding and to identify a functionally important variant will be required, but NOS3 is an intriguing possible contributor to the variable development of airflow obstruction in PI Z subjects.

COPD IN OTHER GENETIC SYNDROMES

Emphysema has been reported in several very rare genetic syndromes. Cutis laxa, also known as generalized elastolysis, is a rare and heterogeneous condition associated with loose and redundant, but inelastic, skin. Both inherited and acquired forms have been described; in some inherited cases an autosomal recessive pattern of inheritance has been noted, while in other cases an autosomal dominant pattern has been observed.[41] Multiple inherited cases of cutis laxa with pulmonary emphysema in infancy and childhood have been described, and rare inherited cases in adults have also been reported.[42,43] Several autosomal dominant cutis laxa cases have been shown to be related to mutations in the terminal exons of the elastin gene; no other specific genetic etiologies have been reported.[44,45]

In Marfan's syndrome, an autosomal dominant disorder related to mutations in the Fibrillin-1 gene, a variety of pulmonary complications have been reported. In a series of 100 patients with Marfan's syndrome, five were reported to have bullae on chest radiographs.[46] However, the etiologic relationship of Marfan's syndrome to COPD is unclear.

RISK TO RELATIVES FOR COPD

Familial aggregation of spirometry and COPD

Several types of studies have suggested that genetic factors other than alpha-1-antitrypsin type may be involved in the susceptibility to develop COPD. We will review the evidence from general population studies and from COPD families.

A variety of studies of pulmonary function measurements performed in the general population and in twins have suggested that genetic factors influence variation in pulmonary function. Redline and colleagues assessed spirometry in 256 monozygotic and 158 dizygotic twins who were not selected for respiratory problems.[47] For FEV_1, higher correlation in monozygotic twins (0.72) than dizygotic twins (0.27) suggested that genetic factors influence variation in pulmonary function. However, such general population studies do not address whether genetic factors influence the development of chronic airflow obstruction.

Studies in relatives of COPD patients also have supported a role for genetic factors. Several studies in the 1970s reported higher rates of airflow obstruction in first-degree relatives of COPD patients than in control subjects. For example, Larson compared spirometry in 156 first-degree relatives of COPD patients to 86 spouse controls with similar pack-years of smoking.[48] Airflow obstruction was found in 23% of first-degree relatives, but only 9% of control subjects. Although this study did show familial aggregation for airflow obstruction, it did have several weaknesses. Alpha-1-antitrypsin deficiency was not rigorously excluded as a potential contributor to airflow obstruction. In addition, a higher percentage of the first-degree relatives than controls were smokers, so at least some of the observed differences may relate to differences in smoking behavior. Nonetheless, genetic predisposition to COPD was suggested by this study.

Kueppers et al. studied 114 subjects with COPD and control subjects matched based on age, gender, occupation and smoking history.[49] Siblings of COPD and control subjects also were included; the mean FEV_1 among siblings of COPD subjects (90% of predicted) was significantly lower than the siblings of control subjects (103% of predicted). This difference in pulmonary function between sibs of COPD and control subjects remained significant after adjustment for smoking history.

A large study of COPD in families was performed at Johns Hopkins.[50,51] Variance components analysis of their data suggested a significant genetic contribution to FEV_1 and the ratio of FEV_1/FVC.[52]

Additional studies have demonstrated familial aggregation for chronic bronchitis. In a survey of 9226 residents of Tecumseh, Higgins and Keller found approximately three-fold higher rates of chronic bronchitis in offspring when at least one parent had chronic bronchitis than if neither parent had chronic bronchitis; this analysis did not include adjustment for cigarette smoking.[53] Speizer et al. analyzed National Health Interview Survey data for chronic respiratory conditions; they found higher rates of bronchitis or emphysema among offspring when at least one parent had bronchitis or emphysema; this effect appeared to be independent of cigarette smoking.[54] Finally, in a study in East Boston, Tager et al. found approximately two-fold higher rates of chronic bronchitis or airflow obstruction in first-degree relatives of probands with chronic bronchitis or airflow obstruction than in first-degree relatives of control probands; this familial aggregation also appeared to be independent of cigarette smoking.[55]

Familial aggregation of severe, early-onset COPD

In an effort to identify novel genetic risk factors for COPD; Silverman and colleagues have focused on subjects with severe, early-onset COPD unrelated to severe alpha-1-antitrypsin deficiency.[56] Probands in this Boston Early-Onset COPD study had FEV_1 less than 40% predicted at age less than 53 years, without severe alpha-1-antitrypsin deficiency.[56] The initial phase of the Boston COPD Study included 44 early-onset COPD probands, with 204 first-degree relatives, 54 second-degree relatives and 20 spouses. In addition, 20 control families with 83 individuals were recruited from previous population-based studies at the Channing Laboratory.

Among first-degree relatives of early-onset COPD probands, highly significant differences in FEV_1 and FEV_1/FVC were found when current or ex-smoking first-degree relatives of early-onset COPD probands were compared to control subjects. No significant differences in age or pack-years of smoking were noted. As shown in Figure 4.4, current or ex-smoking first-degree relatives of early-onset COPD probands had a shift toward lower FEV_1 values, without an apparent bimodal distribution, compared to smoking control subjects.

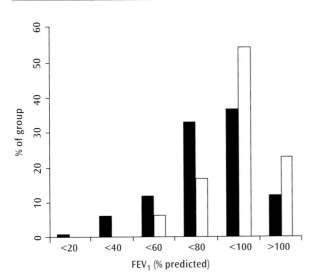

Figure 4.4 *FEV$_1$ in current or ex-smoking first-degree relatives of early-onset COPD probands compared to current or ex-smoking control subjects. Solid bars correspond to first-degree relatives of early-onset COPD probands; open bars correspond to control subjects. The distribution for first-degree relatives is clearly shifted toward low FEV$_1$ values. Although 7% of first-degree relatives had FEV$_1$ values below 40% predicted, this degree of severe impairment was not observed in the control group. (From ref. 56.)*

No significant differences in FEV$_1$ or FEV$_1$/FVC were found when lifelong non-smoking first-degree relatives of early COPD probands were compared to lifelong non-smoking control subjects. In fact, the mean FEV$_1$ values were 93.4% of predicted in both groups of non-smokers. This pattern of smoking-related susceptibility, which was confirmed by multivariate analysis adjusting for age and pack-years of smoking, would be consistent with genetic risk factors which interact with smoking to result in COPD. A similar pattern of smoking-related susceptibility was also seen for chronic bronchitis and bronchodilator responsiveness.[56,57]

A remarkably high percentage of females, 80%, was noted among the early-onset COPD probands.[58] This female predominance differed from previous studies of severe COPD, which had found a male predominance.[59–62] The explanation for the female predominance found by Silverman and colleagues is uncertain, but this study included a group of probands who were younger, more severely affected, and more recently collected than prior series of severe COPD subjects. Reduced survival of male subjects with severe COPD could contribute to the observed female predominance; however, it is certainly possible that there is a biological basis for the increased female susceptibility, due to hormonal or other factors, that could mediate a genotype-by-gender interaction in early-onset COPD pedigrees.

CASE-CONTROL ASSOCIATION STUDIES

A variety of association studies have compared the distribution of variants in genes hypothesized to be involved in the development of COPD in COPD patients and control subjects. We will review the controversy regarding the PI MZ genotype as a risk factor for COPD, and we will also discuss other candidate genes that have been assessed in association studies.

PI MZ

The risk of lung disease in heterozygous PI MZ individuals has been a subject of considerable controversy for many years. PI MZ individuals do have reduced serum alpha-1-antitrypsin concentrations (approximately 60% of PI M levels). However, general population surveys have typically found no difference in pulmonary function between PI MZ and PI M individuals.[63,64] A study by Larsson *et al.* showed that PI MZ individuals who smoke cigarettes show some deficits in sensitive pulmonary function tests compared to smoking PI M subjects, but there was no evidence for increased airflow obstruction in smoking PI MZ subjects (assessed by the ratio of FEV$_1$ to vital capacity).[65] Larsson did not find any significant differences in pulmonary function between non-smoking PI M and PI MZ individuals. However, case-control studies comparing the prevalence of the PI MZ type in patients with COPD and control subjects have usually discovered an excess of PI MZ individuals among COPD patients.[7,66] The basis for these inconsistencies remains unresolved.

A recent study by Sandford and colleagues provides evidence that PI MZ is associated with more rapid pulmonary function decline in COPD patients.[67] Among current smokers in the Lung Health Study, Sandford and colleagues identified 283 COPD patients who demonstrated a rapid pulmonary function decline, and 308 COPD patients who demonstrated no significant pulmonary function decline during a 5-year follow-up. PI MZ subjects were significantly more common in the rapid decliners.

Many of the previous studies that have attempted to assess the potential risk to PI MZ subjects have been limited by small sample size. Seersholm and colleagues matched 1551 PI MZ subjects from the Danish Alpha-1-antitrypsin Deficiency Registry with control subjects from the general population (with 10 controls for each PI MZ subject); using the Danish Hospital Discharge Registry, they compared the rates of hospitalization for obstructive lung diseases among the PI MZ and control subjects.[68] The PI MZ subjects were significantly more likely to be hospitalized for asthma, emphysema and chronic bronchitis than the control subjects; however, this increased risk for hospitalization was limited to the 565 subjects who were first-degree relatives of PI Z subjects with severe COPD.

This study is limited by the lack of data related to smoking history on the PI MZ and control subjects, but the results suggest that the subset of PI MZ subjects who are first-degree relatives of PI Z subjects with COPD may be at increased risk for obstructive lung disease.

Despite several recent studies which have suggested that PI MZ is associated with an increased risk for COPD, the actual risk associated with PI MZ remains unclear. In addition, it is uncertain if PI MZ represents a slight risk for all PI MZ subjects or a significant risk for a subset of PI MZ subjects because of gene–gene or gene–environment interactions.

Other candidate gene studies

A variety of other candidate genetic loci have been studied with the case-control association analysis approach. A partial list of loci that have been associated with COPD is presented in Table 4.1.[7,63,69–84] In addition to PI MZ, other genetic loci in protease/antiprotease pathways have been assessed as possible candidate genes in COPD. For example, a polymorphism in the 3′ region of the PI locus was associated with COPD by Kalsheker and colleagues; however, Sandford and colleagues could not replicate this association.[83,84] Two polymorphisms within alpha-1-antichymotrypsin, another serine protease inhibitor, were associated with COPD in small samples;[81] these associations were not replicated by Sandford and colleagues.[82]

Because of the significant capacity of cigarette smoke to create reactive oxygen species, candidate genes in oxidant/antioxidant pathways have also been examined as potential contributors to the development of COPD. Yamada and colleagues assessed a dinucleotide short tandem repeat polymorphism in the 5′ flanking region of the heme oxygenase 1 gene in emphysema patients and smoking control subjects.[78] The alleles at this polymorphic marker were grouped as S (<25 repeats), M (25–29

repeats) and L (>29 repeats). A higher frequency of class L alleles was noted in emphysema patients (21%) than control subjects (10%). The authors performed transient-transfection assays to assess the functional significance of polymorphism repeat length; they demonstrated upregulation with hydrogen peroxide exposure of the 16 and 20 repeat alleles, but not with the 29 or 38 repeat alleles. Although this study is interesting, it will be important to determine if these findings can be replicated.

Smith and Harrison demonstrated associations between two polymorphisms in the microsomal epoxide hydrolase (mEPHX) gene which have been related to functional differences in enzyme activity with COPD.[79] Based on the postulated functional effects of the genotypes at these two loci, the COPD patients were more likely to include genotypes with reduced mEPHX activity than control subjects. These findings were supported by Sandford and colleagues in the Lung Health Study, in which more rapid decline in pulmonary function of COPD patients was demonstrated for individuals homozygous for the genotype associated with reduced mEPHX activity.[67] However, in a case-control study of 83 COPD patients and 76 smoking control subjects from Korea, Yim and colleagues found no relationship of mEPHX genotype to COPD.[80]

Finally, glutathione S-transferases are a collection of metabolic enzymes potentially involved in the detoxification of tobacco smoke. Ishii and colleagues found an association between a polymorphism in exon 5 of glutathione S-transferase P1 in 53 COPD patients compared with 50 control patients from Japan.[77] This association has not yet been replicated.

Interpretation of case-control association studies with candidate gene loci

As noted above and as shown in Table 4.1, a variety of candidate loci have been assessed with case-control association

Table 4.1 *Case-control genetic association studies in COPD*

Category	Candidate gene	Support association	Do Not support association
Protease/antiprotease	PI MZ	Lieberman (1986)[7]	Bruce (1984)[63]
	AIAT 3′ flanking region	Kalsheker (1990)[83]	Sandford (1997)[84]
	Alpha-1-antichymotrypsin	Poller (1992)[81]	Sandford (1998)[82]
Oxidant/antioxidant	Microsomal epoxide hydrolase	Smith (1997)[79]	Yim (2000)[80]
	Heme oxygenase-1	Yamada (2000)[78]	
	Glutathione S-transferase P1	Ishii (1999)[77]	
Other candidates	CFTR	Gervais (1993)[75]	Artlich (1995)[76]
	ABO blood group	Cohen (1980)[50]	Vestbo (1993)[74]
	ABH secretor status	Cohen (1980)[50]	Vestbo (1993)[74]
	Vitamin D binding protein	Schellenberg (1998)[71]	Kauffmann (1983)[72]
	Tumor necrosis factor α	Sakao (2001)[69]	Higham (2000)[70]

Note: Selected references which support or do not support an association to the specified locus are presented.

studies in COPD. Several factors could contribute to the inconsistent results of case-control genetic association studies in COPD.[85] Genetic heterogeneity, or different genetic mechanisms, in different populations could contribute to difficulty in replicating associations. In addition, false positive or false negative results, potentially related to the small sample sizes that have been used in most COPD genetic association studies, could contribute to inconsistent replication. In addition, case-control association studies are susceptible to supporting associations based purely on population stratification.[86] Population stratification can result from incomplete matching between cases and controls, including differences in ethnicity and geographic origin. No association studies in COPD have been reported which used family-based controls, a study design which is immune to such population stratification effects. Importantly, linkage studies have only recently been published in COPD to identify regions of the genome which are likely to contain COPD susceptibility genes – regions in which association studies with positional candidate genes may be more fruitful. Other methodologic problems in case-control genetic association studies have included the failure to adjust for the multiple statistical comparisons involved in a study of more than one genetic locus. In summary, a variety of candidate genes have been examined with case-control genetic association studies in COPD, but inconsistent results of these studies have limited the identification of novel genetic risk factors for COPD.

ANIMAL MODELS OF COPD

Animal models have played an important role in the determination of emphysema pathophysiology since 1964, when Gross and colleagues observed that intratracheal injection of papain in rats led to the development of severe emphysema.[87] Subsequently, a variety of other elastolytic enzymes, including leukocyte elastase and proteinase 3, have been shown to cause emphysema in rodents following intratracheal instillation.[88] This work has provided critical evidence for the protease-antiprotease hypothesis for the pathogenesis of emphysema. Animal models continue to play an important role in the elucidation of COPD pathophysiology. Molecular genetic analysis of natural mutant strains, transgenic animals that overexpress key proteins, and knockout animals that fail to express certain genes are all providing new insights into potentially important pathways in human COPD.

Several naturally occurring mouse models have emphysema-like features.[89] For example, the tight skin mouse develops enlarged airspaces due to a mutation in fibrillin-1.[90] This fibrillin-1 mutation interferes with elastic fiber assembly and probably represents a developmental defect resulting in airspace enlargement rather than a destructive process of normally developed, mature lung tissue.

Transgenic mice which overexpress interstitial collagenase develop histological evidence for emphysema.[91] However, these interstitial collagenase transgenic mice do not have associated inflammation or a decrease in elastin fibers. Therefore, it is unclear if the collagenase transgenic model represents a failure of alveolar septation in development or if it corresponds to the tissue destruction that presumably leads to adult-onset emphysema. To overcome the potential impact of impaired developmental processes in transgenic models of emphysema, several recent reports have employed transgenic mice with inserted elements that could be activated after key developmental events had occurred. Zheng and colleagues employed inducible overexpression of a transgene including interleukin 13 (IL-13),[92] a cytokine that has been implicated as a key mediator in murine models of asthma.[93] Overexpression of IL-13 was induced at desired time points by including elements of the promoter construct that would only express when exposed to doxycycline; moreover, this doxycycline responsiveness was placed within the Clara Cell 10-kDa protein promoter in order to create lung-specific expression. After the mice reached 1 month of age, IL-13 expression was activated by adding doxycycline to the drinking water. Emphysematous changes rapidly developed in response to IL-13 overexpression, and marked inflammation including macrophages, lymphocytes and eosinophils was noted. Marked mucus metaplasia was also noted in the IL-13 transgenic mice, analogous to chronic bronchitis. Similarly, Wang and colleagues demonstrated that inducible overexpression of interferon gamma (IFN-γ) in transgenic mice led to the development of emphysema and pulmonary inflammation with macrophages and neutrophils. Of interest, the IFN-γ transgenic mice did not develop mucus metaplasia. The importance of IL-13 and IFN-γ in human COPD remains to be demonstrated, but these transgenic models have identified potentially critical pathways in COPD pathophysiology.

In addition to transgenic models that assess the effects of overexpression of certain genes, knockout mouse models, which assess the impact of inactivating gene expression, have also been employed in COPD. Mice which underwent targeted disruption of the platelet-derived growth factor A chain (PDGF-A) developed enlarged airspaces associated with the absence of alveolar septation.[94] This developmental defect resulted from a failure of alveolar development with a lack of elastin fiber production, caused by an absence of alveolar myofibroblast cells.

Macrophages from a macrophage elastase knockout mouse had impaired ability to degrade elastin.[95] Subsequently, Hautamaki and colleagues compared the effects of cigarette smoke exposure on these macrophage elastase knockout mice with their wild-type litter mates.[96] In wild-type animals, macrophage elastase was only expressed in mice that had been exposed to cigarette smoke; these smoke-exposed wild-type mice developed emphysema after 6 months of cigarette smoke exposure. However, macrophage elastase knockout mice did not develop emphysema after 6 months of cigarette smoke exposure.

To demonstrate that the development of emphysema was not simply a reflection of the increased number of lung macrophages in smoke-exposed mice, Hautamaki and colleagues instiled monocyte chemoattractant protein 1 (MCP-1) intratracheally into the macrophage elastase knockout mice. Although the number of pulmonary macrophages increased substantially in response to MCP-1 instillation, the macrophage elastase knockout mice still did not develop emphysema with cigarette smoke exposure. The importance of macrophage elastase in human emphysema remains to be determined, but it is an attractive candidate proteinase in COPD pathophysiology.

Although rodent models have provided important insights into potential biochemical mechanisms of COPD, identification of susceptibility loci using linkage analysis with experimental crosses of relatively susceptible and relatively non-susceptible strains has not yet been reported. Differences in susceptibility between murine strains to the development of smoking-induced COPD may provide unique opportunities to uncover genetic determinants of COPD.[89]

CONCLUSIONS

Severe alpha-1-antitrypsin deficiency is a proven genetic risk factor for COPD. Although considerable insight into the pathogenesis of COPD has been provided by studies of alpha-1-antitrypsin deficiency, fundamental questions about the natural history of alpha-1-antitrypsin deficiency remain unanswered.

Only a small percentage of COPD patients inherit severe alpha-1-antitrypsin deficiency, and additional genetic factors are likely to influence the development of COPD. Further efforts in linkage analysis, association studies and animal models may lead to the identification of such factors. To achieve a complete understanding of COPD pathophysiology, characterization of the interactions between genetic determinants and cigarette smoking (and potentially other environmental factors) will be required. Identification of genetic factors influencing the development of COPD unrelated to alpha-1-antitrypsin deficiency could clarify the biochemical mechanisms causing COPD, allow identification of highly susceptible individuals and lead to new therapeutic interventions for COPD.

ACKNOWLEDGEMENTS

The author would like to thank Dr Scott Weiss for providing helpful comments. E.K.S. is supported by NIH grant R01 HL61575.

REFERENCES

1. Hurst A. Familial emphysema. *Am Rev Respir Dis* 1959; **80**:179–80.
2. Laurell CB, Eriksson S. The electrophoretic α_1-globulin pattern of serum in α_1-antitrypsin deficiency. *Scand J Clin Lab Invest* 1963;**15**:132–40.
3. Burrows B, Knudson RJ, Cline MG, Lebowitz MD. Quantitative relationships between cigarette smoking and ventilatory function. *Am Rev Respir Dis* 1977;**115**:195–205.
4. Auerbach O, Hammond EC, Garfinkel L, Benante C. Relation of smoking and age to emphysema. Whole-lung section study. *New Engl J Med* 1972;**286**:853–7.
5. Petty TL, Ryan SF, Mitchell RS. Cigarette smoking and the lungs. Relation to postmortem evidence of emphysema, chronic bronchitis, and black lung pigmentation. *Arch Environ Health* 1967;**14**:172–7.
6. Gillooly M, Lamb D. Microscopic emphysema in relation to age and smoking habit. *Thorax* 1993;**48**:491–5.
7. Lieberman J, Winter B, Sastre A. Alpha 1-antitrypsin Pi-types in 965 COPD patients. *Chest* 1986;**89**:370–3.
8. Lai EC, Kao FT, Law ML, Woo SL. Assignment of the alpha 1-antitrypsin gene and a sequence-related gene to human chromosome 14 by molecular hybridization. *Am J Hum Genet* 1983;**35**:385–92.
9. Yamamoto Y, Sawa R, Okamoto N, Matsui A, Yanagisawa M, Ikemoto S. Deletion 14q(q24.3 to q32.1) syndrome. Significance of peculiar facial appearance in its diagnosis, and deletion mapping of Pi(alpha 1-antitrypsin). *Hum Genet* 1986;**74**:190–2.
10. Paakko P, Kirby M, du Bois RM, Gillissen A, Ferrans VJ, Crystal RG. Activated neutrophils secrete stored alpha 1-antitrypsin. *Am J Respir Crit Care Med* 1996;**154**:1829–33.
11. Perlmutter DH, Cole FS, Kilbridge P, Rossing TH, Colten HR. Expression of the alpha 1-proteinase inhibitor gene in human monocytes and macrophages. *Proc Natl Acad Sci USA* 1985;**82**:795–9.
12. Fagerhol MK, Laurell CB. The polymorphism of 'prealbumins' and alpha-1-antitrypsin in human sera. *Clin Chim Acta* 1967;**16**:199–203.
13. Brantly M, Nukiwa T, Crystal RG. Molecular basis of alpha-1-antitrypsin deficiency. *Am J Med* 1988;**84**(suppl 6A):13–31.
14. Sifers RN, Brashears-Macatee S, Kidd VJ, Muensch H, Woo SL. A frameshift mutation results in a truncated alpha 1-antitrypsin that is retained within the rough endoplasmic reticulum. *J Biol Chem* 1988;**263**:7330–5.
15. Holmes M, Curiel D, Brantly M, Crystal RG. Characterization of the intracellular mechanism causing the alpha-1-antitrypsin Nullgranite falls deficiency state. *Am Rev Respir Dis* 1989;**140**:1662–7.
16. Brantly M, Lee JH, Hildesheim J, *et al.* Alpha 1-antitrypsin gene mutation hot spot associated with the formation of a retained and degraded null variant. *Am J Respir Cell Mol Biol* 1997;**16**:225–31.
17. Takahashi H, Crystal RG. Alpha 1-antitrypsin Null(isola di procida): an alpha 1-antitrypsin deficiency allele caused by

deletion of all alpha 1-antitrypsin coding exons. *Am J Hum Genet* 1990;**47**:403–13.

18. Frazier GC, Siewertsen MA, Hofker MH, Brubacher MG, Cox DW. A null deficiency allele of alpha 1-antitrypsin, QOludwigshafen, with altered tertiary structure. *J Clin Invest* 1990;**86**:1878–84.

19. Muensch H, Gaidulis L, Kueppers F, *et al.* Complete absence of serum alpha-1-antitrypsin in conjunction with an apparently normal gene structure. *Am J Hum Genet* 1986;**38**:898–907.

20. Cox DW, Levison H. Emphysema of early onset associated with a complete deficiency of alpha-1-antitrypsin (null homozygotes). *Am Rev Respir Dis* 1988;**137**:371–5.

21. Dubel JR, Finwick R, Hejtmancik JF. Denaturing gradient gel electrophoresis of the alpha 1-antitrypsin gene application to prenatal diagnosis. *Am J Med Genet* 1991;**41**:39–43.

22. Martin NG, Clark P, Ofulue AF, Eaves LJ, Corey LA, Nance WE. Does the PI polymorphism alone control alpha-1-antitrypsin expression? *Am J Hum Genet* 1987;**40**:267–77.

23. Silverman EK, Province MA, Campbell EJ, Pierce JA, Rao DC. Family study of alpha 1-antitrypsin deficiency. Effects of cigarette smoking, measured genotype, and their interaction on pulmonary function and biochemical traits. *Genet Epidemiol* 1992;**9**:317–31.

24. Cox DW, Woo SL, Mansfield T. DNA restriction fragments associated with alpha 1-antitrypsin indicate a single origin for deficiency allele PI Z. *Nature* 1985;**316**:79–81.

25. Hutchison DC. Alpha 1-antitrypsin deficiency in Europe. Geographical distribution of Pi types S and Z. *Respir Med* 1998;**92**:367–77.

26. Kellermann G, Walter H. Investigations on the population genetics of the alpha-1-antitrypsin polymorphism. *Humangenetik* 1970;**10**:145–50.

27. Sveger T. Liver disease in alpha 1-antitrypsin deficiency detected by screening of 200 000 infants. *N Engl J Med* 1976;**294**:1316–21.

28. Silverman EK, Miletich JP, Pierce JA, *et al.* Alpha-1-antitrypsin deficiency. High prevalence in the St Louis area determined by direct population screening. *Am Rev Respir Dis* 1989;**140**:961–6.

29. O'Brien ML, Buist NR, Murphey WH. Neonatal screening for alpha 1-antitrypsin deficiency. *J Pediatr* 1978;**92**:1006–10.

30. Dirksen A, Friis M, Olesen KP, Skovgaard LT, Sorensen K. Progress of emphysema in severe alpha-1-antitrypsin deficiency as assessed by annual CT. *Acta Radiol* 1997;**38**:826–32.

31. Janus ED, Phillips NT, Carrell RW. Smoking, lung function, and alpha 1-antitrypsin deficiency. *Lancet* 1985;**i**:152–4.

32. Larsson C. Natural history and life expectancy in severe alpha 1-antitrypsin deficiency, Pi Z. *Acta Med Scand* 1978;**204**:345–51.

33. Tobin MJ, Cook PJL, Hutchison DCS. Alpha 1-antitrypsin deficiency. The clinical and physiological features of pulmonary emphysema in subjects homozygous for Pi type Z. *Br J Dis Chest* 1983;**77**:14–27.

34. Brantly ML, Paul LD, Miller BH, Falk RT, Wu M, Crystal RG. Clinical features and history of the destructive lung disease associated with alpha-1-antitrypsin deficiency of adults with pulmonary symptoms. *Am Rev Respir Dis* 1988;**138**:327–36.

35. Black LF, Kueppers F. Alpha 1-antitrypsin deficiency in nonsmokers. *Am Rev Respir Dis* 1978;**117**:421–8.

36. Silverman EK, Pierce JA, Province MA, Rao DC, Campbell EJ. Variability of pulmonary function in alpha 1-antitrypsin deficiency. Clinical correlates. *Ann Intern Med* 1989;**111**:982–91.

37. Seersholm N, Kok-Jensen A, Dirksen A. Decline in FEV$_1$ among patients with severe hereditary alpha 1-antitrypsin deficiency type PiZ. *Am J Respir Crit Care Med* 1995;**152**:1922–5.

38. Mayer AS, Stoller JK, Bucher Bartelson B, Ruttenber AJ, Sandhaus RA, Newman LS. Occupational exposure risks in individuals with PI*Z alpha(1)-antitrypsin deficiency. *Am J Respir Crit Care Med* 2000;**162**:553–8.

39. Silverman EK, Province MA, Rao DC, Pierce JA, Campbell EJ. A family study of the variability of pulmonary function in alpha 1-antitrypsin deficiency. Quantitative phenotypes. *Am Rev Respir Dis* 1990;**142**:1015–21.

40. Novoradovsky A, Brantly ML, Waclawiw MA, *et al.* Endothelial nitric oxide synthase as a potential susceptibility gene in the pathogenesis of emphysema in alpha 1-antitrypsin deficiency. *Am J Respir Cell Mol Biol* 1999;**20**:441–7.

41. Milewicz DM, Urban Z, Boyd C. Genetic disorders of the elastic fiber system. *Matrix Biol* 2000;**19**:471–80.

42. Van Maldergem L, Vamos E, Liebaers I, *et al.* Severe congenital cutis laxa with pulmonary emphysema: a family with three affected sibs. *Am J Med Genet* 1988;**31**:455–64.

43. Corbett E, Glaisyer H, Chan C, Madden B, Khaghani A, Yacoub M. Congenital cutis laxa with a dominant inheritance and early onset emphysema. *Thorax* 1994;**49**:836–7.

44. Tassabehji M, Metcalfe K, Hurst J, *et al.* An elastin gene mutation producing abnormal tropoelastin and abnormal elastic fibres in a patient with autosomal dominant cutis laxa. *Hum Mol Genet* 1998;**7**:1021–8.

45. Zhang MC, He L, Giro M, Yong SL, Tiller GE, Davidson JM. Cutis laxa arising from frameshift mutations in exon 30 of the elastin gene (ELN). *J Biol Chem* 1999;**274**:981–6.

46. Wood JR, Bellamy D, Child AH, Citron KM. Pulmonary disease in patients with Marfan syndrome. *Thorax* 1984;**39**:780–4.

47. Redline S, Tishler PV, Rosner B, *et al.* Genotypic and phenotypic similarities in pulmonary function among family members of adult monozygotic and dizygotic twins. *Am J Epidemiol* 1989;**129**:827–36.

48. Larson RK, Barman ML, Kueppers F, Fudenberg HH. Genetic and environmental determinants of chronic obstructive pulmonary disease. *Ann Intern Med* 1970;**72**:627–32.

49. Kueppers F, Miller RD, Gordon H, Hepper NG, Offord K. Familial prevalence of chronic obstructive pulmonary disease in a matched pair study. *Am J Med* 1977;**63**:336–42.

50. Cohen BH. Chronic obstructive pulmonary disease. A challenge in genetic epidemiology. *Am J Epidemiol* 1980;**112**:274–88.

51. Cohen BH, Ball WC Jr, Brashears S, *et al.* Risk factors in chronic obstructive pulmonary disease (COPD). *Am J Epidemiol* 1977;**105**:223–32.

52. Beaty TH, Liang KY, Seerey S, Cohen BH. Robust inference for variance components models in families ascertained through probands. II. Analysis of spirometric measures. *Genet Epidemiol* 1987;**4**:211–21.

53. Higgins M, Keller J. Familial occurrence of chronic respiratory disease and familial resemblance in ventilatory capacity. *J Chron Dis* 1975;**28**:239–51.

54. Speizer FE, Rosner B, Tager I. Familial aggregation of chronic respiratory disease. Use of National Health Interview Survey data for specific hypothesis testing. *Int J Epidemiol* 1976;**5**:167–72.

55. Tager I, Tishler PV, Rosner B, Speizer FE, Litt M. Studies of the familial aggregation of chronic bronchitis and obstructive airways disease. *Int J Epidemiol* 1978;**7**:55–62.

56. Silverman EK, Chapman HA, Drazen JM, *et al.* Genetic epidemiology of severe, early-onset chronic obstructive pulmonary disease. Risk to relatives for airflow obstruction and chronic bronchitis. *Am J Respir Crit Care Med* 1998;**157**:1770–8.

57. Celedon JC, Speizer FE, Drazen JM, *et al.* Bronchodilator responsiveness and serum total IgE levels in families of probands with severe early-onset COPD. *Eur Respir J* 1999;**14**:1009–14.

58. Silverman EK, Weiss ST, Drazen JM, *et al.* Gender-related differences in severe, early-onset chronic obstructive pulmonary disease. *Am J Respir Crit Care Med* 2000;**162**:2152–8.

59. O'Donnell DE, Webb KA. Breathlessness in patients with severe chronic airflow limitation. Physiologic correlations. *Chest* 1992;**102**:824–31.

60. Wegner RE, Jorres RA, Kirsten DK, Magnussen H. Factor analysis of exercise capacity, dyspnoea ratings and lung function in patients with severe COPD. *Eur Respir J* 1994;**7**:725–9.

61. Postma DS, Burema J, Gimeno F, *et al.* Prognosis in severe chronic obstructive pulmonary disease. *Am Rev Respir Dis* 1979;**119**:357–67.

62. Damsgaard T, Kok-Jensen A. Prognosis in severe chronic obstructive pulmonary disease. *Acta Med Scand* 1974;**196**: 103–8.

63. Bruce RM, Cohen BH, Diamond EL, *et al.* Collaborative study to assess risk of lung disease in Pi MZ phenotype subjects. *Am Rev Respir Dis* 1984;**130**:386–90.

64. Morse JO, Lebowitz MD, Knudson RJ, Burrows B. Relation of protease inhibitor phenotypes to obstructive lung diseases in a community. *N Engl J Med* 1977;**296**:1190–4.

65. Larsson C, Eriksson S, Dirksen H. Smoking and intermediate alpha 1-antitrypsin deficiency and lung function in middle-aged men. *Br Med J* 1977;**2**:922–5.

66. Bartmann K, Fooke-Achterrath M, Koch G, Nagy I, Schutz I, Weis E, Zierski M. Heterozygosity in the Pi-system as a pathogenetic cofactor in chronic obstructive pulmonary disease (COPD). *Eur J Respir Dis* 1985;**66**:284–96.

67. Sandford AJ, Chagani T, Weir TD, Connett JE, Anthonisen NR, Pare PD. Susceptibility genes for rapid decline of lung function in the LUNG HEALTH STUDY. *Am J Respir Crit Care Med* 2001;**163**:469–73.

68. Seersholm N, Wilcke JT, Kok-Jensen A, Dirksen A. Risk of hospital admission for obstructive pulmonary disease in alpha(1)-antitrypsin heterozygotes of phenotype PiMZ. *Am J Respir Crit Care Med* 2000;**161**:81–4.

69. Sakao S, Tatsumi K, Igari H, Shino Y, Shirasawa H, Kuriyama T. Association of tumor necrosis factor alpha gene promoter polymorphism with the presence of chronic obstructive pulmonary disease. *Am J Respir Crit Care Med* 2001;**163**:420–2.

70. Higham MA, Pride NB, Alikhan A, Morrell NW. Tumour necrosis factor-alpha gene promoter polymorphism in chronic obstructive pulmonary disease. *Eur Respir J* 2000;**15**:281–4.

71. Schellenberg D, Pare PD, Weir TD, Spinelli JJ, Walker BA, Sandford AJ. Vitamin D binding protein variants and the risk of COPD. *Am J Respir Crit Care Med* 1998;**157**:957–61.

72. Kauffmann F, Kleisbauer JP, Cambon-De-Mouzon A, *et al.* Genetic markers in chronic air-flow limitation. A genetic epidemiologic study. *Am Rev Respir Dis* 1983;**127**:263–9.

73. Cohen BH, Bias WB, Chase GA, *et al.* Is ABH nonsecretor status a risk factor for obstructive lung disease? *Am J Epidemiol* 1980;**111**:285–91.

74. Vestbo J, Hein HO, Suadicani P, Sorensen H, Gyntelberg F. Genetic markers for chronic bronchitis and peak expiratory flow in the Copenhagen Male Study. *Dan Med Bull* 1993;**40**: 378–80.

75. Gervais R, Lafitte JJ, Dumur V, *et al.* Sweat chloride and delta F508 mutation in chronic bronchitis or bronchiectasis. *Lancet* 1993;**342**:997 [letter].

76. Artlich A, Boysen A, Bunge S, Entzian P, Schlaak M, Schwinger E. Common CFTR mutations are not likely to predispose to chronic bronchitis in northern Germany. *Hum Genet* 1995;**95**:226–8.

77. Ishii T, Matsuse T, Teramoto S, *et al.* Glutathione *S*-transferase P1 (GSTP1) polymorphism in patients with chronic obstructive pulmonary disease. *Thorax* 1999;**54**:693–6.

78. Yamada N, Yamaya M, Okinaga S, *et al.* Microsatellite polymorphism in the heme oxygenase-1 gene promoter is associated with susceptibility to emphysema. *Am J Hum Genet* 2000;**66**:187–95.

79. Smith CAD, Harrison DJ. Association between polymorphism in gene for microsomal epoxide hydrolase and susceptibility to emphysema. *Lancet* 1997;**350**:630–3.

80. Yim JJ, Park GY, Lee CT, *et al.* Genetic susceptibility to chronic obstructive pulmonary disease in Koreans: combined analysis of polymorphic genotypes for microsomal epoxide hydrolase and glutathione S-transferase M1 and T1. *Thorax* 2000;**55**:121–5.

81. Poller W, Faber JP, Scholz S, *et al.* Mis-sense mutation of alpha 1-antichymotrypsin gene associated with chronic lung disease. *Lancet* 1992;**339**:1538 [letter].

82. Sandford AJ, Chagani T, Weir TD, Pare PD. Alpha 1-antichymotrypsin mutations in patients with chronic obstructive pulmonary disease. *Dis Markers* 1998;**13**:257–60.

83. Kalsheker NA, Watkins GL, Hill S, Morgan K, Stockley RA, Fick RB. Independent mutations in the flanking sequence of the alpha-1-antitrypsin gene are associated with chronic obstructive airways disease. *Dis Markers* 1990;**8**:151–7.

84. Sandford AJ, Spinelli JJ, Weir TD, Pare PD. Mutation in the 3′ region of the alpha-1-antitrypsin gene and chronic obstructive pulmonary disease. *J Med Genet* 1997;**34**:874–5.

85. Silverman EK, Palmer LJ. Case-control association studies for the genetics of complex respiratory diseases. *Am J Respir Cell Mol Biol* 2000;**22**:645–8.

86. Lander ES, Schork NJ. Genetic dissection of complex traits. *Science* 1994;**265**:2037–48.

87. Gross P, Babyak MA, Tolker E, Kaschak M. Enzymatically produced pulmonary emphysema. *J Occup Med* 1964;**6**:481–4.

88. Kao RC, Wehner NG, Skubitz KM, Gray BH, Hoidal JR. Proteinase 3: a distinct human polymorphonuclear leukocyte proteinase that produces emphysema in hamsters. *J Clin Invest* 1988;**82**:1963–73.

89. Shapiro SD. Animal models for chronic obstructive pulmonary disease – age of klotho and marlboro mice. *Am J Respir Cell Mol Biol* 2000;**22**:4–7.

90. Kielty CM, Raghunath M, Siracusa LD, *et al.* The Tight Skin mouse: demonstration of mutant fibrillin-1 production and assembly into abnormal microfibrils. *J Cell Biol* 1998;**140**: 1159–66.

91. D'Armiento J, Dalal SS, Okada Y, Berg RA, Chada K. Collagenase expression in the lungs of transgenic mice causes pulmonary emphysema. *Cell* 1992;**71**:955–61.

92. Zheng T, Zhu Z, Wang Z, *et al.* Inducible targeting of IL-13 to the adult lung causes matrix metalloproteinase- and cathepsin-dependent emphysema. *J Clin Invest* 2000;**106**:1081–93.

93. Wills-Karp M, Luyimbazi J, Xu X, *et al.* Interleukin-13: central mediator of allergic asthma. *Science* 1998;**282**:2258–61.

94. Bostrom H, Willetts K, Pekny M, *et al.* PDGF-A signaling is a critical event in lung alveolar myofibroblast development and alveogenesis. *Cell* 1996;**85**:863–73.

95. Shipley JM, Wesselschmidt RL, Kobayashi DK, Ley TJ, Shapiro SD. Metalloelastase is required for macrophage-mediated proteolysis and matrix invasion in mice. *Proc Natl Acad Sci USA* 1996;**93**:3942–6.

96. Hautamaki RD, Kobayashi DK, Senior RM, Shapiro SD. Requirement for macrophage elastase for cigarette smoke-induced emphysema in mice. *Science* 1997;**277**:2002–4.

97. Seersholm N, Kok-Jensen A, Dirksen A. Survival of patients with severe alpha 1-antitrypsin deficiency with special reference to non-index cases. *Thorax* 1994;**49**:695–8 [published errata appear in *Thorax* 1994;**49**(11):1184 and 1998;**53**(1):78].

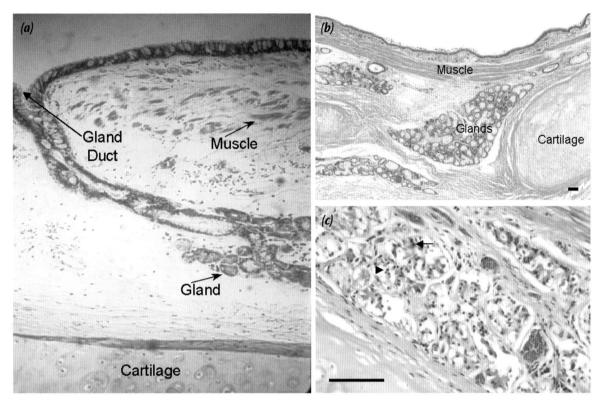

Plate 1 *(a) Histological section of a normal bronchus showing the epithelium lining the airway lumen and a duct leading to a bronchial mucus gland. The opening of the duct, the airway smooth muscle, the gland and the cartilage are labelled for orientation; (b) is a bronchial mucus gland at low power (bar = 100 microns); (c) a bronchial gland at higher power (bar = 200 microns) arrow and arrowhead point to inflammatory cells.*

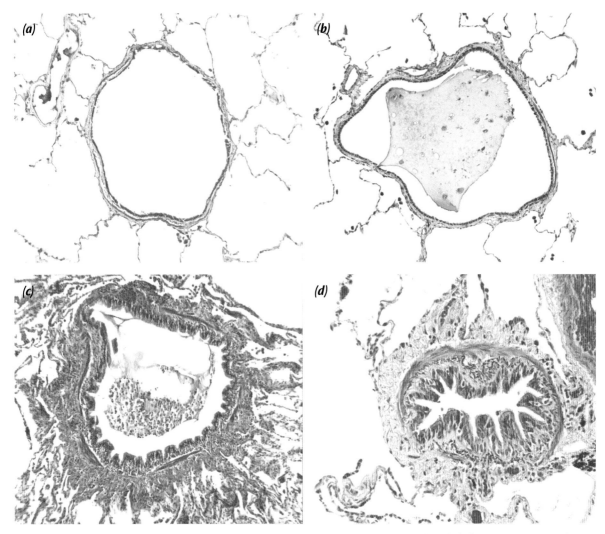

Plate 2 *Comparison of a normal peripheral airway to an airway that is involved by a chronic inflammatory process in the airway wall and lumen. These inflammatory changes are associated with abnormal peripheral airway function and increased peripheral airways resistance – (see text for further discussion) (a) is a normal airway; (b) is an airway containing mucus and a few cells; (c) is an airway with an active inflammatory exudates in the wall and lumen; (d) is an airway with a markedly thickened wall where peri bronchiolar connective tissue deposition apears as though it would restrict the lumen from opening fully as the lung is inflated.*

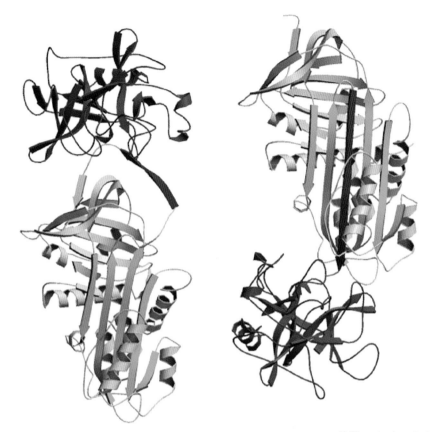

Plate 3 *(a) Serpins such as alpha-1-antitrypsin may be considered to act as mousetraps.[35,97] Following docking (left) the neutrophil elastase (grey) is inactivated by movement from the upper to the lower pole of the protein (right). This is associated with insertion of the reactive loop (red) as an extra strand into beta-sheet A (green).*

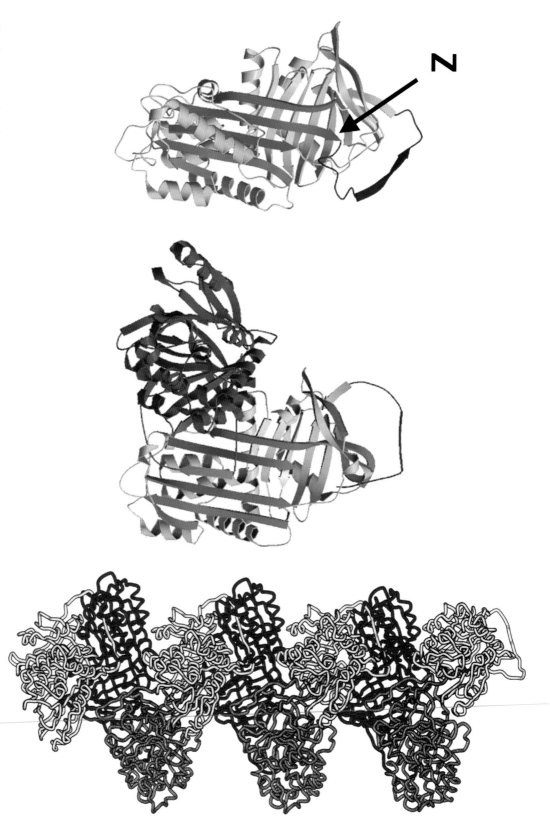

Plate 3 (b) The structural basis of loop-sheet polymerization. The mousetrap mechanism (Fig. 3a) may be triggered spontaneously by point mutations in association with disease. This process is best characterized for the Z variant of alpha-1-antitrypsin (^{342}glutamic acid→lysine at P_{17}) which opens beta-sheet A to favour the insertion of the reactive loop of another molecule. (Left) The reactive loop of alpha-1-antitrypsin (red) is held as a beta-strand that can readily insert into beta-sheet A of a second molecule (green). The linkage is facilitated by the Z mutation which perturbs beta-sheet A thereby making it more receptive to the peptide loop of another molecule of alpha-1-antitrypsin (middle). This process can extend to form chains of polymers (right). Each molecule of alpha-1-antitrypsin is shown in a different colour in the polymer.

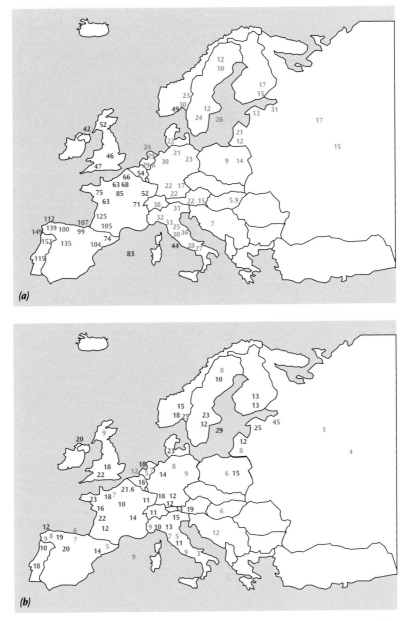

Plate 4 *Distribution of S (a) and Z (b) alleles of alpha-1-antitrypsin in 70 selected European populations. Red figures represent very high frequencies, green intermediate frequencies and brown low frequencies. The greatest frequency of the S allele is the Iberian Peninsula and the value gradually reduces from south to north and from west to east. The greatest frequency of the Z allele is in Northern and Western Europe with the values gradually declining from west to east and from north to south. (From ref. 215 with permission.)*

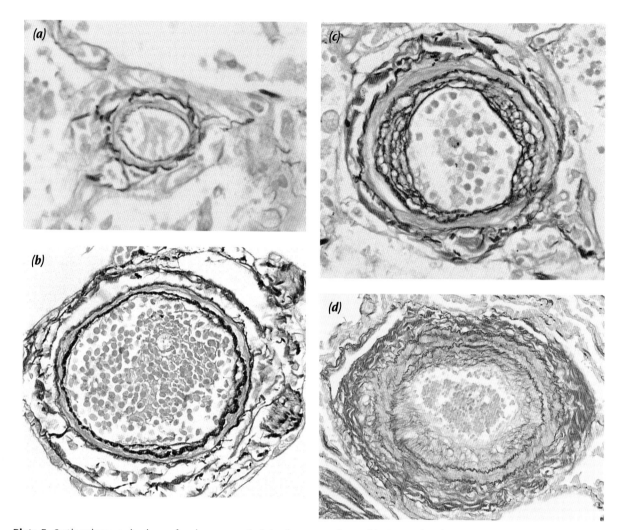

Plate 5 *Optic microscopic views of pulmonary arterioles from a patient with COPD, showing medial hypertrophy (a), intimal longitudinal muscle (b, c) and intimal fibrosis (d). (From M Wilkinson, personal communication.)*

Occupational factors

P SHERWOOD BURGE

Many chapters on occupational COPD start with a long section on how the subject is difficult and how conflicting the evidence is. There will probably be a long section on confounding factors in epidemiologic studies. This chapter will be different, showing how easy it can be and how consistent the evidence is. It all depends on where you start. We will start with whole population samples, and see whether those who have had dust or fume-exposed jobs have different risks for COPD compared with similar people who have worked in cleaner surroundings. This is analogous to the usual methods of investigating the effects of cigarette smoking, starting with populations and looking at the risks in those who smoke and those (who say) that they have not. With all the problems of smoking histories, most smokers at least recognize that they have been smokers, even if they do not tell you. Specific occupational exposures are more of a problem, as many do not know exactly what they have been exposed to, but can tell you whether there were fumes in the work environment, or whether it was dusty. Most of the community-based studies use these two items as indicators of exposure.

Several studies, mostly set up to study atmospheric air pollution, have been used to estimate occupational risks of COPD. Published studies include the general older working population of Beijing,[1] a rural population in Northern Italy,[2] and studies of city dwellers in France[3] and the USA.[4] Others have originated as studies of hypertension in an urban and rural population in Norway,[5] or cardiovascular disease in Holland.[6] Summaries of those studied are shown in Table 5.1. All have come to similar conclusions; that those who have worked in dusty jobs have more COPD than those who have worked in environments that were not dusty; exposure to fume is somewhat less risky. As both smoking and occupational exposures are maximal in those with the best lung function at the start of exposure (the healthy worker or healthy smoker effect), the relative risks will depend on the age groups studied. It is best to estimate the occupational effect in relation to the smoking effect in the same population. Table 5.2 shows the estimates of COPD related to smoking, which increases from 1.3 for those smoking less than 10 cigarettes a day, to 4.5 for those smoking more than 20 a day.

Table 5.1 *Principal community-based studies including analysis of occupational exposures on COPD or longitudinal decline in FEV$_1$*

	Population	Original aim	Age and sex	Years data collected
Zutphen, Holland[6]	Urban	CVS	Older males	1960–85
Bergen, Norway[5]	Urban, rural	BP	Older males	1965–90
Crakow, Poland[7]	Urban	COPD	Males 19–70	1968–81
PAARC, France[3]	Urban	Air pollution	Non-manual 25–59	1975
Six cities, USA[4]	Urban	Air pollution	25–74	1979
Po delta, Italy[2]	Rural	Air pollution	18–64	1981
Beijing, China[1]	Urban	Air pollution	40–69	1986

Table 5.2 *Estimates of relative risk of COPD from smoking, dust and fume exposure from community studies*

	Smoking/day			Exposures		
	<10	10–19	≥20	Dust	Fume	Dust or fume
Zutphen, Holland[6]		2.75	4.62			
Bergen, Norway[5]			3.86			
PAARC, France[3]	1.3	2.47	4.56			1.53
Po delta, Italy[2]						1.43
Six cities, USA[4]				1.53	1.15	
Beijing, China[1]				1.39	1.21	

Similar estimates for gas and/or fume exposure are also shown. The relative risk is lower than for smoking, two studies suggesting that exposure to dust had a higher relative risk than exposure to gases and were similar to smoking 10 cigarettes a day.

EFFECT OF OCCUPATION ON DECLINE IN FEV₁

The role of occupational exposures on FEV_1 decline has been studied in community studies either from cross-sectional measurements (Beijing[1]), or from longitudinal measurements (Crakov,[7] Bergen[5] and Zutphen[6]). FEV_1 decline cannot be estimated reliably from cross-sectional studies. Several cross-sectional studies have estimated FEV_1 decline assuming that the FEV_1 started from the level found in the younger members of the population, who are likely to be part of a healthier population from childhood than the older population. Longitudinal studies have generally shown smaller declines in FEV_1 than estimated from the first cross-sectional part of the study.[8] Longitudinal studies support the role of occupational exposure on FEV_1 decline, giving similar results to the symptom-based studies. Dust exposure resulted in an excess annual decline in FEV_1 of 7 ml/year (smoking 10 ml/year) in the Crakov study.[7]

Some specific occupations have shown increased rates of FEV_1 decline, which in general coincide with known risk factors for airflow obstruction. Workers exposed to quartz or silica were at increased risk in all four longitudinal studies (longitudinal decline in FEV_1 about 60 ml/year[9]). Construction, outdoor or cement-exposed workers were at excess risk in Crakow.[7] Farmers, grain workers, foundry workers (or workers exposed to chromium, nickel or platinum in the Norwegian study), woodworkers and workers exposed to excess heat including furnace workers (who are also likely to have silica exposure) are identified as increased risk groups in several studies. Sulfur dioxide exposure was associated with greater declines in FEV_1 in Bergen.[5] Increasing numbers of occupational exposures

were used as a measure of 'dose' in the Bergen study; they were associated with a greater annual decline in FEV_1,[5] suggesting a dose-related effect. Studies of FEV_1 decline therefore show effects of dust exposure similar to at least 10 cigarettes a day. Similar groups have been identified from questionnaire studies. For instance the Zutphen study[6] identified several jobs as high risk, including construction and cement, farmers, furnace work, wood and paper exposure, transport, textiles and tailors.

ARE SOME DUSTS MORE DANGEROUS THAN OTHERS?

To study individual exposures with any degree of accuracy it is usually necessary to attempt studies based on workforces rather than communities, with all the problems that this entails. There are some jobs where workers are expected to stay for a lifetime, and which are closely associated with the communities in which they live. Mining, cotton spinning and farming are good examples. In these situations the biases are not quite so big. Nevertheless biases are still considerable. Those starting work of any kind are in general more healthy than the general population (the healthy worker effect). There is evidence that workers starting exposure to particularly dusty environments have even higher lung function than the general working population. This is illustrated in Figure 5.1 from the French PAARC study,[3] originally set up to investigate the effects of air pollution. Households whose head was not a manual worker were sampled, the difference between the FEV_1 of workers exposed to dust or fume was compared with age-matched workers without such exposure. The FEV_1 was higher in the younger exposed workers and lower in the older exposed workers. If this population was studied cross-sectionally, a population under 40 years old would have higher levels of FEV_1 if exposed, those about 40 would have no effect, and those over 50 would show an effect of exposure. Longitudinal studies need to include all those starting the study in the follow-up measurements. Studies of specific workforces in particular have

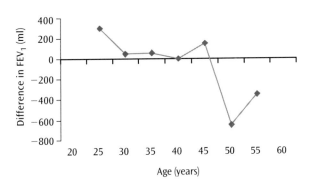

Figure 5.1 *Difference in FEV₁ between unexposed workers and workers exposed to dust or fume from the PAARC community study in France.[3] The younger exposed workers have even better lung function than the average healthy worker; the effects of exposure are only apparent in the older population.*

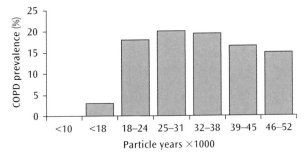

Figure 5.2 *Prevalence of bronchitis (cough and sputum) in South African gold miners related to cumulative silica exposure. There is an increasing prevalence up to 30 000 particle-years, followed by a decrease probably due to a survivor population. Those resistant to the adverse effects of silica are able to tolerate longer exposures.[10]*

a major problem in following up workers who have left employment. There is a preferential loss from the workforce of those who show the greatest effect of FEV₁ decline. Longitudinal studies tend to underestimate any effect, and cross-sectional studies may show a diminishing effect of higher exposures. This is illustrated in a study of silica-exposed gold miners[10] where the prevalence of bronchitis is related to cumulative silica exposure. There was increasing bronchitis with increasing exposures up to 30 000 particle years, then a decrease, probably due to loss of the most affected from the cohort (Figure 5.2). Similar results were obtained in longitudinal studies of British and US coal miners, where those with the highest cumulative coal dust exposure had the lowest rates of longitudinal decline in FEV₁.[11] This is best explained as those most resistant to the effects of coal dust on lung function are able to tolerate the greatest exposures, those who are affected either reducing their exposures or being removed from the cohort.

The effect of only studying survivors has been clearly shown in grain processors,[12] where measurements were repeated in the 50% who were still employed after 5 years. Those who were lost to follow-up had more respiratory symptoms and lower lung function than did the remainder. For those who continued to be exposed, the greatest decline in FEV₁ was in those who had moved from high to lower exposure during the follow-up period (63.7 ml/year, compared with 47.6 ml/year in those remaining in high exposure and 29.5 ml/year in those always in the low exposure group). The result was a reduction in the apparent effect of grain exposure on those who were exposed for the longest.

Cadmium and emphysema

Cadmium fume exposure is the best example of a specific occupational exposure causing a specific variety of COPD, namely emphysema. Cadmium has a very long half-life in the body (4–19 years), allowing total exposure to be estimated reasonably accurately from blood levels many years after exposure has ceased, as it is stored in the liver. The most complete study is of survivors from a foundry manufacturing copper-cadmium alloy. For those with the highest exposure the mean excess loss of FEV₁ (compared with similarly smoking industrial controls) was 398 ml, for DLco the reduction was 1.58 kPa, with a dose/effect gradient for cohorts with lesser exposure. Nineteen per cent of the cadmium workers and 3% of the controls had a gas transfer measurement less than 1.96 SD from the predicted values. Kco correlated significantly with cumulative exposure.[13]

Cotton exposure

Workers exposed to cotton are at increased risk of accelerated loss of FEV₁, which in general is greater in smokers than non-smokers. Cough and sputum are associated with increasing cotton dust exposure,[14] with a relative risk for non-smoking cotton workers over 45 years in comparison with non-smoking man-made fiber workers of 5.3. This is similar to the relative risk of smoking in man-made fiber workers of 4.9, and shows an additive effect with smoking in cotton workers where smokers have a relative risk of 9.3.[15] High levels of cotton dust exposure in former Yugoslavia, India and China have been associated with increasing annual declines in FEV₁ in longitudinal studies.[16,17] In England the loss of FEV₁ was found to be of similar order to that of smoking.[18] In the USA in workers with low exposures an effect of cotton dust on loss of FEV₁ was only seen in smokers.[19] This study showed effects in non-smokers at higher cotton exposure levels.

How the confusion arose that loss of FEV$_1$ was only a feature of complicated coal and silica pneumoconiosis, and was not seen in those with a normal X-ray

Early studies showed that lung function in miners with uncomplicated pneumoconiosis was similar to miners without pneumoconiosis.[20] This was interpreted as implying that silica or coal exposure had no effect on lung function in the absence of progressive massive fibrosis. The community studies have often identified increased risks in workers exposed to silica (foundryworkers, quarrymen, tunneling workers, stonemasons, etc). Silica is one of the few exposures where there are good longitudinal workplace studies, mainly from the South African gold mines. A reasonable number of air measurements have been made from which cumulative personal exposures can be estimated. These studies confirm the lack of effect of radiological uncomplicated pneumoconiosis (Categories 1 to 3) on lung function, but show that increasing silica exposure is associated with reducing levels of FEV$_1$ and FVC; i.e. the effect on lung function is acting independently of the effect of the nodular shadows on the chest X-ray. Similar effects occur with coal dust exposure.

South African gold miners are exposed to mine dust with 30% free silica. Studies have shown reductions in FEV$_1$ in workers with and without silicosis, with the major effects seen in smokers. After controlling for radiologic silicosis the excess annual loss of FEV$_1$ attributed to mining was 8 ml, that due to smoking 20 cigarettes a day was 6.9 ml/year in black miners, who were more heavily exposed to silica and smoked less than white miners.[21,22] The studies on white miners showed that the contribution to FEV$_1$ loss due to silica (236 ml for average lifetime exposure) was estimated to be about half that of smoking 20 cigarettes daily for 30 years (552 ml). The relationship between death from COPD, silica exposure and smoking has suggested that the effect of silica is predominantly in smokers, with 5% of the increased mortality due to dust alone, 34% due to smoking, and 59% due to the interaction of smoking and dust.[23] Like smoking, exposure in early adult life appeared to have more effect than later exposure. It is possible that smoking and silica are acting through the same mechanism, in which neutrophil-derived inflammation is prominent. Silica is ingested by macrophages, which cannot detoxify the silica, which is toxic to the macrophage. The macrophage dies releasing neutrophil chemotactic cytokines, the process being repeated by the re-ingestion of the released silica. This cycle accounts for the high output of pulmonary macrophages and activated neutrophils after relatively brief exposures.[24] Smoking has similar effects,[25] and both are capable of releasing reactive oxygen species into the pulmonary interstitium.[26] Gold miners without silicosis who were non-smokers have been shown to have similar levels of reactive oxygen species in peripheral blood (as measured by luminol enhanced chemiluminescence) to non-exposed controls, suggesting the relative safety of current levels of silica exposure in the absence of smoking.[27]

For the same levels of exposure, coal has much less effect than silica. There is little evidence that coal dust *per se* is particularly toxic, its adverse effects may be related principally to the dust burden retained in the lungs. The evidence favors an additive effect with smoking on FEV$_1$ decline. The attributable risk of dust exposure for an FEV$_1$ of less than 80% predicted is less for smokers than non-smokers, but the attributable risk for an FEV$_1$ less than 65% predicted is about twice as high for smokers as non-smokers.[28,29] (i.e. smoking is more likely to lead to severe airflow obstruction than coal dust exposure, the reverse being true for less severe disease, compatible with an additive effect). It is often argued that the average loss of FEV$_1$ is small in relation to that likely to cause significant disability. It depends on whether all the exposed population decline at a rate close to the mean, or whether there is wide variation, as in the effect of cigarette smoking. The evidence is tending to favor a large clinically significant effect in a few individuals. This has been calculated on the basis of 35 years' exposure to the mean level of exposure per 1000 workers. For coal miners a lifetime exposure of 122.5 g.h/m^3 would result in 80/1000 having a 20% loss attributed to dust and 12/1000 a 35% loss. The comparable attributable risk for smokers is 66/1000 and 23/1000 respectively. The highest group cumulative dust exposure for the South African gold miners was only 21.3 g.h/m^3, a tenth of the highest exposure group of British coal miners. Despite this the attributable risk for an FEV$_1$ smaller than 80% was 4.9 for silica-exposed gold miners versus 1.5 for coal miners.[28]

There is some evidence that coal dust exposure causes centrilobular emphysema, based on post-mortem lung sections, there being a relationship between emphysema score and lung dust burden.[30] The relationship is easier to demonstrate when dust-related fibrosis is present.[31] The relationship between emphysema score and lung dust burden is stronger in non-smokers than smokers.[32]

THE ORIGINS OF OCCUPATIONAL COPD

Acute occupational exposures can cause small changes in FEV$_1$. Changes before and after a workshift are correlated with accelerated FEV$_1$ decline and the development of clinical COPD. It is possible that clinical COPD develops as a consequence of repeated minor airway insults. The changes related to acute exposure are small (often 50–150 ml), and not clinically significant on their own. These changes are seen in workers exposed to cotton dust, especially in the earlier stages of processing in opening and carding. Cotton mill dust contains much endotoxin. Some have found that

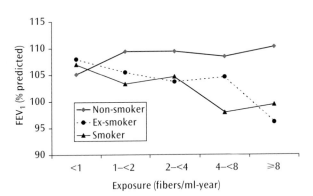

Figure 5.3 *Effect of increasing exposures to ceramic fibers on FEV₁ (exposure to an air level of 1 fiber per milliliter of air for 1 year = 1 fiber/ml-year, similar to cigarette consumption in pack-years). There is no effect in non-smokers, but a dose-related effect in current and ex-smokers.*[39]

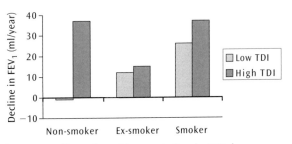

Figure 5.4 *Effect of smoking on decline in FEV₁ in workers manufacturing toluene diisocyanate. (Ref. 40)*

the health effects are more closely related to endotoxin exposures than total dust.[33] Endotoxin is a constituent of many other bioaerosols, including swine confinement building dust, refuse plant aerosols[34] and grain dust.[12] Pig farmers exposed to the aerosols from pigs kept in intensive indoor conditions with poor ventilation have been shown to have small pre-post shift declines in FEV₁, with similar consequences to those seen in cotton workers.

Both smoking and occupational exposures affect some individuals earlier and more severely than others. Exposures to dust may accelerate FEV₁ decline in those with alpha-1-antitrypsin deficiency both in ZZ homozygotes,[35,36] and probably also in MZ heterozygotes[37] in a similar manner to cigarette smoking.[38] Occupational exposures may enhance the effects of cigarette smoking, having their effect predominantly in smokers, or act like cigarettes, having their effects measured more easily in non-smokers. The preferential susceptibility of smokers has been shown in specific industry studies; the effect of ceramic fiber exposure is shown in Figure 5.3.[39] Increasing exposure had no effect in non-smokers, but a dose-related effect in current and ex-smokers. In other situations the burden of the disease appears to be taken by the non-smokers; this was particularly apparent in a study of isocyanate manufacturers (Figure 5.4), after exclusion of those who developed occupational asthma.[40]

Follow-up studies of workers with occupational asthma suggest the development of an element of fixed airflow obstruction.[41] Investigation of non-asthmatic workers with similar exposures may also cause accelerated FEV₁ decline; this has been shown best with isocyanate exposure.[40] Studies with induced sputum in workers exposed to small molecular weight agents who phenotypically have occupational asthma, can be divided into those with sputum eosinophilia and those without.[42] Both groups have increased sputum neutrophils. Those without eosinophilia have less severe disease, less

non-specific reactivity and less bronchodilator responsiveness, i.e. they appear more 'bronchitic'. At least with cotton exposure there is evidence that in the absence of smoking the COPD is not due to emphysema. It is possible that occupational exposures will differentiate between agents capable of causing emphysema (e.g. cadmium) and those causing airway disease and obstructive bronchitis (e.g. cotton), and that there is a disease clinically resembling asthma without sputum eosinophilia which may be the origins of some forms of COPD.

CONCLUSIONS AND CLINICAL IMPLICATIONS

Working can result in large exposures to respirable particulates and gases, second only in importance to the deliberate inhalation of tobacco smoke into the lungs. There is now growing evidence that chronic airflow obstruction (COPD), as well as cough and sputum, are caused by exposures other than tobacco smoke, and that occupational exposures particularly to dusts are amongst such causes. COPD due to occupational exposures and tobacco smoking are clinically indistinguishable. The disease cannot be attributed to smoking with any more confidence than to occupation, particularly when it involves silica, coal or cadmium exposure. It is not clear what turns a smoker without airflow obstruction into one with COPD. Occupational exposures can enhance the effect of smoking, having their principal effect in smokers (such as silica), can act in a similar manner to smoking, having an additive effect with tobacco and having some effect in non-smokers (such as coal), or have their principal effect in non-smokers (such as isocyanates). Some occupational agents may act long after acute exposure ceases, such as silica which is poorly cleared from the lungs. So far there are no good studies relating cessation of occupational exposure to altered rates of decline in FEV₁, unlike the studies of smoking cessation which show that the rate of decline is reduced, but generally remains above that of a lifelong non-smoker.[43] As the working population smokes less the significance of occupational exposures causing COPD will increase. It is now time to extend the observations on miners exposed to coal and silica to other populations with similarly careful studies to define the relationships between exposure and disease.

REFERENCES

1. Xu X, Christiani DC, Dockery DW, Wang L. Exposure–response relationships between occupational exposures and chronic respiratory illness: a community-based study. *Am Rev Respir Dis* 1992;**146**:413–18.

2. Viegi G, Prediletto R, Paoletti P, *et al.* Respiratory effects of occupational exposure in a general population sample in north Italy. *Am Rev Respir Dis* 1991;**143**:510–15.

3. Krzyzanowski M, Kauffmann F. The relation of respiratory symptoms and ventilatory function to moderate occupational exposure in a general population. Results from the French PAARC study of 16 000 adults. *Int J Epidemiol* 1988;**17**: 397–406.

4. Korn RJ, Dockery DW, Speizer FE, Ware JH, Ferris BG Jr. Occupational exposures and chronic respiratory symptoms. A population-based study. *Am Rev Respir Dis* 1987;**136**:298–304.

5. Humerfelt S, Gulsvik A, Skjaerven R, *et al.* Decline in FEV$_1$ and airflow limitation related to occupational exposures in men in an urban community. *Eur Respir J* 1993;**6**:1095–103.

6. Heederik D, Pouwels H, Kromhout H, Kromhout D. Chronic non-specific lung disease and occupational exposures estimated by means of a job exposure matrix: the Zutphen Study. *Int J Epidemiol* 1989;**18**:382–9.

7. Krzyzanowski M, Jedrychowski W, Wysocki M. Factors associated with the change in ventilatory function and the development of chronic obstructive pulmonary disease in a 13-year follow-up of the Cracow Study. Risk of chronic obstructive pulmonary disease. *Am Rev Respir Dis* 1986;**134**:1011–19.

8. Glindmeyer HW, Diem JE, Jones RN, Weill H. Noncomparability of longitudinally and cross-sectionally determined annual change in spirometry. *Am Rev Respir Dis* 1982; **125**:544–8.

9. Kauffmann F, Drouet D, Lellouch J, Brille D. Occupational exposure and 12-year spirometric changes among Paris area workers. *Br J Industr Med* 1982;**39**:221–32.

10. Wiles FJ, Faure MH, Walton WH, McGowan B, eds. *Inhaled Particles*, iv. *Chronic Obstructive Lung Disease in Gold Miners.* Pergamon Press, Oxford, 1977, pp 727–35.

11. Sandhu PS, Bourke SJ, Hendrick DJ, Stenton SC. The effects of cigarette smoking and duration of work on the lung function in coal miners. *Thorax* 1996;**51**(suppl 3):A43.

12. Chan-Yeung M, Dimich-Ward H, Enarson DA, Kennedy SM. Five cross-sectional studies of grain elevator workers. *Am J Epidemiol* 1992;**136**:1269–79.

13. Davison AG, Fayers PM, Newman Taylor AJ, *et al.* Cadmium fume inhalation and emphysema. *Lancet* 1988;**i**:663–7.

14. Imbus HR, Suh MW. Byssinosis – a study of 10 133 textile workers. *Arch Environ Health* 1973;**26**:183–91.

15. Niven RM, Fletcher AM, Pickering CA, *et al.* Chronic bronchitis in textile workers. *Thorax* 1997;**52**:22–7.

16. Zuskin E, Ivankovic D, Schachter EN, Witek TJ Jr. A ten-year follow-up study of cotton textile workers. *Am Rev Respir Dis* 1991;**143**:301–5.

17. Kamat SR, Kamat GR, Salpekar VY, Lobo E. Distinguishing byssinosis from chronic obstructive pulmonary disease. Results of a prospective five-year study of cotton mill workers in India. *Am Rev Respir Dis* 1981;**124**:31–40.

18. Berry G, McKerrow CB, Molyneux MKB, Rossiter CE, Tompleson JBL. A study of the acute and chronic changes in the ventilatory capacity of workers in Lancashire cotton mills. *Br J Industr Med* 1973;**30**:25–36.

19. Glindmeyer HW, Lefante JJ, Jones RN, Rando RJ, Kader HMA, Weill H. Exposure-related declines in the lung function of cotton textile workers. *Am Rev Respir Dis* 1991;**144**:675–83.

20. Irwig LM, Rocks P. Lung function and respiratory symptoms in silicotic and nonsilicotic gold miners. *Am Rev Respir Dis* 1978;**117**:429–35.

21. Cowie RL, Mabena SK. Silicosis, chronic airflow limitation, and chronic bronchitis in South African gold miners. *Am Rev Respir Dis* 1991;**143**:80–4.

22. Hnizdo E. Loss of lung function associated with exposure to silica dust and with smoking and its relation to disability and mortality in South African gold miners. *Br J Industr Med* 1992;**49**:472–9.

23. Hnizdo E. Combined effect of silica dust and tobacco smoking on mortality from chronic obstructive lung disease in gold miners. *Br J Industr Med* 1990;**47**:656–64.

24. Bowden DH, Adamson IY. The role of cell injury and the continuing inflammatory response in the generation of silicotic pulmonary fibrosis. *J Pathol* 1984;**144**:149–61.

25. Hunninghake GW, Crystal RG. Cigarette smoking and lung destruction. Accumulation of neutrophils in the lungs of cigarette smokers. *Am Rev Respir Dis* 1983;**128**:833–8.

26. Richards GA, Theron AJ, Van der Merwe CA, Anderson R. Spirometric abnormalities in young smokers correlate with increased chemiluminescence responses of activated blood phagocytes. *Am Rev Respir Dis* 1989;**139**:181–7.

27. Theron AJ, Richards GA, Myer MS, *et al.* Investigation of the relative contributions of cigarette smoking and mineral dust exposure to activation of circulating phagocytes, alterations in plasma concentrations of vitamin C, vitamin E, and beta carotene, and pulmonary dysfunction in South African gold miners. *Occup Environ Med* 1994;**51**:564–7.

28. Oxman AD, Muir DC, Shannon HS, Stock SR, Hnizdo E, Lange HJ. Occupational dust exposure and chronic obstructive pulmonary disease. A systematic overview of the evidence. *Am Rev Respir Dis* 1993;**148**:38–48.

29. Coggon D, Newman Taylor AJ. Coal mining and chronic obstructive pulmonary disease: a review of the evidence. *Thorax* 1998;**53**:398–407.

30. Cockcroft A, Seal RM, Wagner JC, Lyons JP, Ryder R, Andersson N. Post-mortem study of emphysema in coalworkers and non-coalworkers. *Lancet* 1982;**ii**:600–3.

31. Ruckley VA, Fernie JM, Chapman JS, *et al.* Comparison of radiographic appearances with associated pathology and lung dust content in a group of coalworkers. *Br J Industr Med* 1984;**41**:459–67.

32. Leigh J, Driscoll TR, Cole BD, Beck RW, Hull BP, Yang J. Quantitative relation between emphysema and lung mineral content in coalworkers. *Occup Environ Med* 1994;**51**:400–7.

33. Zejda JE, Barber E, Dosman JA, *et al.* Respiratory health status in swine producers relates to endotoxin exposure in the presence of low dust levels. *J Occup Med* 1994;**36**:49–56.

34. Sigsgaard T, Malmros P, Nersting L, Petersen C. Respiratory disorders and atopy in Danish refuse workers. *Am J Respir Crit Care Med* 1994;**149**:1407–12.

35. Piitulainen E, Tornling G, Eriksson S. Environmental correlates of impaired lung function in non-smokers with severe alpha 1-antitrypsin deficiency. *Thorax* 1998;**53**: 939–43.

36. Mayer AS, Stoller JK, Bucher Bartleson B, Ruttenber A, Sandhaus RA, Newman LS. Occupational exposure risks in

individuals with PI*Z alpha 1-antitrypsin deficiency. *Am J Respir Crit Care Med* 2000;**162**:553–8.

37. Pierre F, Pham QT, Mur JM, Chau N, Martin JP. Respiratory symptoms and pulmonary function in 871 miners according to Pi phenotype: a longitudinal study. *Eur J Epidemiol* 1988;**4**:39–44.

38. Sandford AJ, Chagani T, Weir TD, Connett JE, Anthonisen NR, Pare PD. Susceptibility genes for rapid decline of lung function in the lung health study. *Am J Respir Crit Care Med* 2001;**163**:469–73.

39. Trethowan WN, Burge PS, Rossiter CE, Harrington JM, Calvert IA. Study of the respiratory health of employees in seven European plants that manufacture ceramic fibres. *Occup Environ Med* 1995;**52**:97–104.

40. Diem JE, Jones RN, Hendrick DJ, *et al*. Five-year longitudinal study of workers employed in a new toluene diisocyanate manufacturing plant. *Am Rev Respir Dis* 1982;**126**:420–8.

41. Gannon PF, Weir DC, Robertson AS, Burge PS. Health, employment, and financial outcomes in workers with occupational asthma. *Br J Industr Med* 1993;**50**:491–6.

42. Anees W, Huggins V, Pavord ID, Robertson AS, Burge PS. Occupational asthma due to low molecular weight agents: eosinophilic and non-eosinophilic variants. *Thorax* 2002;**57**: 231–236.

43. Doll R, Peto R, Wheatley K, Gray R, Sutherland I. Mortality in relation to smoking: 40 years observation on male British doctors. *Br Med J* 1994;**309**:901–11.

6

Air pollution

KENNETH DONALDSON AND WILLIAM MACNEE

PAST AND PRESENT AIR POLLUTION

Old air pollution

In the second week of December 1952 London experienced a period of stagnant weather when the wind speed fell to virtually zero for almost 5 days. The attendant accumulation of fog and air pollution produced a smog containing principally particles and sulfur dioxide that reached extremely high airborne concentrations – up to 4 mg/m^3 of particles. This air pollution episode caused more than 4000 deaths in the following few weeks.[1] Such was the severity of the pollution that cattle at an agricultural show died and there were cancellations of theater performances because the audience could not see the stage. Although it was more than 20 years until the term COPD was to be adopted, many of those who died or became ill had chronic bronchitis and no doubt were smokers with COPD. This episode caused a resurgence of public and political concern regarding the issue of air pollution, culminating in 'the clean air acts', legislation that limited the burning of coal in urban areas – the main factor responsible for these pollution episodes. This type of pollution, dominated by sulfur dioxide and smoke particles, was known in the UK for hundreds of years but is now largely a thing of the past.

New air pollution

In the 1950s, when the above events were taking place in Europe, a new type of air pollution was first documented in Los Angeles. Effluent from the large number of road vehicles, together with intense sunlight, leads to the formation of photochemical smog. Release of nitrogen oxides from vehicles during the morning rush hour is followed by the formation of nitrogen dioxide. This then reacts in a complex series of reactions with polluting hydrocarbons in the presence of solar energy to form ozone, amongst other potentially harmful compounds. Modern cities such as London suffer much less from air pollution than they did in the 1950s, and this downward change in the quantity of air pollution has been accompanied by a qualitative change. Modern air pollution is more like the 'new' pollution referred to above, which is a consequence of traffic and industry, rather than fossil fuel burning.[2] However, there is still well-documented and substantial morbidity and mortality arising from air pollution and this is discussed below. Modern statistical methods enable relatively huge populations to be monitored and so quite small effects can be measured as effects on large numbers of people. There is also a suggestion that the traffic-derived carbon-centered particulate air pollution, measured as PM$_{2.5}$ or PM$_{10}$ (see below) has no safe level[3] and causes the majority of the mortality and morbidity.[4] COPD sufferers constitute a substantial proportion of those affected by air pollution.

AIR POLLUTION EPISODES

Atmospheric pollutants tend to accumulate and become concentrated when air movement is stopped by a temperature inversion, as was the case in the London smogs. Usually the air is warmer at the earth's surface and colder above, but during a temperature inversion a layer of warm air forms above and holds down a layer of cool air at the ground. These events that lead to large increases in air pollution are termed 'episodes' as opposed to the day-to-day variation that normally occurs.

Indoor versus outdoor air pollution

Most people spend the majority of their time, up to 95%, indoors and so the indoor environment is likely to be most important in the genesis of respiratory disease. The day-to-day monitoring of pollution on which health effects research is based relies, almost exclusively, on outdoor sampling sites, so far. Outdoor air pollution permeates rather readily indoors where it is added to by the local pollutants generated inside, for example gas cookers. There may also be a risk from specific indoor air pollution such as fungal spores and fungal products or environmental (see references cited in ref. 5). Personal monitoring of some individuals can reveal a much greater personal exposure than is suggested by the levels measured at a local stationary monitor.[6] The paucity of information on indoor air health effects and COPD necessitates that this chapter is based on its relationship with outdoor air pollution.

The main types of outdoor air pollution

Although there are a very large number of components to air pollution and these vary between sites, the main types of pollution normally considered to mediate the adverse health effects are those given below. The components listed in the last row of Table 6.1 are not discussed here.

SULFUR DIOXIDE

SO_2 is released into the atmosphere when coal and oil, which contain significant amounts of sulfur, are burnt, or during industrial processes, as well as from natural sources such as volcanoes and sulfur springs. In the atmosphere, sulfur dioxide can form acidic particles, or react with cloud droplets, producing acid rain.[7] SO_2, and the other pollutant gases, readily enter the lungs and penetrate according to their solubility, with the most sol-

Table 6.1 *The major components of modern air pollution*

Pollutant	Sources
Sulfur dioxide	Domestic homes and power stations burning fossil fuels; industry
Nitrogen dioxide	Burning of fossil fuels; automobile fuel combustion
Ozone	Formed in sunlight by the photochemical reaction of nitrogen oxides and hydrocarbons released by motor vehicles and industry
Particles	Motor vehicles, industry, burning of fossil fuels, large-scale bush/forest fires
Other air pollutants less likely to be involved in COPD	Volatile organic compounds, heavy metals, polycyclic aromatic hydrocarbons, fungal products, etc.

See refs 14–16.

uble compounds dissolving high in the pulmonary tree and the less soluble ones penetrating more deeply. When SO_2 interacts with water in lung-lining fluid it forms sulfite (SO_3^{2-}) and bisulfite (HSO_3^-) ions along with some other compounds.[8] Both bisulfite and sulfite have a lone pair of electrons and so are readily oxidized by biological molecules forming and consuming free radicals such as superoxide anion, hydroxyl radical and sulfoxyl radical. Thus SO_2 exposure can result in free radical production and oxidative stress in lungs.

NITROGEN DIOXIDE

NO_x is the common term for NO_2 and NO, the most potentially harmful of the nitrogen oxides in the atmosphere. NO is formed by the oxidation of atmospheric N_2 at high temperature combustion processes such as internal combustion in motor vehicles, and in industrial processes. In the presence of ozone, NO is converted to NO_2. In the lung fluid, NO and NO_2 dissolve in the form of nitrate, nitrite and nitrous acid.[7] If there is co-exposure to cigarette smoke or smog, both of which contain hydrogen peroxide, then hydroxyl radical forms from the reaction of H_2O_2 with NO_x. Thus NO_x can also lead to free radical generation and oxidative stress in the lungs.

OZONE

Ozone is a powerful oxidant produced by the action of sunlight on NO_2 to produce monatomic oxygen, which forms ozone (triatomic oxygen) by reacting with molecular oxygen. Atmospheric hydrocarbons such as acetylene, benzene, butanes, ethane and hexane, as well as CO, accelerate this photolysis via peroxy radical formation and with concomitant production of hydroxyl radicals.[7] On dissolving in lung-lining fluid ozone forms hydrogen peroxide, hydroxyhydroperoxides and reactive aldehydes by a process known as ozonolysis.[9] In addition to ozone, photochemical smog contains a number of other harmful secondary pollutants such as peroxyacetyl nitrate (PAN) and aldehydes, which are severe irritants. Thus ozone and other components of photochemical smog also cause oxidative stress in lung tissue following deposition.

PARTICLES

Particles of sea salt and dust from soil and volcanic eruptions arise naturally in the atmosphere. Motor vehicles and industry, however, add significantly to the concentration of particles in the atmosphere in cities where many people can be exposed. The particle cloud or aerosol is a complex mixture comprising organic matter, elemental carbon or soot, metals, sea salt, sulfates, nitrates and geologically derived crustal dust.[10] Particles are divided into those that are primary – i.e. formed immediately, such as diesel particles – and secondary – those particles that form from chemical reactions in the atmosphere, for example ammonium nitrate.[11] Particles can be heterogeneous, such as diesel particles that have a carbon core coated with metals, polycyclic aromatic hydrocarbons (PAHs) and sulfates. Particles deposit in the lung depending on their aerodynamic diameter.[12] The sampling conventions for sampling environmental particulate collect all particles that enter the bronchial tree – PM_{10} – or those that can reach the non-ciliated airspaces – $PM_{2.5}$ (see below for details). Once deposited the particle may dissolve if they are salts such as nitrate and sulfate. If the particles release transition metals that undergo Fenton chemistry, then hydroxyl radicals may be produced. If the ubiquitous bacterial product endotoxin is present in association with the particles then lung cells may be stimulated to produce inflammation. All of these effects may lead to oxidative stress.

Particles have a special problem of nomenclature because they are always measured by a sampling convention that collects some fraction of the material suspended in the air. For the purposes of risk assessment the fraction of particles that enters the lungs is clearly the preferred index:

1 Total suspended particulate (TSP) – a TSP monitor captures atmospheric particulate smaller than 40 μm in diameter. This means that it is not representative of the particles that would enter the lungs since large particles that do not enter the lower respiratory tract could be measured.
2 Black smoke – this is the system that was used in the UK and in other countries until the end of the 1980s. Air was drawn through a size-selective filter onto a white paper and the blackness of the 'smudge' was measured. This method obviously is biased towards

black, i.e. carbon-based, particles; there is a variable relationship between particles as measured by black smoke and PM_{10}.
3 PM_{10} – this is a size-selective sampling convention that captures particles of 10 μm with 50% efficiency; it roughly corresponds to the thoracic fraction of particles as defined by the International Standards Organization (ISO).[12]
4 $PM_{2.5}$ – this is a size-selective sampling convention that captures particles of 2.5 μm with 50% efficiency; it roughly corresponds to the respirable fraction of particles as defined by ISO.[12]

THE ADVERSE HEALTH EFFECTS OF AIR POLLUTION

Effects of air pollution in diseases other than COPD

The general effects of air pollution, excluding effects in COPD, are outlined in Table 6.2; the table is based on an amalgam of chamber studies, acute and chronic epidemiology studies for various endpoints in various countries, and refer to exposures to plausible environmental levels. The table shows that the effects are more often seen in susceptible groups such as asthmatics, although effects can sometimes be seen in normals at much higher exposures. Pollution exposures never involve single pollutants but are combined exposures and so interactions between pollutants are to be anticipated, especially since oxidative stress is a likely common final pathway for both gaseous pollutants and particles to deliver harm to the lung. This may explain the common finding that higher exposures are required to obtain an effect in chamber studies than exist generally in the air when adverse effects can be seen in populations.

The adverse effects of air pollutants in COPD patients

The health effects of air pollutants on patients with COPD can be assessed in chamber studies or in epidemiology studies in panels of subjects at risk, studies of hospital admissions or studies of mortality from records.[13] Chamber studies enable very accurately controlled exposures of pollutant to be delivered to volunteers under well-controlled conditions. The disadvantage is that usually these are healthy volunteers or those who only have mild disease, and unlike real-life exposures there is no co-exposure to other pollutants; children are generally not studied for ethical reasons.[13]

Data has also been gathered from epidemiological studies which are concerned with real-life exposures at

Table 6.2 *The main air pollutants found in the UK and their major adverse health effects other than COPD. Average concentrations of pollutants found in an average UK city (Glasgow) are given in parts per billion for the gases (ppb) and micrograms per cubic meter ($\mu g/m^3$) for particles*

Pollutant	Population	Adverse effect
SO_2 3 ppb	Normal Asthmatic	None or very little Increased airways resistance Increased bronchial hyperreactivity Reduced peak flow Increased hospital admissions
	Other susceptibles, e.g. cardiovascular disease	Increased mortality
NO_2 20 ppb	Normal Asthmatic	None or very little Small effect on bronchial responsiveness Enhancement of response to antigen
	Other susceptibles, e.g. cardiovascular disease	Possible increased mortality
Ozone 10 ppb	Normal	Small increases in airways resistance and bronchial hyperreactivity at high exposure Lung function change (FEV, FVC) Increased symptoms of cough and chest discomfort Inflammation caused by high exposures
	Asthmatic	Enhancement of response to antigen Small increases in airway resistance
	Other susceptibles, e.g. cardiovascular disease	Increased mortality
PM_{10} 17 $\mu g/m^3$	Normal	Slight lung function decrease at very high exposure
	Asthmatic	Increased symptoms Increased hospitalizations
	Other susceptibles, e.g. cardiovascular disease	Increased mortality

The above data is derived from the following sources: refs 13,14,9,15,10,8,16.

the population level. These kinds of studies have their own problems, including trying to discriminate which pollutant, out of the many pollutants normally present during a pollution episode, is in fact responsible for any adverse effect. It is also difficult to untangle interactions which might be occurring between air pollutants leading to the adverse effects. However, evidence from epidemiologic studies provides the main basis for the concerns over the adverse heath effect of air pollution in COPD.

Chamber studies

The reader is referred to Table 6.2 for the average levels seen in a typical UK city to compare with the levels of pollutants given for the chamber studies. In general the chamber studies use high concentrations, sometimes more than two orders of magnitude greater than the average environmental exposure.

In the study reported by von Nieding *et al.*,[17] COPD patients were exposed to 1.5 ppm of NO_2 and this produced a small but detectible increase in airway resistance. Vagaggini *et al.*[18] exposed seven COPD subjects to 0.3 ppm NO_2 for 1 hour with moderate intermittent exercise; there were no changes in the nasal lavage or induced sputum inflammatory profile of the COPD subjects following NO_2 exposure but there was a mild decrease in FEV_1 2 hours after NO_2 exposure in these patients and the symptom score showed a mild increase.

EPIDEMIOLOGY STUDIES OF THE EFFECTS OF AIR POLLUTION ON COPD

Mortality

To assess the risk of death, 1845 men and 460 women who had visited emergency rooms because of COPD exacerbations during the period 1985 to 1989 were followed to death.[19] The authors then assessed the acute association between levels of particulate air pollution and death. Particle levels, measured as black smoke, were associated with mortality for all causes but were stronger for respiratory causes (odds ratio = 1.182; 95% confidence intervals = 1.025–1.365). In the recent large-scale APHEA study in Europe the four main pollutants (NO, O_3, SO_2 and particles) were studied for their short-term association with adverse health effects including mortality. The daily number of deaths was associated with increases in the levels of particles, SO_2, ozone and NO_2, and cardiovascular and respiratory deaths were associated with increases in particles, SO_2 and ozone.

Rossi et al.[20] reported an association between a 12% increase in deaths from COPD and the mean level of airborne particulate 3 and 4 days prior to death. In a study in Birmingham, UK,[21] deaths from COPD were significantly associated with the levels of PM_{10} both 24 hours previously and on the same day. A $10 \mu g/m^3$ rise in PM_{10} was also estimated to produce a 1.1% increase in all-cause mortality.

The well-documented 'six cities' study[4] reported that a $10 \mu g/m^3$ increase in 2-day mean $PM_{2.5}$ was associated with a 3.3% increase in deaths from COPD. The relationship with $PM_{2.5}$ suggested that finer combustion-related particles may be important. In a study reported by Xu and coworkers[22] the heavily polluted areas of Beijing which had maxima of $630 \mu g/m^3$ of SO_2 and $1003 \mu g/m^3$ of total suspended particulate were studied. Regressions were carried out on SO_2 and TSP levels against deaths, controlling for the effects of temperature, humidity and day of the week. Significant associations were seen between mortality from COPD and a doubling of SO_2 and a doubling of TSP. In their study of mortality in Philadelphia, Schwartz and Dockery[3] reported that, for a $100 \mu g/m^3$ increase in TSP, COPD deaths increased by 19% (95% confidence interval = 0.42%).

Exacerbations

In the APHEA study[23] hospital emergency room visits for COPD in Barcelona were studied in relation to temporal trends in air pollution. Results showed that a reduction of about $50 \mu g/m^3$ in particles or sulfur dioxide was accompanied by a reduction of about 6% in emergency room visits for COPD. Ozone levels were also associated with emergency room visits for COPD with reductions in O_3 of $50 \mu g/m^3$ being associated with a 4% reduction in emergency room visits for COPD. Morgan et al.[24] studied hospital admissions in Sydney, Australia between 1990 and 1994. An increase in daily maximum concentration of nitrogen dioxide from the 10th to the 90th percentile was associated with an increase of 4.6% (−0.17 to 9.61 confidence intervals) in COPD admissions. A similar

increase in daily maximum 1-hour particulate concentration was associated with an increase of 3.01% (confidence interval 0.38–6.52) in COPD admissions. In a prospective study[25] 40 subjects with COPD who completed symptom diaries twice daily for 3 months during the winter of 1994 were followed. All the subjects lived within a 5 kilometer radius of the regional council's air pollution monitoring site and the daily and hourly mean pollutant levels (PM_{10}, NO_2, SO_2 and CO) were measured at the monitoring site. The pollution levels were low in that year and the only significant association seen was between a rise in the PM_{10} concentration equivalent to the interquartile range and an increase in night-time chest symptoms. A same-day rise in NO_2 concentration equivalent to the interquartile range was associated with increased inhaler use and 24 hour lag NO_2 concentrations with increased nebulizer use. The association between air pollution and hospital admissions for COPD was investigated in Minneapolis–St Paul and Birmingham, Alabama for the period 1986 to 1991.[26] After adjustment for temperature, day of the week and season temporal trends, associations between air pollution and hospital admissions for respiratory causes were seen in Minneapolis–St Paul but not in Birmingham. A 15 ppb increase in O_3 on the previous day was associated with a 5.15% (confidence interval = 2.36–7.94%) increase in admissions. PM_{10}, SO_2 and NO_2 were also associated with hospital admissions although none could be singled out as being more important than the others.

In the APHEA study[27] admissions for COPD in six European cities were examined. For all ages the relative risk of admission to hospital for COPD for a $50 \mu g/m^3$ increase in the daily level of any pollutant were: sulfur dioxide 1.02 (0.08–1.06); black smoke 1.04 (1.01–1.06), total suspended particulate 1.02 (1.00–1.05); nitrogen dioxide 1.02 (1.00–1.05); ozone 1.04 (1.02–1.07). Wordley et al.[21] reported on hospital admissions in Birmingham, UK in relation to particulate air pollution. A $10 \mu g/m^3$ rise in PM_{10} was associated with a 2.4% increase in respiratory admissions and this risk, while low, was linear without evidence of a threshold. Dab et al.[28] reported for the APHEA study on the relationship between air pollution and hospital admissions in Paris between 1987 and 1992. PM_{10} and black smoke were associated with hospital admissions due to all respiratory causes when the black smoke level exceeded its 5th centile value by $100 \mu g/m^3$. SO_2 levels consistently influenced hospital admissions for all respiratory causes including COPD. Schouten et al. reporting for the APHEA study in The Netherlands[29] showed that ozone had a significant effect on respiratory emergency admissions in Rotterdam but not in Amsterdam; although other trends were found none were significant. In a study of 75 patients with either asthma or COPD their peak expiratory flow rates and symptoms, such as wheeze, dyspnea, cough, throat and eye irritation were recorded[30] along with their bronchodilator use. These were then related to pollution levels. On the basis of methacholine sensitivity 36 patients were classified as 'reactors'. There were small but significant increases in PEF variability, bronchodilator use and wheeze with increasing sulfur dioxide level, whilst increased bronchodilator use, dyspnea, eye irritation and minimum PEF recordings were related to ozone levels. In the subgroup of 'reactors', variability in peak flow and increases in wheeze, dyspnea and bronchodilator use were associated with increased levels of both sulfur dioxide and ozone. These associations were seen with pollution levels on the same day as well as delayed by 24 or 48 hours. The relative risk (RR) of an increase of $100 \mu g/m^3$ in daily PM_{10} for hospital admissions was 1.57 (confidence intervals 2.06–1.20). Notably when days exceeding the national ambient air quality standard for PM_{10} were excluded the association remained for COPD admissions (RR = 1.54 confidence intervals = 2.06–1.16).

Schwartz[31] analyzed hospital admissions for the elderly in Birmingham, Alabama in relation to air pollution levels. Inhalable particles were a risk factor for admission for COPD (RR = 1.27, confidence intervals = 1.08–1.50). An increase in ozone exposure of 50 ppb was more weakly associated with admissions for COPD with a one day lag (RR = 1.17, confidence interval = 0.86–1.60). The relationship between air pollution and emergency room admissions for COPD over 5 years in Barcelona, Spain was investigated.[32] An increase of $25 \mu g/m^3$ of sulfur dioxide produced adjusted changes of 6% and 9% in emergency room admissions for COPD during winter and summer respectively. For particulate expressed as black smoke, a similar change was found during winter although the change was smaller in the summer. This association of each pollutant with COPD admissions remained significant after controlling for the other pollutant.

Pulmonary function

The association between long-term exposure to outdoor air pollution and the severity of COPD and the prevalence of bronchial hyperreactivity to $beta_2$-agonists were studied.[33] Two groups of adult patients were chosen with similar ages and similar smoking habits and who lived in a downtown district or in the outer, less polluted suburbs of Marseilles. Regions were similar with respect to sulfur dioxide levels but levels of nitric oxide and PM_{10} were higher in the downtown area than in the suburbs. Airway obstruction, as determined by decrease in FEV_1, mean forced expiratory flow and central airway resistance were measured. Baseline lung function was altered more significantly in both male and female patients who lived in downtown Marseilles than in those who resided in the suburbs. The differences persisted regardless of the

season during which the study occurred. Pope and Kanner[34] assessed the association between PM_{10} and changes in FEV_1, FEV_1/FVC and FVC in smokers with mild to moderate airflow limitation. This spirometric data was obtained from Salt Lake City inhabitants from the Lung Health Study at two screening visits 10–90 days apart following an initial screening visit. Differences in pulmonary function were analyzed and significant association between changes in pulmonary function and PM_{10} were observed. Decreases in FEV_1 and FEV_1/FVC were associated with changes in PM_{10}. On average an increase in PM_{10} equal to $100 \mu g/m^3$ was associated with a decline in FEV_1 equal to approximately 2%. The authors concluded that in current smokers PM_{10} possibly had a small transient negative effect on lung function, not entirely obscured by their smoking habit.

POTENTIAL MECHANISMS FOR THE EFFECTS OF AIR POLLUTANTS ON COPD PATIENTS

There are at least three ways in which pollutants would worsen COPD leading to exacerbation:

1 by enhancing inflammation
2 by injuring or impairing ciliated cells
3 by increasing mucus production in mucous cells.

All four of the principal air pollutants, that is SO_2, NO_2, ozone and PM_{10}, have an impact in COPD. This may supply some clues as to the mechanism whereby they have this effect. Because of the central role of inflammation in COPD with COPD patients, outwith exacerbations possessing some degree of inflammation we may look to the potential mechanisms whereby air pollutants might enhance inflammation. As described earlier, on making contact with lung-lining fluid, all four are liable to cause oxidative stress whilst SO_2 is also likely to generate acid conditions if the exposure is high enough. Particles appear to be the most potent of the urban air pollutants in terms of ability to cause adverse effects with no threshold in many studies.[14] Therefore PM_{10} mechanisms will be discussed more extensively than the other pollutants.

SO_2

When it dissolves in the lungs sulfur dioxide forms sulfate which is toxic to the lung at high exposure and known to cause bronchoconstriction in asthmatics. In addition it has recently been demonstrated that sulfate can considerably potentiate the inactivation of alpha-1-antiprotease by peroxynitrite which is generated at inflammatory sites.[35] It is proposed that the formation of protein-modifying sulfate radicals from the interaction of SO_3^{2-} with peroxynitrite is the mechanism by which

SO_2 lowers the antiproteolytic defences. In addition, SO_2 has been shown in rats to cause dramatic decreases in lung glutathione as well as in other tissues and organs. The underlying mechanism appears to be inhibition of γ-glutamylcysteine synthetase, glutathione peroxidase and glutathione S-transferase in the lung.[36] Based on studies with ibuprofen which reduced hyperreactivity at 24 hours post SO_2 exposure but not immediately after SO_2 exposure,[37] it is suggested that two phases of hyper-reactivity exist following SO_2 exposure. These phases have an immediate effect which possibly involves epithelial cell damage and loss and a later inflammatory phase.

NO₂ and ozone

NO_2 and ozone can directly oxidize lipids and proteins as described earlier. This is likely to occur through deple-tion of antioxidants in lung-lining fluid.[38,39] Epithelial cells of the airways and central lung may then become the targets for the oxidative stress and these may respond with activation of transcription factors such as NF-κB leading to increased transcription of genes for chemokines, inducible nitric oxide synthase, cyclo-oxygenase and other pro-inflammatory mediators.[40]

Particles

PM_{10} has well-documented free radical activity and the potential to produce oxidative stress and inflammation (reviewed in ref. 41).

PM_{10} is a size-selective sampling convention that col-lects and expresses, as mass, particles with a 50% cut off for an aerodynamic diameter of $10\,\mu$m – thus a very low percentage of particles of $15\,\mu$m, 50% of particles of $10\,\mu$m and about 80% of particles of $5\,\mu$m and more than 90% of particles of $1\,\mu$m aerodynamic diameter. This is closely equivalent to the 'thoracic fraction'[12] defined as the mass fraction of airborne particles that penetrates beyond the larynx. The $PM_{2.5}$ sampling convention is roughly equivalent to the respirable fraction,[12] with 50% efficiency for particles of 2–$3\,\mu$m aerodynamic diameter. The PM_{10} sampling convention therefore expresses the mass of particles of interest for COPD, since these par-ticles will deposit in the large and small airways and down to the non-ciliated airways. Any particles in the air within the aerodynamic diameter boundaries described above will be sampled regardless of composition. Therefore local sources of particulate can be very important although transboundary movement of particles is also important. PM_{10} is a complex and heterogeneous mixture which varies depending on the site of the sampler. PM_{10} can be divided into coarse, fine and ultrafine fractions:

- The coarse fraction comprises relatively large inhalable particles ranging from 2.5–10 μm and generally consists of particles derived from soil, re-entrained road dust and other crustal materials from mechanical wear processes.
- The fine fraction is particles within an aerodynamic diameter range of 0.1–2.5 μm. The fine mode fraction comprises a mixture of particles including carbonaceous material such as diesel soot and its aggregates, and secondary aerosols such as ammonium sulfate and ammonium nitrate derived from atmospheric chemical reactions.
- The ultrafine fraction is in the size range 0.1 μm and downwards and is considered to be primarily derived from combustion sources, especially diesel and petrol exhaust and other combustion processes in industry.
- There are a number of other components of PM_{10} that depend largely on local concentrations such as endotoxin fungal spores, environmental tobacco smoke (etc.).

DIRECT EFFECTS OF PARTICLES

From a toxicologic viewpoint it is important to determine which of these components are likely to drive the exacer-bations of COPD. The ability of components to produce oxidative stress and initiate or prolong inflammation is a likely route whereby any particulate fraction might have an effect in COPD. Generally there is little within the coarse fraction that is likely to have this effect. However, in the fine and ultrafine fractions there are potential culprits that might cause oxidative stress when particles deposit in lung-lining fluid and interact with cells.

Transition metals

Oxidative stress can arise directly from the particles them-selves through the localized release of transition metals. For instance in cell-free systems we have shown that both Edinburgh and London PM_{10} have the ability to generate hydroxy radical activity[42] that is inhibited by transition metal chelator. Similar transition metal-mediated free radical generation has been demonstrated for PM from Utah Valley.[43] This is further supported by studies where the addition of particulates such as residual oil fly-ash (ROFA) and PM_{10} to cells in culture cause metal-dependent oxidative stress and expression of genes for pro-inflammatory mediators.[44,45] When the same types of particles are instiled into the lungs of animals again the subsequent inflammation that arises[46] can be driven by transition metals.[47]

Ultrafine particles

Ultrafine particles less than 100 nm are very readily measurable in urban air. Epidemiologic evidence on their role in the adverse effects of PM_{10} is scanty because ultrafine particles are not routinely measured in urban air sampling. However, Peters et al.[48] reported that decre-ments in evening peak flow in a group of asthmatics was best associated with the ultrafine component of the airborne particles during a severe pollution episode; COPD patients might also be at risk from ultrafine particles.

Toxicologic evidence supports the contention that ultrafine particles may be important mediators of adverse effects (reviewed in ref. 49), giving rise to the 'ultrafine hypothesis' of the adverse effects of air pollution particles. Ultrafine particles may also be found in the fine fraction since ultrafine particles aggregate, if they are at high enough concentration, to form secondary particles which have a larger aerodynamic diameter but are in fact composed of multiple ultrafine particles. These may then disaggregate in the lungs.

Singlet ultrafine particles deposit in increased amounts in COPD lung[50] which may contribute to susceptibility in COPD. This greater deposition was presumably due to turbulence in the flow of air, or the speed of airflow through inflamed or partially blocked airways.

Animal studies have extensively demonstrated that ultrafine particles have enhanced pathogenic potential compared to larger respirable particles of the same material (reviewed in ref. 49). Following instilation of ultrafine carbon black and fine carbon black at the same mass there was substantially more inflammation with the ultrafine carbon black than the fine carbon black.[51] Similar results have been shown for other ultrafine materials that are insoluble and non-toxic, including latex and titanium dioxide.[52] Ultrafine particles have a relatively huge surface area compared to the same mass of non-ultrafine particles and so it is important to discriminate whether the ability of ultrafine particles to cause inflammation is merely an ability to release, from their large surface area large local concentrations of transition metals.

Diesel exhaust and other combustion-derived, carbon-centered particles such as ROFA often have high levels of transition metals associated with them. It is therefore important to determine whether the effects of ultrafines are due to transition metals and the ultrafine hypothesis is merely an extension of the transition metal hypothesis. We have demonstrated that, at least in the case of ultrafine carbon black, the inflammation is not mediated by transition metals since treating the ultrafine particles with a transition metal chelator had no effect on the ability of the ultrafine carbon black to cause inflammation.[51] Additionally a soluble extract of the ultrafine carbon black which would contain any transition metals was not inflammogenic. It is therefore necessary to consider ultrafine particles as an additional risk factor over and above the transition metal content of any airborne PM_{10} sample.

The mechanism of inflammation caused by ultrafine particles appears to be mediated by oxidants or free radicals. We have demonstrated that this is not necessarily through a transition metal-mediated mechanism and yet, in cell-free systems ultrafine carbon black and other ultrafine particles oxidize dichlorofluorescein to its fluorescent form. Thus even in the absence of transition metals, ultrafine particles have the ability to cause oxidative stress (unpublished work). The mechanism of this is unknown but may be related to the unique molecular configuration present in the surface of such small particles.

Endotoxin

The ubiquitous gram-negative bacterial product endotoxin (lipopolysaccharide (LPS)) is found in many PM_{10} samples.[53] In some *in vitro* studies the endotoxin has been found to explain the biological activity.[53,54] However many studies show that the major biological activity in a PM sample is not endotoxin but is in fact transition metal (see above). However the multicomponent nature of PM_{10} does not preclude 'networking' between cells in orchestrating an inflammatory response, for example stimulation of macrophage by LPS and stimulation of epithelial cells by metals or ultrafines.

MECHANISMS FOR THE ADVERSE EFFECTS OF AIR POLLUTANTS ON THE CELLS OF THE AIRWAYS

Any effect that pollutants have in promoting airway obstruction would very likely contribute to exacerbations of COPD. A range of studies demonstrate effects of pollutants on the mucociliary clearance system and mucus production by airway cells and these are reviewed in the following section.

Effects of air pollutants on ciliated cells

Kienast *et al.*[55] investigated the influence of SO_2 on epithelial cells from nasal brushings from 12 healthy volunteers. Nasal ciliated cells were exposed to SO_2, and ciliary beat frequency was measured. SO_2 exposure caused a dose-dependent decrease in ciliary beat frequency that ranged from 42.8% with 2.5 ppm SO_2 to 100% inhibition with 12.5 ppm SO_2. Majima *et al.*[56] also demonstrated slowing of mucociliary transport in chickens exposed to 6 ppm SO_2. This appeared to be a result of a change in the recoil distance of mucus caused by SO_2 exposure *in vivo*, and the authors proposed that SO_2 causes the formation of multiple points of adhesion of transit mucus between acinar gland cells and the emergent extracellular mucus; the net effect of this is for mucociliary transport to be retarded. When olfactory epithelium of mice was exposed for up to 120 minutes to 20 ppm SO_2,[57] exposure time, a surrogate for dose, was related to changes in ciliary loss, epithelial thinning and desquamation; the changes were most pronounced 24 hours after exposure. Nikula and Wilson[58] used rat tracheal organ cultures exposed to 1 ppm ozone and reported loss of ciliated cells and ciliated cell damage.

Human respiratory epithelial cells from healthy volunteers were grown on membranes at air–fluid interfaces and exposed to gaseous SO_2 for 30 minutes or 2 hours. Under these conditions the cells exposed to air showed a 20% reduction in ciliary beat frequency whilst exposure to SO_2 (2.5–12.5 ppm) caused a further concentration-dependent decrease in ciliary beat frequency.[59]

In a related study[61] minor morphologic changes were noted in guinea pig trachea exposed to sulfur dioxide for 30 minutes and mucociliary activity was halved. At high exposures there was further slowing of ciliary activity with widespread structural alterations such as sloughing, edema and mitochondrial swelling. Tamaoki *et al.*[61] exposed human bronchial epithelial cells to 3 ppm sulfur dioxide. This rapidly decreased the ciliary beat frequency by 59% and was accompanied by a reduction in intracellular cAMP levels to a quarter. Interestingly this effect was prevented by pretreatment of cells with an antihistamine – azelastine. Carson *et al.*[62] exposed human nasal epithelial cells to 2 ppm NO_2 for 4 hours. The authors reported a trend towards structural alterations in six out of seven nasal epithelial samples, characterized by excess matrix in the cilia, multiple ciliary axonemes and vesiculations of the luminal border of the ciliary membranes. Rats were exposed to 10 ppm NO_2 and O_3 for 7 days and assessed for lung inflammation and morphology, airway microvascular leakage and *in vitro* contractile responses of the main bronchi.[63] Histologic signs of increased inflammation were evident in the respiratory bronchioles and alveoli, and there was loss of cilia from the epithelium of the small airways. No alterations in microvascular permeability or smooth muscle responsiveness were found.

Kakinoki *et al.*[64] exposed rabbits for 24 hours to 3 ppm NO_2 and then assessed ciliary activity, mucociliary transport velocity in the trachea and tracheal permeability. In rabbits exposed to NO_2, ciliary activity was decreased, as was mucociliary transport velocity, whilst epithelial permeability was increased.

In an interesting approach, rats were housed either in the center of Sao Paulo, the largest city in South America, or in a non-polluted area.[65] The rats housed in the polluted area developed secretory cell hyperplasia in their airways, and alterations in cilia at the ultrastructural level and had more rigid mucus; all of these changes contributed to impairment of mucociliary clearance. Additionally the number of inflammatory cells in the bronchoalveolar lavage (BAL) were higher in the air pollution-exposed group than in the group kept in a non-polluted area. Harkema *et al.*[66] exposed Bonnet monkeys to 0.15 or 3 ppm ozone for 6–90 days 8 hours per day. The endpoints selected were quantitative morphologic changes as assessed by light and electron microscopy. Lesions consisting of necrotic ciliated cells, shortened cilia and secretory cell hyperplasia were seen after 6 and 90 days' exposure to both levels of ozone. Some adaptation was present, with inflammatory cell influx being only present at 6 days and not at 90 days.

Effects of air pollutants on mucus cells

Basbaum *et al.*[67] measured steady-state levels of mucin mRNA following exposure to SO_2 in rats. There was an increase in goblet cells from 0 to 4.5/mm in the trachea, from 0.2 to 6.2/mm in the main stem bronchus and from 0.2 to 22.7/mm in the distal airways. Concomitantly mucin mRNA was increased up to ninefold in response to SO_2 exposure. Mucin gene expression was measured in rat airways following exposure to SO_2 and qualitative increases in mRNA reported.[68] In an attempt to more closely mimic realistic exposure to mixtures of pollutants, Abraham *et al.*[69] exposed sheep to a combined ozone and SO_2 cloud and measured tracheal-mucus velocity and ciliary beat frequency. On two separate occasions sheep were exposed to either 0.3 ppm ozone and 3 ppm SO_2 or air. The combination of ozone and SO_2 depressed mucus velocity by 40% compared to the air exposure, with no corresponding change in ciliary beat frequency. Since the ciliary beat frequency was conserved it must be assumed that either the contact between the cilia and the mucus or the mechanical properties of the mucus were changed by the exposure to ozone and SO_2.

Jiang *et al.*[70] utilized a panel of particulate samples which included ROFA, fly ash from a domestic oil burning furnace, ambient PM from St Louis, Ottowa and Washington DC, as well as volcanic ash from Mount St Helen's. All of these were tested for their effects on mucus secretion in guinea-pig tracheal epithelial cells. Only ROFA produced significant stimulation of mucus secretion and studies with antioxidants showed the mechanism to be oxidant mediated. Furthermore, ROFA caused dramatic reductions in glutathione by a transition metal-mediated mechanism. mRNA for the mucus gene MUC2 was increased following ROFA treatment along with the increased secretion of mucus. In a similar study[71] marked upregulation of the MUC5ac and lysozyme genes were seen on exposure to ROFA; vanadium, which comprised 18.8% by weight of the ROFA, mediated the oxidative stress that caused the gene expression. The authors suggest that vanadium acts as a tyrosine phosphatase inhibitor favoring phosphorylation-dependent signaling pathways that lead to mucin and lysozyme secretion.

CONCLUSION

Numerous epidemiologic studies demonstrate that there is a relationship between increases in air pollution and both mortality and morbidity in COPD patients. It is not easy, given the complex nature of air pollution, to ascribe

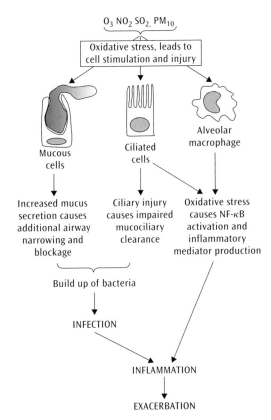

O₃ NO₂ SO₂, PM₁₀

Oxidative stress, leads to cell stimulation and injury

Mucous cells

Ciliated cells

Alveolar macrophage

Increased mucus secretion causes additional airway narrowing and blockage

Ciliary injury causes impaired mucociliary clearance

Oxidative stress causes NF-κB activation and inflammatory mediator production

Build up of bacteria

INFECTION

INFLAMMATION

EXACERBATION

Figure 6.1 *Hypothetical sequence of cellular events regarding the effects of pollution in COPD.*

these effects to a single entity but all of the main components, gaseous and particles, appear to be influential to some degree. However, particles appear to be especially harmful. In terms of a plausible mechanism for the effects of pollutants on COPD, oxidative stress emanating from the interaction of the pollutants with the lung, added to existing oxidative stress from inflammation and smoking, stands out as offering a testable central unifying hypothesis. There are a large number of studies demonstrating *in vitro* and experimental correlates of ciliary damage and stimulation of mucus secretion that offers a plausible pathway from deposition of pollutants to infection that might contribute to exacerbations. Figure 6.1 shows these pathways diagrammatically.

Long-term trends suggest an ongoing reduction in air pollution, and so this factor in the exacerbation and mortality from COPD could become less important. Novel developments in antioxidant therapy again offer hope of interventions that might be effective against pollution-mediated exacerbations.

REFERENCES

1. Wilson R. Introduction. In: R Wilson, J Spengler, eds. *Particles in our Air*. Harvard University Press, 1996, pp 1–14.

2. Williams M. Patterns of air pollution in developed countries. In: ST Holgate, JM Samet, HS Koren, RL Maynard, eds. *Air Pollution and Health*. Academic Press, San Diego, 1999, pp 83–112.

3. Schwartz J, Dockery DW. Increased mortality in Philadelphia associated with daily air pollution concentrations. *Am Rev Respir Dis* 1992;**45**:600–4.

4. Schwartz J, Dockery DW, Neas LM. Is daily mortality associated specifically with fine particles? *J Air Waste Manag Assoc* 1996;**46**:927–39.

5. Samet JM, Spengler JD, eds. *Indoor Air Pollution: A Health Perspective*. The Johns Hopkins University Press, Baltimore, 1991.

6. Watt M, Godden D, Cherrie J, Seaton A. Individual exposure to particulate air pollution and its relevance to thresholds for health effects: a study of traffic wardens. *Occup Environ Med* 1995;**52**:790–2.

7. Wellburn A. *Air Pollution and Climate Change: The Biological Impact*. Longman, New York, 1994.

8. Expert Panel on Air Quality. *Sulphur Dioxide*. HMSO, London, 1995.

9. Expert Panel on Air Quality. *Ozone*. HMSO, London, 1994.

10. Expert Panel on Air Quality. *Particles*. HMSO, London, 1995.

11. Quality of Urban Air Review Group. *Airborne Particulate Matter in the United Kingdom: Third Report of the Quality of Urban Air Review Group*. Quality of Urban Air Review Group. 1996 (prepared at the request of the Department of the Environment; further copies can be obtained from the University of Birmingham).

12. International Standards Organisation. *Air Quality: Particle Size Fraction Definitions for Health-related Sampling*. IS 7708, ISO, Geneva, 1994.

13. Ayres JG. Heath effects of gaseous air pollutants. In: RE Hester, RM Harrison, eds. *Issue in Environmental Science and Technology*. 10. *Air Pollution and Health*. The Royal Society of Chemistry, Cambridge, UK, 1998, pp 1–20.

14. Pope CA, Dockery DW. Epidemiology of particle effects. In: ST Holgate, JM Samet, HS Koren, RL Maynard, eds. *Air Pollution and Health*. Academic Press, San Diego, 1999, pp 673–705.

15. Expert Panel on Air Quality. *Nitrogen Dioxide*. HMSO, London, 1996.

16. Committee on the Medical Effects of Air Pollution and Health. *Handbook on Air Pollution and Health*. HMSO, Norwich, 1997.

17. Nieding GV, Wagner M, Krekeler H, Smidt U, Muysers K. Minimum concentrations of NO₂ causing acute effects on the respiratory gas exchange and airway-resistance in patients with chronic bronchitis. *Int Arch Arbeitsmed* 1971;**27**:338–48.

18. Vagaggini B, Paggiaro PL, Giannini D, *et al.* Effect of short-term NO₂ exposure on induced sputum in normal, asthmatic and COPD subjects. *Eur Respir J* 1996;**9**:1852–7.

19. Sunyer J, Schwartz J, Tobias A, Macfarlane D, Garcia J, Anto JM. Patients with chronic obstructive pulmonary disease are at increased risk of death associated with urban particle air pollution: a case-crossover analysis. *Am J Epidemiol* 2000;**151**:50–6.

20. Rossi G, Vigotti MA, Zanobetti A, Repetto F, Gianelle V, Schwartz J. Air pollution and cause-specific mortality in Milan, Italy, 1980–1989. *Arch Environ Health* 1999;**54**:158–64.

21. Wordley J, Walters S, Ayres JG. Short term variations in hospital admissions and mortality and particulate air pollution. *Occup Environ Med* 1997;**54**:108–16.

22. Xu X, Gao J, Dockery DW, Chen Y. Air pollution and daily mortality in residential areas of Beijing, China. *Arch Environ Health* 1994;**49**:216–22.

23. Tobias GA, Sunyer DJ, Castellsague PJ, Saez PM, Anto JM, Boque JM. [Impact of air pollution on the mortality and emergencies of chronic obstructive pulmonary disease and asthma in Barcelona.] [Spanish]. *Gaceta Sanitaria* 1998;**12**:223–30.

24. Morgan G, Corbett S, Wlodarczyk J. Air pollution and hospital admissions in Sydney, Australia, 1990 to 1994. *Am J Pub Health* 1998;**88**:1761–6.

25. Harre ES, Price PD, Ayrey RB, Toop LJ, Martin IR, Town GI. Respiratory effects of air pollution in chronic obstructive pulmonary disease: a three month prospective study. *Thorax* 1997;**52**:1040–4.

26. Moolgavkar SH, Luebeck EG, Anderson EL. Air pollution and hospital admissions for respiratory causes in Minneapolis–St Paul and Birmingham. *Epidemiology* 1997;**8**:364–70.

27. Anderson HR, Spix C, Medina S, *et al.* Air pollution and daily admissions for chronic obstructive pulmonary disease in 6 European cities: results from the APHEA project. *Eur Respir J* 1997;**10**:1064–71.

28. Dab W, Medina S, Quenel P, *et al.* Short term respiratory health effects of ambient air pollution: results of the APHEA project in Paris. *J Epidemiol Commun Health* 1996;**50**(suppl 1): s42–6.

29. Schouten JP, Vonk JM, de Graaf A. Short term effects of air pollution on emergency hospital admissions for respiratory disease: results of the APHEA project in two major cities in The Netherlands, 1977–89. *J Epidemiol Commun Health* 1996;**50**(suppl 1):s229.

30. Higgins BG, Francis HC, Yates CJ, *et al.* Effects of air pollution on symptoms and peak expiratory flow measurements in subjects with obstructive airways disease. *Thorax* 1995;**50**: 149–55.

31. Schwartz J. Air pollution and hospital admissions for the elderly in Birmingham, Alabama. *Am J Epidemiol* 1994;**139**: 589–98.

32. Sunyer J, Saez M, Murillo C, Castellsague J, Martinez F, Anto JM. Air pollution and emergency room admissions for chronic obstructive pulmonary disease: a 5-year study. *Am J Epidemiol* 1993;**137**:701–5.

33. Jammes Y, Delpierre S, Delvolgo MJ, Humbert-Tena C, Burnet H. Long-term exposure of adults to outdoor air pollution is associated with increased airway obstruction and higher prevalence of bronchial hyperresponsiveness. *Arch Environ Health* 1998;**53**:372–7.

34. Pope CA III, Kanner RE. Acute effects of PM10 pollution on pulmonary function of smokers with mild to moderate chronic obstructive pulmonary disease. *Am Rev Respir Dis* 1993;**147**:1336–40.

35. Reist M, Jenner P, Halliwell B. Sulphite enhances peroxynitrite-dependent alpha-1-antiproteinase inactivation. A mechanism of lung injury by sulphur dioxide? *FEBS Lett* 1998;**423**:231–4.

36. Langley-Evans SC, Phillips GJ, Jackson AA. Sulphur dioxide: a potent glutathione depleting agent. *Comp Biochem Physiol C Pharmacol Toxicol Endocrinol* 1996;**114**:89–98.

37. Norris AA, Jackson DM. Sulphur dioxide-induced airway hyperreactivity and pulmonary inflammation in dogs. *Agents Actions* 1996;**26**:360–6.

38. Menzel DB. Antioxidant vitamins and prevention of lung disease. *Ann NY Acad Sci* 1992;**669**:141–55 [review, 40 refs].

39. Mudway IS, Kelly FJ. Ozone and the lung: a sensitive issue. *Mol Aspects Med* 2000;**21**:1–48.

40. Barnes PJ, Karin M. Nuclear factor-kappaB: a pivotal transcription factor in chronic inflammatory diseases. *New Engl J Med* 1997;**336**:1066–71.

41. MacNee W, Donaldson K. How can ultrafine particles be responsible for increased mortality? *Monaldi Arch Chest Dis* 2000;**55**:135–9.

42. Gilmour PS, Brown DM, Lindsay TG, Beswick PH, MacNee W, Donaldson K. Adverse health effects of PM10 particles: involvement of iron in generation of hydroxyl radical. *Occup Environ Med* 1996;**53**:817–22.

43. Frampton MW, Ghio AJ, Samet JM, Carson JL, Carter JD, Devlin RB. Effects of aqueous extracts of PM(10) filters from the Utah valley on human airway epithelial cells. *Am J Physiol* 1999;**277**:L960-7.

44. Jimenez LA, Thompson J, Brown DA, *et al.* Activation of NF-kappaB by PM(10) occurs via an iron-mediated mechanism in the absence of IkappaB degradation. *Toxicol Appl Pharmacol* 2000;**166**:101–10.

45. Carter JD, Ghio AJ, Samet JM, Devlin RB. Cytokine production by human airway epithelial cells after exposure to an air pollution particle is metal-dependent. *Toxicol Appl Pharmacol* 1997;**146**:180–8.

46. Li XY, Gilmour PS, Donaldson K, MacNee W. *In vivo* and *in vitro* proinflammatory effects of particulate air pollution (PM10). *Environ Health Perspect* 1997;**105**(suppl 5):1279–83.

47. Costa DL, Dreher KL. Bioavailable transition metals in particulate matter mediate cardiopulmonary injury in healthy and compromised animal models. *Environ Health Perspect* 1997;**105**(suppl 5):1053–60.

48. Peters A, Wichmann HE, Tuch T, Heinrich J, Heyder J. Respiratory effects are associated with the number of ultrafine particles. *Am J Respir Crit Care Med* 1997;**155**: 1376–83.

49. Donaldson K, Stone V, MacNee W. The toxicology of ultrafine particles. In: RL Maynard, CV Howard, eds. *Particulate Matter: Properties and Effects upon Health*. Bios, Oxford, 1999, pp 115–27.

50. Anderson PJ, Wilson JD, Hiller FC. Respiratory tract deposition of ultrafine particles in subjects with obstructive or restrictive lung disease. *Chest* 1990;**97**:1115–20.

51. Brown DM, Stone V, Findlay P, MacNee W, Donaldson K. Increased inflammation and intracellular calcium caused by ultrafine carbon black is independent of transition metals or other soluble components. *Occup Environ Med* 2000;**57**: 685–91.

52. Donaldson K, Stone V, Gilmour PS, Brown DM, MacNee W. Ultrafine particles: mechanisms of lung injury. *Phil Trans R Soc Lond* A 2000;**358**:2741–9.

53. Becker S, Soukup JM, Gilmour MI, Devlin RB. Stimulation of human and rat alveolar macrophages by urban air particulates: effects on oxidant radical generation and cytokine production. *Toxicol Appl Pharmacol* 1996; **141**:637–48.

54. Dong WM, Lewtas J, Luster MI. Role of endotoxin in tumor-necrosis-factor-alpha expression from alveolar macrophages treated with urban air particles. *Exp Lung Res* 2000;**22**: 577–92.

55. Kienast K, Riechelmann H, Knorst M, *et al.* Combined exposures of human ciliated cells to different concentrations of sulfur dioxide and nitrogen dioxide. *Eur J Med Res* 1996;**1**:533–6.

56. Majima Y, Swift DL, Bang DG, Bang FB. Mechanism of slowing of mucociliary transport induced by SO_2 exposure. *Ann Biomed Engin* 1985;**13**:515–30.

57. Min YG, Rhee CS, Choo MJ, Song HK, Hong SC. Histopathologic changes in the olfactory epithelium in mice after exposure to sulfur dioxide. *Acta Oto-Laryngol* 1994;**114**: 447–52.

58. Nikula KJ, Wilson DW. Response of rat tracheal epithelium to ozone and oxygen exposure *in vitro*. *Fund Appl Toxicol* 1990;**15**:121–31.

59. Riechelmann H, Kienast K, Schellenberg J, Mann WJ. An *in vitro* model to study effects of airborne pollutants on human ciliary activity. *Rhinology* 1994;**32**:105–8.

60. Riechelmann H, Maurer J, Kienast K, Hafner B, Mann WJ. Respiratory epithelium exposed to sulfur dioxide – functional and ultrastructural alterations. *Laryngoscope* 1994;**105**:295–9.

61. Tamaoki J, Chiyotani A, Sakai N, Takeyama K, Konno K. Effect of azelastine on sulphur dioxide induced impairment of ciliary motility in airway epithelium. *Thorax* 1994;**48**:542–6.

62. Carson JL, Collier AM, Hu SC, Delvin RB. Effect of nitrogen dioxide on human nasal epithelium. *Am J Respir Cell Mol Biol* 1998;**9**:264–70.

63. Chitano P, Rado V, Di Stefano A, *et al*. Effect of subchronic *in vivo* exposure to nitrogen dioxide on lung tissue inflammation, airway microvascular leakage, and *in vitro* bronchial muscle responsiveness in rats. *Occup Environ Med* 1996;**53**:379–86.

64. Kakinoki Y, Ohashi Y, Tanaka A, *et al*. Nitrogen dioxide compromises defence functions of the airway epithelium. *Acta Oto-Laryngol Suppl* 1998;**538**:221–6.

65. Saldiva PH, King M, Delmonte VL, *et al*. Respiratory alterations due to urban air pollution: an experimental study in rats. *Env Res* 1992;**57**:19–33.

66. Harkema JR, Plopper CG, Hyde DM, St George JA, Wilson DW, Dungworth DL. Response of the macaque nasal epithelium to ambient levels of ozone. A morphologic and morphometric study of the transitional and respiratory epithelium. *Am J Pathol* 1987;**128**:29–44.

67. Basbaum C, Gallup M, Gum J, Kim Y, Jany B. Modification of mucin gene expression in the airways of rats exposed to sulfur dioxide. *Biorheology* 1990;**27**:485–9.

68. Jany B, Gallup M, Tsuda T, Basbaum C. Mucin gene expression in rat airways following infection and irritation. *Biochem Biophys Res Commun* 1991;**181**:1–8.

69. Abraham WM, Sielczak MW, Delehunt JC, Marchette B, Wanner A. Impairment of tracheal mucociliary clearance but not ciliary beat frequency by a combination of low level ozone and sulfur dioxide in sheep. *Eur J Respir Dis* 1986;**68**:114–20.

70. Jiang N, Dreher KL, Dye JA, *et al*. Residual oil fly ash induces cytotoxicity and mucin secretion by guinea pig tracheal epithelial cells via an oxidant-mediated mechanism. *Toxicol Appl Pharmacol* 2000;**163**:221–30.

71. Longphre M, Li D, Li J, *et al*. Lung mucin production is stimulated by the air pollutant residual oil fly ash. *Toxicol Appl Pharmacol* 2000;**162**:86–92.

7

Airway responsiveness

A SONIA BUIST

Although hyperresponsiveness has been recognized to be a characteristic of COPD for some time, the question of whether it is a true risk factor (i.e. predates the onset of COPD) or results from the disease process itself has been intensely controversial. Cross-sectional studies, of which there have been many, are unable to disentangle the causal chain in this complex relationship.

Airway hyperresponsiveness is defined as an exaggerated response of the airways to non-specific stimuli, most commonly methacholine or histamine. The key longitudinal studies that have helped to sort out the chicken-or-egg relationship between hyperresponsiveness and COPD will be reviewed here. The two studies that have shed the most light on this complex relationship are the Vlagtwedde–Vlaardingen Cohort Study (VVCS)[1–6] and the Lung Health Study-1 (LHS).[7–10]

Both studies have important strengths that have contributed to our understanding of the natural history of COPD. Major strengths of the VVCS are that it is population based, spans 30 years, and has had outstanding follow-up. Consequently, the external validity of the study is high and the results are generalizable to a broader population. The only disadvantage of the VVCS is the size, since the number of individuals with COPD is somewhat limited. The LHS-1 had the advantages of size (nearly 6000 smokers followed for 5 years), strict standardization of lung function testing, the inclusion of a large number of women smokers and excellent follow-up, but the disadvantage of only including smokers who volunteered for the study. This limits the generalizability of the results but the limitation is probably not likely to distort the findings significantly.

Nevertheless, both studies have accumulated a huge amount of data about airway responsiveness, and are complementary. We are therefore much further ahead in understanding the complex relationship between airway hyperresponsiveness and COPD than we were before the studies were undertaken. The contributions of the two studies to our understanding of hyperresponsiveness and COPD will be described in some detail.

THE VLAGTWEDDE–VLAARDINGEN COHORT STUDY

The Vlagtwedde–Vlaardingen Cohort Study (VVCS) is a cohort study of risk factors for obstructive lung disease performed in random samples of the inhabitants of two Dutch communities.[1–6] The overall study goal has been to identify environmental risk factors in adults that influence the development of mucus hypersecretion and airflow obstruction. The two communities are Vlagtwedde, a rural community in the northeast of The Netherlands, and Vlaardingen, an urban community in the southwest of the country. The study started in 1965 as a random sample of adults in the mid-adult years in both communities: the Vlagtwedde cohort consisted of 450 people aged 40–44 years at recruitment in 1965 and 1793 aged 15–39 years at recruitment in 1967. The Vlaardingen cohort consisted of 859 people aged 40–54 years at recruitment in 1965 and 1590 people aged 15–39 years at recruitment in 1959. After the baseline surveys, the cohorts were followed prospectively every 3 years for a maximum of eight times over a 30-year period.

Longitudinal data spanning 30 years are available from 921 males, providing 2376 paired observations, and 698 females, providing 1682 paired observations. Bronchial responsiveness was assessed using histamine with the threshold value (PC_{10}) defined as the provocative concentration of histamine that caused a decrease of $\geq 10\%$ in the FEV_1 relative to the baseline value. Those with the PC_{10} less than or equal to 8 mg/ml were classified as having increased bronchial hyperresponsiveness.[6]

The key findings of the VVCS are:

- Airway hyperresponsiveness is associated with an accelerated decline in FEV_1.
- Airway hyperresponsiveness is associated with the development and remission of clinical respiratory symptoms.
- Airway hyperresponsiveness predicts mortality from COPD.

The evidence for these conclusions is described below.

Airway hyperresponsiveness is associated with an accelerated decline in FEV$_1$

An analysis of the relationship between airway responsiveness and rate of decline of FEV_1 was carried out after approximately 25 years of follow-up[11] (Table 7.1). These analyses showed that airway hyperresponsiveness was associated with an accelerated decline in FEV_1 in all gender and smoking subgroups. Since these analyses were adjusted for potentially confounding variables such as age, gender, smoking status, baseline FEV_1 and symptom

prevalence, the investigators concluded that airway hyperresponsiveness is significantly and independently associated with an accelerated decline in FEV_1.

Since this was a population-based cohort study and assessment of risk factors and airway responsiveness *preceded* the observation of a decline in lung function, this study provides compelling data that airway responsiveness is indeed a risk factor for an accelerated decline in FEV_1, rather than a result of a disease process. In so far as an accelerated decline in FEV_1 reflects the natural history of COPD, it is reasonable to conclude from these data that airway hyperresponsiveness is a risk factor for the development for COPD.

Airway hyperresponsiveness is associated with the development and remission of chronic respiratory symptoms

In another analysis of the 24-year follow-up data,[6] the investigators explored the relationship between airway responsiveness and the development and remission of chronic respiratory symptoms. The study focused on four respiratory symptoms (cough, phlegm, dyspnea and wheeze) and two diseases (asthma and bronchitis). Standard definitions were used for the respiratory symptoms. This analysis involved data from 1482 men and 1202 women who contributed 7082 observations.

The most striking finding was that individuals with increased airway responsiveness ($PC_{10} \leq 8$ mg/ml histamine) had higher incidence rates for symptoms from the two diseases than those without increased responsiveness

Table 7.1 *Association between airway hyperresponsiveness and decline in FEV_1 ml/yr estimated from multiple linear regression analysis by gender adjusting for FEV_1 residuals, Vlagtwedde–Vlaardingen 1965–1990. (From ref. 11 with permission)*

Smoking status	Male (*n* = 2376)*			Female (*n* = 1682)		
	Coefficient	SEM[†]	*P* value	Coefficient	SEM[†]	*P* value
Hyperresponsiveness	−12.05	3.22	<0.001	−11.50	2.98	0.001
Age 50 yr	−0.33	0.12	<0.001	−0.18	0.14	0.188
Vlaardingen	6.5	2.67	0.016	4.16	2.76	0.133
Former	7.8	4.40	0.076	−0.74	3.54	0.834
Pipe/cigar	−5.69	5.58	0.307	−	−	−
Current <15	−1.59	5.19	0.759	−1.99	4.00	0.619
Current 15–24	−1.51	4.76	0.750	−11.26	4.38	0.010
Current >25	−6.59	5.76	0.253	−8.25	5.68	0.147
Other	11.14	5.75	0.052	3.25	4.94	0.511
Any symptoms[‡]	1.20	3.24	0.711	−0.82	3.88	0.832
FEV_1, 100 ml[§]	−0.025	0.003	0.553	−0.04	0.004	0.254
Intercept	−49.8	5.54	0.171	−28.52	4.20	0.069

*Paired observations.
[†]Standard error of the mean (see 'Methods' in ref. 11).
[‡]For definitions, see 'Methods' in ref. 11.
[§]Residuals of FEV_1 at the beginning of the interval (see 'Methods' in ref. 11).
Current: Cigarettes/day.

(Figure 7.1). The patterns for remission rates were similar except for dyspnea and wheeze for which there was no clear pattern. In a multivariate logistic regression analysis, restricted to participants who did not report any of the four symptoms or two diseases at baseline, adjusted odds ratios for incidence rates for those with and without increased airway responsiveness at baseline were all significant: chronic cough 1.9 (95% CI 1.2–2.9), chronic phlegm 2.0 (95% CI 1.3–3.0), dyspnea ≥ grade 3, 2.3 (95% CI 1.5–3.5), persistent wheeze 2.7 (95% CI 1.7–4.4), asthmatic attacks 3.7 (95% CI 2.2–6.1), bronchitis 1.4 (95% CI 1.0–2.0). The adjusted odds ratios for any symptom was 1.7 (95% CI 1.2–2.3). Interestingly, smokers with increased airway responsiveness were no more susceptible to the development of respiratory symptoms than comparable non-smokers. Adjusted odds ratios for the remission of the same symptoms and diseases were mostly similar, but the confidence intervals were broader.

A question that arises from these data is whether the results are due to the inclusion of individuals with asthma. To evaluate this, all of the analyses were repeated excluding asthmatics. There were no changes in the findings. The investigators conclude from this interesting analysis that airway responsiveness represents a genetic susceptibility to environmental inflammatory stimuli, such as allergens and cigarette smoke exposure.

Airway hyperresponsiveness predicts mortality from COPD

When the VVCS had reached 30 years of follow-up, the investigators were able to explore the relationship between mortality from COPD and airway responsiveness. For this analysis, an additional community, Meppel, was included.[12] Vital status of the cohort was assessed for 99% with only 29 individuals lost to follow-up. Causes of death were obtained from Statistics Netherlands, the national database, with the primary and secondary causes of death coded according to the International Classification of Diseases. The associations of airway responsiveness with all-cause and cause-specific mortality were estimated using Cox's proportional hazards model. Because of the small number of deaths due to COPD when COPD was restricted to the primary cause of death, COPD as a secondary cause of death was also included. The analysis controlled for sex, age, FEV_1% predicted, smoking, body mass index, city, history of asthma attacks, eosinophilia and skin test positivity. Of the 2008 individuals included in this analysis, 30.8% had airway hyperresponsiveness to histamine at the start of the study. Those with severe hyperresponsiveness (threshold 1 mg/ml) had a significantly higher risk of all-cause mortality than those without, relative risk 15.8 (95% CI, 3.72–67.1). Figure 7.2 shows the survival curve for individuals with severe hyperresponsiveness (1 mg/ml) compared to those who had normal responsiveness.

When the analyses were repeated excluding individuals without a history of asthma attacks, the direction and significance of these associations were unchanged.

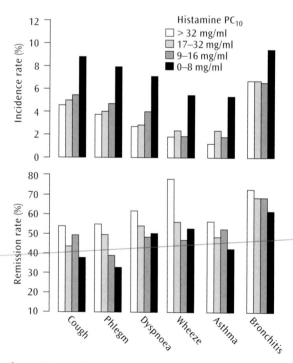

Figure 7.1 *Development and remission of six respiratory symptoms of interest. (From ref. 6.)*

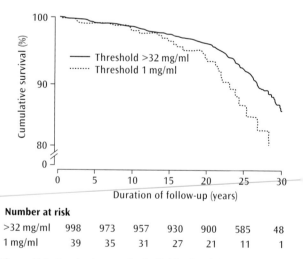

Figure 7.2 *Survival curve for individuals with severe histamine airway hyperresponsiveness and individuals with no histamine threshold, 1964–72. Adjusted for sex, age, smoking, lung function, eosinophilia, positive skin tests, asthma and city (Vlagtwedde, Vlaardingen, Meppel). (From ref. 12.)*

Interestingly, although the trend for increased mortality was more pronounced in smokers, the trend was also present in never-smokers. The investigators calculated that the relative risks for mortality from COPD associated with airway hyperresponsiveness were roughly equivalent to the relative risks associated with cigarette smoking and low lung function. The fact that this trend exists in never-smokers as well as smokers is intriguing and raises many questions about the genes determining airway responsiveness and the subsequent gene–environment interaction.

THE LUNG HEALTH STUDY-1

The Lung Health Study-1 (LHS-1) was a multicenter prospective randomized clinical trial carried out in nine centers in the USA and one in Canada. The LHS-1 was designed to determine if ipratropium bromide and smoking cessation slowed the rate of decline of FEV_1 over 5 years in smokers with mild–moderate COPD.[7,8] The study involved 5887 smokers, aged 35–60 years with an FEV_1/FVC ratio less than 0.7 and $FEV_1\%$ predicted less than 80%. Follow-up was 5 years with annual clinic visits. Methacholine inhalation challenge was performed at baseline and at the 9-month and 33-month follow-up visits.[9,10]

The key findings of the LHS-1 in relation to airway hyperresponsiveness and COPD are:

- Airway hyperresponsiveness occurs in the majority of individuals with mild–moderate COPD.
- Airway hyperresponsiveness is a risk factor for accelerated decline in lung function.
- Airway hyperresponsiveness is more strongly related to rates of decline of lung function in women than men.

Airway hyperresponsiveness occurs in almost all men and women with mild–moderate COPD

Perhaps the most surprising observations stemming from the baseline visit (methacholine challenge data available for 5666 participants) were that the vast majority of study participants had increased airway responsiveness, and that there was a striking gender difference in bronchial responsiveness. When the Lung Health Study was planned, the initial estimate, during the planning phase, was that approximately 25% of eligible participants would demonstrate bronchial hyperresponsiveness (defined as a $\geq 20\%$ decline in FEV_1 in response to ≤ 25 mg/ml methacholine). The finding, therefore, that 87% of women in the LHS-1 and 62.5% of men demonstrated bronchial hyperresponsiveness was unexpected

(Figure 7.3).[13] This gender difference was apparent at all concentrations of methacholine.

The reasons for these gender differences were explored with the Cox proportional-hazards model, using a sequence of models with gender as a covariate in each model. Addition of baseline FEV_1 to the model, as a surrogate for airway caliber, eliminated the gender effect (Table 7.2). The conclusion drawn from this was that airway caliber is an important determinant for airway hyperresponsiveness, and the gender differences in airway caliber explain the gender differences in airway hyperresponsiveness in the LHS.

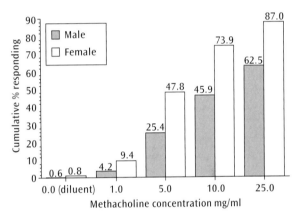

Figure 7.3 *Cumulative percentage of males and females responding to increasing concentrations of methacholine with a positive response at each concentration being defined as a $\geq 20\%$ decline in FEV_1. Baseline was the postdiluent value except for the response to diluent, in which case the prediluent value was used. (From ref. 13.)*

Table 7.2 *Relative risk estimates and 95% confidence intervals for females being more likely than males to react to methacholine according to variables entered into the Cox proportional-hazards model. (From ref. 9 with permission)*

Variables	Relative risk of AHR for female gender	95% confidence interval
Model 1: age, gender, pack-years, height and weight	1.75	(1.60, 1.92)
Model 2: Model 1 plus FEV_1	1.06	(0.96, 1.18)
Model 3: Model 2 plus FVC	1.29	(1.16, 1.43)
Model 4: Model 2 plus FEV_1/FVC	1.31	(1.18, 1.46)

AHR: airway hyperresponsiveness.

Bronchial hyperresponsiveness as a risk factor for accelerated decline in lung function

The question of whether bronchial hyperresponsiveness is a risk factor for an accelerated decline in lung function, or a consequence of the structural changes that occur in the airway walls in COPD, requires longitudinal follow-up of a cohort, preferably from health to disease.[10] The LHS-1 provides part of this, but not all, since all LHS-1 participants already had mild–moderate airflow limitation at the beginning of the study. Within these limitations, the LHS-1 was clearly able to demonstrate that bronchial hyperresponsiveness was a strong predictor of change in FEV_1, after controlling for baseline lung function, age, sex, baseline smoking history and changes in smoking status (Figure 7.4).

In the LHS-1 data set, significant interactions were found between airway responsiveness and smoking behavior. This was manifested by differences between quitters and smokers as a function of airway responsiveness. Participants who quit smoking in the first year showed improvement in FEV_1, whereas those who continued to smoke showed a decline in FEV_1. In subsequent years (one through five) lung function declined in both quitters and continuing smokers, but to a greater extent in those who continued to smoke than in sustained quitters. To illustrate the interaction between airway responsiveness and smoking, continuing smokers in the highest quintile of responsiveness lost 2.2% (women) or 1.7% (men) of FEV_1% predicted from year 1 to year 5, whereas those in the lowest quintile lost only 0.94% (women) or 0.74% (men) of FEV_1% predicted. In comparison, the sustained quitters with the highest baseline reactivity showed considerably less loss in FEV_1% predicted from year 1 to year 5 (men 0.5%; women 0.64%) in comparison to the least reactive continuing smokers. The quitters in the lowest reactivity group showed minimal changes in FEV_1% predicted (men, +0.42%; women, −0.06%).

MECHANISMS OF HYPERRESPONSIVENESS IN COPD

Since airway hyperresponsiveness is not helpful in the diagnosis of COPD, or very helpful in assessing the response to treatment, there has been relatively little attention paid to understanding the underlying mechanisms. Two major hypotheses have been put forward to explain the presence of airway hyperresponsiveness in individuals with COPD.

'The Dutch hypothesis' was first proposed by Orie and Van der Lende in the early 1960s.[14–16] According to this hypothesis, airway hyperresponsiveness reflects a genetic predisposition to excessive airway narrowing in response to inhaled bronchoconstrictor agents, and it is this genetic predisposition that leads to the eventual development of chronic airflow limitation in individuals who are exposed to noxious inhaled particles or gases. This hypothesis has been intensely controversial. This is good because it has stimulated a lot of thought, discussion and studies that have tried to address it. Underlying this hypothesis is the notion that airway hyperresponsiveness, which is a characteristic of asthma, is a risk factor for the development of clinically significant COPD. The causal pathway in this is not, however, clear. For example, is airway hyperresponsiveness related independently to asthma and to COPD, or do asthma genes (including genes for airway hyperresponsiveness) increase risk for COPD?[17]

Mullen and coworkers[18] were the first to show that airway hyperresponsiveness in a group of patients with COPD was related to their baseline FEV_1, and to a semi-quantitative index that measured the inflammation of their peripheral airways. Later work from the same group[19] extended these findings with evidence that airway hyperresponsiveness in COPD is a *result* of the

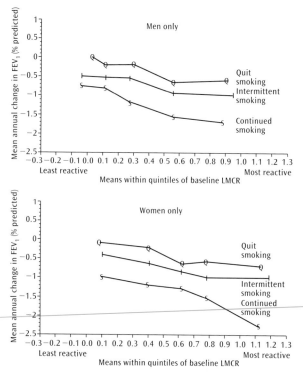

Figure 7.4 *Mean annual change from year 1 to year 5 in FEV_1% predicted versus methacholine reactivity by smoking status at the last annual visit for men and women separately and for all treatment groups combined. LMCR: log methacholine reactivity. (From ref. 10.)*

structural changes within the airway wall, rather than occur in COPD and cause airflow limitation.

This conclusion came from a study in which non-specific bronchial responsiveness to methacholine was assessed in 77 smokers with mild to moderate COPD prior to resection of a pulmonary nodule.[19] When they related airway responsiveness to baseline lung function and to functional and morphometric markers of lung elasticity, and to small airway thickening, they found that airway responsiveness was significantly related to $FEV_1\%$ predicted and lung recoil pressure at total lung capacity (PLmax). After adjusting for these functional parameters, airway responsiveness was inversely related to airway wall thickness. There was also a trend for the most responsive individuals to have fewer alveolar attachments on the airway walls.

SUMMARY

The population-based and morphometric studies described above have brought us a long way towards sorting out the chicken-and-egg relationship of airway responsiveness and COPD. We now know that airway hyperresponsiveness is very strongly dependent on airway diameter in COPD, and that gender differences in airway diameter are largely responsible for gender differences in airway hyperresponsiveness. We also have good evidence now that airway hyperresponsiveness is a *consequence* of the structural changes in the airways and lung parenchyma in COPD. It is therefore a marker of the degree of airway narrowing and of the pathophysiologic changes causing airflow limitation in COPD: airway inflammation and thickening, and loss in lung elastic recoil.

REFERENCES

1. Rijcken B, Schouten JP, Weiss ST, Speizer FE, Van der Lende R. The relationship of nonspecific bronchial responsiveness to respiratory symptoms in random population sample. *Am Rev Respir Dis* 1987;**136**:62–8.
2. Rijcken B, Schouten JP, Weiss ST, Meinesz AF, De Vries K, Van der Lende R. The distribution of bronchial responsiveness to histamine in symptomatic and asymptomatic subjects. A population based analysis of various indices of responsiveness. *Am Rev Respir Dis* 1989;**140**:615–23.
3. Rijcken B, Schouten JP, Weiss ST, Speizer FE, Van der Lende R. The relationship between airway responsiveness to histamine and pulmonary function level in a random population sample. *Am Rev Respir Dis* 1988;**137**:826–32.
4. Xu X, Laird N, Dockery DW, Schouten JP, Rijcken B, Weiss ST. Age, period and cohort effects on pulmonary function in a 24-year longitudinal study. *Am J Epidemiol* 1995;**141**:554–66.
5. Xu X, Weiss ST, Dockery DW, Schouten JP, Rijcken B. Comparing FEV_1 in adults in two community based studies. *Chest* 1995;**108**:656–62.
6. Xu X, Rijcken B, Schouten JP, Weiss ST. Airways responsiveness and development and remission of chronic respiratory symptoms in adults. *Lancet* 1997;**350**:1431–4.
7. Buist AS, Connett JE, Miller RD, Kanner RE, Owens GR, Voelker HT. Chronic obstructive pulmonary disease early intervention trial (Lung Health Study). *Chest* 1993;**103**: 1863–72.
8. Anthonisen NR, Connett JE, Kiley JP, *et al.* Effects of smoking intervention and use of an inhaled anticholinergic bronchodilator on the rate of decline in FEV_1 (The Lung Health Study). *JAMA* 1994;**272**:1497–51.
9. Tashkin DP, Altose MD, Bleecker ER, *et al.* The Lung Health Study: airway responsiveness to inhaled methacholine in smokers with mild to moderate airflow limitation. *Lung Health Study* 1991;**145**:301–10.
10. Tashkin DP, Altose MD, Connett JE, Kanner RE, Lee WW, Wise RA, for the Lung Health Study Research Group. Methacholine reactivity predicts changes in lung function over time in smokers with early chronic obstruction pulmonary disease. *Am J Respir Crit Care Med* 1996;**153**: 1802–11.
11. Rijcken B, Schouten JP, Xu X, Rosner B, Weiss ST. Airway hyperresponsiveness to histamine associated with accelerated decline in FEV_1. *Am J Respir Crit Care Med* 1995;**151**:1377–82.
12. Hospers JJ, Postma DS, Rijcken B, Weiss ST, Schouten JP. Histamine airway hyperresponsiveness and mortality from chronic obstructive disease: a cohort study. *Lancet* 2000;**356**:1313–18.
13. Kanner RE, Connett JE, Altose MD, *et al.* Gender differences in airway hyperresponsiveness in smokers with mild COPD (The Lung Health Study). *Am J Respir Crit Care Med* 1994;**150**: 956–61.
14. Orie NGM, Sluiter HJ, De Vries K, Tammeling GJ, Witkop J. The host factor in bronchitis. *Bronchitis: an international symposium, 27–29 April 1960*. University Groningen. Royal van Gorcum, Assen, 1961;43–59.
15. Postma DS, Kerstjens HA. Characteristics of airway hyperresponsiveness in asthma and chronic obstructive pulmonary disease. *Am J Respir Crit Care Med* 1998;**158**: S187–92.
16. Sluiter HJ, Koeter GH, De Monchy JGR, Postma DS, De Vries K, Orie NGM. The Dutch hypothesis (chronic nonspecific lung disease) revisited. *Eur Respir J* 1991;**4**:479–89.
17. Meyers DA. Genetics of airway responsiveness and atopy. In: ST Weiss, D Sparrow, eds. *Airway Responsiveness and Atopy in the Development of Chronic Lung Disease*. Raven, New York, 1989, pp 157–80.
18. Mullen JBM, Wiggs BR, Wright JL, Hogg JC, Pare PD. Nonspecific airway reactivity in cigarette smokers: relationship to airway pathology and baseline lung function. *Am Rev Respir Dis* 1986;**1**:120–5.
19. Riess A, Wiggs B, Verburgt L, Wright JL, Hogg JC, Pare PD. Morphologic determinants of airway responsiveness in chronic smokers. *Am J Respir Crit Care Med* 1996;**154**:1444–9.

8

Infection

ADAM HILL AND ROBERT A STOCKLEY

INTRODUCTION

The lung has an extensive and sophisticated defence system that ensures that the lower airways remain sterile. In COPD bacteria often colonize the airways and may be associated with inflammation or the development of acute exacerbations. The mechanisms involved and the implications of the bacterial/host interactions are largely unknown. The current chapter outlines these inter-actions and explores the implications for patients with COPD.

ANTIBACTERIAL DEFENCES IN THE NORMAL AIRWAY

The normal respiratory tract is kept sterile despite being exposed daily to 7000 liters of air containing inorganic and organic particulate material as well as potential pathogenic bacteria and viruses. This is achieved initially by the primary host defences including bronchial mucus, the mucociliary escalator and the integrity of the airway epithelium (Figure 8.1). Animal models have shown that primary host defences are able to clear bacterial loads of up to 2×10^5 colony forming units per ml[1] with little or no activation of the secondary host defences. At higher bacterial loads, the secondary host defences are activated,

which is likely to reflect the release of pro-inflammatory mediators, resulting in an acute inflammatory response with recruitment of neutrophils which helps clear the bacteria.[2,3]

Bronchial secretions

The bronchial secretions protect the epithelium by forming a barrier, trapping and removing inhaled particles as a result of ciliary activity, and acting as a vehicle for immunoglobulins and other antibacterial proteins. Bronchial secretions consist of a mucus layer which rests on an aqueous layer and is moved by the insertion of the tips of cilia during the forward phase of beating. The gel phase consists of about 95% water, 1% salt, 1–3% proteins and mucoglycoproteins, and 1–3% proteoglycans and lipids.[4] Many proteins have been identified in the sputum sol phase including plasma proteins, immunoglobulins, antibacterial proteins and cytokines particularly when inflammation is present.

The mucus gel acts as a barrier for bacteria, which adhere to it and can subsequently multiply within it.[5] Mucins have chemical receptors and glycolipids that can bind to the adhesins on many bacteria. The adhesins on common respiratory pathogens include the pilin proteins in fimbriae, mucoid exopolysaccharide, hemagglutinins, internal lectins, exoenzyme S and non-pilus

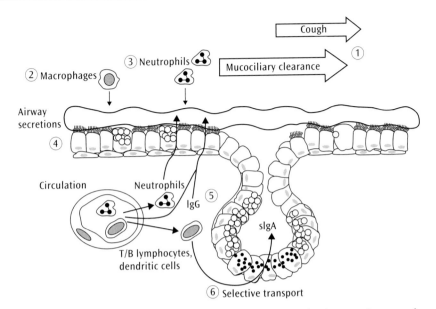

Figure 8.1 *Host defences of the respiratory tract. 1 = mucus secreted by mucous glands trap micro-organisms and are cleared by the mucociliary escalator and cough. Secretions also contain antibacterial proteins such as lysozyme, defensins and SLPI. 2 = Resident airway macrophages clear organisms by phagocytosis but also release complement, β defensins and other pro-inflammatory cytokines including neutrophil chemoattractants. 3 = Neutrophils recruited into the airways play a key role in the secondary host defence. 4 = Epithelial cells restrict colonization and release pro-inflammatory cytokines and chemoattractants. 5 = Protein transudation for passive transport of local and systemic immunoglobulins and other serum proteins including antiproteases. 6 = Specific transport mechanisms for secretory IgA and release of local proteins such as SLPI.*

protein components.[6,7] The respiratory pathogens that bind strongly to mucus include *Streptococcus pneumoniae*, *Haemophilus influenzae*, *Staphylococcus aureus* and *Pseudomonas aeruginosa*. This may facilitate clearance of the bacteria by removing them with the mucus. Alternatively this binding mechanism will also retain bacteria in the airway when clearance is defective.

In recent years a variety of antimicrobial peptides have been identified and shown to play a key role in bacterial killing as well as being mediators of inflammation. They can influence processes as diverse as cell proliferation, wound healing, cell damage, cytokine release and redox homostasis. In the airways β-defensins and the cathelicidin LL-37/h CAP-18 originate from neutrophils and are involved in secondary defence. On the other hand the β-defensins as well as LL-37/h CAP-18 are produced by respiratory epithelial cells and alveolar macrophages and secreted into the airway surface fluids. The β-defensins are 36–42 residues in length and, like all peptides in this class, interact with bacterial cell walls electrostatically resulting in destabilization. At present there are few studies of the β-defensins although they are increased in response to infection[8] and can be generated *in vitro* by epithelial cells in the presence of tumor necrosis factor alpha (TNF-α), interleukin 1β (IL-1β) and bacteria.[9] Other proteins from the lung secretions participate in airway bacterial defence. Transferrin and lactoferrin bind and thus exclude iron from the bacteria

and hence impair their proliferation. Lysozyme is capable of attacking the carbohydrate polymers comprising the external membrane of bacteria and can disrupt the cell wall leading to bacterial death.[10,11] In addition, the lactoperoxidase system is thought to be important in bacterial clearance and functions by forming biocidal compounds.[12,13] The antiprotease secretory leukoprotease inhibitor (SLPI) has a broad spectrum of antibiotic properties that include antiretroviral, bactericidal, and antifungal activity.[14] This protein is produced locally in the lung by epithelial cells,[15] and is present in serous glands[16,17] and Clara cells.[18] A recent study has demonstrated that the antibacterial potency of airway secretions may be the result of synergistic and additive interactions between several antimicrobial factors.[19]

Mucociliary clearance

The tracheobronchial epithelium consists mainly of ciliated cells, although these are reduced in number at the bronchiolar level.[20,21] The clearance of normal mucus with any entrapped material depends mainly on ciliary activity.[22–25] The function of cilia can be impaired by proteases (such as neutrophil elastase released from the activated neutrophil and the elastase from *P. aeruginosa*)[6,26] as well as other bacterial products such as 1-hydroxyphenazine and pyocyanin.[27]

Immune system

The immunoglobulins are relatively large molecules which limits their ability to diffuse from plasma. Thus in the absence of inflammation most of the immunoglobulin detected in lung secretions represents that made locally and secreted by B-lymphocytes around the bronchial glands.[28] There is an active transport mechanism for the passage of dimeric immunoglobulin A into the lumen of the lung. Immunoglobulin A (IgA) is an important component of bronchial mucus and the predominant immunoglobulin in the upper respiratory tract and central airways.[29] On the other hand IgG and IgM contribute little at this site but are the major immunoglobulins in the more peripheral airways.[30]

In the lung most of the IgA is present as a dimer (linked by a peptide called the J chain), 70% is of the IgA 1 subclass and the remainder IgA 2 subclass. The dimeric form is transported across the epithelial cell by the polymeric IgA receptor, which is cleaved at the cell surface releasing the dimer attached to the secretory component of the receptor. IgA can prevent the epithelial adherence of bacteria and viruses but also has other effects such as enhancing macrophage phagocytosis[31] and facilitating antibody-dependent cell-mediated cytotoxicity in synergism with IgG.[32]

Cells

In health, the major phagocyte in the airways is the macrophage and accounts for approximately 95% of the total cells recovered by lung lavage in health.[33] It provides a continuous phagocytic role in the lung and probably initiates and maintains the secondary defence when local defences have been breached. Neutrophils, on the other hand, are rarely found in the airways in health but are rapidly recruited in inflammation for phagocytosis. In addition, monocytes recruited to sites of inflammation may also play an important role in the inflammatory process. A subpopulation (20–30%) of circulating monocytes have neutrophil-like pro-inflammatory properties (P phenotype), including avid adherence to the extracellular matrix, the ability to produce reactive oxygen species, high neutrophil elastase content, and proteolytic activity against elastin and fibronectin.[34,35] These pro-inflammatory monocytes have considerably higher phagocytic activity than other monocytes and also lack the HLA-DR antigen, which means they cannot participate in specific immune responses. It is thought to be this neutrophil-like pro-inflammatory subpopulation that is recruited rapidly by chemoattractants to sites of inflammation, where they can either promote resolution of inflammation or contribute to tissue injury in a similar way to the neutrophil.

Intraepithelial lymphocytes are regularly present alone or in groups in the normal healthy epithelium[36] and function to remove allergenic particles from the airways. They consist of mainly T cells (>90%), with the remainder comprising up to 10% B-lymphocytes and 1% natural killer cells.[37] The T-cell surface markers identified in the normal bronchial epithelium include the universal lymphocyte marker CD3+, as well as the more specific CD4+ and CD8+ cells although the latter predominates[38] unlike in the lamina propria where CD4+ cells predominate.[39] The CD4+ cells activate mononuclear phagocytosis and promote proliferation and differentiation of B cells, whereas the CD8+ cells demonstrate cytotoxic or suppressor activity. The CD8+ cells may limit infection through their cytotoxic activity but can also limit damage caused as a byproduct of prolonged immunity-related inflammation by suppressing the immune response. The immunostimulation of resting T-lymphocytes is thought to require the initial presentation of antigen in association with class II major histocompatibility complex (Ia) molecules expressed by normal dendritic cells.[40]

Airway wall

If the layer of the mucus overlying the epithelium is inadequate to protect the mucosa, the airway epithelium presents the next important barrier.[41,42] Measurement of the permeability of radiolabeled tracers through the epithelium or the airway mucosa supports the view that the epithelium is a major barrier,[43,44] especially to hydrophilic molecules. The epithelium is also a major barrier to macromolecules and, in healthy airways, horseradish peroxidase placed on the apical surface penetrates the epithelium only up to the tight junctions between cells.[45] However, if the tight junctions are opened by the effect of histamine or cigarette smoke, the peroxidase penetrates through the epithelium to the basement membrane.[45,46]

Bacteria are more likely to adhere to mucus than to undisrupted epithelium provided the latter is healthy.[5–7] Most respiratory pathogens, apart from *Mycoplasma pneumoniae* and *Bordatella pertussis*, do not adhere to epithelium until it has been damaged by toxins or proteases.[47,48] However, following damage, airway pathogens such as non-typeable *H. influenzae*, *S. pneumoniae* and *S. aureus* adhere readily to both ciliated and non-ciliated cells.[6,49,50]

PATHOLOGY OF COPD THAT PREDISPOSES TO BACTERIAL COLONIZATION

In patients with COPD there is alteration to the host defences including inflammation of the airway wall,[51] hypersecretion of mucus, goblet cell hyperplasia, enlargement of tracheobronchial submucosal glands and a disproportionate increase in acidic mucus.[52–55] The mucus-secreting goblet cells are increased in the bronchi and bronchioles (which can become blocked by the secretions) but not in the terminal or respiratory bronchioles.[56–57] Other epithelial changes may include atrophy, focal squamous metaplasia, ciliary abnormalities, and decreases in both ciliated cell number and mean ciliary length.[58] The net effect of these changes will be to impair mucociliary clearance[59] and thereby predispose to bacterial colonization.

Inflammation

Patients with COPD have evidence of persistent airway inflammation. Early studies indicated that the inflammatory process in the bronchial mucosa of subjects with COPD was characterized predominantly by macrophages and activated T-lymphocytes.[51,60–62] Bronchial biopsies demonstrated that the inflammatory process often persisted even after smoking cessation, in subjects who continue to have symptoms of chronic bronchitis.[63] More recently Di Stefano and colleagues studied smokers with COPD with a wide range of airflow limitation and found that patients with COPD with severe airflow limitation ($FEV_1 < 50\%$ predicted) also had increased numbers of neutrophils, macrophages and natural killer (NK) lymphocytes in the lamina propria. Furthermore, the FEV_1 correlated inversely with the numbers of neutrophils, macrophages and NK lymphocytes[64] and the authors postulated that neutrophils could be of importance in disease progression.

Increased numbers of neutrophils have been identified in bronchial lavage and bronchoalveolar lavage fluid from patients with COPD.[65,66] Adhesion molecules are critical for neutrophil migration from the vascular space into the lung. Studies of patients with COPD with airway obstruction have shown an increase in the vascular adhesion molecule E-selectin on submucosal vessels, intercellular adhesion molecule 1 (ICAM-1) on bronchial epithelium[67] and β2-integrin (Mac-1) on sputum neutrophils.[68] In addition, Mac-1 expression has been shown to correlate negatively with the FEV_1/VC ratio, and Maestrelli and colleagues suggested that this represented a marker for smokers who develop COPD. Also Riise and colleagues[69] found that patients with COPD had increased levels of soluble ICAM-1 both in serum and in bronchial lavage. These studies generally indicate involvement and activation of adhesion molecules in the pathogenesis of COPD.

Role of the neutrophil

It is generally accepted that patients with COPD have evidence of persistent airway inflammation with neutrophil recruitment. Activation of the neutrophils releases proteolytic enzymes which can impair several of the primary host defences and thus predispose to bacterial colonization. Neutrophil elastase is produced during the early stages of neutrophil differentiation, stored within the azurophil granules,[70] and released when the neutrophil is activated. Both *in vitro* and *in vivo* studies have demonstrated that neutrophil elastase can cause epithelial damage,[71] reduce ciliary beat frequency,[72] produce mucus gland hyperplasia[73] and stimulate mucus secretion.[74] In addition neutrophil elastase can inactivate other more specific lung host defences such as a major phagocytic receptor on the neutrophil itself (C3bi)[75] and immunoglobulins,[76] thereby reducing opsonophagocytosis. Neutrophil elastase can also reduce secretion of its own inhibitor (SLPI) *in vitro*,[77] and this is consistent with data obtained *in vivo*.[78] The net effect not only results in persistence of elastase activity but also reduces any antibacterial or antiviral action of this protein. Indeed recent studies have shown that subjects with recurrent exacerbations (which are often bacterial or viral in origin) have low secretion concentrations of SLPI, supporting the concept that it does play a key role in host defence.[79] Finally neutrophil elastase can amplify the whole inflammatory process by releasing the neutrophil chemoattractants IL-8[80] and leukotriene B4,[81] resulting in continued recruitment of neutrophils and hence further elastase release. Neutrophil elastase therefore can produce many of the pathologic processes seen in COPD and at the same time damage many facets of the host defences resulting in a predisposition to bacterial colonization and infection and thereafter amplify the whole sequence of events further (Figure 8.2).

Smoking

Smoking cigarettes is central to the pathogenesis of COPD in most patients and may be a further mediator to promote bacterial colonization. Smoke also induces mucosal gland hypertrophy[82–84] and increases mucus secretion. This, together with an inhibitory effect of cigarette smoke on the bronchial ciliary blanket reducing tracheal mucus velocity,[85] will predispose to the accumulation of mucus in the bronchial tree.

Cigarette smoke is also associated with an increase in lung neutrophils as seen in bronchoalveolar lavage fluid[86] and this may be the result of several distinct mechanisms. Firstly, cigarette smoke has been shown to stimulate bronchial epithelial cells to produce the important neutrophil chemoattractant IL-8,[87] and indeed current smokers have been found to have raised IL-8 levels in their airway secretions.[88] Secondly, nicotine has been shown to be a neutrophil chemoattractant *in vitro*.[89] Finally, cigarette smoke can stimulate alveolar macrophages to

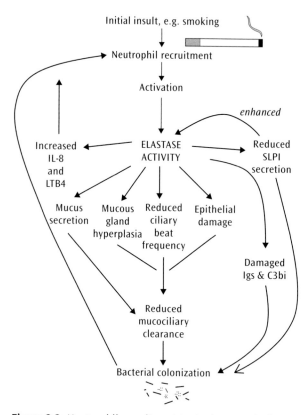

release neutrophil chemoattractants.[86] Whatever the mechanism neutrophils are increased especially in the lungs of smokers with airflow obstruction[64,90] and the number is related to the amount smoked.[91]

Smokers with airflow obstruction also have increased expression of adhesion molecules including E selectin on submucosal vessels,[67] ICAM-1 in bronchial epithelium,[67] and the β2-integrin CD11b/CD18 on airway neutrophils.[68] All these adhesion molecules are likely to be critical in the process of neutrophil migration from the vascular space into the lung. *In vitro* studies have demonstrated that oxidants,[92] but not nicotine,[93] from cigarette smoke can reduce neutrophil deformability, which should restrict the ability of these cells to pass through the pulmonary circulation. This is consistent with *in vivo* studies showing a delay in neutrophil transit time in lungs immediately after smoking.[94] This 'slowing' of neutrophil transit may facilitate endothelial adhesion and migration into the lung in response to local chemoattractants (Figure 8.3).

Summary

Patients with COPD have an ongoing inflammatory response that can be perpetuated by smoking. The neutrophil is thought to be of central importance in this process and patients with COPD have increased neutrophil numbers in the lung with increased expression of adhesion molecules involved in cell migration. The activated neutrophil releases proteases that can potentially impair many aspects of the primary host defences and hence predispose patients to bacterial colonization. Evidence of specific immune defects in COPD is generally lacking, although patients do show impairment of mucociliary clearance *in vivo*.[59] Thus at least this primary defence mechanism is defective and will compromise airway sterilization facilitating bacterial colonization.

Figure 8.2 *Neutrophil recruitment to the lung results in release of neutrophil elastase. The enzyme then has the potential to damage epithelium and ciliary beating whilst causing excess mucus production. The net effect is reduced mucociliary clearance and this facilitates bacterial colonization. At the same time elastase damages other more specific host defences and decreases SLPI secretion thereby facilitating its own activity and decreasing any antibacterial function of SLPI. Bacterial colonization leads to more neutrophil recruitment and this may be amplified by chemoattractant release by the neutrophil and via the activity of elastase resulting in a self-perpetuating cycle of inflammation and damage.*

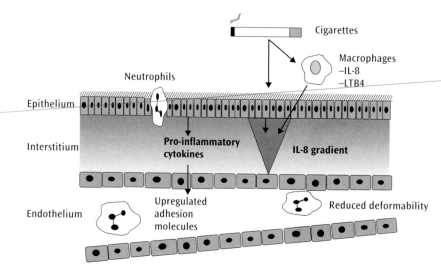

Figure 8.3 *Cigarette smoking promotes neutrophil influx by (i) stimulating the bronchial epithelium to release interleukin 8 (IL-8), (ii) stimulating airway macrophages to release the neutrophil chemoattractants IL-8 and leukotriene B4 (LTB4), (iii) upregulating adhesion molecules, and finally (iv) reducing neutrophil deformity.*

BACTERIAL COLONIZATION IN COPD

Despite the presence of airway inflammation associated with COPD and the presence of an overactive immune system, some patients with COPD are unable to maintain a sterile airway and bacterial colonization occurs. The bacteria isolated are generally considered to be of low pathogenicity (*Haemophilus* species, non-typeable *H. influenzae* and *Haemophilus parainfluenzae*, *S. pneumoniae*, and *Moraxella catarrhalis*) but may themselves facilitate the process of colonization by inactivation of host defences. For instance, bacterial products can interfere with the chemotactic response inhibiting neutrophil migration[95] and thus the antibacterial potential of phagocytosis by these cells. In addition, bacteria may impair other features of the primary host defences, thus facilitating their persistence in the airways. These may include:

- Interference with ciliary function via cilia toxins such as pyocyanin and hydroxyphenazine.[27]
- Production of excess mucus[96] by several bacterial species including *H. influenzae*, *S. aureus*, *S. pneumoniae* and *P. aeruginosa* due to secretion of proteases and rhamnolipids.[97,98] This process could be advantageous to the host if it promotes bacterial binding and greater clearance of mucus from the airway by cough and normal mucociliary clearance. However it could also be a disadvantage if it leads to blockage of the smaller airways, impairment of mucociliary clearance, thereby becoming a reservoir for bacterial multiplication.
- Direct damage to the epithelium by bacterial enzymes thereby facilitating bacterial adherence.[71]
- Inhibition of the immune response as a result of a variety of bacterial products.[99] For instance mucoid exopolysaccharide from *P. aeruginosa* can act as a barrier to phagocytes and inhibit antibody and complement binding; proteolytic enzymes can inactivate opsonophagocytosis; pyocyanin can inhibit lymphocyte proliferation; exotoxin A can both inhibit macrophage and granulocyte progenitor cell proliferation and be cytotoxic to macrophages; leukocidin is cytotoxic to neutrophils and lymphocytes and finally lipase can inhibit monocyte chemotaxis and oxidative burst.
- Evasion of the immune response by changing the antigenic nature of bacteria during colonization[100] thus facilitating their survival.

From collective studies, a current hypothesis is that once significant bacterial colonization of the airways occurs, activation of secondary host defences and the development of inflammation should take place which would normally result in clearance of the bacteria. However, if this secondary response fails to sterilize the bronchial tree, continued bacterial proliferation can occur resulting in a

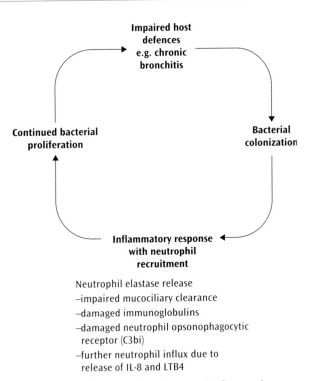

Neutrophil elastase release
–impaired mucociliary clearance
–damaged immunoglobulins
–damaged neutrophil opsonophagocytic receptor (C3bi)
–further neutrophil influx due to release of IL-8 and LTB4

Figure 8.4 *The vicious cycle of bronchial inflammation related to a failure of the inflammatory response to eradicate bacterial colonization.*

vicious circle of tissue damage (Figure 8.4). In this circle, both the bacteria (described earlier) and the inflammatory response itself may play a role in the persistence of bacterial colonization by reducing the efficacy of the host defences further and causing progressive tissue damage indirectly.

Patients who are chronically colonized often have increased serum immunoglobulin concentrations with increased immunoglobulins in their secretions, including IgG_1, IgG_2, IgG_3 and IgG_4 subclasses.[101] The lung tissues contain increased numbers of T-lymphocytes, predominantly of the CD8+ phenotype.[102] This suggests an active but ineffective immune response as the bacterial load exceeds the protective capacity of the immune system. Studies of the immune system have failed to identify any significant immune defects, although in some patients the production of the wrong subclass of immunoglobulin (IgG_2) may actually hinder bacterial clearance by conventional phagocytosis.[103]

BACTERIA ISOLATED FROM PATIENTS WITH STABLE COPD

One of the difficulties in determining the importance of bacterial colonization of the lung is distinguishing lower respiratory tract colonization from contamination of secretions by the upper airway (nasopharyngeal) flora.

Recent studies have used the protective specimen brush (PSB) to avoid this problem, using the flexible fiberoptic bronchoscope. Studies have assumed that isolation of bacterial loads larger than 10^3 colony forming units/ml represent evidence of colonization.

Monso studied 40 patients with stable COPD (mean FEV_1 51% predicted) and found that 25% were colonized[104] with *H. influenzae* and *S. pneumoniae* as the commonest bacteria. A later study by the same author comprising 41 patients with stable chronic bronchitis (11 with normal lung function, 25 with an $FEV_1 > 50$% predicted, and five patients with an $FEV_1 < 50$% predicted) found that 22% were colonized, mainly with non-typeable *H. influenzae*, *Streptococcus viridans* and *S. pneumoniae*.[105] In a different study of 52 patients with stable COPD (28 with mild COPD – $FEV_1 > 50$% predicted; 11 with moderate COPD – FEV_1 35–50% predicted and 13 with severe COPD – $FEV_1 < 35$% predicted), Soler *et al.*[106] found bacterial colonization in 33% of patients and confirmed that *H. influenzae*, *S. viridans*, *S. pneumoniae*, *S. aureus* and *M. catarrhalis* were the most frequent organisms. Finally Zalacain *et al.* studied 88 patients with stable COPD (26 with mild COPD – $FEV_1 > 65$% predicted; 36 with moderate COPD – FEV_1 50–64% predicted; 26 with severe COPD – $FEV_1 < 50$% predicted) and found 41% to have bacterial colonization. Again the authors found *H. influenzae*, *S. viridans*, *S. pneumoniae* and *M. catarrhalis* to be the most frequent organisms isolated.[107] Thus several studies have confirmed that bacterial colonization of the lower airways is a relatively common feature of COPD patients in the stable clinical state.

Studies of spontaneous sputum samples have been less easy to interpret because of the clear problem of oropharyngeal contamination with organisms similar to those identified by PSB. Bacterial culture of samples expectorated by patients whilst in the stable clinical state have isolated an organism from between 22% and 55% of samples.[108–110] The most frequent organisms identified are the same as those identified by PSB including *Haemophilus* species, *M. catarrhalis* and *Streptococcus* species. Although this may represent oropharyngeal contamination, Pye *et al.* found that the number of organisms in sputum was usually greater than 10^5 colony forming units/ml compared with less than 10^4 colony forming units/ml in saliva from the same patient.[111] More recently Stockley *et al.*[109] identified bacteria in 38% of patents with stable COPD with a median value of 10^7 colony forming units/ml, suggesting that oropharyngeal contamination was not influencing the results. Thus both the PSB and sputum data would support the presence of chronic colonization of the lower respiratory tract of 22–55% patients with COPD in the stable state. The implications of this with reference to exacerbations and pathophysiology will be discussed later.

RISK FACTORS FOR LOWER AIRWAYS COLONIZATION IN STABLE COPD

Studies to date have found that current smoking and possibly the severity of airflow obstruction are independent risk factors for lower airways colonization in COPD, although no independent association has been found with age.[105,107]

Studies have shown that 55% of current smokers with COPD are colonized compared with 30% of ex-smokers.[107] Furthermore, current smoking was associated with lower airways bacterial colonization with an odds ratio of 9.8 as compared to ex-smokers (confidence interval 1.2–83.2).[105] The potential mechanisms by which smoking promotes bacterial colonization has been outlined earlier but may also relate to the fact that nicotine is an important growth factor for *H. influenzae*[112] and thus smoking alone may facilitate proliferation of this organism in the lower respiratory tract.

The relationship of colonization to the severity of airflow obstruction is uncertain. Zalacain *et al.*[107] found that 58% of patients with severe airflow obstruction ($FEV_1 < 50$% predicted) were colonized compared to 42% of patients with moderate airflow obstruction (FEV_1 50–64% predicted) and 23% of patients with mild airflow obstruction ($FEV_1 > 65$% predicted), suggesting that airflow obstruction was an important factor in colonization. However, Monso *et al.*[105] found no such association with FEV_1 although a smaller number of patients with severe airflow obstruction were assessed. More recently results from Hill *et al.*[113] also failed to find an association of lower airways bacterial colonization with FEV_1 using spontaneous sputum cultures. Further studies are therefore required to clarify whether and how lower airways bacterial colonization is associated with the severity of airflow obstruction and whether this represents cause/effect or reflects treatment algorithms.

BACTERIAL LOAD AND SPECIES IN STABLE COPD

It is possible that persistent bacterial airway colonization in patients with COPD contributes in important ways to the morbidity of the disease. In particular, the chronic airway bacterial colonization may stimulate secondary host defenses and lead directly to persistent airway inflammation even in the stable clinical state. Recent studies have confirmed that a variety of inflammatory mediators were increased in sputum samples with a positive bacterial culture.[106,114] The implication is that bacterial colonization is not a benign process even in what appears to be the stable clinical state. This provides further support to a mechanism that may play a key role in

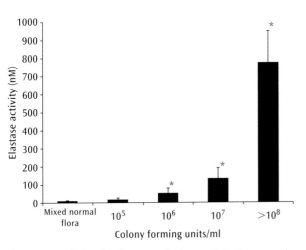

Figure 8.5 *Relationship between elastase activity (mean and standard error) and airway bacterial load. Asterisks indicate significant differences compared to samples containing normal flora alone (*P < 0.001). nM = nano-Molar. (Data from ref. 113.)*

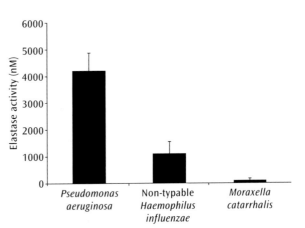

Figure 8.6 *Histograms representing mean (standard error) elastase activity associated with different bacterial species all with a load greater than 10^8 colony forming units/ml. nM = nano-Molar. (Data from ref. 113.)*

airway inflammation in COPD, amplifying tissue damage as shown in Figure 8.2. However interpretation of these studies may be an oversimplification of the results.

In animal models, a low bacterial load instiled into the airways is cleared efficiently by the primary host defense mechanisms alone.[1] However, as an increasing load is instiled, secondary host defenses (including neutrophil recruitment) are activated.[1,2] This is likely to reflect the release of pro-inflammatory mediators, causing an acute inflammatory response characterized by neutrophil infiltration.[2,3] The same process has been demonstrated recently by Stockley *et al.*[109] in acute exacerbations of COPD associated with neutrophil influx. In these patients the median number of organisms recovered was 3.7×10^8 colony forming units/ml compared to 7.5×10^6 colony forming units/ml for samples with little or no neutrophil influx. These results indicated that the size of the bacterial load was more important than colonization alone. However perhaps the clearest demonstration of relationship of bacterial load to inflammation was published recently by Hill *et al.*[113] who studied sputum from 160 patients with stable chronic bronchitis. The authors found the colonizing bacterial load was either absent or ranged to more than 10^8 colony forming units/ml. Bacterial loads less than 10^6 colony forming units/ml had a similar degree of mild airways inflammation to patients not colonized. Airways inflammation, however, increased at bacterial loads of between 10^6 and 10^7 colony forming units/ml, and increased further as the bacterial load increased (Figure 8.5). Of importance, the increase related to the detection of free neutrophil elastase activity which has the potential to cause more airway damage (see earlier). Furthermore, the study revealed that some bacterial species influenced airways inflammation

more than others. For instance, *P. aeruginosa* provoked a more intense inflammatory response than *H. influenzae*, and *H. influenzae*, in turn, stimulated a more intense inflammatory response than *M. catarrhalis* (Figure 8.6). These results challenge conventional thinking about bacterial 'colonization' of the airways in stable patients with COPD. Thus it appears that bacterial colonization alone is not necessarily a stimulus to activate the secondary host defense in the stable state but the magnitude of the bacterial load is the major factor.

BACTERIAL EFFECT ON AIRWAYS INFLAMMATION

The mechanisms by which bacteria stimulate inflammation and neutrophil recruitment are uncertain. However several distinct processes, have been, or can be implicated. Endotoxin from bacterial sources can stimulate airway epithelial cells to release a variety of pro-inflammatory cytokines including IL1β, TNFα and the neutrophil chemoattractant IL-8.[115,116] In addition endotoxin can increase neutrophil adhesion because of an effect on ICAM-1 expression.[116] Bacterial products such as pyocyanin can enhance oxidative metabolism of neutrophils and 1-hydroxyphenazine can enhance the release of elastase by neutrophils.[99] Finally activation of macrophages and neutrophils during bacterial phagocytosis is also associated with the release of other inflammatory mediators as well as the neutrophil chemoattractants IL-8[116–118] and leukotriene B4.[81] These positive effects on inflammation have to be counterbalanced by the ability of some bacteria to release factors that reduce neutrophil migration.[95]

IMPLICATIONS OF BACTERIAL COLONIZATION IN STABLE COPD

The long-term effects of bacterial colonization in the stable state on progression of lung damage is not known and requires appropriate prospective studies. To date there have been no controlled studies of antimicrobial strategies in patients in the stable state with this outcome clearly in mind. Previous placebo-controlled studies have attempted to address whether antibiotic prophylaxis in stable COPD patients can prevent acute exacerbations and whether this affects the decline in FEV_1.

For example one 10-week study in 60 patients with chronic bronchitis compared sulfonamide antibiotic therapy given once weekly with placebo over the winter period of 1965–66 and found less relapses among the treated group, although the level of functional impairment of the patients at baseline was not reported.[119] In another study of 48 patients with chronic bronchitis, sulfonamide antibiotic therapy given once weekly was compared to placebo over a 6-month period. Most patients had severe COPD with type 2 respiratory failure (mean FEV_1 about 1 liter). However, in this study the authors found no benefit of antibiotics for reducing the number of exacerbations.[120]

A longer study (5-year) assessed whether antibiotic therapy could reduce the number of exacerbations in patients with COPD by giving antibiotic prophylaxis during the winter to 79 patients with chronic bronchitis and an FEV_1 of approximately 50% predicted. The study demonstrated a significant reduction in the number of exacerbations among those who had suffered more than one exacerbation each winter. The average rate of decline in FEV_1 over the 5 years was less in the antibiotic-treated group, although this failed to reach statistical significance.[121] A further 5-year study investigated antibiotic chemoprophylaxis in 497 patients with early chronic bronchitis (mean FEV_1 about 2 liters) who had at least two chest illnesses with increased phlegm, and a total absence from work greater than 3 weeks over the preceding 3 years. Oxytetracycline or placebo was given continually from September to April but the study did not demonstrate an effect on the number of exacerbations or rate of decline of FEV_1.[122]

These studies do not demonstrate clearly whether antibiotic prophylaxis has an impact on the number of exacerbations or FEV_1 decline. The studies have limitations, particularly since the patients were poorly characterized, the antibiotics were given to all patients as opposed to only those who were colonized, and the exacerbations were not characterized. Future studies addressing these issues are therefore needed, and it is the size of bacterial colonization that is critical in determining efficacy since this determines the effect on airway inflammation.[113]

EXACERBATIONS OF COPD DUE TO BACTERIA

Acute exacerbations of COPD (AECB) are poorly defined episodes when the patient's symptoms increase. Recently a consensus view has been published[123] which defines an exacerbation as 'a sustained worsening of the patient's condition, from the stable state and beyond normal day-to-day variations, that is acute in onset and necessitates a change in regular medication in a patient with underlying COPD'. These episodes can relate to a variety of physiopathologic changes which may include increased airflow obstruction, viral infection, bacterial infection, mucus plugging, etc.

Previous studies have examined whether 'exacerbations' influence decline in FEV_1 in England,[124] Canada[125] and more recently in the Lung Health Study.[126] The initial studies by Fletcher and Peto[124] and Bates[125] found that deterioration in lung function occurred independently of respiratory infections. Fletcher and Peto[124] in their 8-year prospective study of working men in London found that bronchopulmonary infection caused an acute decline in lung function but that recovery was complete. Although these authors found an association between mucus hypersecretion, increased frequency of infection and lower absolute levels of FEV_1, they concluded that neither mucus hypersecretion nor bronchial infection caused FEV_1 to decline more rapidly (after adjustment for age, smoking and FEV_1 there remained no independent correlation between indices of mucus hypersecretion or bronchial infection and annual decline in FEV_1). On the other hand, the Lung Health Study[126] revealed that over a 5-year period, lower respiratory tract illnesses had a significant effect on the rate of decline in FEV_1 although only in current smokers, suggesting a synergistic effect. These epidemiologic studies were derived mainly from patients with mild COPD. Once obstruction has developed hypersecretion and/or infections may accelerate the subsequent decline in FEV_1. This was demonstrated by a large community study in Copenhagen[127] in which hypersecretion was associated with a relative risk of death from chronic bronchitis of 1.2 if the FEV_1 was 80% (or more) predicted but a risk of 4.2 if the FEV_1 was 40% (or less) predicted. With the known potential for an infection to cause lung tissue damage, it seems likely that such episodes will have some effect on lung function although more focused studies may be required to confirm this possibility.

Nevertheless it is recognized that exacerbations with their broadest definition are associated with ill health and their frequency relates to the patients overall health status.[128] In addition, AECB are an important cause of mortality, particularly in patients with moderate to severe COPD.[129] The role played by bacteria in AECB however has remained controversial, partly because bacteria are not always isolated (see below) and partly because the same bacteria are present in the stable clinical state of a significant proportion of patients (see above).

Bacteria isolated

Studies using the PSB with or without bronchoalveolar lavage have found bacterial pathogens in about 50% of patients with AECB.[104,130–132] The most frequent species isolated are similar to those identified in the stable clinical state, namely non-typeable *H. influenzae*, *M. catarrhalis*, *S. pneumoniae*, and *P. aeruginosa*.[104,130–132] The bacterial isolation rate from sputum has been variable (30–84%) during AECB[108,109,133–135] and the bacteria isolated are also mainly *Haemophilus* species, *M. catarrhalis*, *S. pneumoniae*[109] and *P. aeruginosa*.[135] In the latter study of 91 patients the frequency of isolating potential pathogens was greater in patients with an FEV_1 less than 50% predicted and in current smokers.[135] This is similar to the findings reported by Eller *et al.* in 112 cases of AECB requiring hospital admission,[136] where a relationship was also found between the severity of lung function impairment and the bacterial species isolated from sputum. Enterobacteriacaea and *Pseudomonas* were the predominant pathogens isolated in patients with an FEV_1 less than 35% predicted. However in this latter study most of the patients had already received and failed to respond to one course of antibiotics and many of the patients had received oral corticosteroids, which is likely to have influenced the spectrum of organisms isolated. For instance in a study of 121 AECB cases treated in the community, who had received no prior treatment with antibiotics or oral corticosteroids, the FEV_1 showed no relationship to the organism identified and gram-negative organisms were generally uncommon.[109]

Finally, atypical bacteria have often been implicated in AECB. *Chlamydia pneumoniae* has been associated with symptoms of AECB in 5–10% of cases,[137,138] although a further study found *C. pneumoniae* in 18% of severe exacerbations requiring admission to an intensive care unit.[130] However interpretation of these studies can be difficult as asymptomatic acute acquisition and chronic carriage of the organism can occur and this may affect up to 54% of COPD patients in the stable state.[139–142] *Mycoplasma pneumoniae* infection has generally been found to be an uncommon (<1%) cause of AECB.[130,143,144]

As bacteria are isolated from airway secretions in the stable clinical state, there is clearly controversy concerning their role in AECB. An early longitudinal study assessed sputum bacteriology during remissions and exacerbations and isolated *S. pneumoniae* and/or *H. influenzae* in 9% during remissions and in 40% during

exacerbations.[145] Monso *et al.*[104] using PSB samples found a higher prevalence of bacterial isolation (52%) during exacerbations compared to the stable state (25%), and when present the bacterial load was greater during the exacerbation. This study and the higher incidence of bacterial isolation from sputum during exacerbations suggests bacteria do play a role. However perhaps the clearest information came from a recent study by Stockley *et al.*[109] These authors found that a positive bacterial culture was obtained from 84% of the samples if the sputum was purulent at presentation compared with only 38% if the sputum was mucoid. This finding indicated that purulent sputum (which reflects neutrophil influx) is a clinical observation associated with a high probability of bacterial colonization. However in addition the bacterial load (when present) was higher in these exacerbations than in mucoid exacerbations, suggesting it was the load rather than the presence of bacteria that determined the nature of the episode. In addition the purulent exacerbations were associated with a systemic response as reflected in an elevated serum C reactive protein. Following treatment with antibiotics, only 38% of the patient samples were positive for bacterial culture (odds ratio 8.3; 95% CI, 3.9–18.2), fewer samples yielded a high bacterial growth of greater than 10^7 colony forming units/ml (odds ratio 7.8; 95% CI, 3.7–16.5) and the C reactive protein concentrations returned to normal.[109] However, the patients who presented with mucoid sputum samples improved without antibiotic therapy and the proportion in whom bacteria were isolated from the sputum remained the same (41%) as at the start of the episode. Furthermore, this group was no longer different from the patients who had recovered from a purulent exacerbation. The conclusions were that purulent exacerbations were usually bacterial in origin, either as the result of a new organism or an increase in the number of the stable colonizing organisms sufficient to stimulate a neutrophil response. The mucoid exacerbations occurred in the absence of a neutrophil response even in patients colonized with bacteria and they returned to their stable state with no change in their colonizing state or load.

This concept was supported recently as part of a longitudinal study in patients with COPD with and without alpha-1-antitrypsin deficiency. All exacerbations in this study group were defined as having a deterioration of symptoms, increasing sputum volume and increased sputum purulence. The patients were carefully followed and data was available in the stable state prior to the exacerbation, throughout the exacerbation treated with antibiotic therapy, and in the stable state after the antibiotic therapy. The study demonstrated an increase in bacterial load at the start of the exacerbations, associated with increased airway inflammation and a systemic response (increased C reactive protein). With antibiotic therapy the inflammation resolved and the microbial

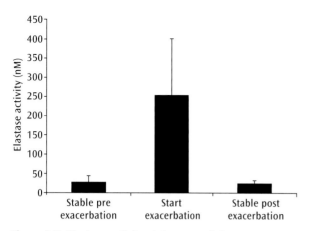

Figure 8.7 *Elastase activity at the start of the exacerbation (increased sputum volume, purulence and symptoms) and in the stable state (pre and post exacerbation) in 11 patients with alpha-1-antitrypsin deficiency. Histograms expressed as mean and standard error. nM = nano-Molar. (Data from ref. 146.)*

load decreased, both to the level found prior to the exacerbation. This change is illustrated for sputum elastase activity in Figure 8.7.[146]

In summary bacteria are frequently isolated with AECB. The proportion of positive cultures is increased primarily in purulent exacerbations where the load is increased and is associated with a neutrophilic inflammatory response in the airway and a systemic response.

The final proof of the role of bacteria in AECB requires evidence that antibiotic therapy has a beneficial effect. Although the data have been controversial bacteria undoubtedly play a role in some exacerbations, as a meta-analysis of placebo-controlled trials by Saint *et al.* found an overall 5% improvement in peak expiratory flow rates from antibiotic therapy for exacerbations compared to placebo.[147] In addition, a retrospective cohort study of 173 patients found that patients who received antibiotics had lower relapse rates than those who did not receive antibiotics.[148] Perhaps, however, the best and most widely quoted study is that by Anthonisen and colleagues.[149] This carefully conducted, placebo-controlled study showed spontaneous resolution of many exacerbations but a significant increase in resolution rate when an antibiotic was given. However, the authors also stratified patients according to the severity of the episode (determined by the number of new symptoms). The study indicated that antibiotics had an overall advantage over placebo, particularly when all three symptoms of increased breathlessness, increased sputum volume and increased sputum purulence were present. This observation is consistent with recent studies where the presence of purulent sputum was 94% sensitive to a positive bacterial culture and suggests that it is this

subset that mainly require and benefit from appropriate antibiotic therapy.[109]

CHOICE OF ANTIBIOTIC

There is an increasing choice of antibiotics available for treating AECB, including β lactams, β lactams with a β lactamase inhibitor (for β lactamase producing organisms), macrolides, trimethoprim/sulfamethoxazole, cephalosporins and quinolones. The choice of antibiotic will vary with the clinical features and will depend on the bacteria isolated, local resistance patterns, efficacy and perhaps cost. The tendency particularly in the UK is to choose an appropriate β lactam as first line therapy (British Thoracic Society guidelines) as most organisms are sensitive.[150] However, the final choice of antibiotic class may depend on factors other than sensitivity. For instance in a recent retrospective study, patients treated with amoxicillin had higher relapse rates than those treated with other antibiotic classes.[148] Furthermore, recent randomized double blind controlled studies have compared antibiotic regimens to determine bacterial eradication rates and the time to the next exacerbation. These studies have compared a quinolone (ciprofloxacin) to a cephalosporin (cefuroxime axetil) and a macrolide (clarithromycin).[151,152] In both studies, the quinolone improved bacterial eradication rates although there was no significant difference in the time to the next exacerbation. However a recent study with a newer quinolone (gemifloxacin) suggested that a longer exacerbation free interval could be obtained following treatment of an acute episode than following a macrolide (clarithromycin).[153] Clearly further studies of the antibiotic response rate and exacerbation-free interval are necessary to determine the most cost-effective therapy. These studies should be confined to purulent exacerbations where a bacterial etiology is highly likely and the effects on health status and progression of COPD should be confirmed.

FUTURE STUDIES

In conclusion bacteria commonly colonize the airways in stable COPD patients and are frequently implicated in exacerbations. Studies are needed to determine why only a proportion of the patients are colonized and the long-term implications of bacterial colonization in stable COPD, including the effect on exacerbation rates, FEV_1 decline and health status. However at present it seems logical to apply the same criteria when assessing airway secretions to those used in assessing urine samples. Antibiotic therapy should be based not just on a positive bacterial culture but also be influenced by the size of the bacterial load and a clear neutrophil response.

REFERENCES

1. Onofrio JM, Toews GB, Lipscomb MF, Pierce AK. Granulocyte–alveolar–macrophage interaction in the pulmonary clearance of *Staphylococcus aureus*. *Am Rev Respir Dis* 1983;**127**:335–41.

2. Vial WC, Toews GB, Pierce AK. Early pulmonary granulocyte recruitment in response to *Streptococcus pneumoniae*. *Am Rev Respir Dis* 1984;**129**: 87–91.

3. Toews GB, Vial WC. The role of C5 in polymorphonuclear leukocyte recruitment in response to Streptococcus pneumoniae. *Am Rev Respir Dis* 1984;**129**:82–6.

4. Boat TF, Cheng PW, Leigh MW. Airway secretion, physiological basis for the control of mucous hypersecretion. In: T Takishima, S Shimura, eds. *Biochemistry of Mucus*. Marcel Dekker, New York, 1994.

5. Puchelle E, Girod-de Bentzmann S, Jacquot, J. Airway defence mechanisms in relation to biochemical and physical properties of mucus. *Eur Respir Rev* 1992;**2**:259–63.

6. Widdicombe JG, Webber SE. Airway mucus secretion. *N Physiol Sci* 1990;**5**:2–5.

7. Girod S, Zahm JM, Plotkowski C, Beck G, Puchelle E. Role of the physiochemical properties of mucus in the protection of the respiratory epithelium. *Eur Respir J* 1992;**5**:477–87.

8. Hiratsuka T, Nakazato M, Date Y, *et al.* Identification of human beta-defensin-2 in respiratory tract and plasma and its increase in bacterial pneumonia. *Biochem Biophys Res Commun* 1998;**249**:943–7.

9. Harder J, Meyer-Hoffert U, Teran LM, *et al.* Mucoid *Pseudomonas aeruginosa*, TNF-alpha, and IL-1beta, but not IL-6, induce human beta-defensin-2 in respiratory epithelia. *Am J Respir Cell Mol Biol* 2000;**22**:714–21.

10. Jacquot J, Puchelle E, Zahm JM, Beck G, Plotkowski MC. Effect of human airway lysozyme on the in vitro growth of type I *Streptococcus pneumoniae*. *Eur J Respir Dis* 1987;**71**: 295–305.

11. Ellison RTD, Giehl TJ. Killing of gram-negative bacteria by lactoferrin and lysozyme. *J Clin Invest* 1991;**88**:1080–91.

12. Gerson C, Sabater J, Scuri M, *et al.* The lactoperoxidase system functions in bacterial clearance of airways. *Am J Respir Cell Mol Biol* 2000;**22**:665–71.

13. Salathe M, Holderby M, Forteza R, Abraham WM, Wanner A, Conner GE. Isolation and characterization of a peroxidase from the airway. *Am J Respir Cell Mol Biol* 1997;**17**: 97–105.

14. Tomee JFC, Koeter GH, Hiemstra PS, Kauffamn HF. Secretory leukoprotease inhibitor: a native antimicrobial protein presenting a new therapeutic option? *Thorax* 1998;**53**: 114–16.

15. Maruyama M, Hay JG, Yoshimura K, Chu CS, Crystal RG. Modulation of secretory leukoprotease inhibitor gene expression in human bronchial epithelial cells by phorbol ester. *J Clin Invest* 1994;**94**:368–75.

16. De Water R, Willems LN, Van Muijen GN, *et al.* Ultrastructural localization of bronchial antileukoprotease in central and peripheral human airways by a gold-labelling technique using monoclonal antibodies. *Am Rev Respir Dis* 1986;**133**: 882–90.

17. Mooren HW, Kramps JA, Franken C, Meijer CJ, Dijkman JA. Localization of a low-molecular-weight bronchial protease inhibitor in the peripheral human lung. *Thorax* 1983;**38**:180–3.

18. Sallenave JM, Silva A, Marsden ME, Ryle AP. Secretion of mucus proteinase inhibitor and elafin by Clara cell and type II pneumocyte cell lines. *Am J Respir Cell Mol Biol* 1993;**8**:126–33.

19. Singh PK, Tack BF, McCray PB Jr, Welsh MJ. Synergistic and additive killing by antimicrobial factors found in human airway surface liquid. *Am J Physiol Lung Cell Mol Physiol* 2000;**279**:L799–805.

20. Shimura S, Takishima T. Airway submucosal gland secretion. In: T Takishima, S Shimura, eds. *Airway Secretion, Physiological Basis for the Control of Mucous Hypersecretion*. Marcel Dekker, New York, 1994.

21. Widdicombe JH, Widdicombe JG. Regulation of human airway surface liquid. *Respir Physiol* 1995;**99**:3–12.

22. Hasani A, Pavia D. Cough as a clearance mechanism. In: PC Braga, L Allegra, eds. *Cough*. New York: Raven Press, 1989.

23. Puchelle E, Zahm JM, Girard F, *et al.* Mucociliary transport *in vivo* and in vitro. Relations to sputum properties in chronic bronchitis. *Eur J Respir Dis* 1980;**61**:254–64.

24. Yeates DB, Aspin N, Levison H, Jones MT, Bryan AC. Mucociliary tracheal transport rates in man. *J Appl Physiol* 1975;**39**:487–95.

25. Pavia D. Lung mucociliary clearance. In: SW Clarke, D Pavia, eds. *Aerosols and the Lung*. Boston, Butterworths, 1984.

26. Wilson R, Cole PJ. The effect of bacterial products on ciliary function. *Am Rev Respir Dis* 1988;**138**:S49–53.

27. Wilson R, Pitt T, Taylor G, *et al.* Pyocyanin and 1-hydroxyphenazine produced by *Pseudomonas aeruginosa* inhibit the beating of human respiratory cilia in vitro. *J Clin Invest* 1987;**79**:221–9.

28. Soutar CA. Distribution of plasma cells and other cells containing immunoglobulin in the respiratory tract of normal man and class of immunoglobulin contained therein. *Thorax* 1976;**31**:158–66.

29. Morgan KL, Hussein AM, Newby TJ, Bourne FJ. Quantification and origin of the immunoglobulins in porcine respiratory tract secretions. *Immunol* 1980;**41**:729–36.

30. Burnett D. Immunoglobulins in the lung. *Thorax* 1986;**41**: 337–44.

31. Richards CD, Gauldie J. IgA-mediated phagocytosis by mouse alveolar macrophages. *Am Rev Respir Dis* 1985;**132**:82–5.

32. Shen L, Lydyard PM, Roitt IM, Fanger MW. Synergy between IgG and monoclonal IgM antibodies in antibody-dependent cell cytotoxicity. *J Immunol* 1981;**127**:73–8.

33. du Bois RM. The alveolar macrophage. *Thorax* 1985;**40**: 321–7.

34. Owen CA, Campbell MA, Boukedes SS, Campbell EJ. Monocytes recruited to sites of inflammation express a distinctive proinflammatory (P) phenotype. *Am J Physiol* 1994;**267**:L786–96.

35. Owen CA, Campbell MA, Boukedes SS, Stockley RA, Campbell EJ. A discrete subpopulation of human monocytes expresses a neutrophil-like proinflammatory (P) phenotype. *Am J Physiol* 1994;**267**:L775–85.

36. McDermott MR, Befus AD, Bienenstock J. The structural basis for immunity in the respiratory tract. *Int Rev Exp Pathol* 1982;**23**:47–112.

37. Pabst R. Localization and dynamics of lymphoid cells in the different compartments of the lung. In: RA Stockley, ed. *Pulmonary Defences*. John Wiley, Chichester, 1997:59–75.

38. Bradley PA, Bourne FJ, Brown PJ. The respiratory tract immune system in the pig. I. Distribution of immunoglobulin-containing cells in the respiratory tract mucosa. *Vet Pathol* 1976;**13**:81–9.

39. Azzawi M, Bradley B, Jeffery PK, *et al.* Identification of activated T lymphocytes and eosinophils in bronchial biopsies in stable atopic asthma. *Am Rev Respir Dis* 1990;**142**:1407–13.

40. Holt PG. Pulmonary dendritic cell populations. *Adv Exp Med Biol* 1993;**329**:557–62.

41. Laitinen LA, Laitinen A, Heino M. Airway hyperresponsiveness, epithelial disruption, and epithelial inflammation. In: SG Farmer, DWP Hay, eds. *The Airway Epithelium*. Marcel Dekker, New York, 1991.

42. Munakata M, Mitzner W. The protective role of the airway epithelium. In: SG Farmer, DWP Hay, eds. *The Airway Epithelium*. Marcel Dekker, New York, 1991.

43. Hanafi Z, Webber SE, Widdicombe JG. Permeability of ferret trachea in vitro to ^{99m}Tc-DTPA and [^{14}C]antipyrine. *J Appl Physiol* 1994;**77**:1263–73.

44. Wells UM, Woods AJ, Hanafi Z, Widdicombe JG. Tracheal epithelial damage alters tracer fluxes and effects of tracheal osmolality in sheep *in vivo*. *J Appl Physiol* 1995;**78**:1921–30.

45. Hogg JC. Mucosal permeability and smooth muscle function in asthma. *Med Clin North Am* 1990;**74**:731–40.

46. Hulbert WC, Walker DC, Jackson A, Hogg JC. Airway permeability to horseradish peroxidase in guinea pigs: the repair phase after injury by cigarette smoke. *Am Rev Respir Dis* 1981;**123**:320–6.

47. Tuomanen E, Hendley JO. Adherence of *Bordetella pertussis* to human respiratory epithelial cells. *J Infect Dis* 1983;**148**:125–30.

48. Bredt W, Feldner J, Klaus B. Adherence of mycoplasmas: phenomena and possible role in the pathogenesis of disease. *Infect* 1982;**10**:199–202.

49. Plotkowski MC, Beck G, Tournier JM, Bernardo-Filho M, Marques EA, Puchelle E. Adherence of *Pseudomonas aeruginosa* to respiratory epithelium and the effect of leucocyte elastase. *J Med Microbiol* 1989;**30**:285–93.

50. Feldman C, Read R, Rutman A, *et al.* The interaction of *Streptococcus pneumoniae* with intact human respiratory mucosa in vitro. *Eur Respir J* 1992;**5**:576–83.

51. Mullen JB, Wright JL, Wiggs BR, Pare PD, Hogg JC. Reassessment of inflammation of airways in chronic bronchitis. *Br Med J* 1985;**291**:1235–9.

52. Reid L. Pathology of chronic bronchitis. *Lancet* 1954; **i**:275–8.

53. Wright JL, Lawson LM, Pare PD, Wiggs BJ, Kennedy S, Hogg JC. Morphology of peripheral airways in current smokers and ex-smokers. *Am Rev Respir Dis* 1983;**127**:474–7.

54. Thurlbeck WM. Pathology of chronic airflow obstruction. *Chest* 1990;**97**(suppl):S6–10.

55. Jeffery PK. Pathology of asthma and COPD: a synopsis. *Eur Respir Rev* 1997;**7**:111–18.

56. Thurlbeck WM. *Chronic Airflow Obstruction in the Lung*. WB Saunders, London, 1976.

57. Lumsden AB, McLean A, Lamb D. Goblet and Clara cells of human distal airways: evidence for smoking induced changes in their numbers. *Thorax* 1984;**39**:844–9.

58. Jeffery PK. Structural and inflammatory changes in COPD: a comparison with asthma. *Thorax* 1998;**53**:129–36.

59. Currie DC, Pavia D, Lopez-Vidriero MT, *et al.* Impaired tracheobronchial clearance in bronchiectasis. *Thorax* 1987;**42**:126–30.

60. Fournier M, Lebargy F, Le Roy Ladurie F, Lenormand E, Pariente R. Intraepithelial T-lymphocyte subsets in the airways of normal subjects and of patients with chronic bronchitis. *Am Rev Respir Dis* 1989;**140**:737–42.

61. Ollerenshaw SL, Woolcock AJ. Characteristics of the inflammation in biopsies from large airways of subjects with asthma and subjects with chronic airflow limitation. *Am Rev Respir Dis* 1992;**145**:922–7.

62. Saetta M, Di Stefano A, Maestrelli P, *et al.* Activated T-lymphocytes and macrophages in bronchial mucosa of subjects with chronic bronchitis. *Am Rev Respir Dis* 1993;**147**:301–6.

63. Turato G, Di Stefano A, Maestrelli P, *et al.* Effect of smoking cessation on airway inflammation in chronic bronchitis. *Am J Respir Crit Care Med* 1995;**152**:1262–7.

64. Di Stefano A, Capelli A, Lusuardi M, *et al.* Severity of airflow limitation is associated with severity of airway inflammation in smokers. *Am J Respir Crit Care Med* 1998;**158**:1277–85.

65. Spurzem JR, Thompson AB, Daughton DM, Mueller M, Linder J, Rennard SI. Chronic inflammation is associated with an increased proportion of goblet cells recovered by bronchial lavage. *Chest* 1991;**100**:389–93.

66. Thompson AB, Daughton D, Robbins RA, Ghafouri MA, Oehlerking M, Rennard SI. Intraluminal airway inflammation in chronic bronchitis. Characterization and correlation with clinical parameters. *Am Rev Respir Dis* 1989;**140**:1527–37.

67. Di Stefano A, Maestrelli P, Roggeri A, *et al.* Upregulation of adhesion molecules in the bronchial mucosa of subjects with chronic obstructive bronchitis. *Am J Respir Crit Care Med* 1994;**149**:803–10.

68. Maestrelli P, Calcagni PG, Saetta M, *et al.* Integrin upregulation on sputum neutrophils in smokers with chronic airway obstruction. *Am J Respir Crit Care Med* 1996;**154**: 1296–300.

69. Riise GC, Larsson S, Lofdahl CG, Andersson BA. Circulating cell adhesion molecules in bronchial lavage and serum in COPD patients with chronic bronchitis. *Eur Respir J* 1994;**7**:1673–7.

70. Sandborg RR, Smolen JE. Biology of disease: early biochemical events in leukocyte activation. *Lab Invest* 1988;**59**:300–20.

71. Amitani R, Wilson R, Rutman A, *et al.* Effects of human neutrophil elastase and *Pseudomonas aeruginosa* proteinases on human respiratory epithelium. *Am J Respir Cell Mol Biol* 1991;**4**:26–32.

72. Smallman LA, Hill SL, Stockley RA. Reduction of ciliary beat frequency in vitro by sputum from patients with bronchiectasis: a serine proteinase effect. *Thorax* 1984;**39**:663–7.

73. Snider GL, Stone PJ, Lucey EC, *et al.* Eglin-c, a polypeptide derived from the medicinal leech, prevents human neutrophil elastase-induced emphysema and bronchial secretory cell metaplasia in the hamster. *Am Rev Respir Dis* 1985;**132**:1155–61.

74. Sommerhoff CP, Nadel JA, Basbaum CB, Caughey GH. Neutrophil elastase and cathepsin G stimulate secretion from cultured bovine airway gland serous cells. *J Clin Invest* 1990;**85**:682–9.

75. Tosi MF, Zakem H, Berger M. Neutrophil elastase cleaves C3bi on opsonized pseudomonas as well as CR1 on neutrophils to create a functionally important opsonin receptor mismatch. *J Clin Invest* 1990;**86**:300–8.

76. Doring G, Goldstein W, Botzenhart K, *et al.* Elastase from polymorphonuclear leucocytes: a regulatory enzyme in immune complex disease. *Clin Exp Immunol* 1986;**64**:597–605.

77. Sallenave JM, Shulmann J, Crossley J, Jordana M, Gauldie J. Regulation of secretory leukocyte proteinase inhibitor (SLPI) and elastase-specific inhibitor (ESI/elafin) in human airway epithelial cells by cytokines and neutrophilic enzymes. *Am J Respir Cell Mol Biol* 1994;**11**:733–41.

78. Hill AT, Bayley D, Stockley RA. The interrelationship of sputum inflammatory markers in patients with chronic bronchitis. *Am J Respir Crit Care Med* 1999;**160**:893–8.

79. Gompertz S, Bayley DL, Hill SL, Stockley RA. Relationship between airway inflammation and the frequency of exacerbations in patients with smoking related COPD. *Thorax* 2001;**56**:36–41.

80. Nakamura H, Yoshimura K, McElvaney NG, Crystal RG. Neutrophil elastase in respiratory epithelial lining fluid of individuals with cystic fibrosis induces interleukin-8 gene expression in a human bronchial epithelial cell line. *J Clin Invest* 1992;**89**:1478–84.

81. Hubbard RC, Fells G, Gadek J, Pacholok S, Humes J, Crystal RG. Neutrophil accumulation in the lung in alpha-1-antitrypsin deficiency. Spontaneous release of leukotriene B4 by alveolar macrophages. *J Clin Invest* 1991;**88**:891–7.

82. Megahed GE, Senna GA, Eissa MH, Saleh SZ, Eissa HA. Smoking versus infection as the aetiology of bronchial mucous gland hypertrophy in chronic bronchitis. *Thorax* 1967;**22**:271–8.

83. Greenberg SD, Boushy SF, Jenkins DE. Chronic bronchitis and emphysema: correlation of pathologic findings. *Am Rev Respir Dis* 1967;**96**:918–28.

84. Thurlbeck WM, Angus GE. The variation of Reid index measurements within the major bronchial tree. *Am Rev Respir Dis* 1967;**95**:551–5.

85. Goodman RM, Yergin BM, Landa JF, Golivanux MH, Sackner MA. Relationship of smoking history and pulmonary function tests to tracheal mucous velocity in non smokers, young smokers, ex-smokers, and patients with chronic bronchitis. *Am Rev Respir Dis* 1978;**117**:205–14.

86. Hunninghake GW, Crystal RG. Cigarette smoking and lung destruction. Accumulation of neutrophils in the lungs of cigarette smokers. *Am Rev Respir Dis* 1983;**128**:833–8.

87. Mio T, Romberger DJ, Thompson AB, Robbins RA, Heires A, Rennard SI. Cigarette smoke induces interleukin-8 release from human bronchial epithelial cells. *Am J Respir Crit Care Med* 1997;**155**:1770–6.

88. Keatings VM, Barnes PJ. Comparison of inflammatory cytokines in chronic obstructive pulmonary disease, asthma and controls. *Eur Respir Rev* 1997;**7**:146–50.

89. Totti ND, McCusker KT, Campbell EJ, Griffin GL, Senior RM. Nicotine is chemotactic for neutrophils and enhances neutrophil responsiveness to chemotactic peptides. *Science* 1984;**223**:169–71.

90. Stanescu D, Sanna A, Veriter C, et al. Airways obstruction, chronic expectoration, and rapid decline of FEV_1 in smokers are associated with increased levels of sputum neutrophils. *Thorax* 1996;**51**:267–71.

91. Bosken CH, Hards J, Gatter K, Hogg JC. Characterization of the inflammatory reaction in the peripheral airways of cigarette smokers using immunocytochemistry. *Am Rev Respir Dis* 1992;**145**:911–17.

92. Drost EM, Selby C, Lannan S, Lowe GD, MacNee W. Changes in neutrophil deformability following in vitro smoke exposure: mechanism and protection. *Am J Respir Cell Mol Biol* 1992;**6**:287–95.

93. Aoshiba K, Nagai A, Konno K. Nicotine prevents a reduction in neutrophil filterability induced by cigarette smoke exposure. *Am J Respir Crit Care Med* 1994;**150**:1101–7.

94. Bosken CH, Doerschuk CM, English D, Hogg JC. Neutrophil kinetics during active cigarette smoking in rabbits. *J Appl Physiol* 1991;**71**:630–7.

95. Cundell DR, Taylor GW, Kanthakumar K, et al. Inhibition of human neutrophil migration in vitro by low-molecular-mass products of nontypeable *Haemophilus influenzae*. *Infect Immun* 1993;**61**:2419–24.

96. Li JD, Dohrman AF, Gallup M, et al. Transcriptional activation of mucin by *Pseudomonas aeruginosa* lipopolysaccharide in the pathogenesis of cystic fibrosis lung disease. *Proc Natl Acad Sci USA* 1997;**94**:967–72.

97. Adler KB, Hendley DD, Davis GS. Bacteria associated with obstructive pulmonary disease elaborate extracellular products that stimulate mucin secretion by explants of guinea pig airways. *Am J Pathol* 1986;**125**:501–14.

98. Somerville M, Taylor GW, Watson D, et al. Release of mucus glycoconjugates by *Pseudomonas aeruginosa* rhamnolipid into feline trachea *in vivo* and human bronchus *in vitro*. *Am J Respir Cell Mol Biol* 1992;**6**:116–22.

99. Buret A, Cripps AW. The immunoevasive activities of *Pseudomonas aeruginosa*. Relevance for cystic fibrosis. *Am Rev Respir Dis* 1993;**148**:793–805.

100. Groeneveld K, van Alphen L, Eijk PP, Jansen HM, Zanen HC. Changes in outer membrane proteins of nontypable *Haemophilus influenzae* in patients with chronic obstructive pulmonary disease. *J Infect Dis* 1988;**158**:360–5.

101. Hill SL, Mitchell JL, Burnett D, Stockley RA. IgG subclasses in the serum and sputum from patients with bronchiectasis. *Thorax* 1998;**53**:463–8.

102. Lapa e Silva JR, Jones JA, Cole PJ, Poulter LW. The immunological component of the cellular inflammatory infiltrate in bronchiectasis. *Thorax* 1989;**44**:668–73.

103. Fick RB Jr, Olchowski J, Squier SU, Merrill WW, Reynolds HY. Immunoglobulin-G subclasses in cystic fibrosis. IgG_2 response to *Pseudomonas aeruginosa* lipopolysaccharide. *Am Rev Respir Dis* 1986;**133**:418–22.

104. Monso E, Ruiz J, Rosell A, et al. Bacterial infection in chronic obstructive pulmonary disease. A study of stable and exacerbated outpatients using the protected specimen brush. *Am J Respir Crit Care Med* 1995;**152**:1316–20.

105. Monso E, Rosell A, Bonet G, et al. Risk factors for lower airway bacterial colonization in chronic bronchitis. *Eur Respir J* 1999;**13**:338–42.

106. Soler N, Ewig S, Torres A, Filella X, Gonzalez J, Zaubet A. Airway inflammation and bronchial microbial patterns in patients with stable chronic obstructive pulmonary disease. *Eur Respir J* 1999;**14**:1015–22.

107. Zalacain R, Sobradillo V, Amilibia J, et al. Predisposing factors to bacterial colonization in chronic obstructive pulmonary disease. *Eur Respir J* 1999;**13**:343–8.

108. McHardy VU, Inglis JM, Calder MA, et al. A study of infective and other factors in exacerbations of chronic bronchitis. *Br J Dis Chest* 1980;**74**:228–38.

109. Stockley RA, Pye A, Hill SL. Relationship of sputum colour to nature and outpatient management of acute exacerbations of COPD. *Chest* 2000;**117**:1638–45.

110. Hill AT, Bayley DL, Campbell EJ, Hill SL, Stockley RA. Airways inflammation in chronic bronchitis: the effects of smoking and alpha-1-antitrypsin deficiency. *Eur Respir J* 2000;**15**:886–90.

111. Pye A. The Assessment and Characterization of Bacterial Load in Chronic Lung Disease. PhD thesis, Birmingham, 1993.

112. Roberts D, Cole P. Effect of tobacco and nicotine on growth of *Haemophilus influenzae in vitro*. *J Clin Pathol* 1979;**32**:728–31.

113. Hill AT, Campbell EC, Hill SL, Bayley DL, Stockley RA. Association between airway bacterial load and markers of airway inflammation in patients with stable chronic bronchitis. *Am J Med* 2000;**109**:288–95.

114. Bresser P, Out TA, van Alphen L, Jansen HM, Lutter R. Airway inflammation in non obstructive and obstructive chronic bronchitis with chronic *Haemophilus influenzae* airway infection. Comparison with noninfected patients with chronic obstructive pulmonary disease. *Am J Respir Crit Care Med* 2000;**162**:947–52.

115. Von Essen S. The role of endotoxin in grain dust exposure and airway obstruction. *Curr Opin Pulm Med* 1997;**3**:198–202.

116. Khair OA, Devalia JL, Abdelaziz MM, Sapsford RJ, Tarraf H, Davies RJ. Effect of *Haemophilus influenzae* endotoxin on the synthesis of IL-6, IL-8, TNF-alpha and expression of ICAM-1 in cultured human bronchial epithelial cells. *Eur Respir J* 1994;**7**:2109–16.

117. Bedard M, McClure CD, Schiller NL, Francoeur C, Cantin A, Denis M. Release of interleukin-8, interleukin-6, and colony-stimulating factors by upper airway epithelial cells: implications for cystic fibrosis. *Am J Respir Cell Mol Biol* 1993;**9**:455–62.

118. Bigby TD, Holtzman MJ. Enhanced 5-lipoxygenase activity in lung macrophages compared to monocytes from normal subjects. *J Immunol* 1987;**138**:1546–50.

119. Pines A. Controlled trials of a sulphonamide given weekly to prevent exacerbations of chronic bronchitis. *Br Med J* 1967;**3**:202–4.

120. Vandenbergh E, Clement J, Van de Woestijne KP. Prevention of exacerbations of bronchitis: trial of a long acting sulphonamide. *Br J Dis Chest* 1970;**64**:58–62.

121. Johnston RN, McNeill RS, Smith DH, *et al*. Five year winter chemoprophylaxis for chronic bronchitis. *Br Med J* 1969;**4**:265–9.

122. Medical Research Council. Value of chemoprophylaxis and chemotherapy in early chronic bronchitis. A report to the Medical Research Council by their working party on trials of chemotherapy in early chronic bronchitis. *Br Med J* 1966;**5499**:1317–22.

123. Rodriguez-Roisin R. Toward a consensus definition for COPD exacerbations. *Chest* 2000;**117**(5 suppl 2):398S–401S.

124. Fletcher C, Peto R. The natural history of chronic airflow obstruction. *Br Med J* 1977;**1**:1645–8.

125. Bates DV. The fate of the chronic bronchitic: a report of the ten-year follow-up in the Canadian Department of Veteran's Affairs co-ordinated study of chronic bronchitis. The J Burns Amberson Lecture of the American Thoracic Society. *Am Rev Respir Dis* 1973;**108**:1043–65.

126. Kanner RE, Anthonisen NR, Connett JE. Lower respiratory illnesses promote FEV_1 decline in current smokers but not ex-smokers with mild chronic obstructive pulmonary disease. *Am J Respir Crit Care Med* 2001;**164**:358–64.

127. Lange P, Nyboe J, Appleyard M, Jensen G, Schnohr P. Relation of ventilatory impairment and of chronic mucus hypersecretion to mortality from obstructive lung disease and from all causes. *Thorax* 1990;**45**:579–85.

128. Seemungal TAR, Donaldson GC, Paul EA, Bestall JC, Jeffries DJ, Wedzicha JA. Effect of exacerbation on quality of life in patients with chronic obstructive pulmonary disease. *Am J Respir Crit Care Med* 1998;**157**:1418–22.

129. Burrows B, Earle RH. Course and prognosis of chronic obstructive lung disease: a prospective study of 200 patients. *New Engl J Med* 1969;**280**:397–404.

130. Soler N, Torres A, Ewig S, *et al*. Bronchial microbial patterns in severe exacerbations of chronic obstructive pulmonary disease (COPD) requiring mechanical ventilation. *Am J Respir Crit Care Med* 1998;**157**(5 Pt 1):1498–505.

131. Fagon JY, Chastre J, Trouillet JL, *et al*. Characterization of distal bronchial microflora during acute exacerbation of chronic bronchitis. Use of the protected specimen brush technique in 54 mechanically ventilated patients. *Am Rev Respir Dis* 1990;**142**:1004–8.

132. Pela R, Marchesani F, Agostinelli C, *et al*. Airways microbial flora in COPD patients in stable clinical conditions and during exacerbations: a bronchoscopic investigation. *Monaldi Arch Chest Dis* 1998;**53**:262–7.

133. Pines A, Raafat H, Greenfield JS, Linsell WD, Solari ME. Antibiotic regimens in moderately ill patients with purulent exacerbations of chronic bronchitis. *Br J Dis Chest* 1972;**66**:107–15.

134. Elmes PC, King TK, Langlands JH, *et al*. Value of ampicillin in the hospital treatment of exacerbations of chronic bronchitis. *Br Med J* 1965;**5467**:904–8.

135. Miravitlles M, Espinosa C, Fernandez-Laso E, Martos JA, Maldonado JA, Gallego M. Relationship between bacterial flora in sputum and functional impairment in patients with acute exacerbations of COPD. Study Group of Bacterial Infection in COPD. *Chest* 1999;**116**:40–6.

136. Eller J, Ede A, Schaberg T, Niederman MS, Mauch H, Lode H. Infective exacerbations of chronic bronchitis: relation between bacteriologic aetiology and lung function. *Chest* 1998;**113**:1542–8.

137. Blasi F, Legnani D, Lombardo VM, *et al*. *Chlamydia pneumoniae* infection in acute exacerbations of COPD. *Eur Respir J* 1993;**6**:19–22.

138. Miyashita N, Niki Y, Nakajima M, Kawane H, Matsushima T. *Chlamydia pneumoniae* infection in patients with diffuse panbronchiolitis and COPD. *Chest* 1998;**114**:969–71.

139. Hammerschlag MR, Chirgwin K, Roblin PM, *et al*. Persistent infection with *Chlamydia pneumoniae* following acute respiratory illness. *Clin Infect Dis* 1992;**14**:178–82.

140. Hyman CL, Roblin PM, Gaydos CA, Quinn TC, Schachter J, Hammerschlag MR. Prevalence of asymptomatic nasopharyngeal carriage of *Chlamydia pneumoniae* in subjectively healthy adults: assessment by polymerase chain reaction-enzyme immunoassay and culture. *Clin Infect Dis* 1995;**20**:1174–8.

141. Bourke SJ, Lightfoot NF. *Chlamydia pneumoniae*: defining the clinical spectrum of infection requires precise laboratory diagnosis. *Thorax* 1995;**50**(suppl 1):S43–8.

142. Wu L, Skinner SJ, Lambie N, Vuletic JC, Blasi F, Black PN. Immunohistochemical staining for *Chlamydia pneumoniae* is increased in lung tissue from subjects with chronic obstructive pulmonary disease. *Am J Respir Crit Care Med* **162**:1148–51.

143. Buscho RO, Saxtan D, Shultz PS, Finch E, Mufson MA. Infections with viruses and *Mycoplasma pneumoniae* during exacerbations of chronic bronchitis. *J Infect Dis* 1978;**137**:377–83.

144. Smith CB, Golden CA, Kanner RE, Renzetti AD Jr. Association of viral and *Mycoplasma pneumoniae* infections with acute respiratory illness in patients with chronic obstructive pulmonary diseases. *Am Rev Respir Dis* 1980;**121**:225–32.

145. Fisher M, Akhtar AJ, Calder MA, *et al*. Pilot study of factors associated with exacerbations in chronic bronchitis. *Br Med J* 1969;**4**:187–92.

146. Hill AT, Campbell EJ, Bayley DL, Hill SL, Stockley RA. Evidence for excessive bronchial inflammation during an acute exacerbation of chronic obstructive pulmonary disease in patients with alpha(1)-antitrypsin deficiency (PiZ). *Am J Respir Crit Care Med* 1999;**160**:1968–75.

147. Saint S, Bent S, Vittinghoff E, Grady D. Antibiotics in chronic obstructive pulmonary disease exacerbations. A meta-analysis. *JAMA* 1995;**273**:957–60.

148. Adams SG, Melo J, Luther M, Anzueto A. Antibiotics are associated with lower relapse rates in outpatients with acute exacerbations of COPD. *Chest* 2000;**117**:1345–52.

149. Anthonisen NR, Manfreda J, Warren CPW, Hershfield ES, Harding GKM, Nelson NA. Antibiotic therapy in

exacerbations of chronic obstructive pulmonary disease. *Ann Intern Med* 1987;**106**:196–204.

150. British Thoracic Society. BTS guidelines for the management of COPD. *Thorax* 1997;**52**(suppl 5):S1–28.

151. Chodosh S, McCarty J, Farkas S, *et al*. Randomized, double-blind study of ciprofloxacin and cefuroxime axetil for treatment of acute bacterial exacerbations of chronic bronchitis. The Bronchitis Study Group. *Clin Infect Dis* 1998;**27**:722–9.

152. Chodosh S, Schreurs A, Siami G, *et al*. Efficacy of oral ciprofloxacin vs. clarithromycin for treatment of acute bacterial exacerbations of chronic bronchitis. The Bronchitis Study Group. *Clin Infect Dis* 1998;**27**:730–8.

153. Ball P, Wilson R, Mandell L, *et al*. Gemifloxacin long term outcomes in bronchitis exacerbations (GLOBE) study – as assessment of health outcome benefits in AECB patients following 5 days gemifloxacin (GEMI) therapy. *40th ICAAC* 2000:A475.

Protease/antiprotease

DAVID A LOMAS

Alpha-1-antitrypsin deficiency was reported in an Alaskan girl who died 800 years ago[1] and may have accounted for the premature death of Frederic Chopin in 1849.[2,3] It was first described as a clinical entity in 1963 by Laurell and Eriksson who noted an absence of the alpha-1 band on serum protein electrophoresis.[4] The major function of alpha-1-antitrypsin is to protect the tissues against the enzyme neutrophil elastase.[5,6] Its role in protecting the lungs against proteolytic attack is underscored by the association of plasma deficiency with early-onset panlobular emphysema.[7] This association of alpha-1-antitrypsin deficiency with early-onset emphysema gave rise to the protease/antiprotease hypothesis of lung disease. In health there is a balance between proteases and antiproteases but when proteases are in excess then tissue destruction will ensue. The protease/antiprotease hypothesis was developed over 35 years ago but still remains central to our understanding of the pathogenesis of lung disease. It has evolved to include a variety of proteases and their inhibitors (Table 9.1) and has been implicated in other lung diseases such as cystic fibrosis,[8] adult respiratory distress syndrome,[9] tumor metastasis[10] and chronic lung infection.[11,12] In this chapter I will review the proteases that contribute to the lung damage in emphysema and then focus on the deficiency of alpha-1-antitrypsin which is associated with obstructive lung disease.

PROTEASES

It is generally accepted that neutrophil elastase is the most important protease in the pathogenesis of emphysema.

This came from the demonstration that elastase could digest elastin *in vitro*[13] and *in vivo*[14–16] and that genetic deficiency of the major serum inhibitor of elastase, alpha-1-antitrypsin, predisposed to emphysema.[4,7] However in recent years there has been growing interest in the role of neutrophil and macrophage metalloproteases.[17] It now seems likely that in individuals with emphysema there is a complex interplay between both of these enzymes, their inhibitors and the structural proteins within the lung.

Serine proteases

The strong link between the deficiency of a protease inhibitor, alpha-1-antitrypsin, and emphysema highlighted the role of serine proteases and their inhibitors in lung disease.[7] This was supported by studies that demonstrated the development of emphysema following the instillation of porcine pancreatic elastase,[18] neutrophil elastase[14–16] and protease 3[19] into the lungs of rodents. Similarly the neutrophil serine protease cathepsin G can cause bronchial disease and elastolysis *in vitro*.[13] The serine proteases, neutrophil elastase, cathepsin G and protease 3 are stored in the azurophil granule of the neutrophil and when released are capable of damaging many of the structural proteins and protease inhibitors within the lung.

There are increased numbers of macrophages and an excess of neutrophils in the small airways of smokers.[20] As neutrophils migrate from the vasculature they use neutrophil elastase to produce a destructive path to facilitate migration.[21] Lung elastin can be repaired but if neutrophil migration is excessive then proteolysis

Table 9.1 *Proteases and their inhibitors in the human lung*

Protease	Protease inhibitor
Serine proteases	*Serpins*
Human neutrophil elastase	Alpha-1-antitrypsin
Protease 3	Alpha-1-
Cathepsin G	antichymotrypsin
Tissue plasminogen activator	PAI-1
Mast cell chymase	*Cheloninians*
Mast cell tryptase	SLPI
	Elafin
	High MW inhibitors
	Alpha-2-
	macroglobulin
Cysteine proteases	*Cystatins*
Cathepsin B	Cystatin A
Cathepsin H	Cystatin B
Cathepsin S	Cystatin C
Cathepsin L	Cystatin D
	Cystatin SN
	L-kininogen
	H-kininogen
Matrix metalloproteases	*Tissue inhibitor of*
(MMP)	*metalloproteases*
Collagenases	*(TIMP)*
Interstitial	TIMP-1
collagenase (MMP-1)	TIMP-2
Neutrophil collagenase	TIMP-3
(MMP-8)	TIMP-4
Collagenase 3 (MMP-13)	*High MW inhibitors*
Gelatinases	Alpha-2-
Gelatinase A (MMP-2)	macroglobulin
Gelatinase B (MMP-9)	
Stromelysins	
Stromelysin-1 (MMP-3)	
Stromelysin-2 (MMP-10)	
Matrilysins (MMP-7)	
Others	
Metalloelastase (MMP-12)	
Stromelysin-3 (MMP-11)	
Membrane type MMP	

Table 9.2 *Substrates of human neutrophil elastase within the lung. Neutrophil elastase has many roles in the inflammatory response including the destruction of structural proteins and protease inhibitors and the activation of pro-enzymes which themselves may cause lung damage*

Structural proteins
Collagen – Types II-IV IX-XI[217,218,219]
Elastin[220]
Fibronectin[221]
Proteoglycans[222]
Laminin[223]
Fibrin[224]
Pro-enzymes
Collagenase[225]
Cathepsin B[226]
Matrix metalloproteases 2, 3 and 9[227,228]
Protein inhibitors
Serpins
Alpha-1-antitrypsin[5,229]
Antithrombin[221]
C1-inhibitor[230]
PAI-1[231]
Alpha-2-macroglobulin[232]
Alpha-2-antiplasmin[221]
Cystatin C[233]
Coagulation factors[234]
Immunoglobulins
IgG[235]
Complement factors
C1,[236] C3,[221,237] C5[238]

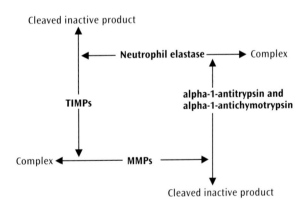

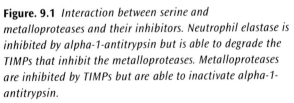

Figure. 9.1 *Interaction between serine and metalloproteases and their inhibitors. Neutrophil elastase is inhibited by alpha-1-antitrypsin but is able to degrade the TIMPs that inhibit the metalloproteases. Metalloproteases are inhibited by TIMPs but are able to inactivate alpha-1-antitrypsin.*

exceeds repair and tissue damage and emphysema ensues. Previous studies have shown a strong relationship between the quantity of neutrophil elastase in the interstitium of the lung and the severity of emphysematous change,[22–25] although these findings have been refuted by other workers.[26] It is uncertain whether the elastase in the interstitium causes disease or whether it is a reaction to tissue damage. Nevertheless free elastase has many destructive effects (Table 9.2). It can: (i) damage epithelial cells;[27] (ii) reduce cillary beat frequency;[28] (iii) reduce the effectiveness of other protease inhibitors such as the tissue inhibitors of metalloproteases (TIMPs); (iv) activate pro-enzymes of the metalloprotease cascade

which can themselves cause lung damage (Figure 9.1); and (v) digest elastin which in turn attracts mononuclear phagocytic cells to the site of injury.[29] Neutrophil elastase that is bound to structural proteins such as elastin may be even more damaging than free enzyme as it is resistant to inhibition by protease inhibitors.[30,31]

The most potent inhibitor of neutrophil elastase is alpha-1-antitrypsin[5] but this is clearly ineffective or overwhelmed in the lungs of patients with emphysema. Inactivated alpha-1-antitrypsin has been detected in the bronchoalveolar lavage of smokers without plasma alpha-1-antitrypsin deficiency.[32,33] This has been attributed to oxidation of the P_1 methionine residue by oxygen free radicals from leukocytes or direct oxidation by cigarette smoke.[5,6] Other investigators have failed to show increased inactivation of alpha-1-antitrypsin in cigarette smokers[34] and thus the role of alpha-1-antitrypsin inactivation in smoking-related emphysema remains unclear. Protease inhibitors such as alpha-1-antitrypsin and alpha-1-antichymotrypsin can also be inactivated by the formation of an inhibitory complex with target proteases[5,35] or by cleavage of the reactive center loop by exogenous metalloproteases.[36,37] In both cases the resulting protein acts as a chemotactic stimulus for the recruitment of more neutrophils to the lung.[36–39] A further explanation for the ineffectiveness of alpha-1-antitrypsin is that the binding of the neutrophil to its substrate excludes protease inhibitors, thereby facilitating the proteolytic effect of neutrophil elastase.[40] The local interaction between enzymes and their inhibitors has been modeled by Liou and Campbell.[41] Sixty-seven thousand molecules of neutrophil elastase are stored in each azurophil granule at a mean concentration of 5.33 mM. This exceeds the pericellular inhibitor concentrations *in vivo* by nearly three orders of magnitude. Diffusion analysis predicts obligate catalytic activity (excess of local enzyme over local inhibitor) that extends 1.33 microns from the site of granule extrusion with a duration of 12 milliseconds in individuals with normal levels of alpha-1-antitrypsin. In individuals with alpha-1-antitrypsin deficiency the radius and duration of the catalytic activity are increased 2.5- and 6.2-fold respectively. Smaller protease inhibitors, such as secretory leukoprotease inhibitor, may be more effective in protecting against tissue damage as they can more readily access the neutrophil–substrate interface.[42]

The physiologic role of the neutrophil and its requirement to release elastase suggest that connective tissue damage and remodeling is a constant and necessary feature of chemotaxis. However only 10–15% of smokers are particularly susceptible to the effects of cigarette smoke.[43] This susceptibility may relate to additional environmental factors,[44–46] diet[47] or previous viral infections.[48] The familial clustering of COPD suggests that it is genetic risk factors that predispose smokers to airflow obstruction.[49–53] Indeed in a recent study the relative risk for the development of airflow obstruction in a smoker was 4.7 if they had a sibling with severe COPD.[53] The genetic factors that render a proportion of smokers

particularly susceptible to COPD have still to be defined. Nevertheless it is possible that susceptible smokers may overproduce inflammatory cytokines such as interleukin 8 (IL-8)[54] or tumor necrosis factor alpha (TNF-α)[55] or have a less effective antiprotease screen or repair mechanism. An alternative explanation is that the neutrophils themselves respond differently in susceptible individuals. Indeed neutrophils from patients with emphysema have an enhanced chemotactic response and increased ability to digest connective tissue when compared to age- and smoking-matched controls.[56] Once again it is difficult to dissect out cause and effect, as neutrophils may be activated as they pass through the inflammatory battlefield that underlies progressive emphysema.

Metalloproteases

The family of matrix metalloproteases (MMPs) can destroy virtually, if not all, the proteins of the extracellular matrix.[57–59] They are characterized by: (i) a common sequence of amino acids; (ii) secretion as inactive proenzymes; (iii) activation by proteolysis; (iv) a zinc residue at the active center; (v) an ability to act at neutral pH and cleave extracellular matrix proteins; and (vi) inhibition by tissue inhibitors of metalloproteases or TIMPs.[59] The MMPs are divided into four main groups which differ in size and substrate specificity: the stromolysins, collagenases, gelatinases and membrane-type metalloproteases (Table 9.1). Two of these proteases, MMP8 and MMP9, are found within the neutrophil and are able to degrade collagen and elastin respectively. MMP9, matrilysin (MMP7) and MMP12 (metalloelastase) are produced in large amounts by the macrophage and are able to degrade elastin.[59] The other metalloproteases are produced by a variety of cells after stimulation by cytokines. The proteolytic substrate of metalloproteases extends beyond extracellular matrix proteins of the lung and includes protease inhibitors such as alpha-1-antitrypsin[60,61] and alpha-1-antichymotrypsin.[37] Indeed there is a complex interplay between the serine and metalloproteases and their inhibitors, the serine protease inhibitors and TIMPs respectively (Figure 9.1). Members of the TIMP family are found in all tissues.[62] They are synthesized by connective tissue cells and bind and inhibit metalloproteases with a 1:1 stoichiometry.[63] TIMP-2 and TIMP-3 are the major inhibitors within the lung with additional protection being provided by α_2-macroglobulin which can inhibit all of the matrix metalloproteases.[58]

The role of metalloproteases in the pathogenesis of emphysema was discovered by serendipity. D'Armiento and colleagues overexpressed the matrix metalloprotease collagenase (MMP-1) in transgenic mice in an attempt to develop a model of hepatic fibrosis. The resulting mice developed emphysema in the absence of inflammation or fibrosis.[64] This developmental model of emphysema prompted an examination of the role of collagenase in animals and humans with emphysema. Collagenase was demonstrated in guinea pig[65] and human[66,67] lung in association with cigarette smoke-induced emphysema. The role of metalloproteases in the pathogenesis of lung disease is supported by an elegant study which showed that removing macrophage metalloelastase (MMP-12) protects mice against cigarette smoke-induced emphysema.[68] MMP-12 is also likely to be important in man as it is expressed in high levels in the alveolar macrophages of cigarette smokers.[69] The conclusion from the study is not that macrophage elastase is the sole protease responsible for human disease, but that macrophages have the capacity to cause emphysema upon recruitment and activation by cigarette smoke.[70]

Mice have also been used to assess the role of IL-13 and interferon gamma (IFN-γ) in the pathogenesis of lung disease. IL-13 drives a Th2 cytokine response that has been strongly implicated in the development of airway hyperreactivity and asthma. Mice that overexpress IL-13 develop emphysema with increased lung volumes, increased compliance, mucus metaplasia and inflammation.[71] IL-13 exerts its effects by inducing the production of MMP-2, -9, -12, -13 and -14 and cathepsins B, S, L and H. The study showed that IL-13 was able to cause emphysema via MMP- and cathepsin-dependent mechanisms. Moreover it illustrates that a common mechanism may underlie the development of COPD and asthma, the so-called 'Dutch hypothesis'. Similar studies have shown that the overexpression of IFN-γ can also cause emphysema in mice.[72] In this case the pathogenesis is driven by activation of MMP-12 and cathepsins B, H, D, S and L.

ANTIPROTEASES

In recent years there have been major advances in our understanding of the structure and function of protease inhibitors within the lung and the mechanism by which they can be inactivated in disease. To date no naturally occurring deficiency mutants of SLPI, elafin, TIMPs or the cystatins have been described in association with lung disease. This chapter will therefore concentrate on the genetics and pathophysiology of two inhibitory serpins whose deficiency has been intimately linked with lung damage: alpha-1-antitrypsin and alpha-1-antichymotrypsin.

Alpha-1-antitrypsin

Alpha-1-antitrypsin is the most abundant circulating protease inhibitor. It is a 394-amino-acid,[73] acute-phase glycoprotein[74] encoded on chromosome 14q31-32.1.[75]

The protein is synthesized in hepatocytes,[76,77] macrophages,[78] intestinal[79] and lung epithelial cells.[80] It has a molecular weight of 52 kDa and circulates at a concentration of 1.9–3.5 mg/ml. The protein was originally named because of its ability to inhibit pancreatic trypsin[81] but was subsequently found to be an effective inhibitor of a variety of proteases including neutrophil elastase,[5] cathepsin G[5] and protease 3.[82] The broad spectrum of protease inhibition gave rise to its alternative name of alpha-1-protease inhibitor.[83]

Alpha-1-antitrypsin deficiency

Alpha-1-antitrypsin deficiency is the most widely recognized abnormality of a protease inhibitor that causes lung disease. Over 70 naturally occurring variants have been described and characterized by their migration on isoelectric focusing gels – the protease inhibitor or PI system.[84] The two most common deficiency variants S and Z result from point mutations in the alpha-1-antitrypsin gene[85–87] and make the protein migrate more slowly than normal M alpha-1-antitrypsin. A recent review of 70 surveys has provided an assessment of the frequency and distribution of the S and Z alpha-1-antitrypsin alleles throughout Europe (Plate 4). The greatest frequency of the S allele is in the Iberian Peninsula with the value gradually reducing from south to north and from west to east. The greatest frequency of the Z allele is in Northern and Western Europe with the value gradually declining from west to east and from north to south. S alpha-1-antitrypsin (^{264}glutamic acid $\rightarrow$ valine) is found in up to 28% of Southern Europeans and although it results in plasma alpha-1-antitrypsin levels that are 60% of the M allele it is not associated with any pulmonary sequelae. The Z variant (^{342}glutamic acid $\rightarrow$ lysine) results in a more severe deficiency which is characterized in the homozygote by plasma alpha-1-antitrypsin levels of 10% of the normal M allele and by levels of 60% in the MZ heterozygote (50% from the M allele and 10% from the Z allele). The Z mutation results in the accumulation of alpha-1-antitrypsin as inclusions in the rough endoplasmic reticulum of the liver. These inclusions predispose the homozygote to juvenile hepatitis, cirrhosis[88,89] and hepatocellular carcinoma.[90] The lack of circulating protein predisposes the homozygote to early-onset panlobular emphysema.

MOLECULAR PATHOLOGY OF ALPHA-1-ANTITRYPSIN DEFICIENCY: CIRRHOSIS

Alpha-1-antitrypsin is the archetypal member of the **ser**ine **p**rotease **in**hibitor or serpin superfamily. The structure of all the members of this family is based on three beta-sheets (A–C) and nine alpha-helices. This scaffold supports an exposed mobile reactive loop that presents a peptide sequence as a pseudosubstrate for the target protease. In the case of alpha-1-antitrypsin the loop presents the P_1–P_1 residues methionine-serine as a 'bait' for neutrophil elastase.[91] After docking the protease is inactivated by a mousetrap action that swings it from the top to the bottom of the protein (Plate 3(a)) in association with the insertion of an extra strand in beta-sheet A.[92,93] This six-stranded protein bound to its target enzyme is then recognized by hepatic receptors and cleared from the circulation.[94]

The structure of alpha-1-antitrypsin is very much a dual-edged sword in that it is central to its role as an effective antiproteases but also renders it liable to undergo conformational change in association with disease. Point mutations can destabilize beta-sheet A to allow incorporation of the loop of another molecule of alpha-1-antitrypsin. Sequential loop insertion results in chains of polymers that are retained within the cell of synthesis. This process is best characterized for the severe Z deficiency variant of alpha-1-antitrypsin that results in protein retention in hepatocytes in association with cirrhosis.[95,96] The Z mutation of alpha-1-antitrypsin is at residue P_{17} (17 residues proximal to the P_1 reactive center) at the head of strand 5 of beta-sheet A and the base of the mobile reactive loop (Plate 3(b)). The mutation opens beta-sheet A thereby favoring the insertion of the reactive loop of a second alpha-1-antitrypsin molecule to form a dimer. This can then extend to form polymers (Plate 3(b)) that tangle in the endoplasmic reticulum of the liver to form inclusion bodies.[97,98] Support for this comes from the demonstration that Z alpha-1-antitrypsin formed chains of polymers when incubated under physiologic conditions.[95,96] The rate was accelerated by raising the temperature to 41°C and could be blocked by peptides that compete with the loop for annealing to beta-sheet A.[95,99] The role of polymerization *in vivo* was clarified by the finding of alpha-1-antitrypsin polymers in inclusion bodies from the livers of Z alpha-1-antitrypsin homozygotes.

Although many alpha-1-antitrypsin deficiency variants have been described, only two other mutants of alpha-1-antitrypsin have similarly been associated with plasma deficiency and hepatic inclusions: alpha-1-antitrypsin Siiyama ([53]serine → phenylalanine;[100]) and alpha-1-antitrypsin Mmalton ([52]phenylalanine deleted[101]). Both of these mutants also destabilize beta-sheet A to allow the formation of loop-sheet polymers *in vivo*.[102,103] The temperature and concentration dependence of polymerization,[104] along with genetic factors,[105,106] may account for the heterogeneity in liver disease amongst individuals who are homozygous for the Z mutation. As alpha-1-antitrypsin is an acute-phase protein the concentration will rise during episodes of inflammation. At these times the formation of polymers is likely to overwhelm the degradative pathway thereby exacerbating the formation of hepatic inclusions and the associated hepatocellular damage. There is anecdotal evidence to support this hypothesis from the prospective study of Sveger in Sweden.[107] They screened 200 000 newborn babies and identified 120 Z homozygotes whom they have followed into late adolescence.[88] Two of these patients developed progressive jaundice during the course of the study; in one this followed appendicitis and in the other severe pneumonia.

Recent investigations have shown that polymerization also underlies the mild plasma deficiency of the S and I ([39]arginine → cysteine) variants of alpha-1-antitrypsin.[108,109] The point mutations that are responsible for these variants have less effect on beta-sheet A than does the Z variant. Thus the rates of polymer formation are much slower than that of Z alpha-1-antitrypsin which results in less retention of protein within hepatocytes, milder plasma deficiency and the lack of a clinical phenotype.[104] However if a mild, slowly polymerizing S or I variant of alpha-1-antitrypsin is inherited with a rapidly polymerizing Z variant then the two can interact to form heteropolymers within hepatocytes, inclusions and cirrhosis.[109] As would be predicted null mutations that result in no production of d_i-antitrpsin are not associated with cirrhosis.

MOLECULAR PATHOLOGY OF ALPHA-1-ANTITRYPSIN DEFICIENCY: EMPHYSEMA

The single most important factor in the development of emphysema in patients with alpha-1-antitrypsin deficiency is smoking.[110,111] The combination of antiprotease deficiency and cigarette smoke can have a devastating effect on lung function,[112,113] presumably by allowing the unopposed action of proteolytic enzymes. Alpha-1-antitrypsin levels are greatly reduced in the lungs of individuals with alpha-1-antitrypsin deficiency.[114] Moreover the alpha-1-antitrypsin that is available to protect the lungs is approximately fivefold less effective at inhibiting neutrophil elastase than normal M alpha-1-antitrypsin.[96,115,116] The inhibitory activity of Z alpha-1-antitrypsin can be further reduced as alpha-1-antitrypsin is susceptible to inactivation by oxidation of the P_1 methionine residue by free radicals from leukocytes or direct oxidation by cigarette smoke.[5,6,32,33] Finally the Z mutation favors the spontaneous formation of alpha-1-antitrypsin loop-sheet polymers within the lung.[117] This conformational transition inactivates the protein, thereby further reducing the already depleted levels of alpha-1-antitrypsin that are available to protect the alveoli (Figure 9.2). An assessment of bronchoalveolar lavage from patients with Z alpha-1-antitrypsin deficiency has revealed an excess number of neutrophils when compared with controls.[118] This may reflect an excess of chemoattractant agents such as leukotriene B4 (LTB4)[119] and IL-8. However recent

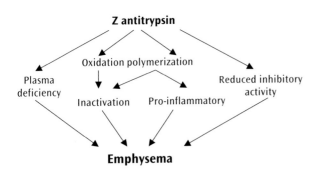

Figure 9.2 *Proposed model for the pathogenesis of emphysema in patients with PiZ alpha-1-antitrypsin deficiency. The plasma deficiency and reduced inhibitory activity of Z alpha-1-antitrypsin are exacerbated by oxidation and polymerization of alpha-1-antitrypsin within the lungs. These processes inactivate the inhibitor thereby further reducing the antiprotease screen. Alpha-1-antitrypsin polymers may also act as a pro-inflammatory stimulus to attract and activate neutrophils thereby increasing tissue damage. (Reproduced from Blanco et al. Alpha-1-antitrypsin PI phenotypes S and Z in Europe: an analysis of the published surveys. Clin. Genet 2001;60: 31–41. With permission from Blackwell Publishing.)*

studies have demonstrated that the polymers are themselves chemotactic for human neutrophils *in vitro*.[120] The relationship of intrapulmonary Z alpha-1-antitrypsin polymers to smoking, infection, cytokine production and rate of decline in lung function in Z homozygotes requires further evaluation in prospective studies.

OTHER SERPINOPATHIES: SERPIN POLYMERIZATION IN THROMBOSIS, ANGIOEDEMA, DEMENTIA AND EMPHYSEMA WITHOUT ALPHA-1-ANTITRYPSIN DEFICIENCY

Alpha-1-antitrypsin is the archetypal member of the serine protease inhibitor or serpin superfamily. This family includes members such as alpha-1-antichymotrypsin, C1 esterase inhibitor, antithrombin and plasminogen activator inhibitor-1 which play an important role in the control of proteases involved in the inflammatory, complement, coagulation and fibrinolytic cascades respectively.[83,121] The family is characterized by more than 30% sequence homology with alpha-1-antitrypsin and conservation of tertiary structure.[73,122] Consequently physiologic and pathologic processes that affect one member may be extrapolated to another. The phenomenon of loop-sheet polymerization is not restricted to alpha-1-antitrypsin and has now been reported in other mutants of other members of the serpin superfamily to cause disease (the serpinopathies). Mutants of C1-inhibitor, antithrombin and alpha-1-antichymotrypsin can also destabilize the serpin architecture to form inactive polymers that are associated with angioedema,

thrombosis and chronic obstructive pulmonary disease respectively (see later).[123–129] The process is most striking in a recently described inclusion body dementia, familial encephalopathy with neuroserpin inclusion bodies (FENIB), that results from polymerization of the neurone-specific serpin, neuroserpin.[130] The dementia has been described in two Caucasian families in the USA.[131,132] In the first family, 95% of affected individuals presented with dementia between the ages of 45 and 56. The second family had an earlier age of onset of symptoms with epilepsy and progressive decline in cognitive function occurring in the second and third decades of life. Both were characterized by eosinophilic neuronal inclusion bodies in the deeper layers of the cerebral cortex and the substantia nigra. The inclusions were PAS positive and diastase resistant (Figure 9.3) but were distinctly different from any previously described entity including Lewy bodies, Pick bodies and Lafora bodies. The inclusion bodies had a striking resemblance to those of Z alpha-1-antitrypsin in the hepatocytes of homozygotes with cirrhosis (Figure 9.3). Biochemical analysis revealed that the inclusions were formed of neuroserpin and that affected individuals carried point mutations that would destabilize the protein to form polymers. Indeed one of the mutations was in the same position as the Siiyama variant which causes hepatic inclusions and profound plasma deficiency of alpha-1-antitrypsin.[102] Structural analysis showed that the mutant neuroserpin had indeed formed intraneuronal polymers that were identical to those of Z alpha-1-antitrypsin.[130] Thus therapies that attenuate serpin polymerization may be useful in a whole range of diseases.

CLINICAL FEATURES OF ALPHA-1-ANTITRYPSIN DEFICIENCY

Neonatal jaundice, juvenile cirrhosis and hepatocellular carcinoma

Z alpha-1-antitrypsin liver disease is characterized by the accumulation of diastase-resistant, periodic acid-Schiff positive inclusions of alpha-1-antitrypsin in the periportal cells[133,134] (Figure 9.3(a),(c)). This insoluble material accumulates within the endoplasmic reticulum of hepatocytes stimulating a massive increase in cellular degradative activity. The PIMZ individuals are able to degrade much of the abnormal alpha-1-antitrypsin but not the PIZ homozygote in whom aggregation overwhelms the degradative process resulting in alpha-1-antitrypsin accumulation, hepatocellular damage and cell death. The accumulation of alpha-1-antitrypsin within hepatocytes is also seen with two other rare mutations: Siiyama (^{53}serine $\rightarrow$ phenylalanine) which is the commonest cause of alpha-1-antitrypsin deficiency in Japan[100,135] and Mmalton (also known as Mnichinan[136] and Mcagliari,[137] deletion of phenylalanine at position 52) which is the commonest cause of alpha-1-antitrypsin

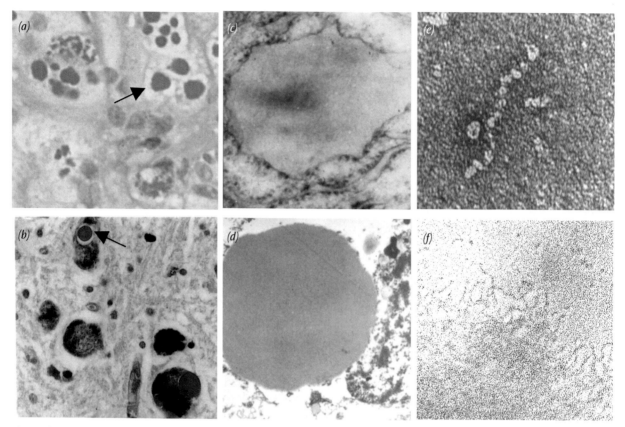

Figure 9.3 *Z alpha-1-antitrypsin is retained within hepatocytes as intracellular inclusions. These inclusions are PAS positive and diastase resistant ((a), arrowed) and are associated with neonatal hepatitis and hepatocellular carcinoma. (c) Electron micrograph of an hepatocyte from the liver of a patient with Z alpha-1-antitrypsin deficiency shows the accumulation of alpha-1-antitrypsin within the rough endoplasmic reticulum. These inclusions are composed of chains of alpha-1-antitrypsin polymers shown here from the plasma of a Siiyama alpha-1-antitrypsin homozygote (e)[102] and from the liver of a Z alpha-1-antitrypsin homozygote (f).[95] Similar mutations in alpha-1-antitrypsin deficiency and neuroserpin encephalopathy result in similar intracellular inclusions of alpha-1-antitrypsin and neuroserpin.[130,131] They are shown here in hepatocytes and neurons with PAS staining ((a) and (b) respectively) and as endoplasmic aggregates of the abnormal proteins on electron microscopy ((c) and (d) respectively). Electron microscopy confirms that the abnormal neuroserpin forms bead-like polymers and entangled polymeric aggregates identical to those shown here with Z alpha-1-antitrypsin ((e) and (f) respectively). (Magnification: (a),(b) ×200; (c),(d) ×20 000; (e),(f) ×220 000.) (From ref. 216.) Copyright © 200 × Mass. Medical Society. All rights reserved.*

deficiency in Sardinia. Both of these point mutations result in perturbations of alpha-1-antitrypsin and the ready formation of loop-sheet polymers. Cirrhosis has also been reported sporadically in SZ[138,139] and IZ[109] heterozygotes in whom the 'polymerogenic' Z and S or I alpha-1-antitrypsin can interlink to form chains of mixed SZ or IZ heteropolymers.

Seventy-three per cent of Z alpha-1-antitrypsin homozygote infants have a raised serum alanine aminotransferase in the first year of life but in only 15% of people is it still abnormal by the age of 12 years.[88,89,107,140] Similarly serum bilirubin is raised in 11% of PIZ infants in the first 2–4 months but falls to normal by 6 months of age. One in ten infants develops cholestatic jaundice and 6% develop clinical evidence of liver disease without

jaundice. These symptoms usually resolve by the second year but approximately 15% of patients with cholestatic jaundice progress to juvenile cirrhosis. The reasons for this variable progression are not known but intercurrent illness, hormonal and genetic factors are likely to be involved. Indeed cholestatic jaundice in infancy is twice as common in boys than girls. The overall risk of death from liver disease in PIZ children during childhood is 2–3%. All PIZ individuals have slowly progressive hepatic damage that is often subclinical and only evident as a minor degree of portal fibrosis.[90] However up to 50% of Z alpha-1-antitrypsin homozygotes present with clinically evident cirrhosis and occasionally with hepatocellular carcinoma.[90] The presence of Z alpha-1-antitrypsin deficiency, including the heterozygous PIMZ and PISZ, should always be considered before making the diagnosis of cryptogenic cirrhosis.

Lung disease

The FEV$_1$ value is a convenient measure of lung function that predicts mortality in patients with COPD.[43] After the age of 30 years in healthy non-smokers, the FEV$_1$ decreases by 35 ml/year, although there is considerable individual variation. By old age, most people will have an appreciable loss of lung function but only occasionally in the non-smoker will this be clinically apparent. The assessment of symptomatic hospital patients has shown that the loss of FEV$_1$ may be accelerated to 80 ml/year in the Z alpha-1-antitrypsin homozygote.[112] As a consequence there is a hastened but still variable onset of emphysema. In this study PIZ non-smokers were free from dyspnea up to the age of 50 years with an average age of death from respiratory disease being 67 years. Again there was considerable individual variation and, particularly in women, there was a good likelihood of a full life span without significant respiratory impairment. The outlook, however, was poor for PIZ alpha-1-antitrypsin homozygotes who were heavy smokers as the loss in FEV$_1$ increased to 300 ml/year. The onset of dyspnea was approximately 30 years, with death from respiratory disease by the age of 50 years. This and other studies[113] are subject to selection bias as patients were identified as the result of impaired respiratory function. The analysis of individuals selected on family studies as well as impaired respiratory function[110,111,141,142] have reported a more favorable outcome. This registry data has shown lower rates of decline in lung function in PIZ homozygotes who are ex- or non-smokers (approximately 50 ml/year). However the studies reinforce the accelerated rate of decline in lung function in PiZ homozygotes who continue to smoke (70–132 ml/year). It is likely that other combinations of alpha-1-antitrypsin deficiency alleles such as SZ,[143] and possibly FZ,[144] also place the smoker at an increased risk of developing emphysema. However the risk is much less than in PIZZ homozygotes.[145]

In addition to smoking, exposure to dust may also accelerate the rate of decline in lung function in patients with alpha-1-antitrypsin deficiency. A study from the Swedish alpha-1-antitrypsin registry found a lower FEV$_1$ in non-smoking PIZZ individuals who were agricultural workers or who used kerosene stoves but not in those who used gas stoves.[146] Non-smoking PIZZ homozygotes were also at increased risk of chronic bronchitis if they were exposed to passive smoking. Analysis of a different cohort concluded that PIZZ homozygotes who were exposed to mineral dusts also had a lower FEV$_1$.[147] The results of this study are more difficult to interpret as smokers were included in the analysis. The precise role of dusts in the pathogenesis of emphysema is uncertain but individuals with alpha-1-antitrypsin defi-

ciency should probably not work in a dusty environment if it can be avoided.

Homozygous Z alpha-1-antitrypsin deficiency makes up only 1–2% of all cases of COPD and there is considerable variability in FEV$_1$ between current and ex-smokers with the same PI Z genotype.[148] This is particularly so if cohorts are analyzed on whether the alpha-1-antitrypsin deficiency was identified in patients with impaired respiratory function or through family studies.[111] Clearly other coexisting genetic factors must predispose to lung disease in Z alpha-1-antitrypsin homozygotes. A logical follow-on from the association of alpha-1-antitrypsin deficiency with emphysema is an assessment of the risk of COPD in heterozygotes who carry an abnormal Z allele and a normal M allele. These individuals have plasma alpha-1-antitrypsin levels that are approximately 65% of normal. A population-based study demonstrated that PI MZ heterozygotes do not have a clearly increased risk of lung damage.[149] However if groups of patients are collected who already have COPD, then the prevalence of PI MZ individuals appears to be elevated.[150] In addition, longitudinal studies have demonstrated that among COPD patients, the PI MZ heterozygotes have a more rapid decline in lung function.[151,152] These data suggest that either all PI MZ individuals are at slightly increased risk for the development of COPD, or that a subset of the PI MZ subjects are at substantially increased risk of pulmonary damage if they smoke.[153] An alternative explanation is that the apparent increased risk among PI MZ subjects reflects ascertainment bias, and the elevated rate of PI MZ subjects among COPD cases reflects the influence of other, as yet unidentified, factors.

Patients with alpha-1-antitrypsin deficiency related emphysema usually present with increasing dyspnea and weight loss, with cor pulmonale and polycythemia occurring late in the course of the disease. Chest radiographs typically show bilateral basal emphysema with paucity and pruning of the basal pulmonary vessels (Figure 9.4). Upper lobe vascularization is relatively normal. Ventilation perfusion radioisotope scans and angiography also show abnormalities with a lower zone distribution.[154] Lung function tests are typical for emphysema with a reduced FEV$_1$/FVC ratio, gas trapping (raised residual volume/total lung capacity ratio) and low gas transfer factor. High resolution CT scans with 1–2 mm collimation are the most accurate method of assessing the distribution of panlobular emphysema and for monitoring progress of the pulmonary disease,[155,156] although this currently has little clinical value outside clinical trials. The severity of lung function abnormalities and health status correlates well with the quantification of emphysema by CT scans.[157]

Plasma deficiency of alpha-1-antitrypsin is associated with an increased prevalence of asthma[158,159] and Wegener's granulomatosis.[160,161] There have also been

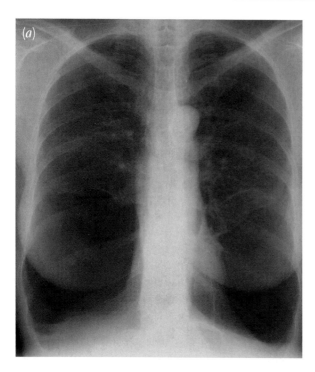

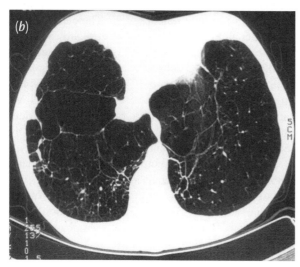

Figure 9.4 *Chest X-ray (a) and high resolution CT scan (b) of the thorax of a patient with alpha-1-antitrypsin deficiency. The radiographs demonstrate the characteristic panlobular basal emphysema seen in patients with alpha-1-antitrypsin deficiency rather than the upper lobe centrilobular disease seen in smokers with normal levels of alpha-1-antitrypsin.*

reports of an increased prevalence of bronchiectasis in individuals with alpha-1-antitrypsin deficiency.[162,163] This was recently investigated in a survey of 202 patients with bronchiectasis. In 121 of these patients the cause of the bronchiectasis was unknown. The allelic frequency of S and Z alpha-1-antitrypsin was no different in the patients with bronchiectasis when compared to healthy

blood donor controls living in the same geographic area.[164] Thus the authors concluded that alpha-1-antitrypsin did not predispose to the development of bronchiectasis. They did however find an overrepresentation of PIZ alleles in patients with bronchiectasis and coexisting emphysema and suggest that the bronchiectasis may be a consequence of emphysema in Z alpha-1-antitrypsin homozygotes rather than a primary effect.

Extrapulmonary conditions associated with alpha-1-antitrypsin deficiency

Panniculitis is a rare complication of alpha-1-antitrypsin deficiency that is characterized by an acute inflammatory infiltrate and fat necrosis. The first case of panniculitis in association with alpha-1-antitrypsin deficiency was described in 1972.[165] Since then there have been 28 case reports with a mean age of almost 40 years and an equal sex distribution (reviewed in ref. 166). Sixty-four per cent of individuals have a PIZZ phenotype and there is strong anecdotal evidence that replacing the deficient alpha-1-antitrypsin brings about a resolution of symptoms.[166,167] The risk of other extrapulmonary conditions has recently been assessed in 605 patients with alpha-1-antitrypsin deficiency enroled in the Danish registry because of respiratory symptoms or through family screening.[168] A case-control analysis revealed that there was an increased risk of liver cirrhosis (relative risk 6.0), pancreatitis (relative risk 3.1) and gall stones (relative risk 1.9) and a reduced risk of cerebrovascular disorders (relative risk 0.5) in individuals with alpha-1-antitrypsin deficiency. This study found no increased risk of vasculitis, rheumatoid arthritis, arterial diseases or aneurysms. This is in contrast to case reports of vascular aneurysms in individuals with MZ and ZZ alpha-1-antitrypsin phenotypes.[169,170]

TREATMENT OF ALPHA-1-ANTITRYPSIN DEFICIENCY

The new understanding of the structural basis of alpha-1-antitrypsin deficiency provides a platform for rational drug design to block polymerization *in vivo* and so attenuate the associated liver disease.[98] Until that time supportive therapy is the only treatment available for the cirrhosis associated with alpha-1-antitrypsin deficiency. The liver disease progresses with varying speed and lacks specific features.[171,172] Liver transplantation provides definitive treatment for patients with end-stage alpha-1-antitrypsin deficiency-related cirrhosis and children who receive a transplant have an excellent clinical outcome.[173]

There is good evidence that many Z alpha-1-antitrypsin homozygotes would develop only mild lung disease if they abstain from smoking.[110,174] Patients with alpha-1-antitrypsin deficiency-related emphysema should receive advice on smoking cessation and where appropriate they should be offered nicotine replacement therapy and/or bupropion.[175] Those patients with airflow obstruction should be assessed with lung function tests followed by trials of bronchodilators and inhaled corticosteroids.[176] Many patients benefit from pulmonary rehabilitation[177] and, where appropriate, assessment for long-term oxygen therapy.[176] The most severely affected individuals should be referred for consideration of lung transplantation. In appropriately selected patients with alpha-1-antitrypsin deficiency-related emphysema, lung transplantation prolongs survival, improves functional capacity and enhances quality of life.[178] However rejection remains an obstacle to better medium-term results and currently heart-lung transplantation has a 5-year survival of approximately 60%. There is anecdotal evidence that patients with alpha-1-antitrypsin deficiency have more postoperative complications following lung transplantation. Assessment of lung lavage from 11 transplant recipients with alpha-1-antitrypsin deficiency revealed minimal or unmeasureable free elastase.[179] However free elastase was detected in three of seven patients during severe respiratory illnesses. The requirement for alpha-1-antitrypsin replacement therapy in patients with alpha-1-antitrypsin deficiency after lung transplantation requires further investigation.

The role of lung volume reduction surgery (LVRS) in patients with alpha-1-antitrypsin is unclear. Cassina and colleagues reported 12 patients with alpha-1-antitrypsin deficiency who had undergone bilateral thoracotomy and lower lobe LVRS.[180] They found a transient improvement in FEV$_1$ and static lung volumes with deterioration to below the starting values by 24 months of follow-up. The only exception was the 6-minute walk distance which was still slightly improved compared to baseline after 24 months. By contrast, Gelb and colleagues reported six patients with alpha-1-antitrypsin deficiency in whom there was a significant improvement in lung function following bilateral lower lobe video-assisted thoracoscopic LVRS.[181] In four of the patients who were followed up for more than 22 months there was a sustained improvement in breathlessness and exercise tolerance.[181] Despite the conflicting reports both authors agree that the benefit from LVRS is far less in patients with alpha-1-antitrypsin deficiency than in individuals with smoking-related upper lobe emphysema with normal levels of alpha-1-antitrypsin.[180,181] Thus LVRS should not be offered routinely in patients with alpha-1-antitrypsin deficiency until further information is available.[182]

The genetic deficiency in the anti-elastase screen may be rectified biochemically by intravenous infusions of alpha-1-antitrypsin.[114] There is registry data to suggest that this therapy may slow the rate of decline in lung function in patients with an FEV$_1$ of 35–49% predicted[142] but this has yet to be proven in randomized controlled trials. The only controlled trial that has assessed alpha-1-antitrypsin replacement therapy showed that infusions of alpha-1-antitrypsin may slow down the progression of emphysema as assessed by HRCT scans but had no effect on decline in FEV$_1$.[183] A larger study is required to confirm these findings[184] and alpha-1-antitrypsin replacement therapy (Prolastin, Bayer) is currently not available in many parts of Europe.

Other treatments at earlier stages of development include gene therapy and the administration of retinoic acid and chemical chaperones. Vectors carrying the alpha-1-antitrypsin gene have been targeted to liver,[185] lung[186] and muscle[187,188] in animals. There is good expression of alpha-1-antitrypsin but further data are required to assess whether this can be achieved in man. In particular it is important to determine the length of time of protein expression and whether the levels of alpha-1-antitrypsin in the epithelial lining fluid of the lung are sufficient to prevent ongoing proteolytic damage. Similarly although the effects of retinoic acid on alveolar regeneration in the rat look promising,[189] they have yet to be demonstrated in patients with emphysema. The most exciting new development is the use of chemical chaperones in an attempt to improve secretion of Z alpha-1-antitrypsin from hepatocytes. The chaperone trimethyamine oxide had no effect on the secretion of Z alpha-1-antitrypsin in cell culture,[190] as it favors the conversion of unfolded Z alpha-1-antitrypsin to polymers.[191] By contrast, 4-phenylbutyrate (4-PBA) increased the secretion of Z alpha-1-antitrypsin from cell lines and transgenic mice.[190] This agent has been used for several years to treat children with urea cycle disorders and more recently 4-PBA has been shown to increase the expression of mutant (ΔF508) cystic fibrosis transmembrane regulator protein *in vitro*[192] and *in vivo*.[193] These encouraging findings have led to a pilot study to evaluate the potential of 4-PBA to promote the secretion of alpha-1-antitrypsin in patients with alpha-1-antitrypsin deficiency.

Alpha-1-antichymotrypsin

Alpha-1-antichymotrypsin is a 374-amino-acid, 64 kDa, acute-phase glycoprotein which is secreted from the liver[194] and human bronchial epithelial cells.[195] The gene has been mapped to chromosome 14q32.1 in close proximity to the alpha-1-antitrypsin gene[75] and alpha-1-antichymotrypsin circulates in the plasma at one-tenth the concentration of alpha-1-antitrypsin. Alpha-1-antichymotrypsin has inhibitory activity against cathepsin G,[5,196,197] mast cell chymase[198] and chymotrypsin.[5]

The association of alpha-1-antichymotrypsin deficiency and lung disease was first reported when five volunteers undergoing health screening were found to have reduced plasma levels and airflow obstruction.[199,200]

Point mutations of the alpha-1-antichymotrypsin gene have now been characterized and are associated with decreased circulating protein in the heterozygote; no patient who is homozygote for alpha-1-antichymotrypsin deficiency mutations has yet been described. The ^{229}proline $\rightarrow$ alanine and ^{55}leucine $\rightarrow$ proline alpha-1-antichymotrypsin mutations have been found in 4%[128,201] and 1.5%[127] respectively of unrelated patients with chronic airflow obstruction but in no healthy controls. The ^{229}proline $\rightarrow$ alanine alpha-1-antichymotrypsin mutation is of particular interest as plasma deficiency is associated with hepatic inclusions of alpha-1-antichymotrypsin which are similar to those of Z alpha-1-antitrypsin.[128] Both the ^{229}proline $\rightarrow$ alanine and ^{55}leucine $\rightarrow$ proline mutations will allow the formation of alpha-1-antichymotrypsin loop-sheet polymers by a mechanism identical to that of the point mutations of alpha-1-antitrypsin.[128,129] However, the association of these two mutations with COPD was not replicated in a study of 168 patients with COPD and 61 control subjects.[202] Moreover, the mutations are uncommon so that even if they do predispose to COPD it will be in relatively few individuals.[202,203]

Two other mutations, ^{389}methionine $\rightarrow$ valine[204] and a two base pair deletions at codon 391,[205] have been described that result in decreased circulating levels of alpha-1-antichymotrypsin but the clinical significance of these mutations has yet to be established. Finally there is evidence of segregation of a signal peptide mutation (−15 threonine $\rightarrow$ alanine), that possibly increases the production of alpha-1-antichymotrypsin, with an increased risk of late onset Alzheimer's disease[206] although this observation has not been confirmed by other groups.[207–211] The role of this polymorphism in chronic lung disease has not been evaluated.

Alpha-1-antichymotrypsin in the lungs of patients with chronic bronchitis and emphysema is intact but inactive.[212] The recent understanding of the conformational transitions of alpha-1-antitrypsin has provided an explanation of the molecular basis for this inactivation. Biochemical evidence from bronchoalveolar lavage suggests that alpha-1-antichymotrypsin adopts an inactive latent conformation.[213] The association of this conformational transition of alpha-1-antichymotrypsin with smoking, infection and decline in lung function remains to be determined in longitudinal studies.

SUMMARY

The protease/antiprotease hypothesis evolved as individuals with alpha-1-antitrypsin deficiency developed emphysema[4,7] and this could be reproduced experimentally by instiling papain into the lungs of rats.[214] After 35 years the

hypothesis still remains central to our understanding of the pathogenesis of lung disease. Many more proteases and antiproteases have been added to the equation and their interaction adds another level of complexity to our understanding of the disease process. The use of animal models has been invaluable in dissecting out the role of proteases in lung disease and we have now entered a new and exciting era with the advent of powerful transgenic technology. On the other side of the balance a more detailed understanding of the structural mechanisms underlying the deficiency of the antiprotease screen should allow the development of novel strategies to prevent disease. Whilst much has been achieved there is still plenty to be done. It is salutary to think that none of the data that have been generated since the evolution of the protease/antiprotease hypothesis have yielded a drug that is proven in clinical trials to be useful in treating the relentless progression of emphysema. Hopefully we will do better in the next 35 years!

REFERENCES

1. Kiernan V. Warm hearts in a cold land. *New Scientist* 1995;**4 March**:10.
2. Kuzemko JA. Chopin's illnesses. *J R Soc Med* 1994;**87**: 769–72.
3. Kubba AK, Young M. The long suffering of Frederic Chopin. *Chest* 1997;**113**:210–16.
4. Laurell C-B, Eriksson S. The electrophoretic alpha-1-globulin pattern of serum in alpha-1-antitrypsin deficiency. *Scand J Clin Lab Invest* 1963;**15**:132–40.
5. Beatty K, Bieth J, Travis J. Kinetics of association of serine proteinases with native and oxidized α-1-proteinase inhibitor and α-1-antichymotrypsin. *J Biol Chem* 1980;**255**: 3931–4.
6. Carrell RW, Jeppsson J-O, Laurell C-B, *et al*. Structure and variation of human alpha-1-antitrypsin. *Nature* 1982;**298**: 329–34.
7. Eriksson S. Studies in alpha-1-antitrypsin deficiency. *Acta Med Scand* 1965;(suppl 432):1–85.
8. Birrer P, McElvaney NG, Rüdeberg A, *et al*. Protease-antiprotease imbalance in the lungs of children with cystic fibrosis. *Am J Respir Crit Care Med* 1994;**150**:207–13.
9. Schraufstatter I, Revak SD, Cochrane CG. Biochemical factors in pulmonary inflammatory disease. *Fed Proc* 1984;**43**:2807–10.
10. Ray JM, Stetler-Stevenson WG. The role of matrix metalloproteases and their inhibitors in tumour invasion, metastasis and angiogenesis. *Eur Respir J* 1994;**7**:2062–72.
11. Cole PJ. A new look at the pathogenesis and management of persistent bronchial sepsis: a "vicious circle" hypothesis and its logical therapeutic connotations. In: RJ Davies, ed. *Strategies for the Management of Chronic Bronchial Sepsis*. Medicine Publishing Foundation, Oxford, 1984, pp 1–20.
12. Stockley RA, Hill SL, Burnett D. Proteinases in chronic lung infection. *Ann NY Acad Sci* 1991;**624**:257–65.
13. Lucey EC, Stone PJ, Breuer R, *et al*. Effect of combined human neutrophil cathepsin G and elastase on induction of secretory cell metaplasia and emphysema in hamsters, with *in vitro*

observations on elastolysis by these enzymes. *Am Rev Respir Dis* 1985;**132**:362–6.

14. Senior RM, Tegner H, Kuhn C, *et al.* The induction of pulmonary emphysema with human leukocyte elastase. *Am Rev Respir Dis* 1977;**116**:469–75.

15. Janoff A, Sloan B, Weinbaum G, *et al.* Experimental emphysema induced with purified human neutrophil elastase: tissue localization of the instilled protease. *Am Rev Respir Dis* 1977;**115**:461–78.

16. Snider GL, Lucey EC, Christensen TG, *et al.* Emphysema and bronchial secretory cell metaplasia induced in hamsters by human neutrophil products. *Am Rev Respir Dis* 1984;**129**:155–60.

17. Tetley TD. Matrix metalloproteinases: a role in emphysema. *Thorax* 1997;**52**:495.

18. Kaplan PD, Kuhn C, Pierce JA. The induction of emphysema with elastase. I. The evolution of the lesion and the influence of serum. *J Lab Clin Med* 1973;**82**:349–56.

19. Kao RC, Wehner NG, Skubitz KM, Gray BH, Hoidal JR. Proteinase 3. A distinct human polymorphonuclear leucocyte proteinase that produces emphysema in hamsters. *J Clin Invest* 1988;**82**:1963–73.

20. Hunninghake GW, Crystal RG. Cigarette smoking and lung destruction. *Am Rev Respir Dis* 1983;**128**:833–8.

21. Owen CA, Campbell MA, Sannes PL, Boukedes SS, Campbell EJ. Cell surface-bound elastase and cathepsin G on human neutrophils: a novel, non-oxidative mechanism by which neutrophils focus and preserve catalytic activity of serine proteinases. *J Cell Biol* 1995;**131**:775–89.

22. Damiano VV, Tsang A, Kucich U, *et al.* Immunolocalization of elastase in human emphysematous lungs. *J Clin Invest* 1986;**78**:482–93.

23. Ge YM, Zhu YJ, Luo WC, Gong YH, Zhang XQ. Damaging role of neutrophil elastase in the elastic fiber and basement membrane in human emphysematous lung. *Chin Med J (Engl)* 1990;**103**:588–94.

24. de Santi MM, Martorana PA, Cavarra E, Lungarella G. Pallid mice with genetic emphysema. Neutrophil elastase burden and elastin loss occur without alteration in the bronchoalveolar lavage cell population. *Lab Invest* 1995;**73**:40–7.

25. Cavarra E, Martorana PA, Gambelli F, de Santi M, van Even P, Lungarella G. Neutrophil recruitment into the lungs is associated with increased lung elastase burden, decreased lung elastin, and emphysema in alpha 1 proteinase inhibitor-deficient mice. *Lab Invest* 1996;**75**:273–80.

26. Fox B, Bull TB, Guz A, Harris E, Tetley TD. Is neutrophil elastase associated with elastic tissue in emphysema? *J Clin Pathol* 1988;**41**:435–40.

27. Amitani R, Wilson R, Rutman A, *et al.* Effects of human neutrophil elastase and *Pseudomonas aeruginosa* proteinases on human respiratory epithelium. *Am J Respir Cell Mol Biol* 1991;**4**:26–32.

28. Smallman LA, Hill SL, Stockley RA. Reduction of ciliary beat frequency *in vitro* by sputum from patients with bronchiectasis: a serine proteinase effect. *Thorax* 1984;**39**:663–7.

29. Senior RM, Griffin GL, Mecham RP. Chemotactic activity of elastin derived peptides. *J Clin Invest* 1980;**66**:859–62.

30. Padrines M, Schneider-Pozzer M, Bieth JG. Inhibition of neutrophil elastase by alpha-1-proteinase inhibitor oxidized by activated neutrophils. *Am Rev Respir Dis* 1989;**139**:783–90.

31. Bangalore N, Travis J. Comparison of properties of membrane bound versus soluble forms of human leukocyte elastase and cathepsin G. *Biol Chem Hoppe-Seyler* 1994;**375**:659–66.

32. Gadek JE, Fells GA, Crystal RG. Cigarette smoking induces functional antiprotease deficiency in the lower respiratory tract of humans. *Science* 1979;**206**:1315–16.

33. Janoff A, Carp H, Lee DK, Drew RT. Cigarette smoke inhalation decreases alpha-1-antitrypsin activity in rat lung. *Science* 1979;**206**:1313–14.

34. Stone P, Calore JD, McGowen SE. Functional alpha-1-antitrypsin in the lower respiratory tract of smokers is not decreased. *Science* 1983;**221**:1187–9.

35. Huntington JA, Read RJ, Carrell RW. Structure of a serpin–protease complex shows inhibition by deformation. *Nature* 2000;**407**:923–6.

36. Banda M, Rice AG, Griffin GL, Senior RM. Alpha-1-proteinase inhibitor is a neutrophil chemoattractant after proteolytic inactivation by macrophage elastase. *J Biol Chem* 1988;**263**:4481–4.

37. Potempa J, Fedak D, Dubin A, Mast A, Travis J. Proteolytic inactivation of alpha-1-anti-chymotrypsin. Sites of cleavage and generation of chemotactic activity. *J Biol Chem* 1991;**266**:21482–7.

38. Banda MJ, Rice AG, Griffin GL, Senior RM. The inhibitory complex of human alpha-1-proteinase inhibitor and human leukocyte elastase is a neutrophil chemoattractant. *J Exp Med* 1988;**167**:1608–15.

39. Stockley RA, Shaw J, Afford SC, Morrison HM, Burnett D. Effect of alpha-1-proteinase inhibitor on neutrophil chemotaxis. *Am J Respir Cell Mol Biol* 1990;**2**:163–70.

40. Campbell EJ, Senior RM, McDonald JA, Cox DL. Proteolysis by neutrophils. Relative importance of cell-substrate contact and oxidative inactivation of proteinase inhibitors *in vitro*. *J Clin Invest* 1982;**70**:845–52.

41. Liou TG, Campbell EJ. Nonisotropic enzyme–inhibitor interactions: a novel nonoxidative mechanism for quantum proteolysis by human neutrophils. *Biochemistry* 1995;**34**:16171–7.

42. Llewellyn-Jones CG, Lomas DA, Stockley RA. Potential role of recombinant secretory leucoprotease inhibitor in the prevention of neutrophil mediated matrix degradation. *Thorax* 1994;**49**:567–72.

43. Fletcher C, Peto R. The natural history of chronic airflow obstruction. *Br Med J* 1977;**1**:1645–8.

44. Kauffmann F, Drouet D, Lellouch J, Brille D. Twelve years spirometric changes among Paris area workers. *Int J Epidemiol* 1979;**8**:201–12.

45. Oxman AD, Muir DCF, Shannon HS, Stock SR, Hnizdo E, Lange HJ. Occupational dust exposure and chronic obstructive pulmonary disease. A systematic overview of the evidence. *Am Rev Respir Dis* 1993;**148**:38–48.

46. Ulvestad B, Bakke B, Melbostad E, Fuglerud P, Kongerud J, Lund MB. Increased risk of obstructive pulmonary disease in tunnel workers. *Thorax* 2000;**55**:277–82.

47. Sargeant LA, Jaeckel A, Wareham NJ. Interaction of vitamin C on the relation between smoking and obstructive airways disease in EPIC-Norfolk. *Eur Respir J* 2000;**16**:397–403.

48. Matsuse T, Hayashi S, Kuwano K, Keunecke H, Jefferies WA, Hogg JC. Latent adenoviral infection in the pathogenesis of chronic airways obstruction. *Am Rev Respir Dis* 1992;**146**:177–84.

49. Larson RK, Barman ML, Kueppers F, Fudenberg HH. Genetic and environmental determinants of chronic obstructive pulmonary disease. *Ann Intern Med* 1970;**72**:627–32.

50. Kueppers F, Miller RD, Gordon H, Hepper NG, Offord K. Familial prevalence of chronic obstructive pulmonary disease in a matched pair study. *Am J Med* 1977;**63**:336–42.

51. Rybicki BA, Beaty TH, Cohen BH. Major genetic mechanisms in pulmonary function. *J Clin Epidemiol* 1990;**43**:667–75.

52. Silverman EK, Chapman HA, Drazen JM, *et al*. Genetic epidemiology of severe, early-onset chronic obstructive pulmonary disease. *Am J Respir Crit Care Med* 1998;**157**: 1770–8.

53. McCloskey SC, Patel BD, Hinchliffe SJ, Reid ED, Wareham NJ, Lomas DA. Siblings of patients with severe chronic obstructive pulmonary disease have a significant risk of airflow obstruction. *Am J Respir Crit Care Med* 2001;**164**: 1419–1424.

54. McCrea KA, Ensor JE, Nall K, Bleecker ER, Hasday JD. Altered cytokine regulation in the lungs of cigarette smokers. *Am J Respir Crit Care Med* 1994;**150**:696–703.

55. Huang S-L, Su C-H, Chang S-C. Tumor necrosis factor-α gene polymorphism in chronic bronchitis. *Am J Respir Crit Care Med* 1997;**156**:1436–9.

56. Burnett D, Chamba A, Hill SL, Stockley RA. Neutrophils from subjects with chronic obstructive lung disease show enhanced chemotaxis and extracellular proteolysis. *Lancet* 1987;**ii**:1043–6.

57. Woessner JF Jr. Matrix metalloproteinases and their inhibitors in connective tissue remodeling. *FASEB J*. 1991;**5**:2145–54.

58. Birkedal-Hansen H, Moore WG, Bodden MK, *et al*. Matrix metalloproteinases:a review. *Crit Rev Oral Biol Med* 1993;**4**:197–50.

59. Cawston T, Carrere S, Catterall J, *et al*. Matrix metalloproteinases and TIMPs: properties and implications for the treatment of chronic obstructive pulmonary disease. In: *Chronic Obstructive Pulmonary Disease: Pathogenesis to Treatment. (Novartis Foundation Symposium 234)*. Wiley, Chichester, 2001, pp 205–28.

60. Winyard PG, Zhang Z, Chidwick K, Blake DR, Carrell RW, Murphy G. Proteolytic inactivation of human alpha-1-antitrypsin by human stromelysin. *FEBS Lett* 1991;**279**:91–4.

61. Liu Z, Zhou X, Shapiro SD, *et al*. The serpin alpha-1-proteinase unhibitor is a critical substrate for gelatinase B/MMP-9 *in vivo*. *Cell* 2000;**102**:647–55.

62. Murphy G, Willenbrock F. Tissue inhibitors of matrix metalloendopeptidases. *Methods Enzymol* 1995;**248**: 496–510.

63. Gomis-Ruth FX, Maskos K, Betz M, *et al*. Mechanism of inhibition of the human matrix metalloproteinase stromelysin-1 by TIMP-1. *Nature* 1997;**389**:77–81.

64. D'Armiento J, Dalal SS, Okada Y, Berg RA, Chada K. Collagenase expression in the lungs of transgenic mice causes pulmonary emphysema. *Cell* 1992;**71**:955–61.

65. Selman M, Montaño M, Ramos C, *et al*. Tobacco smoke-induced lung emphysema in guinea pigs is associated with increased interstitial collagenase. *Am J Physiol* 1996;**271**:L743.

66. Finlay GA, Russell KJ, McMahon KJ, *et al*. Elevated levels of matrix metalloproteinases in bronchoalveolar lavage fluid of emphysematous patients. *Thorax* 1997;**52**:502–6.

67. Finlay GA, O'Driscoll LR, Russell KJ, *et al*. Matrix metalloproteinase expression and production by alveolar macrophages in emphysema. *Am J Respir Crit Care Med* 1997;**156**:240–7.

68. Hautamaki RD, Kobayashi DK, Senior RM, Shapiro S. Requirement for macrophage elastase for cigarette smoke-induced emphysema in mice. *Science* 1997;**277**:2002–4.

69. Shapiro SD. Elastolytic metalloproteinases produced by human mononuclear phagocytes. Potential roles in destructive lung disease. *Am J Respir Crit Care Med* 1994;**150**:S160–4.

70. Shapiro SD. Evolving concepts in the pathogenesis of chronic obstructive pulmonary disease. *Clin Chest Med* 2000;**21**: 621–32.

71. Zheng T, Zhu Z, Wang Z, *et al*. Inducible targeting of IL-13 to the adult lung causes matrix metalloproteinase- and cathepsin-dependent emphysema. *J Clin Invest* 2000;**106**: 1081–93.

72. Wang Z, Zheng T, Zhu Z, *et al*. Interferon gamma induction of pulmonary emphysema in the adult murine lung. *J Exp Med* 2000;**192**:1587–600.

73. Huber R, Carrell RW. Implications of the three-dimensional structure of alpha-1-antitrypsin for structure and function of serpins. *Biochemistry* 1989;**28**:8951–66.

74. Aronsen KF, Ekelund G, Kindmark CO, Laurell C-B. Sequential changes of plasma proteins after surgical trauma. *Scand J Clin Lab Invest* 1972;**29**(suppl 124):127–36.

75. Billingsley GD, Walter MA, Hammond GL, Cox DW. Physical mapping of four serpin genes: alpha-1-antitrypsin, alpha-1-antichymotrypsin, corticosteroid-binding globulin, and protein C inhibitor, within a 280 kb region on chromosome 14q31.1. *Am J Hum Genet* 1993;**52**:343–53.

76. Koj A, Regoeczi E, Toews CJ, Leveille R, Gauldie J. Synthesis of antithrombin III and alpha-1-antitrypsin by the perfused rat liver. *Biochim Biophys Acta* 1978;**539**:496–504.

77. Eriksson S, Alm R, Åstedt B. Organ cultures of human fetal hepatocytes in the study of extra- and intracellular alpha-1-antitrypsin. *Biochim Biophys Acta* 1978; **542**:496–505.

78. Mornex JF, Chytil-Weir A, Martinet Y, Courtney M, LeCocq J, Crystal RG. Expression of the alpha-1-antitrypsin gene in mononuclear phagocytes of normal and alpha-1-antitrypsin-deficient individuals. *J Clin Invest* 1986;**77**:1952–61.

79. Perlmutter DH, Daniels JD, Auerbach HS, *et al*. The alpha-1-antitrypsin gene is expressed in a human intestinal epithelial cell line. *J Biol Chem* 1989;**264**:9485–90.

80. Cichy J, Potempa J, Travis J. Biosynthesis of alpha-1-proteinase inhibitor by human lung-derived epithelial cells. *J Biol Chem* 1997;**272**:8250–5.

81. Schultze HE, Heide K, Haupt H. Alpha-1-antitrypsin aus humanserum. *Klin Wochschr* 1962;**40**:427–9.

82. Rao NV, Wehner NG, Marshall BC, Gray WR, Gray BH, Hoidal JR. Characterization of proteinase-3 (PR-3), a neutrophil serine proteinase. Structure and functional properties. *J Biol Chem* 1991;**266**:9540–8.

83. Potempa J, Korzus E, Travis J. The serpin superfamily of proteinase inhibitors: structure, function, and regulation. *J Biol Chem* 1994;**269**:15957–60.

84. Brantly M, Nukiwa T, Crystal RG. Molecular basis of alpha-1-antitrypsin deficiency. *Am J Med* 1988;**84**(suppl 6A):13–31.

85. Owen MC, Carrell RW, Brennan SO. The abnormality of the S variant of human alpha-1-antitrypsin. *Biochim Biophys Acta* 1976;**453**:257–61.

86. Jeppsson J.-O. Amino acid substitution Glu→Lys in alpha-1-antitrypsin PiZ. *FEBS Lett* 1976;**65**:195–7.

87. Yoshida A, Lieberman J, Gaidulis L, Ewing C. Molecular abnormality of human alpha$_1$-antitrypsin variant (Pi-ZZ) associated with plasma activity deficiency. *Proc Natl Acad Sci USA* 1976;**73**:1324–8.

88. Sveger T. Liver disease in alpha$_1$-antitrypsin deficiency detected by screening of 200 000 infants. *N Engl J Med* 1976;**294**:1316–21.

89. Sveger T. The natural history of liver disease in alpha-1-antitrypsin deficient children. *Acta Paediatr Scand* 1988; **77**:847–51.

90. Eriksson S, Carlson J, Velez R. Risk of cirrhosis and primary liver cancer in alpha$_1$-antitrypsin deficiency. *N Engl J Med* 1986;**314**:736–9.

91. Johnson D, Travis J. Structural evidence for methionine at the reactive site of human α-1-proteinase inhibitor. *J Biol Chem* 1978;**253**:7142–4.

92. Stratikos E, Gettins PGW. Major proteinase movement upon stable serpin–proteinase complex formation. *Proc Natl Acad Sci USA* 1997;**4**:453–8.

93. Wilczynska M, Fa M, Karolin J, Ohlsson P-I., Johansson LB-A, Ny T. Structural insights into serpin–protease complexes reveal the inhibitory mechanism of serpins. *Nat Struct Biol* 1997;**4**:354–7.

94. Mast AE, Enghild JJ, Pizzo SV, Salvesen G. Analysis of the plasma elimination kinetics and conformational stabilities of native, proteinase-complexed, and reactive site cleaved serpins: comparison of alpha-1-proteinase inhibitor, alpha-1-antichymotrypsin, antithrombin III, α$_2$-antiplasmin, angiotensinogen, and ovalbumin. *Biochemistry* 1991;**30**: 1723–30.

95. Lomas DA, Evans DL, Finch JT, Carrell RW. The mechanism of Z alpha-1-antitrypsin accumulation in the liver. *Nature* 1992;**357**:605–7.

96. Lomas DA, Evans DL, Stone SR, Chang W-SW, Carrell RW. Effect of the Z mutation on the physical and inhibitory properties of alpha-1-antitrypsin. *Biochemistry* 1993; **32**:500–8.

97. Elliott PR, Lomas DA, Carrell RW, Abrahams J-P. Inhibitory conformation of the reactive loop of alpha-1-antitrypsin. *Nat Struct Biol* 1996;**3**:676–81.

98. Elliott PR, Abrahams J-P, Lomas DA. Wildtype alpha-1-antitrypsin is in the canonical inhibitory conformation. *J Mol Biol* 1998;**275**:419–25.

99. Skinner R, Chang W-SW, Jin L, *et al.* Implications for function and therapy of a 2.9 Å structure of binary-complexed antithrombin. *J Mol Biol* 1998;**283**:9–14.

100. Seyama K, Nukiwa T, Souma S, Shimizu K, Kira S. Alpha-1-antitrypsin-deficient variant Siiyama (Ser^{53}[TCC] to Phe^{53}[TTC]) is prevalent in Japan. Status of alpha-1-antitrysin deficiency in Japan. *Am Rev Respir Dis* 1995;**152**:2119–26.

101. Roberts EA, Cox DW, Medline A, Wanless IR. Occurrence of alpha-1-antitrypsin deficiency in 155 patients with alcoholic liver disease. *Am. J Clin Pathol* 1984;**82**:424–7.

102. Lomas DA, Finch JT, Seyama K, Nukiwa T, Carrell RW. Alpha-1-antitrypsin Siiyama (Ser^{53}→Phe);further evidence for intracellular loop-sheet polymerisation. *J Biol Chem* 1993;**268**:15333–5.

103. Lomas DA, Elliott PR, Sidhar SK, *et al.* Alpha$_1$-antitrypsin Mmalton (^{52}Phe deleted) forms loop-sheet polymers *in vivo*: evidence for the C sheet mechanism of polymerisation. *J Biol Chem* 1995;**270**:16864–70.

104. Dafforn TR, Mahadeva R, Elliott PR, Sivasothy P, Lomas DA. A kinetic description of the polymerisation of alpha-1-antitrypsin. *J Biol Chem* 1999;**274**:9548–55.

105. Wu Y, Whitman I, Molmenti E, Moore K, Hippenmeyer P, Perlmutter DH. A lag in intracellular degradation of mutant alpha-1-antitrypsin correlates with liver disease phenotype in homozygous PiZZ alpha-1-antitrypsin deficiency. *Proc Natl Acad Sci USA* 1994;**91**:9014–18.

106. Teckman JH, Perlmutter DH. The endoplasmic reticulum degradation pathway for mutant secretory proteins alpha-1-antitrypsin Z and S is distinct from that for an unassembled membrane protein. *J Biol Chem* 1996;**271**:13215–20.

107. Sveger T. Alpha-1-antitrypsin deficiency in early childhood. *Pediatrics* 1978;**62**:22–5.

108. Elliott PR, Stein PE, Bilton D, Carrell RW, Lomas DA. Structural explanation for the dysfunction of S alpha-1-antitrypsin. *Nat Struct Biol* 1996;**3**:910–11.

109. Mahadeva R, Chang W-SW, Dafforn T, *et al.* Heteropolymerisation of S, I and Z alpha-1-antitrypsin and liver cirrhosis. *J Clin Invest* 1999;**103**:999–9.

110. Piitulainen E, Eriksson S. Decline in FEV$_1$ related to smoking status in individuals with severe alpha1-antitrypsin deficiency. *Eur Respir J* 1999;**13**:247–51.

111. Seersholm N, Kok-Jensen A, Dirksen A. Survival of patients with severe alpha-1-antitrypsin deficiency with special reference to non-index cases. *Thorax* 1994;**49**:695–8.

112. Larsson C. Natural history and life expectancy in severe alpha$_1$-antitrypsin deficiency, PiZ. *Acta Med Scand* 1978;**204**:345–51.

113. Janus ED, Phillips NT, Carrell RW. Smoking, lung function, and alpha-1-antitrypsin deficiency. *Lancet* 1985;**i**:152–4.

114. Wewers MD, Casolaro MA, Sellers SE, *et al.* Replacement therapy for alpha$_1$-antitrypsin deficiency associated with emphysema. *N Engl J Med* 1987;**316**:1055–62.

115. Ogushi F, Fells GA, Hubbard RC, Straus SD, Crystal RG. Z-type alpha-1-antitrypsin is less competent than M1-type alpha-1-antitrypsin as an inhibitor of neutrophil elastase. *J Clin Invest* 1987;**80**:1366–74.

116. Llewellyn-Jones CG, Lomas DA, Carrell RW, Stockley RA. The effect of the Z mutation on the ability of alpha-1-antitrypsin to prevent neutrophil mediated tissue damage. *Biochim Biophys Acta* 1994;**1227**:155–60.

117. Elliott PR, Bilton D, Lomas DA. Lung polymers in Z alpha-1-antitrypsin related emphysema. *Am J Respir Cell Mol Biol* 1998;**18**:670–4.

118. Morrison HM, Kramps JA, Burnett D, Stockley R.A. Lung lavage fluid from patients with alpha-1-proteinase inhibitor deficiency or chronic obstructive bronchitis: anti-elastase function and cell profile. *Clinical Science* 1987;**72**:373–81.

119. Hubbard RC, Fells G, Gadek J, Pacholok S, Humes J, Crystal RG. Neutrophil accumulation in the lung in alpha 1-antitrypsin deficiency. Spont   elease of leukotriene B4 by alveolar macrophages. *J Clin Invest* 1991;**88**:891–7.

120. Parmar JS, Mahadeva R, Reed BJ, *et al.* Polymers of alpha-1-antitrypsin are chemotactic for human neutrophils: a new paradigm for the pathogenesis of emphysema. *Am J Respir Cell Mol Biol* 2002;**26**:723–30.

121. Silverman GA, Bird PI, Carrell RW, *et al.* The serpins are an expanding superfamily of structurally similar but functionally diverse proteins. Evolution, novel functions, mechanism of inhibition and a revised nomenclature. *J Biol Chem* 2001;**276**:33293–6.

122. Whisstock JC, Skinner R, Lesk AM. An atlas of serpin conformations. *Trends Biochem Sci* 1998;**23**:63–7.

123. Aulak KS, Eldering E, Hack CE, *et al.* A hinge region mutation in C1-inhibitor (Ala^{436}→Thr) results in nonsubstrate-like behavior and in polymerization of the molecule. *J Biol Chem* 1993;**268**:18088–94.

124. Eldering E, Verpy E, Roem D, Meo T, Tosi M. COOH-terminal substitutions in the serpin C1 inhibitor that cause loop overinsertion and subsequent multimerization. *J Biol Chem* 1995;**270**:2579–87.

125. Bruce D, Perry DJ, Borg J-Y, Carrell RW, Wardell MR. Thromboembolic disease due to thermolabile conformational changes of antithrombin Rouen VI (187 Asn→Asp). *J Clin Invest* 1994;**94**:2265–74.

126. Lindo VS, Kakkar VV, Learmonth M, Melissari E, Zappacosta F, Panico M, Morris HR. Antithrombin-TRI (Ala382 to Thr)

causing severe thromboembolic tendency undergoes the S-to-R transition and is associated with a plasma-inactive high-molecular-weight complex of aggregated antithrombin. *Br J Haematol* 1995;**89**:589–601.

127. Poller W, Faber J-P, Weidinger S, *et al.* A leucine-to-proline substitution causes a defective alpha-1-antichymotrypsin allele associated with familial obstructive lung disease. *Genomics* 1993;**17**:740–43.

128. Faber J-P, Poller W, Olek K, Baumann U, Carlson J, Lindmark B, Eriksson S. The molecular basis of alpha-1-antichymotrypsin deficiency in a heterozygote with liver and lung disease. *J Hepatol* 1993;**18**:313–21.

129. Gooptu B, Hazes B, Chang W-SW, *et al.* Inactive conformation of the serpin alpha-1-antichymotrypsin indicates two stage insertion of the reactive loop; implications for inhibitory function and conformational disease. *Proc Natl Acad Sci USA* 2000;**97**:67–72.

130. Davis RL, Shrimpton AE, Holohan PD, *et al.* Familial dementia caused by polymerisation of mutant neuroserpin. *Nature* 1999;**401**:376–9.

131. Davis RL, Holohan PD, Shrimpton AE, *et al.* Familial encephalopathy with neuroserpin inclusion bodies (FENIB). *Am J Pathol* 1999;**155**:1901–13.

132. Bradshaw CB, Davis RL, Shrimpton AE, *et al.* Cognitive deficits associated with a recently reported familial neurodegenerative disease. *Arch Neurol* 2001;**58**:1429–34.

133. Sharp HL, Bridges RA, Krivit W, Freier EF. Cirrhosis associated with alpha-1-antitrypsin deficiency: a previously unrecognised inherited disorder. *J Lab Clin Med* 1969;**73**:934–9.

134. Eriksson S, Larsson C. Purification and partial characterization of PAS-positive inclusion bodies from the liver in alpha$_1$-antitrypsin deficiency. *N Engl J Med* 1975;**292**:176–80.

135. Seyama K, Nukiwa T, Takabe K, Takahashi H, Miyake K, Kira S. Siiyama (serine 53 (TCC) to phenylalanine 53 (TTC)). A new alpha-1-antitrypsin-deficient variant with mutation on a predicted conserved residue of the serpin backbone. *J Biol Chem* 1991;**266**:12627–32.

136. Matsunaga E, Shiokawa S, Nakamura H, Maruyama T, Tsuda K, Fukumaki Y. Molecular analysis of the gene of the alpha-1-antitrypsin deficiency variant, Mnichinan. *Am J Hum Genet* 1990;**46**:602–12.

137. Sergi C, Consalez GC, Fabbretti G, *et al.* Immunohistochemical and genetic characterization of the M Cagliari α-1-antitrypsin molecule (M-like α-1-antitrypsin deficiency). *Lab Invest* 1994;**70**:130–3.

138. Cruz M, Molina JA, Pedrola D, Muñoz-López F. Cirrhosis and heterozygous alpha-1-antitrypsin deficiency in a 4 year old girl. *Helv Paediatr Acta* 1975;**30**:501–7.

139. Campra JL, Craig JR, Peters RL, Reynolds TB. Cirrhosis associated with partial deficiency of alpha-1-antitrypsin in an adult. *Ann Intern Med* 1973;**78**:233–8.

140. Sveger T, Eriksson S. The liver in adolescents with alpha$_1$-antitrypsin deficiency. *Hepatology* 1995;**22**:514–17.

141. Seersholm N, Dirksen A, Kok-Jensen A. Airways obstruction and two year survival in patients with severe alpha$_1$-antitrypsin deficiency. *Eur Respir J* 1994;**7**:1985–7.

142. The alpha-1-antitrypsin deficiency registry study group. Survival and FEV$_1$ decline in individuals with severe deficiency of alpha-1-antitrypsin. *Am J Respir Crit Care Med* 1998;**158**:49–59.

143. Turino GM, Barker AF, Brantly ML, *et al.* Clinical features of individuals with PI*SZ phenotype of alpha-1-antitrypsin deficiency. *Am J Respir Crit Care Med* 1996;**154**:1718–25.

144. Cockcroft DW, Tennent RK, Horne SL. Pulmonary emphysema associated with the FZ alpha-1-antitrypsin phenotype. *CMA J* 1981;**124**:737–42.

145. Seersholm N, Kok-Jensen A. Intermediate alpha$_1$-antitrypsin deficiency PiSZ: a risk factor for pulmonary emphysema? *Respir Med* 1998;**92**:241–5.

146. Piitulainen E, Tornling G, Eriksson S. Environmental correlates of impaired lung function in non-smokers with severe alpha-1-antitrypsin deficiency (PiZZ). *Thorax* 1998;**53**:939–43.

147. Mayer NS, Stoller JK, Bartelson BB, Ruttenber AJ, Sandhaus RA, Newman LS. Occupational exposure risks in individuals with PI*Z alpha-1-antitrypsin deficiency. *Am J Respir Crit Care Med* 2000;**162**:553–8.

148. Silverman EK, Province MA, Campbell EJ, Pierce JA, Rao DC. Biochemical intermediates in alpha-1-antitrypsin deficiency: residual family resemblance for total alpha-1-antitrypsin, oxidised alpha-1-antitrypsin, and immunoglobulin E after adjustment for the effect of the Pi locus. *Genet Epidemiol* 1989;**7**:137–49.

149. Bruce RM, Cohen BH, Diamond EL, *et al.* Collaborative study to assess risk of lung disease in Pi MZ phenotype subjects. *Am Rev Respir Dis* 1984;**130**:386–90.

150. Lieberman J, Winter B, Sastre A. Alpha1-antitrypsin Pi-types in 965 COPD patients. *Chest* 1986;**89**:370–3.

151. Tarján E, Magyar P, Váczi Z, Lantos Á, Vaszár L. Longitudinal lung function study in heterozygous PiMZ phenotype subjects. *Eur Respir J* 1994;**7**:2199–204.

152. Sandford AJ, Chagani T, Weir TD, Connett JE, Anthonisen NR, Paré PD. Susceptibility genes for rapid decline of lung function in the lung health study. *Am J Respir Crit Care Med* 2001;**163**:469–73.

153. Seersholm N, Torgny J, Wilcke R, Kok-Jensen A, Dirksen A. Risk of hospital admission for obstructive pulmonary disease in alpha-1-antrypsin heterozygotes of phenotype PiMZ. *Am J Respir Crit Care Med* 2000;**2000**:81–4.

154. Stein PD, Leu JD, Welsh MH, Guenter CA. Pathophysiology of the pulmonary circulation in emphysema associated with alpha-1 antitrypsin deficiency. *Circulation* 1971;**43**:227–39.

155. Dirksen A, Holstein-Rathlou N-H, *et al.* Long-range correlations of serial FEV$_1$ measurements in emphysematous patients and normal subjects. *J Appl Physiol* 1998;**85**:259–65.

156. Dirksen A, Friis M, Olesen KP, Skovgaard LT, Sørensen K. Progress of emphysema in severe alpha-1-antitrypsin deficiency as assessed by annual CT. *Acta Radiologica* 1997;**38**:826–32.

157. Dowson LJ, Guest PJ, Hill SL, Holder RL, Stockley RA. High-resolution computed tomography scanning in alpha-1-antitrypsin deficiency: relationship to lung function and health status. *Eur Respir J* 2001;**17**:1097–4.

158. Colp C, Pappas J, Moran D, Lieberman J. Variants of alpha-1-antitrypsin in Puerto Rican children with asthma. *Chest* 1993;**103**:812–15.

159. Eden E, Mitchell D, Khouli H, Nejat M, Grieco MH, Turino GM. Atopy, asthma, and emphysema in patients with severe alpha-1-antitrypsin deficiency. *Am J Respir Crit Care Med* 1997;**156**:68–74.

160. Griffith ME, Lovegrove JU, Gaskin G, Whitehouse DB, Pusey CD. C-antineutrophil cytoplasmic antibody positivity in vasculitis patients is associated with the Z allele of alpha-1-antitrypsin, and P-antineutrophil cytoplasmic antibody positivity with the S allele. *Nephrol Dial Transplant* 1996;**11**:438–43.

161. Baslund B, Szpirt W, Eriksson S, *et al*. Complexes between proteinase 3, alpha-1-antitrypsin and proteinase 3 anti-neutrophil cytoplasmic autoantibodies: a comparison between alpha-1-antitrypsin PiZ allele carriers and non-carriers with Wegener's granulomatosis. *Eur J Clin Invest* 1996;**26**:786–92.

162. King MA, Stone JA, Diaz PT, Mueller CF, Becker WJ, Gadek JE. Alpha-1-antitrypsin deficiency: evaluation of bronchiectasis with CT. *Radiology* 1996;**199**:137–41.

163. Rodriguez-Cintron W, Guntupalli K, Fraire AE. Bronchiectasis and homozygous (PiZZ) alpha-1-antitrypsin deficiency in a young man. *Thorax* 1995;**50**:424–5.

164. Cuvelier A, Muir J-F, Hellot M-F, *et al*. Distribution of alpha-1-antitrypsin alleles in patients with bronchiectasis. *Chest* 2000;**117**:415–19.

165. Warter J, Storck D, Grosshans E, Metais P, Kuntz J-L, Klumpp T. Syndrome de Weber–Christian associe a un deficit en alpha-1-antitrypsine;enquete familiale. *Ann Med Intern (Paris)* 1972;**123**:877–82.

166. O'Riordan K, Blei A, Rao MS, Abecassis M. Alpha-1-antitrypsin deficiency-associated panniculitis. Resolution with intravenous alpha-1-antitrypsin administration and liver transplantation. *Transplantation* 1997;**63**:480–2.

167. Smith KC, Pittelkow MR, Su WPD. Panniculitis associated with severe alpha-1-antitrypsin deficiency. *Arch Dermatol* 1987;**123**:1655–61.

168. Seersholm N, Kok-Jensen A. Extrapulmonary manifestations of alpha-1-antitrypsin deficiency. *Am J Respir Crit Care Med* 2001;**163**:A343.

169. Schievink WI, Prakash UBS, Piepgras DG, Mokri B. Alpha-1-antitrypsin deficiency in intracranial aneurysms and cervical artery dissection. *Lancet* 1994;**343**:452–3.

170. Cox DW. Alpha-1-antitrypsin: a guardian of vascular tissue. *Mayo Clin Proc* 1994;**69**:1123–4.

171. Nemeth A. Liver transplantation in alpha-1-antitrypsin deficiency. *Eur J Pediatr* 1999;**158**(suppl 2):S85–8.

172. Francavilla R, Castellaneta SP, Hadzic N, *et al*. Prognosis of alpha-1-antitrypsin deficiency-related liver disease in the era of paediatric liver transplantation. *J Hepatol* 2000;**32**:986–92.

173. Prachalias AA, Kalife M, Francavilla R, *et al*. Liver transplantation for alpha-1-antitrypsin deficiency. *Transpl Int* 2000;**13**:207–10.

174. Seersholm N, Kok-Jensen A. Clinical features and prognosis of life time non-smokers with severe alpha-1-antitrypsin deficiency. *Thorax* 1998;**53**:265–8.

175. British Thoracic Society. Smoking cessation guidelines and their cost effectiveness. *Thorax* 1998;**53**(suppl 5).

176. British Thoracic Society. BTS guidelines for the management of chronic obstructive pulmonary disease. *Thorax* 1997;**52**:Supplement 5.

177. Lacasse Y, Wong E, Guyatt GH, King D, Cook DJ, Goldstein RS. Meta-analysis of respiratory rehabilitation in chronic obstructive pulmonary disease. *Lancet* 1996;**348**:1115–19.

178. Trulock 3rd EP. Lung transplantation for COPD. *Chest* 1998;**113**(suppl 4):269S–76S.

179. King MB, Campbell EJ, Gray BH, Hertz MI. The protease-antiproteinase balance in α-1-proteinase inhibitor-deficient lung transplant recipients. *Am J Respir Crit Care Med* 1994;**149**:966–71.

180. Cassina PC, Teschler H, Konietzko N, Theegarten D, Stamatis G. Two-year results after lung volume reduction surgery in alpha-1-antitrypsin deficiency versus smoker's emphysema. *Eur Respir J* 1998;**12**:1028–32.

181. Gelb AF, McKenna RJ, Brenner M, Fischel R, Zamel N. Lung function after bilateral lower lobe lung volume reduction surgery for alpha-1-antitrypsin deficiency. *Eur Respir J* 1999;**14**:928–33.

182. Berger RL, Celli BR, Meneghetti AL, *et al*. Limitations of randomized clinical trials for evaluating emerging operations: the case of lung volume reduction surgery. *Ann Thorac Surg* 2001;**72**:649–57.

183. Dirksen A, Dijkman JH, Madsen F, *et al*. A randomised clinical trial of alpha-1-antitrypsin augmentation therapy. *Am J Respir Crit Care Med* 1999;**160**:1468–72.

184. Schluchter MD, Stoller JK, Barker AF, *et al*. Feasibility of a clinical trial of augmentation therapy for alpha-1-antitrypsin deficiency. The alpha-1-antitrypsin deficiency study group. *Am J Respir Crit Care Med* 2000;**161**:796–801.

185. Song S, Embury J, Laipis PJ, Berns KI, Crawford JM, Flotte TR. Stable therapeutic serum levels of human alpha-1 antitrypsin (AAT) after portal vein injection of recombinant adeno-associated virus (rAAV) vectors. *Gene Ther* 2001;**8**:1299–306.

186. Rosenfeld MA, Siegfried W, Yoshimura K, *et al*. Adenovirus-mediated transfer of a recombinant alpha-1 antitrypsin gene to the lung epithelium *in vivo*. *Science* 1991;**252**:431–4.

187. Song S, Morgan M, Ellis T, *et al*. Sustained secretion of human alpha-1-antitrypsin from murine muscle transduced with adeno-associated virus vectors. *Proc Natl Acad Sci USA* 1998;**95**:14384–8.

188. Bou-Gharios G, Wells DJ, Lu QL, Morgan JE, Partridge T. Differential expression and secretion of alpha 1 anti-trypsin between direct DNA injection and implantation of transfected myoblast. *Gene Ther* 1999;**6**:1021–9.

189. Massaro GD, Massaro D. Retinoic acid treatment abrogates elastase-induced pulmonary emphysema in rats. *Nature Med* 1997;**3**:675–7.

190. Burrows JAJ, Willis LK, Perlmutter DH. Chemical chaperones mediate increased secretion of mutant alpha-1-antitrypsin (alpha-1-AT) Z: a potential pharmacological strategy for prevention of liver injury and emphysema. *Proc Natl Acad Sci USA* 2000;**97**:1796–801.

191. Devlin GL, Parfrey H, Tew DJ, Lomas DA, Bottomley SP. Prevention of polymerization of M and Z alpha-1-antitrypsin (alpha-1-AT) with trimethylamine *N*-oxide. Implications for the treatment of alpha-1-AT deficiency. *Am J Respir Cell Mol Biol* 2001;**24**:727–32.

192. Rubenstein RC, Egan ME, Zeitlin PL. In vitro pharmacologic restoration of CFTR-mediated chloride transport with sodium 4-phenylbutyrate in cystic fibrosis epithelial cells containing delta F508-CFTR. *J Clin Invest* 1997;**100**:2457–65.

193. Rubenstein RC, Zeitlin PL. A pilot clinical trial of oral sodium 4-phenylbutyrate (Buphenyl) in deltaF508-homozygous cystic fibrosis patients: partial restoration of nasal epithelial CFTR function. *Am J Respir Crit Care Med* 1998;**157**:484–90.

194. Kurdowska A, Travis J. Acute phase protein stimulation by alpha-1-antichymotrypsin-cathepsin G complexes. Evidence for the involvement of interleukin-6. *J Biol Chem* 1990;**265**:21023–6.

195. Cichy J, Potempa J, Chawla RK, Travis J. Stimulatory effect of inflammatory cytokines on alpha-1-antichymotrypsin expression in human lung-derived epithelial cells. *J Clin Invest* 1995;**95**:2729–33.

196. Rubin H, Wang Z, Nickbarg EB, *et al*. Cloning, expression purification, and biological activity of recombinant native

and variant human alpha-1-antichymotrypsins. *J Biol Chem* 1990;**265**:1199–207.

197. Lomas DA, Stone SR, Llewelyn-Jones C, *et al.* The control of neutrophil chemotaxis by inhibitors of cathepsin G and chymotrypsin. *J Biol Chem* 1995;**270**:23437–43.

198. Schechter NM, Jordan LM, James AM, Cooperman BS, Wang ZM, Rubin H. Reaction of human chymase with reactive site variants of alpha-1-antichymotrypsin. Modulation of inhibitor *versus* substrate properties. *J Biol Chem* 1993;**268**:23626–33.

199. Eriksson S, Lindmark B, Lilja H. Familial alpha-1-antichymotrypsin deficiency. *Acta Med Scand* 1986;**220**: 447–53.

200. Lindmark BE, Arborelius M Jr, Eriksson SG. Pulmonary function in middle-aged women with heterozygous deficiency of the serine protease inhibitor alpha1-antichymotrypsin. *Am Rev Respir Dis* 1990;**141**:884–8.

201. Poller W, Faber J-P, Scholz S, *et al.* Mis-sense mutation of alpha-1-antichymotrypsin gene associated with chronic lung disease. *Lancet* 1992;**339**:1538.

202. Sandford AJ, Chagani T, Weir TD, Paré PD. Alpha-1-antichymotrypsin mutations in patients with chronic obstructive pulmonary disease. *Dis Markers* 1998;**13**:257–60.

203. Benetazzo MG, Gile LS, Bombieri C, *et al.* Alpha-1-antitrypsin TAQ I polymorphism and alpha-1-antichymotrypsin mutations in patients with obstructive pulmonary disease. *Respir Med* 1999;**93**:648–54.

204. Tsuda M, Sei Y, Yamamura M, Yamamoto M, Shinohara Y. Detection of a new mutant α-1-antichymotrypsin in patients with occlusive-cerebrovascular disease. *FEBS Lett* 1992;**304**:66–8.

205. Tsuda M, Sei Y, Ohkubo T, *et al.* The defective secretion of a naturally occurring α-1-antichymotrypsin variant with a frameshift mutation. *Eur J Biochem* 1996;**235**:821–7.

206. Kamboh MI, Sanghera DK, Ferrell RE, DeKosky ST. APOE*4-associated Alzheimer's disease risk is modified by alpha-1-antichymotrypsin polymorphism. *Nature Genet* 1995;**10**:486–8.

207. Christie J, Lamb H, Singleton AB, *et al.* Determination of the alpha-1 anti-chymotrypsin polymorphism in Alzheimer's disease. *Alzheimer's Res* 1996;**2**:201–4.

208. Müller U, Bödeker R-H, Gerundt I, Kurz A. Lack of association between alpha-1-antichymotrypsin polymorphism, Alzheimer's disease, and allele ϵ4 of apolipoprotein E. *Am Acad Neurol* 1996;**47**:1575–7.

209. Haines JL, Pritchard ML, Saunders AM, *et al.* No genetic effect of alpha-1-antichymotrypsin in Alzheimer disease. *Genomics* 1996;**33**:53–6.

210. Haines JL, Pritchard ML, Saunders AM, *et al.* No association between alpha-1-antichymotrypsin and familial Alzheimer's disease. *Ann NY Acad Sci* 1996;**802**:35–41.

211. Murphy GM Jr, Sullivan EV, Gallagher-Thompson D, *et al.* No association between the alpha 1-antichymotrypsin A allele and Alzheimer's disease. *Neurology* 1997;**19**:1313–16.

212. Berman G, Afford SC, Burnett D, Stockley RA. α-1-antichymotrypsin in lung secretions is not an effective proteinase inhibitor. *J Biol Chem* 1986;**261**:14095–9.

213. Chang W-SW, Lomas DA. Latent alpha-1-antichymotrypsin: a molecular explanation for the inactivation of alpha-1-antichymotrypsin in chronic bronchitis and emphysema. *J Biol Chem* 1998;**273**:3695–701.

214. Gross P, Pfitzer EA, Tolker E, Babyak MA, Kaschak M. Experimental emphysema. Its production with papain in normal and silicotic rats. *Arch Environ Health* 1965;**11**:50–8.

215. Blanco I, Fernández E, Bustillo EF. Alpha-1-antitrypsin PI phenotypes S and Z in Europe: an analysis of the published surveys. *Clin Genet* 2001;**60**:31–41.

216. Carrell RW, Lomas DA. Alpha-1-antitrypsin deficiency: a model for the conformational dementias. *N Engl J Med* 2001;**346**:45–53.

217. Kafienah W, Buttle DJ, Burnett D, Hollander AP. Cleavage of native type 1 collagen by human neutrophil elastase. *Biochem J* 1998;**330**:897–902.

218. Pipoly DJ, Crouch EC. Degradation of native type IV procollagen by human neutrophil elastase. Implications for leukocyte-mediated degradation of basement membranes. *Biochemistry* 1987;**26**:5748–54.

219. Gadher SJ, Eyre DR, Duance VC, *et al.* Susceptibility of cartilage collagens type II, IX, X, and XI to human synovial collagenase and neutrophil elastase. *Eur J Biochem* 1988;**175**:1–7.

220. Baugh RJ, Travis J. Human leukocyte granule elastase: rapid isolation and characterization. *Biochemistry* 1976;**15**: 836–41.

221. Björk P, Axelsson L, Bergenfeldt M, Ohlsson K. Influence of plasma protease inhibitors and the secretory leucocyte protease inhibitor on leucocyte elastase-induced consumption of selected plasma proteins *in vitro* in man. *Scand J Clin Lab Invest* 1988;**48**:205–11.

222. Malemud CJ, Janoff A. Identification of neutral proteases in human neutrophil granules that degrade articular cartilage proteoglycan. *Arthritis Rheum* 1975;**18**:361–8.

223. Heck LW, Blackburn WD, Irwin MH, Abrahamson DR. Degradation of basement membrane laminin by human neutrophil elastase and cathepsin G. *Am J Pathol* 1990;**136**:1267–74.

224. Plow EF. The major fibrinolytic proteases of human leukocytes. *Biochim Biophys Acta* 1980;**630**:47–56.

225. Murphy G, Bretz U, Baggiolini M, Reynolds JJ. The latent collagenase and gelatinase of human polymorphonuclear neutrophil leucocytes. *Biochem J* 1980;**192**:517–25.

226. Dalet-Fumeron V, Guinec N, Pagano M. In vitro activation of pro-cathepsin B by three serine proteinases: leucocyte elastase, cathepsin G, and the urokinase-type plasminogen activator. *FEBS Lett* 1993;**332**:251–4.

227. Okada Y, Nakanishi I. Activation of matrix metalloproteinase 3 (stromelysin) and matrix metalloproteinase 2 (gelatinase) by human neutrophil elastase and cathepsin G. *FEBS Lett* 1989;**249**:353–6.

228. Ferry G, Lonchampt M, Pennel L, De Nanteuil G, Canet E, Tucker GC. Activation of MMP-9 by neutrophil elastase in an *in vivo* model of acute lung injury. *FEBS Lett* 1997;**402**: 111–15.

229. Suter S, Chevallier I. Proteolytic inactivation of alpha-1-proteinase inhibitor in infected bronchial secretions from patients with cystic fibrosis. *Eur Respir J* 1991;**4**:40–9.

230. Pemberton PA, Harrison RA, Lachmann PJ, Carrell RW. The structural basis for neutrophil inactivation of C1 inhibitor. *Biochem J* 1989;**258**:193–8.

231. Abe H, Matsuda E, Binder BR. Effect of type-1 plasminogen activator inhibitor on human leukocyte elastase. *Thrombosis Res* 1994;**73**:361–9.

232. Baumstark JS. Studies on the elastase-serum protein interaction. II On the digestion of human α2-macroglobulin, an elastase inhibitor, by elastase. *Biochim Biophys Acta* 1970;**207**:318–30.

233. Abrahamson M, Buttle DH, Mason RW, *et al.* Regulation of cystatin C activity by serine proteinases. *Biomed Biochim Acta* 1991;**50**:587–93.

234. Gillis S, Furie BC, Furie B. Interaction of neutrophils and coagulation proteins. *Semin Haematol* 1997;**34**:336–42.

235. Prince HE, Folds JD, Spitznagel JK. Proteolysis of human IgG by human polymorphonuclear leucocyte elastase produces

an Fc fragment with *in vitro* biological activity. *Clin Exp Immunol* 1979;**37**:162–8.

236. Heinz H-P, Loos M. Activation of the first component of complement, C1: comparison of the effect of sixteen different enzymes on serum C1. *Immunobiology* 1983;**165**:175–85.

237. Taylor JC, Crawford IP, Hugli TE. Limited degradation of the third component (C3) of human complement by human leukocyte elastase (HLE): partial characterization of C3 fragments. *Biochemistry* 1977;**16**:3390–6.

238. Wetsel RA, Kolb WP. Expression of C5a-like biological activities by the fifth component of human complement (C5) upon limited digestion with noncomplement enzymes without release of polypeptide fragments. *J Exp Med* 1983;**157**:2029–48.

Oxidative stress

IRFAN RAHMAN AND WILLIAM MACNEE

INTRODUCTION

Biological systems are continuously exposed to oxidants either generated endogenously by metabolic reactions (e.g. from mitochondrial electron transport during respiration or released from phagocytes) or exogenously, such as air pollutants or cigarette smoke. The tissues are protected against this oxidative challenge by well-developed enzymatic and non-enzymatic antioxidant defence systems.[1]

Oxidative stress occurs when the balance between oxidants and antioxidants shifts in favor of oxidants.[2] This results from either an excess of oxidants and/or depletion of antioxidants. Oxidative stress is thought to play an important role in the pathogenesis of a number of lung diseases,[3] both through its potential to produce direct injurious effects and also by playing a key role in the molecular mechanisms which control lung inflammation, which include modulation of redox-regulated signal transduction, regulation of cell proliferation and apoptosis. Oxidative stress is also considered to be involved in remodeling of extracellular matrix, inactivation of surfactant and the antiprotease screen, and alteration in mitochondrial respiration.

The pathogenesis of Chronic Obstructive Pulmonary Disease (COPD) is strongly linked to the effects of cigarette smoke.[4] Although nearly 90% of all patients with COPD are smokers,[5] for as yet unknown, and probably complex reasons, only a proportion of smokers develop clinically significant COPD. The fact that cigarette smoke contains 10^{17} oxidant molecules per puff,[6,7] together with evidence of increased oxidative stress in smokers and in patients with COPD, has led to the proposal that an oxidant/antioxidant imbalance occurs in COPD, which is important in the pathogenesis of this condition.[8,9] This chapter will review the evidence for the role of oxidative stress in the pathogenesis of COPD, and the mechanisms, responses and consequences of oxidative stress in this condition.

THE OXIDATIVE BURDEN IN THE LUNGS

Oxidants in cigarette smoke

Cigarette smoke is a complex mixture of over 6000 chemical compounds, including free radicals and other oxidants that are present in high concentrations.[6,7] Cigarette smoke has both a gas and a tar phase.[6] Free radicals are present in both the tar and the gas phases of cigarette smoke. The gas phase of cigarette smoke contains approximately 10^{15} radicals per puff, primarily of the alkyl and peroxyl types. Nitric oxide is another oxidant which is present in the gas phase of cigarette smoke in concentrations of 500–1000 ppm.[7] Nitric oxide (NO) reacts quickly with the superoxide anion ($O_2^{\cdot-}$) to form highly reactive peroxynitrite ($ONOO^-$), and with peroxyl radicals to give alkyl peroxynitrites. The gas phase of cigarette smoke also contains organic carbon and oxygen-centered radicals which have short lifetimes, typically of less than 1 second. However, reactions can occur which can prolong the effect of inhaled radicals. An example is the slow oxidation of nitric oxide present in cigarette smoke, to produce reactive nitrogen species such as nitrogen dioxide, which can react with unsaturated compounds, such as isoprene in cigarette smoke to form carbon-centered organic radicals. These radicals react rapidly with oxygen to form peroxyl radicals, which are converted to alkoxyl radicals by reaction with nitric oxide, resulting in more nitrogen dioxide, which can re-enter the reaction.[7] The gas phase of cigarette smoke also contains high concentrations of olefins and dienes.

The tar phase of cigarette smoke contains a high concentration of radicals which are more stable, such as the semiquinone radical, which can reduce oxygen to produce the superoxide anion ($O_2^{\cdot-}$) and the hydroxyl radical (•OH). It also contains reactive oxygen species which are not radicals such as hydrogen peroxide (H_2O_2).[7] The tar phase is also an effective metal chelator and can bind iron to produce tar-semiquinone plus tar-Fe^{2+}, which can generate H_2O_2 continuously.[10,11]

The lung epithelial lining fluid (ELF) and mucus, both of which have antioxidant properties,[12] are the first line of defence in the lungs against inhaled oxidants, by quenching the short-lived free radicals in the gas phase of cigarette smoke. However, cigarette smoke condensate, which forms in the epithelial lining fluid, may continue to produce reactive oxygen species (ROS) for a considerable time. Cigarette smokers deposit up to 20 mg of tar per cigarette smoked, or as much as a gram per day. Tar contains over 6000 different chemical organic compounds from which the water-soluble components, such as aldehydes, catechol and hydroquinone, are extracted out into the ELF.[9] Polyphenols, such as catechols, are not free radicals, however solutions of polyphenols undergo autoxidation and polymerize to form substances which are oxidants.[13,14] Furthermore, since both cigarette tar and lung epithelial lining fluid contain metal ions, such as iron, Fenton chemistry will result in the production of the hydroxyl radical (HO•), which is a very reactive and potent oxidant.

Cell-derived oxidants

Inflammation is a characteristic feature in the lungs of smokers.[15-17] Recent bronchial biopsy studies have clearly shown increased numbers of leukocytes in the airway and distal airspace walls in smokers who develop COPD compared with those who have not developed the condition.[17] The increase in the oxidative burden produced directly by inhaling cigarette smoke is therefore further enhanced in smoker's lungs by the release of ROS from inflammatory leukocytes, both neutrophils and macrophages, which are known to migrate in increased numbers into the lungs of cigarette smokers, compared

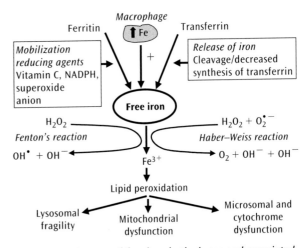

Figure 10.1 *Sources of free iron in the lungs and associated oxidative reactions.*

with non-smokers.[18] Moreover, the lungs of smokers with airway obstruction have more neutrophils than smokers without airway obstruction,[19] with the potential to further increase the oxidative burden.

Alveolar macrophages obtained by bronchoalveolar lavage from the lungs of smokers are more activated compared with those obtained from non-smokers.[20] One manifestation of this is the release of increased amounts of ROS such as $O_2^{\cdot-}$ and H_2O_2.[21-24] Exposure to cigarette smoke *in vitro* has also been shown to increase the oxidative metabolism of alveolar macrophages.[25] Subpopulations of alveolar macrophages with a higher density appear to be more prevalent in the lungs of smokers and are thought to be the source of the increased $O_2^{\cdot-}$ production in airspace macrophages in smokers.[26]

Superoxide anion and H_2O_2 can be generated by the xanthine/xanthine oxidase (X/XO) reaction. XO activity has been shown to be increased in cell-free bronchoalveolar lavage fluid from COPD patients, compared with normal subjects, associated with increased O_2^- and uric acid production.[27] Increased XO activity has also been shown in the lungs in animal models of cigarette smoke exposure.[28]

Iron is a critical element in many oxidative reactions.[29] Free iron in the ferrous form catalyzes the Fenton reaction and the superoxide driven Haber–Weiss reaction, which generate the hydroxyl radical, a free radical which is extremely damaging to all tissues, particularly to cell membranes, producing lipid peroxidation (Figure 10.1). The lung lining fluid in smokers contains more iron than in non-smokers.[30,31] In addition, alveolar macrophages from smokers, particularly those who develop chronic bronchitis, both contain[31] and release more iron[32] than those of non-smokers. Thus the generation of oxidants in epithelial lining fluid may therefore be further enhanced by the presence of increased amounts of free iron in the airspaces in smokers.[33]

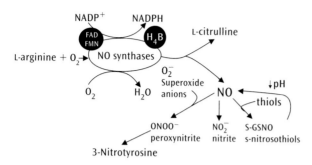

Figure 10.2 *Synthesis of nitric oxide (NO) and NO-related products. S-nitrosothiol (GSNO), flavin adeninedinucleotide (FAD), flavin mononucleotide (FMN).*

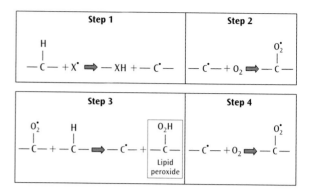

Figure 10.3 *Reactions producing lipid peroxidation.*

Airway epithelial cells are another source of reactive oxygen species.[34] Type II alveolar epithelial cells have been shown to release both H_2O_2 and O_2^- in similar quantities to alveolar macrophages.[35] Indeed the release of ROS from type II cells is able, in the presence of myeloperoxidase, to inactivate alpha-1-antitrypsin *in vitro*.[35]

Recent studies have shown that in response to tumor necrosis factor alpha (TNF-α) and lipopolysaccharide (LPS), which are relevant stimuli in the inflammatory response in COPD, airway epithelial cells can concurrently produce increased amounts of intracellular ROS and reactive nitrogen species (RNS).[36] This intracellular production of oxidants and the subsequent changes in intracellular redox status is important for the molecular events controlling the expression of genes for inflammatory mediators (see below). ROS and RNS species can also be generated intracellularly from several sources such as mitochondrial respiration, the NADPH oxidase system, X/XO and, in the case of RNS, from arginine, by the action of nitric oxide synthetase[34] (Figure 10.2). Depending on the relative amounts of ROS and RNS, and particularly the amounts of O_2^- and NO$^\cdot$, which are almost invariably produced simultaneously at sites of inflammation, these can react together to produce the powerful oxidant peroxynitrite (ONOO$^-$). Since this reaction occurs at a nearly diffusion-limited rate, it is thought that NO$^\cdot$ can outcompete superoxide dismutase (SOD) for reaction with O_2^- and thus ONOO$^-$ will be generated:[37]

$$O_2^{\cdot-} + NO^\cdot \rightarrow ONOO^-$$

The generation of peroxynitrate is thought to prolong the action of NO$^\cdot$ and to be responsible for most of the adverse effects of excess generation of NO.[38] Peroxynitrite is directly toxic to cells or may decompose to produce the hydroxyl radical:

$$ONOO^{-\cdot} + H^+ \rightarrow OH^\cdot + NO_2^\cdot$$

Lipid peroxidation following the reaction of free radicals with polyunsaturated fatty acid side chains in membranes or lipoproteins, is a further reaction which can result in cell damage and has even greater importance in this respect since it is a self-perpetuating process which continues as a chain reaction[39] (Figure 10.3). The presence of lipid peroxides may also have a role in the signaling events involved in the lung inflammation in COPD (see below).

Oxidative stress and the pathogenesis of COPD

The evidence for the presence of increased oxidative stress in smokers and patients with COPD is now overwhelming.[9,40–43] The only direct method to measure excessive free radical activity is by electron spin resonance using spin traps, which cannot be applied to the study of tissues at present. Most studies have therefore relied on indirect measurements of free radical activity in biologic fluids. Although these studies using markers suggest the occurrence of oxidative stress, they do not prove a role in the pathogenesis. There are now numerous studies, using different techniques, which have shown that increased markers of oxidative stress are present in the epithelial lining fluid, in the breath, in the urine and in the blood in cigarette smokers and in patients with COPD.

Evidence of local oxidative stress in the lungs

ANTIOXIDANTS IN LUNG LINING FLUID

The ELF forms the interface between the airspace epithelium and the external environment and therefore forms a critical defence mechanism against inhaled oxidants or those produced by cells in the airspaces.[44] An antioxidant is defined as a substance that when present at low concentrations, compared to those of an oxidizable substrate, significantly delays, or inhibits, oxidation of that substrate.[45] Antioxidants in ELF comprise low molecular weight antioxidants, metal binding proteins, antioxidant

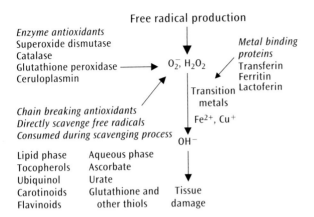

Figure 10.4 *Antioxidant defences.*

Table 10.1 *Antioxidant constituents of epithelial lining fluid*

Antioxidant	Plasma (μM)	ELF (μM)
Ascorbic acid	40	100
Glutathione	1.5	100
Uric acid	300	90
Albumin-SH	500	70
Alpha-tocopherol	25	2.5
Beta-carotene	0.4	–

enzymes, sacrificial reactive proteins and unsaturated lipids (Figure 10.4). The concentrations of non-enzymatic antioxidants vary in ELF, and some are concentrated in ELF compared to plasma, such as glutathione and ascorbate, which may indicate their relative importance[46–49] (Table 10.1). The major antioxidants in ELF include mucin, reduced glutathione, uric acid, protein (largely albumin), ceruloplasmin and ascorbic acid.[44,50]

Mucin is a glycoprotein with a core which is rich in serine and threonine, to which carbohydrates and cysteine residues (sulfydryls) are attached. The antioxidant properties of mucus derive from the abundance of sulfydryl and disulfide moieties in its structure,[51] which effectively scavenge oxidants such as the hydroxyl radical ($^{\cdot}$OH).[52] Mucin also has metal binding properties,[53] which adds to its antioxidant properties in the airways. Oxidant generating systems, such as X/XO have been shown to cause the release of mucus from airway epithelial cells.[54] Relevant to COPD, animal models of elastase-induced emphysema also show features of airways disease with goblet cell hyperplasia.[55] In addition, neutrophil elastase is known to be a potent secretagogue for mucous and therefore both oxidants and elastase may contribute to the hypermucous secretion in chronic bronchitis.[56] Toxic inhalants such as cigarette smoke increase the secretion of mucins, which represents a major protective mechanism in the bronchial tree.

There is limited information on the respiratory epithelial antioxidant defences in smokers, and less for patients with COPD. Several studies have shown that glutathione (GSH) is elevated in bronchoalveolar lavage fluid (BALF) in chronic smokers.[57–59] However, the twofold increase in BALF GSH in chronic smokers may not be sufficient to deal with the excessive oxidant burden during smoking, when acute depletion of GSH may occur.[60–62]

Several studies have suggested that GSH homostasis may play a central role in the maintenance of the integrity of the lung airspace epithelial barrier. Decreasing the levels of GSH in epithelial cells leads to loss of barrier function and increased permeability[61,63] (see below).

Pacht and coworkers[64] demonstrated reduced levels of vitamin E in the BALF of smokers compared with non-smokers, whereas Bui and colleagues[65] found a marginal increase in vitamin C in BALF of smokers, compared to non-smokers. Similarly, alveolar macrophages from smokers have both increased levels of ascorbic acid and augmented uptake of ascorbate.[66] Increased activity of antioxidant enzymes (SOD and catalase) in alveolar macrophages from young smokers has also been reported.[67] However, Kondo and coworkers[68] found that the increased superoxide generation by alveolar macrophages in elderly smokers was associated with decreased antioxidant enzyme activities when compared with non-smokers. The activities of CuZnSOD, glutathione-S-transferase and glutathione peroxidase (GP) are all decreased in alveolar macrophages from elderly smokers. However, this reduced activity was not associated with decreased gene expression, but was due to modification at the post-translational level.[68]

Thus there appears to be no consistent change in antioxidant defences in ELF in smokers. The apparent inconsistencies between these studies in the levels of the different antioxidants in ELF and alveolar macrophages may be due to differences in the smoking histories in chronic smokers, particularly the time of the last cigarette in relation to the sampling of BALF, which is rarely reported in these studies.

The activities of SOD and glutathione peroxidase (GP_x) have been shown to be higher in the lungs of rats exposed to cigarette smoke.[69] McCusker and Hoidal[67] have also demonstrated enhanced antioxidant enzyme activities in alveolar macrophages in hamsters following cigarette smoke exposure, which resulted in reduced mortality when the animals were subsequently exposed to more than 95% oxygen. They speculated that alveolar macrophages undergo an adaptive response to chronic oxidant exposure that may ameliorate potential damage to lung cells from further oxidant stress. The mechanisms for the induction of antioxidant enzymes in erythrocytes,[70] alveolar macrophages[67] and lungs[69] by cigarette smoke exposure are currently unknown.

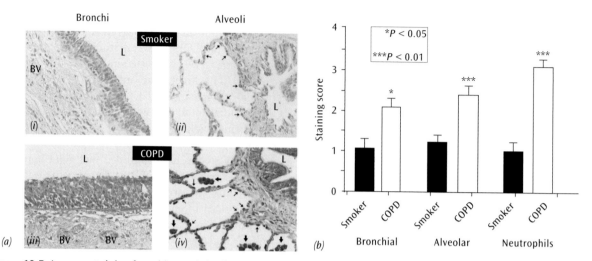

Figure 10.5 *Immunostaining for adducts of the lipid peroxidation product 4-hydroxynonenal (a) in the bronchi and alveoli in smokers without COPD (smoker) and smokers with COPD (COPD). Much greater intensity of staining for 4-hydroxynonenal adducts is seen in both the bronchi and alveoli in patients with COPD. Semiquantitative staining score for the degree of staining is shown (b) to be more intensive in both bronchial and alveolar areas and also in neutrophils from lung of smokers who have developed COPD than smokers who have not developed the disease. (Adapted from ref. 74.)*

Evidence of oxidative stress in lung tissue

There is considerable evidence, demonstrating the presence of oxidative stress locally in the lungs, as measured by increased levels of numerous surrogate markers of oxidative stress. However, the presence of markers of oxidative stress by no means confirms a role for oxidative stress in the pathogenesis of COPD. Support for this link would come from the demonstration of the reaction of reactive oxygen species with target lung molecules, and the presence of these oxidatively modified molecules in increased amounts in the lungs of smokers, particularly those who develop COPD. Increased products of lipid peroxidation have been found in the lungs of cigarette smokers and the levels relate to the length of the smoking history.[71] Furthermore, smoking-associated mitocondrial DNA mutations have been found in the lungs of smokers[71] and, in addition, neutrophils have been shown to cause oxidative DNA damage to alveolar epithelial cells *in vitro*.[72] Thus evidence is accumulating that oxidative stress can induce reactions with target molecules in lung tissue in patients with COPD.

4-Hydroxy-2-nonenal (4-HNE) is a highly reactive aldehyde lipid peroxidation product which has been shown to enter cells and activate MAP kinase signaling pathways.[73] It also acts as a chemoattractant for neutrophils *in vitro* and *in vivo*.[73] Recent data indicate increased 4-HNE-modified protein levels in airway and alveolar epithelial cells, endothelial cells and neutrophils in subjects with airway obstruction compared to subjects without airway obstruction[74] (Figure 10.5). This demonstrates not only the presence of 4-HNE, but that 4-HNE modifies proteins in lung cells to a greater extent in patients with COPD. Levels

of 4-HNE-adducts in alveolar and airway epithelium have been shown to be inversely related to the FEV_1, suggesting a role for 4-HNE in the pathogenesis of COPD.

Evidence of systemic oxidative stress

There has been interest recently in the concept that COPD produces local lung and also systemic manifestations.[75] This relates not only to the systemic effects of hypoxemia, as reflected in peripheral muscle function, but also the concept that inflammation may have systemic effects such as the weight loss which occurs in some patients, which is a predictor of reduced survival.[76]

One manifestation of a systemic effect is the presence of markers of oxidative stress in the blood in patients with COPD. This may be reflected as an increased sequestration of neutrophils in the pulmonary microcirculation during smoking and during exacerbations of COPD which, as described below, may be an oxidant-mediated event.[42,77,78]

Increased production of superoxide anion has been shown from peripheral blood neutrophils obtained from patients during acute exacerbations of COPD.[79,80] Other studies have shown that circulating neutrophils from patients with COPD show upregulation of their surface adhesion molecules, which may also be an oxidant-mediated effect.[81] Activation may be even more pronounced in neutrophils which are sequestered in the pulmonary microcirculation in smokers and in patients with COPD, since neutrophils which are sequestered in the pulmonary microcirculation in animal models of lung inflammation release more reactive oxygen species

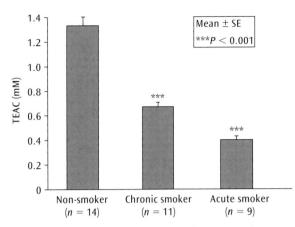

Figure 10.6 *Plasma antioxidant capacity measured as Trolox Equivalent Antioxidant Capacity (TEAC) in healthy non-smokers and healthy chronic smokers who have not smoked for 12 hours and smokers who smoked 2 cigarettes 1 hour prior to measurement (acute smoker) ***P < 0.001 compared with non-smokers. (Adapted from ref. 79.)*

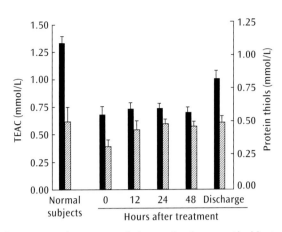

Figure 10.7 *Time course of changes in plasma antioxidant capacity measured by Trolox Equivalent Antioxidant Capacity (TEAC) (solid columns) and protein thiols (hatched columns) in normal subjects and patients during exacerbations of COPD. P < 0.05 for all time points during exacerbations compared with normal subjects. (From ref. 80.)*

than circulating neutrophils.[82] Thus neutrophils, which are sequestered in the pulmonary microcirculation, may be a source of oxidative stress, and may have a role in inducing endothelial adhesion molecule expression in COPD (see below).

Products of lipid peroxidation reactions can be measured in body fluids as thiobarbituric acid reactive substances (TBARS). The levels of TBARS in plasma are significantly increased in healthy smokers and patients with acute exacerbations of COPD, compared with healthy non-smokers.[21,79] Other studies have measured the levels of conjugated dienes of linoleic acid, a secondary product of lipid peroxidation, and have shown that the levels in plasma were elevated in chronic smokers.[83] In addition, elevated circulating levels of F_2-isoprostane, which is a more direct measurement of lipid peroxidation, have been found in smokers.[84]

Changes in the antioxidant capacity in the blood have been measured as a marker of systemic oxidative stress in smokers and patients with acute exacerbations of COPD.[79] One study found that the plasma antioxidant capacity was significantly decreased in chronic smokers when compared with plasma from age-matched non-smoking controls[75] (Figure 10.6). Acute smoking produced a further decrease in plasma antioxidant capacity, which may be due to a profound depletion of plasma protein sulfydryls, as shown following cigarette smoke exposure *in vitro*.[85–88] In exacerbations of COPD the decrease in antioxidant capacity remained low for several days after the onset of the exacerbation, tending to return towards normal values at the time of recovery from the exacerbation[80] (Figure 10.7). The depletion of antioxidant capacity could in part be explained by the increased release of ROS from peripheral blood neutrophils, as shown by a significant negative correlation between

neutrophil superoxide anion release and plasma antioxidant capacity.[79] Depletion of plasma antioxidants will reduce the protection against cigarette smoke-induced plasma membrane peroxidation. Studies showing depletion of total antioxidant capacity in smokers are supported by earlier studies showing decreased levels of the major plasma antioxidants in smokers.[89–95]

Inhalation of NO from cigarette smoke, as well as NO and superoxide anion released by activated phagocytes, react to form peroxynitrite, which has been shown to decrease plasma antioxidant capacity by rapid oxidation of ascorbic acid, uric acid and plasma sulfydryls.[96] Evidence of NO/peroxynitrite activity in plasma has been demonstrated in cigarette smokers.[97] Nitration of tyrosine residues in plasma leads to the production of 3-nitrotyrosine.[97] Higher levels of 3-nitrotyrosine have been found in the plasma in smokers compared with non-smokers[97] and the plasma antioxidant capacity has been shown to be negatively correlated with the levels of 3-nitrotyrosine in smokers.[97]

SURROGATE MARKERS OF OXIDATIVE STRESS IN THE LUNGS

There are now a number of surrogate markers of oxidative stress which have been measured in smokers and patients with COPD. Many of these markers have been measured in breath or breath condensate or in induced or spontaneously produced sputum. Direct measurements of oxidative stress are difficult, since free radicals are highly reactive and thus short lived. An alternative has been to measure markers of the effects of radicals on lung biomolecules such as lipids, protein or DNA, or to measure the stress responses to an increased oxidant burden.

Hydrogen peroxide, measured in exhaled breath, is a direct measurement of the burden of this oxidant in the airspaces. Smokers and patients with COPD have higher levels of exhaled H_2O_2 than normal non-smokers,[98,99] and levels are even higher during exacerbations of COPD.[100] The source of the increased H_2O_2 is unknown but may in part derive from increased release of O_2^- from alveolar macrophages in smokers.[101] However, smoking in one study did not appear to influence the levels of exhaled H_2O_2.[98] The levels of exhaled H_2O_2 in this study correlated with the degree of airflow obstruction as measured by the FEV_1. Nevertheless, the variability of the measurement of exhaled H_2O_2 has led to concerns over its reproducibility as a measure of oxidative stress.

Exhaled nitric oxide (NO) has been used as a marker of airway inflammation and indirectly as a measure of oxidative stress. There have been some reports of increased levels of NO in exhaled breath in patients with COPD, but not to the high levels reported in asthmatics,[102,103] although one other study failed to confirm this result.[104] Smoking decreases NO levels in breath[105] and the reaction of NO with O_2^- limits the usefulness of this marker in COPD, except perhaps to differentiate from asthma.

Carbon monoxide (CO) is another biomarker of oxidative stress which is generated by the induction of the stress responsive protein heme oxygenase 1 (HO-1).[106] HO-1 catalyzes the initial rate-limiting step in the oxidative degradation of heme to bilirubin. HO-1 catalyzes the breakdown of heme to biliverdin; this is then converted by biliverdin reductase to bilirubin which has antioxidant properties (Figure 10.8). The reaction of HO-1 with heme releases iron and carbon monoxide, which can be measured in exhaled breath and has been shown to be elevated in patients with COPD.[107]

Isoprostanes are products of non-enzymatic lipid peroxidation and have therefore been used as markers of oxidative stress.[108] The isoprostanes are free radical catalyzed isomers of arachadinic acid and are stable lipid peroxidation products which circulate in plasma and are excreted in the urine.[108–110] Isoprostane $F_{2\alpha}$ has been shown to be elevated in cigarette smokers and can be reduced by antioxidant vitamin supplimentation.[111]

Urinary levels of isoprostane $F_{2\alpha-3}$ have been shown to be elevated in patients with COPD compared with control subjects (Figure 10.9b) and are even more elevated during exacerbations of COPD.[109] Isoprostane $F_{2\alpha}$ is also elevated in exhaled breath in patients with COPD and does not seem to be influenced by treatment with inhaled corticosteroids[110] (Figure 10.9a). Indirect measurements of lipid peroxidation products, such as thiobarbituric acid reactive substances, have also been shown to be elevated in breath condensate in patients with stable COPD.[112] Thus from a number of studies markers of oxidative stress are elevated in the breath and breath condensate in smokers compared with non-smokers, with higher levels occurring in smokers who develop COPD and even greater levels in exacerbations of COPD.

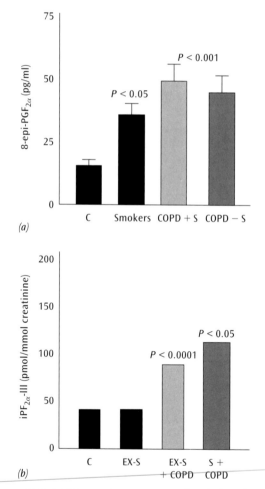

Figure 10.9 *(a) 8-Isoprostane concentrations in breath condensate in healthy non-smokers (control, C), normal smokers (SMOKERS) and patients with COPD who were (COPD + S) or were not (COPD − S) treated with inhaled corticosteroids. (Adapted from ref. 110.) (b) Isoprostane $F_{2\alpha}$-III (iPF$_{2\alpha}$-III) in urine in healthy non-smokers (control, C) in ex-smokers without COPD (EX-S) and in ex-smokers (EX-S + COPD) and smokers with (S + COPD) COPD. (Adapted from ref. 109.)*

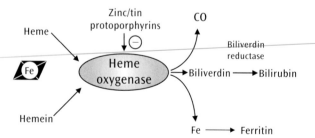

Figure 10.8 *Synthesis and source of carbon monoxide in breath as an indication of heme oxygenase activity in response to oxidative stress.*

AIRSPACE EPITHELIAL INJURY/PERMEABILITY

The airspace epithelial surface of the lungs is particularly vulnerable to the effects of oxidative stress produced by cigarette smoke by virtue of its direct contact with the environment. At least three processes may be responsible for oxidant injury to the respiratory tract epithelial cells from cigarette smoke: (i) a direct toxic interaction with constituents of cigarette smoke (including free radicals) which have penetrated the protective antioxidant shield of the ELF; (ii) damage to the cells by toxic reactive products generated by interaction between cigarette smoke and ELF; and (iii) reactions occurring subsequent to activation of inflammatory-immune processes initiated by (i) and/or (ii).[44,52]

Injury to the epithelium may be an important early event in the inflammation produced by cigarette smoke and results in an increase in airspace epithelial permeability.[113] Lannan and colleagues[114] demonstrated the injurious effect of both the whole and vapor phases of cigarette smoke on human alveolar epithelial cell monolayers in vitro, as shown by increased epithelial cell detachment, decreased cell adherence and increased cell lysis. These effects were in part oxidant-mediated since they were partially prevented by the antioxidant GSH in concentrations (500 μM) which are present in the epithelial lining fluid. Extra- and intra-cellular GSH appears to be critical to the maintenance of epithelial integrity following exposure to cigarette smoke. Studies by Li et al.[60,63] and Rahman et al.[61] demonstrated that the increased epithelial permeability of epithelial cell monolayers in vitro, and in rat lungs in vivo following exposure to cigarette smoke condensate, was associated with profound changes in the antioxidant GSH. Concentrations of GSH were considerably decreased, concomitant with a decrease in the activities of the enzymes involved in the GSH redox cycle such as glutathione peroxidase and glucose-6-phosphate dehydrogenase by cigarette smoke exposure. Furthermore, depletion of lung GSH alone, by treatment with the GSH synthesis inhibitor buthionine sulfoximine, induces increased airspace epithelial permeability both in vitro and in vivo.[61,63,115]

Similar to these in vitro and animal studies, human studies have shown increased epithelial permeability in chronic smokers compared with non-smokers, as measured by increased ^{99m}technetium-diethylenetriamine-pentacetate (^{99m}Tc-DTPA) lung clearance, with a further increase in ^{99m}Tc-DTPA clearance following acute smoking.[57] Thus cigarette smoke has a detrimental effect on alveolar epithelial cell function which is, in part, oxidant mediated, since antioxidants provide protection against this injurious event.

Neutrophil sequestration and migration in the lungs

The recruitment of neutrophils to the distal airspaces is initiated by the sequestration of these cells in the lung microcirculation.[116] Sequestration occurs under normal circumstances in the pulmonary capillary bed, and results from the size differential between neutrophils (average diameter 7 μM) and pulmonary capillary segments (average diameter 5 μM). Thus a proportion of the circulating neutrophils have to deform in order to negotiate the smaller capillary segments.[116] Studies using a variety of techniques, including radiolabeled or fluorescently labeled neutrophils, have supported the idea that the lungs contain a large pool of non-circulating neutrophils, which are either retained or slowly moving within the pulmonary microcirculation. Radiolabeled neutrophil studies in healthy subjects indicate that a proportion of neutrophils are normally delayed in the pulmonary circulation, compared to radiolabeled erythrocytes.[77] In normal subjects, there is a correlation between neutrophil deformability measured in vitro and the subsequent sequestration of these cells in the pulmonary microcirculation following their re-injection – the less deformable the cells the greater the sequestration of these cells occurs in the pulmonary circulation.[117] This provides a mechanism for the creation of a pool of sequestered or non-circulating cells in the pulmonary microcirculation, without the need to invoke margination of neutrophils in the post-capillary venules, which is the mechanism by which a non-circulating pool of cells is present in the systemic circulation.[118] Sequestration of neutrophils in the pulmonary capillaries allows time for the neutrophils to interact with the pulmonary capillary endothelium, resulting in their adherence to the endothelium and thereafter their transmigration across the alveolar capillary membrane to the interstitium and airspaces of the lungs in response to inflammation or infection.

Any condition leading to a decrease in neutrophil deformability will potentially increase neutrophil sequestration in the lungs. Cell activation is associated with decreased neutrophil deformability and occurs due to the assembly of the cytoskeleton, in particular the polymerization of microfilaments (F actin), resulting in cell stiffening. Inhaled oxidants, such as those contained in cigarette smoke and other air pollutants, could influence the transit of cells in the pulmonary capillary bed. Studies in man using radiolabeled neutrophils and red cells show a transient increase in neutrophil sequestration in the lungs during smoking,[77] which returns to normal upon cessation of smoking. Using an in vitro positive pressure cell filtration technique to measure cell stiffness, cells exposed to cigarette smoke in vitro decrease their deformability.[119] A similar decrease in deformability can be demonstrated in vivo for neutrophils obtained from the blood of subjects who are actively smoking,[120] which may be an oxidant-mediated effect of cigarette smoke on neutrophil deformability since it can be prevented by antioxidants.[119]

Recent studies have also shown that cigarette smoke causes the release of neutrophils from the bone marrow and that these neutrophils may have decreased deformability and may thus preferentially sequester in the pulmonary microcirculation.[121] The mechanism of this release of bone marrow neutrophils is as yet unclear, but may be mediated by granulocyte macrophage-colony stimulating factor (GM-CSF).

Thus cigarette smoking increases neutrophil sequestration in the pulmonary microcirculation, at least in part, by decreasing neutrophil deformability.

Once sequestered, components of cigarette smoke can alter neutrophil adhesion to endothelium by upregulating CD18 integrins,[122,123] which is known to upregulate the NADPH oxidase–H_2O_2 generating system.[124] Inhalation of cigarette smoke by hamsters increases neutrophil adhesion to the endothelium of both arterioles and venules.[122] This increased neutrophil adhesion is thought to be mediated by superoxide anion derived from cigarette smoke, since it was inhibited by pretreatment with CuZnSOD.[122] Changes in intracellular GSH redox status in endothelial cells have been shown to alter neutrophil chemotactic and other metabolic functions, such that depletion of GSH enhanced neutrophil endothelial adhesion, an effect which was blocked by increasing intracellular GSH with *N*-acetylcysteine.[125] The mechanism of this change in neutrophil adhesion involves the expression of intracellular adhesion molecule 1 (ICAM-1) and E-selectin involving the activation of the transcription factor nuclear factor kappa B (NF-κB). Increased expression of adhesion molecules on neutrophils and endothelial cells in smoke-exposed animals may result from the secondary inflammatory effects of smoking, through the release of cytokines, since direct smoke exposure *in vitro* does not produce increased expression of neutrophil adhesion molecules, nor does it enhance functional adherence.[126]

Thus several mechanisms involving oxidants cause neutrophil sequestration in the pulmonary microcirculation in smokers. Oxidant-mediated mechanisms may also result in the increased sequestration of neutrophils, which occurs in the pulmonary microcirculation during exacerbations of COPD.[78,80]

Activation of neutrophils sequestered in the pulmonary microvasculature could also induce the release of reactive oxygen intermediates and proteases within the microenvironment with limited access for free radical scavengers and antiproteases. Thus destruction of the alveolar wall, as occurs in emphysema, could result from a proteolytic or oxidant insult from the intravascular space, without the need for the neutrophils to migrate into the airspaces.[127]

Protease/antiprotease imbalance

The development of a protease/antiprotease imbalance in the lungs is a central hypothesis in the pathogenesis of emphysema in smokers. This theory was developed from studies of early onset emphysema in alpha-1-antitrypsin-deficient subjects. In the case of smokers with normal levels of alpha-1-antitrypsin, the elastase burden may be increased as a result of increased recruitment of leukocytes to the lungs and there may be a functional deficiency of alpha-1-antitrypsin, due to oxidative inactivation of alpha-1-antitrypsin in the lungs. This 'functional alpha-1-antitrypsin deficiency' is thought to be due to inactivation of the alpha-1-antitrypsin by oxidation of the methionine residue at its active site[128,129] by oxidants in cigarette smoke. Secretory leukoprotease inhibitor (SLPI), another major inhibitor of neutrophil elastase (NE), can also be inactivated by oxidants released by neutrophils.[130,131]

In vitro studies have also shown loss of alpha-1-antitrypsin inhibitory capacity when treated with oxidants,[132] including cigarette smoke.[133] However, there are also conflicting data on whether alpha-1-antitrypsin function lavage is altered in cigarette smokers,[134–136] as most of the alpha-1-antitrypsin the airspaces in cigarette smokers remains active and is therefore still capable of protecting against the increased protease burden.

The acute effects of cigarette smoking on the functional activity of alpha-1-antitrypsin in bronchoalveolar lavage fluid has also been studied and shows a transient, but non-significant, fall in the antiprotease activity of bronchoalveolar lavage fluid 1 hour after smoking.[137] Thus studies assessing the function of alpha-1-antitrypsin in either chronic or acute cigarette smoking have failed to produce a clear picture.

OXIDATIVE STRESS AND APOPTOSIS

Apoptosis or programed cell death of leukocytes is an important mechanism in the resolution of inflammation.[138] However, structural lung cells may also undergo apoptosis. Hydrogen peroxide can induce apoptosis in airway epithelial cells.[139] Recent evidence from both *in vitro* and *in vivo* studies in animals and in man have shown that apoptosis occurs in smoke-exposed macrophages.[140] The marked decrease in intracellular GSH which occurs upon exposure of cells to cigarette smoke exposure may have a role in the regulation of apoptosis.[141] Recently an hypothesis has been developed that pulmonary capillary endothelial cell apoptosis, induced by cigarette smoking, may be an early event in the process that leads to alveolar wall destruction and emphysema. Studies have shown both *in vivo* and *in vitro* that cigarette smoke exposure produces endothelial cell apoptosis[142,143] and that pulmonary vascular endothelial cell apoptosis is present in emphysematous lungs.[143] Signaling pathways involving of alpha-1-antitrypsin and NF-κB and the downregulation of the vascular endothelial growth factor receptor KDR (VEGF-KDR) have been proposed as part of the mechanism, which may also involve oxidants in cigarette smoke.

REMODELING OF EXTRACELLULAR MATRIX

Oxidative stress has been shown to be involved in the remodeling of extracellular matrix in lung injury.[144] This was supported by two observations: (i) oxidant-induced lung injury was attenuated by the synthetic matrix metalloprotease (MMP) inhibitor BB-3103;[145] and (ii) depletion of intracellular GSH was associated with the activation of MMPs, thereby increasing degradation of the alveolar extracellular matrix in lungs.[146] This breakdown of lung ECM by MMPs was blocked by increasing lung GSH levels.[146] It has been shown that the oxidative stress caused by ozone and lipid peroxides induce MMP-1 gene expression.[147] Other forms of oxidative stress derived from terbutyl hydroperoxide and iron can also modify collagen synthesis, by a mechanism presumably involving a redox sensor/receptor.[148,149]

OXIDATIVE STRESS AND MUSCLE DYSFUNCTION

Dysfunction of the respiratory and of peripheral skeletal muscles is known to occur in patients with severe COPD. The mechanisms underlying muscle dysfunction in COPD are not well understood. Skeletal muscles generate ROS at rest and ROS production increases during contractile activity. Oxidative stress occurs in skeletal muscle during skeletal muscle fatigue, accompanied by an increased load imposed on the diaphragm in patients with severe COPD.[150] This may be due to hypoxia, impaired mitochondrial metabolism and increased cytochrome C oxidase activity in skeletal muscle in patients with COPD.[151] Engelen and coworkers have found reduced muscle glutamate (a precursor of GSH) levels associated with increased muscle glycolytic metabolism in patients with severe COPD.[152] Lowered levels of glutamate were associated with decreased GSH levels, suggesting that an oxidant/antioxidant imbalance is involved in skeletal muscle dysfunction in patients with COPD. A causal relationship between abnormally low muscle redox potential at rest and the alterations of protein metabolism observed in patients with emphysema has been suggested. This is supported by Rabinovich and coworkers who showed decreased muscle redox capacity, probably due to lower ability to synthesize GSH during endurance training in patients with COPD.[153] It may be that oxidative stress plays a central role in mediating muscle mass wasting, particularly in susceptible subsets of patients with COPD. Support for this hypothesis comes from recent studies showing increased skeletal muscle apoptosis in skeletal muscles of patients with weight loss and a low body mass index, associated with increased markers of oxidative stress.[154]

RELATIONSHIP BETWEEN OXIDATIVE STRESS AND THE DEVELOPMENT OF AIRWAYS' OBSTRUCTION

The neutrophil appears to be a critical cell in the pathogenesis of COPD. Previous epidemiologic studies have shown a relationship between circulating neutrophil numbers and the FEV_1.[155] Moreover, a relationship has also been shown between the change in peripheral blood neutrophil count and the increase in airflow limitation over time.[156] Another study has shown a relationship between the release of reactive oxygen species from peripheral blood neutrophil luminol enhanced chemiluminescence and measurements of airflow limitation in young cigarette smokers.[157] Even passive cigarette smoking has been associated with increased peripheral blood leukocyte counts and their enhanced release of oxygen radicals.[158] Oxidative stress, measured as lipid peroxidation products in plasma, has also been shown to correlate inversely with the FEV_1 as a percentage of the predicted value in a population study.[159]

In the general population there is an association between dietary intake of antioxidant vitamins and lung function. Britton and coworkers,[160] in a population study of 2633 subjects, showed an association between dietary intake of the antioxidant vitamin E and lung function, supporting the hypothesis that this antioxidant may have a role in protecting against the development of COPD. Another study has suggested that antioxidant levels in the diet could be a possible explanation for differences in COPD mortality in different populations.[161] Dietary polyunsaturated fatty acids may protect cigarette smokers against the development of COPD,[162,163] although this effect is not supported by some studies.[164] These studies support the concept that dietary antioxidant supplementation may be a possible therapy to prevent the development of COPD. Such intervention studies have been difficult to carry out,[164] but there is at least some evidence to suggest that antioxidant vitamin supplementation reduces oxidant stress in smokers, measured as a decrease in pentane levels in breath as an indication of lipid peroxides in the airways.[165]

OXIDATIVE STRESS AND GENE EXPRESSION

Pro-inflammatory genes

Evidence from a large number of studies indicates that COPD is associated with airway and airspace inflammation, as shown in recent bronchial biopsy studies[16,17] and by the presence of mediators of inflammation, including IL-8 and TNF-α, which are elevated in the sputum of patients with COPD.[166]

Many inflammatory mediator genes, such as those for the cytokines, IL-8 and TNF-α, and for nitric oxide, are regulated by transcription factors, such as NF-κB, which are redox sensitive. Studies *in vitro* show that treatment of macrophages, alveolar and bronchial epithelial cells, with oxidants stimulates the release of inflammatory mediators such as IL-8, IL-1, and nitric oxide. This is associated with increased expression of the mRNA for the genes for these inflammatory mediators, and increased nuclear binding and activation of NF-κB.[167,168] In addition a stimulus that is relevant to exacerbations of COPD, such as particulate air pollution, which has oxidant properties, also activates NF-κB in alveolar epithelial cells.[169]

Thiol antioxidants such as *N*-acetylcysteine and Nacystelyn, which are potential therapies in COPD, have been shown in experiments *in vitro* to block oxidant-mediated release of these inflammatory mediators from epithelial cells and macrophages by a mechanism involving increasing intracellular GSH and decreasing NF-κB activation.[167,169] Intracellular GSH redox status, which is affected by cigarette smoke, therefore plays a critical role in the regulation of transcription factors such as NF-κB and AP-1.[170–172]

Gene transcription is also influenced by changes in the structure of chromatin. In quiescent cells DNA is tightly wound around a core of histone residues which decreases access for transcription factors such as NF-κB to the transcription machinery. Under the action of oxidants, activation of NF-κB results in the formation of a complex with transcription cofactors which has histone acetylase transferase (HAT) activity. This produces acetylation of the core histone residues, causing a change in their charge, resulting in the unwinding of DNA, access for transcription factors to their binding sites on DNA and for RNA polymerase to cause gene transcription (Figure 10.10). Histone deacetylases produce rewinding of DNA and suppression of gene expression. Both increased histone acetylation and decreased deacetylation has been shown to occur in bronchial biopsies in smokers.[173]

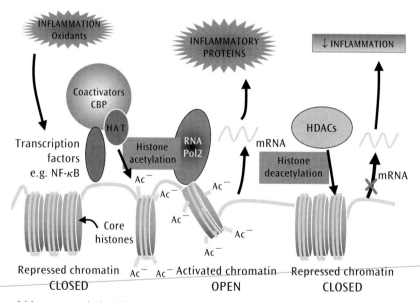

Figure 10.10 *Process of histone acetylation/deacetylation and its role in inflammation. Inflammatory mediators and oxidants activate transcription factors such as NF-κB which form a complex with transcription factor co-activators such as CBP giving the complex histone acetyl transferase activity. This then causes histone acetylation changing the charge on the co-histones resulting in unwinding of DNA and activated open chromatin. This allows access for transcription factors to the nuclear binding sites and also for RNA polymerase and subsequent increased transcription of messenger RNA for inflammatory proteins. This process is reversed by histone deacetylases (HDACs) which deacetylate core histone residues causing binding of DNA and repressed chromatin which decreases transcription for inflammatory proteins and hence decreases inflammation. CBF = cyclic AMP response element binding proteins (CREB)-binding pattern (CPB).*

Antioxidant genes

An important effect of oxidative stress in the lungs is the upregulation of protective antioxidant genes. The antioxidant GSH is concentrated in epithelial lining fluid compared with plasma[44] and has an important protective role, together with its redox enzymes, in the airspaces and intracellularly in epithelial cells. Human studies have shown elevated levels of GSH in epithelial lining fluid in chronic cigarette smokers compared with non-smokers.[50] However, this increase is not present immediately after acute cigarette smoking.[57]

The discrepancy between GSH levels in epithelial lining fluid in chronic and acute cigarette smokers has been investigated in animal models and *in vitro* using cultured epithelial cells.[60–63,174] Exposure of airspace epithelial cells to cigarette smoke condensate (CSC) *in vitro* produces an initial decrease in intracellular GSH with a rebound increase after 12 hours.[175] This effect *in vitro* is mimicked by a similar change in GSH in rat lungs *in vivo* following intratracheal instilation of cigarette smoke condensate.[61] The initial fall in lung and intracellular GSH after treatment with cigarette smoke condensate was associated with a decrease in the activity of gamma-glutamylcysteine synthetase (γGCS), the rate-limiting enzyme for GSH synthesis, with recovery of the activity by 24 hours (Figure 10.11).[174,175] The increased levels of GSH following cigarette smoke condensate exposure has been shown to be due to transcriptional upregulation of the gene for GSH synthesis γGCS by components within cigarette smoke[175,176] (Figure 10.11). The mechanism by which cigarette smoke causes the upregulation of γGCS involves redox-sensitive transcription factors. Using both a gel mobility shift assay and a reporter system in which the promoter region of γGCS gene was transfected into airway epithelial cells, cigarette smoke can be shown to activate the transcription factor activator protein-1 (AP-1).[177,178] Deletion experiments and site-directed mutagenesis in the reporter assay have shown that the proximal AP-1 site on the γGCS gene promotor region is critical for the regulation of γGCS gene expression in response to various oxidants including cigarette smoke.[178] Thus oxidative stress, including that produced by cigarette smoking, causes upregulation of the gene involved in the synthesis of GSH as a protective mechanism against oxidative stress. These events are likely to account for the increased levels of GSH seen in the epithelial lining fluid in chronic cigarette smokers.[21] However, the injurious effects of cigarette smoke may occur repeatedly during and immediately after cigarette smoking when the lung is depleted of antioxidants, including GSH.[21]

Gilks and coworkers[179] have shown that rats exposed to whole cigarette smoke had increased expression of a number of antioxidant genes in the bronchial epithelial cells for up to 14 days. Whereas mRNA of manganese superoxide dismutase (MnSOD) and metallothionein (MT)

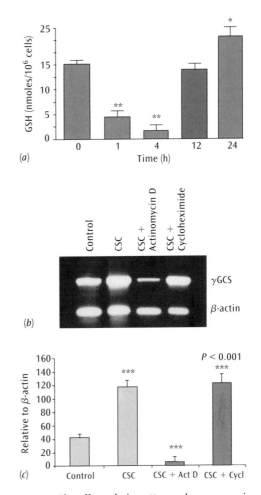

Figure 10.11 *The effect of cigarette smoke exposure in A549 epithelial cells on: (a) glutathione (GSH); (b) gamma-glutamylcysteine synthetase (γGCS) mRNA by RT-PCR; (c) AP-1 nuclear binding by gel mobility shift assay. (With permission from Trends in Molecular Medicine 2001;7:55–62)*

was increased at 1–2 days and returned to normal by 7 days, mRNA for GSH peroxidase did not increase until 7 days' exposure, suggesting the importance of the GSH redox system as a mechanism for chronic protection against the effects of cigarette smoke.[179]

The *cfos* gene belongs to a family of growth and differentiation-related immediate early genes, the expression of which generally represents the first measurable response to a variety of chemical and physical stimuli. Studies in various cell lines have shown enhanced gene expression of the *cfos* in response to cigarette smoke condensate.[180,181] These effects of cigarette smoke condensate can be mimicked by peroxynitrite and smoke-related aldehydes in concentrations that are present in cigarette smoke condensate.[180] This effect can be enhanced by pretreatment of the cells with buthionine sulfoximine to decrease intracellular GSH and can be prevented by treatment with the thiol antioxidant *N*-acetylcysteine.[180] These studies emphasize the importance of intracellular levels of the antioxidant GSH in regulating gene expression.

Thus oxidative stress, including that produced by cigarette smoke, causes increased gene expression of both pro-inflammatory genes, by oxidant-mediated activation of NF-κB, and also activation of protective genes, such as γ-GCS through other transcription factors (AP-1/ARE). A balance may therefore exist between pro- and anti-inflammatory gene expression in response to cigarette smoke, which may be critical to whether cell injury is induced by cigarette smoking. Knowledge of the molecular mechanisms that regulate these events may open new therapeutic avenues in the treatment of COPD.

Oxidative stress and susceptibility to COPD

Only a proportion of cigarette smokers appear to be susceptible to the effects of cigarette smoke. These subjects show a rapid decline in FEV$_1$ and develop COPD.[182] There has been considerable interest in identifying those who are susceptible and the mechanisms of that susceptibility,[182–184] since this would provide an important insight into the pathogenesis of COPD as did the recognition of the association between alpha-1-antitrypsin and COPD.

Polymorphisms of various genes have been shown to be more prevalent in smokers who develop COPD.[183] A number of these polymorphisms may have functional significance, such as the association between the TNF-α gene polymorphism (TNF2), which is associated with increased TNF levels in response to inflammation, and the development of chronic bronchitis.[185] Relevant to the effects of cigarette smoke is a polymorphism in the gene for microsomal epoxide hydrolase, an enzyme involved in the metabolism of highly reactive epoxide intermediates which are present in cigarette smoke.[186] The proportion of individuals with slow microsomal epoxide hydrolase activity (homozygus) was significantly higher in patients with COPD and a subgroup of patients shown pathologically to have emphysema (COPD 22%; emphysema 19%), compared with control subjects (6%).[186] However, these data have not been reproduced in other patient populations.[187] It may be that a panel of 'susceptibility' polymorphisms, of functional significance in enzymes involved in xenobiotic metabolism or antioxidant enzyme genes, may allow individuals to be identified as being susceptible to the effects of cigarette smoke.

PERSPECTIVES FOR THERAPY

There is now convincing evidence for an oxidant/antioxidant imbalance in smokers and a probable role for this imbalance in the pathogenesis of COPD. However,

proof of concept of the role of oxidative stress in the pathogenesis of COPD will come with studies of effective antioxidant therapy.

Various approaches have been tried to redress the oxidant/antioxidant imbalance. One approach is to target the inflammatory response by reducing the sequestration or migration of leukocytes from the circulation into the airspaces. Possible therapeutic options for this are drugs that alter cell deformability, so preventing neutrophil sequestration or the migration of neutrophils, either by interfering with the adhesion molecules necessary for migration, or preventing the release of inflammatory cytokines such as IL-8 or leukotriene B4 which result in neutrophil migration. It should also be possible to use agents to prevent the release of oxygen radicals from activated leukocytes or to quench those oxidants once they are formed, by enhancing the antioxidant screen in the lungs. Recent studies of a phosphodiesterase 4 inhibitor (PDE4) have shown some therapeutic benefit in patients with COPD.[188] The mechanism by which such drugs act is by increasing cAMP which decreases neutrophil activation. In particular the release of ROS by neutrophils may be decreased since increasing cAMP blocks the assembly of NADPH oxidase.[189]

There are various options to enhance the lung antioxidant screen. One approach would be to use specific spin traps such as α-phenyl-N-tert-butyl nitrone to react directly with reactive oxygen and reactive nitrogen species at the site of inflammation. However, considerable work is needed to demonstrate the efficacy of such drugs *in vivo*. Inhibitors which have a double action, such as the inhibition of lipid peroxidation and quenching radicals, could be developed.[190] Another approach could be the molecular manipulation of antioxidant genes, such as glutathione peroxidase or genes involved in the synthesis of GSH, such as γGCS or by developing molecules with activity similar to these or other antioxidant enzymes.

Molecular regulation of GSH synthesis, by targeting γGCS has promise as a means of treating oxidant-medicated injury in the lungs. Recent work has shown that recombinant γGCS in rat hepatoma cells completely protected against the TNF-α-induced activation of NF-κB, AP-1 and the development of inflammation and apoptosis. Cellular GSH may be increased by increasing γGCS activity, which may be possible by gene transfer techniques, although this would be an expensive treatment that may not be considered for a condition such as COPD. However, knowledge of how γGCS is regulated may allow the development of other compounds that may act to enhance GSH.

Recent animal studies have shown that recombinant SOD treatment can prevent the neutrophil influx to the airspaces and IL-8 release induced by cigarette smoking through a mechanism involving downregulation of

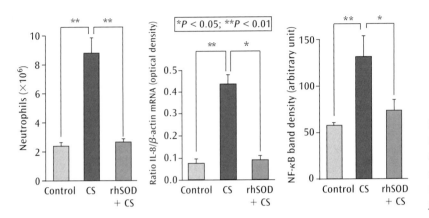

Figure 10.12 *The effect of a recombitant SOD (rhSOD) on cigarette smoke (CS) induced: neutrophil influx; IL-8 mRNA by RT-PCR; NF-κB nuclear binding in guinea pig lungs. (Adapted from ref. 193.)*

NF-κB[192] (Figure 10.12). This holds great promise if compounds can be developed with antioxidant enzyme properties which may be able to act as novel anti-inflammatory drugs by regulating the molecular events in lung inflammation.

Another approach would simply be to administer antioxidant therapy. This has been attempted orally in cigarette smokers using various antioxidants such as vitamin C and vitamin E.[193,194] The results have been rather disappointing, although as described above the antioxidant vitamin E has been shown to reduce oxidative stress in patients with COPD.[165] Attempts to supplement lung GSH have been made using GSH or its precursors.[195] GSH itself is not efficiently transported into most animal cells and in excess may be a source of the thiyl radical under conditions of oxidative stress.[196] Nebulized GSH has also been used therapeutically, but this has been shown to induce bronchial hyperreactivity.[197] The thiol cysteine is the rate-limiting amino acid in GSH synthesis. Cysteine administration is not possible since it is oxidized to cystine which is neurotoxic.[198] The cysteine-donating compound *N*-acetylcysteine (NAC) acts as a cellular precursor of GSH and is de-acetylated in the gut to cysteine following oral administration. It reduces disulfide bonds and has the potential to interact directly with oxidants. The use of *N*-acetylcysteine in an attempt to enhance GSH in patients with COPD has met with varying success.[199,200] NAC given orally in low doses of 600 mg per day, to normal subjects, results in very low levels of NAC in the plasma for up to 2 hours after administration.[199] Bridgeman and colleagues[200] showed after 5 days of NAC 600 mg three times daily, that there was a significant increase in plasma GSH levels. However, there was no associated significant rise in BAL GSH or in lung tissue. These data seem to imply that producing a sustained increase in lung GSH is difficult using NAC in subjects who are not already depleted of GSH. In spite of this, continental European studies have shown that NAC reduces the number of exacerbation days in patients with COPD.[201,202] This was not confirmed in a British Thoracic Society study of NAC.[203] The contradictory results of these studies may result from several reasons; firstly the positive studies of NAC were in patients who had relatively mild COPD, whereas in the British Study the patients had more severe COPD. Secondly, a relatively small dose of *N*-acetylcysteine was given in both studies. However a meta-analysis of studies of the use of NAC has demonstrated positive effects on exacerbations.[204] Recently a study of *N*-isobutyrylcysteine, a derivative of *N*-acetylcysteine, failed to reduce exacerbation rates in patients with COPD.[205]

N-acystelyn (NAL) is a lysine salt of *N*-acetylcysteine. It is a mucolytic and oxidant thiol compound that, in contrast to NAC, which is acidic, has a neutral pH. NAL can be aerosolized into the lung without causing significant side effects.[206] Studies comparing the effects of NAL and NAC found that both drugs enhanced intracellular GSH in alveolar epithelial cells and inhibited hydrogen peroxide and superoxide anion release from neutrophils harvested from peripheral blood from smokers and patients with COPD.[207]

FUTURE PERSPECTIVES

There is now very good evidence for an oxidant/antioxidant imbalance in COPD, and increasing evidence that this imbalance is important in the pathogenesis of this condition. Oxidative stress may also be critical in the inflammatory response to cigarette smoke, through the upregulation of redox-sensitive transcription factors and hence pro-inflammatory gene expression; but it is also involved in the protective mechanisms against the effects of cigarette smoke by the induction of antioxidant genes. Inflammation itself induces oxidative stress in the lungs, and polymorphisms in genes for inflammatory mediators or antioxidant genes may have a role in the susceptibility to the effects of cigarette smoke. Knowledge of the mechanisms of the effects of oxidative stress should the future allow the development of potent antioxidant therapies which can be used to further support the hypothesis that oxidative stress is involved in the pathogenesis of COPD, not only by direct injury to cells, but also as a fundamental factor in the inflammation in smoking-related lung disease.

REFERENCES

1. Halliwell B. Antioxidants in human health and disease. *Ann Rev Nutr* 1996;**16**:33–50.
2. Sies H. *Oxidative Stress*. Academic Press, New York, 1985.
3. Halliwell B. Free radicals, antioxidants, and human disease: curiosity, cause, or consequence? *J Lab Clin Med* 1992;**119**: 598–620.
4. MacNee W, Donaldson K. Pathogenesis of chronic obstructive pulmonary disease. In: AJ Wardlaw and Q Hamid, eds. *Textbook of Respiratory Cell and Molecular Biology* Martin Dunitz Ltd, London 2002;99–132.
5. Peto R, Lopez AD, Boreham J, Thun M, Heatch C. Mortality from tobacco in developed countries: indirect estimation from national vital statistics. *Lancet* 1992;**339**:1268–78.
6. Church T, Pryor WA. Free-radical chemistry of cigarette smoke and its toxicology implications. *Environ Health Perspect* 1985;**64**:111–26.
7. Pryor WA, Stone K. Oxidants in cigarette smoke: radicals hydrogen peroxides, peroxynitrate and peroxynitrite. *Annals NY Acad Sci* 1993;**686**:12–28.
8. Rahman I, MacNee W. Role of oxidants/antioxidants in smoking-induced lung diseases. *Free Rad Biol Med* 1996; **21**:669–81.
9. Repine JE, Bast A, Lankhorst I, and the Oxidative Stress Study Group. Oxidative stress in chronic obstructive pulmonary disease. *Am J Respir Crit Care Med* 1997;**156**:341–57.
10. Zang KY, Stone K, Pryor WA. Detection of free radicals in aqueous extracts of cigarette tar by electron spin resonance. *Free Rad Biol Med* 1995;**19**:161–7.
11. Nakayama T, Church DF, Pryor WA. Quantitative analysis of the hydrogen peroxide formed in aqueous cigarette tar extracts. *Free Rad Biol Med* 1989;**7**:9–15.
12. Cross CE, Van der Vliet A, Eiserich JP, Wong J. Oxidative stress and antioxidants in respiratory tract lining fluids. In: LB Clerch, DJ Massaro, eds. *Oxygen, Gene Expression, and Cellular Function*. Marcel Dekker, New York, 1997, pp 367–98.
13. Beckman JS, Beckman TW, Chen J, Marshall PA, Freeman BA. Apparent hydroxyl radical production by peroxynitrite: implications for endothelial injury from nitric oxide and superoxide. *Proc Natl Acad Sci USA* 1990;**87**:1620–4.
14. Moreno JJ, Foroozesh M, Church DF, Pryor WA. Release of iron from ferritin by aqueous extracts of cigarette smoke. *Chem Res Toxicol* 1992;**5**:116–23.
15. Eidelman D, Saetta MP, Nai-San Wang HG, Hoidal JR, King M,Cosio MG. Cellularity of the alveolar walls in smokers and its relation to alveolar destruction. *Am Rev Respir Dis* 1990;**141**:1547–52.
16. Jeffery PK. Structural and inflammatory changes in COPD: a comparison with asthma. *Thorax* 1998;**53**:129–36.
17. Saetta M, Stefano A, Maestrelli P, *et al*. Activated T-lymphocytes and macrophages in bronchial mucosa of subjects with chronic bronchitis. *Am Rev Respir Dis* 1993;**147**:301–6.
18. Hunninghake GW, Crystal RG. Cigarette smoking and lung destruction: accumulation of neutrophils in the lungs of cigarette smokers. *Am Rev Respir Dis* 1983;**128**:833–8.
19. Bosken CH, Hards J, Gatter K, Hogg JC. Characterization of the inflammatory reaction in the peripheral airways of cigarette smokers using immunocytochemistry. *Am Rev Respir Dis* 1992;**145**:911–17.
20. Costabel U, Guyman J. Effect of smoking on bronchoalveolar lavage constituents. *Eur Respir J* 1992;**5**:776–9.
21. Morrison D, Rahman I, Lannan S, MacNee W. Epithelial permeability, inflammation and oxidant stress in the air spaces of smokers. *Am J Respir Crit Care Med* 1999;**159**: 473–9.
22. Hoidal JR, Fox RB, LeMarbe PA, Perri R, Repine JE. Altered oxidative metabolic responses *in vitro* of alveolar macrophages from asymptomatic cigarette smokers. *Am Rev Respir Dis* 1981;**123**:85–9.
23. Nakashima H, Ando M, Sugimoto M, Suga M, Soda K, Araki S. Receptor-mediated O_2^- release by alveolar macrophages and peripheral blood monocytes from smokers and nonsmokers. *Am Rev Respir Dis* 1987;**136**:310–15.
24. Schaberg T, Haller H, Rau M, Kaiser D, Fassbender M, Lode H. Superoxide anion release induced by platelet-activating factor is increased in human alveolar macrophages from smokers. *Eur Respir J* 1992;**5**:387–93.
25. Drath DB, Larnovsky ML, Huber GL. The effects of experimental exposure to tobacco smoke on the oxidative metabolism of alveolar macrophages. *J Reticul Soc* 1970; **25**:597–604.
26. Schaberg T, Klein U, Rau M, Eller J, Lode H. Subpopulation of alveolar macrophages in smokers and nonsmokers: relation to the expression of CD11/CD18 molecules and superoxide anion production. *Am J Respir Crit Care Med* 1995;**151**:1551–8.
27. Pinamonti S, Muzzuli M, Chicca C, *et al*. Xanthine oxidase activity in bronchoalveolar lavage fluid from patients with chronic obstructive lung disease. *Free Rad Biol Med* 1996;**21**:147–55.
28. Toth KM, Burton LL, Berger EM, *et al*. Cigarette smoke exposure increases erythrocyte (RBC) and lung antioxidant levels and lung xanthine oxidase (XO) activities. *Clin Res* 1987;**35**:172A.
29. Halliwell B, Gutteridge JMC. Role of free radicals and catalytic metal ions in human disease: an overview. *Methods Enzymol* 1990;**186**:1–85.
30. Pacht ER, Davis WB. Role of transferring and ceruloplasmin in antioxidant activity of lung epithelial lining fluid. *J Appl Physiol* 1988;**64**:2092–9.
31. Thompson AB, Bohling T, Heires A, Linder J, Rennard SI. Lower respiratory tract iron burden is increased in association with cigarette smoking. *J Lab Clin Med* 1991;**117**:494–9.
32. Wesselius LJ, Nelson ME, Skikne BS. Increased release of ferritin and iron by iron loaded alveolar macrophages in cigarette smokers. *Am J Respir Crit Care Med* 1994;**150**:690–5.
33. Mateos F, Brock JF, Perez-Arellano JL. Iron metabolism in the lower respiratory tract. *Thorax* 1998;**53**:594–600.
34. Halliwell B, Gutteridge JMC, Cross CE. Free radicals, antioxidants, and human disease: Where are we now? *J Lab Clin Med* 1992;**119**:598–620.
35. Wallaert B, Gressier B, Marquette CH, *et al*. Inactivation of alpha 1-proteinase inhibitor by alveolar inflammatory cells from smoking patients with or without emphysema. *Am Rev Respir Dis* 1993;**147**:1537–43.
36. Rochelle LG, Fischer BM, Adler KB. Concurrent production of reactive oxygen and nitrogen species by airway epithelial cells *in vitro*. *Free Rad Biol Med* 1998;**24**:863–8.
37. van der Vliet A, Eiserich JP, Shigenaga MK, Cross CE. Reactive nitrogen species and tyrosine nitration in the respiratory tract. *Am J Respir Crit Care Med* 1999;**160**:1–9.
38. Beckman JS, Koppenol WH. Nitric oxide, superoxide, and peroxynitrite: the good, the bad, and the ugly. *Am J Physiol* 1996;**271**:C1424–37.

39. Gutteridge JMC. Lipid peroxidation and antioxidants as biomarkers of tissue damage. *Clin Chem* 1995;**41/12**: 1819–28.

40. MacNee W. Oxidants/antioxidants and chronic obstructive pulmonary disease: pathogenesis to therapy. *Novartis Foundation Symp 2* 2001;**34**:169–88.

41. MacNee W. Oxidative stress and lung inflammation in airways disease. *Eur J Pharmacol* 2001;**429**:195–207.

42. MacNee W. Chronic obstructive pulmonary disease from science to the clinic: role of glutathione in oxidant–antioxidant balance. *Monaldi Arch Chest Dis* 1997;**52**:479–85.

43. Rahman I, MacNee W. Oxidant/antioxidant imbalance in smokers and in chronic obstructive pulmonary disease. *Thorax* 1996;**51**:348–50.

44. Cross CE, van der Vliet A, O'Neill CA, Louie S, Halliwell B. Oxidants, antioxidants, and respiratory tract lining fluids. *Environ Health Perspect* 1994;**102**:185–91.

45. Gutteridge JMC. Biological origin of free radicals, and mechanisms of antioxidant protection. *Chemico-Biol Interact* 1994;**91**:133–40.

46. Hatch GE. Comparative biochemistry of the airway lining fluid. In: RA Parent, ed. *Treatise on Pulmonary Toxicology*, vol 1, *Comparative Biology of the Normal Lung*. CRC Press, Boca Raton, FL, 1991, pp 617–32.

47. Sies H, Stahl W, Sundquist AR. Antioxidant functions of vitamins (vitamins E and C, beta-carotene, and other carotenoids). In: LF Machlin, HE Sauberlich, eds. Beyond deficiency: new views on the function and health benefits of vitamins. *Ann NY Acad Sci* 1992;**669**:7–20.

48. Halliwell B, Gutteridge JMC. The antioxidants of human extracellular fluids. *Arch Biochem Biophys* 1990;**280**:1–8.

49. Frei B, Stocker R, Smes BN. Small molecule antioxidant defenses in human extracellular fluids. In: J Scandalois, ed. *The Molecular Biology of Free Radical Scavenging Systems*. Cold Spring Harbor Laboratory Press, Cold Spring Harbor, NY, 1992, pp 23–45.

50. Cantin AM, Fells GA, Hubbard RC, Crystal RG. Antioxidant macromolecules in the epithelial lining fluid of the normal human lower respiratory tract. *J Clin Invest* 1990;**86**:962–71.

51. Gum JR. Mucin genes and the proteins they encode: structure, diversity and regulation. *Am J Respir Cell Mol Biol* 1992;**7**:557–64.

52. Cross CE, Halliwell B, Allen A. Antioxidant protection: a function of tracheobranchial and gastrointestinal mucus. *Lancet* 1984;**i**:1328–30.

53. Cooper B, Creeth JM, Donald ASR. Studies of the limited degradation of mucus glycoproteins: the mechanism of the peroxide reaction. *Biochem J* 1985;**228**:615–26.

54. Adler KB, Holden-Stauffer WJ, Repine JE. Oxygen metabolites stimulate release of high-molecular-weight glycoconjugates by cell and organ cultures of rodent respiratory epithelium via an arachidonic acid-dependent mechanism. *J Clin Invest* 1990;**85**:75–85.

55. Lucey EC, Stone PJ, Breuer R, *et al.* Effect of combined human neutrophil cathepsin G and elastase on induction of secretory cell metaplasia and emphysema in hamsters with *in vitro* observations on elastolysis by these enzymes. *Am Rev Respir Dis* 1985;**132**:362–6.

56. Sommerhoff CP, Nadel JA, Basbaum CB, Caughey GH. Neutrophil elastase and cathepsin G stimulate secretion from cultured bovine airway gland serous cells. *J Clin Invest* 1990;**85**:682–9.

57. Morrison D, Lannan S, Langridge A, Rahman I, MacNee W. Effect of acute cigarette smoking on epithelial permeability, inflammation and oxidant status in the airspaces of chronic smokers. *Thorax* 1994;**49**:1077.

58. Cantin AM, North SL, Hubbard RC, Crystal RG. Normal alveolar epithelial lung fluid contains high levels of glutathione. *J Appl Physiol* 1987;**63**:152–7.

59. Linden M, Hakansson L, Ohlsson K, *et al.* Glutathione in bronchoalveolar lavage fluid from smokers is related to humoral markers of inflammatory cell activity. *Inflammation* 1989;**13**:651–8.

60. Li XY, Donaldson K, Rahman I, MacNee W. An investigation of the role of glutathione in the increased epithelial permeability induced by cigarette smoke *in vivo* and *in vitro*. *Am J Respir Crit Care Med* 1994;**149**:1518–25.

61. Rahman I, Li XY, Donaldson K, MacNee W. Cigarette smoke, glutathione metabolism and epithelial permeability in rat lungs. *Biochem Soc Trans* 1995;**23**:235S.

62. Rahman I, Li XY, Donaldson K, Harrison DJ, MacNee W. Glutathione homeostasis in alveolar epithelial cells *in vitro* and lung *in vivo* under oxidative stress. *Am J Physiol: Lung Cell Mol Biol* 1995;**269**:L285–92.

63. Li XY, Rahman I, Donaldson K, MacNee W. Mechanisms of cigarette smoke induced increased airspace permeability. *Thorax* 1996;**51**:465–71.

64. Pacht ER, Kaseki H, Mohammed JR, Cornwell DG, Davis WR. Deficiency of vitamin E in the alveolar fluid of cigarette smokers influence on alveolar macrophage cytotoxicity. *J Clin Invest* 1988;**77**:789–96.

65. Bui MH, Sauty A, Collet F, Leuenberger P. Dietary vitamin C intake and concentrations in the body fluids and cells of male smokers and nonsmokers. *J Nutr* 1992;**122**:312–36.

66. McGowan SE, Parenti CM. Hoidal JR, Niewoehner DW. Differences in ascorbic acid content and accumulation by alveolar macrophages from cigarette smokers and non-smokers. *J Lab Clin Med* 1984;**104**:127–34.

67. McCusker K, Hoidal J. Selective increase of antioxidant enzyme activity in the alveolar macrophages from cigarette smokers and smoke-exposed hamsters. *Am Rev Respir Dis* 1990;**141**:678–82.

68. Kondo T, Tagami S, Yoshioka A, Nishimura M, Kawakami Y. Current smoking of elderly men reduces antioxidants in alveolar macrophages. *Am J Respir Crit Care Med* 1994; **149**:178–82.

69. York GK, Pierce TH, Schwartz LS, Cross CE. Stimulation by cigarette smoke of glutathione peroxidase system enzyme activities in rat lung. *Arch Environ Health* 1976;**31**:286–90.

70. Toth KM, Berger EM, Buhler CJ, Repine JE. Erythrocytes from cigarette smokers contain more glutathione and catalase and protect endothelial cells from hydrogen peroxide better than do erythrocytes from non-smokers. *Am Rev Respir Dis* 1986;**134**:281–4.

71. Fahn HJ, Wang LS, Kao SH, Chang SC, Huang MH, Wei YH. Smoking-associated mitochondrial DNA mutations and lipid peroxidation in human lung tissues. *Am J Respir Cell Mol Biol* 1998;**19**:901–9.

72. Knaapen ADM, Seiler F, Schilderman PA, *et al.* Neutrophils cause oxidative DNA damage in alveolar epithelial cells. *Free Rad Biol Med* 1991;**27**:234–40.

73. Schaur RJ, Dussing G, Kink E, *et al.* The lipid peroxidation product 4-hydroxynonenal is formed by – and is able to attract – rat neutrophils *in vivo*. *Free Rad Res* 1994;**20**: 365–73.

74. Rahman I, van Schadewijk AA, Crowther AJ, *et al.* 4-Hydroxy-2-nonenal, a specific lipid peroxidation product, is elevated in lungs of patients with chronic obstructive pulmonary diease. *Am J Respir Crit Care Med* 2002;**166**:490–5.

75. Agusti AG. Systemic effects of chronic obstructive pulmonary disease. *Novartis Found Symp* 2001;**234**:242–9;discussion 250–4.

76. Schols AM, Slangen J, Volovics L, Wouters EF. Weight loss is a reversible factor in the prognosis of chronic obstructive pulmonary disease. *Am J Respir Crit Care Med* 1998;**157**:1791–7.

77. MacNee W, Wiggs B, Belzberg AS, Hogg JC. The effect of cigarette smoking on neutrophil kinetics in human lungs. *N Engl J Med* 1989;**321**:924–8.

78. Selby C, Drost E, Lannan S, Wraith PK, MacNee W. Neutrophil retention in the lungs of patients with chronic obstructive pulmonary diseases. *Am Rev Respir Dis* 1991;**143**:1359–64.

79. Rahman I, Morrison D, Donaldson K, MacNee W. Systemic oxidative stress in asthma, COPD, and smokers. *Am J Respir Crit Care Med* 1996;**154**:1055–60.

80. Rahman I, Skwarska E, MacNee W. Attenuation of oxidant/antioxidant imbalance during treatment of exacerbations of chronic obstructive pulmonary disease. *Thorax* 1997;**52**:565–8.

81. Noguera A, Busquets X, Sauleda J, *et al.* Expression of adhesion molecules and g-proteins in circulating neutrophils in COPD. *Am J Respir Crit Care Med* 1998;**158**:1664–8.

82. Brown DM, Drost E, Donaldson K, MacNee W. Deformability and CD11/CD18 expression of sequestered neutrophils in normal and inflamed lungs. *Am J Respir Cell Mol Biol* 1995;**13**:531–9.

83. Duthie GG, Arthur JR, James WPT. Effects of smoking and vitamin E on blood antioxidant status. *Am J Clin Nutr* 1991;**53**:1061S–3S.

84. Morrow JD, Frei B, Longmire AW, *et al.* Increase in circulating products of lipid peroxidation (F_2-isoprostanes) in smokers. *New Engl J Med* 1995;**332**:1198–203.

85. O'Neill CA, Halliwell B, Van der Vliet A, *et al.* Aldehyde-induced protein modifications in human plasma: protection by glutathione and dihydrolipoic acid. *J Lab Clin Med* 1994;**124**:359–70.

86. Reznick AZ, Cross CE, Hu ML, *et al.* Modification of plasma proteins by cigarette smoke as measured by protein carbonyls formation. *Biochem J* 1992;**286**:607–11.

87. Cross CE, O'Neill CA, Reznick AZ, *et al.* Cigarette smoke oxidation of human plasma constitutents. *Ann NY Acad Sci USA* 1993;**686**:72–90.

88. Eiserich JP, Vossen V, O'Neil CA, Halliwell B, Cross CE, Van der Viliet A. Molecular mechanisms of damage by excess nitrogen oxides: nitration of tyrosine by gas-phase cigarette smoke. *FEBS Lett* 1994;**353**:53–6.

89. Petruzzelli S, Hietanen E, Bartsch H, *et al.* Pulmonary lipid peroxidation in cigarette smokers and lung patients. *Chest* 1990;**98**:930–5.

90. Bridges AB, Scott NA, Parry GJ, Belch JJF. Age, sex, cigarette smoking and indices of free radical activity in healthy humans. *Eur J Med* 1993;**2**:205–8.

91. Duthie GG, Arthur JR, James WPT. Effects of smoking and vitamin E on blood antioxidant status. *Am J Clin Nutr* 1991;**53**:1061S–3S.

92. Mezzetti A, Lapenna D, Pierdomenico SD, *et al.* Vitamins E, C and lipid peroxidation in plasma and arterial tissue of smokers and non-smokers. *Atherosclerosis* 1995;**112**:91–9.

93. Antwerpen LV, Theron AJ, Myer MS, Richards GA, Wolmarans L, Booysen U. Cigarette smoke-mediated oxidant stress, phagocytes, vitamin C, vitamin E and tissue injury. *Ann NY Acad Sci USA* 1993;**686**:53–65.

94. Pelletier O. Vitamin C status of cigarette smokers and nonsmokers. *Am J Clin Nutr* 1970;**23**:520–8.

95. Chow CK, Thacker R, Bridges RB, Rehm SR, Humble J, Turbek J. Lower levels of vitamin C and carotenes in plasma of cigarette smokers. *J Am Coll Nutr* 1986;**5**:305–12.

96. Van der Vliet A, Smith D, O'Neill CA, *et al.* Interactions of peroxynitrite and human plasma and its constituents: oxidative damage and antioxidant depletion. *Biochem J* 1994;**303**:295–301.

97. Petruzzelli S, Puntoni R, Mimotti P, *et al.* Plasma 3-nitrotyrosine in cigarette smokers. *Am J Respir Crit Care Med* 1997;**156**:1902–7.

98. Nowak D, Kasielski M, Pietras T, Bialasiewicz P, Antczak A. Cigarette smoking does not increase hydrogen peroxide levels in expired breath condensate of patients with stable COPD. *Monaldi Arch Chest Dis* 1998;**53**:268–73.

99. Nowak D, Antczak A, Krol M, *et al.* Increased content of hydrogen peroxide in expired breath of cigarette smokers. *Eur Respir J* 1996;**9**:652–7.

100. Dekhuijzen PNR, Aben KKH, Dekker I, *et al.* Increased exhalation of hydrogen peroxide in patients with stable and unstable chronic obstructive pulmonary disease. *Am J Respir Crit Care Med* 1996;**154**:813–16.

101. Hill AT, Bayley D, Stockley RA. The interrelationship of sputum inflammatory markers in patients with chronic bronchitis. *Am J Respir Crit Care Med* 1999;**160**:893–8.

102. Maziak W, Loukides S, Culpitt S, Sullivan P, Kharitonov SA, Barnes PJ. Exhaled nitric oxide in chronic obstructive pulmonary diease. *Am J Respir Crit Care Med* 1998;**157**: 998–1002.

103. Corradi M, Majori M, Cacciani GC, Consigli GF, de'Munari E, Pesci A. Increased exhaled nitric oxide in patients with stable chronic obstructive pulmonary disease. *Thorax* 1999;**54**:576–680.

104. Rutgers SR, van der Mark TW, Coers W, *et al.* Markers of nitric oxide metabolism in sputum and exhaled air are not increased in chronic obstructive pulmonary disease. *Thorax* 1999;**54**:576–680.

105. Robbins RA, Millatmal T, Lassi K, Rennard S, Daughton D. Smoking cessation is associated with an increase in exhaled nitric oxide. *Chest* 1997;**112**:313–18.

106. Choi AM, Alam J. Heme oxygenase-1: function, regulation, and implication of a novel stress-inducible protein in oxidant-induced lung injury. *Am J Respir Cell Mol Biol* 1996;**15**:9–19.

107. Montuschi P, Kharitonov SA, Barnes PJ. Exhaled carbon monoxide and nitric oxide in COPD. *Chest* 2001;**120**:496–501.

108. Morrow JD, Roberts LJ. The isoprostanes: unique bioactive products of lipid peroxidation. *Prog Lipid Res* 1997;**36**: 1–21.

109. Pratico D, Basili S, Vieri M, Cordova C, Violi F, FitzGerald GA. Chronic obstructive pulmonary disease is associated with an increase in urinary levels of isoprostane $F_{2\alpha}$-III, an index of oxidant stress. *Am J Respir Crit Care Med* 1998;**158**:1709–14.

110. Montaschi P, Collins P, Ciabattoni G, Lazzeri N, Corradi M, Kharitonov SA, Barnes PJ. Exhaled 8-isoprostane as *in vivo* biomarker of lung oxidative stress in patients with COPD and healthy smokers. *Am J Respir Crit Care Med* 2000;**162**: 1175–7.

111. Reilly M, Delanty N, Lawson JA, FitzGerald GA. Modulation of oxidant stress *in vivo* in chronic cigarette smokers. *Circulation* 1996;**94**:19–25.

112. Nowark D, Kasielski M, Antczak A, Pietras T, Bialasiewicz P. Increased content of thiobarbiturate reactive acid substances in hydrogen peroxide in the expired breath condensate of patients with stable chronic obstructive pulmonary disease: no significant effect of cigarette smoking. *Resp Med* 1999;**93**:389–96.

113. Jones JG, Lawler P, Crawley JCW, Minty BD, Hulands G, Veall N. Increased alveolar epithelial permeability in cigarette smokers. *Lancet* 1980;**1**:66–8.

114. Lannan S, Donaldson K, Brown D, MacNee W. Effects of cigarette smoke and its condensates on alveolar cell injury *in vitro. Am J Physiol* 1994;**266**:L92–100.

115. Li XY, Donaldson K, Brown D, MacNee W. The role of tumour necrosis factor in increased airspace epithelial permeability in acute lung inflammation. *Am J Resp Cell Mol Biol* 1995;**13**:185–95.

116. MacNee W, Selby C. Neutrophil traffic in the lungs: role of haemodynamics, cell adhesion, and deformability. *Thorax* 1993;**48**:79–88.

117. Selby C, Drost E, Wraith PK, MacNee W. *In vivo* neutrophil sequestration within the lungs of man is determined by *in vitro* 'filterability'. *J Appl Physiol* 1991;**71**:1996–2003.

118. Selby C, MacNee W. Factors affecting neutrophil transit during acute pulmonary inflammation: minireview. *Exp Lung Res* 1993;**19**:407–28.

119. Drost EM, Selby C, Lannan S, Lowe GDO, MacNee W. Changes in neutrophil deformability following *in vitro* smoke exposure : mechanism and protection. *Am J Respir Cell Mol Biol* 1992;**6**:287–95.

120. Drost E, Selby C, Bridgeman MME, MacNee W. Decreased leukocyte deformability following acute cigarette smoking in smokers. *Am Rev Respir Dis* 1993;**148**:1277–83.

121. Terashima T, Klut ME, English D, Hards J, Hogg JC, van Eeden SF. Cigarette smoking causes sequestration of polymorphonuclear leukocytes released from the bone marrow in lung microvessels. *Am J Respir Cell Mol Biol* 1999;**20**:171–7.

122. Lehr HA, Kress E, Menger MD, *et al.* Cigarette smoke elicits leukocyte adhesion to endothelium in hamsters: inhibition by CuZnSOD. *Free Rad Biol Med* 1993;**14**:573–81.

123. Klut DE, Doerschuk CM, Van Eeden JF, Burns AF, Hogg JC. Activation of neutrophils within the pulmonary microvasculature of rabbits exposed to cigarette smoke. *Am J Respir Cell Mol Biol* 1993;**39**:82–90.

124. Nathan C, Srimal S, Farber C, *et al.* Cytokine-induced respiratory burst of human neutrophils, dependence on extracellular matrix proteins and CD11/CD18 integrins. *J Cell Biol* 1989;**109**:1341–9.

125. Kokura S, Wolf RE, Yoshikawa T, Granger DN, Aw TY. Molecular mechanisms of neutrophil-endothelial cell adhesion induced by redox imbalance. *Circ Res* 1999;**84**:516–24.

126. Selby C, Drost E, Brown D, Howie S, MacNee W. Inhibition of neutrophil adherence and movement by acute cigarette smoke exposure. *Exp Lung Res* 1992;**18**:813–27.

127. Brumwell ML, MacNee W, Doerschuk CM, Wiggs B, Hogg JC. Neutrophil kinetics in normal and emphysematous regions of human lungs. *Ann NY Acad Sci* 1991;**624**:30–9.

128. Carp H, Janoff A. Inactivation of bronchial mucous proteinase inhibitor by cigarette smoke and phagocyte-derived oxidants. *Exp Lung Res* 1980;**1**:225–37.

129. Hubbard RC, Ogushi F, Fells GA, *et al.* Oxidants spontaneously released by alveolar macrophages of cigarette smokers can inactivate the active site of alpha-1-antitrypsin rendering it ineffective as an inhibitor of neutrophil elastase. *J Clin Invest* 1987;**80**:1289–95.

130. Kramps JA, Rudolphus A, Stolk J, Willems LNA, Dijkman JH. Role of antileukoprotease in the lung. *Ann NY Acad Sci USA* 1991;**624**:97–108.

131. Kramps JA, van Twisk C, Dijkman DH. Oxidative inactivation of antileukoprotease is triggered by polymorphonuclear leucocytes. *Clin Sci* 1988;**75**:53–62.

132. Johnson D, Travis J. The oxidative inactivation of human alpha-1-proteinase inhibitor. Further evidence for methionine at the reactive center. *J Biol Chem* 1979;**254**:4022–6.

133. Carp H, Janoff A. Possible mechanisms of emphysema in smokers: *in vitro* suppression of serum elastase-inhibitory capacity by fresh cigarette smoke and its prevention by anti-oxidants. *Am Rev Respir Dis* 1978;**118**:617–21.

134. Carp H, Miller F, Hoidal JR, Janoff A. Potential mechanisms of emphysema: alpha-1-proteinase inhibitor recovered from lungs of cigarette smokers contains oxidised methionine and has decreased elastase inhibitory capacity. *Proc Natl Acad Sci USA* 1982;**79**:2041–5.

135. Stone P, Calore JD, McGowan SE, Bernardo J, Snider GL, Franzblau C. Functional alpha-1-protease inhibitor in the lower respiratory tract of smokers is not decreased. *Science* 1983;**221**:1187–9.

136. Boudier C, Pelletier A, Pauli G, Bieth JG. The functional activity of alpha-1-proteinase inhibitor in bronchoalveolar lavage fluids from healthy human smokers and non smokers. *Clin Chim Acta* 1983;**131**:309–15.

137. Abboud RT, Fera T, Richter A, Tabona MZ, Johal S. Acute effect of smoking on the functional activity of alpha-1-protease inhibitor in bronchoalveolar lavage fluid. *Am Rev Respir Dis* 1985;**131**:1187–9.

138. Rossi AG, Haslett C. Inflammation, cell injury, and apoptosis. In: SI Said, ed. *Lung Biology in Health and Disease. Proinflammatory and Antiinflammatory Peptides.* Marcel Dekker, New York, 1998, p 9.

139. Nakajima Y, Aoshiba K, Yasui S, Nagai A. H_2O_2 induces apoptosis in bovine tracheal epithelial cells *in vitro*. *Life Sci* 1999;**64**:2489–96.

140. Aoshiba K, Yasui S, Nagai A. Apoptosis of alveolar macrophages by cigarette smoke. *Chest* 2000;**117**:320S.

141. Hall AG. Review: the role of glutathione in the regulation of apoptosis. *Eur J Clin Invest* 1999;**29**:238–45.

142. Tuder RM, Wood K, Taraseviciene L, Flores S, Voelkel NF. Cigarette smoke extract decreases the expression of vascular endothelial growth factor by cultured cells and triggers apoptosis of pulmonary endothelial cells. Proceedings of Aspen Lung Conference 1999. *Chest* (in press).

143. Kasahara Y, Tuder RM, Cool C, Voelkel NF. Expression of 15-lipoxygenase and evidence for apoptosis in the lungs from patients with COPD. *Chest* 2000;**117**:260S.

144. Tyagi SC. Homocysteine redox receptor and regulation of extracellular matrix components in vascular cells. *Am J Physiol* 1998;**274**:C396–405.

145. Lois M, Brown LA, Moss IM, Roman J, Guidot DM. Ethanol ingestion increases activation of matrix metalloproteinases in rat lungs during acute endotoxemia. *Am J Respir Crit Care Med* 1999;**160**:1354–60.

146. Fod HD, Rollo EE, Brown P, *et al.* Attenuation of oxidant-induced lung injury by the synthetic matrix metalloproteinase inhibitor BB-3103. *Ann NY Acad Sci* 1999;**878**:650–3.

147. Choi AM, Elbon CL, Bruce SA, Bassett DJ. Messenger RNA levels of lung extracellular matrix proteins during ozone exposure. *Lung* 1994;**172**:15–30.

148. Hagen K, Zhu C, Melefors O, Hultcrantz R. Susceptibility of cultured rat hepatocytes to oxidative stress by peroxides and iron. The extracellular matrix affects the toxicity of ter-butyl hydroperoxide. *Int J Biochem Cell Biol* 1999;**31**:499–508.

149. Siwik DA, Pagano PJ, Colucci WS. Oxidative stress regulates collagen xynthesis and matrix metalloproteinase activity in cardiac fibroblasts. *Am J Physiol: Cell Physiol* 2001;**280**: C53–60.

150. Heunks LM, Dekhuijzen PN. Respiratory muscle function and free radicals: from cell to COPD. *Thorax* 2000;**55**:704–16.

151. Sauleda J, Garcia-Palmer F, Wiesner RJ, *et al.* Cytochrome oxidase activity and mitochondrial gene expression in skeletal muscle of patients with chronic obstructive

pulmonary disease. *Am J Respir Crit Care Med*
1998;**157**:1413–17.

152. Engelen MP, Schols AM, Does JD, Deutz NE, Wouters EF.
Altered glutamate metabolism is associated with reduced
muscle glutathione levels in patients with emphysema.
Am J Respir Crit Care Med 2000;**161**:98–103.

153. Rabinovich RA, Ardite E, Trooster T, *et al*. Reduced muscle
redox capacity after endurance training in patients with
chronic obstructive pulmonary disease. *Am J Respir Crit
Care Med* 2001;**164**:1114–18.

154. Agusti AG, Sauleda J, Miralles C, *et al*. Skeletal muscle
apoptosis and weight loss in chronic obstructive pulmonary
disease. *Am J Respir Crit Care Med* 2002;**15**:485–9.

155. Chan-Yeung M, Dybuncio A. Leucocyte count, smoking and
lung function. *Am J Med* 1984;**76**:31–7.

156. Chan-Yeung M, Abboud R, Dybuncio A, Vedal S. Peripheral
leucocyte count and longitudinal decline in lung function.
Thorax 1988;**43**:426–68.

157. Richards GA, Theron AJ, van der Merwe CA, Anderson R.
Spirometric abnormalities in young smokers correlate with
increased chemiluminescence responses of activated blood
phagocytes. *Am Rev Respir Dis* 1989;**139**:181–7.

158. Anderson R, Theron AJ, Richards GA, Myer MS,
van Rensburg AJ. Passive smoking by humans sensitizes
circulating neutrophils. *Am Rev Respir Dis* 1991;**144**:570–4.

159. Schunemann HJ, Muti P, Freudenheim JL, *et al*. Oxidative
stress and lung function. *Am J Epedemiol* 1997;**146**:939–48.

160. Britton JR, Pavord ID, Richards KA, *et al*. Dietary
antioxidant vitamin intake and lung function in the general
population. *Am J Respir Crit Care Med* 1995;**151**:1383–7.

161. Grievink L, Smit HA, Ocke MC, van't Veer P, Kromhout D.
Dietary intake of antioxidant (pro)-vitamins, respiratory
symptoms and pulmonary function: the MORGEN study.
Thorax 1998;**53**:166–71.

162. Shahar E, Folsom AR, Melnick SL, *et al*. Dietary n-3
polyunsaturated fatty acids and smoking-related chronic
obstructive pulmonary disease. Atherosclerosis Risk in
Communities Study Investigators. *N Engl J Med* 1994;**331**:
228–33.

163. Shahar E, Boland LL, Folsom AR, Tockman MS, McGovern
PG, Eckfeldt JH. Docosahexaenoic acid and smoking related
chronic obstructive pulmonary disease. Atherosclerosis Risk
in Communities Study Investigators. *Am J Respir Crit Care
Med* 1999;**159**:1780–5.

164. Sridhar MK, Galloway A, Lean MEJ, Banham SW. An outpatient nutritional supplementation programme in COPD
patients. *Eur Respir J* 1994;**7**:720–4.

165. Steinberg FM, Chait A. Antioxidant vitamin
supplementation and lipid peroxidation in smokers. *Am J
Clin Nutr* 1998;**68**:319–27.

166. Keatings VM, Collins PD, Scott DM, Barnes PJ. Differences in
interleukin 8 and tumour necrosis factor-α in induced
sputum from patients with chronic obstructive pulmonary
disease or asthma. *Am J Respir Crit Care Med* 1996;**153**:
530–4.

167. Parmentier M, Hirani N, Rahman I, Drost EM, MacNee W,
Antonicelli F. Regulation of LPS-mediated interleukin-1β
release by *N*-acetylcysteine in THP-1 cells. *Eur Respir J*
2000;**16**:933–9.

168. Antonicelli F, Parmentier M, Drost EM, Hirani N, Rahman I,
Donaldson K, MacNee W. Nacystelyn inhibits oxidant-
mediated interleukin-8 expression and NF-κB nuclear
binding in alveolar epithelial cells. *Free Radic Biol Med*
2002;**32**:492–502.

169. Jimenez LA, Thompson J, Brown DA, Rahman I, *et al*.
Activation of NF-κB by PM(10) occurs via an iron-mediated

mechanism in the absence of 1-κB degradation. *Toxico Appl
Pharmacol* 2000;**166**:101–10.

170. Galter D, Mihm S, Droge W. Distinct effects of glutathione
disulphide on the nuclear transcription factor kappa B and
the activator peotein-1. *Eur J Biochem* 1994;**221**: 639–48.

171. Ginn-Pease ME, Whisler RL. Optimal NF kappa B mediated
transcriptional responses in Jurkat T cells exposed to
oxidative stress are dependent on intracellular glutathione
and costimulatory signals. *Biochem Biophys Res Commun*
1996;**226**:695–702.

172. Cho S, Urata Y, Iida T, *et al*. Glutathione downregulates the
phosphorylation of I kappa B: autoloop regulation of the
NF-kappa B-mediated expression of NF-kappa B subunits by
TNF-alpha in mouse vascular endothelial cells. *Biochem
Biophys Res Commun* 1998;**253**:104–8.

173. Ito K, Lim S, Caramori G, Chung KF, Barnes PJ, Adcock IM.
Cigarette smoking reduces histone descetylase 2 expression,
enhances cytokine expression, and inhibits glucocorticoid
actions in alveolar macrophages. *FASEB J* 2001;**15**:1110–12.

174. Rahman I, Li XY, Donaldson K, Harrison DJ, MacNee W.
Glutathione homeostasis in alveolar epithelial cells *in vitro*
and lung *in vivo* under oxidative stress. *Am J Physiol: Lung
Cell Mol Biol* 1995;**269**:L285–92.

175. Rahman I, Smith CAD, Lawson M, Harrison DJ, MacNee W.
Induction of gamma-glutamylcysteine synthetase by
cigarette smoke condensate is associated with AP-1 in
human alveolar epithelial cells. *FEBS Lett* 1996;**396**:21–5.

176. Rahman I, Bel A, Mulier B, *et al*. Transcriptional regulation
of γ-glutamylcysteine synthetase-heavy subunit by oxidants
in human alveolar epithelial cells. *Biochem Biophys Res
Commun* 1996;**229**:832–7.

177. Rahman I, Smith CAD, Antonicelli F, MacNee W.
Characterization of γ-glutamylcysteine synthetase-heavy
subunit promoter: a critical role for AP-1. *FEBS Lett*
1998;**427**:129–33.

178. Rahman I, Antonicelli F, MacNee W. Molecular mechanisms
of the regulation of glutathione synthesis by tumour
necrosis factor-α and dexamethasone in human alveolar
epithelial cells. *J Biol Chem* 1999;**274**:5088–96.

179. Gilks CB, Price K, Wright JL, Churg A. Antioxidant gene
expression in rat lung after exposure to cigarette smoke.
Am J Pathol 1998;**152**:269–78.

180. Muller T, Gebel S. The cellular stress response induced by
aqueous extracts of cigarette smoke is critically dependent
on the intracellular glutathione concentration.
Cardiogenesis 1998;**19**:797–801.

181. Muller T. Expression of c-fos in quiescent Swiss 3T3 exposed
to aqueous cigarette smoke fractions. *Cancer Res* 1995;
55:1927–32.

182. Silverman EK, Speizer FE. Risk factors for the development
of chronic obstructive pulmonary disease. *Med Clin N Am*
1996;**80**:501–22.

183. Sandford AJ, Weir TD, Pare PD. Genetic risk factors for
chronic obstructive pulmonary disease. *Eur Respir J*
1997;**10**:1380–91.

184. Barnes PJ. Genetics and pulmonary medicine. 9. Molecular
genetics of chronic obstructive pulmonary disease. *Thorax*
1999;**54**:245–52.

185. Huang S-L, Su C-H, Chang S-C. Tumour necrosis factor-α
gene polymorphism in chronic bronchitis. *Am J Respir Crit
Care Med* 1997;**156**:1436–9.

186. Smith CAD, Harrison DJ. Associaton between polymorphism
in gene for microsomal epoxide hydrolase and susceptibility
to emphysema. *Lancet* 1997;**350**:630–3.

187. Yim JJ, Park GY, Lee CT, *et al*. Genetic susceptibility to
chronic obstructive pulmonary disease in Koreans: combined

analysis of polymorphic genotypes for microsomal epoxide hydrolase and glutathione *S*-transferase M1 and T1. *Thorax* 2000;**55**:121–125.

188. Compton CH, Gubb J, Cedar E, *et al*. SB 207499, a second generation oral PDE4 inhibitor, first demonstration of efficacy in patients with COPD. *Eur Respir J* 1999;**14**(suppl 30):281s.

189. Torphy TJ. Phosphodiesterase isozymes. *Am J Respir Crit Care Med* 1998;**157**:351–70.

190. Chabrier P-E, Auguet M, Spinnewyn B, *et al*. BN 80933, a dual inhibitor of neuronal nitric oxide synthase and lipid peroxidation: A promising neuroprotective strategy. *Proc Natl Acad Sci USA* 1999;**96**:10824–9.

191. Manna SK, Tien Kuo M, Aggarwal BB. Overexpression of γ-glutamylcysteine synthetase suppresses tumor necrosis factor-induced apoptosis and activation of nuclear transcription factor-kappa B and activator protein-1. *Oncogene* 1999;**18**:4371–82.

192. Nishikawa M, Kakemizu N, Ito T, *et al*. Superoxide mediates cigarette smoke-induced infiltration of neutrophils into the airways through nuclear factor-κB activation and IL-8 mRNA expression in guinea pigs *in vivo*. *Am J Respir Cell Mol Biol* 1999;**20**:189–98.

193. Clausen J. The influence of antioxidants on the enhanced respiratory burst reaction in smokers. *Ann NY Acad Sci* 1991;**629**:337–41.

194. Hoshino E, Shariff R, Ban Gossum A. Vitamin E suppresses increased lipid peroxidation in cigarette smokers. *J Parenter Enter Nutr* 1990;**40**:300–5.

195. MacNee W, Bridgeman MME, Marsden M, *et al*. The effects of *N*-acetylcysteine and glutathione on smoke-induced changes in lung phagocytes and epithelial cells. *Am J Med* 1991;**90**:60s–6s.

196. Ross D, Norbeck K, Moldeus P. The generation and subsequent fate of glutathionyl radicals in biological systems. *J Biol Chem* 1985;**260**:15028–32.

197. Marrades RM, Roca J, Barbera JA, *et al*. Nebulized glutathione induces bronchoconstriction in patients with mild asthma. *Am J Respir Crit Care Med* 1997;**156**:425–30.

198. Meister A, Anderson ME. Glutathione. *Ann Rev Biochem* 1983;**52**:711–60.

199. Bridgeman MME, Marsden M, MacNee W, *et al*. Cysteine and glutathione concentrations in plasma and bronchoalveolar lavage fluid after treatment with *N*-acetylcysteine. *Thorax* 1991;**46**:39–42.

200. Bridgemen MME, Marsden M, Selby C, Effect of *N*-acetyl cysteine on the concentrations of thiols in plasma bronchoalveolar lavage fluid and lining tissue. *Thorax* 1994;**49**:670–5.

201. Bowman G, Backer U, Larsson S, *et al*. Oral acetylcysteine reduces exaceration rate in chronic bronchitis. *Eur J Respir Dis* 1983;**64**:405–15.

202. Rasmusse JB, Glennow C. Reduction in days of illness after long-term treatment with *N*-acetylcysteine controlled-release tablets in patients with chronic bronchitis. *Eur J Respir Dis* 1988;**1**:351–5.

203. British Thoracic Society Research Committee. Oral *N*-acetylcysteine and exacerbation rates in patients with chronic bronchitis and severe airways obstruction. *Thorax* 1985;**40**:823–35.

204. Grandjean EM, Berthet P, Ruffmann R, Leuenberger P. Efficacy of oral long-term *N*-acetylcysteine in chronic bronchopulmonary disease: a meta-analysis of published double-blind, placebo-controlled clinical trials. *Clin Ther* 2000;**22**:209–21.

205. Ekberg-Jansson A, Larson M, MacNee W, *et al*. for the *N*-isobutyrylcysteine Study Group. *N*-isobutyrylcysteine, a donor of systemic thiols, does not reduce the exacerbation rate in chronic bronchitis. *Eur Respir J* 1999;**13**:829–34.

206. Gillissen A, Jaworska M, Orth M, *et al*. Nacystelyn a novel lysine salt of *N*-acetylcysteine to augment cellular antioxidant defence *in vitro*. *Respir Med* 1997;**91**:159–68.

207. Nagy AM, Vanderbist F, Parij N, *et al*. Effect of the mucoactive drug Nacystelyn on the respiratory burst of human blood polymorphonuclear neutrophils. *Pulm Pharmacol Ther* 1997;**10**:287–92.

Inflammation

PETER J BARNES

INTRODUCTION

It is now well established that inflammation is of critical importance in asthma and this has been a major impetus to changing the management of asthma, with emphasis on the early use of anti-inflammatory treatments. Inflammation is also important in COPD; chronic inflammation is present in the airways and lung parenchyma of patients with COPD, although the pathophysiologic significance of this inflammation is currently uncertain. The inflammatory process in COPD differs in most respects from that in asthma in terms of inflammatory cells, inflammatory mediators, inflammatory responses and response to corticosteroid therapy.[1] However, some patients with COPD ($\approx 10\%$) also have asthma and therefore may share inflammatory features. Cigarette smoking itself induces an inflammatory response and the inflammatory changes described in COPD appear to be an exaggeration of the normal inflammatory response to an irritant.[2] More comparisons between COPD patients and individuals with normal lung function who are matched for smoking exposure are needed. It is also important to differentiate COPD from asthma, and a negative trial of corticosteroids is recommended in selecting suitable patients for study. There is little information about the inflammatory process in patients with COPD that is not due to smoking.[3]

MEASUREMENT OF INFLAMMATION IN COPD

Several approaches have been used to characterize the inflammatory response in COPD.

Pathology

Detailed histologic examination of pathologic specimens of lung obtained at post-mortem, during surgical lobectomy or lung volume reduction surgery have demonstrated inflammatory changes in the airways and lung parenchyma in patients with COPD.[4–8] In the airway mucosa of large and small airways there is an increase in macrophages and T-lymphocytes, particularly CD8+ T cells. Similar changes are found in lung parenchyma in association with emphysema.

Bronchoalveolar lavage

Bronchoalveolar lavage may reflect inflammation in the lung periphery and is characterized by a marked increase in the numbers of macrophages and neutrophils.[9–12]

Bronchial biopsy

Fiberoptic bronchial biopsies are restricted to proximal airways and show an increase in macrophages and T cells, particularly CD8+ cells, thus reflecting the changes in peripheral airways.[13] In smokers and patients with mild COPD neutrophils do not appear to be increased,[13,14] but are increased in patients with severe COPD.[14] The inflammatory changes in bronchial biopsies are also present in ex-smokers, suggesting that the inflammatory response in COPD may persist even in the absence of causal mechanisms.[15,16] Increased numbers of eosinophils have also been reported in the airways of some patients with COPD, although these patients may have coexisting asthma[10,17] and in other studies no increase in the numbers of airway eosinophils has been reported.[13] In addition, increased numbers of eosinophils have been reported in the airways during acute exacerbations of COPD.[18,19]

Induced sputum

Induction of sputum with nebulized hypertonic saline can be safely performed even in patients with severe COPD ($FEV_1 < 40\%$ predicted) and is a useful means of investigating airway inflammation in COPD. Induced sputum in COPD shows an increase in total cell numbers, indicating an increase in macrophages and there is an increase in the proportion of neutrophils but not eosinophils.[20,21] This is matched by an increase in myeloperoxidase (MPO) and human neutrophil lectin (HNL), reflecting neutrophil activation.[22] In normal cigarette smokers there is an increase in the proportion of neutrophils compared with age-matched non-smoking subjects, but this is less than seen in COPD patients. There is an inverse correlation between the proportion of neutrophils and % predicted FEV_1.[20,21] Although the numbers of eosinophils are not increased in sputum in stable COPD, there is a surprising increase in both eosinophil cationic protein (ECP) and eosinophil peroxidase (EPO), suggesting that eosinophils may have been degranulated.[22] It is possible that neutrophil elastase derived from activated neutrophils in sputum may be responsible for degranulating these eosinophils.[23]

Exhaled markers

There is a need to develop non-invasive markers of airway inflammation and there has been particular interest in measurement of volatile markers of inflammation in the breath and exhaled condensates. Exhaled nitric oxide (NO) has been most extensively investigated and is clearly elevated in patients with asthma. Exhaled NO levels are much lower in COPD than in asthma and have been reported to be only slightly increased or normal in stable COPD[24–26] and increased during exacerbations.[24] This is partly because cigarette smoking itself reduces exhaled NO levels.[27] Levels of exhaled carbon monoxide (CO) are increased in patients with COPD, although this measurement is affected by cigarette smoking. However, the levels of exhaled CO are increased even in ex-smokers with COPD.[28] Markers of oxidative stress, including hydrogen peroxide (H_2O_2), ethane and 8-isoprostane are increased in expired condensates of patients with COPD.[29–31]

INFLAMMATORY CELLS

Many inflammatory cells are increased and/or activated in COPD, but their contribution to disease progression is largely unknown. There are clearly interactions between the inflammatory cells involved in COPD (Figure 11.1).

Neutrophils

Increased numbers of activated neutrophils are found in sputum and bronchoalveolar lavage (BAL) fluid of patients with COPD,[9,11,20,21] yet are little increased in the airways or lung parenchyma.[4,13] This may reflect their rapid transit through the airways and parenchyma. Neutrophils secrete several proteases, including neutrophil elastase (NE), cathepsin G and protease-3, which may contribute to parenchymal destruction. NE and protease-3 are potent mucus stimulants.[32] Neutrophil recruitment to the airways and parenchyma involves adhesion to endothelial cells and the adhesion molecule E-selectin is upregulated on endothelial cells in the

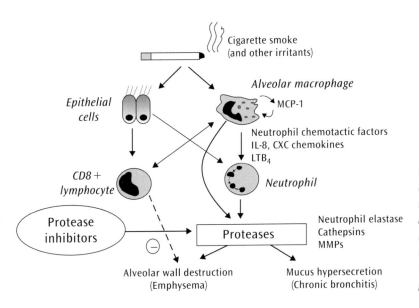

Figure 11.1 *Cellular mechanisms in COPD. Activation of macrophages leads to recruitment of neutrophils and both cells release proteases which may result in emphysema and chronic bronchitis if not counteracted by antiproteases. MCP-1 = Macrophage chemotactic protein-1.*

airways of COPD patients[33] (Figure 11.2). Circulating neutrophils show upregulation of Mac-1 (CD11b/CD18) in stable COPD patients. Adherent neutrophils then migrate into the respiratory tract under the direction of neutrophil chemotactic factors, which include the chemokine interleukin 8 (IL-8) and leukotriene B4 (LTB4). Neutrophil survival in the respiratory tract may be increased by cytokines, such as granulocyte-macrophage colony stimulating factor (GM-CSF). The role of neutrophils in COPD is not yet clear. Neutrophil numbers in bronchial biopsies and induced sputum are correlated with COPD disease severity[14,20,34] and the numbers of neutrophils in BAL fluid and sputum are markedly increased during acute exacerbations of COPD.[35] BAL neutrophils are increased in patients with COPD who have never smoked, whereas macrophage numbers are not increased, emphasizing the importance of neutrophils in COPD.[3] However, while neutrophils have the capacity to cause elastolysis this is not a significant feature of other pulmonary diseases where chronic airway

neutrophilia is prominent, including cystic fibrosis and bronchiectasis. This suggests that additional factors must be involved. It is likely that neutrophilia is linked to mucus hypersecretion in chronic bronchitis, however.

Macrophages

There is an increase in the numbers of macrophages in airways, lung parenchyma, BAL fluid and sputum in patients with COPD. Furthermore, macrophages are localized to sites of alveolar wall destruction in patients with emphysema[4] and in the epithelium of small airways.[8] There is a correlation between macrophage numbers in the airways and severity of COPD.[14] Macrophages may be activated by cigarette smoke to release inflammatory mediators, including tumor necrosis factor alpha (TNF-α), IL-8 and LTB4, providing a cellular mechanism that links cigarette smoking with inflammation in COPD (Figure 11.3). Macrophages are likely to play an

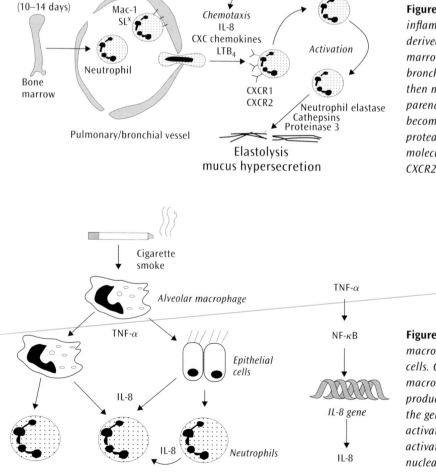

Figure 11.2 *Mechanism of neutrophil inflammation in COPD. Neutrophils derived from promyeloblasts in the bone marrow adhere to endothelial cells in the bronchial and pulmonary circulations, then move into the airways or parenchyma, where they survive and become activated to release serine proteases. ICAM-1: intercellular adhesion molecule 1. CXCR1 = CXC receptor-1; CXCR2 = CXC receptor-2.*

Figure 11.3 *Interaction between macrophages, neutrophils and epithelial cells. Cigarette smoke activates macrophages and epithelial cells to produce TNF-α, which in turn switches on the gene for IL-8, which recruits and activates neutrophils. This is via the activation of the transcription factor nuclear factor-kappa B (NF-κB).*

important orchestrating role in the inflammation of COPD, but little is yet understood about different types of macrophage in the respiratory tract. Alveolar macrophages are also likely to be an important cellular source of elastolytic enzymes, including cathepsins and matrix metalloproteases. The mechanisms that result in macrophage accumulation in COPD are not yet understood. It is likely that chemokines such as monocyte chemotactic protein 1 (MCP-1) recruit macrophages from circulating monocytes, although local production of macrophages in the lung may also be important. Elastin degradation products may also be important as chemotactic stimuli for macrophages in the lung parenchyma.[36]

T-lymphocytes

There is an increase in the total numbers of T-lymphocytes in lung parenchyma, peripheral and central airways of patients with COPD, with the greatest increase in CD8+ (cytotoxic) cells.[4,7,13] There is a correlation between the numbers of T cells and the amount of alveolar destruction and the severity of airflow obstruction.[4,13] However, the role of T cells in pathophysiology is not yet certain. CD8+ cells have the capacity to cause cytolysis and apoptosis of alveolar epithelial cells through release of perforin and granzyme-B and by the release of TNF-α.[37] An increased number of natural killer (NK) cells has also been reported in patients with severe COPD.[14]

Eosinophils

The role of eosinophils in COPD is uncertain. Reports of increased eosinophils in the airways of some patients with COPD might be due to coexisting asthma. However, an increase in eosinophils during exacerbations of COPD[18,19] may be important. Surprisingly the levels of ECP and EPO in induced sputum are as elevated in COPD as in asthma, despite the absence of visible eosinophils, suggesting that they may have degranulated and are no longer recognizable by light microscopy.[22] Perhaps this is due to the high levels of NE that degranulate eosinophils.[23]

Epithelial cells

Airway epithelial cells play a critical role in asthma and may be a major source of inflammatory mediators. Airway epithelial cells are characteristically shed in asthmatic airways and have weakened attachments. The role of airway epithelial cells in COPD is uncertain. Epithelial cells may be an important source of chemokines, such as IL-8.

INFLAMMATORY MEDIATORS

While many inflammatory mediators have been identified in asthma,[38] there is much less information about the production and role of mediators in COPD, although it is certain that many mediators are involved and mediator antagonists have potential as new therapies for COPD. Inflammatory mediators are derived from several cell types in the respiratory tract and these mediators are likely to mediate several inflammatory effects (Figure 11.4).

Leukotrienes

LTB4 is a potent chemoattractant of neutrophils and is increased in the sputum and exhaled condensates of patients with COPD.[34,39] It is probably derived mainly from alveolar macrophages, which secrete greater amounts of LTB4 in patients with COPD. Several potent LTB4 receptor antagonists have been developed for clinical studies and should elucidate the role of this mediator in COPD. There is no evidence that cysteinyl-leukotrienes (LTC4, LTD4, LTE4) are involved in COPD and levels of LTE4 in exhaled breath condensates are not increased, but studies with antileukotrienes in COPD are currently underway.

Prostaglandins

The role of prostaglandins in COPD is unknown. Oxidative stress may result in the non-enzymatic formation of novel prostanoid mediators, isoprostanes, directly from arachidonic acid without the involvement of cyclooxygenase. There is increased formation of 8-isoprostane in COPD as measured in urine and in expired condensate.[40,41] 8-Isoprostane is a potent constrictor of human airways. The levels of PGE_2 are increased in exhaled breath condensates of patients with COPD.[39]

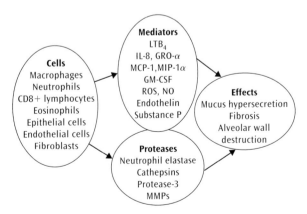

Figure 11.4 *Multiplicity of cells and mediators involved in the inflammatory response in COPD.*

Platelet-activating factor

PAF enhances the release of LTB4 from activated neutrophils, indicating that it might have an amplifying effect on neutrophilic inflammation.[42] Whether PAF is released from alveolar macrophages in patients with COPD is not yet certain.

Reactive oxygen species

There is compelling evidence for increased oxidative stress in patients with COPD.[43] Cigarette smoke contains a high concentration of reactive oxygen species (ROS) (10^{17} moles/puff) and inflammatory cells, such as activated macrophages and neutrophils, also contribute. Evidence for increased oxidative stress in COPD is provided by demonstration of increased concentrations of H_2O_2 in expired condensates, particularly during exacerbations,[29] increased 8-isoprostane levels in urine and expired condensate.[30,40] The increased oxidative stress in COPD may have several deleterious effects; oxidation of antiproteases, such as α_1-antitrypsin and secretory leukoprotease inhibitor (SLPI) may reduce the antiprotease shield, and may directly activate matrix metalloproteases, resulting in increased proteolysis. H_2O_2 directly constricts airway smooth muscle *in vitro* and hyroxyl radicals (OH^-) potently induce plasma exudation in airways. Oxidants also activate the transcription factor nuclear factor-κB (NF-κB) which orchestrates the expression of multiple inflammatory genes, including IL-8 and TNF-α. Superoxide anions (O_2^-) rapidly combine with nitric oxide (NO) to form the potent radical peroxynitrite, which itself generates OH^-. Peroxynitrite reacts with tyrosine residues in proteins to form stable 3-nitrotyrosine residues and there is evidence that 3-nitrotyrosine immunoreactivity is increased in inflammatory cells in induced sputum in patients with COPD.[44] ROS also induce lipid peroxidation, resulting in the formation of additional mediators, such as isoprostanes and the volatile hydrocarbons pentane and ethane, as well as inducing DNA damage. Exhaled ethane levels are markedly elevated in patients with COPD.[31]

ROS are normally counteracted by endogenous (glutathione, uric acid, bilirubin) and exogenous (vitamin C and vitamin E from diet) antioxidants. There is evidence for a reduction in antioxidant defences in patients with COPD.[43]

Chemokines

IL-8 is selectively chemoattractant to neutrophils and is present in high concentrations in induced sputum of patients with COPD.[20,45] Indeed, there is a good correlation between the levels of IL-8 and the degree of neutrophilia in sputum.[20,45] IL-8 concentrations are also increased in BAL fluid of patients with COPD and this is also correlated with neutrophil counts.[12] IL-8 may be secreted by macrophages, neutrophils and by airway epithelial cells. Other related (CXC) chemokines, such as GRO-α and GRO-β, are also increased in COPD.[46]

The CC-chemokine MCP-1 is increased in BAL fluid of patients with COPD and healthy smokers, whereas another CC-chemokine macrophage inflammatory protein-1β (MIP-1β) is increased in COPD compared to normal subjects and healthy smokers.[47] MCP-1 is a potent chemoattractant of monocytes and may be involved in macrophage recruitment into the lungs in smokers. The CC-chemokine MIP-1α shows increased expression in airway epithelial cells and might contribute to the macrophage activation in COPD.[14]

Cytokines

TNF-α is present in high concentration in the sputum of COPD patients[20] and is detectable in bronchial biopsies from patients with COPD.[17] TNF-α activates the transcription factor nuclear factor-κB (NF-κB), which switches on the transcription of the IL-8 gene in epithelial cells and macrophages. Serum levels of TNF-α and stimulated TNF-α production from peripheral blood monocytes are increased in weight-losing COPD patients, suggesting that it may play a role in the cachexia of severe COPD.[48]

The concentrations of GM-CSF in BAL fluid are increased in stable COPD but markedly elevated during exacerbations.[35] The number of GM-CSF-immunoreactive macrophages is increased in sputum of patients with COPD.[49] GM-CSF is important for neutrophil survival and may play an enhancing role in neutrophilic inflammation.

Growth factors

Transforming growth factor beta (TGF-β) and epidermal growth factor (EGF) show increased expression in epithelial cells and submucosal cells (eosinophils and fibroblasts) in patients with COPD and might play a role in the structural changes in the airways.[50] EGF may play an important role in amplifying mucus secretion in COPD.[51]

Endothelins

There is an increased concentration of endothelin 1 (ET-1) in induced sputum of patients with COPD.[52] Plasma levels of ET-1 are elevated in patients with severe COPD and this is likely to be related to chronic hypoxia in these patients.[53] There is increased expression of ET-1 in pulmonary endothelial cells of patients with COPD who have secondary pulmonary hypertension,[54] suggesting that ET-1 may contribute to the vascular remodeling associated with hypoxic pulmonary hypertension.

Neuropeptides

Several neuropeptides have potent effects on vascular function and mucus secretion. An increase in the concentration of substance P (SP) is found in sputum of patients with chronic bronchitis.[55] However, no significant differences in the number of nerves immunoreactive for SP, calcitonin gene-related peptide or vasoactive intestinal peptide (VIP) are found in bronchial biopsies from patients with COPD,[56] although there is a slight decrease in the expression of neuropeptide Y in airway smooth muscle. Another study reports an increase in VIP-immunoreactive nerves in the vicinity of submucosal glands in bronchial biopsies of patients with chronic bronchitis, so that this neuropeptide may play a role in mucous hypersecretion.[57]

Proteases

Several enzymes that degrade matrix proteins are released in COPD and appear to be the underlying mechanism for alveolar destruction in emphysema. It is likely that they also result in mucous hypersecretion in chronic bronchitis. Proteases differ in their substrate specificity, but the combination of proteases increased in COPD is capable of degrading collagens and elastin, and therefore of destroying alveolar walls. Elastin may be the most important target for these enzymes as there is a loss of elasticity in the lung parenchyma and elastin.

Neutrophil Elastase (NE), a neutral serine protease, is a major constituent of lung elastolytic enzyme activity; it may well not be the major elastolytic enzyme in smoking-related COPD, and it is important to consider other enzymes as targets for inhibition.

Neutrophil cathepsin G and proteinase 3 also have elastolytic activity and may need to be inhibited together with neutrophil elastase. Cathepsins (cathepsins B, L and S) are also released from macrophages.

Matrix metalloproteases (MMP) are a group of over 20 closely related endopeptidases that are capable of degrading all of the components of the extracellular matrix of lung parenchyma, including elastin, collagen, proteoglycans, laminin and fibronectin. They are produced by neutrophils, alveolar macrophages and airway epithelial cells.[58] Increased levels of collagenase (MMP-1), gelatinase A (MMP-2) and gelatinase B (MMP-9) have been detected in BAL fluid and induced sputum of patients with COPD.[59,60] Lavaged macrophages from patients with emphysema express more MMP-9 and MMP-1 than cells from control subjects, suggesting that these cells, rather than neutrophils, may be a major

cellular source.[61] Alveolar macrophages also express a unique MMP, macrophage metalloelastase (MMP-12).[58] MMP-12 knockout mice do not develop emphysema and do not show the expected increases in lung macrophages after long-term exposure to cigarette smoke,[62] but there are doubts about the relevance of MMP-12 in humans.[61] Immunocytochemical studies of emphysematous lungs indicate increased expression of MMP-9 and MMP-2, but not NE or MMP-12 at sites of alveolar destruction.[63]

For many years it has been proposed that there is an imbalance between proteases and endogenous antiproteases in COPD. Serine antiprotease (serpins) include alpha-1-antitrypsin, which is the major antiproteinase in plasma and the lung parenchyma, and SLPI, which is the major antiprotease in airways. Both are effective inhibitors of NE. Oxidative stress may oxidize sulfydryl groups on methionine in these antiproteases and impair their efficiency, or there may be genetic polymorphisms that reduce the production of antiproteases. Tissue inhibitors of MMPs (TIMPs) are the major inhibitors of MMPs and there is evidence for a reduced ratio of TIMP-1:MMP-9 in sputum of patients with COPD.[64]

RESPONSE TO ANTI-INFLAMMATORY TREATMENTS

Since inflammation is a feature of COPD, it follows that anti-inflammatory therapies may have clinical benefit in controlling symptoms, preventing exacerbations and reducing the progression of the disease. This has provided a rationale for the use of corticosteroids in asthma therapy.

Corticosteroids

While the value of oral corticosteroids in the management of acute exacerbations of COPD has been established in controlled trials, there is little evidence for the clinical benefit of inhaled corticosteroids in preventing disease progression.[65] There have been few studies of the effects of corticosteroids on the inflammatory response in COPD. Neither high doses of oral or inhaled corticosteroids reduce the numbers of neutrophils or macrophages, the concentrations of cytokines (IL-8, TNF-α), granule proteins (MPO, ECP, EPO) or proteases (NE, MMPs) in induced sputum in patients with severe COPD.[60,66] In one study an inhibitory effect of corticosteroids on neutrophils was reported, but is difficult to interpret, as there was a high baseline eosinophilia in these patients, suggesting that they may be asthmatic.[67] An increase in sputum eosinophils (>3% total) and exhaled NO is predictive of a response to oral steroids in patients with severe COPD,[68,69] which is likely to indicate that there is coexisting asthma. A high dose of inhaled corticosteroids for three months had no effect on inflammatory cells in bronchial biopsies of COPD patients, apart from a small reduction in the CD8+: CD4+ ratio in the epithelium.[70] The reasons for the lack of anti-inflammatory effects of corticosteroids is not yet known; neutrophilic inflammation may not be responsive to corticosteroids as steroids prolong the survival of neutrophils whereas they decrease the survival of eosinophils. A high dose of inhaled corticosteroid has no effect on ozone-induced airway neutrophilia in normal subjects, indicating the resistance of airway neutrophilic inflammation to corticosteroids in humans.[71] Another possibility is that there is resistance to the anti-inflammatory effects of corticosteroids in COPD; there is evidence that cigarette smoking inhibits the anti-inflammatory effects of corticosteroids in asthmatic patients.[72] Cigarette smoking appears to inhibit histone deacetylases, the enzymes that reverse the acetylation of core histones that regulate the expression of inflammatory genes, such as TNF-α and IL-8.[73]

Other anti-inflammatory treatments

There are surprisingly few trials of other potentially anti-inflammatory treatments in COPD, although several new drugs, including LTB4 antagonists and phosphodiesterase (PDE) inhibitors, are now in progress.[74] Theophylline, a weak PDE inhibitor that may have other anti-inflammatory effects, reduces the neutrophilic inflammation and neutrophil activation in induced sputum in COPD patients, in contrast to the lack of effect of corticosteroids in a similar patient population.[75] Recently a selective PDE4 inhibitor, cilomilast, has been found to increase lung function and reduce symptoms in patients with moderate to severe COPD, but it is not yet known whether this is associated with a reduction in inflammation.[76] PDE4 inhibitors potently inhibit neutrophilic inflammation and also have an inhibitory effect on macrophage and CD8+ T-cell function.

DIFFERENCES FROM ASTHMA

There are striking differences in the inflammatory response between COPD and asthma, although in some patients there is an overlap as both diseases may coexist (Table 11.1).

COPD is characterized by a neutrophilic airway inflammation, a large increase in macrophages and a preponderance of CD8+ cells in airways and lung parenchyma, but asthma is typified by an increase in active eosinophils, a preponderance of CD4+ Th2 cells, a small increase in macrophages and mast cell activation.[1,5] Whereas in COPD the predominant mediators are LTB$_4$, IL-8 and TNF-α, in asthma LTD4, histamine, eotaxin, IL-4 and IL-5 are prominent. The inflammatory consequences between the two diseases is also different; in COPD there is squamous metaplasia of the epithelium, whereas in asthma the epithelium is fragile. The characteristic thickening of the basement membrane in asthma is not seen in COPD. There is parenchyma destruction in COPD that does not occur in asthma. Finally the response to corticosteroids differs markedly between asthma and COPD, with an inhibitory effect of corticosteroids in asthmatic inflammation which is not seen in COPD.

Table 11.1 *Differences between COPD and asthma*

Inflammation	Asthma	COPD
Inflammatory cells	Mast cells Eosinophils CD4+ cells (Th2) Macrophages +	Neutrophils CD8+ cells (Tc) Macrophages +++
Inflammatory mediators	LTD$_4$, histamine IL-4, IL-5, IL-13 Eotaxin, RANTES Oxidative stress +	LTB$_4$ TNF-α IL-8, GRO-α Oxidative stress +++
Inflammatory effects	All airways Airway hyperresponsiveness +++ Epithelial shedding Fibrosis + No parenchymal involvement Mucus secretion +	Peripheral airways Airway hyperresponsiveness + Epithelial metaplasia Fibrosis ++ Parenchymal destruction Mucus secretion +++
Response to corticosteroids	+++	$\pm$

LT: leukotriene; IL: interleukin.

REFERENCES

1. Barnes PJ. Mechanisms in COPD: differences from asthma. *Chest* 2000;**117**:10S–14S.
2. Barnes PJ. Chronic obstructive pulmonary disease. *New Engl J Med* 2000;**343**:269–80.
3. Lusuardi M, Capelli A, Cerutti CG, Spada EL, Donner CF. Airways inflammation in subjects with chronic bronchitis who have never smoked. *Thorax* 1994;**49**:1211–16.
4. Finkelstein R, Fraser RS, Ghezzo H, Cosio MG. Alveolar inflammation and its relation to emphysema in smokers. *Am J Respir Crit Care Med* 1995;**152**:1666–72.
5. Jeffery PK. Structural and inflammatory changes in COPD: a comparison with asthma. *Thorax* 1998;**53**:129–36.
6. Saetta M, Di Stefano A, Maestrelli P, *et al*. Activated T-lymphocytes and macrophages in bronchial mucosa of subjects with chronic bronchitis. *Am Rev Respir Dis* 1993;**147**:301–6.
7. Saetta M, Di Stefano A, Turato G, *et al*. CD8+ T-lymphocytes in peripheral airways of smokers with chronic obstructive pulmonary disease. *Am J Respir Crit Care Med* 1998;**157**:822–6.
8. Saetta M, Turato G, Baraldo S, *et al*. Goblet cell hyperplasia and epithelial inflammation in peripheral airways of smokers with both symptoms of chronic bronchitis and chronic airflow limitation. *Am J Respir Crit Care Med* 2000;**161**:1016–21.
9. Thompson PB, Daughton D, Robbins GA, Ghafouki MA, Oehlerking M, Rennard SI. Intramural airway inflammation in chronic bronchitis. Characterization and correlation with clinical parameters. *Am Rev Respir Dis* 1989;**140**:1527–37.
10. Lacoste JY, Bousquet J, Chanez P. Eosinophilic and neutrophilic inflammation in asthma, chronic bronchitis and chronic obstructive pulmonary disease. *J Allergy Clin Immunol* 1993;**92**:537–48.
11. Pesci A, Majori M, Cuomo A, *et al*. Neutrophils infiltrating bronchial epithelium in chronic obstructive pulmonary disease. *Respir Med* 1998;**92**:863–70.
12. Pesci A, Balbi B, Majori M, *et al*. Inflammatory cells and mediators in bronchial lavage of patients with chronic obstructive pulmonary disease. *Eur Respir J* 1998;**12**:380–6.
13. O'Shaughnessy TC, Ansari TW, Barnes NC, Jeffery PK. Inflammation in bronchial biopsies of subjects with chronic bronchitis: inverse relationship of CD8+ T lymphocytes with FEV$_1$. *Am J Respir Crit Care Med* 1997;**155**:852–7.
14. Di Stefano A, Capelli A, Lusuardi M, *et al*. Severity of airflow limitation is associated with severity of airway inflammation in smokers. *Am J Respir Crit Care Med* 1998;**158**:1277–85.
15. Turato G, Di Stefano A, Maestrelli P, *et al*. Effect of smoking cessation on airway inflammation in chronic bronchitis. *Am J Respir Crit Care Med* 1995;**152**:1262–7.
16. Rutgers SR, Postma DS, ten Hacken NH, *et al*. Ongoing airway inflammation in patients with COPD who do not currently smoke. *Thorax* 2000;**55**:12–18.
17. Mueller R, Chanez P, Campbell AM, Bousquet J, Heusser C, Bullock GR. Different cytokine patterns in bronchial biopsies in asthma and chronic bronchitis. *Respir Med* 1996;**90**:79–85.
18. Saetta M, Distefano A, Maestrelli P, *et al*. Airway eosinophilia in chronic bronchitis during exacerbations. *Am J Respir Crit Care Med* 1994;**150**:1646–52.
19. Saetta M, Di Stefano A, Maestrelli P, *et al*. Airway eosinophilia and expression of interleukin-5 protein in asthma and in exacerbations of chronic bronchitis. *Clin Exp Allergy* 1996;**26**:766–74.
20. Keatings VM, Collins PD, Scott DM, Barnes PJ. Differences in interleukin-8 and tumor necrosis factor-α in induced sputum from patients with chronic obstructive pulmonary disease or asthma. *Am J Respir Crit Care Med* 1996;**153**:530–4.
21. Peleman RA, Rytila PH, Kips JC, Joos GF, Pauwels RA. The cellular composition of induced sputum in chronic obstructive pulmonary disease. *Eur Respir J* 1999;**13**:839–43.
22. Keatings VM, Barnes PJ. Granulocyte activation markers in induced sputum: comparison between chronic obstructive pulmonary disease, asthma and normal subjects. *Am J Respir Crit Care Med* 1997;**155**:449–53.
23. Liu H, Lazarus SC, Caughey GH, Fahy JV. Neutrophil elastase and elastase-rich cystic fibrosis sputum degranulate human eosinophils *in vitro*. *Am J Physiol* 1999;**276**:L28–34.
24. Maziak W, Loukides S, Culpitt S, Sullivan P, Kharitonov SA, Barnes PJ. Exhaled nitric oxide in chronic obstructive pulmonary disease. *Am J Respir Crit Care Med* 1998;**157**:998–1002.
25. Corradi M, Majori M, Cacciani GC, Consigli GF, de'Munari E, Pesci A. Increased exhaled nitric oxide in patients with stable chronic obstructive pulmonary disease. *Thorax* 1999;**54**:572–5.
26. Rutgers SR, Van der Mark TW, Coers W, *et al*. Markers of nitric oxide metabolism in sputum and exhaled air are not increased in chronic obstructive pulmonary disease. *Thorax* 1999;**54**:576–80.
27. Kharitonov SA, Robbins RA, Yates D, Keatings V, Barnes PJ. Acute and chronic effects of cigarette smoking on exhaled nitric oxide. *Am J Respir Crit Care Med* 1995;**152**:609–12.
28. Culpitt SV, Paredi P, Kharitonov SA, Barnes PJ. Exhaled carbon monoxide is increased in COPD patients regardless of their smoking habit. *Am J Respir Crit Care Med* 1998;**157**:A287.
29. Dekhuijzen PNR, Aben KHH, Dekker I, *et al*. Increased exhalation of hydrogen peroxide in patients with stable and unstable chronic obstructive pulmonary disease. *Am J Respir Crit Care Med* 1996;**154**:813–16.
30. Montuschi P, Collins JV, Ciabattoni G, *et al*. Exhaled 8-isoprostane as an *in vivo* biomarker of lung oxidative stress in patients with COPD and healthy smokers. *Am J Respir Crit Care Med* 2000;**162**:1175–7.
31. Paredi P, Kharitonov SA, Leak D, Ward S, Cramer D, Barnes PJ. Exhaled ethane, a marker of lipid peroxidation, is elevated in chronic obstructive pulmonary disease. *Am J Respir Crit Care Med* 2000;**162**:369–73.
32. Witko-Sarsat V, Halbwachs-Mecarelli L, Schuster A, *et al*. Proteinase 3, a potent secretagogue in airways, is present in cystic fibrosis sputum. *Am J Respir Cell Mol Biol* 1999;**20**:729–36.
33. Di Stefano A, Maestrelli P, Roggeri A, *et al*. Upregulation of adhesion molecules in the bronchial mucosa of subjects with chronic obstructive bronchitis. *Am J Respir Crit Care Med* 1994;**149**:803–10.
34. Hill AT, Bayley D, Stockley RA. The interrelationship of sputum inflammatory markers in patients with chronic bronchitis. *Am J Respir Crit Care Med* 1999;**160**:893–8.
35. Balbi B, Bason C, Balleari E, *et al*. Increased bronchoalveolar granulocytes and granulocyte/macrophage colony-stimulating factor during exacerbations of chronic bronchitis. *Eur Respir J* 1997;**10**:846–50.
36. Mecham RP, Broekelmann TJ, Fliszar CJ, Shapiro SD, Welgus HG, Senior RM. Elastin degradation by matrix metalloproteinases. Cleavage site specificity and mechanisms of elastolysis. *J Biol Chem* 1997;**272**:18071–6.
37. Liu AN, Mohammed AZ, Rice WR, *et al*. Perforin-independent CD8(+) T-cell-mediated cytotoxicity of alveolar epithelial cells is preferentially mediated by tumor necrosis factor-alpha: relative insensitivity to Fas ligand. *Am J Respir Cell Mol Biol* 1999;**20**:849–58.
38. Barnes PJ, Chung KF, Page CP. Inflammatory mediators of asthma: an update. *Pharmacol Rev* 1998;**50**:515–96.

39. Montuschi P, Kharitonov SA, Carpagnano E, *et al.* Exhaled prostaglandin E$_2$: a new marker of airway inflammation in COPD. *Am J Respir Crit Care Med* 2000;**161**:A821.

40. Pratico D, Basili S, Vieri M, Cordova C, Violi F, Fitzgerald GA. Chronic obstructive pulmonary disease is associated with an increase in urinary levels of isoprostane F$_{2\alpha}$-III, an index of oxidant stress. *Am J Respir Crit Care Med* 1998;**158**:1709–14.

41. Montuschi P, Ciabattoni G, Corradi M, *et al.* Increased 8-isoprostane, a marker of oxidative stress, in exhaled condensates of asthmatic patients. *Am J Respir Crit Care Med* 1999;**160**:216–20.

42. Shindo K, Koide K, Fukumura M. Enhancement of leukotriene B4 release in stimulated asthmatic neutrophils by platelet activating factor. *Thorax* 1997;**52**:1024–9.

43. Repine JE, Bast A, Lankhorst I. Oxidative stress in chronic obstructive pulmonary disease. *Am J Respir Crit Care Med* 1997;**156**:341–57.

44. Ichinose M, Sugiura H, Yamagata S, Koarai A, Shirato K. Increase in reactive nitrogen species production in chronic obstructive pulmonary disease airways. *Am J Respir Crit Care Med* 2000;**160**:701–6.

45. Yamamoto C, Yoneda T, Yoshikawa M, *et al.* Airway inflammation in COPD assessed by sputum levels of interleukin-8. *Chest* 1997;**112**:505–10.

46. Traves SL, Culpitt S, Russell REK, Barnes PJ, Donnelly LE. Elevated levels of the chemokines GRO-α and MCP-1 in sputum samples from COPD patients. *Thorax* 2002;**57**:590–5.

47. Capelli A, Di Stefano A, Gnemmi I, *et al.* Increased MCP-1 and MIP-1β in bronchoalveolar lavage fluid of chronic bronchitis. *Eur Respir J* 1999;**14**:160–5.

48. de Godoy I, Donahoe M, Calhoun WJ, Mancino J, Rogers RM. Elevated TNF-alpha production by peripheral blood monocytes of weight-losing COPD patients. *Am J Respir Crit Care Med* 1996;**153**:633–7.

49. Hoshi H, Ohno I, Honma M, *et al.* IL-5, IL-8 and GM-CSF immunostaining of sputum cells in bronchial asthma and chronic bronchitis. *Clin Exp Allergy* 1995;**25**:720–8.

50. Vignola AM, Chanez P, Chiappara G, *et al.* Transforming growth factor-beta expression in mucosal biopsies in asthma and chronic bronchitis. *Am J Respir Crit Care Med* 1997;**156**:591–9.

51. Takeyama K, Dabbagh K, Lee HM, *et al.* Epidermal growth factor system regulates mucin production in airways. *Proc Natl Acad Sci USA* 1999;**96**:3081–6.

52. Chalmers GW, Macleod KJ, Sriram S, *et al.* Sputum endothelin-1 is increased in cystic fibrosis and chronic obstructive pulmonary disease. *Eur Respir J* 1999;**13**:1288–92.

53. Fujii T, Otsuka T, Tanaka S, *et al.* Plasma endothelin-1 level in chronic obstructive pulmonary disease: relationship with natriuretic peptide. *Respiration* 1999;**66**:212–19.

54. Giaid A, Yanagisawa M, Langleben D, *et al.* Expression of endothelin in the lungs of patients with pulmonary hypertension. *New Engl J Med* 1993;**328**:1732–9.

55. Tomaki M, Ichinose M, Miura M, *et al.* Elevated substance P content in induced sputum from patients with asthma and patients with chronic bronchitis. *Am J Respir Crit Care Med* 1995;**151**:613–17.

56. Chanez P, Springall D, Vignola AM, *et al.* Bronchial mucosal immunoreactivity of sensory neuropeptides in severe airway diseases. *Am J Respir Crit Care Med* 1998;**158**:985–90.

57. Lucchini RE, Facchini F, Turato G, *et al.* Increased VIP-positive nerve fibers in the mucous glands of subjects with chronic bronchitis. *Am J Respir Crit Care Med* 1997;**156**:1963–8.

58. Shapiro SD. Elastolytic metalloproteinases produced by human mononuclear phagocytes. Potential roles in destructive lung disease. *Am J Respir Crit Care Med* 1994;**150**:S160–4.

59. Finlay GA, Russell KJ, McMahon KJ, *et al.* Elevated levels of matrix metalloproteinases in bronchoalveolar lavage fluid of emphysematous patients. *Thorax* 1997;**52**:502–6.

60. Culpitt SV, Nightingale JA, Barnes PJ. Effect of high dose inhaled steroid on cells, cytokines and proteases in induced sputum in chronic obstructive pulmonary disease. *Am J Respir Crit Care Med* 1999;**160**:1635–9.

61. Finlay GA, O'Driscoll LR, Russell KJ, *et al.* Matrix metalloproteinase expression and production by alveolar macrophages in emphysema. *Am J Respir Crit Care Med* 1997;**156**:240–7.

62. Hautamaki RD, Kobayashi DK, Senior RM, Shapiro SD. Requirement for macrophage metalloelastase for cigarette smoke-induced emphysema in mice. *Science* 1997;**277**:2002–4.

63. Ohnishi K, Takagi M, Kurokawa Y, Satomi S, Konttinen YT. Matrix metalloproteinase-mediated extracellular matrix protein degradation in human pulmonary emphysema. *Lab Invest* 1998;**78**:1077–87.

64. Vignola AM, Riccobono L, Mirabella A, *et al.* Sputum metalloproteinase-9/tissue inhibitor of metalloproteinase-1 ratio correlates with airflow obstruction in asthma and chronic bronchitis. *Am J Respir Crit Care Med* 1998;**158**:1945–50.

65. Barnes PJ. Inhaled corticosteroids are not helpful in chronic obstructive pulmonary disease. *Am J Respir Crit Care Med* 2000;**161**:342–4.

66. Keatings VM, Jatakanon A, Worsdell YM, Barnes PJ. Effects of inhaled and oral glucocorticoids on inflammatory indices in asthma and COPD. *Am J Respir Crit Care Med* 1997;**155**:542–8.

67. Confalonieri M, Mainardi E, Della Porta R, *et al.* Inhaled corticosteroids reduce neutrophilic bronchial inflammation in patients with chronic obstructive pulmonary disease. *Thorax* 1998;**53**:583–5.

68. Pizzichini E, Pizzichini MM, Gibson P, *et al.* Sputum eosinophilia predicts benefit from prednisone in smokers with chronic obstructive bronchitis. *Am J Respir Crit Care Med* 1998;**158**:1511–17.

69. Papi A, Romagnoli M, Baraldo S, *et al.* Partial reversibility of airflow limitation and increased exhaled NO and sputum eosinophilia in chronic obstructive pulmonary disease. *Am J Respir Crit Care Med* 2000;**162**:1773–7.

70. Hattotuwa K, Ansari T, Gizycki M, Barnes N, Jeffery PK. A double-blind placebo-controlled trial of the effect of inhaled corticosteroids on the immunopathology of COPD. *Am J Respir Crit Care Med* 1999;**159**:A523.

71. Nightingale JA, Rogers DF, Chung KF, Barnes PJ. No effect of inhaled budesonide on the response to inhaled ozone in normal subjects. *Am J Respir Crit Care Med* 2000;**161**:479–86.

72. Pedersen B, Dahl R, Karlstrom R, Peterson CG, Venge P. Eosinophil and neutrophil activity in asthma in a one-year trial with inhaled budesonide. The impact of smoking. *Am J Respir Crit Care Med* 1996;**153**:1519–29.

73. Ito K, Lim S, Caramori G, Chung KF, Barnes PJ, Adcock IM. Cigarette smoking reduces histone deacetylase 2 expression, enhances cytokine expression and inhibits glucocorticoid actions in alveolar macrophages. *FASEB J* 2001;**15**:1100–2.

74. Barnes PJ. Effect of beta agonists on inflammatory cells. *J Allergy Clin Immunol* 1999;**104**:10–17.

75. Culpitt S, Maziak W, Loukides S, Keller A, Barnes PJ. Effect of theophylline on induced sputum inflammatory indices in COPD patients. *Am J Respir Crit Care Med* 1997;**157**:A797.

76. Torphy TJ, Barnette MS, Underwood DC, *et al.* Ariflo (SB 207499), a second generation phosphodiesterase 4 inhibitor for the treatment of asthma and COPD: from concept to clinic. *Pulm Pharmacol Ther* 1999;**12**:131–6.

12

Repair

STEPHEN I RENNARD

INTRODUCTION

Injury followed by repair is common to many lung diseases. In some conditions such as the adult respiratory distress syndrome, lung injury is acute and massive, and both the injury and the exuberant repair response which follows can compromise lung function. In pulmonary emphysema, chronic low-grade tissue injury exceeds the capacity of the lung for repair, and net tissue destruction results. In chronic bronchitis, current concepts suggest that injury of the airways followed by attempts at repair leads to a number of consequences. These include metaplasia of the airway epithelium with alterations in mucus production and mucociliary clearance as well as development of fibrosis in the airway wall. Contraction of these fibrotic scars results in airway narrowing which can compromise airflow. COPD, therefore, is characterized both by inadequate repair in emphysema and excessive or disordered repair in bronchitis. This chapter will review current understanding of repair processes in the lung, particularly as they apply to COPD.

AIRWAYS

Repair following mechanical wounding

In an elegant series of studies subsequently confirmed and extended by several investigators,[1–4] Wilhelm demonstrated, in the 1950s, that mechanical injury of the rat trachea is followed by an orderly sequence of repair events[5]

(Figure 12.1). Following denudation of the trachea by a mechanical probe, epithelial cells migrate onto the wound surface. These cells acquire a markedly flattened shape and form junctions, thus re-establishing a thin, but intact, epithelial barrier. Within 24 hours, the wounded area becomes filled with proliferating epithelial cells. These cells are rounded, stratified and do not resemble any of the cells normally present in the airway epithelium. The wave of epithelial cell proliferation stops over the next several days, although there is the accumulation of mesenchymal cells beneath the wounded area. These mesenchymal cells also undergo a burst of proliferation which is maximal at about 72 hours, a time when epithelial cell proliferation has largely ceased[2,6] (Figure 12.2). The accumulated epithelial cells acquire a columnar shape and re-establish a pseudo-stratified epithelium over the next several weeks. Eventually a normal ciliated epithelium with a relatively normal distribution of cell types results. Accumulated mesenchymal cells are eventually lost, and normal airway architecture can be re-established. It is likely that these processes are also accompanied by the formation and resorption of vascular structures in the injured airway, although vascular events are less well studied.

The initial events in the repair process appear to occur within minutes. The first event may be leakage of plasma proteins onto the airway surface.[7] Polymerization of fibrinogen with incorporation of fibronectin into an insoluble gel can establish a provisional matrix which may be crucial in supporting repair events. Within 15 minutes of wounding, epithelial cells at the edge of the wound have detached from their neighbors and can be observed streaming across the wounded surface.[6] The molecular

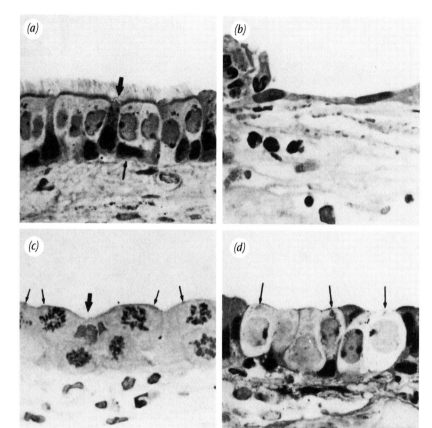

Figure 12.1 *(a) Normal hamster airway epithelium. (b) Twelve hours post-injury: flattened epithelial cells migrated into the wound and completely cover the wounded area restoring epithelial integrity. (c) Twenty-four hours post-injury. All cells present within the wound are undergoing mitosis. Note that the cells are stratified and their morphology does not correspond to any cell present in the normal epithelium. (d) Seventy-two hours post-injury. Cells are assuming a columnar shape and beginning to differentiate into recognizable airway epithelial cells. See text for details. (From ref. 2.)*

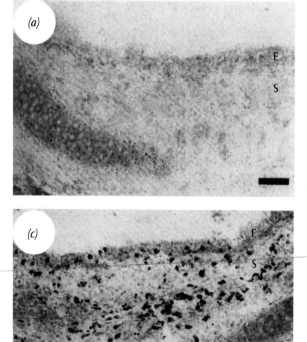

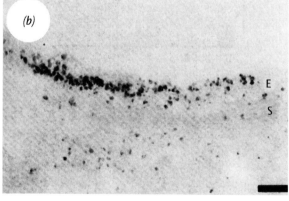

Figure 12.2 *Autoradiography demonstrating cellular proliferation in injured rat airway epithelium. (a) Normal epithelium. Note that neither the epithelium (E) nor the subepithelial tissues (S) take up the label indicating no proliferative activity. (b) Thirty hours post-injury. Note the marked stimulation of proliferation in the epithelial cells in the wounded area. (c) Seventy hours post-injury. Note that the epithelial cell proliferation is diminishing while there is increasing proliferation in the subepithelial tissue. See text for details. (Reproduced from ref. 6 with permission.)*

events which lead to detachment of cells from their neighbors and which lead to reattachment of cells to each other in order to re-establish the epithelial barrier remain undetermined.

It is unclear which cells serve as a source for the migrating cells in the early repair events. When assessed 12 hours after wounding, migrating cells were noted to express cytokeratin 14.[3] This cytoskeletal protein is characteristically present in basal cells but not in other cells of the airway epithelium. While this suggests that basal cells may be the source of migrating cells in the wound, it is possible that the migrating cells could represent de-differentiated columnar cells which have induced the expression of cytokeratin 14. Expression of other genes is induced in epithelial cells participating in the repair response (see below). Columnar cells as a source of cells for early repair is appealing for several reasons, as these cells are present at all levels in the airway, in contrast to basal cells which are relatively common in the proximal airways but increasingly rare to absent in the more distal airways.[8,9] A progenitor cell population located in gland ducts also may play a role in repair (see below), but is unlikely to account for the cells initially recruited to cover a wound.[10] The cell source for migrating cells during repair, therefore, remains unestablished.

Cytokeratin 14 expression persists in cells proliferating in the wounded airway.[3] Expression is also noted as the epithelial cells differentiate into columnar cells, although it is eventually lost over the next few weeks when the cells become fully differentiated expressing cilia and mucins. By contrast, cytokeratin 18, a cytokeratin characteristically expressed in columnar cells in the airway but absent from basal cells, is lacking in the epithelial cells present early within a wound, becoming expressed only as the cells differentiate. Whether these events represent a process of de-differentiation of columnar cells followed by re-differentiation or whether they represent recruitment and transdifferentiation of basal cells or, alternatively, recruitment and initiation of a repair response from other cells present within the airway epithelium, it is clear that an orderly sequence of molecular events characterizes the repair response in the airway. Disruption of this process could result in anatomic abnormalities and functional derangment (Figure 12.3).

Molecular mediators of repair

While the molecular events which regulate the repair process remain to be fully defined, a number of *in vitro*

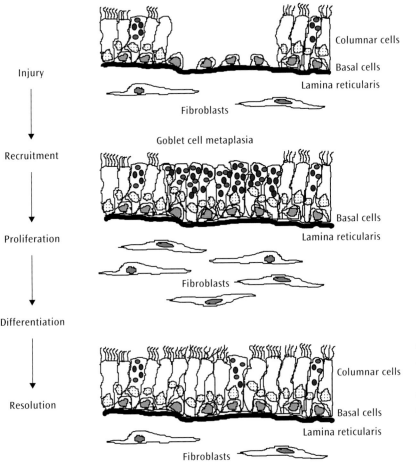

Injury

Recruitment

Proliferation

Differentiation

Resolution

Columnar cells
Basal cells
Lamina reticularis
Fibroblasts

Goblet cell metaplasia
Basal cells
Lamina reticularis
Fibroblasts

Columnar cells
Basal cells
Lamina reticularis
Fibroblasts

Figure 12.3 *Tissue alterations consequent to repair following injury. Injury is followed by cellular recruitment, proliferation, differentiation and resolution. Either excessive accumulation of cells and matrix or failure of resolution could result in formation of scar tissue with the potential for loss of function.*

and *in vivo* studies suggest candidate mediators. In this regard, epithelial cell migration has been evaluated in several *in vitro* systems. Shoji and colleagues[11] demonstrated that bovine bronchial epithelial cells can migrate in response to chemotactic stimuli using the blindwell Boyden chamber technique in which cells migrate through holes in a membrane. Insulin-like growth factor 1 (IGF-1),[11] fibronectin[12] and fragments of extracellular matrix[13] were capable of driving epithelial cell chemotaxis.

Several investigators have utilized an *in vitro* 'wound repair' technique in which cells are removed from a small area of a culture dish, and the ability of cells to migrate into and fill the resulting defect can be assessed.[14,15] Using this method, Zahm *et al.*[14] and Kim *et al.*[16] have demonstrated that endothelial growth factor (EGF) can augment epithelial-cell mediated 'wound closure'. The EGF receptor is upregulated in the injured epithelium in asthma and inhibition of EGF receptor signaling blocks wound closure *in vitro* by a human airway epithelial cell line.[17] Interestingly, there is an associated increase in transforming growth factor beta (TGF-β) production (see below). Taken together, these data suggest a key role for EGF in augmenting epithelial repair. Other mediators may play similar roles. Tumor necrosis factor alpha (TNF-α),[18] hepatocyte growth factor (HGF),[19] keratinocyte growth factor (KGF)[20] and prostaglandin E (PGE)[21] have all been demonstrated to accelerate epithelial cell migration in similar assay systems.

Production and release of factors which can drive epithelial cell recruitment is likely to be increased at sites of injury. IGF-1 is a growth factor released by a number of cell types including inflammatory cells recruited into an injured area.[22] Fibronectin is a multifunctional glycoprotein also produced by many cell types within the airway.[23,24] Its production by both epithelial cells[25,26] and fibroblasts[27] is greatly augmented by TGF-β, a cytokine thought to play a key role in regulating repair responses. It is unlikely, however, that production of fibronectin or polypeptide growth factors could account for the initial chemotaxis of epithelial cells which develops in minutes, particularly if inflammatory cell recruitment and/or induction of new gene expression is required.

Matrix and proteases

The matrix over which epithelial cells migrate probably also plays an important role in epithelial repair. In this regard, epithelial cells have been noted to migrate more rapidly over surfaces composed of interstitial collagens rather than basement membrane collagen.[28] Proteolytic cleavage of extracellular matrix, moreover, has the potential to expose novel binding sites for cell surface integrins.[29] Interestingly, epithelial cells can also migrate more rapidly across protease-treated extracellular matrix.[28] Matrilysin

(MMP-7) may be particularly important in this regard. It is expressed in normal airway epithelium, and expression increases in cells mediating repair in an *in vitro* model.[30] Inhibition of MMPs inhibits epithelial repair in explants of human tracheas *in vitro*. While several MMPs are expressed by epithelial cells in skin wounds including MMP-1, MMP-3, MMP-9 and MMP-10, MMP-7 was the only MMP among those tested that was prominent in human airway epithelial cells. Similarly, the MMP-7 knockout mouse has markedly deficient epithelial repair, further supporting the role of MMP-7 in epithelial repair in the airway.

Increased expression of MMP-3[31] as well as MMP-9 and MMP-2,[32] however, has also been noted in other *in vitro* models of airway epithelial injury. The expression of these MMPs appears to correlate with migration ability.[33] Moreover, exogenous MMP-9 increases migration while, in contrast, exogenous MMP-2 inhibits migration.[34] Induction of uPA (urine type plasminogen activator) has been noted at the leading edge of a wound.[35] As uPA can activate MMP-9 and blocking uPA activity decreases migration, interactions among these proteases seems likely. Taken together, the available data suggest that proteases are likely to play a crucial role in airway epithelial repair, particularly with regard to migration. It seems likely that the proteases involved will be multiple, may vary with the nature of the injury, the stage of repair and, possibly, with species. Regulation of protease expression in airway epithelial cells, therefore, is likely to be a key feature of repair. Conversely, abnormal regulation of proteases may be a key feature in pathologic processes. Increased expression of MMPs, for example, has been associated with malignant transformation and the acquisition of metastatic potential.[36]

Proteolytic generation of chemotactic factors for airway epithelial cells is an appealing mechanism for their rapid generation. Other mechanisms are also possible. Formation of eicosinoids and release of pre-formed mediators are mechanisms which could, in part, account for rapid increases in epithelial cell movement.[21] Peptides derived from nerves and from neuroendocrine cells can increase epithelial cell migration *in vitro*.[37] Depletion of neuropeptides can slow the initial phase but not the eventual repair, suggesting a role for neuropeptides in early repair events.[38] Serum is also a potent chemotactic stimulus, although the responsible moieties are not fully established.[12] Nevertheless, it is possible that the leakage of plasma and generation of a provisional matrix[7] also generates chemotactic factors which contribute to epithelial cell recruitment.

Wound closure

Early after wounding in the rat trachea, the migrating cells can be observed as individual cells streaming away from the wounded edge.[6] This contrasts with the pattern of migration observed in many of the *in vitro* 'wound closure' assays noted above. In those assay systems, the epithelial cells commonly migrate as a 'sheet' in which cells at the leading edge are attached both to each other and to their neighbors.[14,18] Interestingly, the cytokine HGF, sometimes termed 'scatter factor', can induce epithelial cell detachment from their neighbors and migration as individual cells,[39] and it can increase the rate of closure of 'wounds' *in vitro*.[19] As noted below, HGF can have important effects in alveolar repair following bleomycin injury. Whether it plays a role in airway repair following mechanical injury or in COPD, however, remains to be established.

The receptors through which migrating epithelial cells interact with extracellular matrix are also not yet established. In cultured airway epithelial cells *in vitro*, antibodies to $\alpha2$, $\alpha3$ and $\alpha6$ integrins blocked wound closure on type IV collagen but not on laminin while antibodies to $\beta1$ integrin blocked closure on all surfaces tested.[40] This suggests several integrins interacting with multiple substrates may play roles. Following wounding, epithelial cells at the edge of a mechanical wound have been reported to express $\alpha5$, αV, $\beta5$ and $\beta6$ integrins, integrins not highly expressed in the normal epithelium.[41] Using the *in vitro* cultured epithelial cell system, in contrast, Herard reported increased epithelial cell expression of $\alpha_5 \beta_1$ integrin and fibronectin, but no change in the expression of αV, $\alpha2$ or $\alpha3$ integrin.[42] Experimental differences including culture conditions, the nature of the wound and the species may account for these differences in induced integrin expression. It is clear, however, that airway epithelial cells are capable of expressing several integrins and that the expression of integrins can be modulated in the face of injury. It is likely, therefore, that migrating cells can interact with matrix using a different repertoire of receptors than do cells in the normal airway. Interestingly, αV$\beta6$ integrin is also able to activate TGF-β by inducing a confirmational change in the latent TGF-β molecule.[43] This suggests additional functions for integrins induced in epithelial cells during the repair response.

Undoubtedly the marked phenotypic changes observed in epithelial cells participating in the wound repair response is accompanied by changes in the expression of many genes and gene products. The full spectrum of such changes remains to be established. In addition to induction of integrins and expression of proteases, alterations in cell surface expression of isoforms of CD44 have been described which play a role in regulating the process of migration.[44] Alterations in cell surface receptor expression likely changes the susceptibility of the repairing epithelium to pathogens. Bacteria, for example, may adhere to epithelial cells through fibronectin, and the increased fibronectin receptor expression on airway epithelial cells may lead to increased bacterial adherence and airway colonization.[45] Similarly, cytokines present in the repairing milieu may increase epithelia cell expression of intercellular adhesion molecule 1 (ICAM-1).[46] By serving as an adhesion receptor for inflammatory cells, this could increase the susceptibility of the airway epithelium to collateral damage during an inflammatory response.[47]

Proliferation and differentiation

Recruitment of epithelial cells is followed by their subsequent proliferation and re-differentiation. The factors which regulate epithelial cell proliferation and differentiation during repair are also not established. Fibroblasts,[48] epithelial cells[49–51] and mononuclear phagocytes[52] are all potential sources of epithelial cell growth factors, and a number of potential epithelial cell growth factors have been identified.[49,53] Some factors including IGF-1,[54] EGF,[50] HGF[51] and fibronectin[55] which can stimulate epithelial cell recruitment can also serve as epithelial cell growth promoters. Which factors induce the wave of epithelial cell proliferation following mechanical injury, however, is undefined. Similarly, the role of specific factors in the airway in bronchitis is also undefined. Importantly, the mechanisms which terminate the 'wave' of proliferation and induce subsequent differentiation are also undefined.

In cultures *in vitro*, epithelial cells maintained on the surface of a filter in growth supporting medium will proliferate and form a layer of cells several cells thick.[56] Proliferation, however, will spontaneously stop even in the continuous presence of a growth stimulatory medium. If such cultures are transferred to an air–liquid interface, differentiation will 'spontaneously' take place with the formation of both ciliated cells and mucin-expressing cells resembling goblet cells. The signals induced by the air–liquid interface culture technique remain to be defined. It seems likely, however, at least in this culture system, that the epithelial cells themselves can produce the mediators which regulate proliferation and can undergo complex differentiation of several cell types without an external source of mediators.

Differentiation, however, is also probably regulatable by external mediators. EGF, for example, is a potent inducer of mucin gene expression.[57,58] The EGF receptor, moreover, may be activated not only by exogenous factors, but also by non-ligand-mediated mechanisms.[59] Importantly, inflammatory cells can induce EGF-receptor activation and lead to mucin gene expression by an oxidant-dependent process.[60] It is likely, therefore, that the inflammatory response present in the airways in COPD can modify repair responses by altering differentiation signals.

ALVEOLAR EPITHELIAL REPAIR

It is probable that processes analogous to those described in the airways are involved in alveolar epithelial repair.

While the alveoli are not accessible for mechanical injury, chemical toxins, particularly bleomycin, have been used to induce diffuse alveolar damage after which repair processes can be assessed. In addition, *in vitro* culture systems have also been used to assess alveolar type 2-like cells; in particular the A549 alveolar carcinoma-derived cell line has been used extensively. As with airway cells, HGF and KGF have been suggested to promote epithelial cell recruitment and proliferation following injury.[61,62] HGF can also induce the expression of uPA.[63] Interestingly, HGF can reduce the severity of fibrosis as indicated by collagen deposition following bleomycin injury,[63] and KGF can reduce the severity of allogeneic injury in a bone marrow model[64] consistent with the concept that these mediators promote re-epithelialization and inhibit fibrotic scarring. Moreover, both mediators are present after bleomycin injury.[65] In addition, other cytokines probably contribute. IL-1, for example, increases alveolar cell migration perhaps by stimulating TNF-α and EGF.[66]

Vasculature

The pulmonary capillary bed is also injured in processes which damage alveoli. Loss of pulmonary capillary bed is a defining feature of emphysema, and inadequate maintenance of the pulmonary vascular bed has been suggested to be a primary cause of emphysema.[67] Vascular endothelial growth factor (VEGF) is believed to play an important role in the development of pulmonary vessels and in the regulation of pulmonary vessels in the lung both during normal physiology and following injury. It has been suggested, however, that different VEGF splice variants are expressed during normal events and following repair,[68] perhaps providing one mechanism for incomplete restoration of normal architecture following some injuries. The role of VEGF in maintaining vascular integrity within alveolar structures has led to the suggestion that VEGF deficiency can lead to emphysema. Consistent with this, blockade of VEGF signaling can induce endothelial cell apoptosis and the formation of emphysema in rats.[69] In human lungs, increased apoptosis of endothelial cells as well as epithelial cells and decreased expression of VEGF has been assessed histologically.[70]

Mesenchymal cells

In addition to epithelial cells and endothelial cells, the mesenchymal cells also are recruited and activated during repair following injury. As noted above, mechanical injury of the airway is associated with accumulation of mesenchymal cells beneath the injured area in a wave of recruitment and proliferation which follows by a few days that of the epithelial cells.[6] Many of the same mediators

which drive epithelial cell recruitment and proliferation such as TGF-β, fibronectin and EGF are also potent stimuli for fibroblast recruitment and proliferation. In addition, interactions between epithelial cells and fibroblasts are essential for normal lung morphogenesis.[71] It seems likely that many of the interactions which regulate development are, to some extent, recapitulated during repair following injury.[72] In this regard, the epithelial cells of the lung are sources of several potential fibroblast growth factors including fibronectin,[73] IGF-1,[74] endothelin[75] and PDGF.[76] Epithelial cell production of TGF-β[77] may be particularly important in regulating mesenchymal cell activity. Conversely, fibroblasts, as noted above, are a potent source of epithelial cell growth factors.[48] Other structural cells present in the airway, including chondrocytes,[78] are also potentially important sources of mediators which can regulate the repair response. Whether attempts at repair result in restoration of normal structure or in dysfunctional fibrotic scar probably depends on the balance between epithelial and mesenchymal cell stimulation.

While the role that mesenchymal cells play in normal repair remains to be established, it is clear that overabundant recruitment of mesenchymal cells can result in fibrosis. The development of peribronchiolar fibrosis together with the contraction that characterizes fibrotic tissues is likely to account for airway narrowing and airflow limitation in many patients with COPD.[79] Fibrosis of alveolar structures results in severe physiologic compromise in interstitial lung diseases.[80] A similar process can result from massive alveolar injury in the acute respiratory distress syndrome.[81] It is likely that pulmonary emphysema is also characterized by increased activation of mesenchymal cells as, at least in the early stages, increased total lung collagen content[82,83] and focal areas of increased deposition of collagen[84] are characteristically present within the alveolar structures.

Repair in emphysema

Experimental evidence also supports a role for repair in emphysema (Figure 12.4). Infusion of elastase intertracheally results in the development of emphysema in animals.[85] Associated with this is a marked acute decrease in lung elastin content. This is followed, however, by an increase in elastin and collagen synthesis such that elastin concentrations are returned to normal over several weeks. Inhibition of elastin synthesis with agents which block elastin crosslinking exacerbates the development of emphysema.[85] Cigarette smoke (see also below) can also impair elastin crosslinking and also exacerbates elastase-induced emphysema.[86]

Elegant studies by Shapiro *et al.* have suggested that elastin in the normal adult human lung turns over very little throughout an individual's lifetime.[87] This does not

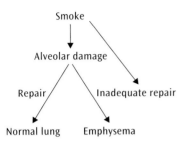

Figure 12.4 *Diagram of the events in the development of emphysema. Injury of the alveolar wall results from cigarette smoke or other insult. This leads to damage of the airway wall. If repair mechanisms are effective, normal architecture can be restored. If these mechanisms are ineffective, alveolar defects can develop. Over time, these may progress to emphysema. Smoke can not only cause alveolar damage, but can interfere with alveolar repair (see text for details).*

preclude, however, elastin turnover in individuals who have lung injury. The concept that elastin, once synthesized, cannot undergo repair remodeling, moreover, has come into question. *In vitro* studies suggest that elastic fibers can undergo repair.[88] Indeed, during lung growth remodeling of elastic fibers must take place. Increased urinary desmosines, while not specific for lung elastin, suggest increased elastin turnover in smokers and individuals with COPD.[89] Taken together, these data support the concept that lung connective tissue structures including both elastic fibers and collagen are participating in repair responses in COPD.

Emphysema was reported in the lungs of previously healthy individuals who were starved during the famine in the Warsaw ghetto during the second world war.[90] Starvation can also induce loss of lung elastic recoil in animal models and can greatly potentiate the development of elastase-induced emphysema in animals.[91,92] Intraperitoneal injection of TNF-α has also been associated with the development of emphysema-like changes.[93] These data support the concept that the catabolic state, perhaps by interfering with lung repair processes, can lead to the development of pulmonary emphysema.

The role for mesenchymal cells in 'normal repair' of alveolar structures has been suggested from studies of intra-alveolar pores. These structures were once suggested to be the anatomic correlates of collateral alveolar ventilation.[94] Such a function, however, has been suggested to be unlikely as the pores are usually too small to be covered with surfactant and, not likely to be functional as transfer structures.[95,96] Rather, alveolar pores are likely to represent small defects in alveolar walls.[97–99] Their repair would presumably require new connective tissue synthesis and remodeling including contraction around the edges of the pore. Increases in intra-alveolar pore

number and size characterize senile emphysema in animals[95] and human emphysema[100] as well as the emphysema which occurs in cigarette smokers.[99] While the mechanisms and mediators which may serve to effectively repair alveolar pores remain unknown, it is likely that the mesenchymal cells of the alveolar wall play an important role.

Fibrosis

The mediators responsible for determining whether fibroblast recruitment and activation leads to permanent fibrosis or restitution of normal airway architecture, remains to be determined. A number of mediators, however, have been described which can modify mesenchymal cells during repair. TGF-β in particular is believed to have a particularly important role. This cytokine is a potent inducer of fibroblast matrix production,[101] can stimulate fibroblast proliferation and differentiation into myofibroblasts[102] (cells more commonly present in fibrotic lesions), and can drive fibroblast contraction of extracellular matrices,[103] potentially leading to the contraction which results in tissue distortion and physiological derangement. TGF-β is present in the airway in increased amounts in asthma and in COPD,[104] as well as in the alveolar structures following bleomycin injury.[105] Inhibition of TGF-β activity can inhibit fibrosis in model systems.[106]

Cytokines

It is likely that other cytokines can play similar roles. PDGF, for example, has been suggested to play an important role in the development of intra-alveolar fibrosis.[107] PDGF is also present in the airways, although levels in asthma have been reported to be no different from normals.[108] Cytokines probably present in the airway in asthma and COPD; however, they can modulate fibroblast activities. IL-4, for example, can stimulate TGF-β production by airway epithelial cells[109] and can also stimulate fibroblast chemotaxis,[110] collagen synthesis[111] and contraction of extracellular matrices.[112] IL-4, therefore, could contribute to mesenchymal cell activity during repair and fibrosis. IL-1 and TNF-α can also directly affect fibroblasts. Both are capable of inducing PGE and NO production in human fibroblasts[113] and of inducing the production of several matrix metalloproteases. NO and PGE can function to inhibit fibroblast chemotaxis,[114] proliferation,[115] apoptosis[116] and matrix production[117] and tissue reorganization.[113] The MMPs induced by IL-1 and TNF-α, while released in latent form, can be activated and can lead to degradation of extracellular matrix.[118] IL-1 and TNF-α, therefore, while capable of inducing an inflammatory response, may also serve to limit the severity of subsequent fibroblast-mediated fibrosis.

IMPLICATIONS OF ALTERED REPAIR IN PATHOGENESIS AND TREATMENT OF COPD

Pathogenesis

Inflammatory cells are potent sources of mediators which can contribute to the regulation of repair responses. Many of the mediators discussed above which are capable of stimulating epithelial or mesenchymal cell participation in repair responses can be produced by inflammatory cells. It is likely, therefore, that the nature of the inflammatory process in an injured tissue can have major effects on the character of the repair response. COPD is characterized by chronic inflammatory process in both the airways and the alveolar structures of the lung.[119] Superimposed on this are probable episodes of acute inflammation associated with exacerbations.[120] It seems likely, therefore, that the mediators released by these inflammatory cells will contribute to the altered repair which characterizes COPD.

Several additional mechanisms could contribute to altered repair in chronic obstructive pulmonary disease. First, cigarette smoking is the most important risk factor for the development of COPD,[121] and cigarette smoke can affect repair processes in multiple ways. Cigarette smoke, for example, can directly inhibit epithelial cell migration and attachment as assessed in assays in vitro.[122] Smoke, moreover, can result in a markedly impaired repair response following naphthalene-induced injury in mice.[123] These effects of smoke, therefore, may lead to incomplete re-epithelialization following injury and, hence, could lead to abnormal restoration of tissue structure. Interestingly, viral infections may have similar effects.[124] This suggests there may be multiple mechanisms for altered epithelial repair in individuals with COPD.

Smoke can also have adverse effects on mesenchymal cell participation in repair. It can directly inhibit fibroblast chemotaxis and proliferation.[125] Smoke, moreover, inhibits fibroblast contraction of three-dimensional collagen gels, an effect mediated through the inhibition of fibronectin production.[126] Cigarette smoke can also inhibit lysyloxidase,[127] an enzyme essential in the formation of elastin and collagen crosslinks. Through such an effect, elastin re-synthesis can be inhibited by cigarette smoke. Any of these mechanisms could contribute to the development of emphysema in smoke-exposed animals and to smoke potentiation of elastase damage.[86] Inhibition of repair could, therefore, represent an additional mechanism by which cigarette smoking can lead to the development of emphysema. Interestingly, cadmium can also impair mesenchymal repair responses, perhaps accounting, in part, for cadmium-induced emphysema.[128]

TREATMENT

The possibility that altered repair contributes to the pathogenesis of COPD raises the possibility of new therapeutic strategies. Peribronchiolar fibrosis and associated airway narrowing appears to be a major contributor to fixed airflow limitation in chronic bronchitis.[129] Inhibition of this process has the potential to alter the relentlessly progressive loss of function which characterizes COPD. Several approaches show promise in this regard. A number of agents have been suggested which can block the release of pro-fibrotic mediators. Alternatively, agents which directly inhibit pro-fibrotic responses may be of benefit. In this regard, elevation of cyclic AMP inhibits many pro-fibrotic responses including chemotaxis proliferation,[115] matrix production[130] and matrix remodeling.[131] Prostaglandin E, in particular, appears to be an important endogenous regulator of fibroblast activity in systems in vitro. PGE, moreover, appears to augment epithelial repair processes.[21] PGE, or agents which act through similar mechanistic pathways, therefore, has the potential to augment epithelial repair while inhibiting fibrotic responses. While PGE can act through several mechanisms, many of its effects appear to depend on increasing intracellular levels of cyclic AMP. Pharmacologic manipulation of cyclic AMP levels can be achieved with the use of alternative agonists which activate adenyl cyclase or by inhibitors of the phosphodiesterases responsible for grading cyclic AMP.[132] Finally, it may be possible to reverse the accumulation of fibrotic lesions. It is likely that fibrotic tissue which accumulates in a wound can undergo resorption, and the cells undergo apoptosis similar to that which occurs in the resolution of granulation tissue.[133] The concept that fibrosis, in some circumstances, results from failed apoptosis has been suggested.[134] In this context, agents which stimulate fibroblast apoptosis have been suggested as potential therapeutic strategies.[135] Whether such agents would be applicable to the peribronchiolar fibrosis in COPD remains to be determined.

Stimulation of normal repair with the generation of new alveolar structures is a particularly exciting possibility for the treatment of emphysema. In this regard, retinoic acid appears to play a crucial role in the process of alveolar septation. Alveolar fibroblasts contain high concentrations of retinoids and alveolar epithelial cells express high levels of retinoic acid receptors in animals undergoing alveolarization. Exogenous retinoic acid can augment formation of alveoli in the neonatal rat.[136] In adult animals following elastase-induced emphysema, Massaro and Massaro demonstrated that retinoic acid can induce the formation of new alveolar wall.[137] Whether such effects can be observed in human emphysema is currently the subject of intense basic and clinical investigation. That alveolar repair can be induced in the adult mammal, however, seems likely. The development of a practical means for regenerating functional alveolar tissues in human emphysema would, obviously, represent a huge therapeutic advance.

SUMMARY

COPD has long been recognized as a chronic inflammatory disorder in which the airways and the alveolar structures of the lung are damaged. Both exogenous agents such as cigarette smoke and endogenously released mediators such as those derived from inflammatory cells contribute to this damage. It is also clear that the lung has considerable capacity to repair in the face of damage. The anatomic lesions which develop in COPD and which eventually result in physiologic compromise and in patient symptoms depend on a balance between tissue injury and repair. While the current understanding of repair processes is limited, it is likely that normal repair processes are not only initiated but also altered in COPD. Understanding the nature of normal repair in the lung, and specifically understanding the nature of altered repair in COPD, should create new opportunities for therapeutic intervention to alter the usually relentlessly progressive decline in lung function which characterizes COPD.

REFERENCES

1. Lane BP, Gordon R. Regeneration of rat tracheal epithelium after mechanical injury. *Exp Biol Med* 1974;**145**:1139–44.
2. Keenan KP, Combs JW, McDowell EM. Regeneration of hamster tracheal epithelium after mechanical injury. *Virchows Arch* 1982;**41**:193–214.
3. Shimizu T, Nishihara M, Kawaguchi S, Sakakura Y. Expression of phenotypic markers during regeneration of rat tracheal epithelium following mechanical injury. *Am J Respir Cell Mol Biol* 1994;**11**:85–94.
4. Erjefalt JS, Persson CG. Airway epithelial repair: breathtakingly quick and multipotentially pathogenic. *Thorax* 1997;**52**:1010–12.
5. Wilhelm DL. Regeneration of tracheal epithelium. *J Pathol Bacteriol* 1953;**55**:543–50.
6. Erjefalt JS, Erjefalt I, Sundler F, Persson GA. *In vivo* restitution of airway epithelium. *Cell Tissue Res* 1995;**281**:305–16.
7. Erjefalt JS, Erjefalt I, Sundler F, Persson CGA. Microcirculation-derived factors in airway epithelial repair in vivo. *Microvasc Res* 1994;**48**:161–78.
8. Breeze RG, Wheeldon EB. The cells of the pulmonary airways. *Am Rev Respir Dis* 1977;**116**:705–20.
9. Plopper CG, Mariassy AT, Wilson DW, Alley JL, Nishio SJ, Nettesheim P. Comparison of nonciliated tracheal epithelial cells in six mammalian species: ultrastructure and population densities. *Exp Lung Res* 1983;**5**:281–94.
10. Borthwick DW, Shahbazian M, Krantz QT, Dorin JR, Randell SH. Evidence for stem-cell niches in the tracheal epithelium. *Am J Respir Cell Mol Biol* 2001;**24**:662–70.
11. Shoji S, Ertl RF, Linder J, Koizumi S, Duckworth WC, Rennard SI. Bronchial epithelial cells respond to insulin and insulin-like growth factor-I as a chemoattractant. *Am J Respir Cell Mol Biol* 1990;**2**:553–7.
12. Shoji S, Ertl RF, Linder J, Romberger DJ, Rennard SI. Bronchial epithelial cells produce chemotactic activity for bronchial epithelial cells: possible role for fibronectin in airway repair. *Am Rev Respir Dis* 1990;**141**:218–25.
13. Rickard KA, Taylor J, Rennard SI, Spurzem JR. Migration of bovine bronchial epithelial cells to extracellular matrix components. *Am J Respir Cell Mol Biol* 1993;**8**:63–8.
14. Zahm JM, Chevillard M, Puchelle E. Wound repair of human surface respiratory epithelium. *Am J Respir Cell Mol Biol* 1991;**5**:242–8.
15. Herard AL, Zahm JM, Pierrot D, Hinnrasky J, Fuchey C, Puchelle E. Epithelial barrier integrity during *in vitro* wound repair of the airway epithelium. *Am J Respir Cell Mol Biol* 1996;**15**:624–32.
16. Kim JS, McKinnis VS, Nawrocki A, White SR. Stimulation of migration and wound repair of guinea-pig airway epithelial cells in response to epidermal growth factor. *Am J Respir Cell Mol Biol* 1998;**18**:66–74.
17. Puddicombe SM, Polosa R, Richter A, et al. Involvement of the epidermal growth factor receptor in epithelial repair in asthma. *FASEB J* 2000;**14**:1362–74.
18. Ito H, Rennard SI, Spurzem JR. Mononuclear cell conditioned medium enhances bronchial epithelial cell migration but inhibits attachment to fibronectin. *J Lab Clin Med* 1996;**127**:494–503.
19. Zahm JM, Debordeaux C, Raby B, Klossek JM, Bonnet N, Puchelle E. Motogenic effect of recombinant HGF on airway epithelial cells during the *in vitro* wound repair of the respiratory epithelium. *J Cell Physiol* 2000;**185**:447–53.
20. Waters CM, Savla U. Keratinocyte growth factor accelerates wound closure in airway epithelium during cyclic mechanical strain. *J Cell Physiol* 1999;**181**:424–32.
21. Savla U, Appel HJ, Sporn PH, Waters CM. Prostaglandin E^2 regulates wound closure in airway epithelium. *Am J Physiol: Lung Cell Mol Physiol* 2001;**280**:L421–31.
22. Rom WN, Paakko P. Activated alveolar macrophages express the insulin-like growth factor-I receptor. *Am J Respir Cell Mol Biol* 1991;**4**:432–9.
23. Miyamoto S, Katz BZ, Lafrenie RM, Yamada KM. Fibronectin and integrins in cell adhesion, signaling, and morphogenesis. *Ann NY Acad Sci* 1998;**857**:119–29.
24. Romberger DJ. Fibronectin. *Int J Biochem Cell Biol* 1997;**29**:939–43.
25. Romberger DJ, Beckmann JD, Claassen L, Ertl RF, Rennard SI. Modulation of fibronectin production of bovine bronchial epithelial cells by transforming growth factor-beta. *Am J Respir Cell Mol Biol* 1992;**7**:149–55.
26. Wang A, Cohen DS, Palmer E, Sheppard D. Polarized regulation of fibronectin secretion and alternative splicing by transforming growth factor. *J Biol Chem* 1991;**266**:15558–60.
27. Tegner H, Ohlsson K, Toremalm N, Von Mecklenburg C. Effect of human leucocyte enzymes on tracheal mucous and its mucociliary activity. *Rhinology* 1979;**17**:199–206.
28. Rickard KA, Taylor J, Spurzem JR, Rennard SI. Extracellular matrix and bronchial epithelial cell migration. *Chest* 1992;**101**:17S–18S.
29. Yokosaki Y, Matsuura N, Sasaki T, et al. The integrin alpha(9)beta(1) binds to a novel recognition sequence (SVVYGLR) in the thrombin-cleaved amino-terminal fragment of osteopontin. *J Biol Chem* 1999;**274**:36328–34.
30. Dunsmore SE, Saarialho-Kere UK, Roby JD, et al. Matrilysin expression and function in airway epithelium. *J Clin Invest* 1998;**102**:1321–31.
31. Buisson AC, Gilles C, Polette M, Zahm JM, Birembaut P, Tournier JM. Wound repair-induced expression of

a stromelysins is associated with the acquisition of a mesenchymal phenotype in human respiratory epithelial cells. *Lab Invest* 1996;**74**:658–69.

32. Lynch DA, Newell J, Hale V, *et al.* Correlation of CT findings with clinical evaluations in 261 patients with symptomatic bronchiectasis. *AJR* 1999;**173**:53–8.

33. Legrand C, Gilles C, Zahm JM, *et al.* Airway epithelial cell migration dynamics. MMP-9 role in cell-extracellular matrix remodeling. *J Cell Biol* 1999;**146**:517–29.

34. de Bentzmann S, Polette M, Zahm JM, *et al. Pseudomonas aeruginosa* virulence factors delay airway epithelial wound repair by altering the actin cytoskeleton and inducing overactivation of epithelial matrix metalloproteinase-2. *Lab Invest* 2000;**80**:209–19.

35. Legrand C, Polette M, Tournier JM, *et al.* uPA/plasmin system-mediated MMP-9 activation is implicated in bronchial epithelial cell migration. *Exp Cell Res* 2001;**264**:326–36.

36. Stamenkovic I. Matrix metalloproteinases in tumor invasion and metastasis. *Semin Cancer Biol* 2000;**10**:415–33.

37. Kim JS, McKinnis VS, White SR. Migration of guinea pig airway epithelial cells in response to bombesin analogues. *Am J Respir Cell Mol Biol* 1997;**16**:259–66.

38. Kim JS, McKinnis VS, Adams K, White SR. Proliferation and repair of guinea pig tracheal epithelium after neuropeptide depletion and injury *in vivo. Am J Physiol* 1997;**273**(6 Pt 1): L1235–41.

39. Stoker M. Effect of scatter factor on motility of epithelial cells and fibroblasts. *J Cell Physiol* 1989;**139**:565–9.

40. White SR, Dorscheid DR, Rabe KF, Wojcik KR, Hamann KJ. Role of very late adhesion integrins in mediating repair of human airway epithelial cell monolayers after mechanical injury. *Am J Respir Cell Mol Biol* 1999;**20**:787–96.

41. Pilewski JM, Latoche JD, Arcasoy SM, Albelda SM. Expression of integrin cell adhesion receptors during human airway epithelial repair *in vivo. Am J Physiol* 1997;**273**:L256–63.

42. Herard AL, Pierrot D, Hinnrasky J, *et al.* Fibronectin and its alpha 5 beta 1-integrin receptor are involved in the wound-repair process of airway epithelium. *Am J Physiol* 1996; **21**:L726–33.

43. Munger JS, Huang X, Kawakatsu H, *et al.* The integrin alpha v beta 6 binds and activates latent TGF beta 1: a mechanism for regulating pulmonary inflammation and fibrosis. *Cell* 1999;**96**:319–28.

44. Leir SH, Baker JE, Holgate ST, Lackie PM. Increased CD44 expression in human bronchial epithelial repair after damage or plating at low cell densities. *Am J Physiol Lung Cell Mol Physiol* 2000;**278**:L1129–37.

45. de Bentzmann S, Roger P, Puchelle E. *Pseudomonas aeruginosa* adherence to remodelling respiratory epithelium. *Eur Respir J* 1996;**9**:2145–50.

46. Striz I, Mio T, Adachi Y, *et al.* IL-4 induces ICAM-1 expression in human bronchial epithelial cells and potentiates TNF-α. *Am J Physiol* 1999;**277**:L58–64.

47. DeRose V, Robbins RA, Snider RM, *et al.* Substance P increases neutrophil adhesion to bronchial epithelial cells. *J Immunol* 1994;**152**:1339–46.

48. Shoji S, Rickard KA, Takizawa H, Ertl RF, Linder J, Rennard SI. Lung fibroblasts produce growth stimulatory activity for bronchial epithelial cells. *Am Rev Respir Dis* 1990;**141**: 433–9.

49. Robbins RA, Rennard SI. Biology of airway epithelial cells. In: RG Crystal, JB West, ER Weibel, PJ Barnes, eds. *The Lung: Scientific Foundations*, vol 1, 2nd edn. Lippincott-Raven, Philadelphia, 1997, pp 445–57.

50. Tsao MS, Zhu H, Viallet J. Autocrine growth loop of the epidermal growth factor receptor in normal and

51. Tsao MS, Zhu H, Giaid A, Viallet J, Nakamura T, Park M. Hepatocyte growth factor/scatter factor is an autocrine factor for human normal bronchial epithelial and lung carcinoma cells. *Cell Growth Differ* 1993;**4**:571–9.

52. Takizawa H, Beckmann J, Shoji S, *et al.* Pulmonary macrophages can stimulate cell growth of bovine bronchial epithelial cells. *Am J Respir Cell Mol Biol* 1990;**2**:245–55.

53. Jetten AM, Vollberg TM, Nervi C, George MD. Positive and negative regulation of proliferation and differentiation in tracheobronchial epithelial cells. *Am Rev Respir Dis* 1990;**142**:S36–9.

54. Oyamada H, Kayaba H, Kamada Y, *et al.* An optimal condition of bronchial cell proliferation stimulated by insulin-like growth factor-I. *Int Arch Allergy Immunol* 2000;**122**(suppl 1): 59–62.

55. Aoshiba K, Rennard SI. Fibronectin supports bronchial epithelial cell adhesion and survival in the absence of growth factors. *Am J Physiol* 1997;**273**:L684–93.

56. Whitcutt MJ, Adler KB, Wu R. A biphasic chamber system for maintaining polarity of differentiation of cultured respiratory tract epithelial cells. *In-vitro Cell Dev Biol* 1988;**24**:420.

57. Takeyama K, Dabbagh K, Lee HM, *et al.* Epidermal growth factor system regulates mucin production in airways. *Proc Natl Acad Sci USA* 1999;**96**:3081–6.

58. Guzman K, Randell SH, Nettesheim P. Epidermal growth factor regulates expression of the mucous phenotype of rat tracheal epithelial cells. *Biochem Biophys Res Commun* 1995;**217**:412–18.

59. Hill AT, Bayley D, Stockley RA. The interrelationship of sputum inflammatory markers in patients with chronic bronchitis. *Am J Respir Crit Care Med* 1999;**160**:893–8.

60. Takeyama K, Dabbagh K, Jeong Shim J, Dao-Pick T, Ueki IF, Nadel JA. Oxidative stress causes mucin synthesis via transactivation of epidermal growth factor receptor: role of neutrophils. *J Immunol* 2000;**164**:1546–52.

61. Michelson PH, Tigue M, Panos RJ, Sporn PH. Keratinocyte growth factor stimulates bronchial epithelial cell proliferation *in vitro* and *in vivo. Am J Physiol* 1999;**277** (4 Pt 1):L737–42.

62. Ohmichi H, Matsumoto K, Nakamura T. *In vivo* mitogenic action of HGF on lung epithelial cells: pulmotrophic role in lung regeneration. *Am J Physiol* 1996;**270**(6 Pt 1):L1031–9.

63. Dohi M, Hasegawa T, Yamamoto K, Marshall BC. Hepatocyte growth factor attenuates collagen accumulation in a murine model of pulmonary fibrosis. *Am J Respir Crit Care Med* 2000;**162**:2302–7.

64. Panoskaltsis-Mortari A, Taylor PA, Rubin JS, *et al.* Keratinocyte growth factor facilitates alloengraftment and ameliorates graft-versus-host disease in mice by a mechanism independent of repair of conditioning-induced tissue injury. *Blood* 2000;**96**:4350–6.

65. Adamson IY, Bakowska J. Ralationship of keratinocyte growth factor and hepatocyte growth factor levels in rat lung lavage fluid to epithelial cell regeneration after bleomycin. *Am J Pathol* 1999;**155**:949–54.

66. Geiser T, Jarreau PH, Atabai K, Matthay MA. Interleukin-1β augments *in vitro* alveolar epithelial repair. *Am J Physiol: Lung Cell Mol Physiol* 2000;**279**:L1184–90.

67. Liebow AA. Pulmonary emphysema with special reference to vascular changes. *Am Rev Respir Dis* 1959;**80**:67–93.

68. Watkins RH, D'Angio CT, Ryan RM, Patel A, Maniscalco WM. Differential expression of VEGF mRNA splice variants in newborn and adult hyperoxic lung injury. *Am J Physiol: Lung Cell Mol Physiol* 1999;**276**:L858–67.

immortalized human bronchial epithelial cells. *Exp Cell Res* 1996;**223**:268–73.

69. Kasahara Y, Tuder RM, Taraseviciene-Stewart L, *et al.* Inhibition of VEGF receptors causes lung cell apoptosis and emphysema. *J Clin Invest* 2000;**106**:1311–19.

70. Kasahara Y, Tuder RM, Cool CD, Lynch DA, Flores SC, Voelkel NF. Endothelial cell death and decreased expression of vascular endothelial growth factor and vascular endothelial growth factor receptor 2 in emphysema. *Am J Respir Crit Care Med* 2001;**163**(3 Pt 1):737–44.

71. Cardoso WV. Molecular regulation of lung development. *Annu Rev Physiol* 2001;**63**:471–94.

72. Holgate ST, Davies DE, Lackie PM, Wilson SJ, Puddicombe SM, Lordan JL. Epithelial–mesenchymal interactions in the pathogenesis of asthma. *J Allergy Clin Immunol* 2000; **105**(2 Pt 1):193–204.

73. Shoji S, Rickard KA, Ertl RF, Robbins RA, Linder J, Rennard SI. Bronchial epithelial cells produce lung fibroblast chemotactic factor: fibronectin. *Am J Respir Cell Mol Biol* 1989;**1**:13–20.

74. Harrison NK, Dawes KE, Kwon OJ, Barnes PJ, Laurent GJ, Chung KF. Effects of neuropeptides on human lung fibroblast proliferation and chemotaxis. *Am J Physiol* 1995;**268**: L278–3.

75. Endo T, Uchida Y, Matsumoto H, *et al.* Regulation of endothelin-1 synthesis in cultured guinea pig airway epithelial cells by various cytokines. *Biochem Biophys Res Commun* 1992;**14**:1594–9.

76. Shimizu S, Gabazza EC, Hayashi T, Ido M, Adachi Y, Suzuki K. Thrombin stimulates the expression of PDGF in lung epithelial cells. *Am J Physiol: Lung Cell Mol Physiol* 2000;**279**:L503–10.

77. Sacco O, Romberger D, Rizzino A, Beckmann J, Rennard SI, Spurzem JR. Spontaneous production of transforming growth factor beta 2 by primary cultures of bronchial epithelial cells: effects on cell behavior *in vitro. J Clin Invest* 1992;**90**:1379–85.

78. Hicks W Jr, Sigurdson L, Gabalski E, *et al.* Does cartilage down-regulate growth factor expression in tracheal epithelium? *Arch Otolaryngol Head Neck Surg* 1999;**125**:1239–43.

79. Niewoehner DE. Anatomic and pathophysiological correlations in COPD. In: GL Baum, JD Crapo, BR Celli, JB Karlinsky, eds. *Textbook of Pulmonary Diseases.* Lippincott-Raven, Philadelphia, 1998, pp 823–42.

80. McEwan IJ, Wright AP, Gustafsson JA. Mechanism of gene expression by the glucocorticoid receptor: role of protein–protein interactions. *Bioessays* 1997;**19**:153–60.

81. Bitterman PB, Polunovsky VA, Ingbar DH. Repair after acute lung injury. *Chest* 1994;**105**(3 suppl):118S–21S.

82. Pierce JA, Hocott JB, Ebert RV. The collagen and elastin content of the lung in emphysema. *Ann Intern Med* 1961;**55**:210–21.

83. Lang MR, Fiaux GW, Gillooly M, Stewart JA, Hulmes DJS, Lamb D. Collagen content of alveolar wall tissue in emphysematous and non-emphysematous lungs. *Thorax* 1994;**49**:319–26.

84. Vlahovic G, Russell ML, Mercer RR, Crapo JD. Cellular and connective tissue changes in alveolar septal walls in emphysema. *Am J Respir Crit Care Med* 1999;**160**: 2086–92.

85. Snider G, Lucey E, Stone P. Animal models of emphysema. *Am Rev Respir Dis* 1986;**133**:149–69.

86. Osman M, Cantor JO, Roffman S, Keller S, Turino GM, Mandl I. Cigarette smoke impairs elastin resynthesis in lungs of hamsters with elastase-induced emphysema. *Am Rev Respir Dis* 1985;**132**:640–3.

87. Shapiro SD, Endicott SK, Province MA, Pierce JA, Campbell EJ. Marked longevity of human lung parenchymal elastic fibers deduced from prevalence of D-aspartate and nuclear weapons-related radiocarbon. *J Clin Invest* 1991;**87**:1828–34.

88. Stone PJ, Morris SM, Thomas KM, Schuhwerk K, Mitchelson A. Repair of elastase-digested elastic fibers in acellular matrices by replating with neonatal rat-lung lipid interstitial fibroblasts or other elastogenic cell types. *Am J Respir Cell Mol Biol* 1997;**17**:289–301.

89. Stone PJ, Gottlieb DJ, O'Connor GT, *et al.* Elastin and collagen degradation products in urine of smokers with and without chronic obstructive pulmonary disease. *Am J Respir Crit Care Med* 1995;**151**:952–9.

90. Stein J, Fenigstein H. Anatomie pathologique de la maladie de famine. In: E Apfelbaum, ed. *Maladie de famine.* American Joint Distribution Committee, 1946, pp 21–7.

91. Sahebjami H, Vassallo CL. Effects of starvation and refeeding on lung mechanics and morphometry. *Am Rev Respir Dis* 1979;**119**:443–51.

92. Sahebjami H, Vassallo CL. Influence of starvation on enzyme-induced emphysema. *J Appl Physiol* 1980;**48**:284–8.

93. Sulkowska M, Sulkowski S, Terlikowski S, Nowak HF. Tumor necrosis factor-alpha induces emphysema-like pulmonary tissue rebuilding. Changes in type II alveolar epithelial cells. *Pol J Pathol* 1997;**48**:179–88.

94. Menkes H, Traystman R, Terry P. Collateral ventilation. *Fed Proc* 1979;**38**:22–6.

95. Gillett NA, Gerlach RF, Muggenburg BA, Harkema JR, Griffith WC, Mauderly JL. Relationship between collateral flow resistance and alveolar pores in the aging beagle dog. *Exp Lung Res* 1989;**15**:709–19.

96. Kawakami M, Takizawa T. Distribution of pores within alveoli in the human lung. *J Appl Physiol* 1987;**63**:1866–70.

97. Parra SC, Gaddy LR, Takaro T. Early ultrastructural changes in papain-induced experimental emphysema. *Lab Invest* 1980;**42**:277–89.

98. Takaro T, Gaddy LR, Parra S. Thin alveolar epithelial partitions across connective tissue gaps in the alveolar wall of the human lung: ultrastructural observations. *Am Rev Respir Dis* 1982;**126**:326–31.

99. Cosio MG, Shiner RJ, Saetta M, *et al.* Alveolar fenestrae in smokers. Relationship with light microscopic and functional abnormalities. *Am Rev Respir Dis* 1986;**133**:126–31.

100. Freedman LP, Luisi BF. On the mechanism of DNA binding by nuclear hormone receptors: a structural and functional perspective. *J Cell Biochem* 1993;**51**:140–50.

101. Fine A, Goldstein RH. The effect of transforming growth factor-beta on cell proliferation and collagen formation by lung fibroblasts. *J Biol Chem* 1987;**262**:3897–902.

102. Vaughan MB, Howard EW, Tomasek JJ. Transforming growth factor-beta1 promotes the morphological and functional differentiation of the myofibroblast. *Exp Cell Res* 2000;**257**:180–9.

103. Montesano R, Orci L. Transforming growth factor-β stimulates collagen-matrix contraction by fibroblasts: Implication for wound healing. *Proc Natl Acad Sci USA* 1988;**85**:4894–7.

104. Vignola AM, Chanez P, Chiappara G, *et al.* Transforming growth factor-β expression in mucosal biopsies in asthma and chronic bronchitis. *Am J Respir Crit Care Med* 1997;**156**:591–9.

105. Khalil N, Bereznay O, Sporn M, Greenberg AH. Macrophage production of transforming growth factor beta and fibroblast collagen synthesis in chronic pulmonary inflammation. *J Exp Med* 1989;**170**:727–37.

106. Yehualaeshet T, O'Connor R, Begleiter A, Murphy-Ullrich JE, Silverstein R, Khalil N. A CD36 synthetic peptide inhibits bleomycin-induced pulmonary inflammation and connective tissue synthesis in the rat. *Am J Respir Cell Mol Biol* 2000;**23**:204–12.

107. Snyder LS, Hertz MI, Peterson MS, *et al*. Acute lung injury. Pathogenesis of intraalveolar fibrosis. *J Clin Invest* 1991;**88**:663–73.

108. Chanez P, Vignola M, Stenger R, Vic P, Michel FB, Bousquet J. Platelet-derived growth factor in asthma. *Allergy* 1995;**50**:878–83.

109. Wen FQ, Kohyama T, Liu XD, Zhu YK, Spurzem JR, Rennard SI. IL-4 and IL-13 enhanced TGF-β2 production in cultured human bronchial epithelial cells is attenuated by IFNγ. *Am J Resp Crit Care Med* 2001;**163**:A911.

110. Postlethwaite AE, Seyer JM. Fibroblast chemotaxis induction by human recombinant interleukin-4. *J Clin Invest* 1991;**87**:2147–52.

111. Fertin C, Nicolas JF, Gillery P, Kalis B, Banchereau J, Maquart FX. Interleukin-4 stimulates collagen synthesis by normal and scleroderma fibroblasts in dermal equivalents. *Cell Mol Biol* 1991;**37**:823–9.

112. Liu XD, Zhu YK, Wang H, *et al*. Cytokine regulation of Type I collagen gel contraction mediated by human airway cells. *Am J Respir Crit Care Med* 2000;**161**:A440.

113. Zhu YK, Liu X-D, Skold CM, *et al*. Cytokine inhibition of fibroblast-induced gel contraction is mediated by PGE$_2$ and NO Acting through separate parallel pathways. *Am J Respir Cell Mol Biol* 2001;**25**:245–53.

114. Kohyama T, Ertl RF, Valenti V, *et al*. Prostaglandin E$_2$ inhibits fibroblast chemotaxis. *Am J Physiol* 2001;**281**:L1257–63.

115. Bitterman P, Rennard S, Ozaki T, Adelberg S, Crystal RG. PGE$_2$: a potential regulator of fibroblast replication in the normal alveolar structures. *Am Rev Respir Dis* 1983;**127**:A271.

116. Zhang HY, Gharaee-Kermani M, Phan SH. Regulation of lung fibroblast alpha-smooth muscle actin expression, contractile phenotype, and apoptosis by IL-1beta. *J Immunol* 1997;**158**:1392–9.

117. Rennard SI, Stier LE, Moss J, Oberpriller JC, Hom B, Crystal RG. Prostaglandin E modulation of fibroblast fibronectin production: an interaction between inflammatory cells and the production of connective tissue matrix. *Am Rev Respir Dis* 1982;**125**:167.

118. Zhu YK, Liu XD, Sköld CM, *et al*. Collaborative interactions between neutrophil elastase and metalloproteinases in extracellular matrix degradation in three-dimensional collagen gels. *Respir Res* 2001;**2**:300–5.

119. Piquette CA, Rennard SI, Snider GL. Chronic bronchitis and emphysema. In: JF Murray, JA Nadel, eds. *Textbook of Respiratory Medicine*, vol 2. WB Saunders, Philadelphia, 2000, pp 1187–245.

120. Saetta M, Di Stefano A, Maestrelli P, *et al*. Airway eosinophilia in chronic bronchitis during exacerbations. *Am J Respir Crit Care Med* 1994;**150**(6 Pt 1):1646–52 [see comments].

121. Buist AS, Vollmer WM. Smoking and other risk factors. In: JF Murray, JA Nadel, eds. *Textbook of Respiratory Medicine*. WB Saunders, Philadelphia, 1994, pp 1259–87.

122. Cantral DE, Sisson JH, Veys T, Rennard SI, Spurzem JR. Effects of cigarette smoke extract on bovine bronchial epithelial cell attachment and migration. *Am J Physiol* 1995;**268**:L723–8.

123. Van Winkle LS, Evans MJ, Brown CD, Willits NH, Pinkerton KE, Plopper CG. Prior exposure to aged and diluted sidestream cigarette smoke impairs bronchiolar injury and repair. *Toxicol Sci* 2001;**60**:152–64.

124. Spurzem JR, Raz M, Ito H, *et al*. Bovine herpesvirus-1 infection reduces bronchial epithelial cell migration to extracellular matrix proteins. *Am J Physiol* 1995;**268**:L214–20.

125. Nakamura Y, Romberger DJ, Tate L, *et al*. Cigarette smoke inhibits lung fibroblast proliferation and chemotaxis. *Am J Respir Crit Care Med* 1995;**151**:1497–503.

126. Carnevali S, Nakamura Y, Mio T, *et al*. Cigarette smoke extract inhibits fibroblast-mediated collagen gel contraction. *Am J Physiol* 1998;**247**:L591–8.

127. Laurent P, Janoff A, Kagan HM. Cigarette smoke blocks cross-linking of elastin *in vitro*. *Am Rev Respir Dis* 1983;**127**:189–92.

128. Liu XD, Umino T, Zhu YK, *et al*. A study on the effect of cadmium on human lung fibroblasts. *Chest* 2000;**117**:247S.

129. Kuwano K, Bosken CH, Pare PD, Bai TR, Wiggs BR, Hogg JC. Small airways dimensions in asthma and in chronic obstructive pulmonary disease. *Am Rev Respir Dis* 1993;**148**:1220–5.

130. Rennard SI, Saltzman L, Moss J, *et al*. Modulation of fibroblast production of collagen types I and III: effects of PGE$_1$ and isoproterenol. *Fed Proc* 1981;**40**:1813.

131. Mio T, Liu X, Adachi Y, *et al*. Human bronchial epithelial cells modulate collagen gel contraction by fibroblasts. *Am J Physiol* 1998;**274**:L119–26.

132. Torphy TJ. Phosphodiesterase isozymes: molecular targets for novel antiasthma agents. *Am J Respir Crit Care Med* 1998;**157**:351–70.

133. Spiteri MA, Clarke SW, Poulter LW. Isolation of phenotypically and functionally distinct macrophage subpopulations from human bronchoalveolar lavage. *Eur Respir J* 1992;**5**:717–26.

134. Polunovsky VA, Chen B, Henke C, *et al*. Role of mesenchymal cell death in lung remodeling after injury. *J Clin Invest* 1993;**92**:388–97.

135. Barnes PJ, Adcock IM. *Glucocorticoid Receptors. The Lung*, 2nd edn. 1997, pp 37–54.

136. Massaro GD, Massaro D. Postnatal treatment with retinoic acid increases the number of pulmonary alveoli in rats. *Am J Physiol* 1996;**270**:L305–10.

137. Massaro G, Massaro D. Retinoic acid treatment abrogates elastase-induced pulmonary emphysema in rats. *Nature Med* 1997;**3**:675–7.

Lung mechanics

NB PRIDE AND J MILIC-EMILI

Changes in the mechanical properties of the airways and airspaces are central to the disability in COPD. Increases in airway resistance, decreases in dynamic compliance and loss of lung recoil lead to hyperinflation of the lungs and chest wall and greatly increase the work of breathing. The unequal distribution of these changes leads to abnormal distribution of ventilation and is responsible for much of the inefficiency of the lungs as exchangers of O_2 and CO_2. In this chapter changes in lung mechanics in COPD will be considered at three stages: (i) mild disease as found in population studies of smokers; (ii) moderate to severe disease studied in the stable state; (iii) acute respiratory failure, defined as a significant deterioration of oxygenation from the chronic, stable state. A fuller bibliography of work on stable COPD up to 1985 is published elsewhere.[1]

In stable COPD, great reliance is placed on assessing lung mechanics by simple measurements made during a forced expiratory maneuver, but assessment during exercise, sleep or in the intensive care unit requires measurements during tidal breathing, to derive resistance (or its reciprocal, conductance), compliance and work of breathing. In this chapter the changes in lung distensibility and airway function which determine maximum expiratory flow will be described mainly in the section on moderate and severe disease, while measurements during tidal breathing will be described mainly in the section on acute respiratory failure.

MILD DISEASE

The pathologic changes in smokers leading to airflow obstruction are thought to be predominantly in the small bronchi and bronchioles, so investigations into mild COPD have concentrated on examining peripheral lung function,[2] which may be abnormal[3] when there are few symptoms, no abnormal physical or radiographic signs and total airways conductance, spirometry and exercise capacity remain within normal limits. Consequently mild changes in lung mechanics in smokers can be detected best by tests which show non-uniform behavior of the lungs, such as enhanced airway closure or frequency dependence of lung mechanics. Mild changes can also be detected by the shape of the maximum expiratory flow–volume curve and the response to helium-oxygen breathing.

Enhanced airway closure

The size and patency of the airways are determined by the interaction between airway transmural pressure and the intrinsic properties of the airway wall. Transmural pressures are reduced as lung volume is reduced, but normal peripheral airways are stabilized against closure by the low surface tension of the airway lining liquid;[4] in healthy young subjects significant airway closure does not occur until lung volume is reduced below functional residual capacity (FRC).[5] An early change in disease is enhanced airway closure at low lung volume. This has been assessed by determining the lung volume ('closing volume') at which a sudden increase in expired gas concentration has been observed during a slow deflation from total lung capacity (TLC) (Figure 13.1). In healthy non-smokers, closing volume in seated young adults is usually about 5–10% vital capacity (VC), rising to about 25–30% VC (and thus close to FRC) in old age. Increases in closing volume have been shown in asymptomatic young adult smokers with normal spirometry,[6] but it is not certain that differences between smokers and non-smokers

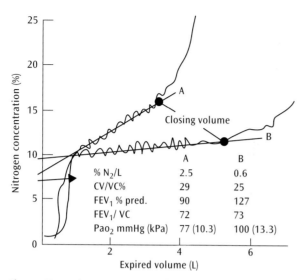

	A	B
% N_2/L	2.5	0.6
CV/VC%	29	25
FEV_1 % pred.	90	127
FEV_1/ VC	72	73
Pao_2 mmHg (kPa)	77 (10.3)	100 (13.3)

Figure 13.1 *Nitrogen concentration plotted against expired volume following a single vital capacity breath of 100% oxygen for two healthy middle-aged smokers. Greater slope (percentage N_2/L) in subject A indicates more uneven distribution of ventilation and asynchronous emptying. Abrupt change of slope at the closing volume (CV) indicates the volume at which some lung units in the most dependent lung zones stop emptying. Note arterial Po_2 (Pao_2) is lower in subject A suggesting ventilation-perfusion mismatching on basis of uneven distribution of ventilation.*

increase in middle age. Sometimes the closing volume has been assessed as an absolute volume (closing capacity (CC) which is closing volume plus residual volume (RV)), expressed as a ratio of TLC (CC/TLC). With more severe airway disease it becomes impossible to define a closing volume because expired N_2 rises continuously through the breath. Areas of closure could however be detected by imaging inhaled radioactive aerosols as has been done in asthma.[7] The slope of expired N_2 versus volume has also been used as an indicator of disease.

Frequency-dependent falls in compliance and resistance

In healthy non-smokers there may be some frequency dependence of compliance resulting from the visco-elastic behavior of lung tissue. A much greater frequency dependence is shown by many smokers, values of dynamic compliance falling progressively below the value of static inspiratory compliance as the breathing frequency increases.[8] This change has been observed consistently in smokers with few other abnormalities of lung function and with normal values for spirometry and total airway resistance. The mechanism is thought to be increased inequality of time constants in the lung which could result from changes in either the compliance or resistance of the various parallel lung compartments, changes in the serial distribution of compliance between central airways

and the periphery of the lung, or arise from the delay imposed on ventilation if some airspaces were only ventilated via collateral channels with long time constants. Measuring dynamic compliance is technically demanding; a more practical technique is to measure the fall in total respiratory resistance (lung and chest wall) with increasing frequency by using the forced oscillation technique applied at the mouth.[9] Because the resistance offered by the peripheral airways is normally less than one-third of the total airways resistance, this technique is probably less sensitive than frequency dependence of compliance in detecting minor abnormalities.

Reductions in maximum expiratory flow and in density dependence of maximum flow

Theory suggests that if narrowing first involves the peripheral airways, the earliest changes in maximum flow should occur in the termination of the maximum expiratory flow–volume (MEFV) curve toward residual volume (RV). Several studies have shown decreased flow confined to the lower 50% of VC in asymptomatic smokers, but this finding is not universal, other investigators having found maximum flow at large volumes is also decreased in young smokers and even that abnormalities in maximum flow are more common at large volumes than at small volumes.[2]

There is a wide variation in normal MEFV curves[10] so that a useful method for detecting mild abnormalities in an individual is to compare the differences in MEFV curves breathing air and after equilibration with a low-density gas mixture of 80% He and 20% O_2. Density dependence of maximum flow (assessed by comparing maximum expiratory flow at 50% VC, $\Delta\dot{V}max_{50}$) is determined by the ratio of density-independent lateral pressure losses (due to laminar flow regimes) to density-dependent lateral pressures losses (due to turbulence and convective acceleration) between alveoli and the site of flow limitation. In some asymptomatic smokers there is a reduction in $\Delta\dot{V}max_{50}$, suggesting a greater contribution of density-independent flow regimes (presumably in peripheral airways) to the pressure drop between alveoli and flow-limiting airways. With increasing age $\Delta\dot{V}max_{50}$ on average does not change in non-smokers but decreases in smokers.[11,12] Unfortunately, reduction in $\Delta\dot{V}max_{50}$ has not been closely related to pathologic changes in peripheral airways in subjects who underwent lobectomy[13] or in lungs studied post-mortem.[14] Furthermore some patients with advanced COPD retain normal $\Delta\dot{V}max_{50}$,[15] possibly because the site of flow limitation remains in central airways; therefore measuring $\Delta\dot{V}max_{50}$ is unlikely to be a consistently reliable method for detecting mild COPD.

Prognostic significance of changes in peripheral lung function

Probably most smokers develop some abnormality of peripheral lung function relatively early in their smoking history, but most do not progress to disabling COPD. The combination of a high N_2 slope and a low $FEV_1/VC\%$ apparently identifies the high-risk, susceptible subject,[6,16,17] while an abnormal slope without reduced $FEV_1/VC\%$ appears to carry no unfavorable prognosis.[18] With mild airway disease, some smoking-related changes appear reversible in the first weeks after stopping smoking. Reductions in frequency dependence of dynamic lung compliance, in the slope of the single breath nitrogen (SBN_2) test, and in closing volume, small improvements in spirometry or indices from air–MEFV curves, and an increased density dependence of maximum flow, have all been described.[19] The tests used generally could not distinguish whether changes were in the peripheral airways or in the airspaces or indeed whether they were reversible or irreversible. In recent years interest in these 'sensitive' tests has waned; in part because change in FEV_1 appears to provide an adequate index of progression of mild disease in smokers. 'Sensitive' tests probably have a role in detecting the early stages of obstructive bronchiolitis developing after lung or bone marrow transplant.

MODERATE AND SEVERE DISEASE

When abnormal breathlessness on exertion develops in COPD, standard tests of overall lung mechanics, such as FEV_1 and airway resistance, are usually abnormal and there are increases in RV and FRC. In some patients there are also increases in TLC and in static lung compliance and loss of lung recoil pressure at a standard volume. The changes are distributed unevenly and frequency dependence of lung compliance and resistance persist. The increase in FRC potentially places the inspiratory muscles at a mechanical disadvantage due to their decreased resting length.

Changes in static lung volumes and distensibility

Studies in the 1930s with multibreath gas equilibration or washout methods established that RV and FRC were consistently increased in patients with COPD. With the introduction of the body plethysmograph technique for measuring thoracic gas volume, larger increases in FRC were found.[20,21] Originally these differences were explained on the basis that the standard gas-dilution methods only measured the gas that communicates with the airway, whereas plethysmography also measured trapped gas; however, it was shown subsequently that if gas dilution was prolonged sufficiently, the communicating gas volume in most patients with COPD was similar to that measured by plethysmography.[22] In the early 1980s various possible errors in the plethysmographic technique

used in patients with increased airway resistance were identified. The major source of error appears to be that swings in mouth pressure during panting can underestimate true swings in alveolar pressure, so that values of TLC derived from mouth pressure are higher than values based on swings in esophageal pressure. The tendency to overestimate TLC based on mouth pressure swings increases with increasing panting frequency and can probably be removed by panting at 1 Hz or less.[23,24] Despite the tendency to overestimate TLC with plethysmography, undoubtedly increases in TLC occur in some patients, particularly those with severe emphysema. This has been shown in emphysematous lungs studied postmortem, and an acquired increase in TLC in life is suggested by chest radiographs taken at full inflation, which frequently show an abnormally low position of the diaphragm sometimes with loss of its normal curvature and exposure of its costal attachments.

Changes in the static volume–pressure (VP) curve of the lungs are partly responsible for the changes in lung volumes. The characteristic changes are an increase in static compliance, reduction in static transpulmonary pressure (PL, syn. lung recoil pressure) at a standard volume, and decreased PL at TLC (Figure 13.2). Such changes are not found in all patients with COPD and are generally regarded as indicating severe generalized emphysema and, in particular, panacinar emphysema.[25] A few studies have compared various indices of lung distensibility with morphologic changes in lungs post-mortem or removed at surgery. In such comparisons, usually only one lung or even a single lobe is available; thus it is desirable to use measurements of distensibility that are independent of the volume, relative expansion and maximum distending pressure of the lung. This can be achieved either by measuring PL at a standard percentage of TLC (or equivalent for a single lung or lobe) or by modeling the volume–pressure curve as a single exponential and fitting the curve with the equation:

$$V = Vmax - Ae^{-kP}$$

where Vmax represents the extrapolated volume at infinite pressure, A is a constant related to the intercept on the volume axis, and the parameter k is a shape factor, which when pressure (PL) is measured in cmH_2O has the dimensions cmH_2O^{-1} (Figure 13.2). The parameter k is particularly useful because it describes the shape of the curve independently of the absolute volume and VC of the lung and the precise positioning of the VP curve on its axes. In human lungs k rises slightly with increasing age,[26–28] reflecting increased concavity of the VP curve to the pressure axis; increases in k in vivo are also found in patients diagnosed as having severe emphysema by conventional clinical criteria, although the extent of increase observed has been variable. The value of k in normal human lungs examined post-mortem appears to be greater

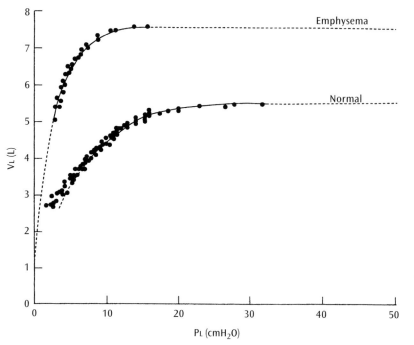

Figure 13.2 *Representative static expiratory volume–pressure (VP) curves of lungs in a subject with severe emphysema compared with a normal subject. Lung volume measured by body plethysmography. Solid lines through experimental points were derived by exponential curve-fitting procedure. Broken lines: extrapolation of curve to infinite pressure and to volume axis at zero pressure. Values of k (cmH₂OL⁻¹): for emphysema, 0.325: normal, 0.143. (Adapted from ref. 27.)*

than *in vivo*, but, allowing for this change, Greaves and Colebatch[29] found a good relation between an increase in k and the presence of relatively severe emphysema in seven lungs studied post-mortem. Subsequent studies have shown a significant but loose relationship between k or PL at 90% TLC and a macroscopic assessment of emphysema in surgical or post-mortem specimens[30,31] and also a relation between abnormalities in the VP curve and the mean number of alveolar attachments to small airways.[32,33] That the relationships are not tighter is not surprising because the static VP curve represents the lumped characteristics of all lung units contributing to VC. Although early in the progression of disease there may be occasional patients with a VC greater than their predicted value, in the great majority of patients with emphysema relative volume expansion (i.e. VC/RV ratio) between RV and TLC is reduced, because increase in RV outweighs any accompanying increase in TLC. The overall reduction in VC/RV ratio conceals large local differences in relative volume expansion. In centrilobular emphysema the affected spaces have a high RV and are less compliant than normal lung tissue and the surrounding lung, which is less severely affected by emphysema.[34] In general, as local emphysematous changes become more severe, the 'VC' of these regions falls and their contribution to the overall VP curve of the lung declines. In the extreme case, areas of lung destroyed by severe macroscopic emphysema, such as a bulla, may not change volume at all during a VC maneuver and contribute to the static VP curve only by displacing it to larger absolute volumes. Hence, similarly to tests of CO transfer, the VP curve is weighted by the proportionately larger volume contribution of the most

normal surviving lung. This idea led to the hypothesis ('the doughnut not the hole'[35]) that changes in the VP curve in emphysema are dominated, not by the often localized macroscopic changes, but by changes in overall microscopic lung structure that accompany (and possibly precede) the macroscopic changes. This has been indirectly confirmed by studies of the relation between 'microscopic' emphysema and CO transfer coefficient,[36,37] but equivalent studies are not available for the VP curve.

The implication is that the distribution of emphysematous changes has a major influence on the extent of changes in the VP curve. When the distribution is very irregular, as in centrilobular emphysema, changes in k and static compliance may be small even in the presence of considerable macroscopic disease.[25] By contrast, when emphysematous change is uniform, as found in panacinar emphysema,[25] considerable changes in the VP curve may be found even when macroscopic emphysema is less obvious.

Studies of asymptomatic subjects, mainly suffering from homozygous alpha-1-antitrypsin deficiency, which is known to be associated with panacinar emphysema, confirm that considerable[38,39] and progressive[40] (Figure 13.3) changes in the VP curve can be found before the development of severe airflow limitation and apparently at an early stage in the natural history of emphysema. The subsequent changes in VP curves as disease continues to progress have not been directly followed in individual patients; but the major change in severe emphysema is a great increase in RV, whereas PL at full inflation, which is largely determined by the extent of any increase in TLC and the consequent reduced ability of the inspiratory

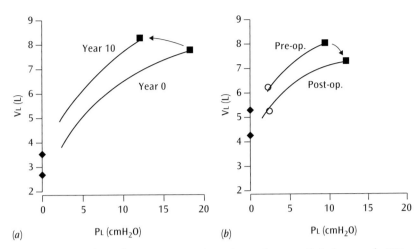

Figure 13.3 *(a) Change over 10 years in expiratory VP curve in early emphysema. Note increase in TLC and reduction in P$_L$ at TLC, with leftward shift of VP curve. No change was found in Cst,L in tidal range. Mean FEV$_1$ was 3.03 L (87% predicted) at year 0 and 2.15 L (67% predicted) at year 10. (Based on data in ref. 40.) (b) VP curve before and 6 months after lung volume reduction surgery. Note similar TLC and P$_L$ at TLC pre-LVRS to those at year 10 in (a), but much larger RV. Post LVRS the VP curve is displaced to smaller volumes with extension of the curve to a higher P$_L$ at the new TLC. Mean FEV$_1$ was 0.69 L (24% predicted) pre-LVRS and 0.85 L (28% predicted) post-LVRS. (Based on data in ref. 43.) In both plots filled square indicates TLC, open circle FRC and filled diamond RV.*

muscles to lower pleural surface pressure, has been found to average about 10 cmH$_2$O (Figure 13.3).[41–43] Reductions in VC due to loss of contributing units also attenuates any increase in static lung compliance.

Loss of lung recoil pressure increases the neutral position of the respiratory system (i.e. relaxation volume, Vr), and this may be enhanced by accompanying reductions in chest wall recoil pressure.[44] However, because of the slow expiratory flow rates caused by airway narrowing, FRC may be determined dynamically in patients with severe COPD; expiration is terminated by the initiation of the next inspiration before the respiratory system has sufficient time to reach its relaxation volume (see 'Dynamic hyperinflation' below). A combination of airway changes and loss of lung recoil probably also accounts for the increase in RV. Loss of lung recoil pressure results in airway closing pressures developing at larger lung volumes, but RV probably is also determined dynamically; in severe COPD the time to empty the lung is greatly prolonged with expiratory flow continuing at very low levels, presumably through dynamically narrowed airways, until RV is essentially limited by the breath-holding ability.

Airway function

In clinical practice, changes in lung mechanics are usually assessed by measurements made during forced vital capacity maneuvers, with much more emphasis on expiratory than inspiratory maneuvers. These tests can be applied in the outpatient clinic, in primary care or at the bedside. By contrast, direct measurements of resistance or conductance usually require a body plethysmograph or introduction of an esophageal balloon-catheter, although simpler methods are being developed.

DETERMINANTS OF CONDUCTANCE AT LOW FLOW

The relation between driving pressure (alveolar pressure Palv) and flow ($\dot{V}$) may be expressed either as airways resistance (Raw, ΔPalv/$\Delta\dot{V}$) or its reciprocal, airway conductance (Gaw, $\Delta\dot{V}$/ΔPalv). Both measurements are highly dependent on the lung volume (V$_L$) at which it is measured, but whereas the relation of Raw to V$_L$ is curvilinear, the relation between Gaw and V$_L$ is linear in both normal and diseased subjects (Figure 13.4). Often specific conductance (SGaw, Gaw/absolute V$_L$) is reported, but while this is a good way for comparing individuals of different height or gender, SGaw does not completely correct for the effect of lung volume because the conductance–volume slope intercepts around RV on the volume axis (Figure 13.4).

Gaw or Raw is usually measured during shallow panting around FRC in a body plethysmograph. Reduced Gaw, as found in COPD, indicates a reduction in overall airway dimensions under near-static conditions, which may be due to intrinsic disease of the airway wall or lumen, or to loss of the normal forces distending the airways which, at least in normal lungs, are closely related to P$_L$. In theory, it is possible to dissect out the roles of intrinsic airway abnormality and loss of recoil by determining the Gaw/P$_L$ ratio at FRC. In practice a much better resolution can be obtained by studying the relation

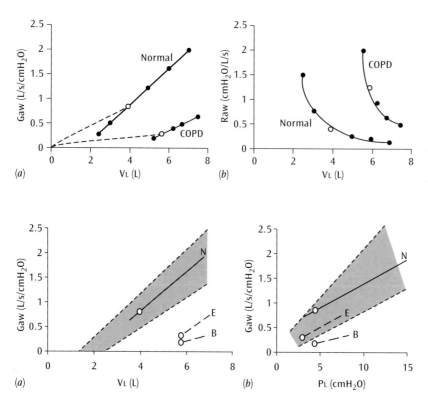

Figure 13.4 *Relation of conductance (Gaw) (a) and resistance (Raw) (b) to lung volume (VL) in normal subjects and severe COPD. Because the ΔGaw/Δ VL slope intercepts on the VL axis, specific conductance (SGaw, Gaw/absVL) indicated by the slope from the origin to FRC (open circle) increases as VL is increased. (Data from ref. 45.)*

Figure 13.5 *Plots of Gaw vs. VL (a) and PL (b) in normal subjects, seven COPD patients with predominant emphysema (E) (FEV₁ 1.40 L) and 10 COPD patients with predominant airway disease (B) (FEV₁ 0.84 L). In both E and B, Gaw is reduced at a given VL but Gaw vs. PL lies within the normal range in E. Values at FRC indicated by open circle. Shaded area shows normal ranges. (Data from ref. 45.)*

between Gaw and P$_L$ over a range of lung volumes, because the increase in P$_L$ as lung volume is increased is a major determinant of the normal increase in Gaw as the lung is inflated.[21,45,46,47] The characteristic change in COPD is a reduced ΔGaw/Δ V$_L$ slope: however, in some patients, the relation between Gaw and P$_L$ is normal (Figure 13.5).[45,46,48] Such patients usually show radiologic and functional evidence of emphysema. But in most patients with severe COPD, Gaw is reduced at a standard P$_L$ and abnormality of the airways is present. The precise airway abnormality cannot be deduced; a reduced Gaw/P$_L$ slope could be caused by loss of parallel airways, smaller dimensions of the airways at low distending pressure, or reduced airway compliance.

There are practical problems in measuring pressure–flow relations during panting in patients with COPD because of looping of these plots, particularly on expiration; in experimental studies pressure–flow relations are usually assessed at 0–0.5 L/s on inspiration. Another problem is frequency-dependence of pressure–flow relations leading to a fall in resistance as breathing frequency is increased;[49] even at the usual panting frequency of 1–2 Hz, differences in resistance between normal subjects and patients with COPD are considerably less than during tidal breathing.

In severe COPD, the best way to measure resistance (or conductance) is during normal tidal breathing, using an esophageal balloon-catheter. The measured resistance (total lung resistance, R$_L$) usually is averaged over a

breath and so includes a component from dynamic narrowing on expiration, which may be large if there is expiratory flow limitation. Although R$_L$ then does not reflect 'fixed' airway dimensions in the same way as inspiratory resistance measured in the body plethysmograph, it does indicate correctly the contribution of increased resistance to the total work of breathing. Non-invasive methods, such as the standard method of applying forced oscillation at the mouth, or airflow interruption, which both rely on measuring pressure at the mouth, considerably underestimate true resistance in severe disease.[50] However this underestimate is less when forced oscillation is applied via the nose so that reliable results may be obtained during non-invasive ventilation.[48] In intubated patients in the intensive care unit, the problem of dissipation of pressure in the compliant upper airway is no longer relevant and accurate measurements at the airway opening can be obtained using forced oscillation or airflow interruption techniques (see 'Acute respiratory failure' below).

SITE OF AIRFLOW RESISTANCE DURING TIDAL BREATHING

In mild disease, studies with a wedged bronchoscope have shown an increase in peripheral lung resistance may be present while total airway function remains within the normal range.[3] When moderate airway obstruction (mean FEV₁ 50–60% of predicted) has developed,

Table 13.1 *Peripheral lung resistance (Rp) as a percentage of total lung resistance (RL) in normal subjects and COPD*

Subjects (no.)	n	Mean age (yr)	FEV$_1$ (% predicted)	RL (cmH$_2$O/L/s)	Rc (cmH$_2$O/L/s)	Rp (cmH$_2$O/L/s)	Rp/RL (%)
Baseline measurements[51]							
Normal	5	56	88	3.1	2.4	0.7	24
COPD							
Chronic bronchitis	7	64	51	8.7	3.9	4.8	55
Emphysema	8	63	39	5.9	2.9	3.0	50
Response to inhaled atropine[57]							
COPD	7						
Before		58	57	7.8	3.6	4.2	54
After		–	–	4.6	1.6	3.0	65
% A/B		–	–	59	44	71	

Total lung resistance (RL) measured during tidal breathing with an esophageal balloon-catheter was divided into peripheral and central components by measuring airway pressure in a 3-mm-diameter airway with an intrabronchial catheter. Peripheral lung resistance (Rp) is the sum of the resistance of the airways smaller than 3 mm diameter and lung tissue resistance. Central resistance (Rc) includes the extrathoracic airway. With this technique RL in normal subjects is about 1 cmH$_2$O/L/s higher than without an airway catheter. Baseline measurements were made after withdrawal of all bronchodilator treatment.

studies using an intrabronchial catheter have found that slightly more than half the total pulmonary resistance resides in airways of less than 3 mm internal diameter (Table 13.1).[51] This proportion was similar for a group with predominant airway disease ('chronic bronchitis') and for a group with physiological evidence (increased static compliance, reduced CO transfer coefficient) of emphysema; despite a lower FEV$_1$ in the emphysema group, total lung resistance was lower than in the chronic bronchitis group.[51]

For severe disease the best information comes from study of lungs at necroscopy using the forced oscillation technique. Most of the increase in resistance in lungs of patients dying with COPD is in the peripheral airways of less than 2 mm diameter; on average these account for 75% of the total resistance at lung volumes and flows comparable with those during tidal breathing in life.[52–55] Despite obvious pathologic changes in their walls, the resistance of central airways is increased in only a minority of lungs[52] and even then it is associated with a proportionally greater increase in peripheral airway resistance. Inspiratory as well as expiratory resistance is increased, indicating that it was due to 'fixed' changes in the peripheral airways, not to a 'check-valve' phenomenon. These post-mortem studies imply a reduction in peripheral airway dimensions at a standard PL. This could result from intrinsic disease of the airways (obliteration and narrowing of airway lumina by scarring, wall thickening, inflammation, mucus plugs) or from loss of airway distension caused by loss or breaks of the attached alveolar walls.

There is an additional labile component to resistance in most patients presumably resulting from bronchial muscle contraction which responds to bronchodilators, or in hypoxic patients breathing oxygen.[56] In contrast to asthma, the response to inhaled anticholinergic drugs is similar to (some would say superior to) that to beta-agonists. This suggests that most of the reversible component in COPD is due to vagal tone, and, because vagal motor innervation does not extend to the most peripheral airways, involves more central airways than those in which the major fixed obstructive changes occur. A study using an intra-airway catheter has confirmed that atropine has a larger dilator effect in central than in peripheral (<3 mm diameter) airways.[57] It is uncertain whether cholinergic 'tone' is greater in COPD than in normal subjects; the absolute increment in FEV$_1$ after cholinergic treatment is similar in COPD and normal subjects and a study of sensory stimulation of the nose failed to show an enhanced vagally induced bronchoconstriction in COPD compared with normal subjects.[58] There is, however, considerable day-to-day variation[59] in the size of the bronchodilator response, possibly reflecting variation in basal cholinergic tone.

COLLATERAL VENTILATION

In advanced COPD there is great parallel inhomogeneity of airway narrowing (and also of alveolar destruction) and many airways can be completely occluded. This would be expected to lead to the development of atelectasis or non-ventilated airspaces acting as effective right-to-left shunt. Yet neither atelectasis nor increase in shunt are features of advanced COPD except in patients in acute respiratory failure (see Chapter 14); this is probably due to a reduction in the resistance to collateral ventilation

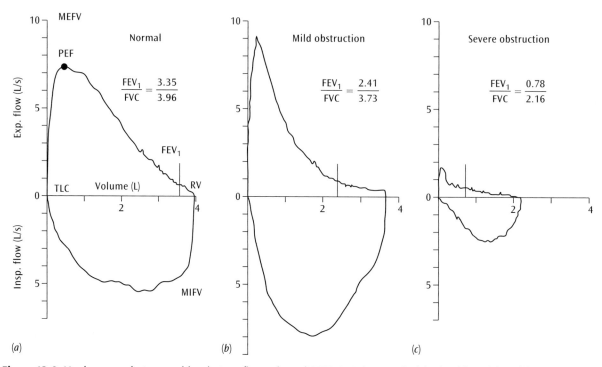

Figure 13.6 *Maximum expiratory and inspiratory flow-volume (MEFV, MIFV) curves in (a) a healthy subject, (b) a subject with mild intrathoracic airways obstruction, (c) advanced intrathoracic airways obstruction. FEV_1 indicated on volume axis by vertical bar. TLC: total lung capacity; RV: residual volume; FVC: forced vital capacity. Note the development of convexity of flow to volume axis in mild obstruction which gives a diagnostic contour despite preservation of a large peak expiratory flow, FVC and only small reduction in FEV_1/FVC ratio. In advanced disease there is severe shrinkage on both volume and flow axes.*

related to the increase in FRC and destruction of alveolar walls in emphysema.[60,61]

DETERMINANTS OF MAXIMUM EXPIRATORY FLOW

Tidal breathing at rest and during exercise has to take place within the confines of the maximum flow–volume envelope. The extreme compression of the whole maximum flow–volume envelope as COPD progresses is shown in Figure 13.6. Characteristically the MEFV curve breathing air becomes increasingly convex toward the volume axis with the greatest proportionate reduction in maximum flow close to RV. Reductions in maximum inspiratory flow are less severe, especially in emphysema where levels may be nearly normal.[62] Maximum flow–volume curves reflect a complex interaction between dynamic airway function, lung recoil and the forces applied to the lung surface by the respiratory muscles; all these aspects of respiratory mechanics are themselves strongly influenced by changes in lung volume. The usefulness of maximum flow–volume curves and derived measurements such as FEV_1, $FEV_1/FVC\%$ probably reflects their ability to integrate all these changes into a simple measurement which itself is related to the maximum breathing capacity.

Isovolume pressure–flow curves

Pressure–flow relations are highly dependent on lung volume and are best analyzed by constructing an isovolume pressure–flow curve (IVPF) from many breaths made with varying efforts (Figure 13.7).[63] Ideally such curves are constructed at the same thoracic gas volume (as measured in a variable-volume body plethysmograph) rather than at a particular expired volume below TLC because the hyperinflation and reduced expiratory flow in patients with severe airflow limitation results in reduction in thoracic gas volume due to gas compression on forceful expiration being considerably larger than the volume expired at the mouth.[64] IVPF curves based on thoracic gas volume usually show a plateau of flow in both normal subjects and patients with COPD at mid-VC. Compared with normal subjects, patients show a reduced maximum expiratory flow, the plateau of maximum expiratory flow is reached at lower driving pressure, and the $\Delta\dot{V}/\Delta P$ slope (conductance) is reduced at low flow (Figure 13.7).[63,65] This initial $\Delta\dot{V}/\Delta P$ slope reflects the lumped static dimensions of the airways. Often there is also a reduced lung recoil pressure. A further difference from normal subjects is that plateaux of maximum expiratory flow develop at large lung volumes. Changes on the inspiratory limb of the IVPF curve are

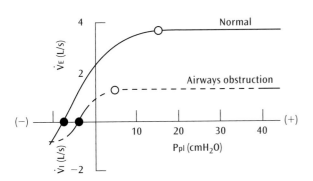

Figure 13.7 *Schematic isovolume pressure-flow (IVPF) curves at 50% VC for normal subject and patient with COPD. Compared with normal subject, in COPD airway conductance at low flow (•–•), the lowest pleural pressure (Ppl) at which maximum flow is achieved (open circle), maximum expiratory flow (solid line) and lung recoil pressure (indicated by distance from • to zero Ppl) are all reduced. V̇E: expiratory flow; V̇I: inspiratory flow. There is no plateau of maximum inspiratory flow in either normal subject or COPD patient.*

less striking and both in normal subjects and patients with COPD maximum inspiratory flow does not show a plateau, the highest values being associated with the most negative pleural pressure.

Roles of static airway dimensions, dynamic airway narrowing and loss of lung recoil

As implied by such IVPF curves, the factors determining maximum flow are only indirectly related to the overall static dimensions of the airways. The airway narrowing found at low flow rates (or during breath holding) results from disease of the airway wall or lumen or from loss of the normal forces distending the airways. Additional dynamic narrowing of the airways develops on forced expiration. In normal subjects pressure losses down the airways on expiration reduce airway distending pressures below the pressure present at the same lung volume during breath holding or inspiration. This leads to dynamic narrowing of all intrathoracic airways, which is most pronounced in the large intrathoracic airways. In COPD reduction in lung recoil pressure (reducing extra-airway distending pressure and effective driving pressure) and airway narrowing (increasing pressure losses down the airways for a given flow) both enhance dynamic narrowing of large intrathoracic airways on expiration. Hence the enhanced dynamic compression of central airways found in COPD does not necessarily indicate altered compliance of these airways (although atrophic changes and loss of cartilage have been described), but is commonly due to more peripheral airway or airspace disease. The functional consequence of these dynamic effects is much greater reduction in maximum expiratory flow than in maximum inspiratory flow.

The role of loss of lung recoil in reducing maximum expiratory flow can be assessed by examining the relation between maximum expiratory flow and static lung recoil pressure (P_L) on maximum flow-static recoil (MFSR) curves (Figure 13.8).[38,45,65,66] These curves may be analyzed in two slightly different ways. In the analysis of Mead et al.,[66] V̇max/P_L is termed the upstream conductance (Gus). In the analysis of Pride et al.[65] a third factor is introduced, the critical transmural pressure of the airways (Ptm'), which is an index of airways collapsibility (see legend to Figure 13.8); the conductance of the airways on the alveolar side of flow limiting segments during forced expiration (Gs) is indicated by the ΔV̇max/ΔP_L slope, not the absolute value of V̇max/P_L. In normal subjects these two analyses are similar because the intercept of the V̇max/ΔP_L slope is very close to the origin, but in COPD there is often an increase in Ptm', giving a positive intercept of the V̇max/ΔP_L slope on the P_L axis. In a few patients with mild or moderate airflow limitation however, the relation between V̇max and P_L remains normal and has an intercept close to the origin, so that both Gus and Gs remain normal. These patients usually have alpha-1-antitrypsin deficiency[38] or other evidence of emphysema. When airflow limitation is more severe (FEV_1 < 50% predicted value), maximum flow is almost always reduced at a standard P_L with both a decrease in Gs and an increase in Ptm' (Figure 13.8).[45] This could be a result of any pathologic change that reduces the total cross-sectional area of the static lumen of the airways; in addition, an enhanced collapsibility of airways at or on the alveolar side of flow-limiting segments could have a similar effect even if resting dimensions are normal.[65]

SITE OF EXPIRATORY FLOW LIMITATION

In normal subjects measurements of intrabronchial pressure suggest that equal pressure points (points in the tracheobronchial tree where lateral airway pressure equals pleural surface pressure) are in the central intrathoracic airways until ~75% of VC has been expired; at smaller lung volumes, equal pressure points move toward the periphery of the lung beyond the large bronchi in which luminal pressure measurements are possible.[67] Probably there is a similar change in the sites of flow limitation. In patients with COPD, Macklem et al.[68] found variable results with some subjects in whom equal pressure points were in central airways over much of the VC, whereas in others equal pressure points were in airways peripheral to the bronchial catheter even at volumes greater than 50% VC.

As discussed above, there is an analogous variability in the density dependence of maximum expiratory flow in COPD.[15] Overall, preservation of density dependence becomes increasingly uncommon as expiratory airflow limitation becomes more severe; nevertheless density

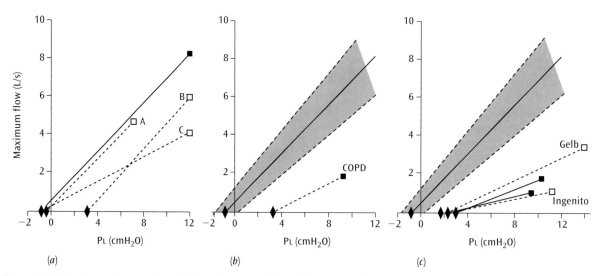

Figure 13.8 *Maximum flow-static recoil (MFSR) curves. (a) Possible mechanisms of reduction in maximum expiratory flow (V̇max) visualized on schematic linearized MFSR curves. According to the equation V̇max = (PL − Ptm')/Gs,[47] [where PL = lung recoil pressure, Gs = ΔV̇max/ΔPL, conductance of the airways on the alveolar side of flow limiting airways during forced expiration, and Ptm' = the critical transmural pressure at which the flow limiting airways narrow sufficiently to restrict flow] V̇max close to full inflation (filled square) may be reduced by loss of PL (A), by increase in Ptm' which displaces the Gs slope to higher pressures with a more positive intercept (filled diamond) on the PL axis (B), or by reduction in slope Gs due to intrinsic airway disease (C). (b) Comparison of mean MFSR slope in normal subjects and in 17 patients with severe COPD, mean FEV₁ 1.02 L. The patients have a combination of all three changes, reduced PL, reduced Gs and increased Ptm' (filled diamond). Changes in these subgroups with predominant emphysema and normal Gaw/PL slopes and those with reduced Gaw/PL slopes (see Figure 13.5(b)) were virtually identical and so are not shown. Shaded area indicates normal range. (Data from ref. 45.) (c) Comparison of mean MFSR slopes before and 6 months after lung volume reduction surgery in two separate studies. In the Gelb study[42] there was an increase in Gs and PL at TLC leading to a large increase in notional V̇max at TLC. The mean FEV₁ increased from 0.69 to 1.16 L. In the study of Ingenito,[43] initial Gs slope was lower and the major postoperative change was extension of the MFSR curve – to larger PL at TLC. Change in notional V̇max at TLC was much smaller. In this study mean FEV₁ increased from 0.69 to 0.85 L. Pre-LVRS TLC is indicated by filled squares and post-LVRS TLC by open squares. See text for further discussion. Note: In each case MFSR curves have been simplified by extending the slope observed in mid-vital capacity to zero flow and to larger lung volume (arbitrary PL of 12 cmH₂O in (a) and to mean observed PL at TLC in (b) and (c)). These conventions assume a one-compartment model with Gs and Ptm' unchanged over the VC and the change in VP curve confined to extension to a higher PL at postoperative TLC.*

dependence is preserved in a minority of patients, possibly because central airways are flow limiting.

SUMMARY

The usual major site of fixed airway narrowing in COPD during tidal breathing appears to be the peripheral airways that are less than 2–3 mm diameter. There may be individual patients in whom obstructive changes in the central airways are of greater importance. Loss of lung recoil plays a role in many patients (particularly those with panacinar emphysema) by reducing the distending force on all intrathoracic airways, but is rarely the sole cause of severe airflow limitation. Static airway narrowing due to intrinsic disease of the airways and loss of lung recoil both enhance expiratory dynamic compression so that flow limitation develops at lower driving pressures and flows. In addition, atrophic changes in the airways and loss of support from surrounding lung may alter airway compliance, enhancing dynamic compression and the development of flow limitation. The site of flow limitation in the upper part of the VC may be more peripheral in many patients with COPD than in normal subjects. The large differences between maximum inspiratory and maximum expiratory flow at the same lung volume (far in excess of the expected hysteresis of airway dimensions and lung recoil pressure) emphasize the large role of dynamic factors in determining expiratory airflow limitation.

Tests of overall airway function, such as airways conductance or FEV₁, reflect the lumped dimensions of all the airways arranged in series and in parallel but do not provide direct evidence on whether large or small airways are the site of airway narrowing. Because the resistance of peripheral airways in normal lungs is low, for the last 30 years such tests (and even more peak expiratory flow, PEF) have been correctly regarded as mainly reflecting large airway function in normal subjects. But, examining the relative changes in maximum expiratory flow on MEFV curves at large versus small volume provides useful information about the site of airway narrowing only when function is nearly normal. Once obvious airflow obstruction has developed, even when the predominant site of airway narrowing is in peripheral airways, as in COPD, this is reflected in reduced values of conductance, FEV_1 and PEF. This is most clearly indicated by the original studies of the lungs studied at necropsy by Hogg and colleagues[52] and characterized by increased peripheral airway resistance; the patients in life had had severe reductions in FEV_1.

Thus, reductions in tests of overall airway function in moderate COPD breathing air do not provide any evidence on whether large or small airways are the site of increased resistance. Indeed the value of the FEV_1 in assessing the abnormality of lung mechanics is that it integrates information on dynamic dimensions of all generations of airways and changes in lung recoil, providing a summary of 'effective' lung size and the maximum rate of lung emptying. Because the pathologic changes in COPD are mainly irreversible, FEV_1 can be regarded as providing a 'structural' summary of their effects on pulmonary mechanics, which probably contributes to its value in assessing progression and prognosis of disease. As discussed above, although derived from the highly artificial maneuver of forced expiration from TLC, values of maximum expiratory flow are relatively independent of the muscle force applied. The FEV_1, as a surrogate of the MEFV curve, is not related directly to mechanics during tidal breathing, even although there may be overall loose connections between FEV_1 and RL or FEV_1 and FRC/TLC. Obviously changes in symptoms or exercise performance will be more related to respiratory mechanics during tidal breathing; furthermore FEV_1 does not indicate the degree of hyperinflation of the subject, nor the load on the inspiratory muscles during exercise. It is therefore hardly surprising that the relation of FEV_1 to exercise performance and dyspnea is weak. As discussed below, the simple addition of measuring inspiratory capacity enhances the information obtained from spirometry.

Contributions of emphysema and intrinsic disease of the airways to alterations in lung mechanics

Many studies of lung mechanics in COPD have attempted to distinguish changes due to primary disease of the airways from those due to emphysematous changes in the terminal bronchioles and airspaces. The most characteristic change in lung mechanics associated with severe emphysema is marked loss of recoil pressure but patients with COPD thought to be due to primary bronchial

disease also show some loss of lung recoil and increase in TLC.[47] It is not clear whether this is because of a direct effect of airway obstruction alone or whether it reflects the presence of lesser or inhomogeneous emphysema among patients thought on clinical and functional grounds to have primary airway disease. In general, emphysema becomes increasingly common and severe as airways obstruction worsens in COPD. As discussed above, some patients thought to have emphysema have shown preservation of a normal relation between total lung conductance and lung recoil pressure (Figure 13.5),[45,46] and, less commonly, between maximum expiratory flow and lung recoil pressure.[38,45,47] Usually, however, emphysema and intrinsic disease of the airways coexist and both relations are abnormal. In part this may be because the value of PL does not reflect all the changes expected with emphysema, particularly if it is distributed very irregularly. Thus selective loss of alveolar wall attachments to the perimeter of airways – particularly peripheral airways – could reduce airway distension disproportionately to the measured reduction in lung recoil pressure. Even if this resulted only in a short stenotic segment,[69] the resistance of the whole pathway could be greatly increased. Overdistension of surrounding airspaces could compress and distort the contained airways even if there was no 'intrinsic' disease of the airway walls themselves.[70] Both changes would result in a reduced maximum expiratory flow at a given PL.

Characteristically patients with severe airflow limitation who develop chronic hypercapnia show low values of dynamic lung compliance, have an increased inspiratory flow resistance and a small tidal volume during resting breathing. These changes have been claimed to be characteristic of intrinsic disease of the airways rather than emphysema.

EFFECTS OF LUNG VOLUME REDUCTION SURGERY (LVRS) ON LUNG MECHANICS AND MAXIMUM EXPIRATORY FLOW

The distinction between airway and alveolar disease in causing abnormalities in lung mechanics may be particularly relevant to the selection of patients suitable for LVRS. As discussed in Chapter 32, selection depends on a full appraisal of clinical, imaging and functional features; apart from spirometry, important functional features include blood gases, CO transfer, respiratory muscle function, cardiac function and exercise performance. This section discusses only mechanisms by which spirometry may improve after LVRS; many studies suggest that improvement in spirometry is usually found when LVRS leads to clinical benefit.

The most predictable effect of LVRS is to reduce RV by the removal of non- or poorly ventilated lung. Reductions vary between subjects, but a typical value is 1.35 L. TLC is also reduced but usually by a smaller volume ($\sim$0.90 L), so that VC increases. The increase in VC occurs because when TLC is greatly enlarged, there is a reduced P_L at TLC caused by the inability of the shortened inspiratory muscles to generate as negative a pleural pressure with a maximum effort as in normal subjects. Improving the mismatch between chest wall and lung size enables a more negative pleural pressure to be generated, increasing P_L at TLC and allowing greater expansion of the remaining lung (Figure 13.5). The size of the increase in VC depends on lung compliance (close to TLC) and the relation between lung volume and the minimum pleural pressure generated with a maximum inspiratory effort, but typically VC increases by 0.4–0.5 L, which is about twice the accompanying increase in FEV_1. Because FRC is determined dynamically, the decrease after LVRS is not easy to predict, but has been found to average approximately 1.0 L. Reported increases in inspiratory capacity (IC) have been less consistent and smaller than the increases in VC, but should allow the generation of a slightly larger V_T during exercise (see Chapters 18 and 33).

Several model approaches to analyze changes after LVRS have been published.[71–73] That of Fessler and Permutt[72] proposed that the most important factor increasing maximum expiratory flow and FEV_1 was the increase in VC resulting from reduction in the mismatch between chest wall and lung volume. Further implications of their model were that the effects on VC did not depend on whether disease was homogenous or not, and that postoperative FEV_1/VC would not necessarily change. In a later study[74] they have reported how results from two surgical centers fitted their model; while increase in VC was a very important factor in postoperative increase in FEV_1, usually there was also some increase in FEV_1/VC, as observed in most other studies.[75]

In studies using an esophageal balloon-catheter, a small increase in mean P_L at TLC, ranging from 2.1 to 4.3 cmH$_2$O, has been consistently observed after LVRS;[41,42,43] but there has been no accompanying change in static compliance,[42,43] so this increase in P_L probably only indicates an extension of the preoperative VP curve without change in the rest of the curve (Figure 13.5). By contrast, several studies have shown a decrease in airflow resistance (Raw or R_L) in the tidal breathing range following LVRS.

Expansion of the remaining ventilated lung to a larger volume with wider airways by an increase in P_L would itself increase maximum expiratory flow at large volumes close to TLC. Two groups[42,43,76] have used MFSR curves[65] to examine the mechanisms increasing maximum expiratory flow after LVRS (Figure 13.8). Both Gelb and colleagues[42] and Ingenito and colleagues[43] found 6 months after operation small reductions in Ptm′ and increases in P_L at TLC, but whereas Ingenito [43] found no change in mean Gs (pre 0.12, post 0.11 L/s/cmH$_2$O), the patients described by Gelb[42] had a higher Gs before surgery

(0.20 L/s/cmH$_2$O) which rose in each subject (mean 0.27 L/s/cmH$_2$O) accounting for the unusually large increase in mean FEV_1 in their study (0.47 L) which was nearly three times as large in the study of Ingenito (0.16 L) (Figure 13.8). The reasons for this difference in baseline values and in effect of operation are not clear. Earlier, Ingenito and colleagues[77] had observed that a near normal inspiratory R_L preoperatively predicted a good increase in FEV_1 with operation, and confirmed this later with larger numbers of patients.[75] Combining this observation with their finding that an increase in P_L at TLC was the most significant postoperative change in patients who showed an improvement in FEV_1, they suggested that only when resistance preoperatively was low did the increase in maximum expiratory flow caused by increase in P_L reach useful levels (Figure 13.8).[43] They concluded that patients who had a large emphysematous, and a lesser airway component, to their disease, were more likely to improve after LVRS.[43,75,77] While these studies have given insight into the mechanical changes underlying improvements in maximum expiratory flow, they do not explain why improvements are so variable in size after successful volume reduction.

Flow, volume and pressure during tidal breathing

REST

Pattern of breathing

Although minute ventilation at rest in patients with severe airflow limitation is usually normal or slightly increased, maintaining this ventilation requires increased swings in pleural pressure to overcome increased airflow resistance and reduced dynamic compliance. Furthermore inspiration is initiated from an increased FRC, which adds an inspiratory threshold load. Hence it is not surprising that activation of the inspiratory muscles, particularly the diaphragm, is increased at rest in COPD patients.[78,79] The increase in FRC and reduction in IC restricts increase in tidal volume so that any increase in ventilation tends to be produced by increase in frequency rather than in tidal volume (V_T).[80] In some patients inspiratory time (T_I) is a lower proportion of total breath duration (T_{TOT}).[81] Patients with severe COPD and chronic hypercapnia tend to have smaller tidal volume both at rest[81] and during exercise[82] than those who maintain a normal P_{CO_2}. These altered patterns of breathing ultimately depend on neurologic control mechanisms but are clearly constrained by the alterations in lung mechanics, particularly expiratory flow limitation.

Expiratory flow limitation

In normal subjects expiratory flows generated during tidal breathing at rest are much below maximum expiratory flow and only reach maximum levels during exercise at the highest workloads. However, when maximum expiratory flow is reduced in COPD, this limit may be reached during mild exercise and, when disease is severe, even at rest.

Expiratory flow limitation (EFL) has been most commonly assessed by a comparison of tidal expiratory flow–volume curves with forced expiratory flow–volume curves. Patients in whom, at comparable absolute lung volumes, tidal flows are similar or higher than those obtained during the forced expiratory maneuver are considered to have EFL. Although this technique has been used to develop most of our present understanding of EFL, it has important practical limitations. Because of thoracic gas compression during forced expiration, tidal and maximum effort flow–volume curves have to be measured in a body plethysmograph to ensure accurate comparison at isovolume. Even then, if the forced expiration is started from TLC the volume and time history of the forced expiration differs from that of the tidal flow–volume curve. This affects the pattern of lung emptying, particularly in the presence of disease; also there are time-dependent changes in viscoelastic properties which tend to reduce maximum expiratory flow at isovolume.[83] These effects can be reduced by starting forced expiration from the end-tidal volume (partial expiratory flow–volume (PEFV) curves). Recently, a simple technique has been introduced to detect tidal expiratory flow limitation.[84–86] In this method a negative expiratory pressure (NEP) of -3 to -5 cmH$_2$O is applied at the airway opening during tidal

expiration and the resultant flow compared with the preceding control breath (Figure 13.9). EFL is present if applying NEP does not increase tidal flow on expiration. With this technique the volume and time history, as well as the intrathoracic pressures, during the expiration with NEP are the same as in the preceding control breath. This method does not require elaborate equipment or patient cooperation and coordination, and can be applied in any desired body position at rest, during exercise and during mechanical ventilation.[87] Because EFL is highly dependent on lung volume it is important to link the NEP technique with measurement of inspiratory capacity so that the position of the tidal volume within the VC is known. This is particularly important when comparing sitting and supine measurements.

The effects of EFL during tidal breathing may be reduced by decreasing TI/TTOT (allowing more time for expiration) and, more effectively, by breathing tidally closer to TLC, where airway size, and consequently maximum expiratory flow, is greater. However, both these adaptations increase the work of the inspiratory muscles: the former by increasing the mean inspiratory flow needed to sustain a given total ventilation, the latter by increasing the elastic work required to inflate the lungs and chest wall.

Thus, although airflow limitation is predominantly expiratory, compensation is achieved by increased work by the inspiratory muscles; most of the increased tidal swings in pleural (esophageal) pressures in these patients are inspiratory.

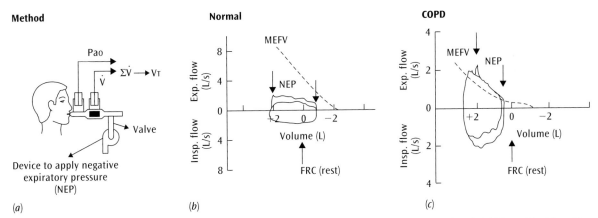

Figure 13.9 Detection of expiratory flow limitation by applying negative expiratory pressure (NEP). (a) The subject breathes initially through a pneumotachograph screen which records flow (V̇), which is integrated to obtain tidal volume (VT). After recording baseline VT, NEP of −5 cmH₂0 is applied during the next VT, reducing pressure at the airway opening (Pao) by 5 cmH₂0. (b,c) Both results were obtained during moderate intensity exercise. In the normal subject (b) expiratory flow increases but apart from a transient spike of flow there is no change in a patient with COPD (c). The flow and volume scales are different in the two panels. Note the rectangular shape of the tidal flow–volume curve in the normal, contrasting with the shape in COPD. Change in volume is referred to FRC at rest: note the decrease in normal and increase in COPD during exercise. The dashed diagonal lines show the position of the complete MEFV curves obtained in a body plethysmograph. There are considerable reserves of expiratory flow capacity in the normal subject. In the COPD subject at baseline, tidal expiratory flow exceeds that on the MEFV curve at the same volume. (Adapted from ref. 85.)

Dynamic hyperinflation

In normal subjects at rest, the end-expiratory lung volume (FRC) corresponds to the relaxation volume (Vr) of the respiratory system, i.e. the lung volume at which the elastic recoil pressure of the total respiratory system is zero (Figure 13.10). Pulmonary hyperinflation is defined as an increase of FRC above predicted normal. This may be caused by increased Vr due to loss of elastic recoil of the lung (e.g. emphysema) or by dynamic pulmonary hyperinflation which is present when the FRC exceeds Vr. Dynamic hyperinflation exists whenever the duration of expiration is insufficient to allow the lungs to deflate to Vr prior to the next inspiration. This tends to occur when expiratory flow is impeded (e.g. increased airway resistance) or when the expiratory time is shortened (e.g. increased breathing frequency). Expiratory flow may also be slowed by persistent contraction of the inspiratory muscles during expiration or by expiratory narrowing of the glottic aperture. Most commonly, however, dynamic pulmonary hyperinflation is observed in patients who exhibit expiratory flow limitation during resting breathing.

Intrinsic positive end-expired pressure (PEEPi)

Under normal conditions when end-expired volume equals Vr, the end-expiratory elastic recoil pressure of the total respiratory system (lungs and chest wall) is zero (case A in Figure 13.10). In this instance, as soon as the inspiratory muscles contract, the alveolar pressure becomes subatmospheric and gas flows into the lungs. When breathing takes place at lung volumes higher than Vr, the end-expiratory elastic recoil pressure is positive (15 cmH$_2$O in case B of Figure 13.10). The elastic recoil pressure present at end-expiration has been termed occult PEEP, auto PEEP, or intrinsic PEEP (PEEPi). When PEEPi is present, the onset of inspiratory muscle activity and inspiratory flow are not synchronous: inspiratory flow starts only when the pressure developed by the inspiratory muscles exceeds PEEPi because only then does alveolar pressure become subatmospheric. In this respect, intrinsic PEEP acts as an inspiratory threshold load which increases the static elastic work of breathing. This places a significant extra burden on the inspiratory muscles, which are operating under disadvantageous force–length conditions and abnormal thoracic geometry.

Patients with severe COPD may contract their abdominal muscles in the second half of expiration raising end-expired abdominal and pleural pressures, which fall rapidly with relaxation of abdominal muscles after the start of inspiration.[88] In spontaneously breathing patients who are not increasing pleural pressure at the end of tidal expiration by contracting abdominal muscles, PEEPi can be estimated as the negative deflection in esophageal pressure from the start of inspiratory effort to the onset of inspiratory flow. This pressure is termed dynamic PEEPi. Values of dynamic PEEPi are usually lower than those of static PEEPi obtained by the end-expiratory occlusion technique used during mechanical ventilation.[89]

Work of breathing

In 1954 McIlroy and Christie[90] observed that the mechanical work of breathing was increased in stable COPD patients, which they attributed to increased airway and 'viscous' resistance of the lung. In later studies it was suggested that in COPD patients there is an increase of work of breathing also as a result of time constant inequality within the lung which causes an increase of effective dynamic pulmonary elastance and flow resistance,[91] and intrinsic PEEP.[92]

If PEEPi is absent and static elastance of the respiratory system (Est,rs) is linear over the volume change considered (ΔV), the static inspiratory work per breath is given by

$$W_I,st,rs = 0.5\ Est,rs\ \Delta V \qquad (1)$$

If PEEPi is present, equation 1 becomes

$$W_I,st,rs = 0.5\ Est,rs\ \Delta V + PEEPi\ \Delta V \qquad (2)$$

Figure 13.10 illustrates the static elastic work required from the inspiratory muscles for the same tidal volume inhaled from Vr and from a higher lung volume. As shown by the hatched areas, W$_I$,st,rs increases markedly

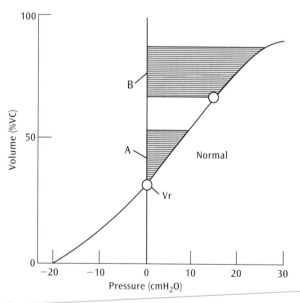

Figure 13.10 *Volume–pressure diagram of the relaxed respiratory system showing the increase in static elastic work caused by dynamic hyperinflation. VC: vital capacity; Vr: relaxation volume of the respiratory system; hatched area A: elastic work for a breath that starts from relaxation volume; hatched area B: elastic work for a similar breath that starts from a volume 29% VC higher than Vr. In case B, the intrinsic PEEP is 15 cmH₂O, as indicated by the upper circle, and W$_{PEEPi}$ is given by PEEPi × tidal volume.*

when the breath is taken at a higher lung volume. In this example, the increase in WI,st,rs is due mainly to PEEPi, though an increase in Est,rs (as reflected by the decreased slope of the static VP curve at the higher lung volume) also plays a role. Clearly, during spontaneous breathing dynamic hyperinflation implies an increase of static inspiratory work, and hence in inspiratory muscle effort. Furthermore, as lung volume increases there is a decrease in effectiveness of the inspiratory muscles as pressure generators, because the inspiratory muscle fibers become shorter and their geometrical arrangement changes. In addition to these increases in static elastic work, resistive work on inspiration is invariably increased due to airway obstruction. The effectiveness of nasal positive-pressure ventilation in exacerbations of COPD is largely due to relief of some of this increased load on the inspiratory muscles.

Relationship of FEV_1 to expiratory flow limitation at rest

Figure 13.11 depicts the relationship between FEV_1 (% predicted) and EFL in 117 stable COPD patients.[84] Expiratory flow limitation was determined during resting breathing in sitting and supine positions. Though, on average, the patients who had EFL both seated and supine had a significantly lower FEV_1 (% predicted) than those without EFL, there was marked scatter of the data. Indeed, 60% of the non-EFL group had an FEV_1 below 49% predicted and would be classified as having severe to very severe airway obstruction. Although a patient with a low FEV_1 and severe impairment of maximum expiratory flow throughout the VC is potentially more prone to show EFL, whether this is present at rest depends on the total ventilation, breathing pattern and absolute end-inspired

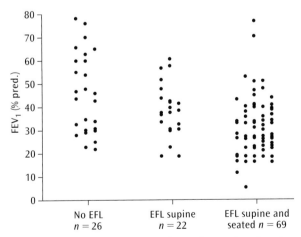

Figure 13.11 *Individual values of FEV_1 (% predicted) and tidal expiratory flow limitation (EFL) of 117 chronic obstructive pulmonary disease patients while seated and supine at rest. *P < 0.002 for non-EFL versus EFL both seated and supine. (From ref. 84 with permission.)*

and end-expired lung volumes, as well as the maximum flow capacity over the chosen tidal volume range.

EXERCISE

Maximum exercise ventilation – prediction from measurements at rest

The highest pulmonary ventilation that a subject can achieve is ultimately limited by the highest flows that can be generated, which in turn are determined by the maximum expiratory and inspiratory flow–volume envelope. Because strenuous exercise is accompanied by some bronchodilatation,[93] the relevant flow–volume envelope is probably that obtained after bronchodilators. Attempts to predict maximum exercise ventilation from resting measurements are only approximations, so it has been difficult to be certain that a truly maximum ventilation is reached at the limits of exercise in COPD. Multiplying the FEV_1 (liters) by 35 or 40 to estimate maximum breathing capacity considerably underestimates the maximum exercise ventilation achieved by patients with the most severe expiratory airflow limitation.[80,94] Measuring maximum voluntary ventilation over 15 seconds, entails a breathing pattern of smaller tidal volumes, more rapid frequency of breathing and larger pressure swings than are used during exercise.[95] Maximum exercise ventilation can be predicted better by measuring the maximum voluntary ventilation that can be sustained for 4 minutes[96] while maintaining isocapnia. Indirect methods incorporating maximum inspiratory flow and pressure have also been proposed.[97]

Expiratory flow limitation and dynamic hyperinflation

A useful way to examine ventilatory limitations to exercise in COPD is to compare the tidal flow–volume curves as workload is increased with the maximum inspiratory and expiratory flow–volume envelope.[95] In this way the presence of EFL, the 'flow reserve' at different volumes on inspiration and expiration, and the effects of moving tidal breathing to larger lung volumes, can all be visualized, indicating the necessity for patients with COPD and EFL at rest to develop further dynamic hyperinflation when the requirement for ventilation is increased by exercise. A full account of the breathing strategy adopted by patients with COPD on exercise and how it differs from that of normal subjects is given in Chapter 18.

Lung mechanics, exercise performance and dyspnea

In COPD there are only loose relations between FEV_1, exercise performance and the sensation of dyspnea. This is hardly surprising, because FEV_1 is only indirectly related to the increased inspiratory load during exercise. A somewhat better relation has been found between EFL at rest as measured with the NEP technique, and chronic dyspnea in COPD[84]. But this relationship in turn probably reflects the association of EFL with dynamic hyperinflation and an increased FRC and reduced IC. Several recent studies have shown there is a somewhat stronger correlation between exercise capacity and IC than with FEV_1[98–101] and that an important effect of bronchodilators is increase in IC. This reflects that in these patients the maximal tidal volume (and hence ventilation) is necessarily closely related to the impairment of IC; during exercise end-expiratory volume increases and end-inspired volume approaches TLC. The increase in end-expiratory volume is achieved exclusively by an increase in ribcage volume;[102] as in normal subjects, there is a small decrease in end-expired abdominal volume. This change in chest cage configuration assists diaphragm function by minimizing the decrease in its length that would otherwise occur with increase in end-expired volume. At the breaking point of exercise, tidal inspiratory flow also approaches maximum levels. These changes in breathing pattern are achieved by increased tidal swings in pleural pressure, which are predominantly due to more negative inspiratory pressures, at least until approaching the breaking point of exercise when more positive pleural pressures in the range $15–20\,cmH_2O$ are generated. Some studies have suggested that the sensation of dyspnea during exercise is related to the generation of more negative inspiratory pressures.

These observations emphasize the importance of the ability to sustain inspiratory muscle force during exercise and have provoked many experiments to examine whether muscle fatigue occurs. These are discussed in Chapter 15. During strenuous exercise in COPD patients, the O_2 requirements of the respiratory muscles have been estimated to be as much as 40% of the observed O_2 consumption;[103] thus, in contrast to normal subjects, there is significant competition between limb and respiratory muscles for the available O_2 (see Chapter 18) for further discussion).

ACUTE RESPIRATORY FAILURE

Until recently few studies have been made of the changes in lung mechanics in exacerbations of disease in COPD and it is only in the last years that adequate studies have been made during the most severe episodes, requiring assisted ventilation. For the purposes of this section we define acute respiratory failure as worsening arterial oxygenation and acute ventilatory failure as an increase in arterial Pco_2; implicitly these exacerbations will have occurred on the background of considerable and persistent underlying abnormalities in lung mechanics.

Origins of increased work of breathing
Acute ventilatory failure in COPD patients is commonly triggered by airway infection. As a result, there is an acute increase in airway resistance which causes increased resistive work of breathing, and promotes dynamic hyperinflation. The latter is further exacerbated by the tachypnea which is invariably present in COPD patients with acute respiratory failure (ARF). Expiratory flow limitation is present during tidal breathing. Dynamic hyperinflation promotes an increase in the static elastic work of breathing which can be due both to PEEPi and decreased lung compliance (Figure 13.8). The highest values of PEEPi observed in stable COPD patients are in the order of $7–9\,cmH_2O$,[104] but with ARF values up to $13\,cmH_2O$ during spontaneous breathing[92] and $22\,cmH_2O$ during mechanical ventilation[105] have been reported. As a result the work of breathing is markedly increased. This increase in work of breathing, in association with the impaired inspiratory muscle performance, produces a heavy load on the inspiratory muscles (Figure 13.12). As a result, the patient may need to be mechanically ventilated.

The average inspiratory work of the respiratory system (WI,rs) and its components in 10 mechanically ventilated sedated paralyzed COPD patients with ARF are shown in Figure 13.13 together with the corresponding values obtained in 18 anaesthetized paralyzed normal subjects.[106] The measurements were obtained during constant-flow inflation with tidal volume of 0.73 L, frequency of 12.5 breaths per minute and inspiratory duration of 0.92 seconds. WI,rs was twofold greater in COPD patients than in normal subjects, the difference reflecting an increase of both static (WI,st,rs) and dynamic (WI,dyn,rs) work. The increase in WI,st,rs in these COPD

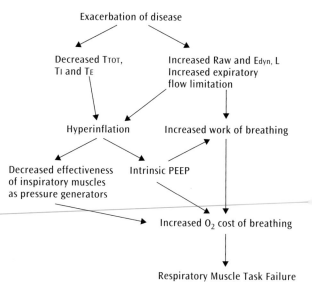

Figure 13.12 *Scheme of the pathophysiology causing acute ventilatory failure in COPD patients. T_{TOT}: total breathing cycle duration; T_I and T_E: inspiratory and expiratory times; Raw: airway resistance; Edyn,L: dynamic lung elastance.*

patients was due almost entirely to the work due to PEEPi (WI,PEEPi) which represented 57% of the overall increase in WI,rs exhibited by the COPD patients relative to normal subjects. These studies agree with those of Guérin *et al.*[107] and Tantucci *et al.*[108] in finding normal values of Est,rs in COPD patients with ARF. By contrast, Broseghini *et al.*,[105] who studied COPD patients during the first day of mechanical ventilation, found increased values of Est,rs (Table 13.2). This was due in part to the fact that these patients had a more marked degree of dynamic pulmonary hyperinflation, and hence their ΔV during mechanical ventilation impinged into the flatter part of their static VP curves (Figure 13.8). Even in these patients, however, most of the increase of static work was due to PEEPi.

In the COPD patients in Figure 13.13, the increase in WI,dyn,rs accounted for 43% of the overall increase in inspiratory work. Airway resistive work (WI,aw) was, on

average, 3.3 times higher than in the normal subjects, and contributed 34% of the overall increase in WI,rs. The increase in WI,aw in the COPD patients reflects increased airway resistance (Raw); according to Guérin *et al.* [107] and Tantucci *et al.* [108] at similar inflation volume and flow, Raw in COPD patients with ARF was about 3.5 times higher than in normal subjects (Table 13.2). Higher values of Raw were found by Broseghini *et al.*,[105] presumably because their patients were studied on the first day of ARF. The results in Figure 13.13 do not include the resistive work done on the endotracheal tubes which is relatively high. With an endotracheal tube size 7 this work amounted to 4.8 cmH₂O/L and even with tube size 9 was 2.0 cmH₂O/L, compared to a value of 3.8 cmH₂O/L for WI,aw due to the lungs themselves.

The remainder of the increase in WI,dyn,rs was accounted for by an increase in the additional work done

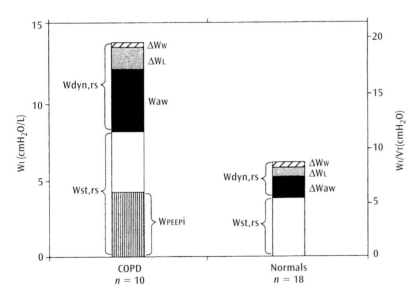

Figure 13.13 *Average values of inspiratory work (WI) done on the respiratory system and its components in 10 COPD patients and 18 normal anaesthetized paralyzed subjects with inflation flow of 0.8 L/s and tidal volume of 0.73 L. Wst,rs: total static work of respiratory system; WPEEPi: static work due to intrinsic PEEP; Wdyn,rs: total dynamic work of respiratory system; Waw: airway resistive work; ΔWw: viscoelastic work of chest wall; ΔWL: work of lung due to time constant inequality and/or viscoelastic pressure dissipations. Work per liter of inspired volume (WI/VT) is shown on right ordinate. (Reproduced from ref. 106 with permission.)*

Table 13.2 *Mean values (±SE) of baseline ventilatory settings and respiratory mechanics in mechanically ventilated COPD patients with ARF*

Authors	n	Time (days)	ΔV (L)	V̇ (L/s)	TI (s)	TE (s)	PEEPi (cmH₂O)	ΔFRC (L)	Est,rs (cmH₂O/L)	Raw (cmH₂O/L/s)	ΔRrs (cmH₂O/L/s)	Rrs (cmH₂O/L/s)
Broseghini *et al.*[105]	8	1	0.69 ±0.03	0.62 ±0.01	1.20 ±0.05	2.14 ±0.05	13.6 ±0.8	0.66 ±0.10	17.9 ±0.01	15.6 ±3.1	10.8 ±2.0	26.4 ±4.7
Tantucci *et al.*[108]	6	1–4	0.80 ±0.04	1.01 ±0.03	0.93 ±0.04	3.35 ±0.04	4.6 ±0.9	0.42 ±0.18	11.1 ±0.01	8.0 ±1.8	5.5 ±1.0	13.5 ±1.0
Guérin *et al.*[107]	10	1–16	0.73 ±0.02	0.80 ±0.03	0.92 ±0.01	3.98 ±0.20	5.7 ±0.9	0.34 ±0.06	12.6 ±0.7	7.2 ±0.6	5.6 ±0.5	12.8 ±1.1

n: number of patients studied; time: days from onset of ARF; ΔV: tidal volume; V̇: inspiratory flow; TI: inspiratory time; TE: expiratory time; PEEPi: intrinsic end-expiratory positive pressure; ΔFRC: difference between the end-expiratory lung volume during mechanical ventilation and the relaxation volume; Est,rs: static elastance of respiratory system; Raw: airway resistance; ΔRrs: additional resistance due to time constant inequality and/or viscoelastic behavior; Rrs: total resistance of respiratory system.

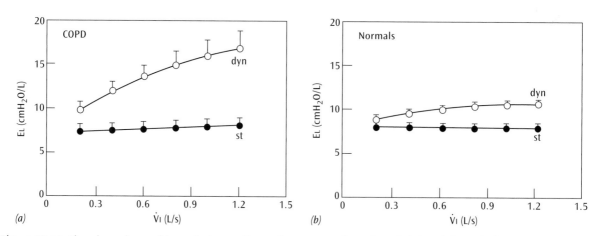

Figure 13.14 *Flow dependence of lung elastance. Change in average values of static (st) and dynamic (dyn) elastance of the lungs (EL) at constant inflation volume (ΔV = 0.73 L) delivered at varying inspiratory flow (V̇I) in 10 COPD patients with ARF[68] (a) and 18 normal subjects[70] (b). Because ΔV was constant, increasing V̇I corresponds to shortening TI. Scale bars = SE. (Reproduced from ref. 107 with permission.)*

on the lung ($\Delta W_{I,L}$); the dynamic work due to the tissues of the chest wall ($\Delta W_{I,W}$) was similar in COPD patients to that of normal subjects. $\Delta W_{I,L}$ is the additional work done on the lung as a result of pressure dissipations caused by viscoelastic behavior of pulmonary tissue and/or time constant inequality.[91,106,107] As originally proposed by Mount[109] in 1955 to explain the decline in dynamic pulmonary compliance with increasing frequency of breathing, $\Delta W_{I,L}$ in normal subjects predominantly reflects viscoelastic behavior of the lungs which 'confers time-dependency of the elastic properties'.[110,111] By contrast, in COPD patients $\Delta W_{I,L}$ should include a substantial component due to time constant inequality.[91,106] This probably explains the higher values of $\Delta W_{I,L}$ found in the COPD patients with ARF in whom $\Delta W_{I,L}$ was, on average, 2.3 times higher than in normal subjects. This increase of $\Delta W_{I,L}$, however, represented only 9% of the overall increase in $W_{I,rs}$ observed in the COPD patients.

Predictably, the increase of $\Delta W_{I,L}$ in COPD patients is associated with more marked time-dependency of pulmonary elastance than in normal subjects, as shown in Figure 13.14 which depicts the relationship of static and dynamic elastance of the lung ($E_{dyn,L} = 1/C_{dyn,L}$) to inspiratory flow obtained at a fixed inflation volume ($\Delta V = 0.73$ L) in 10 COPD patients with ARF[107] and 18 normal subjects.[110] Because inflation volume was fixed, an increase in inspiratory flow ($\Delta V̇I$) implies a shorter duration of inspiration (TI), $\Delta V̇I$ being proportional to 1/TI, so the data in Figure 13.14 actually depict TI dependence of elastic properties. While $E_{st,L}$ was independent of TI and $\Delta V̇I$ in both COPD patients and normal subjects, $E_{dyn,L}$ increased progressively with increasing $\Delta V̇I$, or, more appropriately, with decreasing

duration of inspiration (TI). In COPD patients the increase in $E_{dyn,L}$ with increasing flow was greater than in normal subjects because of time-constant inequality.[107] In normal lungs the time-dependency of pulmonary elastance is due almost entirely to viscoelastic behavior.[110,111]

Table 13.2 depicts the 'effective' additional resistance (ΔR_{rs}) due to time-constant inequality within the lung and viscoelastic behavior of pulmonary and chest wall tissue in COPD patients with ARF. In this instance, ΔR_{rs} represented about 40% of the total resistance of the respiratory system (R_{rs}) and was substantially higher than normal. It should be noted, however, that ΔR_{rs} exhibits marked time-dependency, decreasing progressively with decreasing TI. The values of ΔR_{rs} in Table 13.2 pertain to experimental TI ranging from 0.9 to 1.2 seconds.

Figure 13.15 depicts the average relationships between total respiratory resistance (R_{rs}) and inspiratory flow obtained at fixed inflation volume ($\Delta V = 0.5$ L) in six COPD patients with ARF[108] and 16 normal subjects.[111] At all comparable flow rates, R_{rs} was about threefold higher in the COPD patients. In both normals and COPD patients R_{rs} ($= R_{aw} + \Delta R_{rs}$) was highest at the lowest flow and decreased progressively with $\Delta V̇I$ up to 1 L/s. At this V̇I, R_{rs} had a minimal value. This phenomenon is due to the fact that as V̇I decreased there was a greater decrease of ΔR_{rs} as compared to the concomitant increase of R_{aw}. At V̇I > 1 L/s, R_{rs} tended to increase slightly in the COPD patients, reflecting the fact that over this range of V̇I the increase of R_{aw} becomes predominant. The initial decrease in R_{rs} with increasing flow represents a clinically important aspect because it occurs in the inflation flow range commonly used in the ICU setting (0.5–1 L/s). Fuller accounts of $\Delta W_{I,L}$ and $\Delta W_{I,WL}$ can be found elsewhere.[106,107]

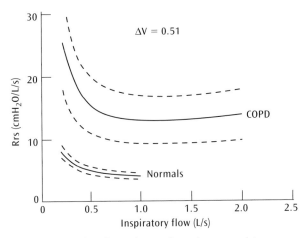

Figure 13.15 *Flow dependence of respiratory resistance. Average ± SEM relationship between total respiratory system resistance (Rrs) and inspiratory flow at constant inflation volume of 0.5 L in six sedated paralysed COPD patients and 16 normal anaesthetized and paralyzed subjects. (From ref. 108 with permission.)*

Implications of PEEPi during mechanical ventilation (see also Chapter 28)

The putative role of patient-triggered, assisted mechanical ventilation is to reduce the activity of the inspiratory muscles to tolerable levels. This end is not always achieved because the pressure which has to be generated by the patient to trigger the ventilator necessarily includes PEEPi. If this is high, the inspiratory effort required by the patient may be excessive.[112] By contrast, during controlled mechanical ventilation all of the work of breathing is done by the ventilator. Nevertheless, PEEPi must be taken into account for correct measurement of respiratory compliance[113] and, more importantly, in terms of its adverse effects on cardiac output. In fact, PEEPi may severely decrease venous return and cardiac output, depending upon intravascular volume status, myocardial function and other factors. Because patients with COPD on mechanical ventilation usually have EFL on passive deflation, care has to be taken that the chosen duty cycle allows sufficient time for passive deflation without further increase in FRC.

Patients with high levels of PEEPi and EFL are difficult to wean from mechanical ventilation and may become ventilator dependent.[114]

Monitoring PEEPi

Fundamental in the management of the mechanically ventilated COPD patients is to monitor PEEPi. Indeed, measurement of PEEPi should be a part of routine monitoring in mechanically ventilated patients, particularly those with airways obstruction. This allows reliable measurement and interpretation of other frequently determined cardiopulmonary variables, such as respiratory

system compliance, pulmonary capillary wedge pressure, etc. The potential adverse effects of PEEPi require that, in addition, management should be specifically directed towards those factors contributing to the development of PEEPi. This includes medical therapy aimed at reducing the severity of airflow obstruction as well as excessive minute ventilation (due to fever, metabolic acidosis, inadequate pain relief, etc.). The inspiratory flow settings should be adjusted such as to maximize the time available for passive expiration.

A simple way to detect the presence of dynamic hyperinflation, and hence of PEEPi, is to monitor the expiratory flow–time profile. When PEEPi is absent, there is a period of zero flow prior to the next spontaneous or mechanical lung inflation. By contrast, when PEEPi is present there is flow throughout expiration, which is abruptly terminated by the next spontaneous breath or by mechanical lung inflation (Figure 13.16(a)).

In mechanically ventilated patients, PEEPi will not normally register on the ventilator manometer. During exhalation, the ventilator manometer is exposed to ambient pressure as the exhalation valve is open. Only the expiratory pressure dissipations due to the valve resistance or the applied PEEP will register on the ventilator manometer. Despite the fact that the alveolar pressure may be positive throughout exhalation, the manometer will not reflect the increased pressure unless the expiratory port is occluded. If the expiratory port is occluded at end-expiration, alveolar pressure and circuit pressure equilibrate, and PEEPi is seen on the ventilator manometer.[115] Figure 13.16(b) illustrates this method to determine PEEPi in a COPD patient during controlled mechanical ventilation. End-expiratory occlusion was done using the end-expiratory hold button on a Siemens 900C Servo ventilator. Following occlusion, the airway pressure rises until it reaches a plateau which corresponds to PEEPi. It should be noted, however, that most ventilators are not equipped with an end-expiratory hold button.

During controlled mechanical ventilation the magnitude of dynamic hyperinflation can be determined by inserting a prolonged expiratory time during steady-state mechanical ventilation[105,116] (Figure 13.16(b)). In this way ΔFRC (i.e. the difference between the end-expiratory lung volume during steady-state mechanical ventilation and Vr) is obtained.

Strategies to reduce the inspiratory load caused by PEEPi

As implied in Figure 13.12, treatment of COPD patients with respiratory failure should be aimed toward increasing the expiratory duration as well as decreasing respiratory flow resistance. To the extent that tachypnea is due to fever and/or airway infection, resolution of these by antibiotic treatment should be beneficial.

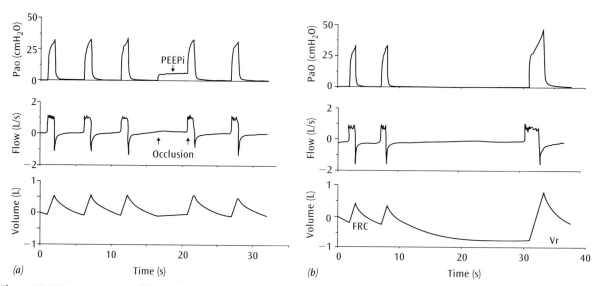

Figure 13.16 *Measurement of intrinsic PEEP and dynamic hyperinflation during mechanical ventilation. (a) Records of pressure at the airway opening (Pao), flow and changes in lung volume during mechanical ventilation in a sedated paralyzed COPD patient. Note that flow continues throughout expiration and is abruptly terminated by the onset of the next breath, indicating the presence of dynamic hyperinflation and PEEPi. PEEPi is measured by end-expiratory airway occlusion (indicated by the first arrow). Upon occlusion, flow drops to zero and airway pressure rises and reaches a plateau that corresponds to the static end-expiratory elastic recoil pressure of the respiratory system (=PEEPi). In this patient PEEPi was 5.5 cmH$_2$O. (b) Records as in (a), illustrating the measurement of ΔFRC which is the difference between end-expiratory lung volume during steady-state mechanical ventilation (FRC) and the relaxation volume of the respiratory system (Vr). A prolonged expiratory time was inserted during steady-state mechanical ventilation that allowed the patient to exhale to Vr. ΔFRC in this patient amounted to 0.67 L. (From ref. 116.)*

Bronchodilator treatment. Effective bronchodilator administration may be useful in reducing both flow resistance and PEEPi. Recent studies have shown that in spontaneously breathing patients, bronchodilators increase IC in those patients who are hyperinflated due to EFL[117,118] and that this change is associated with reduction of dyspnea both at rest and during light exercise and with increased exercise performance.[98,99,118] Hence bronchodilator response, particularly in severe COPD, should be assessed by change in IC as well as by FEV$_1$. Because performance of IC precedes the expiratory FVC maneuver, IC can be recorded easily on many spirometers, but unfortunately at present some devices are only set up for expiratory maneuvers.

The response to bronchodilators can also be assessed during mechanical ventilation. When they are given to relaxed patients receiving mechanical ventilation with a fixed tidal volume and expiratory time, there is an increased expiratory flow at isovolume which results in a decrease in end-expired volume and intrinsic PEEP and the establishment of a new equilibrium at a smaller operating volume.[119] Usually inspiratory resistance is still decreased at this smaller volume; when constant flow inspiration is used, the combined effect of these two changes are reflected in a reduced peak pressure at the airway opening (Pao peak). If an end-inspiratory pause is applied and plateau pressure at the airway opening measured (Pao plat) before and after bronchodilators, ΔPao peak can be divided into the fall due to reduction in end-inspired volume (ΔPao plat) and due to decrease in inspiratory airflow resistance (ΔPao peak − ΔPao plat).

Pressure support. A promising approach to deal with PEEPi is to apply continuous positive airway pressure (CPAP) through a face or nasal mask (often accompanied by positive pressure ventilation) to spontaneously breathing patients with severe COPD during exacerbations or during weaning after a period of mechanical ventilation.[120–122] Application of external PEEP during patient-triggered mechanical ventilation can be used to counterbalance and reduce the inspiratory load imposed by PEEPi.[112] These techniques are described in detail in Chapters 27 and 28.

ACKNOWLEDGEMENTS

The financial support of the Canadian Medical Research Council and Imperial Cancer Research Fund is gratefully acknowledged. The authors would like to thank Angie Bentivegna and Mrs Jan Marshall for typing the manuscript.

REFERENCES

1. Pride NB, Macklem PT. Lung mechanics in disease. In: PT Macklem, J Mead, eds. *Handbook of Physiology, Mechanics of Breathing*, sect 3, vol 3. American Physiological Society, Bethesda, MD. 1986, pp 659–92.

2. Macklem PT, Permutt S, eds. *Lung Biology in Health and Disease. The Lung in Transition Between Health and Disease*, vol. 12. Dekker, New York, 1979.

3. Wagner EM, Bleecker ER, Permutt S, Liu MC. Peripheral airways resistance in smokers. *Am Rev Respir Dis* 1992;**146**:92–5.

4. Macklem PT, Proctor DF, Hogg JC. The stability of peripheral airways. *Respir Physiol* 1970;**8**:191–203.

5. Leblanc P, Ruff F, Milic-Emili J. Effects of age and body position on 'airway closure' in man. *J Appl Physiol* 1970;**28**:448–51.

6. Buist AS, Vollmer WM, Johnson LR, McCamant LE. Does the single-breath N2 test identify the smoker who will develop chronic airflow limitation? *Am Rev Respir Dis* 1988;**137**:293–301.

7. King GG, Eberl S, Salome CM, Young IH, Woolcock AJ. Differences in airway closure between normal and asthmatic subjects measured with single-photon emission computed tomography. *Am J Respir Crit Care Med* 1998;**158**:1900–06.

8. Woolcock AJ, Vincent NJ, Macklem PT. Frequency dependence of compliance as a test for obstruction in the small airways. *J Clin Invest* 1969;**48**:1097–106.

9. Coe CI, Watson A, Joyce H, Pride NB. Effects of smoking on changes in respiratory resistance with increasing age. *Clin Sci* 1989;**76**:487–94.

10. Black LF, Offord K, Hyatt RE. Variability in the maximal expiratory flow volume curve in asymptomatic smokers and in non-smokers. *Am Rev Respir Dis* 1974;**110**:282–92.

11. Dosman J, Bode F, Urbanetti J, Martin R, Macklem PT. The use of a helium-oxygen mixture during maximum expiratory flow to demonstrate obstruction in small airways in smokers. *J Clin Invest* 1975;**55**:1090–9.

12. Hutcheon M, Griffin P, Levison H, Zamel N. Volume of isoflow. A new test in detection of mild abnormalities of lung mechanics. *Am Rev Respir Dis* 1974;**110**:458–65.

13. Cosio M, Ghezzo H, Hogg JC, *et al.* The relations between structural changes in small airways and pulmonary function tests. *N Engl J Med* 1978;**298**:1277–81.

14. Berend N, Thurbeck WM. Correlations of maximum expiratory flow with small airway dimensions and pathology. *J Appl Physiol Respir Environ Exercise Physiol* 1982;**52**:346–51.

15. Meadows JA III, Rodarte JR, Hyatt RE. Density dependence of maximal expiratory flow in chronic obstructive pulmonary disease. *Am Rev Respir Dis* 1980;**121**:47–54.

16. Oloffson J, Bake B, Svardsudd K, Skoogh BE. The single breath N2-test predicts the rate of decline in FEV1: the study of men born in 1913 and 1923. *Eur J Respir Dis* 1986;**69**:46–56.

17. Stanescu DC, Rodenstein DO, Hoeven C, Robert A. 'Sensitive tests' are poor predictors of the decline in forced expiratory volume in one second in middle-aged smokers. *Am Rev Respir Dis* 1987;**135**:585–90.

18. Stanescu D, Sanna A, Veriter C, Robert A. Identification of smokers susceptible to development of chronic airflow limitation. *Chest* 1998;**114**:416–25.

19. Cherniack RM, McCarthy DS. Reversibility of abnormalities of pulmonary function. In: PT Macklem, S Permutt, eds. *Lung Biology and Health Disease. The Lung in the Transition between Health and Disease*, vol 12. Dekker, New York, 1979, pp 329–42.

20. Bedell GN, Marshall R, DuBois AB, Comroe JH Jr. Plethysmographic determination of the volume of gas trapped in the lungs. *J Clin Invest* 1956;**35**:664–70.

21. Butler J, Caro CG, Alcala R, DuBois AB. Physiological factors affecting airway resistance in normal subjects and in patients with obstructive respiratory disease. *J Clin Invest* 1960;**39**:584–91.

22. Tierney DF, Nadel JA. Concurrent measurements of functional residual capacity by three methods. *J Appl Physiol* 1962;**17**:871–3.

23. Rodenstein DO, Stanescu DC. Reassessment of lung volume measurement by helium dilution and by body plethysmography in chronic airflow obstruction. *Am Rev Respir Dis* 1982;**126**:1040–4.

24. Shore SA, Huk O, Mannix S, Martin JG. Effect of panting frequency on the plethysmographic determination of thoracic gas volume in chronic obstructive pulmonary disease. *Am Rev Respir Dis* 1983;**128**:54–9.

25. Kim WD, Eidelman DH, Izquierdo JL, Ghezzo H, Saetta MP, Cosio MG. Centrilobular and panlobular emphysema in smokers. Two distinct morphologic and functional entities. *Am Rev Respir Dis* 1991;**144**:1385–90.

26. Colebatch HJH, Greaves IA, Ng CKY. Exponential analysis of elastic recoil and aging in healthy males and females. *J Appl Physiol Respir Environ Exercise Physiol* 1979;**47**:683–91.

27. Gibson GJ, Pride NB, Davis J, Schroter RC. Exponential description of the static pressure–volume curve of normal and diseased lung. *Am Rev Respir Dis* 1979;**120**:799–811.

28. Knudson RJ, Kaltenhorn WT. Evaluation of lung elastic recoil by exponential curve analysis. *Respir Physiol* 1981;**46**:29–42.

29. Greaves IA, Colebatch HJH. Elastic behaviour and structure of normal and emphysematous lungs post-mortem. *Am Rev Respir Dis* 1980;**121**:127–36.

30. Paré PD, Brooks LA, Bates J. Exponential analysis of the lung pressure – volume curve as a predictor of pulmonary emphysema. *Am Rev Respir Dis* 1982;**126**:54–61.

31. Nagai A, Yamawaki I, Thurlbeck WM, Takizawa T. Assessment of lung parenchymal destruction by using routine histological tissue sections. *Am Rev Respir Dis* 1989;**139**:313–19.

32. Saetta M, Ghezzo H, Won Dong K, *et al.* Loss of alveolar attachments in smokers. *Am Rev Respir Dis* 1985;**132**:894–900.

33. Petty TL, Silvers GW, Stanford RE. Radial traction and small airways disease in excised human lungs. *Am Rev Respir Dis* 1986;**133**:132–5.

34. Hogg JC, Nepszy SJ, Macklem PT, Thurlbeck WM. Elastic properties of the centrilobular emphysematous space. *J Clin Invest* 1969;**48**:1306–12.

35. Nagai A, Thurlbeck WM. Scanning electron microscopic observations of emphysema in humans. *Am Rev Respir Dis* 1991;**144**:901–8.

36. McLean A, Warren PM, Gillooly M, MacNee W, Lamb D. Microscopic and macroscopic measurements of emphysema: relation to carbon monoxide gas transfer. *Thorax* 1992;**47**:144–9.

37. Gevenois PA, De Vuyst P, de Maetelaer V, *et al.* Comparison of computed density and microscopic morphometry in pulmonary emphysema. *Am J Respir Crit Care Med* 1996;**154**:187–92.

38. Black LF, Hyatt RE, Stubbs SE. Mechanism of expiratory airflow limitation in chronic obstructive pulmonary disease associated with alpha1-antitrypsin deficiency. *Am Rev Respir Dis* 1972;**105**:891–9.

39. Eidelman DH, Ghezzo H, Kim WD, Hyatt RE, Cosio MG. Pressure–volume curves in smokers. Comparison with alpha-1-antitrypsin deficiency. *Am Rev Respir Dis* 1989;**139**:1452–8.

40. Demedts M, Aumann J. Early emphysema. Ten years' evolution. *Chest* 1988;**94**:337–42.

41. Sciurba FC, Rogers RM, Keenan RJ, *et al*. Improvement in pulmonary function and elastic recoil after lung reduction surgery for diffuse emphysema. *N Engl J Med* 1996;**334**:1095–9.

42. Gelb AF, Zamel N, McKenna J Jr, Brenner M. Mechanism of short-term improvement in lung function after emphysema resection. *Am J Respir Crit Care Med* 1996;**154**:945–51.

43. Ingenito EP, Loring SH, Moy ML, Mentzer SJ, Swanson SJ, Reilly JJ Jr. Interpreting improvement in expiratory flows after lung volume reduction surgery in terms of flow limitation theory. *Am J Respir Crit Care Med* 2001;**163**:1074–80.

44. Sharp JT, Van Lith P, Vej Nuchprayoon C, Briney R, Johnson FN. The thorax in chronic obstructive lung disease. *Am J Med* 1968;**44**:39–46.

45. Leaver DG, Tattersfield AE, Pride NB. Contributions of loss of lung recoil and of enhanced airways collapsibility to the airflow obstruction of chronic bronchitis and emphysema. *J Clin Invest* 1973;**52**:2117–28.

46. Colebatch HJH, Finucane KE, Smith MM. Pulmonary conductance and elastic recoil relationships in asthma and emphysema. *J Appl Physiol* 1973;**34**:143–53.

47. Leaver DG, Tattersfield AE, Pride NB. Bronchial and extrabronchial factors in chronic airflow obstruction. *Thorax* 1974;**29**:394–400.

48. Farré R, Gavela E, Ferrer M, Roca J, Navajas D. Noninvasive assessment of respiratory resistance in chronic respiratory patients with nasal CPAP. *Eur Respir J* 2000;**15**:314–19.

49. Grimby G, Takishima T, Graham W, Macklem P, Mead J. Frequency dependence of flow resistance in patients with obstructive lung disease. *J Clin Invest* 1968;**47**:1455–65.

50. Phagoo SB, Watson RA, Silverman M, Pride NB. Comparison of four methods of assessing airflow resistance before and after induced airway narrowing in normal subjects. *J Appl Physiol* 1995;**79**:518–25.

51. Yanai M, Sekizawa K, Ohrui T, *et al*. Site of airway obstruction in pulmonary disease: direct measurements of intrabronchial pressure. *J Appl Physiol* 1992;**72**:1016–23.

52. Hogg JC, Macklem PT, Thurlbeck WM. Site and nature of airway obstruction in chronic obstructive lung disease. *N Engl J Med* 1968;**278**:1355–60.

53. Silvers GW, Maisel JC, Petty TL, Filley GF, Mitchell RS. Flow limitation during forced expiration in excised human lungs. *J Appl Physiol* 1974;**36**:737–44.

54. Van Brabandt H, Cauberghs M, Verbeken E, Moerman P, Lauweryns JM, Van de Woestijne KP. Partitioning of pulmonary impedance in excised human and canine lungs. *J Appl Physiol Respir Environ Exercise Physiol* 1983;**55**:1733–42.

55. Verbeken EK, Cauberghs M, Mertens I, Lauweryns JM, Van De Woestijne KP. Tissue and airway impedance of excised normal, senile and emphysematous lungs. *J Appl Physiol* 1992;**72**:2343–53.

56. Coe CI, Pride NB. Effects of correcting arterial hypoxaemia on respiratory resistance in patients with chronic obstructive pulmonary disease. *Clin Sci* 1993;**84**:325–9.

57. Ohrui T, Tanai M, Sekizawa K, *et al*. Effective site of bronchodilation by beta-adrenergic and anticholinergic agents in patients with chronic obstructive pulmonary disease: direct measurement of intrabronchial pressure with a new catheter. *Am Rev Respir Dis* 1992;**146**:88–91.

58. On LS, Boonyongsunchai P, Webb S, *et al*. Function of pulmonary neuronal M (2) muscarinic receptors in stable chronic obstructive pulmonary disease. *Am J Respir Crit Care Med* 2001;**163**:1320–5.

59. Nisar M, Earis JE, Pearson MG, Calverley PMA. Acute bronchodilator trials in chronic obstructive pulmonary disease. *Am Rev Respir Dis* 1992;**146**:555–9.

60. Hogg JC, Macklem PT, Thurlbeck WM. The resistance of collateral channels in excised human lungs. *J Clin Invest* 1969;**48**:421–31.

61. Terry PB, Traystman RJ, Newball HH, Batra G, Menkes HA. Collateral ventilation in man. *N Engl J Med* 1978;**298**:10–15.

62. Stanescu D, Veriter C, Van de Woestijne KP. Maximal inspiratory flow rates in patients with COPD. *Chest* 2000;**118**:976–80.

63. Fry DL, Hyatt RE. Pulmonary mechanics: a unified analysis of the relationship between pressure, volume, and gas flow in the lungs of normal and diseased subjects. *Am J Med* 1960;**29**:672–89.

64. Ingram RH Jr, Schilder DP. Effect of gas compression on pulmonary pressure, flow, and volume relationships. *J Appl Physiol* 1966;**21**:1821–6.

65. Pride NB, Permutt S, Riley RL, Bromberger-Barnea B. Determinants of maximal expiratory flow from the lungs. *J Appl Physiol* 1967;**23**:646–62.

66. Mead J, Turner JM, Macklem PT, Little JB. Significance of the relationship between lung recoil and maximum expiratory flow. *J Appl Physiol* 1967;**22**:95–108.

67. Macklem PT, Wilson NJ. Measurement of intrabronchial pressure in man. *J Appl Physiol* 1965;**20**:653–63.

68. Macklem PT, Fraser RG, Brown WG. Bronchial pressure measurements in emphysema and bronchitis. *J Clin Invest* 1965;**44**:897–905.

69. Wilson AG, Massarella GR, Pride NB. Elastic properties of airways in human lungs post-mortem. *Am Rev Respir Dis* 1974;**110**:716–29.

70. Verbeken EK, Cauberghs M, Van de Woestijne KP. Membranous bronchioles and connective tissue network of normal and emphysematous lungs. *J Appl Physiol* 1996;**81**:2468–80.

71. Hoppin FG Jr. Theoretical basis for improvement following reduction pneumoplasty in emphysema. *Am J Respir Crit Care Med* 1997;**155**:520–5.

72. Fessler HE, Permutt S. Lung volume reduction surgery and airflow limitation. *Am J Respir Crit Care Med* 1998;**157**:715–22.

73. Loring SH, Leith DE, Connolly MJ, *et al*. Model of functional restriction in chronic obstructive pulmonary disease, transplantation, and lung reduction surgery. *Am J Respir Crit Care Med* 1998;**160**:821–8.

74. Fessler HE, Scharf SM, Permutt S. Improvement in spirometry following lung volume reduction surgery. *Am J Respir Crit Care Med* 2002;**165**:34–40.

75. Ingenito EP, Loring SH, Moy ML, *et al*. Comparison of physiological and radiological screening for lung volume reduction surgery. *Am J Respir Crit Care Med* 2001;**163**:1068–73.

76. Gelb AF, Brenner M, McKenna RJ, Rischel R, Zamel N, Schein MJ. Serial lung function and elastic recoil 2 years after lung volume reduction surgery for emphysema. *Chest* 1999;**113**:1497–506.

77. Ingenito EP, Evans RB, Loring SH, *et al*. Relation between preoperative inspiratory lung resistance and the outcome of

lung-volume-reduction surgery for emphysema. *N Engl J Med* 1998;**338**:1181–5.

78. Gandevia SC, Leeper JB, McKenzie DK, De Troyer A. Discharge frequencies of parasternal intercostal and scalene motor units during breathing in normal and COPD subjects. *Am J Respir Crit Care Med* 1996;**153**:622–8.

79. De Troyer A, Leeper JB, McKenzie DK, Gandevia SC. Neural drive to the diaphragm in patients with severe COPD. *Am J Respir Crit Care Med* 1997; **155**:1335–40.

80. Spiro SG, Hahn HL, Edwards RHT, Pride NB. An analysis of the physiological strain of submaximal exercise in patients with chronic obstructive bronchitis. *Thorax* 1975;**30**:415–25.

81. Sorli J, Grassino A, Lorange G, Milic-Emili J. Control of breathing in patients with chronic obstructive lung disease. *Clin Sci Mol Med* 1978;**54**:295–304.

82. Montes de Oca M, Celli BR. Respiratory muscle recruitment and exercise performance in eucapnic and hypercapnic severe chronic obstructive pulmonary disease. *Am J Respir Crit Care Med* 2000;**161**:880–5.

83. D'Angelo E, Prandi E, Marazzini L, *et al*. Dependence of maximal flow–volume curves on time-course of preceding inspiration in patients with chronic obstructive pulmonary disease. *Am J Respir Crit Care Med* 1994;**150**:1581–6.

84. Eltayara L, Becklake MR, Volta CA, *et al*. Relationship of chronic dyspnea and flow limitation in COPD patients. *Am J Respir Crit Care Med* 1996;**154**:1726–34.

85. Koulouris NG, Dimopoulou I, Valta P, *et al*. Detection of expiratory flow limitation during exercise in COPD patients. *J Appl Physiol* 1997;**82**:723–31.

86. Boczkowski J, Murciano D, Pichot M-H, *et al*. Expiratory flow limitation in stable asthmatic patients during resting breathing. *Am J Respir Crit Care Med* 1997;**156**:752–7.

87. Valta P, Corbeil C, Campodonico R, *et al*. Detection of expiratory flow limitation during mechanical ventilation. *Am J Respir Crit Care Med* 1994;**150**:1311–17.

88. Ninane V, Yernault, J-C, de Troyer A. Intrinsic PEEP in patients with chronic obstructive pulmonary disease: role of expiratory muscles. *Am Rev Respir Dis* 1993;**148**:1037–42.

89. Petrof BJ, Legare M, Goldberg P, *et al*. Continuous positive airway pressure reduces work of breathing and dyspnea during weaning from mechanical ventilation in severe chronic obstructive pulmonary disease. *Am Rev Respir Dis* 1990;**141**:281–9.

90. McIlroy MB, Christie RV. The work of breathing in emphysema. *Clin Sci* 1954;**13**:147–54.

91. Otis AB, Mckerrow CB, Bartlett RA, *et al*. Mechanical factors in distribution of pulmonary ventilation. *J Appl Physiol* 1956;**8**:427–43.

92. Fleury B, Murciano D, Talamo C, *et al*. Work of breathing in patients with chronic obstructive pulmonary disease in acute respiratory failure. *Am Rev Respir Dis* 1985; **131**:822–7.

93. Warren JB, Jennings SJ, Clark TJH. Effect of adrenergic and vagal blockade on the normal human airway response to exercise. *Clin Sci* 1984;**66**:79–85.

94. Jones NL, Jones G, Edwards RHT. Exercise tolerance in chronic airway obstruction. *Am Rev Respir Dis* 1971;**103**:477–94.

95. Johnson BD, Weisman IM, Zeballos RJ, Beck KC. Emerging concepts in the evaluation of ventilatory limitation during exercise. *Chest* 1999;**116**:488–503.

96. Freedman S. Sustained maximum voluntary ventilation. *Respir Physiol* 1970;**8**:230–44.

97. Dillard TA, Hnatiuk OW, McCumber TR. Maximum voluntary ventilation. Spirometric determinants in chronic obstructive pulmonary disease patients and normal subjects. *Am Rev Respir Dis* 1993;**147**:870–5.

98. Belman MJ, Botnick WC, Shin JW. Inhaled bronchodilators reduce dynamic hyperinflation during exercise in patients with chronic obstructive pulmonary disease. *Am J Respir Crit Care Med* 1996;**153**:967–75.

99. O'Donnell DE, Lam M, Webb KA. Spirometric correlates of improvement in exercise performance after anticholinergic therapy in chronic obstructive pulmonary disease. *Am J Respir Crit Care Med* 1999;**160**:542–9.

100. Marin JM, Carrizo SJ, Gascon M, Sanchez A, Gallego B, Celli BR. Inspiratory capacity, dynamic hyperinflation, breathlessness, and exercise performance during the 6-minute-walk test in chronic obstructive pulmonary disease. *Am J Respir Crit Care Med* 2001;**163**:1395–9.

101. Diaz O, Villafranca C, Ghezzo H, *et al*. Role of inspiratory capacity on exercise tolerance in COPD patients with and without tidal flow limitation at rest. *Eur Respir J* 2000; **16**:269–75.

102. Grimby G, Elgefors B, Oxhoj H. Ventilatory levels and chest wall mechanics during exercise in obstructive lung disease. *Scand J Respir Dis* 1973;**54**:45–52.

103. Levison H, Cherniack RM. Ventilatory cost of exercise in chronic obstructive pulmonary disease. *J Appl Physiol* 1968;**25**:21–7.

104. Haluszka J, Chartrand DA, Grassino AE, *et al*. Intrinsic PEEP and arterial Pco_2 in stable patients with chronic obstructive pulmonary disease. *Am Rev Respir Dis* 1990;**141**:1194–7.

105. Broseghini C, Brandolese R, Poggi R, *et al*. Respiratory mechanics during the first day of mechanical ventilation in patients with pulmonary edema and chronic airway obstruction. *Am Rev Respir Dis* 1988;**138**:355–61.

106. Coussa ML, Guérin C, Eissa NT, *et al*. Partitioning of work of breathing in mechanically ventilated COPD patients. *J Appl Physiol* 1993;**75**:1711–19.

107. Guérin C, Coussa M-L, Eissa NT, *et al*. Lung and chest wall mechanics in mechanically ventilated COPD patients. *J Appl Physiol* 1993;**74**:1570–80.

108. Tantucci C, Corbeil C, Chassé M, *et al*. Flow resistance in patients with chronic obstructive pulmonary disease in acute respiratory failure. *Am Rev Respir Dis* 1991;**144**:384–9.

109. Mount LE. The ventilation flow-resistance and compliance of rat lungs. *J Physiol (Lond)* 1955;**127**:157–67.

110. D'Angelo E, Robatto FM, Calderini E, *et al*. Pulmonary and chest wall mechanics in anaesthetized paralyzed humans. *J Appl Physiol* 1991;**70**:2602–10.

111. D'Angelo E, Calderini E, Torri G, *et al*. Respiratory mechanics in anesthetized paralyzed humans: effect of flow, volume and time. *J Appl Physiol* 1989;**67**:2556–64.

112. Smith TC, Marini JJ. Impact of PEEP on lung mechanics and work of breathing in severe airflow obstruction. *J Appl Physiol* 1988;**65**:1488–99.

113. Rossi A, Gottfried SB, Zocchi L, *et al*. Measurement of static compliance of the total respiratory system in patients with acute respiratory failure during mechanical ventilation. *Am Rev Respir Dis* 1985;**131**:672–7.

114. Kimball WR, Leith DE, Robbins AG. Dynamic hyperinflation and ventilator dependence in chronic obstructive pulmonary disease. *Am Rev Respir Dis* 1982;**126**:991–5.

115. Pepe PE, Marini JJ. Occult positive end-expiratory pressure in mechanically ventilated patients with airflow obstruction. *Am Rev Respir Dis* 1982;**126**:166–70.

116. Eissa NT, Milic-Emili J. Modern concepts in monitoring and management of respiratory failure. *Anesthesiol Clin N Am* 1991;**9**:199–218.

117. Tantucci C, Duguet A, Similowski T, Zelter M, Derenne J-P, Milic-Emili J. Effect of salbutamol on dynamic

hyperinflation in chronic obstructive pulmonary disease patients. *Eur Respir J* 1998;**12**:799–804.

118. Boni E, Corda L, Franchini D, *et al.* Volume effect and exertional dyspnoea after bronchodilator in patients with COPD with and without expiratory flow limitation at rest. *Thorax* 2002;**57**:528–32.

119. Gay PC, Rodarte JR, Tayyab M, Hubmayr RD. Evaluation of bronchodilator responsiveness in mechanically ventilated patients. *Am Rev Respir Dis* 1987;**136**:880–5.

120. Petrof BJ, Kimoff RJ, Cheong TH, *et al.* Continuous positive airway pressure reduces work of breathing and dyspnea during weaning from mechanical ventilation. *Am Rev Respir Dis* 1990;**141**:281–9.

121. Appendini L, Patessio A, Zanaboni S, *et al.* Physiological effects of positive end-expiratory pressure and mask pressure support during exacerbations of chronic obstructive pulmonary disease. *Am J Respir Crit Care Med* 1994;**149**:1069–76.

122. Appendini L, Purro A, Patessio A, *et al.* Partitioning of inspiratory muscle workload and pressure assistance in ventilator-dependent patients. *Am J Respir Crit Care Med* 1996;**154**:1301–9.

14

Pulmonary gas exchange

R RODRIGUEZ-ROISIN, JA BARBERÀ AND J ROCA

INTRODUCTION

The ultimate goal of the respiratory system is to exchange oxygen (O_2) and carbon dioxide (CO_2), to meet the metabolic needs of the body. In order to effectively transfer both gases, ventilation and blood flow must be adequately apportioned and matched within the lungs. Of the four classic mechanisms determining abnormal arterial blood respiratory gases – i.e. alveolar hypoventilation, impaired alveolar-end capillary diffusion to O_2, increased intrapulmonary shunt and ventilation–perfusion ($\dot{V}_A/\dot{Q}$) mismatching – the last is by far the most common cause of impaired pulmonary gas exchange in respiratory disease. All the abnormalities alluded to above except alveolar hypoventilation may be viewed as intrapulmonary determinants of pulmonary gas exchange. Other key extrapulmonary factors of respiratory blood gases include the fractional concentration of O_2 in the inspired gas, the hemodynamic status (cardiac output) and the metabolic demands (O_2 consumption) of the body.[1]

The underlying structural abnormalities in COPD, which include widespread airway narrowing with varying degrees of parenchymal and vascular structural abnormalities, are at the root of the maldistribution of alveolar ventilation and pulmonary blood flow resulting in abnormal respiratory arterial blood gases and, ultimately, chronic respiratory failure. Ventilation–perfusion imbalance is the principal determinant of pulmonary gas exchange under both acute and chronic conditions even although alveolar hypoventilation often emerges as a key mechanism producing hypercapnia.[2,3] By contrast, only

a mild to moderate increased intrapulmonary shunt is present in acute respiratory insufficiency, or during its recovery, and diffusion limitation to O_2 plays no role.

This chapter reviews the evidence of pulmonary gas exchange in COPD patients predominantly using the results obtained with the multiple inert gas elimination technique (MIGET) over the last quarter of the last century.[4–6] This technique provided a quantum leap forward in the assessment of gas exchange abnormalities. We will first review the different clinical presentations of COPD to gain insight into the correlations between structure and function. Subsequently, the response to exercise and the effects of the breathing of 100% O_2 and those induced by drugs on pulmonary gas exchange will be addressed.

MULTIPLE INERT GAS ELIMINATION TECHNIQUE

The potential and limitations of the MIGET have been explored extensively[4–6] and will not be discussed here. It has three major advantages. Firstly, it gives both quantitative and qualitative estimates of the distributions of $\dot{V}_A/\dot{Q}$ ratios. Secondly, it does so without itself changing the airway caliber or pulmonary vascular tone, because there is no need to alter inspired O_2 concentrations during measurements. Thirdly, it facilitates the interpretation of the complex interplay between intrapulmonary (abnormal $\dot{V}_A/\dot{Q}$ relationships, intrapulmonary shunt and diffusion limitation to O_2) and extrapulmonary (namely, inspired O_2 concentration, total ventilation, cardiac output and O_2 consumption) factors influencing pulmonary gas exchange.[1]

Furthermore, the extent of $\dot{V}A/\dot{Q}$ inequality detected by MIGET exceeds that derived from topographical measurements such as radioactive tracer gas scans, computed tomograms or positron emission tomography (PET), in particular when used in patients with chronic, generalized lung disease, such as COPD.[7] The latter techniques all have a limited spatial resolution which grossly underestimates the intraregional $\dot{V}A/\dot{Q}$ abnormalities.

Full technical details of MIGET have been reported at length elsewhere[1,4–6,8] and will only be summarized here. The arterial, mixed venous and mixed expired concentrations of six infused inert gases, measured with gas chromatography, are used to calculate the ratio of arterial to mixed venous pressures (retention) and the ratio of mixed expired or alveolar to mixed venous pressure (excretion). Retention and excretion are then used to compute a multicompartment $\dot{V}A/\dot{Q}$ distribution. These six gases include a wide spectrum of solubilities (from the more insoluble gas, sulfur hexafluoride, to the most soluble, acetone, through those of intermediate solubility, i.e. ethane, cyclopropane, enfluorane or halothane, and ether). The use of inert gases has two major advantages: firstly, the limitations due to a non-linear dissociation curve on gas exchange, genuine for O_2 and CO_2, are not present; secondly, a large range of solubilities is used. It is known that the gas exchange behavior of any gas in the face of $\dot{V}A/\dot{Q}$ abnormalities is a function of its solubility.[6,8,9] Figure 14.1 depicts a typical distribution of $\dot{V}A/\dot{Q}$ ratios in a young, healthy non-smoker at rest, in a semirecumbent position, breathing room air. The amounts (distributions) of alveolar ventilation and of pulmonary perfusion (y-axis) are plotted against a wide range of 50 $\dot{V}A/\dot{Q}$ ratios (from 0 to infinity) on a log scale (x-axis). Each data point represents a particular amount of alveolar ventilation or pulmonary blood flow, the lines having been drawn to facilitate visual interpretation. Total blood flow or total alveolar ventilation correspond to the sum of all data points of their respective distributions. The logarithmic rather than linear axis of $\dot{V}A/\dot{Q}$ ratios is based on established practice in the field of pulmonary gas exchange. A logarithmic normal distribution of ventilation and blood flow is one of the simplest distributions and allows the spread to be defined by a simple variable, that is the standard deviation on a log scale.

Both distributions are unimodal with three major common findings: symmetry, location around a mean $\dot{V}A/\dot{Q}$ ratio of 1.0 and a narrow dispersion (between 0.1 and 10.0). Thus, in young healthy subjects there is no blood flow diverted to the left to a zone of low $\dot{V}A/\dot{Q}$ ratios (poorly ventilated lung units) nor ventilation distributed to the right to a zone of high $\dot{V}A/\dot{Q}$ ratios (incompletely perfused, but still finite, lung units). Intrapulmonary shunt as detected by MIGET is defined as areas with zero $\dot{V}A/\dot{Q}$ ratio (in practice less than 0.005). Postpulmonary shunt (which corresponds to bronchial and Thebesian circulations) is not detected by MIGET. Consequently shunt measured by MIGET is lower than the conventional venous admixture ratio ($\dot{Q}s/\dot{Q}T$) (1–2% of cardiac output) breathing room air. When breathing 100% O_2 the influence of poorly ventilated units with low $\dot{V}A/\dot{Q}$ ratios is considerably decreased by washout of nitrogen and so the difference between shunt measured by MIGET and 100% O_2 is greatly reduced. The normal value of inert gas physiologic deadspace (infinite $\dot{V}A/\dot{Q}$ ratio, in practice above 100) (approximately 30% of overall alveolar ventilation) is also slightly less than that computed with the traditional Bohr's equation. While the Bohr's formula includes the deadspace-like effects of all lung units whose alveolar PCO_2 values are less than the arterial PCO_2, the

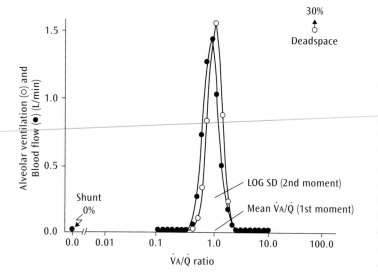

Figure 14.1 *Distributions of alveolar ventilation (open symbols) and pulmonary blood flow (closed symbols) (y-axis) plotted against $\dot{V}A/\dot{Q}$ ratio on a log scale (x-axis) from a healthy, young individual at rest, breathing room air. The first moment of each distribution corresponds to its mean $\dot{V}A/\dot{Q}$ ratio (blood flow $\dot{Q}$, or ventilation, $\dot{V}$) and the dispersion (second moment) of each distribution, expressed as the standard deviation on a log scale, is known as log SD $\dot{Q}$ (blood flow) or log SD $\dot{V}$ (ventilation). These indices are two of the most common markers used to assess $\dot{V}A/\dot{Q}$ mismatch.*

inert gas measurement represents only the deadspace-like effects of those alveoli whose $\dot{V}_A/\dot{Q}$ ratios are greater than 100.

The first moment of each distribution, i.e. the mean $\dot{V}_A/\dot{Q}$ ratio of each distribution, and the second moment (or dispersion), log SD, are commonly used to quantitate the degree of $\dot{V}_A/\dot{Q}$ mismatch. The second moment (square root) of the pulmonary blood flow (log SD $\dot{Q}$) and that of alveolar ventilation (log SD $\dot{V}$) distributions reflects the variance (standard deviation) of $\dot{V}_A/\dot{Q}$ ratios about the mean. In a perfectly homogenous lung, log SD $\dot{Q}$ and log SD $\dot{V}$ should be zero. In practice, in a normal healthy individual they range between 0.30 and 0.60, in young individuals, and 0.70 and 0.75 in older ones.[10] By computing a multicompartmental lung model with a log normal distribution of pulmonary perfusion or alveolar ventilation, or both, West[11] earlier demonstrated that log SD $\dot{Q}$ or log SD $\dot{V}$ values of 1.0 and 1.5 imply moderate and severe degrees of $\dot{V}_A/\dot{Q}$ mismatch, respectively. The degree of $\dot{V}_A/\dot{Q}$ inequality can also be expressed as the total percentage of ventilation and perfusion in defined regions of the $\dot{V}_A/\dot{Q}$ spectrum. Thus, the percentage of blood flow distributed in areas of $\dot{V}_A/\dot{Q}$ ratios below 0.1 and above 0.005 (and, therefore, excluding shunt) is conventionally named 'low $\dot{V}_A/\dot{Q}$ mode' and the amount of ventilation distributed to the region of $\dot{V}_A/\dot{Q}$ ratios located between 10.0 and 100 (and, therefore, excluding deadspace) is regarded as 'high $\dot{V}_A/\dot{Q}$ mode'.[1,6] Using this technique no more than three modes of a distribution can be recovered and only smooth distributions can be obtained. Arterial–alveolar difference averaged for the group of inert gas indices also can be calculated and used to give indirect estimates of the degree of $\dot{V}_A/\dot{Q}$ abnormalities.[12,13] Besides, the amount of $\dot{V}_A/\dot{Q}$ inequality can be assessed qualitatively by describing the morphologic pattern of each distribution, which can be narrowly or broadly unimodal, or clearly bimodal.

MIGET can also assist in addressing the potential presence of diffusion limitation for O_2 because equilibration of inert gases is in practice not diffusion limited.[1,6] Ventilation–perfusion mismatch has been shown to fully explain the measured PaO_2 in patients with COPD.[13]

GAS EXCHANGE PATHOPHYSIOLOGY IN STABLE COPD

With the use of MIGET, different degrees of $\dot{V}_A/\dot{Q}$ inequality have been demonstrated which are by and large consistent with the degree of clinical severity of COPD. Increased intrapulmonary shunt is practically absent in stable conditions, and even during exacerbations rarely exceeds 10% of total pulmonary blood flow even in the presence of abundant, viscous bronchial secretions.[13] In spite of the common finding of a reduced gas transfer factor (TLco) in the most severe cases, all of the studies using MIGET have consistently excluded the presence of alveolar–endcapillary diffusion limitation for O_2 at rest or during exercise, as an additional intrapulmonary mechanism causing hypoxemia.

Severe stage

Combining measurements of arterial blood respiratory gases and routine pulmonary function tests and certain clinical features, Burrows et al.[14] in the mid 1960s were able to subdivide COPD patients into two distinct presentations: Type A and Type B patients. Wagner et al.[15] in the late 1970s, in choosing 23 stable patients with advanced COPD for study (FEV_1 range, 19–58% predicted), with mild to severe gas exchange disturbances (PaO_2 range, 38–71 mmHg; $PaCO_2$ range, 25–64 mmHg; TLco range, 17–157% predicted) aimed to find stable patients who reflected as closely as possible the two classic clinical phenotypes suggested by Burrows and colleagues. In this series of patients $\dot{V}_A/\dot{Q}$ distributions were remarkably abnormal and displayed three distinct $\dot{V}_A/\dot{Q}$ patterns (Figure 14.2). The first $\dot{V}_A/\dot{Q}$ profile showed the presence of lung units with very high $\dot{V}_A/\dot{Q}$ ratios or a 'high $\dot{V}_A/\dot{Q}$ mode' (type H). With this pattern most of its ventilation was located in the zone of higher $\dot{V}_A/\dot{Q}$ ratios. The second pattern was characterized by a mode including a large proportion of blood flow perfusing lung units with very poor low $\dot{V}_A/\dot{Q}$ units or a 'low $\dot{V}_A/\dot{Q}$ mode' (type L), most of the blood flow being into areas of lower $\dot{V}_A/\dot{Q}$ ratios. Finally, the third pattern was a mixed 'high-low $\dot{V}_A/\dot{Q}$ mode' (type H–L), including additional modes above and below the main body. Overall, the dispersions of blood flow or ventilation, or both, were moderately to severely increased (above 1.0, each).

These results suggested that patients with COPD of the Type A variety were very likely to have high $\dot{V}_A/\dot{Q}$ areas, and were unlikely to have distinct low $\dot{V}_A/\dot{Q}$ areas unless they had clinical evidence of Type B COPD as well. It was postulated that pattern H was likely to be produced by continued ventilation of regions with reduced blood flow. Conceivably, these regions might represent emphysematous regions where destruction of the alveolar walls results in the loss of the pulmonary vasculature. By contrast, patients of the Type B variety commonly have distinct low or high $\dot{V}_A/\dot{Q}$ areas, or both, although there is clearly much more variability within this group. Thus, pattern L was likely to represent regions subtended by airways partially blocked by mucus secretions and plugging, smooth muscle hypertrophy, wall edema, bronchospasm, distortion, or some combination of all these abnormalities. Other findings of interest were: the essential absence of increased intrapulmonary shunt, suggesting that collateral ventilation and hypoxic vasoconstriction are very active and that complete airways occlusion does not occur, and a mild to moderate increase in deadspace (range 30–42% of alveolar ventilation) present in most of the patients.

Of further interest was the lack of correlation between spirometry (FEV$_1$) and respiratory blood gases. Similarly, the three patterns of $\dot{V}A/\dot{Q}$ ratio distributions did not correlate with spirometry (Figure 14.3), airways resistance, arterial blood gases or transfer factor. There was, however, some correlation between the loss of elastic recoil (or increased static compliance) and the presence of the type H pattern.

Subsequently, more than a dozen studies,[16–31] including more than 100 patients with stable severe or very severe airflow obstruction (mean FEV$_1$ equal to or below 36% predicted), many of them with hypoxemia (with or without chronic hypercapnia) and some pulmonary hypertension, have been reported. Most of them documented $\dot{V}A/\dot{Q}$ patterns similar to those reported originally by Wagner et al., although the relationship shown with the clinical COPD types could not be established as clearly as in the

study reported by Wagner et al.[15] The amounts of blood flow or ventilation distributed to regions with low or high $\dot{V}A/\dot{Q}$ ratios, respectively, were modest (range equal to or below 10% of cardiac output) in all but a few of the reports. Broad unimodal blood flow and ventilation distributions were shown in 45% of patients, a bimodal blood flow distribution in 23%, a bimodal ventilation distribution in 18%, and in the remaining 14% of patients, it was shown both bimodal blood flow and ventilation distribution patterns.[2] As in the original study of Wagner et al.,[15] the correlation between spirometric and gas exchange indices was very poor.

We have to be aware of the potential influence of an increased CO$_2$ production on PaCO$_2$. Malnutrition is an important clinical and therapeutic problem in COPD patients, and this is receiving progressive attention.[32] Normally, the amount of CO$_2$ produced per minute is a function of the metabolic rate and the substrate used for fuel. In healthy individuals, the absorption and metabolism of carbohydrate loads causes an increase in CO$_2$ output (of the order of 70–100% of the O$_2$

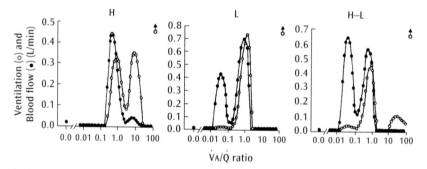

Figure 14.2 *Typical $\dot{V}A/\dot{Q}$ distributions in patients with advanced COPD (from left to right and from top to bottom): Type H (high $\dot{V}A/\dot{Q}$ mode) represents a $\dot{V}A/\dot{Q}$ pattern characterized by a substantial amount of ventilation distributed to high $\dot{V}A/\dot{Q}$ regions; type L (low $\dot{V}A/\dot{Q}$ mode) depicts a $\dot{V}A/\dot{Q}$ profile in which a marked amount of blood flow is diverted to low $\dot{V}A/\dot{Q}$ areas; and, type H–L illustrates both former abnormal $\dot{V}A/\dot{Q}$ patterns. Whilst shunt (left closed symbol) is trivial, deadspace (right open symbol with arrow) is always moderately increased in all three patterns. (From ref. 15.)*

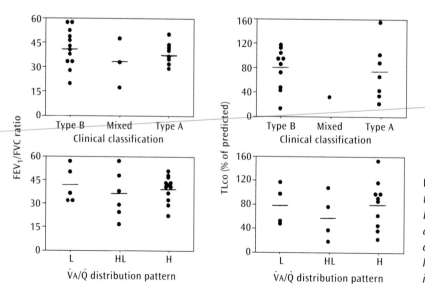

Figure 14.3 *Plots of spirometry and transfer factor (TLco) (y-axes) versus Burrows' clinical classification (top) and $\dot{V}A/\dot{Q}$ patterns (bottom) (x-axes). No correlation was found between routine lung function tests and clinical data or inert gas measurements. (From ref. 15.)*

consumed), as the whole body fuel utilization is shifted from predominantly fat to essentially carbohydrate and also from the thermogenic effect of food *per se*. Some degree of malnutrition is common in COPD patients and has been related to adverse effects that may contribute to complications and increased mortality.[32] A variety of contributing factors, such as increased resting and total energy expenditure, systemic inflammatory response and anorexia, have been proposed as underlying mechanisms of malnutrition in COPD patients. Body weight and body composition need to be considered in nutrition assessment in this population, since loss of fat-free mass occurs not only in the majority of underweight COPD patients, but also in some of the normal weight patients.[33] Different approaches with nutritional support have not always been followed by improvements in anthropometric measures or functional exercise capacity among patients with stable COPD. A substantial number of patients, mainly those with important systemic inflammatory response, failed to respond to the nutritional support. Likewise, the possible implications in pulmonary function of nutritional regimens with high percentage of fat over carbohydrates in hospitalized COPD patients are contradictory. Total caloric intake is probably a more important determinant of the magnitude of added V_{CO_2} than the proportion of carbohydrate.[34]

Mild stage

Barberà *et al.*[25] studied 23 patients with a mild obstructive ventilatory pattern (mean FEV_1, 76% predicted) (see below

'Structure and function'). All but two patients had normal TL_{CO} and total lung capacity was within normal range. Mean Pa_{O_2} and Pa_{CO_2} were normal, but mean alveolar-arterial PO_2 difference was moderately increased (>15 mmHg). Overall, the dispersions of ventilation and blood flow were mildly abnormal (log SD $\dot{Q}$ below 1.0, each), intrapulmonary shunt was absent and deadspace was normal. Blood flow distributions were broadly unimodal in two-thirds of the patients and modestly bimodal in the remaining one-third. By contrast, the ventilation distributions were never bimodal and were devoid of regions of very high $\dot{V}_A/\dot{Q}$ ratios.

In summary, the patterns of $\dot{V}_A/\dot{Q}$ distributions are not uniform in COPD patients. An analysis of 94 patients in a stable clinical condition, including the large clinical spectrum of COPD severity, identified four different patterns of $\dot{V}_A/\dot{Q}$ distribution:[35] broad unimodal distributions of both blood flow and ventilation (45% of the patients); bimodal distribution of blood flow, with both normal and low $\dot{V}_A/\dot{Q}$ areas ('low' pattern) (23% of patients); bimodal distribution of ventilation, with normal and high $\dot{V}_A/\dot{Q}$ areas ('high' pattern) (18% of patients); and both bimodal blood flow and ventilation distribution patterns ('high and low' pattern) (14% of patients). This diversity in the $\dot{V}_A/\dot{Q}$ distribution pattern presumably reflects the heterogeneity of pulmonary pathologic abnormalities as well as the efficiency of compensatory mechanisms. Means and 95% interval confidences of all these data are included in Table 14.1.

Table 14.1 *Ventilation–perfusion distributions in healthy individuals and COPD patients (means and 95% interval confidence)[†] (Reproduced from ref. 35 with permission.)*

	Healthy subjects[10] (*n* = 43)	COPD patients [24,25,29–31,38]		
		Stage I (*n* = 19)	Stage II (*n* = 27)	Stage III (*n* = 44)
Arterial blood gases				
Pa_{O_2} (mmHg)	100 (97–102)	77 (72–81)	67 (64–71)	61 (57–64)
Pa_{CO_2} (mmHg)	37 (35–38)	40 (36–44)	39 (37–41)	47 (45–50)
Aa_{PO_2} (mmHg)	6.4 (3.8–9.0)	28 (24–32)	34 (30–39)	33 (30–36)
Ventilation–perfusion distributions				
Shunt (% cardiac output)	0.3 (0.2–0.5)	0.9 (0.4–1.4)	1.3 (0.5–2.1)	1.3 (0.6–2.3)
Low V_A/Q (% cardiac output)	0 (<0.1)	1.7 (0.4–2.9)	3.3 (1.4–5.2)	3.7 (0.6–6.8)
Log SD Q	0.42 (0.38–0.45)	0.83 (0.74–0.92)	1.05 (0.97–1.13)	1.00 (0.91–1.09)
Log SD V	0.45 (0.40–0.51)	0.76 (0.63–0.88)	0.88 (0.82–0.95)	1.10 (1.01–1.18)
High V_A/Q (% ventilation)	0 (<0.1)	0.8 (0–1.7)	1.5 (6.8–27.0)	4.7 (1.9–7.5)
Deadspace (% ventilation)	24 (21–27)	35.5 (29–42)	36 (32–40)	40 (36–44)
DISP R-E*	2.5 (2.1–2.8)	7.9 (6.2–9.6)	12.6 (11.1–13.9)	14.3 (13.0–15.5)

[†]ATS Staging[36]: stage I, $FEV_1 \geqslant 50\%$ predicted; stage II, FEV_1 35–49% predicted; stage III, $FEV_1 < 35\%$ predicted.
Aa_{PO_2}: alveolar to arterial oxygen gradient; shunt: perfusion to alveolar units with V_A/Q ratio <0.005; low V_A/Q: perfusion to alveolar units with V_A/Q ratios between 0.005 and 0.1; log SD Q: dispersion of blood flow distribution; log SD V: dispersion of ventilation distribution; high V_A/Q: ventilation to alveolar units with V_A/Q ratios between 10 and 100; dead space: ventilation to units with V_A/Q ratios >100; DISP R-E*: dispersion of retention minus excretion of inert gases corrected by deadspace.

Small airways disease

In the only study to date, Barberà *et al.*[37] studied seven patients with functional criteria compatible with small airways disease (mean FEV$_1$, above 80% predicted but abnormalities of maximum mid-expiratory flow and single breath N$_2$ test). These data were compared to six individuals with normal lung function and also to 22 others with FEV$_1$ below 80% predicted. Patients with small airways dysfunction, with normal PaO$_2$, showed a small but significant increase in alveolar–arterial PO$_2$ difference and milder V̇A/Q̇ mismatch, as expressed by modest increases in the dispersions of both blood flow and ventilation (log SD Q̇ below 1.0, each), compared to controls. However, there were no differences in these parameters between patients with mild airway dysfunction and those with early COPD and greater airflow obstruction. Although the interpretation of these data remains speculative, it is akin with the concept, at least theoretically, that functional abnormalities in peripheral airways can produce maldistribution of ventilation and V̇A/Q̇ mismatching in the face of a normal PaO$_2$.

GAS EXCHANGE PATHOPHYSIOLOGY DURING EXACERBATIONS

We have shown that the severity of V̇A/Q̇ abnormalities and their patterns during episodes of exacerbation of COPD may improve substantially over a period of few weeks of adequate treatment.[38] In this sequential study of

patients with acute hypercapnic respiratory failure not needing mechanical ventilation (Figure 14.4), one month after the onset of study, all spirometric and gas exchange indices had improved substantially. Thus, while PaO$_2$ increased and PaCO$_2$ decreased some distributions of V̇A/Q̇ inequalities became unimodal. These data suggest that part of the V̇A/Q̇ abnormalities during exacerbations are related to partially reversible pathophysiologic abnormalities of airway narrowing, such as mucus plugging, bronchial wall edema, bronchoconstriction, increased intrinsic positive end-expiratory pressure (PEEP) and/or air trapping.

Additional studies of COPD patients needing mechanical support for exacerbation of the disease have shown essentially similar qualitatively V̇A/Q̇ patterns, although quantitatively more severe, to those documented in those breathing spontaneously.[39–41] The main difference was the presence of intrapulmonary shunt, which was always slightly increased (range 4–10% of cardiac output). This suggests that some airways were completely occluded, possibly by inspissated bronchial secretions. However, if a patient with COPD shows a substantial increase in intrapulmonary shunt despite a normal chest X-ray, excluding atelectasis, pneumonia, lung collapse or pulmonary edema, then the possibility of a reopening of the foramen ovale due to increase in right atrial pressure should be considered. In the presence of a true shunt, breathing of 100% O$_2$ for 30 minutes or more fails to increase PaO$_2$ (>300–350 mmHg).

Worsening of pulmonary gas exchange during exacerbations not needing mechanical support is primarily produced by increased V̇A/Q̇ mismatching, an effect that

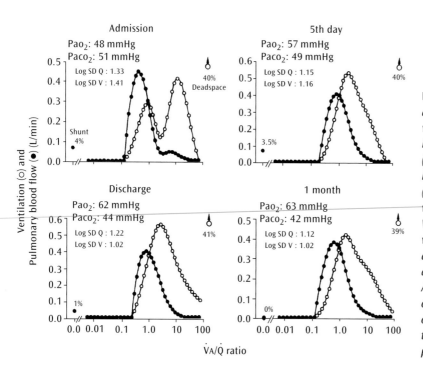

Figure 14.4 *Outcome of V̇A/Q̇ distributions in a representative patient with COPD and acute respiratory failure breathing spontaneously (FIO$_2$ = 0.24) (from left to right and from top to bottom): On admission, V̇A/Q̇ inequalities (log SD Q and log SD V ranges, 1.0–1.5) were moderately to severely abnormal. With appropriate medical care there was a progressive, although partial, amelioration both in V̇A/Q̇ distributions and arterial blood respiratory gases. A modest shunt (less than 5% of cardiac output) is observed during the first days of the acute exacerbation; note also that the bimodal blood flow distribution is present on admission only. (From ref. 38.)*

is amplified by the decreased mixed venous O_2 tension that results from greater O_2 consumption, presumably because of increased work of the respiratory muscles.[38] Interestingly, the increased cardiac output partially counterbalanced the effect of greater O_2 consumption on mixed venous Po_2 (Figure 14.5).

A further finding was the crucial role of both cardiac output and ventilatory pattern in influencing gas exchange when patients were discontinued from mechanical ventilation[39] or were treated with non-invasive mechanical ventilation.[41] During weaning, while cardiac output increased considerably due to the abrupt increase in

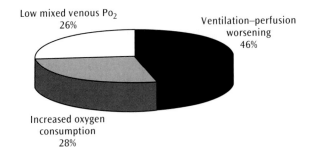

Figure 14.5 *Estimated mechanisms of several determinants of arterial oxygenation during an episode of COPD exacerbation in patients not needing mechanical support. The deterioration of $\dot{V}A/\dot{Q}$ imbalance, an intrapulmonary factor, explains almost half of the arterial deoxygenation shown at the most acute phase of the exacerbation (i.e. 46% of the fall of the Pao_2 to Fio_2 ratio). The other half is caused by an extrapulmonary factor, increased O_2 consumption, which in turn decreases mixed venous Po_2. The latter not only minimizes directly Pao_2, but also indirectly by amplifying the effect of the underlying $\dot{V}A/\dot{Q}$ mismatch on arterial oxygenation. (Reproduced from ref. 35 with permission.)*

venous return (following the reduction of intrathoracic pressure) and total ventilation was maintained, tidal volume was reduced and respiratory frequency increased and became less efficient (Figure 14.6). As a result, both the dispersion of alveolar ventilation and the overall $\dot{V}A/\dot{Q}$ heterogeneity increased resulting in further $\dot{V}A/\dot{Q}$ mismatch. A striking observation was that there was only a small non-significant increase in intrapulmonary shunt from mechanical ventilation to spontaneous breathing (from 3 to 9% of cardiac output) despite the substantial increases in cardiac output and mixed venous Po_2. This is at variance with the well-known, although poorly understood, strong linear relationship between increase in pulmonary blood flow and shunt fraction, commonly observed in patients with acute lung injury.[42] Combining inert gas data and isotopic scans, Beydon *et al.* complemented and extended these data by showing that the critical alteration of the ventilation during weaning led to the development of basal regions of very low $\dot{V}A/\dot{Q}$ ratios.[43]

Another striking finding in the weaning study[39] was that respiratory blood gases remained unaltered despite increases in mixed venous Po_2 and O_2 delivery (arterial O_2 content times cardiac output). In other words, the potentially beneficial effect of the increased cardiac output on Pao_2 was offset by the deleterious influence of the change in ventilatory pattern on Pao_2. Despite these problems, weaning in these patients was successful. When patients were removed from the ventilator in this study,[39] O_2 consumption (calculated according to the Fick principle) did not change. Lemaire and coworkers[44] also stressed the importance of cardiac output variations and other hemodynamic changes together with an increase in O_2 consumption as a cause of unsuccessful weaning, in a similar group of patients with severe COPD in the face of myocardial infarction and left ventricular dysfunction. In the latter[44] and other studies,[45] however, it has been

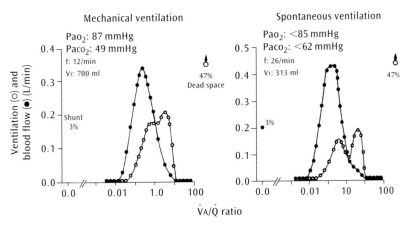

Figure 14.6 *$\dot{V}A/\dot{Q}$ distributions during weaning in a representative patient with COPD, after 9 days of mechanical ventilation. During spontaneous ventilation there was more hypercapnia secondary to an abnormal ventilatory pattern dysfunction (rapid and shallow breathing), which further deteriorated $\dot{V}A/\dot{Q}$ relationships. Cardiac output increased abruptly (not shown) resulting in increased mixed venous Po_2 and, consequently, in less hypoxemia. (From ref. 39 with permission.)*

shown that O_2 consumption usually increases during weaning which could tend to induce a decrease in PaO_2. Subsequently, Rossi *et al.*[40] have investigated the effects of PEEP and those of intrinsic PEEP (PEEPi) on $\dot{V}A/\dot{Q}$ imbalance in mechanically ventilated patients with chronic airflow obstruction (seven out of eight had a diagnosis of COPD), the rationale being that low levels of PEEP can improve rather than impair lung mechanics as PEEP can replace PEEPi. It was shown that the application of PEEP equivalent to 50% of the initial PEEPi improved pulmonary gas exchange without deleterious effects on lung mechanics nor on hemodynamics. Moreover, the use of 'controlled hypoventilation' in conjunction with low PEEPi values significantly reduced alveolar pressure, while increasing cardiac output and systemic O_2 delivery, could be recommended during exacerbations.

The acute effects of non-invasive mechanical ventilation, a progressively demanding therapeutic approach for acute respiratory failure due to COPD, with an undoubted cost-benefit outcome, have also been investigated in our environment.[41] We clearly demonstrated that the beneficial effect on pulmonary gas exchange, namely the combination of decreased hypercapnia, increased PaO_2 and pH improvement, was essentially due to a more optimal ventilatory pattern, i.e. less shallow and slower breathing, without any beneficial influence on the underlying $\dot{V}A/\dot{Q}$ inequalities. It is of note that the significant decrease in cardiac output during the application of mechanical support, because of increased intrathoracic pressure, did not result in any detrimental effect on arterial oxygenation.

Very recently, it has been shown that the combined use of long-term oxygen therapy and nocturnal non-invasive mechanical ventilation in advanced COPD patients with hypercapnic respiratory failure improved substantially arterial blood gases.[46] Moreover, the common descriptors of $\dot{V}A/\dot{Q}$ mismatching ameliorated remarkably, showing a trend to normality. Although it is too early to draw firm conclusions from these preliminary

data, these unique findings suggest that $\dot{V}A/\dot{Q}$ abnormalities may considerably improve possibly due to a structure–function remodeling under some special controled circumstances.

In summary, taken together all these findings point to the view that respiratory gas disturbances (arterial hypoxemia and hypercapnia) are the integrative end-point of $\dot{V}A/\dot{Q}$ abnormalities plus the interaction of overall indices of gas exchange, namely total alveolar ventilation, cardiac output, O_2 consumption and CO_2 production.

STRUCTURE AND FUNCTION

Airways and pulmonary parenchyma

Only one study[25] has investigated the influence of the morphologic changes of both pulmonary emphysema and small airway abnormalities on $\dot{V}A/\dot{Q}$ inequalities. In this study with mild COPD, emphysema was the morphologic variable that correlated best with the respiratory gas indices. The emphysema severity correlated positively with the alveolar–arterial PO_2 difference ($AaPO_2$) and negatively with PaO_2 (Figure 14.7).

Further, emphysema severity was significantly positively related to the dispersion of blood flow and that of alveolar ventilation (Figure 14.7). The more severe the degree of emphysema, the more abnormal the $\dot{V}A/\dot{Q}$ mismatch. The degree of abnormality in the dispersion of pulmonary perfusion suggests the development of areas of lower than normal $\dot{V}A/\dot{Q}$ ratios. These findings suggest that poorly ventilated lung units associated with emphysema may be one of the structural determinants of hypoxemia in these patients. Thus, it can be hypothesized that the loss of alveolar attachments of bronchiolar walls observed in emphysema may result in both distortion and narrowing of the lumen of bronchioles. The latter may cause reduced alveolar ventilation in the dependent

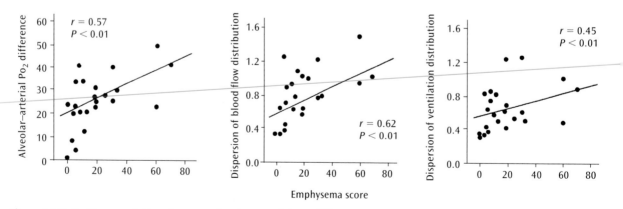

Figure 14.7 *Positive correlations between alveolar–arterial PO_2 difference and blood flow and alveolar ventilation dispersions (y-axes) and emphysema score (x-axes) in patients with early COPD. (From ref. 25 with permission.)*

alveolar units, and hence low $\dot{V}_A/\dot{Q}$ ratios. Likewise, it has been shown that centrilobular emphysema areas have a greater residual volume and a lower compliance leading therefore to a decreased ventilation-to-volume ratio. This is an additional mechanism to account for a reduction in effective ventilation in peripheral alveoli. Reduction in ventilation of some areas produces lung units with continued blood flow and thus low $\dot{V}_A/\dot{Q}$ areas. Accordingly, this abnormality in $\dot{V}_A/\dot{Q}$ relationships becomes evident in the dispersion of blood flow.

The correlation between emphysema and abnormalities in the dispersion of alveolar ventilation (Figure 14.7) may be, at least in part, related to the loss of pulmonary capillary network of emphysematous spaces (namely, wasted ventilation). This would lead to the development of lung units with high $\dot{V}_A/\dot{Q}$ ratios, hence increasing dispersion of ventilation. Accordingly, the bimodal pattern of the ventilation distribution, with a large amount of ventilation diverted to high $\dot{V}_A/\dot{Q}$ ratios (type H) alluded to above in patients with advanced Type A COPD, would be an extension of this phenomenon likely reflecting large areas of destroyed parenchyma.

Despite the lack of any relationship between chronic abnormalities in small airways and the respiratory gas indices, a finding consistent with the absence of correlation between these structural changes and the dispersion of blood flow, bronchiolar lesions were associated with $\dot{V}_A/\dot{Q}$ imbalance as shown by the significant correlation between the airway inflammation score and the dispersion of ventilation (Figure 14.8). One explanation for this correlation could be that airway narrowing secondary to bronchiolar damage produces a heterogeneous distribution of inspired air. This would account for the increased dispersion of ventilation, which is particularly

evident when the latter is broadly unimodal and devoid of very high $\dot{V}_A/\dot{Q}$ ratios as is the case here.

The absence of a correlation between small airways abnormalities and both the dispersion of blood flow and the percentage of perfusion to low $\dot{V}_A/\dot{Q}$ ratios cannot be extrapolated to the usual $\dot{V}_A/\dot{Q}$ findings in patients with more advanced COPD, particularly during exacerbations.[38–41] Under these conditions, a bimodal blood flow pattern distribution may be more common and be attributed to an acute superimposition of airway changes which are potentially reversible, such as bronchial wall edema or mucus plugging, on the chronic airways abnormalities.

These data suggest that there is a spectrum of $\dot{V}_A/\dot{Q}$ abnormalities in patients with COPD. At one end of the spectrum lie those patients with mild to moderate airflow obstruction and little or no arterial blood gas abnormal abnormality, whose $\dot{V}_A/\dot{Q}$ mismatch is mild, and characterized by broadly unimodal profiles of the dispersions of blood flow and alveolar ventilation. At the other end, are those patients with severe advanced disease and marked gas exchange abnormalities. These individuals will show dramatic $\dot{V}_A/\dot{Q}$ inequalities, with bimodal profiles of blood flow or alveolar ventilation distributions, or both, according to clinical conditions, reflecting different degrees of progression of disease. Conceivably, historic Type B patients with high $\dot{V}_A/\dot{Q}$ areas share lesions of emphysema as well as of chronic bronchitis, but Type A COPD patients with areas of low $\dot{V}_A/\dot{Q}$ units are rarely observed. These patients with severe COPD show always increased deadspace and occasionally modest levels of increased intrapulmonary shunt, particularly during exacerbations. In between would be many patients, including different degrees of $\dot{V}_A/\dot{Q}$ mismatch, depending on evolution, clinical condition and therapeutic regimen.

Pulmonary circulation

We have assessed the potential correlation between the pulmonary vascular abnormalities and the $\dot{V}_A/\dot{Q}$ relationships in COPD patients prior to lobectomy for solitary lesions.[47] We found that the lower the degree of pulmonary vascular reactivity to the breathing of 100% O_2, the greater was the thickness of the intimal layer of the pulmonary vascular arteries. Further, the thickness of the intimal layer was related to abnormal gas exchange indices, such as PaO_2 and the degree of $\dot{V}_A/\dot{Q}$ inequality, as reflected by both the dispersion of alveolar ventilation and an overall descriptor of $\dot{V}_A/\dot{Q}$ imbalance, and also to the degree of bronchiolar inflammation. Obviously, this is crucial to the development of further $\dot{V}_A/\dot{Q}$ worsening. Moreover, thickening in small pulmonary arteries can interfere with the adaptability of these vessels to various O_2 concentrations and the maintenance of $\dot{V}_A/\dot{Q}$ matching. It appears that in patients with mild COPD the

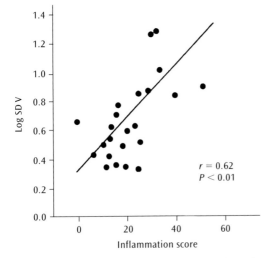

Figure 14.8 *Positive correlation between the dispersion of alveolar ventilation (y-axis) and inflammatory bronchial changes (x-axis) in patients with early COPD. (From ref. 25 with permission.)*

enlargement of the intimal layer in pulmonary muscular arteries is associated with a higher degree of $\dot{V}A/\dot{Q}$ mismatching, and that intimal thickening in small arteries seems to minimize the response of the pulmonary vasculature to different oxygen concentrations.

It has been shown in a multivariate analysis that two of the best independent predictors of hospitalization for exacerbations in patients with moderate to severe COPD were a pulmonary artery pressure above 18 mmHg and a $PaCO_2$ above 44 mmHg.[48] Thus, pulmonary artery pressure could be a marker of the deleterious effects of alveolar hypoxia on the pulmonary circulation, reflecting the individual's susceptibility to arterial hypoxemia and the variability of the hypoxia-induced abnormalities of the pulmonary vasculature. Moreover, both structural and dysfunctional disturbances in the pulmonary circulation that result in pulmonary hypertension are hallmarks of the natural history of COPD. Potential mechanisms of pulmonary hypertension in COPD include remodeling of pulmonary vessels, hypoxic pulmonary vasoconstriction, polycythemia and emphysematous destruction of the capillary network. Pulmonary vascular remodeling appears to be the principal causative factor of pulmonary hypertension in COPD, as suggested by its failure to resolve after arterial hypoxemia correction with acute or continuous administration of oxygen. This remodeling is apparent in COPD patients with a wide range of disease severity. Structural changes of pulmonary vasculature in COPD preferentially affects the pulmonary muscular arteries as well as the precapillary vessels. In patients with end-stage COPD, the media was normal or atrophic while the intima was thickened by deposition of longitudinal muscle, fibrosis and elastosis in pulmonary muscular arteries.[49] At the precapillary level, the formation of a medial coat of circular smooth muscle bounded by a new internal elastic lamina, and sometimes the lumen, was subdivided into parallel tubes.

In a seminal study, Dinh-Xuan and coworkers[50] demonstrated that endothelial pulmonary vascular dysfunction in patients with end-stage COPD undergoing lung transplantation was related linearly to pretransplantation PaO_2. This indicated that chronic hypoxemia may impair endothelial cell metabolism and possibly the synthesis of endogenous nitric oxide (NO), processes that may play a vital role in the remodeling of pulmonary vessels in COPD. Although chronic hypoxemia may account for the impairment of endothelial dysfunction in advanced COPD, the mechanisms operating in mild non-hypoxemic COPD patients remain to be settled.

Peinado and associates[51] have shown that endothelial dysfunction of pulmonary arteries is already present in mild COPD patients undergoing lung resection. They studied non-smokers, smokers with normal spirometry and patients with mild COPD, and expressed the changes in muscle tension of pulmonary arteries, expressed as percent reduction from pre-contraction with L-phenylephrine chloride in response to cumulative concentrations of adenosine diphosphate (ADP). Compared with both smokers and non-smokers, there was a significant reduction in the maximal relaxation in response to ADP; similar findings were seen with acetylcholine (ACh). Thus relaxation of pulmonary artery rings induced by NO-dependent vasodilators, such as ACh and ADP, is diminished early in the natural history of COPD. These maximal relaxations induced by ADP and ACh were linearly correlated with the FEV_1/FVC ratio, suggesting that endothelial dysfunction may be enhanced by disease progression. This is consistent with the findings already alluded to[50] in end-stage COPD but extends them to a stage of the disease when arterial hypoxemia is absent. Remarkably, when compared with non-smokers, both patients with COPD and smokers with normal lung function showed the same severity of intimal thickening in pulmonary arteries.

In summary, although the intensity of the enlargement of the intima of the pulmonary artery wall was similar in both COPD patients and smokers without airflow obstruction and higher than in non-smokers, the degree of maximal relaxation was lowest in patients with COPD alone; smokers lay in between the two populations studied. These findings suggest that structural vascular changes might be initiated well before the impairment of pulmonary vascular reactivity and of lung function and that cigarette smoke may be associated with structural abnormalities of the pulmonary vasculature related to the remodeling process, even though airflow limitation is not present yet.

The intensity of intimal thickening in the pulmonary arteries in COPD patients correlates with the severity of the inflammatory infiltrate in small airways, suggesting a common inflammatory process affecting both structural abnormalities.[47] This could explain why, in some populations of patients with mild to moderate COPD, the presence of gas exchange disturbances may be out of proportion to the severity of airflow obstruction.

Compared with non-smokers, Peinado and coworkers[52] have also shown in both mild COPD patients and smokers with normal lung function that there are an increased number of inflammatory cells in the adventitia of pulmonary muscular arteries. This is largely composed of activated T-lymphocytes, with a predominance of the CD8+ T-cell subset. The reduced CD4/CD8 ratio is akin to that shown in both large and peripheral airways and also in the alveolar septa by other groups.[53,54] Interestingly, the greater the severity of the inflammatory response of the pulmonary vascular wall the more profound is the degree of airflow obstruction, as assessed by the FEV_1/FVC ratio, and the greater the endothelium dysfunction, and intensity of intimal thickening in the walls of the pulmonary vessels. Unlike non-smokers and smokers with normal spirometry, patients with mild COPD expressed less endothelial NO synthase (NOS) in their pulmonary arteries, as assessed by immunochemistry and Western blot analysis.[55] Again smokers without airflow obstruction were an intermediate group between non-smokers and patients with early but already established COPD. This suggests that a diminished synthesis or release of NO by the pulmonary endothelium may contribute to the structural and functional abnormalities of the pulmonary vasculature shown in the early stages of COPD.

Altogether these data suggest that cigarette smoke is involved in the pathogenesis of pulmonary vascular abnormalities in COPD. This is consistent with the hypothesis that a chronic inflammatory process, mainly driven by CD8+ Tcells, and involving the release of inflammatory mediators (such as interleukin 8 (IL-8), leukotriene B_4, tumor necrosis factor), underlies the structural and functional disturbances of the pulmonary vasculature in mild COPD. Alternatively, a direct effect of cigarette smoke might produce the thickening of the intima through a cell proliferation process. This could result in pulmonary vascular remodeling that ultimately leads to pulmonary hypertension. As disease progresses, the coexistence of chronic hypoxemia in more advanced COPD may further amplify and/or enhance this deleterious process.

GAS EXCHANGE DURING EXERCISE

In normal man at maximum exercise, O_2 transport can increase as much as 15–20 times compared to resting

conditions.[56] By contrast, in patients with severe COPD O_2 consumption at maximum symptom-limited exercise only increases by three to four times resting levels to approximately 1 liter per minute. Such limitation is basically due to the inability of the lungs to match pulmonary O_2 uptake and elimination of CO_2 to the higher levels of whole-body metabolic O_2 consumption and CO_2 production that accompany exercise. Physical deconditioning also plays a role limiting exercise performance in these patients. The behavior of both PaO_2 and $PaCO_2$ during exercise in these patients rely on complex interactions between intrapulmonary (essentially $\dot{V}A/\dot{Q}$ mismatching) and extrapulmonary factors (i.e. cardiac output, total ventilation and O_2 consumption) modulating respiratory gases (Figure 14.9). As during weaning, during exercise PaO_2 and $PaCO_2$ do not necessarily reflect parallel variations in $\dot{V}A/\dot{Q}$ inequality because of these extrapulmonary factors.

The original MIGET study of Wagner et al.[15] performed in patients with severe COPD during exercise, showed a complete absence of systematic changes in the measured respiratory gases and in $\dot{V}A/\dot{Q}$ distributions; likewise, there was no evidence of a diffusion defect for O_2. A later study,[21] in a smaller series of patients with similarly advanced COPD, showed the same results for intrapulmonary determinants of respiratory gases ($\dot{V}A/\dot{Q}$ relationships and diffusion limitation) but falls in PaO_2 and mixed venous PO_2 and a rise in $PaCO_2$ occurred during exercise. These results, if explained by an inadequate ventilatory response resulting in increased hypercapnia, decreased mixed venous PO_2 – secondary to an increased O_2 consumption with its subsequent impact on the

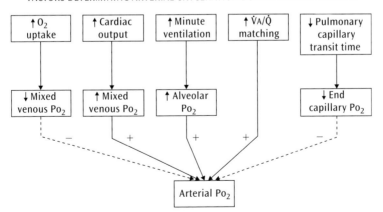

FACTORS DETERMINING ARTERIAL OXYGENATION DURING EXERCISE IN COPD

Figure 14.9 *Arterial PO_2 increases because either cardiac output and/or minute ventilation (extrapulmonary determinants) increase, or $\dot{V}A/\dot{Q}$ mismatching (intrapulmonary determinant) improves; other extrapulmonary factors, such as increased O_2 uptake (consumption) and decreased pulmonary capillary blood transit time (due to increased cardiac output in the absence of pulmonary capillary recruitment/distensibility), may tend to reduce PaO_2. Arterial PO_2 is thus the end-point variable of the complex interaction between all these elements. Similar interplay is observed in other situations, such as discontinuing from mechanical ventilation or after the administration of vasoactive drugs.*

end-capillary P_{O_2} of areas with alveoli with low $\dot{V}_A/\dot{Q}$ ratios – and further hypoxemia, were considered the most likely mechanisms of arterial blood gas abnormalities.

Two further studies[24,57] have assessed the effects of submaximal exercise (approximately at 60% of maximal O_2 consumption) in patients with COPD, with severe airflow obstruction, mild to moderate impairment of gas exchange and no pulmonary hypertension. In the first study,[24] it was shown that, unlike patients with more advanced disease, exercise had a beneficial effect on $\dot{V}_A/\dot{Q}$ distributions with a reduced dispersion of ventilation and a more homogeneous distribution of pulmonary blood flow; as expected, inert gas deadspace fell significantly. It was hypothesized that these improvements were related to less severe structural abnormalities.

In the second study Barberà et al.[57] showed, in patients with even milder COPD, that, as a group, both Pa_{O_2} and AaP_{O_2} improved during exercise without significant changes in Pa_{CO_2}. The main mechanism of adaptation of gas exchange was a relatively greater rise in minute ventilation than in cardiac output. This accounted for a shift of blood flow distribution to higher $\dot{V}_A/\dot{Q}$ ratios, hence optimizing the efficiency of the lung as a gas exchanger. Furthermore, the greater the structural derangement of the airways, as assessed by the total pathologic score of the membranous bronchioles, the more the improvement in the dispersion of alveolar ventilation from resting to maximum symptom-limited exercise conditions. This reduction in the dispersion of ventilation post-exercise suggests a preferential diversion of ventilation to alveolar units with normal $\dot{V}_A/\dot{Q}$ ratios. Conceivably, normal areas with an adequate $\dot{V}_A/\dot{Q}$ matching are more sensitive to ventilation or blood flow changes, or both, than are alveolar units with abnormal $\dot{V}_A/\dot{Q}$ ratios. A complementary explanation for the improvement in the distribution of ventilation could be related to pulmonary mechanical changes during exercise. It can be speculated that lung volume increases due to an increased internal diameter of the membranous bronchioles, hence leading to an increased functional residual capacity, thereby enhancing a more homogeneous distribution of ventilation. In other words, there is an increase in and a more efficient distribution of ventilation that results in an overall improvement in pulmonary gas exchange in these patients.

From a clinical viewpoint, it is important to stress the relevance of invasive exercise testing with gas exchange and pulmonary hemodynamic measurements in patients with COPD at a high risk for lung resection.[58] In this setting, the FEV_1 combined with the extent of parenchymal resection and perfusion of the affected lung remain the most useful parameters to identify patients at greatest risk of postoperative complications in those undergoing lung surgical resection. Interestingly, whereas pulmonary hemodynamics do not appear to have a discriminatory value, gas exchange measurements during exercise may help identify patients with higher mortality risk, as non-survivors had a greater fall in Pa_{O_2} during exercise than survivors. This is consistent with other studies[59] which show that a decreased arterial oxygen saturation during exercise is useful in the prediction of postoperative complication.

GAS EXCHANGE RESPONSE TO OXYGEN

The response to high oxygen concentrations in patients with COPD is broadly similar irrespective of the clinical severity of the disease. With little $\dot{V}_A/\dot{Q}$ mismatch, Pa_{O_2} rises almost linearly as the inspired O_2 is increased. As the severity of $\dot{V}_A/\dot{Q}$ inequality worsens, the rate of rise of Pa_{O_2} is reduced and becomes more curvilinear. We have shown in patients with COPD and acute respiratory failure needing mechanical ventilation that full nitrogen washout of alveolar units, even in patients with poorly ventilated alveolar units with low or very low $\dot{V}_A/\dot{Q}$ ratios, is rapid and that steady-state conditions are easily reached even before 30 minutes.[60] The coexistence of a modest increased intrapulmonary shunt, however, further decreases the elevation of Pa_{O_2}. In clinical practice, however, physicians administer low inspired O_2 concentrations (either 0.24 or 0.28) delivered through high flow masks to patients with COPD and acute respiratory failure. This provides modest but effective increases in Pa_{O_2} (of the order of 10–15 mmHg) without inducing detrimental CO_2 retention, to optimize O_2 delivery to peripheral tissues.

Although $\dot{V}_A/\dot{Q}$ inequality is no longer a barrier to O_2 exchange when 100% O_2 is breathed, 100% O_2 always worsens $\dot{V}_A/\dot{Q}$ mismatch, as assessed by a significant increase in the dispersion of blood flow, without changes in intrapulmonary shunt nor in the dispersion of alveolar ventilation (Figure 14.10); by contrast, pulmonary arterial pressure and pulmonary vascular resistance remains essentially unchanged. The impairment in $\dot{V}_A/\dot{Q}$ relationships indicates release or abolition of hypoxic pulmonary vasoconstriction. The total absence of further increases in intrapulmonary shunt indicates that reabsorption atelectasis does not take place, suggesting that either collateral ventilation is very efficient or regional airway obstruction is never complete. By contrast, in patients with ARDS a mild to moderate increase in shunt without release of hypoxic pulmonary vasoconstriction results following 100% oxygen administration.[60] This response suggests the presence of critical alveolar units (with low inspired $\dot{V}_A/\dot{Q}$ ratios) unstable and vulnerable to high O_2 concentrations over time. These units tend to easily collapse, hence leading to the development of reabsorption atelectasis.[61] When there is no release of hypoxic vasoconstriction, the amount of shunt is always greater, irrespective of the $F_{I_{O_2}}$.

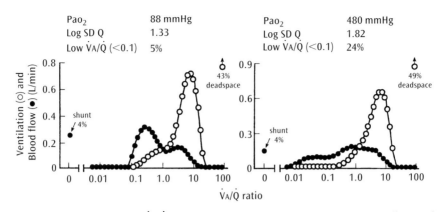

Figure 14.10 *Effect of 100% O_2 breathing on $\dot{V}A/\dot{Q}$ distributions during a COPD exacerbation needing mechanical support (FIO_2, 1.0).[60] Compared to low inspired O_2 concentrations (FIO_2, 0.34, left) the most striking finding was the increase in the dispersion of pulmonary blood flow (log SD $\dot{Q}$), suggesting that hypoxic pulmonary vasoconstriction was reduced. Note that PaO_2 increased to considerable levels indicating full nitrogen washout, whilst shunt remained constant and deadspace increased minimally only. (Data correspond to mean values of four patients.)*

The contention is that alveolar units with poorly ventilated $\dot{V}A/\dot{Q}$ ratios are not able to redistribute blood flow if their vascular resistance remains unaltered. Alternatively, it has been shown, in patients with COPD, that breathing high inspired O_2 concentrations reduces the degree of airways resistance.[62] This should tend to improve the distribution of ventilation, other factors being equal, thus reducing the amount of areas with low $\dot{V}A/\dot{Q}$ ratios and, consequently, the dispersion of pulmonary blood flow.

An intriguing finding is that, irrespective of the FIO_2, inert gas shunt is always less than venous admixture ratio; there are no differences, however, between the latter variable and the sum of inert gas shunt plus the percentage of blood flow diverted to low $\dot{V}A/\dot{Q}$ ratios.[60] At low levels of FIO_2, this is explained because the inert shunt and the low $\dot{V}A/\dot{Q}$ areas are incorporated into the measurement of venous admixture ratio. By contrast, when breathing 100% O_2 shunt and venous admixture ratio should be equal because the washout of nitrogen abolishes all alveolar units with poorly ventilated $\dot{V}A/\dot{Q}$ ratios. Although the reasons for such difference remain to be elucidated, release of hypoxic vasoconstriction in the pulmonary circulation, whilst 100% O_2 breathing could be an explanation.

Using traditional gas exchange measurements, such as the Bohr's dead space, Aubier *et al.*[63] concluded that, in patients with COPD and acute on chronic respiratory insufficiency, the administration of 100% O_2 breathing spontaneously resulted in a remarkable increase in PaCO_2. Since the respiratory muscles maintained ventilation at nearly the same level as when breathing room air, they suggested that the increase in PaCO_2 was mainly attributed to an increased deadspace; additional mechanisms included a small reduction in both tidal volume and the Haldane effect, namely the changes in the CO_2 dissociation

curve facilitating the release of CO_2 from bicarbonate and also from that directly bound as carbamate during 100% O_2. This conclusion has been disputed by Stradling[64] who advocated that the increase in PaCO_2 could be explained entirely by the latter two mechanisms together with that from flattening the slope of the CO_2 pressure/content relationship with a rise in PaCO_2. Our group has also shown an increase in PaCO_2 during 100% O_2 breathing in COPD patients needing mechanical support.[60] Conceivably, the increased deadspace and the experimental evidence that increased $\dot{V}A/\dot{Q}$ disturbances can worsen not only the O_2 transfer but also CO_2 exchange are responsible for this increase. Nevertheless, the Haldane effect could also enhance the ratio of PCO_2 to blood CO_2 content. We estimated however that the hyperoxia-induced increments of PaCO_2 in this subset of patients could be attributed almost entirely to the simultaneous increased deadspace, thereby indicating a marginal role of the Haldane effect. This was further supported by the persistence of hypercapnia when maintenance FIO_2 was restarted. The increased deadspace suggests redistribution of pulmonary blood flow from high $\dot{V}A/\dot{Q}$ ratios to poorly perfused but still ventilated units (low $\dot{V}A/\dot{Q}$ ratios).

An alternative or complementary mechanism could be bronchodilation secondary to the hypercapnia, as postulated by Robinson *et al.*[65] in patients with COPD during exacerbations breathing spontaneously. A similar conclusion was reached when data derived from a computer model of the pulmonary circulation were compared with data from a case series of patients with COPD.[66] In this study, changes in physiologic deadspace were sufficient to account for the hypercarbia developed by patients with exacerbations of COPD when treated with supplemental oxygen.

Robinson *et al.*[65] also found that in hyperoxia-induced CO_2-retaining patients with COPD during exacerbations, ventilation fell by an average of 20% and the dispersion of alveolar ventilation, a reflection of an inert gas measurement of alveolar deadspace, increased by about 25% when breathing 100% O_2. Likewise, patients who were CO_2 retainers showed a significant increase in alveolar deadspace, indicating a higher CO_2 retention, perhaps related to bronchodilation. Moreover, there was an increase in the dispersion of pulmonary blood flow (i.e. areas with low $\dot{V}A/\dot{Q}$ ratios) due to the release of hypoxic vasoconstriction, irrespective of the presence or absence of CO_2 retention.

THE EFFECTS OF DRUGS

Bronchodilators

Ringstedt *et al.*[23] explored the role of the pulmonary vascular tone in modulating gas exchange by studying a small group of patients with advanced COPD and mild respiratory failure, before and after a continuous intravenous infusion of terbutaline (beta$_2$-agonist bronchodilator). After terbutaline, cardiac output increased and systemic blood pressure and pulmonary vascular resistance decreased. In addition, while PaO_2 decreased and mixed venous PO_2 and O_2 delivery increased, $PaCO_2$ remained unchanged. There was further $\dot{V}A/\dot{Q}$ worsening, as assessed by increases both in the perfusion to low $\dot{V}A/\dot{Q}$ ratios and in the dispersion of blood flow. Although FEV_1 and minute ventilation increased, these increments were not significant. Thus, the $\dot{V}A/\dot{Q}$ worsening could have resulted from an increased dispersion of pulmonary blood flow and/or a decrease in the overall $\dot{V}A/\dot{Q}$ ratio due to the increased cardiac output, that was not fully counterbalanced by the simultaneous rise in minute ventilation. The concomitant increase in mixed venous PO_2 may have also contributed to further worsen $\dot{V}A/\dot{Q}$ mismatch by releasing hypoxic pulmonary vasoconstriction. However these data cannot differentiate between an increased cardiac output, increasing pulmonary blood flow dispersion, or an active reduction in pulmonary vascular tone. In the same study[23] in another small group of COPD patients who had more airflow obstruction, hypoxemia, hypercapnia and also more pulmonary hypertension, cardiac output increased without changes in pulmonary artery pressure or pulmonary vascular resistance. Although minute ventilation increased modestly there was no improvement in the airflow obstruction, arterial blood gases or the underlying $\dot{V}A/\dot{Q}$ abnormalities. In summary, although terbutaline increased cardiac output and mixed venous PO_2 by a similar degree to that seen in mild disease, it did not modify the gas exchange of the more severely affected patients. Conceivably, the hypoxic vascular response could have modulated pulmonary gas exchange before and after the drug, with patients with more severe COPD having a reduced or even absent hypoxic vascular response. This could be related to either chronic alveolar hypoxia or to structural changes in the pulmonary circulation coupled with areas of parenchymal destruction due to emphysema, or both. This is in keeping with the concept that the progressive increase of pulmonary vascular resistance seen in advanced COPD not only is due to irreversible structural vascular lesions but also includes a reversible vascular component. This interpretation would also be consistent with the work of Barberà *et al.*,[57] investigating the influence of the structure of pulmonary arteries and the contribution of the hypoxic vascular response in preserving an adequate matching of ventilation and blood flow in patients with mild COPD.

The acute effects of salmeterol, a long-acting beta$_2$-adrenergic agonist in stable patients with COPD, have been compared with those of salbutamol and the anticholinergic agent ipratropium, given in recommended dosages, using conventional arterial blood gas measurements.[67] Arterial blood gases were measured at baseline and at intervals to 120 minutes on separate days in a double-blinded, crossover design. The decline in PaO_2 following salmeterol was of lesser magnitude but more prolonged, of about -2.75 mmHg at 30 minutes, than that after salbutamol, of about -3.5 mmHg at 20 minutes; after ipratropium, the corresponding change was about -1.3 mmHg at 20 minutes. These marginal decrements of PaO_2, almost entirely explained by increases in the alveolar-arterial PO_2 difference, hence suggesting further $\dot{V}A/\dot{Q}$ worsening, were more evident in those patients with higher baseline PaO_2 values. The study concluded that despite small negative changes in PaO_2 after each of the three bronchodilators, the decreases were marginal, transient and, above all, of doubtful clinical relevance.

We have also compared the short-term effect on gas exchange of fenoterol, a selective beta$_2$-agonist, against that of ipratropium bromide, both given by inhalation, in a double-blind, placebo-controlled study in a series of patients with severe COPD and mild to moderate hypoxemia.[29] We found that fenoterol slightly decreased mean PaO_2 (about 6 mmHg) due to a worsening in the dispersion of pulmonary blood flow; gas exchange remained unaltered after ipratropium. Although pulmonary hemodynamics were not measured, pulmonary vascular tone was probably decreased, hence inducing further $\dot{V}A/\dot{Q}$ mismatch. This is at variance with the effects of intravenous salbutamol given to patients with acute severe asthma,[68] in whom PaO_2 remained unchanged despite marked increases in cardiac output and similar changes in $\dot{V}A/\dot{Q}$ inequality. This suggests that fenoterol may have a greater direct effect on the pulmonary vasculature, producing the decreases in the vascular tone. At doses similar to those used in clinical practice, fenoterol causes more adverse effects (namely, cardiac, metabolic and systemic) than salbutamol or terbutaline in patients with mild asthma.[69] The most likely explanation is that fenoterol has been marketed at a higher dose than the other two beta$_2$-agonists, despite having *in vitro* the same potency as isoproterenol; furthermore, it is suggested that fenoterol may be less selective for beta$_2$-receptors.

Vasodilators

Since severe pulmonary hypertension may worsen the prognosis of COPD, attempts have been made to lower pulmonary hypertension in these patients by means of continuous oxygen therapy and/or pulmonary vasodilator treatment. However, a major adverse effect of systemic vasodilators on the pulmonary circulation is the inhibition of hypoxic pulmonary vasoconstriction, hence exerting a negative impact on the underlying $\dot{V}A/\dot{Q}$ abnormalities. A good example of the influence of pulmonary vascular tone on gas exchange is given by the administration of oral nifedipine in patients with COPD and chronic respiratory failure.[17] After nifedipine there was a reduction in mean systemic arterial pressure and also in systemic vascular resistance. While cardiac output increased, pulmonary vascular resistance decreased without accompanying changes in pulmonary artery pressure. Similarly, Pa_{O_2} decreased and there was further deterioration of $\dot{V}A/\dot{Q}$ relationships: blood flow was redistributed to areas with low $\dot{V}A/\dot{Q}$ units such that the dispersion of pulmonary perfusion increased. These changes suggest partial release of hypoxic pulmonary vasoconstriction and represent, in part, a real concern regarding the use of vasodilating drugs for the therapy of pulmonary vasonconstriction due to COPD. Similar results were shown by our group[24] in patients with COPD with mild hypoxemia and less severe disease.

In another study,[26] felodipine, a calcium antagonist vasodilator, was administered to patients with advanced COPD and chronic respiratory failure as an adjuvant to long-term oxygen therapy. Short-term infusion of the drug produced similar pulmonary gas exchange alterations to the two previous studies using nifedipine,[17,24] explained also by a reduction of hypoxic vasoconstriction. Interestingly, while long-term oral administration of felodipine over a period of several weeks induced systemic and pulmonary hemodynamic changes similar to those produced during short-term therapy, there was no further $\dot{V}A/\dot{Q}$ worsening.[26] Although the exact mechanism is still to be elucidated, a redistribution of ventilation to areas with low $\dot{V}A/\dot{Q}$ ratios receiving simultaneously an increased amount of blood flow appears to be the most likely explanation. Similar detrimental effects on gas exchange have been shown following the use of vasoactive agents, such as dopamine and dobutamine, in patients

with COPD and acute respiratory failure needing artificial ventilation,[70] prostaglandin E$_1$,[71] atrial natriuretic factor[72] and acetylcholine.[73]

Administration of inhaled NO exerts a selective vasodilator effect on pulmonary circulation.[74] The lack of systemic vasodilatation when NO is given by inhalation is due to its inactivation when combined with hemoglobin, for which it has a very high affinity. Moreover, in patients with acute respiratory distress syndrome (ARDS) the administration of inhaled NO produces a significant improvement in arterial oxygenation, due to the reduction of intrapulmonary shunting.[75] The effect of inhaled NO in COPD was first investigated by Adnot et al.,[73] who carried out a dose–response study on hemodynamic and gas exchange effects of acutely inhaled NO, and compared with intravenous acetilcholine. It was shown that inhaled NO produced a significant decrease in pulmonary artery pressure at concentrations as low as 5 parts per million (ppm), and that higher concentrations resulted in a further decrease in pulmonary artery pressure in a dose-dependent manner. By contrast, changes in Pa_{O_2} (from 57 to 60 mmHg), were negligible and were observed only at concentrations of 40 ppm (but not at lower concentrations). Moinard et al.[76] evaluated the effect of 15 ppm NO, for a short period, in COPD patients with severe airflow obstruction using MIGET. Pulmonary artery pressure decreased moderately with NO, whereas Pa_{O_2} remained unchanged and this was consistent with the lack of changes in $\dot{V}A/\dot{Q}$ balance. This lack of effect of NO on gas exchange could be explained by the low dose of NO given. However, in both the study by Adnot et al.[73] and that by Moinard et al.[76] the individual responses were quite variable, with some patients showing a decreased Pa_{O_2} during NO inhalation.

To further investigate the potential effects of inhaled NO on hypoxic pulmonary vasoconstriction, we investigated patients with advanced COPD while breathing NO (40 ppm) and 100% O_2.[30] NO inhalation produced a moderate decrease of pulmonary artery pressure and also of Pa_{O_2}. The latter resulted from further worsening of $\dot{V}A/\dot{Q}$ mismatching, as shown by a greater dispersion of blood flow perfusion and an increased proportion of lung units with low $\dot{V}A/\dot{Q}$ ratios. Interestingly, 100% O_2 breathing reduced pulmonary artery pressure to a lesser extent than NO whilst provoking greater $\dot{V}A/\dot{Q}$ imbalance. Baseline intrapulmonary shunt on room air was trivial and did not change while breathing NO or 100% O_2. This deleterious effect of inhaled NO on gas exchange in COPD has been confirmed by other clinical studies,[77] including exacerbations needing mechanical support,[78] and also experimentally in a canine model,[79] and has been also attributed to the inhibition of hypoxic pulmonary vasoconstriction in lung areas with alveolar units with low $\dot{V}A/\dot{Q}$ ratios, to which the gas has also access, hence exerting an effect similar to that of systemic vasodilators. In this regard,

Frostell et al.[80] showed that in healthy subjects the inhalation of 40 ppm NO abolished completely the increase in pulmonary vascular tone induced by breathing a hypoxic mixture (FIO_2 12%). A potential clinical implication of these findings is that in patients in whom hypoxemia is caused essentially by $\dot{V}A/\dot{Q}$ inequality rather than by increased intrapulmonary shunt, as is the case in COPD, inhaled NO can worsen gas exchange by impairing the hypoxic regulation of ventilation and perfusion matching. This may help in predicting which patients with acute respiratory failure will show the greatest improvement of gas exchange with inhaled NO. Patients without pre-existing chronic lung disease, in whom increased intrapulmonary shunt is the principal determinant of hypoxemia (i.e. ARDS, pneumonia), appear to be those most likely to benefit from NO inhalation. The combined use of low levels of inhaled NO (2 ppm) together with low flow supplemental oxygen (1 L/min), in patients with stable moderate to severe COPD, produced remarkable reductions in pulmonary artery pressures and improved gas arterial oxygenation.[81] Conceivably, the combined administration of O_2 and NO in these patients offset the detrimental release of hypoxic vasoconstriction in areas with alveolar units with low $\dot{V}A/\dot{Q}$ ratios in which NO had also access. These data have been complemented and extended recently in patients with advanced COPD requiring long-term oxygen therapy (2 L/min via nasal cannula).[82] This strategy of continuous oxygen therapy and relatively low doses of inhaled NO (25 ppm) can be safely administered for 24 hours, showing a significant improvement in pulmonary vascular resistance.[82] Circulating hemoglobin contributes substantially to vascular reactivity in patients with chronic lung diseases, including COPD, and polycythemia is associated with a loss of NO-mediated endothelium-dependent vasodilator response to acetilcholine.[83]

Studies on the hemodynamic and gas exchange effects of inhaled NO in COPD patients during exercise have also been performed.[31] Nine patients with moderate to severe airflow obstruction were studied at rest and during steady-state submaximal exercise, while breathing room air and 40 ppm NO. NO inhalation reduced pulmonary vascular resistance both at rest and during exercise. However, the effects of NO on pulmonary gas exchange were different during exercise than those at rest.[30] Whereas PaO_2 decreased during exercise whilst breathing room air, no change occurred during NO inhalation. Furthermore, whereas at rest NO inhalation worsened $\dot{V}A/\dot{Q}$ distributions,[30] during exercise $\dot{V}A/\dot{Q}$ imbalance improved while breathing both room air and NO, such that perfusion of poorly ventilated alveolar units with low $\dot{V}A/\dot{Q}$ ratios was similar under both conditions.[31] Accordingly, from rest to exercise the proportion of blood flow to low $\dot{V}A/\dot{Q}$ units decreased significantly with NO, whereas it did not vary while breathing room air.

These findings indicate that, in stable COPD patients, the inhalation of NO while exercising reduces pulmonary hypertension and, unlike the resting data, it may prevent the development of exercise-induced hypoxemia. The latter effect is likely explained by a preferential distribution of NO during exercise to well ventilated alveolar units with faster time constants, more efficient in terms of pulmonary gas exchange. From a clinical viewpoint, these findings imply that if inhaled NO could be delivered specifically to those alveolar units that are better ventilated and have faster time constants, possibly by adjusting the ventilator settings or by minimizing the inhalation of NO with breath by breath delivery of spikes of concentrated gas, the beneficial effect of NO would not be offset by its detrimental impact on gas exchange.[84] A preliminary study using the spike delivery of inhaled NO in stable advanced COPD patients has provided evidence that the underlying $\dot{V}A/\dot{Q}$ imbalance improves significantly,[85] hence supporting the view that NO reaches more adequately well-preserved alveolar units, with faster time constants.

Other drugs

There have been three studies[16,20,86] in patients with COPD and different degrees of ventilatory respiratory failure reporting the effect of oral almitrine bismesylate, a peripheral chemoreceptor stimulant. They illustrate the key role that pulmonary vascular tone plays in improving pulmonary gas exchange. In the first report[16] of relatively few patients (some with hypercapnic respiratory failure), arterial blood gases improved significantly due to $\dot{V}A/\dot{Q}$ amelioration. The only associated hemodynamic change was a modest increase in pulmonary vascular resistance without increases in pulmonary artery pressure. In another study,[20] in patients requiring mechanical ventilation because of severe respiratory failure, conventional and inert gas exchange indices improved significantly together with a small but significant decrease in cardiac output and a mild increase in pulmonary vascular resistance. In all three studies, there was essentially a redistribution of pulmonary blood flow from regions of low $\dot{V}A/\dot{Q}$ units to areas with normal $\dot{V}A/\dot{Q}$ ratios. An even more dramatic improvement in pulmonary gas exchange, by markedly reducing the amount of shunt (of an order of magnitude much greater than that induced by NO),[75] has been shown in patients with ARDS following intravenous almitrine.[87] In both disorders, COPD and ARDS, it was suggested that enhancement of hypoxic pulmonary vasoconstriction explained the overall improvement in pulmonary gas exchange. However, this beneficial effect on gas exchange in patients with COPD does not counterbalance against some of the unwanted side effects of almitrine, such as peripheral neuropathy and body weight loss, particularly if a long-term administration of the drug is contemplated.

ACKNOWLEDGEMENTS

This work was supported by grant 2001/SGR 00386 from the Departament d'Universitats, Recerca i Societat de la Informació (Generalitat de Catalunya).

REFERENCES

1. Glenny R, Wagner PD, Roca J, Rodriguez-Roisin R. Gas exchange in health: rest, exercise, and aging. In: J Roca, R Rodriguez-Roisin, PD Wagner, eds. *Pulmonary and Peripheral Gas Exchange in Health and Disease*. Marcel Dekker, New York, 2000, pp 121–48.

2. Barberà JA. Chronic obstructive pulmonary disease. In: J Roca, R Rodriguez-Roisin, PD Wagner, eds. *Pulmonary and Peripheral Gas Exchange in Health and Disease*. Marcel Dekker, New York, 2000, pp 229–61.

3. Bégin P, Grassino A. Inspiratory muscle dysfunction and chronic hypercapnia in chronic obstructive pulmonary disease. *Am Rev Respir Dis* 1992;**143**:905–12.

4. Wagner PD, Saltzman HA, West JB. Measurements of continuous distributions of ventilation–perfusion ratios: theory. *J Appl Physiol* 1974;**36**:588–99.

5. Evans JW, Wagner PD. Limits on $\dot{V}_A/\dot{Q}$ distributions from analysis of experimental inert gas elimination. *J Appl Physiol* 1977;**42**:889–98.

6. Roca J, Wagner PD. Contribution of multiple inert gas elimination technique to pulmonary medicine – 1: Principles and information content of the multiple inert gas elimination technique. *Thorax* 1994;**49**:815–24.

7. Brudin LH, Rhodes CG, Valind SO, Buckingham PD, Jones T, Hughes JMB. Regional structure–function correlations in chronic obstructive lung disease measured with positron emission tomography. *Thorax* 1992;**47**:914–21.

8. Wagner PD, Laravuso RB, Uhl RR, West JB. Continuous distributions of ventilation–perfusion ratios in normal subjects breathing air and 100% O_2. *J Clin Invest* 1974; **54**:54–68.

9. Kety S. The theory and applications of the exchange of inert gas at the lungs and tissues. *Pharmacol Rev* 1951;**3**:1–41.

10. Cardús J, Burgos F, Diaz O, *et al.* Increase in pulmonary ventilation–perfusion inequality with age in healthy individuals. *Am J Respir Crit Care Med* 1997;**156**:648–53.

11. West JB. Ventilation–perfusion inequality and overall gas exchange in computer lung models of the lung. *Respir Physiol* 1969;**7**:88–110.

12. Gale GE, Torre-Bueno J, Moon RE, Saltzamn HA, Wagner PD. Ventilation–perfusion inequality in normal humans during exercise. *J Appl Physiol* 1985;**58**:978–88.

13. Hlastala MP, Robertson HT. Inert gas elimination characteristics of the normal and abnormal lung. *J Appl Physiol* 1978;**44**:258–66.

14. Burrows BE, Fletcher CM, Heard BE, Jones NL, Wootliff JS. The emphysematous and bronchial tyoes of chronic airways obstruction. A clinicopathological study of patients in London and Chicago. *Lancet* 1966;**1**:830–5.

15. Wagner PD, Dantzker DR, Dueck R, Clausen JL, West JB. Ventilation–perfusion inequality in chronic obstructive pulmonary disease. *J Clin Invest* 1977;**59**:203–16.

16. Mélot C, Naeije R, Rothschild T, Mertens PH, Mols P, Hallemans R. Improvement in ventilation–perfusion matching by almitrine in COPD. *Chest* 1983;**83**:528–33.

17. Mélot C, Hallemans R, Naeije R, Mols P, Lejeune PH. Deleterious effect of nifedipine on pulmonary gas exchange in chronic obstructive pulmonary disease. *Am Rev Respir Dis* 1984;**130**:612–16.

18. Marthan R, Castaing Y, Manier G, Guénard H. Gas exchange alterations in patients with chronic obstructive lung disease. *Chest* 1985;**87**:470–5.

19. Castaing Y, Manier G, Guénard H. Effect of 26% oxygen breathing on ventilation and perfusion distribution in patients with COLD. *Bull Eur Physiopathol Respir* 1985; **21**:17–23.

20. Castaing Y, Manier G, Guénard H. Improvement in ventilation–perfusion relationships by almitrine in patients with chronic obstructive pulmonary disease during mechanical ventilation. *Am Rev Respir Dis* 1986;**134**:910–16.

21. Dantzker DR, D'Alonzo GE. The effect of exercise on pulmonary gas exchange in patients with severe chronic obstructive pulmonary disease. *Am Rev Respir Dis* 1986; **134**:1135–9.

22. Roca J, Montserrat JM, Rodriguez-Roisin R, *et al.* Gas exchange response to naloxone in chronic obstructive pulmonary disease with hypercapnic respiratory failure. *Bull Eur Physiopathol Respir* 1987;**23**:249–54.

23. Ringstedt CV, Eliasen K, Andersen JB, Heslet L, Qvist J. Ventilation–perfusion distributions and central hemodynamics in chronic obstructive pulmonary disease. *Chest* 1989;**96**:976–83.

24. Agustí AGN, Barberà JA, Roca J, Wagner PD, Guitart R, Rodriguez-Roisin R. Hypoxic pulmonary vasoconstriction and gas exchange in chronic obstructive pulmonary disease. *Chest* 1990;**97**:268–75.

25. Barberà JA, Ramirez J, Roca J, Wagner PD, Sánchez-Lloret J, Rodriguez-Roisin R. Lung structure and gas exchange in mild chronic obstructive pulmonary disease. *Am Rev Respir Dis* 1990;**141**:895–901.

26. Bratel T, Hedenstierna G, Nyquist O, Ripe E. The use of a vasodilator, felodipine, as an adjuvant to long-term oxygen treatment in COLD patients. *Eur Respir J* 1990;**3**:46–54.

27. Gunnarson L, Tokics L, Lundquist H, *et al.* Chronic obstructive pulmonary disease and anaesthesia: formation of atelectasis and gas exchange impairment. *Eur Respir J* 1991;**4**:1106–16.

28. Barberà JA, Reyes A, Roca J, Montserrat JM, Wagner PD, Rodriguez-Roisin R. Effect of intravenously administered aminophylline on ventilation/perfusion inequality during recovery from exacerbations of chronic obstructive pulmonary disease. *Am Rev Respir Dis* 1992;**145**:1328–33.

29. Viegas CA, Ferrer A, Montserrat JM, Barberà JA, Roca J, Rodriguez-Roisin R. Ventilation–perfusion response after fenoterol in hypoxemic patients with stable COPD. *Chest* 1996;**110**:71–7 (erratum 1997;**111**:258).

30. Barberà JA, Roger N, Roca J, Rovira I, Higenbottam TW, Rodriguez-Roisin R. Worsening of pulmonary gas exchange with nitric oxide inhalation in chronic obstructive pulmonary disease. *Lancet* 1996;**347**:436–40.

31. Roger N, Barberà JA, Roca J, Rovira I, Gómez FP, Rodriguez-Roisin R. Nitric oxide inhalation during exercise in chronic obstructive pulmonary disease. *Am J Respir Crit Care Med* 1997;**156**:800–6.

32. Schols AMWJ, Slangen J, Volovics L, Wouters EFM. Weight loss is a reversible factor in the progression of chronic obstructive

pulmonary disease. *Am J Respir Crit Care Med* 1998;**157**: 1791–7.

33. Wouters EFM. Nutrition and metabolism in COPD. *Chest* 2000;**117**:274S–80S.

34. Talpers S, Romberger D, Bunce S, Pingleton S. Nutritionally associated increased carbon dioxide production: excess total calories vs high proportion of carbohydrate calories. *Chest* 1992;**102**:551–5.

35. Barberà JA, Rodriguez-Roisin R. Ventilation–perfusion mismatch. In: NF Voelkel, W MacNee, eds. *Chronic Obstructive Pulmonary Diseases*. BC Decker, Hamilton, 2002, pp 292–306.

36. American Thoracic Society. Standards for the diagnosis and care of patients with chronic obstructive pulmonary disease. *Am J Respir Crit Care Med* 1995;**152**:S77–121.

37. Barberà JA, Roca J, Rodriguez-Roisin R, Ussetti P, Wagner PD, Agustí-Vidal A. Gas exchange in patients with small airways dysfunction (abstract). *Eur Respir J* 1988;**1**:27s.

38. Barberà JA, Roca J, Ferrer A, *et al.* Mechanisms of worsening gas exchange during acute exacerbations of chronic obstructive pulmonary disease. *Eur Respir J* 1997;**10**:1285–91.

39. Torres A, Reyes A, Roca J, Wagner PD, Rodriguez-Roisin R. Ventilation–perfusion mismatching in chronic obstructive pulmonary disease during ventilator weaning. *Am Rev Respir Dis* 1989;**140**:1246–50.

40. Rossi A, Santos C, Roca J, Torres A, Félez MA, Rodriguez-Roisin R. Effects of PEEP on $\dot{V}A/\dot{Q}$ mismatching in ventilated patients with chronic airflow obstruction. *Am J Respir Crit Care Med* 1994;**149**:1077–84.

41. Diaz O, Iglesia R, Ferrer M, *et al.* Effects of noninvasive ventilation on pulmonary gas exchange and hemodynamics during acute hypercapnic exacerbations of chronic obstructive pulmonary disease. *Am J Respir Crit Care Med* 1997;**156**:1840–5.

42. Wagner PD, Rodriguez-Roisin R. Clinical advances in pulmonary gas exchange. *Am Rev Respir Dis* 1991;**143**:883–8.

43. Beydon L, Cinotti L, Rekik N, *et al.* Changes in the distribution of ventilation and perfusion associated with separation from mechanical ventilation in patients with obstructive pulmonary disease. *Anesthesiology* 1991; **75**:730–8.

44. Lemaire F, Teboul JL, Cinotti L, *et al.* Acute left ventricular dysfunction during unsuccessful weaning from mechanical ventilation. *Anesthesiology* 1988;**69**:171–9.

45. Hubmayr RD, Loosbrock LM, Gillespie DJ, Rodarte JR. Oxygen uptake during weaning from mechanical ventilation. *Chest* 1988;**94**:1148–55.

46. Robinson TD, Collins ER, Sullivan CE, Young IH. Long-term nocturnal non-invasive ventilation (NIV) improves hypercapnia in patients with COPD by reducing alveolar dead space. *Am J Respir Crit Care Med* 2001;**163**:A501 (abstract).

47. Barberà JA, Riverola A, Roca J, *et al.* Pulmonary vascular abnormalities and ventilation–perfusion relationships in patients with mild chronic obstructive pulmonary disease. *Am Rev Respir Dis* 1994;**149**:423–9.

48. Kessler R, Faller M, Fourgaut G, Mennecier B, Weitzemblum E. Predictive factors of hospitalization for acute exacerbation in a series of 64 patients with chronic obstructive pulmonary disease. *Am J Respir Crit Care Med* 1999;**159**:158–64.

49. Wilkinson M, Langhorme CA, Heath D, Barer GR, Howard P. A pathophysiological study of 10 cases of hypoxemic cor pulmonale. *Q J Med* 1988;**249**:65–85.

50. Dinh-Xuan AT, Higenbottam T, Clelland C, *et al.* Impairment of endothelium-dependent pulmonary-artery relaxation in chronic obstructive pulmonary disease. *N Engl J Med* 1991;**324**:1539–47.

51. Peinado VI, Barberà JA, Ramirez J, *et al.* Endothelial dysfunction in pulmonary arteries of patients with mild COPD. *Am J Physiol* 1998;**274**:L908–13.

52. Peinado VI, Barberà JA, Abatte P, *et al.* Inflammatory reaction in pulmonary muscular arteries of patients with mild chronic obstructive pulmonary disease. *Am J Respir Crit Care Med* 1999;**159**:1605–11.

53. O'Shaughnessy TC, Ansari TW, Barnes NC, Jeffery PK. Inflammation of bronchial biopsies of subjects with chronic bronchitis: inverse relationship of $CD8^{+}$ T lymphocytes with FEV_1. *Am J Respir Crit Care Med* 1997;**155**:852–7.

54. Saetta M, Turat G, Facchini FM, *et al.* Inflammatory cells in the bronchial glands of smokers with chronic bronchitis. *Am J Respir Crit Care Med* 1997;**156**:1633–9.

55. Barberà JA, Peinado VI, Santos S, Ramírez J, Roca J, Rodriguez-Roisin R. Reduced expression of endothelial nitric oxide synthase in pulmonary arteries of smokers. *Am J Respir Crit Care Med* 2001;**164**:709–31.

56. Roca J, Hogan MC, Story D, Bebout DE, Haab P, González O, *et al.* Evidence for tissue diffusion limitation of $\dot{V}O_{2max}$ in normal humans. *J Appl Physiol* 1989;**67**:291–9.

57. Barberà JA, Roca J, Ramirez J, Wagner PD, Ussetti P, Rodriguez-Roisin R. Gas exchange during exercise in mild chronic obstructive pulmonary disease. Correlation with lung structure. *Am Rev Respir Dis* 1991;**144**:520–5.

58. Ribas J, Díaz O, Barberà JA, *et al.* Invasive exercise testing in the evaluation of patients at a high-risk for lung resection. *Eur Respir J* 1999;**12**:1429–35.

59. Pierce RJ, Copland JM, Sharpe K, Barter CE. Preoperative risk evaluation for lung cancer resection: predicted postoperative product as a predictor of surgical mortality. *Am J Respir Crit Care Med* 1994;**150**:947–55.

60. Santos C, Ferrer M, Roca J, Torres A, Hernández C, Rodriguez-Roisin R. Pulmonary gas exchange response to oxygen breathing in acute lung injury. *Am J Respir Crit Care Med* 2000;**161**:26–31.

61. Dantzker DR, Wagner PD, West JB. Instability of lung units with low $\dot{V}A/\dot{Q}$ ratios during O_2 breathing. *J Appl Physiol* 1975;**38**:886–95.

62. Astin TW. The relationships between arterial blood oxygen saturation, carbon dioxide tension, and pH on airway resistance during 30 percent oxygen breathing in patients with chronic bronchitis with airway obstruction. *Am Rev Respir Dis* 1970;**102**:382–7.

63. Aubier M, Murciano D, Milic-Emili J, *et al.* Effects of the administration of O_2 on ventilation and blood flow gases in patients with chronic obstructive pulmonary disease during acute respiratory failure. *Am Rev Respir Dis* 1980;**122**: 747–54.

64. Stradling J. Effects of the administration of O_2 on ventilation and blood flow gases in patients with chronic obstructive pulmonary disease during acute respiratory failure. *Am Rev Respir Dis* 1987;**135**:274 (letter).

65. Robinson TD, Freiberg DB, Regnis JA, Young IH. The role of hypoventilation and ventilation–perfusion redistribution in oxygen-induced hypercapnia during acute exacerbations of chronic obstructive pulmonary disease. *Am J Respir Crit Care Med* 2000;**161**:1524–9.

66. Hanson CW, Marshall BE, Frasch HF, Marshall C. Causes of hypercarbia with oxygen therapy in patients with chronic obstructive pulmonary disease. *Crit Care Med* 1996; **24**:23–8.

67. Khoukaz G, Gross N. Effects of salmeterol on arterial blood gases in patients with stable chronic obstructive pulmonary disease. *Am J Respir Crit Care Med* 1999;**160**:1028–30.

68. Ballester E, Reyes A, Roca J, Guitart R, Wagner PD, Rodriguez-Roisin R. Ventilation–perfusion mismatching in

acute severe asthma: effects of salbutamol and 100% oxygen. *Thorax* 1989;**44**:258–67.

69. Wong CS, Pavord ID, Williams J, Britton JR, Tattersfield AE. Bronchodilator, cardiovascular, and hypokalaemic effects of fenoterol, salbutamol, and terbutaline in asthma. *Lancet* 1990;**336**:1396–9.

70. Rennotte MT, Reynaert M, Clerbaux TH, *et al.* Effects of two inotropic drugs, dopamine and dobutamine, on pulmonary gas exchange in artificially ventilated patients. *Intensive Care Med* 1989;**15**:160–5.

71. Guénard H, Castaing Y, Mélot C, Naeije R. Gas exchange during acute respiratory failure in patients with chronic obstructive pulmonary disease. In: JP Derenne, WA Whitelaw, T Similowski (eds). *Acute Respiratory Failure in Chronic Obstructive Pulmonary Disease.* Marcel Dekker, New York, 1996, pp 227–66.

72. Andrivet P, Chabrier PE, Defouilloy C, Brun-Buisson C, Adnot S. Intravenously administered atrial natriuretic factor in patients with COPD. Effects on ventilation–perfusion relationships and pulmonary hemodynamics. *Chest* 1994;**106**:118–24.

73. Adnot S, Kouyoumdjian C, Defouilloy C, *et al.* Hemodynamic and gas exchange responses to infusion of acetylcholine and inhalation of nitric oxide in patients with chronic obstructive lung disease and pulmonary hypertension. *Am Rev Respir Dis* 1993;**148**:310–16.

74. Pepke-Zaba J, Higenbottam TW, Dinh-Xuan AT, Stone D, Wallwork J. Inhaled nitric oxide as a cause of selective pulmonary vasodilation in pulmonary hypertension. *Lancet* 1991;**338**:1173–4.

75. Rossaint R, Falke KJ, López FA, Slama K, Pison U, Zapol W. Inhaled nitric oxide for the adult respiratory distress syndrome. *N Engl J Med* 1993;**328**:399–405.

76. Moinard J, Manier G, Pillet O, Castaing Y. Effect of inhaled nitric oxide on hemodynamics and $\dot{V}_A/\dot{Q}$ inequalities in patients with chronic obstructive pulmonary disease. *Am J Respir Crit Care Med* 1994;**149**:1482–7.

77. Katayama Y, Higenbottam TW, Diaz de Atauri MJ, *et al.* Inhaled nitric oxide and arterial oxygen tension in patients with chronic obstructive pulmonary disease and severe pulmonary hypertension. *Thorax* 1997;**52**:120–4.

78. Blanch LL, Joseph D, Fernández R, *et al.* Hemodynamic and gas exchange responses to inhalation of nitric oxide in patients with the acute respiratory distress syndrome and in hypoxemic patients with chronic obstructive pulmonary disease. *Intensive Care Med* 1997;**23**:51–7.

79. Hopkins SR, Johnson EC, Richardson RS, Wagner H, De Rosa M, Wagner PD. Effects of inhaled nitric oxide on gas exchange in lungs with shunt or poorly ventilated areas. *Am J Respir Crit Care Med* 1997;**156**:484–91.

80. Frostell C, Blomqvist H, Hedenstierna G, Lundberg J, Zapol WM. Inhaled nitric oxide selectively reverses human hypoxic pulmonary vasoconstriction without causing systemic vasodilation. *Anesthesiology* 1993;**78**:427–35.

81. Yoshida M, Taguchi O, Gabazza EC, *et al.* Combined inhalation of nitric oxide and oxygen in chronic obstructive pulmonary disease. *Am J Respir Crit Care Med* 1997;**155**:526–9.

82. Ashutosh K, Phadke K, Fragale J, Steele D. Use of nitric oxide inhalation in chronic obstructive pulmonary disease. *Thorax* 2000;**55**:109–13.

83. Defouilly C, Teiger E, Sediame S, *et al.* Polycythemia impairs vasodilator response to acetylcholine in patients with chronic obstructive pulmonary disease. *Am J Respir Crit Care Med* 1998;**157**:1452–6.

84. Katayama Y, Higenbottam TW, Cremona G, *et al.* Minimizing the inhaled dose of NO with breath-by-breath delivery of spikes of concentrated gas. *Circulation* 1998;**98**:2429–32.

85. Siddons TE, Asif M, Higenbottam T. Does the method of delivery of inhaled nitrix oxide influence oxygenation and $\dot{V}_A/\dot{Q}$ patterns in severe COPD? *Eur Respir J* 2000;**16**:267s (abstract).

86. Castaing Y, Manier G, Varène N, Guénard H. Effects of oral almitrine on the distribution of $\dot{V}_A/\dot{Q}$ ratio in chronic obstructive pulmonary disease. *Bull Eur Physiopath Resp* 1981;**17**:917–32.

87. Reyes A, Roca J, Rodriguez-Roisin R, Torres A, Ussetti P, Wagner PD. Effect of almitrine on ventilation–perfusion distribution in adult respiratory distress syndrome. *Am Rev Respir Dis* 1988;**137**:1062–7.

15

Respiratory muscles

MICHAEL I POLKEY AND JOHN MOXHAM

INTRODUCTION

The main function of the respiratory system is to maintain oxygen and carbon dioxide homostasis. Hypercapnic respiratory failure may, in the absence of failure of respiratory control, be viewed as an imbalance between the load placed on the respiratory muscle pump and its capacity. Hypercapnia, both acute[1] and chronic,[2] carries a poor prognosis in COPD. Whilst load is increased in COPD (for the reasons covered elsewhere in this volume), theory predicts that the capacity of the respiratory muscle pump to develop inspiratory pressure and, in turn, volume change might also be diminished in COPD. An overview of the influences acting on the respiratory muscle pump is shown in Figure 15.1.

HISTORICAL

Austin Flint, also known for his studies in cardiology, observed that the lateral chest wall may move (paradoxically) inward during inspiration, an observation which later became known as Hoover's sign.[3] However neither Flint nor Hoover considered inspiratory muscle dysfunction to be a feature of COPD, and even in 1951 Dayman[4] formed a view that the problem was entirely expiratory, inspiration being 'relatively unimpeded'.

Although respiratory pressures had been previously measured,[5] it was only at this time that it became appreciated that these pressures were a function of lung volume.[6] In 1968 Sharp *et al.*[7] and Byrd and Hyatt[8] published the first data regarding inspiratory pressures in COPD. In

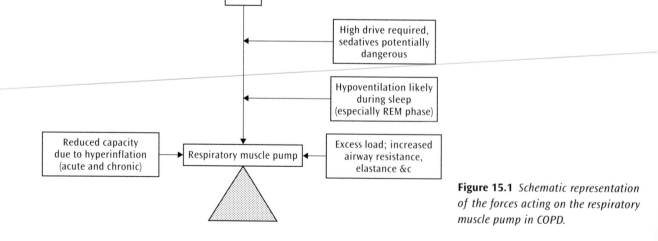

Figure 15.1 *Schematic representation of the forces acting on the respiratory muscle pump in COPD.*

many ways these publications initiated a debate which continues, for Sharp and coworkers emphasized the marked reduction in inspiratory pressure generation available to COPD patients while Byrd and Hyatt argued that, allowing for lung volume, no diminution in strength was present.

Subsequent studies have continued to address this question and raised new questions (which will be addressed in this chapter) regarding the geometrical alignment of the diaphragm, its composition, its performance under load and its contribution to exercise limitation. As a consequence, a variety of therapeutic maneuvers including drugs, hormones, nutrition, ventilatory support and lung volume reduction surgery have been proposed as methods of augmenting diaphragm function. The expiratory muscles are frequently active in patients with COPD[9] and their function will also be considered. Peripheral skeletal muscle function is recognized to be of increasing importance in COPD and although this is covered in Chapters 18 and 30, recent progress in the assessment of peripheral muscle strength is included in this chapter.

OVERVIEW OF NORMAL RESPIRATORY MUSCLE PHYSIOLOGY

Anatomy

The diaphragm is the most important inspiratory muscle in man, accounting for approximately 70% of ventilation at rest.[10] It consists of a central tendon into which insert the two portions, costal and crural, of the diaphragm muscle. Although the two portions have different actions, they are both innervated by the phrenic nerves and available data suggests that they act in concert during respiration.[11] When the diaphragm contracts a negative pressure is created in the thorax by two mechanisms, one of which is simply expansion in lung volume caused by caudal descent of the dome of the diaphragm. However diaphragm descent also causes an increase in pressure in the abdominal compartment which is transmitted outwards through the area where the lower rib cage overlies the diaphragm muscle (the zone of apposition), causing rib cage expansion.[12]

Inspiratory action is also provided by muscles of the upper thorax. Some of these muscles are active even during quiet respiration (e.g. the scalenes), while others are only recruited when minute ventilation is increased (e.g. the sternomastoid).[13] Histologically the diaphragm and other respiratory muscles are skeletal muscles and therefore similar to, for example, the quadriceps muscle; the fiber-type composition is approximately 50% Type I and 25% each Type IIa and IIb.[14] In normal humans the expiratory muscles may contribute to ventilation,[15] but their role in patients with flow limitation remains controversial

(see below). Few, human data concern the extradiaphragmatic muscles, and therefore necessarily this chapter focuses on the diaphragm.

Physiology

The tension generated by muscle is a function of the number of motor units recruited, the frequency of stimulation, the length of the muscle and the velocity of shortening. Force output may also be influenced by the presence of fatigue;[16] this problem is discussed below. In the human respiratory system force is generally assessed as pressure; this may be either esophageal pressure to reflect global inspiratory muscle activity or transdiaphragmatic pressure to reflect diaphragm tension generation. Similarly lung volume is regarded as a clinically accessible surrogate for length.

Force–frequency relationship

The force developed by striated muscle increases as the stimulation frequency is increased until the stimulation frequency reaches approximately 50 Hz beyond which further increases in stimulation frequency produce progressively smaller increases in tension. This relationship has been demonstrated *in vivo* for the human sternomastoid and diaphragm (Figure 15.2). The physiologic firing frequency is approximately 10 Hz in normal man, and, though it is increased in patients with COPD,[17] remains on the steep portion of the force–frequency curve. No human

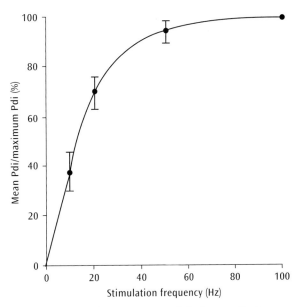

Figure 15.2 *Force–frequency curve of the human diaphragm in vivo. Pdi: transdiaphragmatic pressure. (From ref. 16 with permission.)*

data have addressed phrenic nerve firing rates during exercise, but it is reasonable to assume that discharge rate would increase; it is unknown whether the increase might then be sufficient to reach the plateau portion of the curve. The shape of the force–frequency curve may be altered by length (and therefore lung volume) or fatigue and thus, it is hypothesized, these factors may lead to a requirement for increased neural drive to sustain tension which may, in turn, contribute to dyspnea.

Pressure–volume relationship

Hyperinflation is a frequent finding in COPD and causes inspiratory muscle shortening,[18] which is most pronounced in the diaphragm. Mammalian skeletal muscles have a preferred length with regard to force production, the optimal length L_o. Numerous human studies have shown that the optimal lung volume for the human diaphragm lies below residual volume (RV).[19,20] However the relationship between transdiaphragmatic pressure (Pdi) and lung volume is also dependent on the frequency of stimulation. Thus recent data[21] show that Pdi is disproportionately diminished by an increase in lung volume when the stimulation frequency is 10 Hz, which, of note, is close to the *in vivo* firing frequency.

Hyperinflation also adversely affects the orientation of the diaphragm. In particular increasing hyperinflation results in a progressive and linear decline in the area of the zone of apposition in both normal subjects and patients with COPD, as shown in Figure 15.3.[22] This

results in inefficient translation of transdiaphragmatic pressure to intrathoracic pressure change (Figure 15.4), to the extent that at full inflation diaphragm contraction may fail to create a negative intrathoracic pressure.[20,21,23]

Animal models (most commonly elastase-induced emphysema) have been used to investigate chronic hyperinflation. These studies show that sarcomere loss occurs with the adoption of a new L_o (Figure 15.5) and increased tension generating capacity at a given lung volume.[24–26] Interestingly the diaphragm of the emphysematous hamster has increased fatigue resistance *in vitro*.[26] The relevance of this to the human diaphragm remains, to some extent controversial. In particular the predominant process in human disease appears to be sarcomere shortening rather than loss.[27]

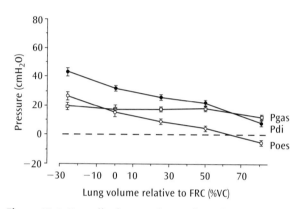

Figure 15.4 *Transdiaphragmatic, esophageal and gastric pressure produced by single bilateral supramaximal phrenic nerve stimulation in normal subjects. Increasing lung volume results in a progressive diminution in Tw Poes. Note that in this case a subatmospheric Poes is expressed positively. (Data modified from ref. 21.)*

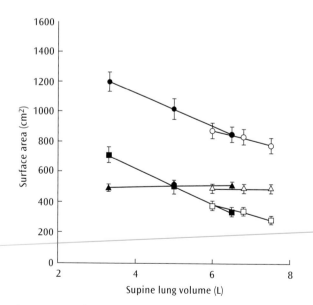

Figure 15.3 *Influence of hyperinflation on diaphragm dimensions in patients with COPD (open symbols) and normal subjects (closed symbols). The total surface area is represented by circles, the area of the dome by triangles and the zone of apposition by squares. (From ref. 22.)*

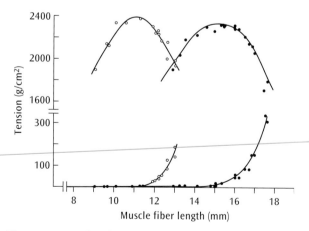

Figure 15.5 In vitro *length–tension curves for the diaphragms of emphysematous (open circles: left hand curves) and control (solid circles: right hand curves) hamsters. Top curves show active tension, bottom curves show passive tension. (Data from ref. 24.)*

Fatigue

When skeletal muscle is subjected to increased load, a reduction in force output may occur which recovers with rest; this physiologic process is termed fatigue.[28] The form of fatigue considered to be of most relevance to clinical practice is low frequency fatigue (LFF), in which the force-response is diminished in response to low frequencies of stimulation, but preserved to high frequencies. LFF of the diaphragm may be produced in the laboratory[29,30] and it has been hypothesized (without data) that the development of such fatigue during exacerbations of COPD could lead to a requirement for mechanical ventilation. The mechanism underlying diaphragm fatigue has not been fully elucidated, but it is clear that loads which cause low-frequency fatigue also cause ultrastructural muscle damage. *In vivo* the optimal method to detect diaphragm fatigue is, in theory, to stimulate the phrenic nerve at supramaximal intensity at varying frequencies. In practice however this method is too painful for patients (and indeed the majority of normal volunteers) to accept, and the currently favored method is to measure the transdiaphragmatic pressure in response to a single bilateral magnetic stimulation of the phrenic nerves.[31] Characteristically low-frequency fatigue is evident by a fall in the twitch transdiaphragmatic pressure (of $>10\%$), which is reversible by rest in the presence of a preserved action potential amplitude. In practice measurement of action potential amplitude may be technically difficult.[32,33] The duration of recovery is usually greater than 60 minutes and may exceed 24 hours.[34,35]

RESPIRATORY MUSCLE PHYSIOLOGY IN COPD

Anatomy

Recent studies using computerized tomography have demonstrated that patients with COPD accommodate to the hyperinflation inherent in the condition by increasing the anterior–posterior diameter over the lower portion of the rib cage. By contrast, upper rib cage dimensions are similar (in absolute terms) between COPD patients and normal controls.[36] As expected diaphragm length is reduced in COPD patients, but not more than would be expected for the degree of hyperinflation.[22] These changes are partially restored by lung volume reduction surgery.[37]

Physiology

Recent advances in cellular biology have disclosed important changes in the diaphragm of patients with emphysema. The most important changes are that patients with COPD have a greater proportion of fatigue-resistant Type I fibers than control subjects, a change achieved at the expense of Type II fibers.[38,39] Of note these changes are the opposite to those observed in peripheral musculature where Type I fiber atrophy occurs[40] and suggest that whereas the locomotor muscles are subject to disuse atrophy,[41] the diaphragm (and by inference the other inspiratory muscles) are subject to a training effect. This concept is supported by the finding that, compared with controls, the diaphragm of COPD patients exhibits an increased mitochondrial density.[27] In addition, this study also found evidence of sarcomere shortening in COPD patients, in contrast to the process of sarcomere loss observed in animal models.[25] This, as well as the modest correlation between sarcomere shortening and FEV_1, suggests that the animal model of emphysema may not faithfully reflect the human disease.

Strength data

As noted in the introduction, early studies[78] in patients with COPD using pressure measured at the mouth during a maximal static effort failed to resolve the question of whether, at a given lung volume, COPD patients could generate a greater inspiratory pressure than control subjects. Gibson *et al.*[42] measured transdiaphragmatic pressure and concluded that inspiratory pressure generation was preserved at high lung volumes. However these and other studies have used voluntary maneuvers which, to some extent, limits their conclusions.

Three studies have used the pressure elicited by phrenic nerve stimulation to investigate diaphragm function in COPD. In the first study Similowski *et al.* used electrical stimulation to study the behavior of seven patients with COPD over a range of lung volumes. The mean twitch transdiaphragmatic pressure (Tw Pdi) was greater at any absolute lung volume in patients than controls. Polkey *et al.*[43] used cervical magnetic stimulation to study 20 patients with COPD and concluded that, allowing for lung volume, diaphragm strength was neither more nor less than expected. Wanke *et al.* investigated COPD patients undergoing single or double lung transplantation.[44] Had such patients undergone significant adaptation then, if the postoperative residual volume had been less than the preoperative L_o, the postoperative sniff Pdi at low lung volume might have been expected to be less than the postoperative sniff Pdi at FRC, but this was not observed. Overall our view is that the tension-generating capacity of the diaphragm in patients with COPD is diminished to a degree appropriate to the hyperinflation, but the data do not clearly support the view that this diminution is greater or less than expected.

The attempt to relate diaphragm strength to lung volume has to a degree been compounded by the fact that diaphragm strength in healthy humans[45] and patients with COPD[46] is very variable. The new therapy of lung volume surgery (LVRS)[47] has provided a further model to examine the impact of chronic hyperinflation on diaphragm strength in COPD. Neural drive to the diaphragm is reduced after LVRS, suggesting that the diaphragm is in a more favorable position,[48] though this does not of itself distinguish between length and orientation. Lahrmann *et al.*[48] studied 14 patients undergoing LVRS. One month after surgery diaphragm strength was increased whereas lung volume was reduced, however after 6 months lung volumes were increased again while sniff transdiaphragmatic pressure had also increased. Similarly the Philadelphia group found the effect of LVRS on diaphragm strength to be poorly correlated with diaphragm length[49] and to have no correlation with lung volume.[50] A final possibility is that LVRS allows a greater contribution to be made by the diaphragm; supporting this concept are data showing that the ratio of gastric to transdiaphragmatic pressure during resting breathing is increased after LVRS.[51] This is best explained by relative derecruitment of extradiaphragmatic inspiratory muscles.

Action of the diaphragm

A unifying explanation for these observations would be that static diaphragm strength is less important than the ability of the diaphragm to reduce intrathoracic pressure during tidal breathing. In this context it should be noted that, as with acute hyperinflation,[20] patients with chronic hyperinflation have a disproportionately diminished ability to translate transdiaphragmatic pressure into negative intrathoracic pressure. Thus in our own study[43] we found that the ratio of esophageal pressure change to transdiaphragmatic pressure change elicited by bilateral phrenic nerve stimulation (Tw Poes : Tw Pdi) was 0.4 compared with 0.64 in normal subjects, and occasionally the Tw Poes elicited by bilateral phrenic nerve stimulation was expiratory in nature (Figure 15.6). A mechanism for these observations is clearly provided by the reduction in the area of apposition which accompanies severe hyperinflation.[22]

DYNAMIC DIAPHRAGM PERFORMANCE

Although there has been considerable debate as to how effectively the diaphragm compensates for hyperinflation, the data considered are usually gathered from patients studied at rest. Since an important clinical problem encountered by patients is exertional dyspnea, it is relevant to consider the function of the respiratory muscles during exercise. It is recognized that high levels of ventilation lead to heightened awareness of respiratory effort,[52] and the presence of respiratory muscle fatigue in

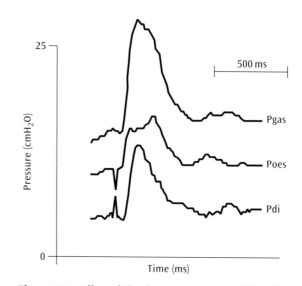

Figure 15.6 *Effect of diaphragm contraction elicited by magnetic stimulation in a patient with extreme hyperinflation (FRC) 228% predicted. Note that the esophageal pressure change is positive (expiratory) instead of negative (inspiratory) as normal. (Modified from ref. 43.)*

patients with COPD has been sought in a number of studies.

What happens in exercise?

During exercise patients with more severe COPD have expiratory flow limitation[53] and to meet their ventilatory requirements end-expiratory lung volume (EELV) increases (see Chapter 18). This is in contrast to normal subjects who drive their EELV below FRC when they exercise. In patients with advanced disease the increase in EELV may be 500–1000 ml.[54] This hyperinflation has the effect of reducing the maximal force output of the diaphragm (see above), yet the generation of an increased minute ventilation requires an increased force output, and potentially increased velocity of contraction if expiratory time is prolonged. Thus, in patients with advanced disease the pressure–time product of the diaphragm during brisk walking is typically 250–300 cmH₂O/s/min compared with around 600 cmH₂O/s/min during voluntary maximal hyperventilation.[55,56] These observations, as well as studies with static efforts,[46] suggest that patients with COPD are likely to exceed the fatigue threshold and if fatigue occurred this could contribute to the sensation of dyspnea.

Do the respiratory muscles fatigue during exercise?

An attempt to answer this question requires a definition of fatigue. Fatigue can be defined as a loss of force generating capacity resulting from activity under load which is reversible by rest.[28] Muscle loading causes other physiologic changes which have been documented in COPD patients undergoing exercise, for example a reduction in the high/low frequency ratio of the EMG[57,58] and slowing of the relaxation rate of inspiratory muscles.[59,60] Nevertheless these observations do not provide direct evidence of respiratory muscle fatigue during exercise in COPD because tension generation was unimpaired.

The technique currently considered most sensitive for the detection of low-frequency fatigue of the diaphragm is measurement of twitch Pdi after bilateral supramaximal phrenic nerve stimulation.[28] This technique has been used to demonstrate low-frequency fatigue in normal volunteers in laboratory studies.[29,30] We used this technique in patients with severe COPD to seek diaphragm fatigue after exhaustive treadmill exercise[61] and voluntary hyperventilation,[56] but it did not occur. This observation could be partially explained by the fatigue-resistant properties arising from the change in diaphragm fiber type subsequently demonstrated by Levine *et al.* and Mercadier *et al.*[38,39] Nevertheless another cause of fatigue resistance is likely to be the shortening inherent in both tasks because of hyperinflation associated with hyperventilation. It has sometimes been considered that shortening would predispose to the development of fatigue,[62] but data from peripheral muscle clearly shows the converse. Specifically, *in vivo* studies of human limb muscle show that if the muscle is subjected to a fatiguing protocol while shortened then the force decrement after the protocol when the muscle is tested at L_o is less than if the muscle is subjected to the same protocol at L_o.[63] Sacco *et al.* repeated and confirmed this study and showed using ^{31}P-labeled nuclear magnetic resonance spectroscopy that this was because of intramuscular activation failure.[64] If such a study could be devised it would be of physiological interest to compare *in vivo* the fatiguability of the diaphragm at static FRC in patients with COPD and age-matched controls, but such a study has not yet been done, although pilot data from our laboratory suggests that it is possible to generate diaphragm fatigue in COPD patients if hyperinflation is avoided.[65]

Do the respiratory muscles contribute to exercise limitation?

The cause of exercise limitation in COPD is likely to be multifactorial. Nevertheless we have shown that exhaustive exercise in patients with severe COPD is accompanied by physiologic changes conventionally considered to represent respiratory failure,[66] specifically a rise in $PaCO_2$ (mean 1 kPa) and fall in pH (mean 0.51 pH units). In the broadest sense this must represent an imbalance between the load placed on the respiratory muscle pump and its capacity. Furthermore, the use of inspiratory pressure support during exercise extends walking distance,[67] reduces inspiratory muscle tension generation[55] and attenuates the physiologic changes (specifically inspiratory muscle relaxation rate) indicative of inspiratory muscle loading.[60] Whether these changes are achieved by direct reduction of tension generation or simply by reducing the load (e.g. by dilating airways) is presently undetermined.

DIAPHRAGM DYSFUNCTION DURING SLEEP

Ventilatory failure is a feature of advanced COPD; as with other forms of ventilatory failure this may be manifest initially at night when the physiologic diminution of the drive to breathe may render the capacity of the respiratory muscle pump inadequate to meet the need placed upon it. By their nature large-scale studies are difficult, but it is likely that COPD patients have an increased frequency of obstructive events of the upper airway but do also have central events[68] which could be viewed as a manifestation of reduced physiologic drive. One study has reported an improvement in nocturnal oxygenation following flow training.[69]

TREATING DIAPHRAGM DYSFUNCTION IN COPD

Drugs

A number of drugs increase skeletal muscle contractility *in vitro*. For patients with COPD there has been particular interest in beta$_2$-agonists and methylxanthines; these drugs are routinely given in clinical practice for their bronchodilating properties. Digoxin has been considered to have an inotropic effect in acute decompensated COPD,[70] but this study has not been repeated, and benefits were not confirmed in a clinical trial of oral digoxin in ambulant COPD patients.[71] Some details are given below but more detail on this topic is provided elsewhere.[72]

METHYLXANTHINES

Methylxanthines have been studied in normal humans. Aubier *et al.*[73] studied eight normal subjects during intravenous aminophylline sufficient to generate a serum level of 13 mg/L. Aminophylline increased the Pdi elicited by voluntary contractions of comparable amplitude as judged by electrical activity (Edi). However Moxham *et al.* using phrenic nerve stimulation to measure the 1 Hz Tw Pdi during aminophylline infusion[74] were unable to demonstrate any benefit with aminophylline despite achieving mean levels of 13.8 mg/L and, in one subject, of 20 mg/L. Although this study did not examine high stimulation frequencies, the same group subsequently failed to show an increase in the Pdi elicited during a maximal voluntary sniff,[75] a maneuver assumed to require a short high-frequency stimulus, during oral aminophylline therapy. DeGarmo *et al.* also failed to show a benefit for intravenous theophylline on inspiratory muscle strength.[76] Subsequent studies also considered lung volume; Wanke *et al.*[77] studied 10 normal subjects using Tw Pdi and Sniff Pdi at lung volumes between residual volume (RV) and 90% total lung capacity (TLC) in both the fresh and fatigued diaphragm. In the fatigued diaphragm only a significant improvement was seen in both Tw Pdi and Sniff Pdi with the effect becoming increasingly pronounced at high lung volume.[77,78] In conclusion, data from normal subjects suggest that, at doses tolerable in man, methylxanthines do not improve the contractile properties of the human diaphragm at FRC. Nevertheless the possibility remains that methylxanthines may have a minor benefit at lung volumes approaching TLC, particularly if there is fatigue.

Similarly data from studies conducted in COPD patients have failed to confirm a role for methylxanthines in improving muscle strength in patients with COPD. For example Murciano *et al.* performed a double-blind randomized crossover study using oral theophylline (10 mg/kg in two divided doses).[79] Compared with the other results the most striking improvement was an increase in the esophageal pressure (Pes) generated during a maximal inspiratory effort from 38 cmH$_2$O to 47 cmH$_2$O (22%), though there were minor improvements in both FEV$_1$ and FVC too. These data are in contrast to the data reported by Foxworth *et al.*[80] and Cooper *et al.*,[81] neither of which showed improvements in inspiratory muscle strength after methylxanthines administration. Thus in conclusion methylxanthines have not been shown to reproducibly improve inspiratory muscle strength in stable COPD; even if a small benefit is conferred the effect is not sufficiently strong to be detectable in patients.

BETA$_2$-AGONISTS

To our knowledge beta$_2$-agonists have not been demonstrated to have any benefit on fresh diaphragm contractility in animal studies. However an increase in the Pdi elicited by low stimulation frequencies in the fatigued diaphragm has been reported for some beta$_2$-agonists,[82–84] although not for salbutamol.[84,85] The reason why beta$_2$-agonists should preferentially benefit low-frequency pressure generation in the fatigued diaphragm is unknown but is of potential interest in that it raises the possibility that a similar benefit might occur at high lung volumes where low stimulation frequencies are also disproportionately affected.

No effect has been shown for beta$_2$-agonists in normal subjects with respect to either limb or diaphragm muscle strength.[86,87] Three studies have investigated beta$_2$-agonists in patients with chronic COPD. Stoller *et al.*[88] and Nava *et al.*[89] failed to show an improvement in inspiratory muscle strength with beta$_2$-agonists.[89] Hatipoglu *et al.* investigated the effect of salbutamol on twitch transdiaphragmatic pressure in patients with COPD. There was an increase in Tw Pdi, but this was wholly explained by a decrease in end-expiratory lung volume.[90] We conclude that beta$_2$-agonists have no demonstrable effect on inspiratory muscle strength in animals, normal subjects or patients with COPD. In animals they enhance recovery from fatigue but the relevance of this property to patients with COPD remains undetermined.

HORMONES

Patients with advanced COPD frequently have a cachexic syndrome and weight loss is recognized to carry a poor prognosis in COPD. The relationship and importance of this syndrome to peripheral muscle function is covered elsewhere, but the same concept has been considered in relation to the respiratory muscles.

Early data supported the concept that nutrition and body weight are determinants of diaphragm muscle mass. For example diaphragm mass was found to be increased in manual laborers and reduced in patients dying from protracted illnesses[91] and, in patients with emphysema, reduced diaphragm muscle mass correlated with disease severity.[92] Nevertheless, the null hypothesis is that weight loss and inspiratory muscle weakness are epiphenomena of advancing disease which is also the explanation for the poor prognosis. Growth hormone and anabolic steroids are two hormonal approaches that have been used in attempts to increase diaphragm mass and, therefore, improve function.

Growth hormone (GH) is a potent anabolic hormone which is normally secreted by the pituitary gland. Among other functions it enhances protein synthesis, nitrogen retention and muscle growth. Aside from case reports,[93] three studies have examined its effects in COPD.[94–96] In an uncontrolled study Suchner *et al.* administered parenteral nutrition to six malnourished patients for a week and followed this with parenteral nutrition and GH in combination for a week. No effect was observed with either therapy on maximal static inspiratory or expiratory pressures.[94] A contradictory result was obtained in a second uncontrolled study in which seven subjects received a defined diet alone followed by diet and GH together for 3 weeks.[95] The investigators found a striking increase in maximal static inspiratory pressure (27%). Burdet *et al.* conducted a prospective double-blind randomized controlled study in which 16 patients received either recombinant GH (0.15 IU/kg daily) or placebo.[96] The patients were participating in an inpatient pulmonary rehabilitation program and were therefore receiving a diet. Although lean body mass increased (by a mean of 2 kg) there was no difference between the groups in maximal static mouth pressures or handgrip strength. In summary therefore available data do not support the use of GH in patients with COPD.

As athletes are aware, supraphysiologic doses of testosterone administered intramuscularly over a period of weeks cause an increase in limb muscle mass and strength[97] and such observations have prompted two studies with anabolic analogues in COPD patients. Schols *et al.*[98] compared nutrition and nandrolone decanoate with nutrition and placebo and with placebo alone in a three way trial in 233 patients. Patients were additionally defined either as nutritionally depleted or non-depleted. Nandrolone decanoate (or placebo) was given at 2, 4 and 6 weeks. An increase in maximal static inspiratory pressure was observed in nutritionally depleted patients receiving both nandrolone and nutrition but it was small in magnitude ($<10\,cmH_2O$ compared with placebo) and not significantly different from nutrition alone. Ferreira *et al.*[99] randomized 23 patients with COPD in a placebo-controlled study of 6 months oral stanozolol against the background of an exercise program. The study group showed a 41% increase in maximal static inspiratory pressure; however this increase was not statistically different from baseline (or from the 20% increase observed in the placebo group). Thus this study could be interpreted as showing the poor value of maximal static inspiratory pressure as a test of respiratory muscle function. Further caution should be exercised in the interpretation of this study because only 17 of the 23 patients finished the study and a reduced maximal static inspiratory pressure was one of the entry criteria (making the data likely to show an improvement as a result of the learning effect alone).

Recent data suggests that, at least as judged by body weight, the presence of systemic catabolism is linked to the presence of a systemic inflammatory response;[100] manipulation of this response may offer future therapeutic opportunities.

Inspiratory muscle training

The role of inspiratory muscle training in COPD, or indeed in patients with other respiratory disease or athletes, remains controversial. Enthusiasts feel that under some circumstances inspiratory muscle training can increase inspiratory muscle strength (e.g. ref. 101), but evaluation of inspiratory muscle training is confounded by the problem that very often the technique purporting to train the inspiratory muscles is very similar to the one used to evaluate them. In particular the maximal static inspiratory mouth pressure maneuver closely resembles the maneuver required to use some proprietary inspiratory muscle trainers. It has long been speculated that this may give rise to a learning effect and a mechanism for this has recently become evident by the observation that even a short inspiratory muscle training program leads

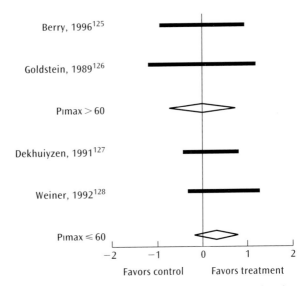

Figure 15.7 *Weighted summary effect sizes of functional exercise capacity (standard deviation units) for the studies with general exercise reconditioning plus inspiratory muscle training. Subgroups were divided on the basis of their baseline $P_{I}max$ ($>60\,cmH_2O$ or $\leqslant 60\,cmH_2O$). Horizontal line indicates the 95% confidence interval of the outcome. Diamonds indicate the weighted summary effect sizes of the group without inspiratory muscle weakness and with inspiratory muscle weakness, respectively. (From refs 124–128.)*

to a significant increase in the cortical excitability of the diaphragm motor area.[102] At least two studies have recently attempted to address the 'learning effect' problem in normal subjects. Sonnetti *et al.* used volitional tests to assess respiratory muscle function in elite athletes before and after inspiratory muscle training.[103] Great care was taken to ensure maximality of the voluntary effort and a credible control intervention was used. Although a trivial increase in inspiratory mouth pressure was observed no performance benefit was observed. In a simpler study from our laboratory we used both the maximal static inspiratory mouth pressure maneuver and the twitch transdiaphragmatic pressure (Pdi) elicited by magnetic phrenic nerve stimulation to evaluate both active and sham inspiratory muscle training.[104] Interestingly, although we found a statistically significant rise in mouth pressure no change was seen in twitch Pdi.

No truly methodologically satisfactory studies have been conducted in patients with COPD, but a recent meta-analysis of existing trials concluded that inspiratory muscle training might have a benefit in the subgroup of patients with COPD related inspiratory muscle weakness (Figure 15.7). Of course this group would also be the group most likely to receive a learning effect and a study that evaluated the effect of inspiratory muscle training using a non-volitional approach would be welcomed.

Ventilatory support

Ventilatory support in COPD is covered elsewhere in this volume, but suffice to say that non-invasive mechanical ventilation is now proven to improve survival in acute acidotic exacerbations of COPD.[105,106] In chronic hypercapnic respiratory failure due to COPD, however, the position of domiciliary non-invasive positive pressure ventilation is less clear, although the therapy is sometimes provided to palliate symptoms of dyspnea. Only one study has randomized such patients;[107] although this study provided some evidence of physiologic improvement it was insufficiently powered to discern differences in 'harder' outcomes.

The relevance to respiratory muscle physiology is that it was once hypothesized that chronic ventilatory failure might arise because of chronic respiratory muscle fatigue and that resting the muscles might relieve this fatigue. This hypothesis is now considered less tenable. In part this is because it has become recognized to be difficult to elicit diaphragm fatigue in normocapnic patients with COPD.[56] However currently ongoing studies are expected to resolve this question definitively in the next few years.

Geometrical considerations

Historically a variety of approaches have been considered to improve diaphragm function in emphysema.[108] Like lung volume reduction surgery, which is enjoying a recent renaissance, these techniques are worthy of recording in case they can be successfully adapted in the future.

Two approaches were described to lengthen the diaphragm. In the first an abdominal belt was used to apply pressure through the anterior abdominal wall to push the diaphragm cranially. A similar approach involved the creation of a pneumoperitoneum. Neither of these approaches is currently used, but it is probably a fair comment that neither has been critically re-evaluated.

THE ABDOMINAL MUSCLE QUESTION

In normal humans the abdominal muscles are recruited in response to minimal increases in ventilation, or even with changes in posture.[109] The function of the abdominal muscles in this situation is to increase expiratory flow and so drive end-expired lung volume (EELV) below FRC. Reduction in EELV lengthens the diaphragm thus increasing the force-output during the subsequent inspiration, which is also aided by the outward recoil of the chest wall and the gravitationally assisted descent of abdominal viscera, which have been pushed cranially by abdominal muscle action.

Abdominal muscles are also important for the generation of cough,[110] which is considered to protect against respiratory tract infection. The simplest method of assessing expiratory muscle function is to measure the mouth pressure during a maximal static expiratory effort,[111] but a non-invasive alternative is the whistle mouth pressure.[112] Magnetic stimulation of the thoracic nerve roots may also be used to evaluate abdominal muscle function non-volitionally and, although it is not a technique which offers supramaximal stimulation, it can be used to seek abdominal muscle fatigue.[113]

Patients with severe COPD are flow limited but yet have significant and substantial abdominal muscle activity[55,114] during exercise. Since these patients are flow limited the function of this activity is unclear; unless there is a mechanism that would allow such activity to be helpful it must be wasteful energetically and should be detrimental. Some authorities hold that this activity is simply a vestigial reflex response to an increased ventilatory requirement,[115] while others believe that there must be a mechanism of action which is presently undetermined. One candidate mechanism could be that of gas compression within the thoracic cavity, permitting lengthening the diaphragm,[116] though the magnitude of this effect is theoretically small if the pressure is uniformly distributed through the thorax. In any event the use of inspiratory pressure support during exercise largely prevents the normally observed increase in expiratory muscle activity.[55]

Abdominal muscle activity is also relevant when assessing respiratory muscle activity in patients with COPD. In essence because such patients are prone to hyperinflation they commonly have an increased end-expiratory esophageal pressure (EEPL). This may be due in part to hyperinflation but can also arise due to abdominal muscle activity.

MEASURING STRENGTH IN THE PERIPHERAL MUSCLES

In recent years there has been recognition that the locomotor muscles of patients with COPD demonstrate myopathic changes which result from disuse, hypoxia and possibly a systemically mediated inflammatory response.[40,41,117] These processes are covered in detail elsewhere but highlight the need to measure contractile function in peripheral muscles.

Of these muscles the most important is probably the quadriceps and this is the one also most amenable to biopsy. The traditional method of measuring quadriceps strength is to use a specially adapted chair and ask the patient to make a maximal voluntary effort.[118] However tests which rely on the patient making a maximal voluntary effort have the disadvantage in clinical practice that the patient may (and often does[119]) fail to make a truly maximal effort. To overcome this problem we have developed the technique of measuring the twitch tension elicited by a single supramaximal twitch applied to the femoral nerve (Figure 15.8), using a modification of the original

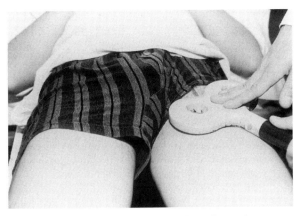

Figure 15.8 *Magnetic stimulation of the femoral nerve. The coil is placed high in the femoral triangle just lateral to the palpated femoral artery.*

recording chair described by Edwards *et al.*[35] This approach was suggested by the successful introduction of magnetic phrenic nerve stimulation for the evaluation of diaphragm function (for reviews see ref. 120). This technique has proved acceptable to patients with COPD, and other serious medical problems,[121] and has been recently used to demonstrate low-frequency quadriceps fatigue after exercise in COPD patients.[122] Magnetic stimulation can also be applied to the ulnar nerve to measure the adductor pollicus twitch tension; this technique has proved acceptable even in the operating room and intensive care unit.[123]

CONCLUSION

It is likely that the diaphragm and other respiratory muscles respond to the increased load imposed by COPD with a compensatory response which resembles a training effect. However the value of this change is likely to be compromised both by changes in diaphragm orientation inherent in chronic hyperinflation, as well as the acute additional hyperinflation which accompanies exercise or an acute exacerbation. With the exception of LVRS, no currently available therapies improve respiratory muscle function in COPD, but modulation of the inflammatory response could offer future therapeutic opportunities.

REFERENCES

1. Moser K, Luchsinger P, Adamson J, *et al.* Respiratory stimulation with intravenous doxapram in respiratory failure. *N Engl J Med* 1973;**288**:427–31.
2. Burrows B, Earle RH. Course and prognosis of chronic obstructive lung disease. A prospective study of 200 patients. *N Engl J Med* 1969;**280**:397–404.
3. Hoover C. The diagnostic significance of inspiratory movements of the costal margins. *Am J Med Sci* 1920;**159**:633–46.
4. Dayman H. Mechanics of breathing in health and emphysema. *J Clin Invest* 1951;**30**:1175–90.
5. Hutchinson J. On the capacity of the lungs and on the respiratory functions. *Med Chir Trans* 1846;**29**:137–252.
6. Rahn H, Otis AB, Chadwick LE, Fenn WO. The pressure–volume diagram of the *Thorax* and lung. *Am J Physiol* 1946;**146**:161–78.
7. Sharp JT, Van Lith P, Nuchprayoo CV, Briney R, Johnson FN. The *Thorax* in chronic obstructive lung disease. *Am J Med* 1968;**44**:39–46.
8. Byrd RB, Hyatt RE. Maximal respiratory pressures in chronic obstructive lung disease. *Am Rev Respir Dis* 1968;**98**: 848–56.
9. Christie RV. The elastic properties of the emphysematous lung and their clinical significance. *J Clin Invest* 1934; **13**:295–319.
10. Mead J, Loring SH. Analysis of volume displacement and length changes of the diaphragm during breathing. *J Appl Physiol* 1982;**53**:750–55.
11. De Troyer A, Sampson M, Sigrist S, Macklem PT. The diaphragm: two muscles. *Science* 1981;**213**:237–8.
12. Urmey WF, De Troyer A, Kelly KB, Loring SH. Pleural pressure increases during inspiration in the zone of apposition of diaphragm to rib cage. *J Appl Physiol* 1988;**65**:2207–12.
13. De Troyer A, Estenne M. Coordination between rib cage muscles and diaphragm during quiet breathing in humans. *J Appl Physiol* 1984;**57**:899–906.
14. Mizuno M. Human respiratory muscles: fibre morphology and capillary supply. *Eur Respir J* 1991;**4**:587–601.
15. Ogilvie CM, Stone RW, Marshall R. The mechanics of breathing during the maximum breathing capacity test. *Clin Sci* 1955;**14**:101–7.
16. Moxham J, Morris AJ, Spiro SG, Edwards RHT, Green M. Contractile properties and fatigue of the diaphragm in man. *Thorax* 1981;**36**:164–8.
17. De Troyer A, Leeper JB, McKenzie DK, Gandevia SC. Neural drive to the diaphragm in patients with severe COPD. *Am J Respir Crit Care Med* 1997;**155**:1335–40.
18. Braun NMT, Arora NS, Rochester DF. Force–length relationship of the normal human diaphragm. *J Appl Physiol* 1982;**53**:405–12.
19. Wanke T, Schenz G, Zwick H, Popp W, Ritschka L, Flicker M. Dependence of maximal sniff generated mouth and transdiaphragmatic pressures on lung volume. *Thorax* 1990;**45**:352–5.
20. Smith J, Bellemare F. Effect of lung volume on *in vivo* contraction characteristics of human diaphragm. *J Appl Physiol* 1987;**62**:1893–900.
21. Polkey MI, Hamnegard C-H, Hughes PD, Rafferty GF, Green M, Moxham J. Influence of acute lung volume change on contractile properties of the human diaphragm. *J Appl Physiol* 1998;**85**:1322–8.
22. Cassart M, Pettiaux N, Gevenois PA, Paiva M, Estenne M. Effect of chronic hyperinflation on diaphragm length and surface area. *Am J Respir Crit Care Med* 1997;**156**: 504–8.
23. Hamnegård C-H, Wragg S, Mills GH, *et al.* The effect of lung volume on transdiaphragmatic pressure. *Eur Respir J* 1995;**8**:1532–6.
24. Supinski GS, Kelsen SG. Effect of elastase-induced emphysema on the force-generating ability of the diaphragm. *J Clin Invest* 1982;**70**:978–88.

25. Farkas GA, Roussos C. Diaphragm in emphysematous hamsters: sarcomere adaptability. *J Appl Physiol* 1983;**54**:1635–40.

26. Oliven A, Supinski G, Kelsen SG. Functional adaptation of diaphragm to chronic hyperinflation in emphysematous hamsters. *J Appl Physiol* 1986;**60**:225–31.

27. Orozco-Levi M, Gea J, Lloreta JL, Felez M, Minguella J, Serrano S, *et al.* Subcellular adaptation of the human diaphragm in chronic obstructive pulmonary disease. *Eur Respir J* 1999;**13**:371–8.

28. NHLBI Workshop summary. Respiratory muscle fatigue. Report of the Respiratory Muscle Fatigue Workshop Group. *Am Rev Respir Dis* 1990;**142**:474–80.

29. Hamnegård C-H, Wragg SD, Kyroussis D, Mills GH, Polkey MI, Moran J, *et al.* Diaphragm fatigue following maximal ventilation in man. *Eur Respir J* 1996;**9**:241–7.

30. Johnson BD, Babcock MA, Suman OE, Dempsey JA. Exercise-induced diaphragmatic fatigue in healthy humans. *J Physiol (Lond)* 1993;**460**:385–405.

31. Polkey MI, Green M, Moxham J. Measurement of respiratory muscle strength. *Thorax* 1995;**50**:1131–5.

32. Luo YM, Polkey MI, Johnson LC, Lyall RA, Harris ML, Green M, Moxham J. Diaphragm EMG measured by cervical magnetic and electrical phrenic nerve stimulation. *J Appl Physiol* **85**:2089–99.

33. Luo YM, Polkey MI, Lyall RA, Moxham J. Effect of brachial plexus co-activation on phrenic nerve conduction time. *Thorax* 1999;**54**:765–70.

34. Laghi F, D'Alfonso N, Tobin MJ. Pattern of recovery from diaphragmatic fatigue over 24 hours. *J Appl Physiol* 1995;**79**:539–46.

35. Polkey MI, Kyroussis D, Hamnegard C-H, Mills GH, Green M, Moxham J. Quadriceps strength and fatigue assessed by magnetic stimulation of the femoral nerve in man. *Muscle Nerve* 1996;**19**:549–55.

36. Cassart M, Gevenois PA, Estenne M. Rib cage dimensions in hyperinflated patients with severe chronic obstructive pulmonary disease. *Am J Respir Crit Care Med* 1996;**154**:800–5.

37. Lando Y, Boiselle P, Shade D, Travaline JM, Furukawa S, Criner GJ. Effect of lung volume reduction surgery on bony thorax configuration in severe COPD. *Chest* 1999;**116**:30–9.

38. Levine S, Kaiser L, Leferovich J, Tikunov B. Cellular adaptations in the diaphragm in chronic obstructive pulmonary disease. *N Engl J Med* 1997;**337**:1799–806.

39. Mercadier J-J, Schwartz K, Schiaffino S, *et al.* Myosin heavy chain gene expression changes in the diaphragm of patients with chronic lung hyperinflation. *Am J Physiol: Lung Cell Mol Physiol* 1998;**274**:L527–34.

40. Jakobsson P, Jorfeldt L, Brundin A. Skeletal muscle metabolites and fibre types in patients with advanced chronic obstructive pulmonary disease, with and without chronic respiratory failure. *Eur Respir J* 1990;**3**:192–6.

41. Bernard S, LeBlanc P, Whittom F, *et al.* Peripheral muscle weakness in patients with chronic obstructive pulmonary disease. *Am J Respir Crit Care Med* 1998;**158**:629–34.

42. Gibson GJ, Clark E, Pride NB. Static transdiaphragmatic pressures in normal subjects and in patients with chronic hyperinflation. *Am Rev Respir Dis* 1981;**124**:685–9.

43. Polkey MI, Kyroussis D, Hamnegard C-H, Mills GH, Green M, Moxham J. Diaphragm strength in chronic obstructive pulmonary disease. *Am J Respir Crit Care Med* 1996;**154**:1310–17.

44. Wanke T, Merkle M, Formanek D, *et al.* Effect of lung transplantation on diaphragmatic function in patients with chronic obstructive pulmonary disease. *Thorax* 1994;**49**:459–64.

45. Polkey MI, Harris ML, Hughes PD, *et al.* The contractile properties of the elderly human diaphragm. *Am J Respir Crit Care Med* 1997;**155**:1560–4.

46. Bellemare F, Grassino A. Force reserve of the diaphragm in patients with chronic obstructive pulmonary disease. *J Appl Physiol* 1983;**55**:8–15.

47. Geddes D, Davies M, Koyama H, *et al.* Effect of lung–volume reduction surgery in patients with severe emphysema. *N Engl J Med* 2000;**343**:239–45.

48. Lahrmann H, Wild M, Wanke T, *et al.* Neural drive to the diaphragm after lung volume reduction surgery. *Chest* 1999;**116**:1593–600.

49. Lando Y, Boiselle PM, Shade D, *et al.* Effect of lung volume reduction surgery on diaphragm length in severe chronic obstructive pulmonary disease. *Am J Respir Crit Care Med* 1999;**159**:796–805.

50. Criner G, Cordova FG, Leyenson V, *et al.* Effect of lung volume reduction surgery on diaphragm strength. *Am J Respir Crit Care Med* 1998;**157**:1578–85.

51. Laghi F, Jubran A, Topeli A, *et al.* Effect of lung volume reduction surgery on neuromechanical coupling of the diaphragm. *Am J Respir Crit Care Med* 1998;**157**:475–83.

52. Gandevia SC, Killian KJ, Campbell EJM. The effect of respiratory muscle fatigue on respiratory sensations. *Clin Sci* 1981;**60**:463–6.

53. Potter WA, Olafsson S, Hyatt RE. Ventilatory mechanics and expiratory flow limitation during exercise in patients with obstructive lung disease. *J Clin Invest* 1971;**50**:910–19.

54. Dodd D, Brancatisano T, Engel L. Chest wall mechanics during exercise in patients with severe chronic airflow obstruction. *Am Rev Respir Dis* 1984;**129**:33–8.

55. Kyroussis D, Polkey MI, Hamnegard CH, Mills GH, Green M, Moxham J. Respiratory muscle activity in patients with COPD walking to exhaustion with and without pressure support. *Eur Respir J* 2000;**15**:649–55.

56. Polkey MI, Kyroussis D, Hamnegard C-H, *et al.* Diaphragm performance during maximal voluntary ventilation in chronic obstructive pulmonary disease. *Am J Respir Crit Care Med* 1997;**155**:642–8.

57. Grassino A, Gross D, Macklem PT, Roussos C, Zagelbaum G. Inspiratory muscle fatigue as a factor limiting exercise. *Bull Eur Pathophysiol Resp* 1979;**15**:105–11.

58. Bye PT, Esau SA, Levy RD, *et al.* Ventilatory muscle function during exercise in air and oxygen in patients with chronic air-flow limitation. *Am Rev Respir Dis* 1985;**132**:236–40.

59. Kyroussis D, Polkey MI, Keilty SEJ, *et al.* Exhaustive exercise slows inspiratory muscle relaxation rate in chronic obstructive pulmonary disease. *Am J Respir Crit Care Med* 1996;**153**:787–93.

60. Polkey MI, Kyroussis D, Mills GH, *et al.* Inspiratory pressure support reduces slowing of inspiratory muscle relaxation rate during exhaustive treadmill walking in severe COPD. *Am J Respir Crit Care Med* 1996;**154**:1146–50.

61. Polkey MI, Kyroussis D, Keilty SEJ, *et al.* Exhaustive treadmill exercise does not reduce twitch transdiaphragmatic pressure in patients with COPD. *Am J Respir Crit Care Med* 1995;**152**:959–64.

62. Roussos C, Fixley M, Gross D, Macklem PT. Fatigue of the inspiratory muscles and their synergic behaviour. *J Appl Physiol* 1979;**46**:897–904.

63. Fitch S, McComas AJ. Influence of human muscle length on fatigue. *J Physiol* 1985;**362**:205–13.

64. Sacco P, McIntyre DB, Jones DA. Effects of length and stimulation frequency on fatigue of the human tibialis anterior muscle. *J Appl Physiol* 1994;**77**:1148–54.

65. Nickoletou D, Man WD, Polkey MI, Moxham J, Johnson PH. Diaphragm fatigue after threshold loading in patients with moderate to severe COPD. *Thorax* 2001;**56**(S3):iii50.

66. Polkey MI, Hawkins P, Kyroussis D, Ellum SG, Sherwood R, Moxham J. Inspiratory pressure support prolongs exercise induced lactataemia in severe COPD. *Thorax* 2000; **55**:547–9.

67. Keilty SE, Ponte J, Fleming TA, Moxham J. Effect of inspiratory pressure support on exercise tolerance and breathlessness in patients with severe stable chronic obstructive pulmonary disease. *Thorax* 1994;**49**:990–4.

68. White JE, Drinnan MJ, Smithson AJ, Griffiths CJ, Gibson GJ. Respiratory muscle activity during rapid eye movement (REM) sleep in patients with chronic obstructive pulmonary disease. *Thorax* 1995;**50**:376–82.

69. Heijdra YF, Dekhuijzen PN, van Herwaarden CL, Folgering HT. Nocturnal saturation improves by target-flow inspiratory muscle training in patients with COPD. *Am J Respir Crit Care Med* 1996;**153**:260–5.

70. Aubier M, Murciano D, Viires N, *et al.* Effects of digoxin on diaphragmatic strength generation in patients with chronic obstructive pulmonary disease during acute respiratory failure. *Am Rev Respir Dis* 1987;**135**:544–8.

71. Liberman D, Brami JL, Bark H, Pilpel D, Heimer D. Effect of digoxin on respiratory muscle performance in patients with COPD. *Respiration* 1991;**58**:29–32.

72. Polkey MI, Moxham J. Pharmacotherapy and hormone therapy of the respiratory muscles in stable COPD. In: T Similowski, WA Whitelaw, J-P Derenne, eds. *Clinical Management of Stable COPD*. Marcel Dekker, New York, 2002;659–80.

73. Aubier M, De Troyer A, Sampson M, Macklem PT, Roussos C. Aminophylline improves diaphragm contractility. *N Engl J Med* 1981;**305**:249–52.

74. Moxham J, Miller J, Wiles CM, Morris AJR, Green M. Effect of aminophylline on the human diaphragm. *Thorax* 1985;**40**: 288–92.

75. Brophy C, Mier A, Moxham J, Green M. The efect of aminophylline on respiratory and limb muscle contractility in man. *Eur Respir J* 1989;**2**:652–5.

76. DeGarmo C, Cerny F, Conboy K, Ellis EF. *In vivo* effects of theophylline on diaphragm, bicep and quadricep strength and fatiguability. *J Allergy Clin Immunol* 1988; **82**:1041–6.

77. Wanke T, Merkle M, Zifko U, *et al.* The effect of aminophylline on the force–length characteristics of the diaphragm. *Am J Respir Crit Care Med* 1994;**149**:1545–9.

78. Gauthier A, Yan S, Suwinski P, Macklem P. Effects of fatigue, fiber length and aminophylline on human diaphragm contractility. *Am J Respir Crit Care Med* 1995;**152**:204–10.

79. Murciano D, Auclair M-H, Pariente R, Aubier M. A randomized controlled trial of theophylline in patients with severe chronic obstructive pulmonary disease. *N Engl J Med* 1989;**320**:1521–5.

80. Foxworth JW, Reisz GR, Knudson SM, Cuddy PG, Pyszczynski DR, Emory CE. Theophylline and diaphragmatic contractility. Investigation of a dose–response relationship. *Am Rev Respir Dis* 1988;**138**:1532–4.

81. Cooper CB, Davidson AC, Cameron IR. Aminophylline, respiratory muscle strength and exercise tolerance in chronic obstructive airway disease. *Bull Eur Physiopathol Respir* 1987;**23**:15–22.

82. Derom E, Janssens S, Gurrieri G, Tjandramaga TB, Decramer M. Effects of broxaterol and theophylline on fatigued

canine diaphragm *in vivo*. A randomized, controlled study. *Am Rev Respir Dis* 1992;**146**:22–5.

83. Aubier M, Viires N, Murciano D, Medrano G, Lecocguic Y, Pariente R. Effects and mechanism of action of terbutaline on diaphragmatic contractility and fatigue. *J Appl Physiol: Respir Environ Exercise Physiol* 1984;**56**:922–9.

84. Numata H, Suzuki S, Miyashita A, Suzuki M, Okubo T. Effects of beta$_2$-agonists on the contractility of fatigued canine diaphragm *in vivo*. *Resp Physiol* 1993;**94**:25–34.

85. Howell S, Fitzgerald RS, Roussos C. Effects of neostigmine and salbutamol on diaphragmatic fatigue. *Resp Physiol* 1985;**62**:15–29.

86. Lanigan C, Howes TQ, Borzone G, Vianna LG, Moxham J. The effects of beta$_2$-agonists and caffeine on respiratory and limb muscle performance. *Eur Respir J* 1993;**6**:1192–6.

87. Javaheri S, Thomas JP, Guilfoile TD, Donovan EF. Albuterol has no efffect on diaphragmatic fatigue in humans. *Am Rev Respir Dis* 1988;**137**:197–201.

88. Stoller JK, Wiedemann HP, Loke J, Snyder P, Virgulto J, Matthay RA. Terbutaline and diaphragm function in chronic obstructive pulmonary disease: a double blind randomized clinical trial. *Br J Dis Chest* 1988;**82**:242–50.

89. Nava S, Crotti P, Gurrieri G, Fracchia C, Rampulla C. Effect of a beta$_2$-agonist (broxaterol) on respiratory muscle strength and endurance in patients with COPD with irreversible airway obstruction. *Chest* 1992;**101**:133–40.

90. Hatipoglu U, Laghi F, Tobin MJ. Does inhaled albuterol improve diaphragmatic contractility in patients with chronic obstructive pulmonary disease? *Am J Respir Crit Care Med* 1999;**160**:1916–21.

91. Arora NS, Rochester DF. Effect of body weight and muscularity on human diaphagm muscle mass, thickness, and area. *J Appl Physiol* 1982;**52**:64–70.

92. Thurlbeck WM. Diaphragm and body weight in emphysema. *Thorax* 1978;**33**:483–7.

93. Felbinger TW, Suchner U, Goetz AE, Briegel J, Peter K. Recombinant human growth hormone for reconditioning of respiratory muscle after lung volume reduction surgery. *Crit Care Med* 1999;**27**:1634–8.

94. Suchner U, Rothkopf MM, Stanislaus G, Elwyn DH, Kvetan V, Askanazi J. Growth hormone and pituitary disease. Metabolic effects in patients receiving parenteral nutrition. *Arch Intern Med* 1990;**150**:1225–30.

95. Pape GS, Friedman M, Underwood LE, Clemmons DR. The effect of growth hormone on weight gain and pulmonary function in patients with chronic obstructive lung disease. *Chest* 1991;**99**:1495–500.

96. Burdet L, de Muralt B, Schutz Y, Pichard C, Fitting J-W. Administration of growth hormone to underweight patients with chronic obstructive pulmonary disease. A prospective randomized controlled study. *Am J Respir Crit Care Med* 1997;**156**:1800–6.

97. Bhasin S, Storer TW, Berman N, *et al.* The effects of supraphysiologic doses of testosterone on muscle size and strength in normal men. *N Engl J Med* 1996;**335**:1–7.

98. Schols AMW, Soeters PB, Mostert R, Pluymers RJ, Wouters EFM. Physiologic effects of nutritional support and anabolic steroids in patients with chronic obstructive pulmonary disease. A placebo-controlled randomized trial. *Am J Respir Crit Care Med* 1995;**152**:1268–74.

99. Ferreira I, Verreschi I, Nery L, *et al.* The influence of 6 months of oral anabolic steroids on body mass and respiratory muscles in undernourished COPD patients. *Chest* 1998;**114**:19–28.

100. Creutzberg EC, Schols AM, Weling-Scheepers CA, Buurman WA, Wouters EF. Characterization of nonresponse to high

caloric oral nutritional therapy in depleted patients with chronic obstructive pulmonary disease. *Am J Respir Crit Care Med* 2000;**161**:745–52.

101. Koessler W, Wanke T, Winkler G, *et al*. 2 Years' experience with inspiratory muscle training in patients with neuromuscular disorders. *Chest* 2001;**120**:765–9.

102. Demoule A, Verin E, Derenne J-P, Similowski T. Plasticity of the human motor cortical representation of the diaphragm. *Am J Respir Crit Care Med* 2001;**163**:A46.

103. Sonetti DA, Wetter TJ, Pegelow DF, Dempsey JA. Effects of respiratory muscle training versus placebo on endurance exercise performance. *Resp Physiol* 2001;**127**:185–99.

104. Hart N, Sylvester K, Ward S, Cramer D, Moxham J, Polkey MI. Evaluation of an inspiratory muscle trainer in healthy humans. *Respir Med* 2001;**95**:526–31.

105. Brochard L, Mancebo J, Wysocki M, *et al*. Noninvasive ventilation for acute exacerbations of chronic obstructive pulmonary disease. *N Engl J Med* 1995;**333**:817–22.

106. Plant PK, Owen JL, Elliott MW. Early use of non-invasive ventilation for acute exacerbations of chronic obstructive pulmonary disease on general respiratory wards: a multicentre randomised controlled trial. *Lancet* 2000;**355**:1931–5.

107. Meecham-Jones D, Paul E, Jones P, Wedzicha J. Nasal pressure support ventilation plus oxygen compared with oxygen therapy alone in hypercapnic COPD. *Am J Respir Crit Care Med* 1995;**152**:538–44.

108. Deslauriers J. History of surgery for emphysema. *Semin Thorac Cardiovasc Surg* 1996;**8**:43–51.

109. Campbell EJM, Green JH. The behaviour of the abdominal muscles and the intraabdominal pressure during quiet breathing and increased pulmonary ventilation. A study in man. *J Physiol (Lond)* 1955;**127**:423–6.

110. Polkey MI, Lyall RA, Green M, Leigh PN, Moxham J. Expiratory muscle function in amyotrophic lateral sclerosis. *Am J Respir Crit Care Med* 1998;**158**:734–41.

111. Black LF, Hyatt RE. Maximal respiratory pressures: normal values and relationships to age and sex. *Am Rev Respir Dis* 1969;**99**:696–702.

112. Chetta A, Harris ML, Lyall RA, *et al*. Whistle mouth pressure as test of expiratory muscle strength. *Eur Respir J* 2001;**17**:688–95.

113. Kyroussis D, Mills GH, Polkey MI, *et al*. Abdominal muscle fatigue after maximal ventilation in humans. *J Appl Physiol* 1996;**81**:1477–83.

114. Ninane V, Yernault JC, de Troyer A. Intrinsic PEEP in patients with chronic obstructive pulmonary disease. Role of expiratory muscles. *Am Rev Respir Dis* 1993;**148**:1037–42.

115. Estenne M, Derom E, De Troyer A. Neck and abdominal muscle activity in patients with severe thoracic scoliosis. *Am J Respir Crit Care Med* 1998;**158**:452–7.

116. Ingram RH, Schilder DP. Effect of gas compression on pulmonary pressure, flow and volume relationship. *J Appl Physiol* 1966;**21**:1821–6.

117. Maltais F, Simard A-A, Simard C, *et al*. Oxidative capacity of the skeletal muscle and lactic acid kinetics during exercise in normal subjects and in patients with COPD. *Am J Respir Crit Care Med* 1996;**153**:288–93.

118. Edwards RHT, Young A, Hosking GP, Jones DA. Human skeletal muscle function: description of tests and normal values. *Clin Sci* 1977;**52**:283–90.

119. Polkey MI, Kyroussis D, Harris ML, Hughes PD, Green M, Moxham J. Are voluntary manoeuvres maximal in routine clinical testing? *Am J Respir Crit Care Med* 1996;**153**:A785.

120. Polkey MI, Moxham J. Clinical aspects of respiratory muscle dysfunction in the critically ill. *Chest* 2001;**119**:926–39.

121. Harris ML, Polkey MI, Bath PMW, Moxham J. Quadriceps weakness following acute hemiplegic stroke. *Clin Rehab* 2001;**15**:274–81.

122. Mador MJ, Kufel TJ, Pineda L. Quadriceps fatigue after cycle exercise in patients with chronic obstructive pulmonary disease. *Am J Respir Crit Care Med* 2000;**161**:447–53.

123. Harris ML, Luo YM, Watson AC, *et al*. Adductor pollicis twitch tension assessed by magnetic stimulation of the ulnar nerve. *Am J Respir Crit Care Med* 2000;**162**:240–5.

124. Lötters F, van Tol B, Kwakkel G, Gosselink R. Effects of controlled inspiratory muscle training in patients with chronic obstructive pulmonary disease: a meta analysis. *Eur Respir J* 2002;**20**:570–6.

125. Berry MJ, Adair NE, Sevensky KS, Quinby A, Lever HM. Inspiratory muscle and whole body reconditioning in Chronic Obstructive Pulmonary Disease. A Controller Randomised Trial. *Am J Respir Crit Care Med* 1996;**153**:1812–6.

126. Goldstein R, De Rosie J, Long S, Dolmage T, Avendano MA. Applicability of a threshold loading device for inspiratory muscle testing and training in patients with COPD. *Chest* 1989;**96(3)**:564–71.

127. Dekhuijzen PN, Folgering HT, van Herwaarden CL. Target-flow inspiratory muscle training during pulmonary rehabilitation in patients with COPD. *Chest* 1991;**99(1)**:128–33.

128. Weiner P, Azgad Y, Ganam R. Inspiratory muscle training combined with general exercise reconditioning in patients with COPD. *Chest* 1992;**102(5)**:1351–6.

16

Ventilatory control and breathlessness

PETER MA CALVERLEY

The progress of ideas in respiratory physiology has often been accelerated by the need for practical solutions. Thus the clinical problems of gasmask design in the first world war led Haldane and coworkers to further study the stimulant effects of respiratory gases, whilst the hypoxia of high altitude experienced by second world war fighter pilots generated new research about the chemical regulation of human breathing. The subsequent rise in the incidence of and mortality from chronic obstructive pulmonary disease gave a new clinical dimension to these problems. The dangers of high concentrations of oxygen during acute exacerbations of COPD were soon recognized[1] and led Campbell to apply new technologies to first identify the physiologic problem (hypercapnia), then hypothesize a mechanism for its production (reduced hypercapnic ventilatory drive) and finally suggest a practical solution (low-flow oxygen treatment by Venturi mask).[2]

About the same time Dornhorst's almost apocryphal (and certainly unreferenced) description of the two extremes of advanced COPD – 'pink and puffing' or 'blue and bloated' – launched a debate about whether these patients could not breathe or would not breathe when confronted with progressive lung disease, a controversy that continues in new forms to the present day. Meanwhile, Campbell and colleagues in a series of pioneering studies had begun the systematic investigation of respiratory sensation in general and breathlessness in particular. Their initial views were set out in a landmark symposium[3]

whilst progress or lack of it has been reviewed more recently on a similar occasion.[4]

This chapter will review some of the evidence underlying the ebb and flow of these ideas. More than most areas of respiratory medicine, studies of ventilatory control and dyspnea have been conditioned by the available technology and especially the problems of data handling. However, subtle and often unstated assumptions about the primary importance of blood gas tensions and the irrelevance of respiratory sensation and consciousness, have had a major effect on the hypotheses tested. These assumptions have now been challenged and hopefully the new approaches to these areas which have resulted will prove more useful to physiologists and clinicians alike.

ORGANIZATION OF VENTILATORY CONTROL

Conventional approaches envisage a hierarchy of command for ventilatory control,[5,6] although there is considerably less agreement about whether the output of the control system is regulated to optimize ventilation or breathing pattern however analyzed.[7,8] Inevitably most data about underlying mechanisms have involved animal studies where stimulation and ablation experiments are performed under anesthesia.[5,9] Whilst these establish that a neural connection exists, they do little to elucidate the integrated action of the system under conditions when mechanical and chemical homostasis is disturbed, as in COPD.

Respiration persists in these animals when the brainstem is sectioned at the pons or medulla.[10] The resulting metronomically regular breathing pattern is seldom seen in man except during deep general anesthesia[11] or stage 3/4 sleep.[12] It is believed to result from the interaction of three groups of tightly interconnected neurones:[5,6]

1 The dorsal respiratory group (DRG) which lies in the ventrolateral nucleus of the tractus solitarius and receives afferent impulses via the glossopharyngeal and vagus nerves from peripheral chemoreceptors and mechanoreceptors. The neurones here are mainly inspiratory but not all are influenced by stretch-receptor inputs. They project onto both the other neural groups and the phrenic nerve nucleus in the cervical cord.

2 The ventral respiratory group (VRG) extends throughout the medulla and includes neurones in the nucleus ambiguus, para-ambiguus and retrofacialis. The rostral neurones are thought to be inspiratory and the caudal ones expiratory. There are no direct connections with neural afferents from outside the CNS.

3 The pontine respiratory group corresponds to the neurones in the nucleus parabrachialis and the Kollicker–Fuse nucleus. These were thought to comprise the phase-spanning neurones that fire in late inspiration and early expiration. Recent data suggest they are a heterogeneous group of neurones rather than belonging to a specific type.[13]

Neurones from the DRG and VRG synapse with phrenic and intercostal neurones in the spinal cord where neuronal firing can be further modified by multiple proprioceptive impulse principally from chest wall mechanoreceptors.[14]

Respiratory rhythm is thought to rely on a central pattern generator[6,14] which acts as a rhythmic oscillator. Several models of how the central pattern generator might work have been suggested, largely based on the simplified neural network of the mollusc *Lymnaea stagnalis*.[15] The favored approach is a conditional oscillator in which oscillations in inspiratory and expiratory firing occur but on top of a tonic input from hypoxic stimulation. Only when a discrete ventilatory pump develops does CO_2 sensitivity become important in the control of respiration.

The precise siting and nature of these respiratory pacemaker cells is still to be identified but extensive studies of the effects of lung inflation at different phases in the respiratory cycle in anesthetized animals have revealed characteristic patterns in neuronal firing in both inspiration and expiration. These data have modified the way in which we analyze breathing patterns with an increased emphasis on the role of inspiratory time (TI)

and total cycle duration (TTOT) as well as tidal volume. Minute ventilation, traditionally expressed as VT × f (respiratory frequency) can now be represented by:

$$VT/TI \times TI/TTOT \times 60$$

where VT/TI is the mean inspiratory flow which approximates to inspiratory neural drive assuming a linear increase in neural output and no mechanical restriction; and TI/TTOT is the proportion of each breath spent in inspiration (respiratory duty cycle). This approach has been helpful in analyzing the breathing pattern of COPD patients (see below).

Phasic respiratory motor output also controls the pharyngeal and laryngeal dimensions, which has considerable importance for patients with COPD. Coordinated genoglossus activation before inspiration is essential if pharyngeal patency is to be maintained.[16] One group has reported that COPD patients with smaller upper airway dimensions are more likely to become hypercapnic, possibly because of an increase in pharyngeal resistance during sleep,[17,18] although this is probably an unusual cause of hypercapnia.[19] Laryngeal braking of expiratory airflow appears to be an important mechanism for stabilizing expiratory lung volume which is a particular problem in COPD patients with hyperinflation.[20] The role of purse-lip breathing and its neurologic basis as an adjunct to this remains uncertain.[21]

FACTORS THAT MODULATE RESPIRATORY OUTPUT

Three major influences modify respiratory motor output, namely chemoreceptor, mechanoreceptor and cortical factors. The relative importance of these will vary depending upon the situation.

Chemoreceptor inputs

The peripheral chemoreceptors in man lie in the carotid body at the junction of the common and external carotid arteries, the aortic bodies having little demonstrable effect on human ventilation. Although only 15 mg in weight, these bodies have a blood flow equivalent to 2 liters per 100 g of tissue and are ideally sited to 'taste' the arterial gas tension of blood going to the brain. Local autonomic regulation of blood flow can further modify the chemoreceptor output.[22] Hypoxia produces a hyperbolic increase in carotid sinus nerve discharge,[23] which may be signaled by intracellular changes in ADP or calcium. Carotid chemoreceptors are hypertrophied in some hypoxemic patients with COPD[24] but this does not seem to have functional significance.

Hypercapnia increases carotid sinus neural traffic linearly, probably due to local changes in pH.[25] The hypoxic and hypercapnic signals affect each other locally in a multiplicative way and travel in the glossopharyngeal nerves to the DRG where they are integrated with other inputs.

Peripheral chemoreceptor inputs contribute approximately 15% to resting ventilation and can be largely abolished by hyperoxia[26] which is thought to explain the beneficial role of supplementary oxygen in normoxic COPD patients (see Chapter 18). The relatively large falls in arterial PO_2 needed before chemoreceptor response occurs suggests that in most patients hypoxia is unimportant in eupneic ventilatory control. Chemoreceptor response to short-term hypoxemia is better related to O_2 saturation (Figure 16.1), an important determinant of tissue oxygen delivery. Thus, chemoreceptor detection of hypoxemia is an important respiratory 'defence mechanism' which is very relevant at altitude when inspired O_2 tension falls and also enhances the effects of small changes in CO_2 tension at least when these occur acutely.

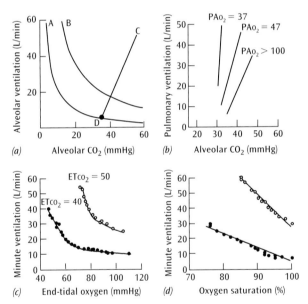

(a)
(b)
(c)
(d)

Figure 16.1 *Classical concepts of the chemical control of breathing in normal subjects. The relationship between alveolar ventilation and alveolar CO_2 tensions are shown in (a). The higher curve (B) represents a greater metabolic CO_2 production and line (C) the effects of adding inspired CO_2. These apply to steady-state conditions only. (b) Shows data obtained during CO_2 rebreathing at three different levels of arterial hypoxia. Note the critical dependence of the VE/Pco$_2$ slope on the oxygen tension. The converse is shown in (c), which also illustrates the curvilinearity of the isocapnic hypoxic response. This can be corrected for by plotting arterial oxygen saturation (Sao$_2$) (d) on the abscissa as is now conventionally done when saturation is measured non-invasively.*

Changes in CO_2 tension produce a linear increase in ventilation, largely due to central chemoreceptor stimulation (Figure 16.1). Unlike the anatomically discrete peripheral chemoreceptors, the central chemoreceptors are disappointingly diffuse with continued disagreement about their exact site and nature. The classical studies of Pappenheimer[27] showed that perfusing the ventrolateral surface of the medulla with hydrogen ions increases ventilation. Changes in hydrogen ion rather than CO_2 are thought to be the major respiratory stimulus,[28] although there is now some evidence that CO_2 has a more complex effect than that expected from changes in pH alone[29] and that other sites can respond to CO_2.[30] Tonically discharging cells responding to limb flexion[31] or peripheral chemoreceptor stimulation[28] are found in this area intermingled with vasomotor neurones, as might be expected from the tight coupling of changes in ventilation and of circulation.

Traditionally hypoxia has been believed to act solely via its stimulant effects on peripheral chemoreceptors. However, when the chemoreceptors are removed in animals and more recently during extended periods of isocapnic hypoxemia in man, hypoxia has been shown to exhibit a central depressant effect.[32] This is probably mediated by the local production of adenosine, one of a range of neurotransmitters which can modify central ventilatory output.[33] Thus, studies in normal subjects before and after aminophylline, a specific adenosine antagonist, found that the fall in ventilation during sustained hypoxia was blocked.[34] Apart from the rather remote relevance of this to the clinical actions of theophylline, these observations may explain the occasional paradoxical falls in PacO$_2$ seen after correction of hypoxemia during acute exacerbations of ventilatory failure, as an increase in medullary PaO$_2$ may increase ventilation more than the simultaneous reduction of peripheral chemoreceptor hypoxic stimulation.[35]

Interpretation of the effects of altered blood gas tensions on the ventilatory control system is clearly complex and likely to be influenced by both the apneic threshold, i.e. the level of CO_2 below which respiration ceases,[36,37] and the amount of metabolic CO_2 production,[38–43] both of which have been little studied in COPD.

Mechanoreceptor inputs

Afferent inputs from mechanoreceptors can augment or terminate inspiration in many animal models but their relevance to conscious man and particularly COPD patients is much less clear. Three major groups have been identified, all travelling in the vagus nerve:[44,45]

1 **Stretch-receptors.** These slowly adapting receptors lie within the airway smooth muscle of the more distal airways and are stimulated by inflation and

changes in gas tensions. They terminate inspiration, stimulate expiratory activity and are responsible for the Hering-Bruer reflex.

2 **Rapidly adapting receptors (RASR).** These lie in the epithelial and submucosa of the larger airways and respond to stimulation by dust or ammonia by producing bronchoconstriction, cough and laryngeal narrowing. Increases in inspiratory airflow augment inspiratory neural activity via these receptors. Unlike the stretch-receptors which have a vasodepressor action, stimulation of RASR produces a vasopressor response.

3 **Bronchial C and J receptors.** These unmyelinated fibers are probably true irritant receptors and the bronchial ones are responsible for cough and the response to capsacin. Like the RASR above their stimulation promotes a rapid shallow breathing pattern. C fiber afferents are thought to be responsible for this pattern when these juxtacapillary receptors are stimulated during pulmonary edema.

Other reflex inputs include those from the rib cage and diaphragmatic muscle spindles which also project to the cortex[31,46] in addition to their well-recognized action at a spinal level. Spindle numbers are relatively low in the diaphragm which may be relevant to respiratory sensation (see below). Less well studied inputs include those in the rib cage joints and from the upper airways. Many of the latter appear to be state dependent, and can only be elicited during sleep. However, pharyngeal stimulation with cold air can reduce the ventilatory response to CO_2 in normal subjects,[47] whilst breathing chilled air during exercise can reduce minute ventilation for a given workload in COPD patients without change in spirometry[48] (Figure 16.2).

The role of intrapulmonary receptors in respiratory regulation in conscious man is probably very small. Vagally mediated regulation of lung volumes which is present in the neonatal lung up to 8 weeks of age[16] can be detected during anesthesia.[49,50] In patients undergoing heart/lung transplantations the ventilatory responses to hypoxia and hypercapnia,[51] exercise and the tidal volume response to added loads[52,53] are unaffected by total pulmonary denervation. One study has suggested some reduction in ventilatory response in patients after double lung transplantation,[54] but this is probably explained by the postoperative mechanical limitations to breathing rather than the loss of reflex regulation.

Cortical influences

The ability of the human respiratory system to modify automatic respiratory control so as to subserve the needs of speech or swallowing has long been recognized[55] but largely ignored because of the problems it creates in

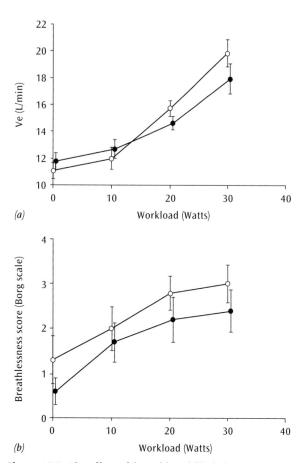

(a)

(b)

Figure 16.2 *The effect of breathing chilled air on exercise ventilation (Ve) and breathlessness in stable COPD. Open circles represent room air breathing; closed circles chilled air breathing. These effects are most marked at the highest work levels in these severe patients. (From ref. 48.)*

analyzing respiratory mechanisms. Studies by Newsom-Davis and Stagg were among the first to confirm the spontaneous breath-to-breath variations in normal human breathing.[56] This may be influenced by breathing route which appears to be selected largely for mechanical reasons[57] but the principal determinant is the level of consciousness. There is a progressive fall in breath-to-breath variability as sleep deepens from 12% during wakefulness to 4% during stage 4 sleep. When cortical activity increases once more in REM sleep, substantial variation to breathing returns especially in phasic REM and tidal volume falls as well.[58] When automatic control of breathing is lost, profound nocturnal hypoventilation occurs as in Ondine's curse.[59] Even during wakefulness differences in the degree of concentration can affect breathing pattern. Thus Rigg *et al.* found that mental arithmetic did not influence the slope of the CO_2 response but the breathing pattern adopted during it, a finding similar to those of Mador and Tobin studying unstimulated breathing at rest.[58,60] These data support the view that cortical

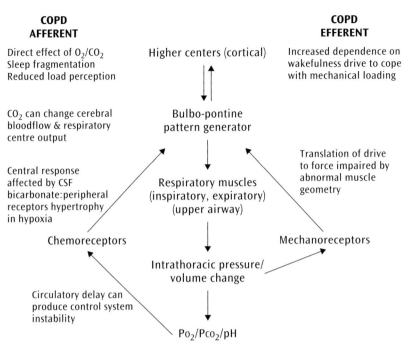

**COPD
AFFERENT**

Direct effect of O_2/CO_2
Sleep fragmentation
Reduced load perception

CO_2 can change cerebral
bloodflow & respiratory
centre output

Central response
affected by CSF
bicarbonate:peripheral
receptors hypertrophy
in hypoxia

Higher centers (cortical)

Bulbo-pontine
pattern generator

Respiratory muscles
(inspiratory, expiratory)
(upper airway)

Chemoreceptors

Intrathoracic pressure/
volume change

Circulatory delay can
produce control system
instability

$Po_2/Pco_2/pH$

**COPD
EFFERENT**

Increased dependence on
wakefulness drive to cope
with mechanical loading

Translation of drive
to force impaired by
abnormal muscle
geometry

Mechanoreceptors

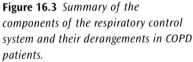

Figure 16.3 *Summary of the
components of the respiratory control
system and their derangements in COPD
patients.*

factors can regulate breathing pattern without the subject being aware of this.

Ventilatory control – a unifying hypothesis

This summary highlights the multiplicity of mechanisms which influence ventilation and which might be disturbed in diseases such as COPD. Conventionally such schemes have been integrated into a complex series of feedback loops (Figure 16.3), which assume that the principal output variable is the maintenance of blood gas homostasis as in the classical model of Grodin.[61] This is clearly not the case as the apparent redundancy of hypoxic drive at rest demonstrates. Changes in Paco₂ oscillations may influence chemoreceptors but seem unlikely to explain the immediate increase in ventilation that accompanies exercise[39] and, in any case, such changes are relatively well buffered in normal subjects let alone COPD patients as short-term hypoventilation studies demonstrate.[62]

One of the earliest attempts at explaining the integrated activity of the respiratory system came in 1965 when Priban and Fincham suggested that the system was regulated to minimize energy consumption.[63] There are now ample data to support this view. The most powerful model so far developed is that of Poon and colleagues at MIT.[64,65]

Using conventional equations of steady-state gas exchange, lung mechanics and chemosensitivity together with a more recent analysis of inspiratory neural drive,[66]

this model has successfully predicted the pattern of breathing seen at rest, during exercise and with mechanical loading in normal subjects.[66] The key feature is the use of an optimizing function for medullary respiratory output such that the product of mechanical and chemical 'cost of breathing' is minimized. The model still has limitations as it makes no allowance for active expiratory muscle activity or the viscoelastic mechanical behavior of the respiratory system. Nonetheless, it fits well with developing ideas about the role of respiratory sensation in ventilatory control. (see below)

SPECIFIC PROBLEMS OF VENTILATORY CONTROL IN COPD

Ventilatory control in COPD is only measureably deranged when respiratory impedance increases significantly, although changes in breathing pattern and ventilation during maximal exercise have been reported in fit elderly people with a physiologic loss of lung elastic recoil.[67] Several factors affect ventilatory control in the COPD patient (Figure 16.3):

1 Gas exchange is impaired in COPD with prolonged time constants for gas mixing (see Chapter **14**). Differences in lung O_2 and blood CO_2 stores will blunt immediate changes in gas tensions as ventilatory stimulants. Conversely, end-tidal gas tensions are imperfect markers of blood gas status in tests of chemical control of breathlessness.

2 COPD is a complex mixture of internal resistive and elastic mechanical loads.[68] The resulting prolongation of the mechanical time constant (the product of resistance and compliance (see Chapter 13)) is particularly sensitive to changes in respiratory frequency. Thus the total respiratory impedance is not constant but changes when ventilation increases, for example during exercise.

3 Pulmonary hyperinflation has a dynamic as well as a passive component and is associated with intrinsic PEEP (see Chapters 13 and 19). This acts as a threshold inspiratory load to breathe. The overinflated chest produces changes in chest wall configuration such that neither intercostals nor diaphragm muscle operates at their optimal length. Although sarcomere numbers may adapt to hyperinflation tending to restore optimum force-generating capacity,[69] the geometric disadvantages of hyperinflation persist (see 'Respiratory Muscle Fatigue' below). Thus respiratory center output must be higher for an equivalent level of ventilation in the face of hyperinflation and airflow resistance.

4 The combination of arterial hypoxemia and increase in ventilatory demand during an acute exacerbation may precipitate respiratory muscle fatigue. The ability of the ventilation control system to choose the breathing pattern that minimizes this risk is vital to the patient's survival.

ASSESSMENT OF VENTILATORY CONTROL IN COPD

A range of techniques has been used to study ventilatory control but each has significant disadvantages in the COPD patient (Table 16.1). The most widely used methods of inducing relatively rapid changes in blood gas tensions, often by rebreathing techniques, may not yield physiologically relevant data. Use of ventilation as a measure of respiratory center output is limited by abnormal lung mechanics. Many of these problems can be overcome by using the mouth occlusion pressure $(P_{0.1})$[70] but even this may not be representative of intrathoracic pressure swings in severe COPD.[71] Occlusion pressure is also influenced by posture[72] and by lung volume which may change during exercise or during rebreathing tests. The strengths and limitations of this approach have been reviewed.[73] In some studies of COPD patients, mouth occlusion pressure has been a particularly poor index of respiratory muscle activation,[74] although these appear to be a minority. Despite these drawbacks, a large amount of data has accumulated about the results of such tests in COPD patients.

CHEMICAL CONTROL OF BREATHING IN COPD

Most studies of chemical control of breathing in COPD have tried to answer one or more of the following questions:

1 Is the response to chemical stimuli abnormal?
2 Is this explicable solely by the increased mechanical load imposed on the respiratory system by the disease or does it reflect an inherent reduction in respiratory chemosensitivity?
3 Do patients who are 'blue and bloated' have different responses to hypoxia and/or CO_2 than those who are 'pink and puffing'?

While the answer to the first question is undoubtedly yes, the response to the other two is still confused reflecting the different methodologies employed in the patient groups studied.

It is over five decades since Donald and Christie noted that patients with severe obstructive lung disease had a reduced ventilatory response to CO_2.[75] Many subsequent studies have confirmed this, mainly using CO_2 re-breathing and with ventilation and/or $P_{0.1}$ as their output variables[76–86] (Figure 16.4). There is a surprisingly good agreement in the severity of ventilatory depression between the groups, at least as compared with normals studied in the same fashion.

Early studies noted that normal subjects breathing against external inspiratory resistances showed similar falls in $\dot{V}E/P{CO_2}$ to those seen in COPD.[87] This is associated with a compensatory increase in $P_{0.1}$, although this is insufficient to maintain ventilation at the initial level (Figure 16.4). These data show very similar $\dot{V}E/P{CO_2}$ and $P_{0.1}/P{CO_2}$ slopes to those seen at rest in patients with chronic mechanical loading due to COPD studied in the same laboratory (Figure 16.4). One way of allowing for the effects of mechanical loading is to plot change in ventilation against change in $P_{0.1}$ which can be derived as the ratio of $\dot{V}E/P{CO_2}:P{CO_2}$ slopes. The values are remarkably consistent between studies and appear to be similar whether or not the patients are hypercapnic. If the data are expressed as a percentage of the maximum voluntary ventilation (derived from the FEV_1) with either $P{CO_2}$ or $P_{0.1}$ as the denominator, then most eucapnic COPD patients fall within the normal range of ventilation responses suggesting that the mechanical load explains the apparent reduction in chemosensitivity.

Further support for the presence of a high central drive to breathe in COPD comes from direct measurement of phrenic nerve activity in single motor units of the diaphragm of COPD patients which showed a significantly greater degree of activation than in normal subjects.[88] This agrees with earlier data reporting a greater integrated diaphragmatic EMG response to hypercapnia in normocapnic COPD patients compared with control

Table 16.1 *Methods of assessing ventilatory control – relevance to COPD*

Test	Method	Result in COPD	Comment
Steady-state CO_2 response	Ventilation measured at 2 stable CO_2 tensions; $\dot{V}/P_{CO_2}$ slope reflects CO_2 'sensitivity' or 'gain' of the system	Variable reduction	Time-consuming 'classical' technique. Depends on adequate gas equilibration in blood and CSF – not easy in severe COPD. Chronic changes in blood buffering may affect this
Hyperoxic CO_2 rebreathing	Rebreathing from O_2-enriched closed system; rapid equilibration of blood/CSF CO_2 content. $\dot{V}/P_{CO_2}$ slope has 14-fold normal variability	Variable reduction	Quick, reproducible test. Ventilation may be limited mechanically, not by reduced drive. Ratio of free-breathing and loaded slope a measure of load compensation
Steady state of CO_2 at 2 levels of oxygen tension	Ratio of hypoxic: hyperoxic $\dot{V}/P_{CO_2}$ slopes gives an index of hypoxic drive	Normal or reduced	Demanding for patient and operator. Does allow for 'hypoxic depression' and CO_2 interaction. Seldom done
Progressive isocapnic hypoxia	Relatively rapid (4–10′) test where ventilation is related to P_{O_2} (or Sa_{O_2}) with CO_2 held constant	Normal or reduced	Usually expressed as $\dot{V}/Sa_{O_2}$ as this is a linear plot. Useful for acute drug studies but hard to interpret when Pa_{O_2} already low; no allowance for hypoxic depression
Transient hypoxia/ hyperoxic test	Rapid change in Pa_{O_2} will stimulate/suppress peripheral chemoreceptors hence ventilation	No good data	Not applicable to COPD
Mouth occlusion pressure ($P_{0.1}$)	Pressure developed 100 ms after inspiration from FRC against a closed airway – should overcome problems of changing airflow/ lung volume – relates to respiratory center output	Variable increase at rest – $P_{0.1}/P_{CO_2}$ slope may be reduced, hypoxic response more so	Influenced by posture, lung volume and probably $P_{I max}$. Mouth pressure may not reflect pleural $P_{0.1}$. Muscle shortening DOES occur after occlusion. Abdominal muscle activity increases $P_{0.1}$ for any given 'drive'. Still the best test in COPD
Integrated electromyogram (usually diaphragm)	Recorded from surface/ esophageal electrodes. Expressed in arbitrary units; reflects activation of muscle recorded	Increased for any given Ppl in COPD. Increased by acute CO_2	Hard to interpret and technically very difficult. Surface electrodes influenced by diaphragm position/lung volume. Esophageal electrodes may move or other muscles may be activated. Not a routine test

subject.[89] Comparing patients and healthy subjects at similar levels of hypercapnia, Gribbin *et al.* found that the minimum pleural pressure swing at a P_{CO_2} of 60 mmHg was only slightly less than normal in 10 COPD patients compared with 10 healthy controls. However this represented 47% of the patient's static Ppl compared with 26% of the maximum pressure generation available to the controls.[85]

The relationship between respiratory drive and muscle weakness was explored by Gorini *et al.* who studied $P_{0.1}$ and integrated diaphragm EMG in normocapnic and hypercapnic COPD and normal subjects.[90] The hypercapnic patients had lower $P_{0.1}$ and higher EMGdi values, suggesting that their central drive was high and the ability to develop pressure limited, a finding supported by their low Pimax values compared to normocapnic patients. The relative importance of impaired lung mechanics or an intrinsically low hypercapnic response remains contentious, however it is assessed. This is seen in the study of Scano and colleagues where the conclusions drawn differed depending on the method of expressing the results. Comparing the diaphragm EMG response to hypercapnia did not distinguish chronically hypercapnic COPD from those with normocapnia, while the EMG at a specific level of ventilation was less if hypercapnia was a clinical finding.[91] The conclusion that both factors contribute seems reasonable.

It is likely that the onset of hypercapnia is a slow adaptive response (see later) and more likely to occur when the intrinsic load on the respiratory system is increased. Thus normocapnic COPD patients who developed CO_2 retention during acute ventilatory loading had a higher FRC and a lower Pdi for any level of diaphragm activation.[92] This is analogous to the intermittent CO_2 retention seen in some, but not all, COPD patients admitted with hypercapnic respiratory failure.[93]

The role of reduced peripheral chemoreceptor responses in promoting hypercapnia remains speculative

at best. Although early studies suggested that the occlusion pressure response to isocapnic hypoxia was reduced in COPD,[94] differences in baseline lung function and CO_2 tension as well as the relatively brief nature of the test make these data hard to interpret. To overcome these difficulties, studies of family members unaffected by lung disease have been conducted.[95,96] These have shown reductions in both hypercapnic and hypoxic drives to breathing in individuals whose relatives subsequently develop hypercapnic but less frequently in those who do not. However, there must be some doubt about the method of subject selection, and larger numbers of both cases and control subjects are needed to validate this approach. Although hypoxemia may be important in some patients and chemoreceptor-mediated hypoventilation can occur with high concentrations of oxygen during exacerbations,[97] differences in chemoreceptor output are unlikely to explain the development of hypercapnia in most patients.

Thus most evidence suggests that the apparent reduction in ventilatory responsiveness in COPD, irrespective of the stimulus applied, results from mechanical factors and involves the use of a greater percentage of the inspiratory muscle pressure-generating capacity. However,

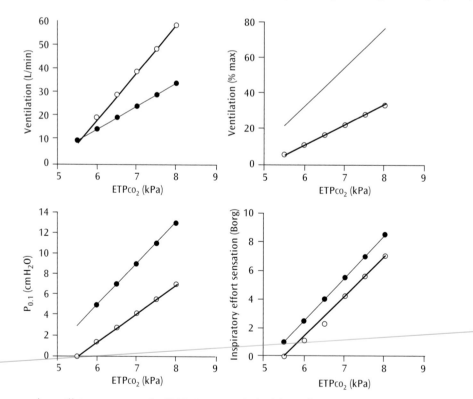

Figure 16.4 *Hypercapnic ventilatory responses in COPD. Data are derived from the mean values of each data point from a group of 12 normocapnic COPD patients studied when stable (mean FEV_1 0.92 L) (closed circles) and are compared to the matched group of control subjects (open circles). COPD patients have a reduced ventilatory response to increase in end-tidal Pco_2 ($ETPco_2$) but a higher occlusion pressure response slope. However, when ventilation is expressed as a percentage of the maximum voluntary ventilation, they are seen to use more of their ventilatory capacity in response to CO_2. The relationships between inspiratory effort sensation and CO_2 are similar in slope in both normal subjects and COPD patients but have a higher initial value in COPD subjects and move in parallel with changes in $P_{0.1}$.*

despite much effort, a role for an intrinsic ventilatory drive in some cases cannot be excluded.

RESPIRATORY MUSCLE FATIGUE AND LUNG VOLUME IN COPD

Studies in healthy subjects[98–101] and in patients during weaning from mechanical ventilation[102] have shown that with continued severe mechanical loading the respiratory muscles fail to develop and maintain the expected force to sustain ventilation, a process described as respiratory muscle fatigue. Elegant biochemical and electrophysiological studies have explored the mechanisms that underlie this process.[6,103] The reduction in maximum respiratory pressure in COPD reduces the denominator of the tension-time index of these muscles and largely explains why these patients are closer to the notional fatigue threshold than are healthy individuals.[104] The observation that daytime hypercapnia in COPD could be relieved by non-invasive ventilation[105] raised hopes that this therapy might relieve the 'chronic respiratory muscle fatigue' presumed to be present. However when a large trial of non-invasive negative pressure ventilation was unsuccessful in lowering $PaCO_2$[106] the problem of muscle fatigue and hypercapnia was re-assessed and an alternative explanation suggested (Figure 16.5).

Most COPD patients have evidence of an increased FRC and the ratio of the pulmonary resistance to the maximum inspiratory pressure is high in those who retain CO_2.[107] When bronchoconstriction is induced in COPD patients by methacholine challenge, FRC rises and maximum inspiratory pressures fall.[108] Although the

$\dot{V}E/PCO_2$ slope is reduced, $P_{0.1}/PCO_2$ is unchanged, as in spontaneously hypercapnic patients. When normal subjects were studied at equivalent lung volumes their ability to develop pressure voluntarily or during electrical stimulation was similar to that of the COPD patients (Figure 16.5),[98] excluding respiratory muscle fatigue as a cause of their abnormal blood gas tensions.

BREATHING PATTERN IN COPD

Studies on the impact of respiratory muscle loading in healthy individuals and new approaches to the neurophysiology of normal breathing[5,9] have led to renewed interest in the pattern of breathing in COPD which has proven more helpful than data acquired during stimulated breathing studies. The range of responses to any increase in respiratory impedance is limited and has been reviewed in detail:[109,110]

1 An increase in the stiffness of the chest wall by immediate respiratory muscle contraction. This will reduce the effect of subsequent changes in impedance and has been described as an operational length-compensating mechanism.[68]

2 Changes in inspiratory timing. These may involve either inspiratory duration (TI), total cycle duration (TTOT) or both. Lengthening TI without changing TTOT reduces mean inspiratory flow and will ultimately cause hypoventilation and CO_2 retention. Optimum breathing patterns may be determined so as to minimize respiratory frequency, respiratory muscle oxygen consumption or 'the discomfort of breathing'.

3 An increase in inspiratory drive. This is the most widely adopted response to increases in impedance but is usually insufficient to completely offset the effects of the added load unless it is a small one. It is conventionally represented by $P_{0.1}$, although this has its own limitations (Table 16.1).

In normal subjects the response to increased respiratory resistance is to prolong TI and reduce VT. This occurs in COPD patients given a similar load to breathe but is not representative of their usual breathing patterns.[83,111–115] In general, minute ventilation is normal or even slightly higher than normal at rest whether instrumented with facemask or noseclip and mouthpiece or whether free breathing where the minute ventilation and breathing pattern are recorded using inductive plethysmography.[115] The overall pattern is rapid and shallow but there are no differences in either minute ventilation or CO_2 production between those who develop CO_2 and those who do not (Figure 16.6). Central drive as reflected by $P_{0.1}$ is high especially during disease exacerbations but can be reduced by administration of relatively high flow oxygen

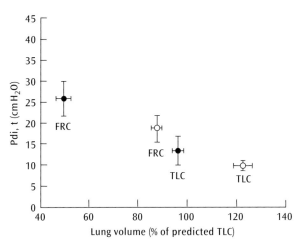

Figure 16.5 *Diaphragm twitch pressure (Pdi, t) at different lung volumes in normal subjects (closed circles) and COPD patients (open circles). These data show that COPD patients can activate their diaphragms just as well as normal subjects, if not better, once allowance is made for their altered geometry. (Adapted from ref. 112.)*

(5 L/min).[112] Patients retaining CO_2 have lower tidal volumes and shorter respiratory times together with a somewhat higher $P_{0.1}$.[83,111] These changes in breathing pattern are load dependent as is seen when acute inspiratory resistive load is performed in stable COPD patients.[116] In this study there was a strong inverse correlation between changes in VT and changes in TI and the tendency to retain CO_2 ($r = -0.91$ and -0.87 respectively). Although it is an oversimplification of the complexities of gas exchange, falls in tidal volumes can be considered to encroach upon the fixed deadspace of these patients and increase the VD/VT ratio and hence P_{CO_2}.[111,113]

Confirmation of the role of mechanical factors in mediating these changes in breathing pattern have come from two studies by the group in Florence. They studied 30 stable COPD patients with a range of resting P_{CO_2} values which were inversely related to tidal volume during spontaneous breathing and positively correlated with respiratory frequency ($r = 0.66$, $P < 0.001$).[117] In these patients the intrinsic positive end-expiratory pressure, which has been related to the presence of arterial hypercapnia in COPD,[118] did not differ between eucapnic and hypercapnic patients and neither did the mean inspiratory flow (VT/TI). Tidal volume and the maximum pleural pressure swing (an index of respiratory muscle strength) accounted for 70% of the variance in Pa_{CO_2}.

Thus hypercapnia in stable disease was associated with rapid shallow breathing as suggested previously and with a reduced capacity of the respiratory muscles to develop pressure (Figure 16.7). The same authors found that increases in tidal volume and reductions in respiratory frequency after a bronchodilator were closely related to reductions in the pleural pressure swing.[119] These changes occurred without any change in minute ventilation, a finding we have confirmed.[120]

How these adaptive changes occur is less clear. Initial studies using naloxone infusion to block endogenous opiate production in the brain found that the response to loading but not chemical stimuli was increased after this therapy in COPD.[121] Interpretation of these data is affected by differences in the initial $P_{0.1}/P_{CO_2}$ between the responder and non-responder groups and others have not been able to replicate them.[122]

The dependence of breathing pattern on the respiratory load is a useful way of unifying the different studies which have related load-related variables to Pa_{CO_2} in COPD. All this seems to justify the original observation of one of the pioneers of respiratory physiology, Richard

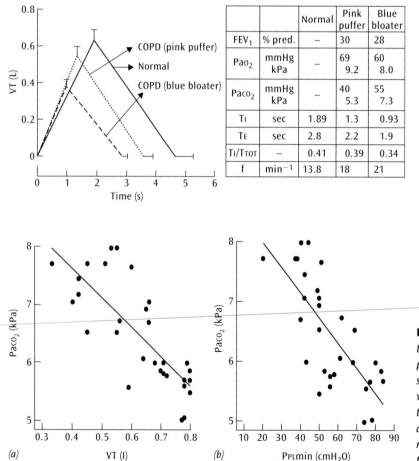

		Normal	Pink puffer	Blue bloater
FEV$_1$	% pred.	–	30	28
Pao$_2$	mmHg kPa	–	69 9.2	60 8.0
Paco$_2$	mmHg kPa	–	40 5.3	55 7.3
TI	sec	1.89	1.3	0.93
TE	sec	2.8	2.2	1.9
TI/TTOT	–	0.41	0.39	0.34
f	min^{-1}	13.8	18	21

Figure 16.6 *Schematic data comparing the breathing pattern in COPD with and without CO_2 retention and in normal subjects. (Data based on ref. 90.)*

Figure 16.7 *Relationship between the tidal volume (a) and minimum pleural pressure (b) and arterial CO_2 tension in severe COPD. The lower the tidal volume the higher is the CO_2, likewise the lower the minimum pressure developed, an index of inspiratory muscle strength, the higher the CO_2 tension. (Data from ref. 117.)*

Riley, that 'hypercapnia is an adaptive mechanism by which the body tolerates an increase in work of breathing which would otherwise be intolerable'.[123] The mechanism by which this compromise is produced is the subject of the remainder of this chapter.

RESPIRATORY SENSATION AND DYSPNEA

Although breathlessness is the principal complaint of patients with COPD, its scientific study is relatively recent. This reflects the difficulties of applying a numerical dimension to a sensory term, a problem that has been reviewed in detail,[124–126] as have the mechanisms underlying dyspnea and their clinical relevance.[10,127] In this section the basic processes relevant to sensory perception in COPD will be reviewed before considering the more limited number of studies in COPD patients.

What is breathlessness?

The semantics of breathlessness have proven at least as difficult as those terms used to define COPD (see Chapter 1). Medically, breathlessness is described as dyspnea – the sensation of difficulty in breathing. However, studies in normal subjects using cluster analysis statistical methods have shown that different stimuli are associated with different sensations.[128] These studies have been extended to a diverse group of patients including those with COPD, who were asked to relate their sensations to 45 different questions. COPD patients are more likely to describe their dyspnea as breathing discomfort and, along with asthmatics, associate it with increased breathing effort and an inability to breathe deeply enough.[129]

Measurement of breathlessness

Uncertainties about the quantitative nature of sensory responses lead early investigators to assess sensation in terms of a sensory threshold. This was measured by the 'just noticeable difference' method,[130] i.e. the intensity of stimulus which was detected on 50% of presentations. Here a sensation was either present or not but this method could not define the sensory intensity when the stimulus increased beyond this threshold value. These studies are examples of psychophysical techniques that quantitatively relate the characteristics or dimensions of a physical stimulus to the magnitude or attributes of the sensory response associated with it. Psychophysics has elucidated the sensory correlates of visual, auditory and kinesthetic responses[125,131] and has been central to the understanding of the mechanisms of breathlessness.

Scaling techniques, both nominal and ordinal, have been developed to assess suprathreshold sensory stimuli. Open magnitude scales relate sensory magnitude to stimulus intensity by assigning an arbitrary value to the magnitude which changes proportionately with the stimulus.[126] They are useful in defining variables that influence sensation but are time consuming to use, not suitable for repeated measures and involve log–log plotting of data to define the subjects' perceptual sensitivity. More widely used is the visual analogue scale (VAS), a form of cross-modality testing. The subject marks the sensory intensity along a 10-cm line with descriptors at each end, usually 'not breathless at all' to 'extreme or worst imaginable breathlessness'. It is relatively simple to use, reproducible, and does not need to be anchored at its upper extremes to an induced level of severe breathlessness. However, it does not have ratio properties.

The most widely used and versatile dyspnea scale is the category scale devised by Borg[132] (Figure 16.8(a)). The scale employs descriptors which in its modified form are spaced so that a doubling of numerical rating is associated with a doubling of sensory intensity. It allows easy comparison of absolute levels of sensation at a given intensity among a group of subjects and is amenable to parametric statistical analysis.[133]

Comparisons between these scales show that VAS and Borg[134,135] are valid measures in normal subjects but the Borg scale tends to have a better reproducibility between days. Studies in COPD have confirmed the reproducibility of VAS,[133] but there is concern about the between-day reproducibility of Borg scaling.[136]

These scales can be clinically useful in assessing the intensity of inspiratory effort or breathlessness at a particular time, for example before or after a corridor walk.[137] They are exquisitely dependent on the question asked and the degree to which the patient understands what is wanted of him and so require some explanation before use. They are sensitive to changes induced by physiologically relevant interventions, for example muscle training[138] or bronchodilators,[137] but do not give an overall impression of patient disability due to dyspnea. This has been assessed using a different questionnaire-based approach. The earliest attempt was the British MRC Dyspnea scale[139] where symptom severity was scored on a five-point scale. This has had a number of modifications, one version being that in Figure 16.8(b). This scale captures the impact of dyspnea on the patient's daily activity and differences between grades are associated with significant differences in health status.[11,140] This approach has been extremely useful epidemiologically but is not sensitive to small changes within an individual. Mahler and colleagues have developed two indices of breathlessness, the baseline dyspnea index (BDI) and the transitional dyspnea index (TDI).[141] These questionnaires assessed three

0	Nothing at all		Grade 1:	Not troubled by breathlessness, except on strenuous exertion
0.5	Very, very slight (just noticeable)			
1	Very slight			
2	Slight		Grade 2:	Short of breath when hurrying on the level or walking up a slight hill
3	Moderate			
4	Somewhat severe		Grade 3:	Have to walk slower than most people on the level
5	Severe			
6				
7	Very severe		Grade 4:	Have to stop for breath after walking about 100 yards on the level
8				
9	Very, very severe (almost maximal)		Grade 5:	Too breathless to leave the house, or breathless after undressing
10	Maximal			

(a) *(b)*

Figure 16.8 *Scales for assessing the degree of breathlessness. (a) The modified Borg category scale, which can be reported in terms of whole integers or using interval points. (b) An example of one of the several variants of the MRC breathlessness scale. This indicates the degree to which breathlessness occurs during specific activities rather than assessing the intensity of the sensation at a particular point in time as is done with the Borg scale. (Adapted from ref. 134.)*

different attributes – functional impairment, magnitude of task and magnitude of effort. The BDI correlates well ($r = 0.6$) with distance covered in a 12-minute-walk test and with scores from the oxygen-cost diagram, a type of VAS where the descriptors relate to every day activity. The TDI was designed to assess changes after some intervention over time and is related to the initial BDI assessment. These instruments take longer to administer than VAS or Borg scales and give a broader view of the impact of dyspnea on the patient's life over time. They appear less suited to single-dose pharmacologic testing but do not give such a comprehensive picture of disability as more formal quality of life scores. Their use has shown that breathlessness is a separate defining characteristic of COPD patients in addition to other aspects of lung function such as spirometry and maximum inspiratory pressure generation.[142] However their clinical application remains difficult (see Chapter 20).

MECHANISMS OF DYSPNEA

Like the blind man describing an elephant, respiratory physiologists have groped for the mechanisms underlying dyspnea for the last 75 years.[143] Certain findings are now widely accepted. There is no single stimulus which uniquely produces the sensation neither is there specific dyspnea receptor in the muscles or the lung parenchyma. Conflicting results from reputable investigators are likely to reflect subtle differences in the protocol adopted or the questions asked rather than entirely different neurophysiologic mechanisms (for an example of this see Killian et al.[4] pp. 121–3). Many of the same stimuli applied to studying ventilatory control have been adapted to study dyspnea, while changes in the sense

of respiratory effort has been the most asked sensory outcome. Fortunately this is a characteristic symptom in COPD.

STUDIES OF AFFERENT INPUTS

These include both mechanoreceptor and chemoreceptor pathways. Among the former are vagally mediated pulmonary stretch reflexes, tendon organs which are mainly in the diaphragm and sense force and muscle spindles which monitor muscle length. As in studies of ventilatory control, vagal blockade either by local anesthesia[144] or iatrogenically during lung transplantation does not affect respiratory sensation.[53] Tendon organs may register certain kinds of sensation, for example volume, and their stimulation can inhibit medullary inspiratory activity. Chest wall vibration can either increase or reduce the sensation of breathlessness in asthmatic subjects or in normal subjects breathing against resistive loads although minute ventilation is maintained, and this is thought to be due to stimulation of muscle spindle afferents.[46,145] Stimulation of the intercostal muscles can inhibit inspiration[146] and evoke cortical potential,[147] and so a pathway exists to signal information from the intercostals not only to the mid-brain but also to higher centers. Whether these are the only pathways is still debated as spinal anesthesia up to the T1 level does not impair load detection.

Initially it was believed that active inspiratory muscle contraction was necessary for the perception of inspiratory effort to occur.[148] Subsequent studies that have used muscle relaxants to induce complete respiratory muscle paralysis have shown that increasing the Pa_{CO_2} does increase the sense of air hunger.[149]

An elevated arterial CO_2 does not, of itself, relate to the intensity of dyspnea at rest or during exercise. Even in healthy subjects dyspnea is more closely related to the level of ventilation than the prevailing CO_2 tension.[150] Similarly isocapnic voluntary ventilation produced equivalent increases in respiratory effort to that induced by hypercapnic ventilatory stimulation.[151] However when chest wall movement is restrained and CO_2 allowed to rise, breathlessness also increases,[152] a finding mimicked clinically when patients undergoing mechanical ventilation receive insufficiently large tidal breaths.

Studies with hypoxia are harder to interpret as the response is very dependent on the preceding CO_2 tension and the oscillatory studies of Lane are technically more challenging.[153] Nonetheless, it seems probable that neither hypoxia nor acidosis[153,154] cause breathlessness independent of their effects on ventilation.

STUDIES OF RESPIRATORY MUSCLES

Respiratory muscles are shortened and pressure generation capacity reduced by hyperinflation, and studies at different lung volumes have confirmed that sensation increases at a given ventilation as FRC rises.[155,156] Moreover, these authors felt that the sense of inspiratory effort (IES) was the best correlate of breathlessness in these normal subjects rather than the sense of muscle tension.[124,157] When muscle function was compromised by sustaining a fatiguing contraction for a prolonged time, effort sensation rose and the ability to scale the load was impaired.[158] This led to the suggestion that inspiratory muscle fatigue may cause breathlessness and would be more likely when hyperinflation was present as in COPD. This is only likely to be true if low-frequency fatigue were common and this is not so. Bradley et al. showed that diaphragm fatigue and sensation are clearly dissociated[159] whilst more recently Clague et al. have shown in normal subjects that increases in effort sensation occur well before critical diaphragmatic tension–time index (TTdi) is reached at least during CO_2 rebreathing.[160] These latter studies show that IES was best related to ribcage tension time indices (TTrc) and that rebreathing ceased when critical levels of TTrc were reached and respiratory sensation was maximum. High levels of inspiratory effort sensation may act as a physiologic monitor of impending muscle overload (Figure 16.8).

Similarly, studies at lung volumes below FRC show that chest wall restriction may also increase the intensity of breathlessness.[152] Distortion of the chest wall can increase the acitivity of the inspiratory muscles and change into a more favorable chest wall configuration, for example leaning forward may reduce breathlessness.[161] The inability of some COPD patients to carry even light loads may reflect the loss of their pectoral muscles as accessory respiratory muscles which stabilize the chest wall.[162]

Studies at rest and during exercise report consistent relationships between Ppl, a marker of inspiratory muscle contraction, and breathlessness. During loading the integrated electrical activity of the sternomastoid muscle appears to be as good or better index than Ppl, suggesting that total respiratory drive is important.[163] During exercise respiratory timing can modify the sense of breathlessness and in patients with a variety of lung diseases, the duration of inspiration and respiratory frequency appear to have a small but independent effect from Ppl on overall breathlessness intensity.[164] Comparisons of the sensation produced by elastic and resistive load suggest that breathing is regulated to minimize inspiratory pressure development.[157] Whether the other timing-related variables integrated together equate to TTrc is less clear at present although the limited studies available would support this.[160]

STUDIES OF CENTRAL SENSORY PROCESSING

That sensory information from the integrated action of the respiratory system reaches the cortex is shown by the detection of cortical evoked responses after airway occlusions.[165,166] These appear maximal over the C4 EEG placement area which corresponds very approximately to the area of the sensory cortex thought to be innervated by the diaphragm.[167] The adjacent motor cortex shows enhanced metabolic activity during increases in ventilation as assessed by PET scanning and also increases in intensity when ventilation rises during exercise. Thus the motor and sensory cortex appear to be activated when ventilation increases and sensation is perceived. It is still unclear whether this activation occurs secondarily to some prior assessment of ventilatory stimulus in the mid-brain or whether the proposed comparatory function is itself cortical. Animal studies suggests that the peak intensity of the integrated diaphragm EMG during resistive loading was reduced after decerebration and favors the latter explanation.[168]

These observations provide the physiologic basis for the monitoring of the central respiratory drive. Rostral projections from the brainstem respiratory neurones have been described which could act as the link between these areas.[169,170] The sense of effort increases in parallel with respiratory drive and is proportional to the pressure developed by the inspiratory muscles.[171] This provides an important link with the fatiguing process (see above).

There is considerable debate about the existence of a separate mechanism controlling voluntary ventilation. Although the studies of isocapnic voluntary ventilation do not support this,[151] the Charing Cross group have found significant differences during exercise in the intensity of breathlessness compared with equivalent levels of ventilation where the subjects copy a preset breathing pattern.[172] Following their observations on cortical activation,[167] they suggest that a separate voluntary pathway of corticospinal phrenic motorneurones exist which can override normal control mechanisms and modify the resulting sensation.

One attractive approach to integrating these diverse observations has come from the length-tension hypothesis of Howell and Campbell.[3] They suggested that dyspnea arose when the change in length of the respiratory muscles was inappropriate for the tension developed. Clearly this cannot explain the changes seen when the respiratory muscles are inactive as occurred during paralysis. Nonetheless it forms the basis of the neuromechanical[173–175] or efferent-reafferent explanations of this sensation[176] which relate the intensity of the respiratory afferent information arising from a range of sources to the central motor command output.

This work has striking parallels with the model of ventilatory control proposed by Poon, in which mechanical loading is associated with a rapid shallow breathing pattern. It is unlikely to be accidental that this is also the best way of minimizing inspiratory effort sensation[64] for a given level of loaded ventilation.

Breathlessness in COPD

Many of the mechanisms outlined above operate in COPD at rest and during exercise. As with ventilatory control, the dominant abnormality appears to be mechanical, with changes in lung volume producing secondary respiratory muscle activation that probably parallels the increased sensation of respiratory effort. Several investigators have shown a good relationship between indices that combine pressure, usually derived from the pleural pressure swing, and tidal volume with the intensity of respiratory effort[117,168,174] (Figure 16.9). These data support the neuromechanical explanation of dyspnea proposed above.

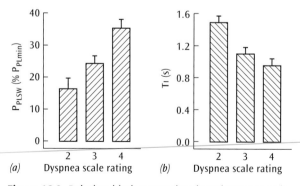

(a) Dyspnea scale rating
(b) Dyspnea scale rating

Figure 16.9 *Relationship between the pleural pressure swing (a) and inspiratory time (b) and dyspnea rating on the MRC scale in patients with severe COPD. The greater the pleural pressure swing expressed as a percentage of the maximum possible the greater the degree of breathlessness. Conversely, the shorter the inspiratory time the greater is the degree of exercise limitation by dyspnea. (From ref. 117.)*

Improvements in these measurements after administration of a bronchodilator are accompanied by reductions in respiratory effort sensation.[118] However there is an equal or better relationship between sensory intensity and change in end- expiratory or end-inspiratory lung volume change during exercise[173] (see Chapter 18). These changes have been demonstrated in patients with more severe COPD where tidal flow limitation is more likely to produce these volume changes. Reduction in the degree of hyperinflation by bronchodilators can reduce perceived dyspnea at rest in the more severe cases.[120]

Changes in chest wall geometry that accompany these altered lung volumes reduce the capacity of the inspiratory muscles to develop pressure and a reduced PImax does predict those COPD patients complaining of dyspnea.[117] The importance of lung mechanical abnormalities and especially elastic loading secondary to hyperinflation has been confirmed by the effect of lung volume reduction surgery on resting and exercise dyspnea.[19,20,177,178] (see Chapter 32). Reductions in lung volume are accompanied by an increased ability to develop inspiratory pressure and a decreased tension time index of the respiratory muscles,[21,179] while in selected patients $PaCO_2$ improves.[22,180] Thus impairment in lung mechanics appears central in generating dyspnea in COPD.

A specific role for blood gas changes is difficult to establish, although COPD patients do increase their perceived effort as $PaCO_2$ rises (Figure 16.4). Whether this is mediated more directly than just by increasing ventilatory effort has not been resolved. Hypoxia appears to be less important in producing breathlessness, and changes in oxygen saturation during exercise do not relate to the subsequent intensity of dyspnea.[181–183]

Two further processes are relevant to the COPD patient. The perception of dyspnea is influenced significantly by the individual's mood and attitudes as is their exercise capacity.[184] One of the collateral benefits of pulmonary rehabilitation is the secondary improvement in mood that usually accompanies it. Conversely the development of COPD is a gradual process and patients adapt to the chronic increase in respiratory system loading. Psychophysical studies have shown that the ability to discriminate an added load is inversely proportional to the background intensity of loading (Weber's law).[185] This may explain why some patients do not notice their dyspnea until their disease is at an advanced stage.

VENTILATORY CONTROL AND DYSPNEA – A SYNTHESIS

It is increasingly clear that ventilatory control and respiratory sensations are intimately connected, although perhaps not in the way initially envisaged. Mental activity can modify breathing pattern at rest and a loss of cortical input during sleep can produce an increase in tidal volume and a fall in frequency.[186] Breathing patterns during CO_2 rebreathing can change with mental activity and have been related to personality,[187,188] whilst there seems to be an inverse relationship between the sensation during CO_2 rebreathing and the slope of the CO_2 response.[189] Moreover, those subjects with the greatest ability to perceive increases in ventilation show the smallest prolongation of inspiratory time when loaded with an external resistance and adopt a rapid shallow breathing pattern.[189] Although initial data in COPD suggested that patients with the lowest sensory magnitude exponents were those most likely to retain CO_2,[190] more recent studies of external loading have shown much the same as in normal subjects, namely that those who perceive sensation most easily to loads compensate by developing rapid shallow breathing.[191] Thus breathing pattern is regulated by similar cortical mechanisms to those determining the intensity of respiratory sensation. Increasing the degree of alertness or cortical activity favors a rapid shallow breathing pattern, which is the one associated with the lowest intensity of sensory discomfort. Respiratory sensation in general, including dyspnea, appears to be well placed to act as the controller signal, the intensity of which must be minimized to optimize respiratory system function.

THERAPEUTIC IMPLICATIONS

Since ventilatory control is intimately connected to respiratory sensation, it is unlikely that changes in the one can be accomplished without affecting the other. There is abundant evidence that changes in intensity of breathlessness reflect changes in ventilation rather than changes in perceptual intensity. Thus, naloxone can reduce the intensity of sensation during acute inspiratory loads but does not alter the relationship between breathlessness and ventilation or mouth pressure.[192] The principal exception appears to be treatment which changes lung mechanics either by increasing respiratory muscle strength or reducing respiratory system loading (see above). The main drugs which do this are the bronchodilators and their actions are reviewed elsewhere, as are the clinical effects of surgical therapy. Three other treatment approaches relevant to ventilatory control and breathlessness remain:

1 **Chemical stimulation of breathing.** Ventilatory stimulants act to increase minute ventilation, secondarily improving gas exchange by increasing the neural traffic from peripheral chemoreceptors, central chemoreceptors or both. The current therapies available have been reviewed.[193] Clinically their use is restricted to acute respiratory failure (see elsewhere) where they can help maintain CO_2 tensions and avoid the use of intermittent positive pressure ventilation (IPPV). Doxapram hydrochloride is the most widely used drug and is given intravenously in a dose titrated to the clinical response.[194] It acts on both central and peripheral chemoreceptors[195] contrary to earlier claims and has a generalized arousal effect which may help the narcotized patient to cope with physiotherapy.

Almitrine bismethylate is an investigational drug available in parts of Europe that is a highly specific peripheral chemoreceptor stimulant[196] which also modifies local ventilation and perfusion matching (see Chapter 14). It improves hypoxemia by day and night in chronically hypoxic patients,[197] but is associated with significant pulmonary hypertension during exercise which may limit exercise performance.[198] It has been given orally in multicenter studies of COPD to see if it affects morbidity and mortality,[199,200] but its use has been limited by peripheral neuropathy which may be dose dependent or simply unmasked by the drug.

Medroxyprogesterone acetate has been used as a central chemostimulant which produces modest changes in CO_2 tensions in COPD[201] but the estrogen-like side effects have limited its practical use. The long-term use of oral ventilatory stimulants is less popular with increasing evidence of CO_2 retention determined by mechanical factors and any increase in overall ventilation is likely to increase symptoms. Whether a subset of relatively chemoinsensitive COPD patients with less severe mechanical problems exist is unclear. If they do, then they will be the ones most likely to benefit from any new oral ventilatory stimulant therapy.

2 **Non-pharmacologic improvements in ventilatory capacity.** Pulmonary rehabilitation produces clinically important improvements in dyspnea without changing lung mechanics or blood gas tensions (see Chapter 30) Reducing respiratory muscle loading by pressure support reduces dyspnea in short-term studies[202,203] and this has been assessed during trials of non-invasive positive pressure ventilation. Although changes occur during treatment for acute exacerbations the chronic effect is disappointing (see Chapter 26)

3 **Reductions in respiratory sensation.** The idea of a specific 'anti-dyspnea' drug is attractive but most unlikely. Mitchell-Heggs reported a rather confused study in four 'pink puffers' who appeared to have reduced symptoms after taking 20 mg per day of diazepam.[204] These data have not been repeated with other benzodiazepines in COPD patients.[205] The similarities between dyspnea and pain, as well as the

involvement of endogenous opiodes in ventilatory control,[206] have led to clinical trials of several opiodes analgesics. Woodcock et al.[207] reported short-term improvement in breathlessness and exercise tolerance after l mg/kg dihydrocodeine together with reduced ventilation and resting oxygen consumption. Johnson et al. found that 15 mg dihydrocodeine tds increased treadmill walking distance by 16% and reduced breathlessness by 18%, although these effects may not be sustained with regular treatment.[208] Oral morphine 0.8 mg/kg increased exercise capacity by 19% in 13 patients with COPD for a comparable level of breathlessness[209] and may alter the intensity of breathlessness for a given level of ventilation. However, these results have not been found by all workers.[210] In all studies side effects (particularly constipation and sedation) limited the regular use of these drugs. For many patients these side effects outweighed the benefits of the modest reductions in breathlessness.

Since mental state has a major effect on the perception of breathlessness, it is reasonable to consider antidepressant treatment in any breathless COPD patient with other factors to suggest even a reactive depressive illness, and such treatment can achieve as much as more aggressive therapy with opiates. Likewise, good counseling and support can be very helpful in symptom control. Occasionally, for the patient in extremis with breathlessness during acute exacerbation, parenteral opiates for a short period can produce a dramatic improvement in both symptoms and breathing pattern which may allow time for other treatments to work. However, such a drastic step can only be considered as a last resort of the experienced clinician.

Because oxygen reduces minute ventilation in normal subjects, it is not surprising that it improves breathlessness in COPD by similar mechanisms. Following initial studies by Woodcock and Geddes who found an increase in exercise tolerance after oxygen compared with compressed air,[211] Davidson et al. showed a significant improvement in exercise tolerance and reduction in breathlessness in a controlled trial of oxygen treatment.[212] The greatest changes were seen with endurance exercise tests, but more recently the same group have shown a modest 'dose–response' effect using self-paced walking tests where high flows of oxygen produced somewhat greater changes in exercise performance.[212,213] Most of the effect of oxygen during exercise is attributable to the reduction in ventilation[214] (see Chapter 18). Stimulation of upper airway receptors by cold air may also diminish breathlessness[215] and improve exercise capacity.[48] Whether this explains the otherwise idiosyncratic benefits of nebulizer treatment in patients who show no spirometric or lung function improvement remains to be determined. Short burst oxygen therapy is

widely used to help patients with severe COPD cope with dyspnea induce by daily activities. Oxygen does decrease the intensity of dyspnea during loading at rest[216] and limited data have confirmed that it can lessen dyspnea intensity post stair climbing. Whether this is due to the oxygen itself or the flow of cold gas on the face is not known.[217]

At present, treatment options for breathlessness are limited. Careful assessment of the patient's potential response to bronchodilator drugs and corticosteroids, their suitability for a rehabilitation program and/or home oxygen is likely to produce the greatest long-term benefit. Dyspnea remains the symptom most feared by COPD patients and is still the hardest one to treat effectively.

REFERENCES

1. Donald KW. Neurological effects of oxygen. *Lancet* 1949;**ii**:1056–7.
2. Campbell EJM. The management of acute respiratory failure in chronic bronchitis and emphysema. *Am Rev Respir Dis* 1967;**96**:626–39.
3. Howell JBL, Campbell EJM. *Breathlessness*. Blackwell Scientific, Oxford, 1966.
4. Jones NL, Killian KJ. *Breathlessness: The Campbell Symposium.* Boehringer Ingelheim, Hamilton, Canada, 1992.
5. von Euler C. Brainstem mechanisms for generation and control of breathing pattern. In: Cherniack NS, Widdicombe JG, eds. *Handbook of Physiology*, vol 2, part II, section 3, *Control of Breathing*. American Physiology Society, Bethesda, 1986, pp 1–67.
6. Long S, Duffin J. The neuronal determinants of respiratory rhythm. *Prog Neurobiol* 1986;**27**:101–82.
7. Mead J. Control of respiratory frequency. *J Appl Physiol* 1960;**15**:325–36.
8. Otis AB. The work of breathing. *Physiol Rev* 1954;**34**:449–58.
9. Clark FJ, von Euler C. On the regulation of depth and rate of breathing. *J Physiol (Lond)* 1972;**222**:267–95.
10. Berger AJ, Mitchell RA, Severinghaus JW. Regulation of respiration. *N Engl J Med* 1977;**297**:92–7.
11. Derenne J-Ph, Couture J, Iscoe S, Whitelaw WA, Milic-Emili J. Regulation of breathing in anaesthetized human subjects. *J Appl Physiol* 1976;**40**:804–14.
12. Shea SA, Horner RL, Beuchetrit G, Guz A. The persistence of a respiratory 'personality' into Stage IV sleep in man. *Respir Physiol* 1990;**80**:33–44.
13. Issa FG, Remmers JE. Identification of a subsurface area in the ventral medulla sensitive to local changes in Pco_2. *J Appl Physiol* 1992;**72**:439–46.
14. Richter DW. Generation and maintenance of the respiratory rhythm. *J Exp Biol* 1982;**100**:93–107.
15. Remmers JE. Central neural control of breathing. In: MD Altose, Y Kawakami, eds. *Control of Breathing in Health and Disease*. Marcel Dekker, New York, 1999, pp 1–35.
16. Rabbette PS, Costelve KL, Stocks J. Persistence of the Hering-Breur reflex beyond the neonatal period. *J Appl Physiol* 1991;**71**:474–80.
17. Chan CS, Grunstein RR, Bye PTP, Woolcock AJ, Sullivan CE. Obstructive sleep apnoea with severe chronic airflow limitation: comparisons of hypercapnic and eucapnic patients. *Am Rev Respir Dis* 1989;**140**:1274–8.

18. Chan CS, Bye PTP, Woolcock AJ, Sullivan CE. Eucapnia and hypercapnia in patients with chronic airflow limitation. *Am Rev Respir Dis* 1990;**141**:861–5.

19. Jalleh R, Fitzpatrick MF, Jan MA, MacNee W, Douglas NJ. Alcohol and cor pulmonale in chronic bronchitis and emphysema. *Br Med J* 1993;**306**:374.

20. Martin JG, De Troyer A. The thorax and control of functional residual capacity. In: C Roussos, PT Macklem, eds. *The Thorax*. Marcel Dekker, New York, 1985, pp 899–922.

21. Ingram RH, Schilder DP. Effect of pursed lips expiration on the pulmonary pressure-flow relationship in obstructive lung disease. *Am Rev Respir Dis* 1967;**96**:381–7.

22. Biscoe TJ, Purves MJ. Factors affecting the cat carotid chemoreceptor and cervical sympathetic activity with special reference to passive hind limb movements. *J Physiol (Lond)* 1967;**190**:425–41.

23. Biscoe TJ, Bradley GW, Purves MJ. The relation between carotid body chemoreceptor discharge, carotid sinus pressure and carotid body venous flow. *J Physiol (Lond)* 1970;**208**:99–120.

24. Calverley PMA, Howatson R, Flenley DC, Lamb D. Clinicopathological correlations in cor pulmonale. *Thorax* 1992;**47**:494–8.

25. Pallot DJ. The mammalian carotid body. *Adv Anat Embryol Cell Biol* 1987;**102**:1–90.

26. Dejours P. Control of respiration by arterial chemoreceptors. *Ann NY Acad Sci* 1963;**109**:682–95.

27. Pappenheimer JR, Fencl V, Hersey SR, Held D. Role of cerebral fluids in control of respiration as studied in unanesthetized goats. *Am J Physiol* 1965;**208**:436–50.

28. Bledsoe SW, Hornbein TF. Central chemoreceptors and the regulation of their chemical environment. In: TF Hornbein, ed. *Regulation of Breathing*. Marcel Dekker, New York, 1981, pp 347–406.

29. Davidson TL, Sullivan MP, Swanson KE, Adams JM. Cl⁻ replacement alters the ventilatory response to central chemoreceptor stimulation. *J Appl Physiol* 1992;**74**:280–5.

30. Bruce EN, Cherniack NS. Central chemoreceptors. *J Appl Physiol* 1987;**62**:389–402.

31. Shannon R. Reflexes from respiratory muscles and costovertebral joints. In: NS Cherniack, JG Widdicombe, eds. *Handbook of Physiology; Control of breathing*, Vol 2, Part 1, Section 3. American Physiology Society, Bethesda, 1986, pp 431–48.

32. Easton PA, Slykerman LJ, Anthonisen NR. Ventilatory response to sustained hypoxia in normal adults. *J Appl Physiol* 1986;**61**:906–11.

33. Parsons ST, Griffiths TL, Christie JML, Holgate ST. Effect of theophylline and dipyridamole on the respiratory response to isocapnic hypoxia in normal human subjects. *Clin Sci* 1991;**80**:107–12.

34. Easton PA, Slykerman LJ, Anthonisen NR. Ventilatory response to sustained hypoxia after pretreatment with aminophylline. *J Appl Physiol* 1988;**64**:1445–50.

35. Rudolf M, Banks RA, Semple SJG. Hypercapnia during oxygen therapy in acute exacerbations of chronic respiratory failure. *Lancet* 1977;**ii**:483–6.

36. Prechter GC, Nelson SR, Hubmayr RD. The ventilatory recruitment threshold for carbon dioxide. *Am Rev Respir Dis* 1990;**141**:758–64.

37. Parisi RA, Edelman NH, Santiago TV. Central respiratory carbon dioxide chemosensitivity does not decrease during sleep. *Am Rev Respir Dis* 1992;**145**:832–6.

38. Wasserman DH, Whipp BJ. Coupling of ventilation to pulmonary gas exchange during non steady-state work in men. *J Appl Physiol* 1983;**54**:587–93.

39. Wasserman KB, Whipp BJ, Casaburi R. Respiratory control during exercise. In: NS Cherniack, JG Widdicombe, eds. *Handbook of Physiology*, vol 2, part 2, section 3. American Physiology Society, Bethesda, 1986, pp 595–619.

40. Band DM, Wolff CB, Ward J, Cochrane GM, Prior J. Respiratory oscillations in arterial carbon dioxide tensions as a control signal in exercise. *Nature* 1980;**283**:84–5.

41. Wasserman K, Whipp BJ, Kogal SN, Cleary MG. Effect of carotid body resection on ventilatory and acid-base control during exercise. *J Appl Physiol* 1975;**39**:354–8.

42. Phillipson EA, Duffin J, Cooper JD. Critical dependence of respiratory rhythmicity on metabolid CO₂ load. *J Appl Physiol* 1981;**50**:45–54.

43. DeBacker WA, Heyrman RM, Wittesaele WM, Waeleghem J-P van, Vermeire PA, Broe ME de. Ventilation and breathing patterns during hemodialysis-induced carbon dioxide unloading. *Am Rev Respir Dis* 1987;**136**:406–10.

44. Paintal AS. Vagal sensory receptors and their reflex effects. *Physiol Rev* 1973;**53**:159–227.

45. Coleridge HM, Coleridge JCG. Reflexes evoked from tracheobronchial tree and lungs. In: NS Cherniack, JG Widdicombe, eds. *Handbook of Physiology; Control of Breathing*, vol 2, part 2, section 3. American Physiology Society, Bethesda, 1986, pp 395–430.

46. Homma I, Obata T, Sibuya M, Uchida M. Gate mechanisms in breathlessness caused by chest wall vibration in humans. *J Appl Physiol* 1984;**56**:8–11.

47. Burgess KR, Whitelaw WA. Reducing ventilatory response to carbon dioxide by breathing cold air. *Am Rev Respir Dis* 1984;**129**:687–90.

48. Spence DPS, Graham DR, Ahmed J, Rees K, Pearson MG, Calverley PMA. Does cold air affect exercise capacity and dyspnoea in stable chronic obstructive pulmonary disease? *Chest* 1993;**103**:693–6.

49. Gautier H, Bonora M, Gaudy JH. Breuer-Hering inflation reflex and breathing pattern in anesthetized humans and cats. *J Appl Physiol* 1981;**51**:1162–8.

50. Zin WA, Behrakis PK, Luijoudijk SCM, *et al.* Immediate response to resistive loading in anaesthetised humans. *J Appl Physiol* 1986;**60**:506–12.

51. Sanders MH, Owens GR, Sciurba FC, *et al.* Ventilation and breathing pattern during progressive hypercapnia and hypoxia after human heart-lung transplantation. *Am Rev Respir Dis* 1989;**140**:38–40.

52. Kagawa FT, Duncan SR, Theodore J. Inspiratory timing of heart-lung transplant recipients during progressive hypercapnia. *J Appl Physiol* 1991;**71**:945–50.

53. Tapper DP, Duncan SR, Kraft S, Kagawa FT, Marshall S, Theodore J. Detection of inspiratory resistive loads by heart-lung transplant recipients. *Am Rev Respir Dis* 1992;**145**:458–60.

54. Frost AE, Zamel N, McClean P, Grossman R, Patterson GA, Maurer JR. Hypercapnic ventilatory response in recipients of double-lung transplants. *Am Rev Respir Dis* 1992;**146**:1610–12.

55. Hugelin A. Supraportine control of respiratory movement. In: JL Feldman, AJ Berger, eds. *Proceedings of International Symposium: Central Neural Production of Periodic Respiratory Movements. Lake Bluff, Illinois*, 1982, pp 60–3.

56. Newsom-Davies J, Stagg D. Interrelationships of the volume and time components of individual breaths in normal man. *J Physiol (Lond)* 1975;**245**:481–8.

57. Wheatley JR, Amis TC, Engel LA. Oronasal partitioning of ventilation during exercise in humans. *J Appl Physiol* 1991;**71**:546–51.

58. Mador MJ, Tobin MJ. Effect of alterations in mental activity on the breathing pattern in healthy subjects. *Am Rev Respir Dis* 1991;**144**:481–7.

59. Severinghaus JW, Mitchell RA. Ondine's curse – failure of respiratory centre automaticity while awake. *Clin Res* 1962;**10**:122.

60. Rigg JRA, Inman EM, Saunders NA, Leeder SR, Jones NL. Interaction of mental factors with hypercapnic ventilatory drive in man. *Clin Sci* 1977;**52**:264–75.

61. Grodins FS. Analysis of factors concerned in regulation of breathing in exercise. *Physiol Rev* 1950;**30**:220–39.

62. Catterall JR, Calverley PMA, MacNee W, *et al.* Mechanisms of transient nocturnal hypoxaemia in hypoxic chronic bronchitis and emphysema. *J Appl Physiol* 1985;**59**:1698–703.

63. Priban IP, Fincham WF. Self-adaptive control and the respiratory system. *Nature* 1965;**208**:339–43.

64. Poon CS. Ventilatory control in hypercapnia and exercise: optimization hypothesis. *J Appl Physiol* 1987;**62**:2447–59.

65. Poon CS. Effects of inspiratory resistive load on respiratory control in hypercapnia and exercise. *J Appl Physiol* 1989;**66**:2391–9.

66. Poon CS, Lin S-L, Knudson OB. Optimization character of inspiratory neural drive. *J Appl Physiol* 1992;**72**:2005–17.

67. Johnson BD, Saupe KW, Dempsey JA. Mechanical constraints on exercise hyperpnea in endurance atheletes. *J Appl Physiol* 1992;**73**:874–86.

68. Mead J. Responses to loaded breathing. *Bull Physiopathol Respir* 1979;**15**(suppl):61–71.

69. Farkas GA, Roussos C. Diaphragm in emphysematous hamsters: Sarcomere adaptability. *J Appl Physiol* 1983;**54**:1635–40.

70. Whitelaw WA, Derenne J-P, Milic-Emili J. Occlusion pressure as a measure of respiratory center output in conscious man. *Respir Physiol* 1975;**23**:181–99.

71. Murciano D, Aubier M, Bussi S, Derenne J-P, Pariente R, Milic-Emili J. Comparison of esophageal, tracheal and mouth occlusion pressure in patients with chronic obstructive pulmonary disease during respiratory failure. *Am Rev Respir Dis* 1982;**126**:37–41.

72. Grassino AE, Derenne J-P, Almirall J, Milic-Emili J, Whitelaw WA. Configuration of the chest wall and occlusion pressures in awake humans. *J Appl Physiol* 1981;**50**:134–42.

73. Whitelaw WA, Derenne J-P. Airway occlusion pressure. *J Appl Physiol* 1993;**74**:1475–83.

74. Elliot MW, Mulvey DA, Green M, Moxham J. An evaluation of $P_{0.1}$ measured in mouth and oesophagus, during carbon dioxide rebreathing in COPD. *Eur Respir J* 1993;**6**:1055–9.

75. Donald KW, Christie RV. The respiratory response to carbon dioxide and anoxia in emphysema. *Clin Sci* 1949;**8**:33–44.

76. Park SS. Factors responsible for carbon dioxide retention in chronic obstructive lung disease. *Am Rev Respir Dis* 1965; **92**:245–54.

77. Lane DJ, Howell JBL. Relationship between sensitivity to carbon dioxide and clinical features in chronic airways obstruction. *Thorax* 1970;**25**:150–8.

78. Flenley DC, Millar JS. Ventilatory response to oxygen and carbon dioxide in chronic respiratory failure. *Clin Sci* 1967;**33**:319–34.

79. Flenley DC, Millar JS. The effects of carbon dioxide inhalation on the inspiratory work   thing in chronic ventilatory failure. *Clin Sci* 1968;**34**:385–95.

80. Flenley DC, Franklin DH, Millar JS. The hypoxic drive to breathing in chronic bronchitis and emphysema. *Clin Sci* 1970;**38**:503–18.

81. Altose MD, McCauley WC, Kelsen SG, Cherniack NS. Effects of hypercapnia and flow resistive loading on respiratory activity in chronic airways obstruction. *J Clin Invest* 1977;**59**:500–7.

82. Gelb AF, Kkein E, Schiffman P, Lugliani R, Aronstam P. Ventilatory response and drive in acute and chronic obstructive pulmonary disease. *Am Rev Respir Dis* 1977;**116**:9–16.

83. Bradley CA, Fleetham JA, Anthonisen NR. Ventilatory control in patients with hypoxaemia due to obstructive lung disease. *Am Rev Respir Dis* 1979;**120**:21–30.

84. Fleetham JA, Bradley CA, Kryger MH, Anthonisen NR. The effect of low flow oxygen therapy on the chemical control of ventilation in patients with hypoxaemic COPD. *Am Rev Respir Dis* 1980;**122**:833–40.

85. Gribbin HR, Gardiner IT, Heinz GJ, Gibson GJ, Pride NB. Role of impaired inspiratory muscle function in limiting the ventilatory response to carbon dioxide in chronic airflow obstruction. *Clin Sci* 1983;**64**:487–95.

86. Chonan T, Hida W, Kikuchi Y, Shindoh C, Takishima T. Role of CO_2 responsiveness and breathing efficiency in determining exercise capacity of patients with chronic airway obstruction. *Am Rev Respir Dis* 1988;**138**:1488–93.

87. Cherniack RM, Snidal DP. The effect of obstruction to breathing on the ventilatory response to CO_2. *J Clin Invest* 1956;**35**:1286–90.

88. De Troyer A, Leeper JB, McKenzie DK, Gandevia SC. Neural drive to the diaphragm in patients with severe COPD. *Am J Respir Crit Care Med* 1997;**155**:1335–40.

89. Lourenco RV, Miranda JM. Drive and performance of the ventilatory apparatus in chronic obstructive lung disease. *N Engl J Med* 1968;**279**:53–9.

90. Gorini MD, Spinelli A, Duranti R, Gigliotti F, Scano G. Neural respiratory drive and neuromuscular coupling in patients with chronic obstructive pulmonary disease (COPD). *Chest* 1990;**98**:1179–86.

91. Scano G, Spinelli A, Duranti R, *et al.* Carbon dioxide responsiveness in COPD patients with and without chronic hypercapnia. *Eur Respir J* 1995;**8**:78–85.

92. Lopata M, Onal E, Cromydas G. Respiratory load compensation in chronic airway obstruction. *J Appl Physiol* 1985;**59**:1947–54.

93. Costello R, Deegan P, Fitzpatrick M, McNicholas WT. Reversible hypercapnia in chronic obstructive pulmonary disease: a distinct pattern of respiratory failure with a favorable prognosis. *Am J Med* 1997;**102**:239–44.

94. Jamal K, Fleetham JA, Thurlbeck WM. Cor pulmonale: correlation with central airway lesions, peripheral airway lesions, emphysema and control of breathing. *Am Rev Respir Dis* 1990;**141**:1172–7.

95. Mountain R, Zwillich CW, Weil J. Hypoventilation in obstructive lung disease. The role of familial factors. *N Engl J Med* 1978;**298**:521–5.

96. Fleetham JA, Arnup ME, Anthonisen NR. Familial aspects of ventilatory control in patients with chronic obstructive pulmonary disease. *Am Rev Respir Dis* 1984;**129**:3–7.

97. Robinson TD, Freiberg DB, Regnis JA, Young IH. The role of hypoventilation and ventilation-perfusion redistribution in oxygen-induced hypercapnia during acute exacerbations of chronic obstructive pulmonary disease. *Am J Respir Crit Care Med* 2000;**161**:1524–9.

98. Similowski T, Yan S, Gauthier AP, Macklem PT, Bellemare F. Contractile properties of the human diaphragm during chronic hyperinflation. *N Engl J Med* 1991;**325**: 917–23.

99. Moxham J, Edwards RHT, Aubier M, *et al.* Changes in EMG power spectrum (high to low ratio) with force fatigue in humans. *J Appl Physiol* 1982;**53**:1094–9.

100. Goldstone JC, Green M, Moxham J. Maximum relaxation rate of the diaphragm during weaning from mechanical ventilation. *Thorax* 1994;**49**:54–60.

101. Levy RD, Esau SA, Bye PTP, Pardy RL. Relaxation rate of mouth pressure with sniffs at rest and with inspiratory muscle fatigue. *Am Rev Respir Dis* 1984;**130**:38–41.

102. Cohen CA, Zagelbaum G, Gross D, Roussos C, Macklem PT. Clinical manifestations of respiratory muscle fatigue. *Am J Med* 1982;**73**:308–16.

103. McKenzie DK, Bellemare F. Respiratory muscle fatigue. *Adv Exp Med Biol* 1995;**384**:401–14.

104. Bellemare F, Grassino A. Force reserve of the diaphragm in patients with chronic obstructive pulmonary disease. *J Appl Physiol* 1983;**55**:8–15.

105. Gutierrez M, Beroiza T, Contreras G, *et al*. Weekly cuirass ventilation improves blood gases and inspiratory muscle strength in patients with chronic airflow limitation and hypercarbia. *Am Rev Respir Dis* 1988;**138**:617–23.

106. Shapiro SH, Ernst P, Gray-Donald K, *et al*. Effect of negative pressure ventilation in severe pulmonary disease. *Lancet* 1992;**340**:1425–9.

107. Begin P, Grassino AE. Inspiratory muscle dysfunction and chronic hypercapnia in chronic obstructive pulmonary disease. *Am Rev Respir Dis* 1991;**143**:905–12.

108. Oliven A, Cherniack NS, Deal EC, Kelsen SG. The effects of acute bronchoconstriction on respiratory activity in patients with chronic obstructive pulmonary disease. *Am Rev Respir Dis* 1985;**131**:236–41.

109. Cherniack NS, Altose MD. Respiratory responses to loading. In: TK Hornbein, ed. *The Regulation of Breathing*, part II. Marcel Dekker, New York, 1981, pp 905–64.

110. Cherniack NS, Milic-Emili J. Mechanical aspects of loaded breathing. In: Ch Roussos, PT Macklem, eds. *Lung Biology in Health and Disease. The Thorax*, part B. Marcel Dekker, New York, 1985, pp 905–64.

111. Sorli J, Grassino A, Lorange G, Milic-Emili J. Control of breathing in patients with chronic obstructive lung disease. *Clin Sci Mol Med* 1978;**54**:295–304.

112. Aubier M, Murciano D, Fournier M, Milic-Emili J, Pariente R, Derenne J-P. Central respiratory drive in acute respiratory failure of patients with chronic obstructive pulmonary disease. *Am Rev Respir Dis* 1980;**122**:191–9.

113. Parot S, Saunier C, Gautier H, Milic-Emili J, Sadoul P. Breathing pattern and hypercapnia in patients with obstructive pulmonary disease. *Am Rev Respir Dis* 1980;**121**:985–91.

114. Javaheri S, Blum J, Kazemi H. Pattern of breathing and carbon dioxide retention in chronic obstructive pulmonary disease. *Am J Med* 1981;**71**:228–34.

115. Loveridge B, West P, Anthonisen NR, Kryger MH. Breathing pattern in patients with chronic obstructive pulmonary disease. *Am Rev Respir Dis* 1984;**130**:730–3.

116. Oliven A, Kelsen SG, Deal EC, Cherniack NS. Mechanisms underlying CO_2 retention during flow-resistive loading in patients with chronic obstructive pulmonary disease. *J Clin Invest* 1983;**71**:1442–9.

117. Gorini M, Misuri G, Corrado A, *et al*. Breathing pattern and carbon dioxide retention in severe chronic obstructive pulmonary disease. *Thorax* 1996;**51**:677–83.

118. Haluszka J, Chartrand DA, Grassino A, Milic-Emili J. Intrinsic PEEP and arterial P_{CO_2} in stable patients with chronic obstructive pulmonary disease. *Am Rev Respir Dis* 1990;**141**:1194–7.

119. Duranti R, Misuri G, Gorini M, Goti P, Gigliotti F, Scano G. Mechanical loading and control of breathing in patients with severe chronic obstructive pulmonary disease. *Thorax* 1995;**50**:127–33.

120. Hadcroft J, Calverley PM. Alternative methods for assessing bronchodilator reversibility in chronic obstructive pulmonary disease. *Thorax* 2001;**56**:713–20.

121. Santiago TV, Remolina C, Scoles V, Edelman NH. Endorphins and the control of breathing. Ability of naloxone to restore flow-resistive load compensation in chronic obstructive pulmonary disease. *N Engl J Med* 1981;**304**:1190–5.

122. Simon PM, Pope A, Lahive K, *et al*. Naloxone does not alter response to hypercapnia or resistive loading in chronic obstructive pulmonary disease. *Am Rev Respir Dis* 1989;**139**:134–8.

123. Riley RL. The work of breathing and its relation to respiratory acidosis. *Ann Intern Med* 1954;**41**:172–6.

124. Katz-Salamon M. Respiratory psychophysics: a methodological overview. In: C von Euler, M Katz-Salamon, eds. *Respiratory Psychophysiology*. Stockton Press, New York, 1988, pp 65–78.

125. Stubbing DG, Ramsdale EH, Killian KJ, Campbell EJM. Psychophysics of inspiratory muscle force. *J Appl Physiol* 1983;**54**:1216–21.

126. Mahutte CK, Campbell EJM, Killian KJ. Theory of resistive load detection. *Respir Physiol* 1983;**51**:131–9.

127. American Thoracic Society. Dyspnea. Mechanisms, assessment, and management: a consensus statement. *Am J Respir Crit Care Med* 1999;**159**:321–40.

128. Simon PM, Schwartzstein RM, Weiss JW, *et al*. Distinguishable sensations of breathlessness induced in normal volunteers. *Am Rev Respir Dis* 1989;**140**:1021–9.

129. Elliot MW, Adams L, Cockcroft A, MacRae KD, Murphy K, Guz A. The language of breathlessness: use of verbal descriptions by patients with cardiopulmonary disease. *Am Rev Respir Dis* 1991;**144**:826–32.

130. Campbell EJM, Freedman S, Smith PS, Taylor ME. The ability to detect added elastic loads to breathing. *Clin Sci* 1961; **20**:222–31.

131. McCloskey DI, Ebeling P, Goodwin GM. Estimation of weights and tensions and apparent involvement of a sense of effort. *Exp Neurol* 1974;**42**:220–32.

132. Borg G. Psychophysical basis of perceived exertion. *Med Sci Sports Exer* 1982;**14**:377–81.

133. Clague JE, Carter J, Pearson MG, Calverley PMA. Relationship between inspiratory drive and perceived inspiratory effort in normal man. *Clin Sci* 1990;**78**:493–6.

134. Muza SR, Silverman MT, Gilmore CG, Hellerstein HK, Kelsen SG. Comparisons of scales used to quantitate the sense of effort to breathe in patients with chronic obstructive pulmonary disease. *Am Rev Respir Dis* 1990;**141**:909–13.

135. Wilson RC, Jones PW. A comparison of the visual analogue scale and modified Borg scale for the measurement of dyspnoea during exercise. *Clin Sci* 1989;**76**:277–82.

136. Mador MJ, Kufel TJ. Reproducibility of visual analog scale measurements of dyspnea in patients with chronic obstructive pulmonary disease. *Am Rev Respir Dis* 1992;**146**:82–7.

137. Hay JG, Stone P, Carter J, *et al*. Bronchodilator reversibility, exercise performance and breathlessness in stable chronic obstructive pulmonary disease. *Eur Respir J* 1992;**5**:659–64.

138. Larson JL, Kim MJ, Sharp JT, *et al*. Inspiratory muscle training with a pressure threshold device in patients with chronic obstructive pulmonary disease. *Am Rev Respir Dis* 1988;**138**:689–96.

139. MRC Committee on Research into Chronic Bronchitis. *Instructions for Use of the Questionaire on Respiratory Symptoms*. WJ Holman, Devon, UK, 1966.

140. Bestall JC, Paul EA, Garrod R, Garnham R, Jones PW, Wedzicha JA. Usefulness of the Medical Research Council (MRC) dyspnoea scale as a measure of disability in patients with chronic obstructive pulmonary disease. *Thorax* 1999;**54**:581–6.

141. Mahler DA, Weinberg DH, Wells CK, Feinstein AR. The measurement of dyspnoea: contents, interobserver

agreement and physiologic correlates of two new clinical indices. *Chest* 1984;**85**:751–8.

142. Mahler DA, Harver A. A factor analysis of dyspnea ratings, respiratory muscle strength and lung function in patients with chronic obstructive pulmonary disease. *Am Rev Respir Dis* 1992;**145**:467–70.

143. Cournand A, Richards DW. Pulmonary insufficiency. *Am Rev Tubercl* 1941;**44**:26–41.

144. Eisele J, Trenchard D, Burki N, Guz A. The effect of chest wall block on respiratory sensation and control in man. *Clin Sci* 1969;**35**:23–33.

145. Manning HL, Basner R, Ringler J, *et al.* Effect of chest wall vibration on breathlessness in normal subjects. *J Appl Physiol* 1991;**71**:175–81.

146. Remmers JE. Inhibition of inspiratory activity by intercostal muscle afferents. *Respir Physiol* 1970;**10**:358–83.

147. Gandevia SC, Macefield G. Projection of low threshold afferents from human intercostal muscles to the cerebral cortex. *Respir Physiol* 1989;**77**:201–14.

148. Campbell EJM, Godfrey S, Clark TJH, Freedman S, Norman J. The effect of muscular paralysis induced by tubocurarine on the duration and sensation of breath holding during hypercapnia. *Clin Sci* 1969;**36**:323–8.

149. Banzett RB, Lansing RW, Brown R, *et al.* 'Air hunger' from increased P_{CO_2} persists after complete neuromuscular block in humans. *Respir Physiol* 1990;**81**:1–18.

150. Adams L, Lane R, Shea SA, Cockcroft A, Guz A. Breathlessness during different forms of ventilatory stimulation: a study of mechanisms in normal subjects and respiratory patients. *Clin Sci* 1985;**69**:663–72.

151. Chonan T, Mulholland MB, Leitner J, Altose MD, Cherniack NS. Sensation of dyspnea during hypercapnia, exercise and voluntary hyperventilation. *J Appl Physiol* 1990;**68**:2100–6.

152. Chonan T, Mulholland MB, Cherniack NS, Altose MD. Effect of voluntary constraining of thoracic displacement during hypercapnia. *J Appl Physiol* 1987;**63**:1822–8.

153. Lane R, Adams L, Guz A. The effects of hypoxia and hypercapnia on perceived during exercise in humans. *J Physiol (Lond)* 1990;**429**:579–93.

154. Lane R, Adams L, Guz A. Acidosis and breathlessness in normal subjects. *Eur Respir J* 1990;**3**:142S.

155. Killian KJ, Mahutte CK, Howell JBL, Campbell EJM. Effect of timing, flow, lung volume and threshold pressures on resistive load detection. *J Appl Physiol* 1980;**49**:958–63.

156. Killian KJ, Gandevia SC, Summers E, Campbell EJM. Effect of increased lung volume on perception of breathlessness, effort and tension. *J Appl Physiol* 1984;**57**:686–91.

157. Killian KJ, Bucens DD, Campbell EJM. The effect of patterns of breathing on the perceived magnitude of added loads to breathing. *J Appl Physiol* 1982;**52**:578–84.

158. Gandevia SC, Killian KJ, Campbell EJM. The effect of respiratory muscle fatigue in respiratory sensations. *Clin Sci* 1981;**60**:463–6.

159. Bradley TD, Chartrand DA, Fitting JW, Killian KJ, Grassino A. The relation of inspiratory effort sensation to fatiguing patterns of the diaphragm. *Am Rev Respir Dis* 1986;**134**:1119–24.

160. Clague JE, Carter J, Pearson MG, Calverley PMA. Physiological determinants of inspiratory effort sensation during CO_2 rebreathing in normal subjects. *Clin Sci* 1993;**85**:637–42.

161. Sharp JT, Druz WS, Moisan T, Foster J, Machnach W. Postural relief of dyspnea in severe COPD. *Am Rev Respir Dis* 1980;**122**:201–11.

162. Celli BR, Rassulo J, Make B. Dyssynchronous breathing during arm but not leg exercise in patients with chronic airflow obstruction. *N Engl J Med* 1986;**314**:1485–90.

163. Ward ME, Eidelman D, Stubbing DG, Bellemare F, Macklem PT. Respiratory sensation and pattern of respiratory muscle activation during diaphragm fatigue. *J Appl Physiol* 1988;**65**:2181–9.

164. Leblanc P, Bowie DM, Summers E, Jones NL, Killian KJ. Breathlessness and exercise in patients with cardiorespiratory disease. *Am Rev Respir Dis* 1986;**133**:21–5.

165. Zechman FW, Muza SR, Davenport PW, Wiley RL, Shelton R. Relationship of transdiaphragmatic pressure and latencies for detecting added inspiratory loads. *J Appl Physiol* 1985;**58**:236–43.

166. Davenport PW, Friedman WA, Thompson FJ, Franzen O. Respiratory-related cortical potentials evoked by inspiratory occlusion in humans. *J Appl Physiol* 1986;**60**:1843–8.

167. Murphy K, Mier A, Adams L, Guz A. Putative cerebral cortical involvement in the ventilatory response to inhaled CO_2 in conscious man. *J Physiol* 1990;**420**:1–18.

168. Xu F, Taylor RF, McLarney T, Lee L-Y, Frazier DT. Respiratory load compensation.1 Role of the cerebrum. *J Appl Physiol* 1993;**74**:853–8.

169. Chen Z, Eldridge FL, Wagner PG. Respiratory-associated thalamic activity is related to level of respiratory drive. *Resp Physiol* 1992;**90**:99–113.

170. Chen Z, Eldridge FL, Wagner PG. Respiratory-associated rhythmic firing of midbrain neurones in cats: relation to level of respiratory drive. *J Physiol* 1991;**437**:305–25.

171. el Manshawi A, Killian KJ, Summers E, Jones NL. Breathlessness during exercise with and without resistive loading. *J Appl Physiol* 1986;**61**:896–905.

172. Lane R, Cockcroft A, Guz A. Voluntary isocapnic hyperventilation and breathlessness during exercise in normal subjects. *Clin Sci* 1987;**73**:519–23.

173. O'Donnell DE, Webb KA. Exertional breathlessness in patients with chronic airflow limitation. The role of lung hyperinflation. *Am Rev Respir Dis* 1993;**148**:1351–7.

174. O'Donnell DE, Bertley JC, Chau LK, Webb KA. Qualitative aspects of exertional breathlessness in chronic airflow limitation: pathophysiologic mechanisms. *Am J Respir Crit Care Med* 1997;**155**:109–15.

175. Belman MJ, Botnick WC, Shin JW. Inhaled bronchodilators reduce dynamic hyperinflation during exercise in patients with chronic obstructive pulmonary disease. *Am J Respir Crit Care Med* 1996;**153**:967–75.

176. Hamilton AL, Killian KJ, Summers E, Jones NL. Muscle strength, symptom intensity, and exercise capacity in patients with cardiorespiratory disorders. *Am J Respir Crit Care Med* 1995;**152**:2021–31.

177. Young J, Fry-Smith A, Hyde C. Lung volume reduction surgery (LVRS) for chronic obstructive pulmonary disease (COPD) with underlying severe emphysema. *Thorax* 1999;**54**:779–89.

178. Martinez FJ, De Oca MM, Whyte RI, Stetz J, Gay SE, Celli BR. Lung-volume reduction improves dyspnea, dynamic hyperinflation, and respiratory muscle function. *Am J Respir Crit Care Med* 1997;**155**:1984–90.

179. Tschernko EM, Gruber EM, Jaksch P, *et al.* Ventilatory mechanics and gas exchange during exercise before and after lung volume reduction surgery. *Am J Respir Crit Care Med* 1998;**158**:1424–31.

180. Shade DJ, Cordova F, Lando Y, *et al.* Relationship between resting hypercapnia and physiologic parameters before and after lung volume reduction surgery in severe chronic obstructive pulmonary disease. *Am J Respir Crit Care Med* 1999;**159**:1405–11.

181. Swinburn CR, Wakefield JM, Jones PW. Relationship between ventilation and breathlessness during exercise in chronic obstructive airways disease is not altered by prevention of hypoxaemia. *Clin Sci* 1984;**67**:515–19.

182. Mak VHF, Bugler JR, Roberts CM, Spiro SG. Effect of arterial oxygen desaturation on six minute walk distances, perceived effort and perceived breathlessness in patients with airflow limitation. *Thorax* 1993;**48**:33–8.

183. Spence DPS, Hay JG, Carter J, Pearson MG, Calverley PMA. Oxygen desaturation and breathlessness during corridor walking in chronic obstructive pulmonary disease: effect of oxitropium bromide. *Thorax* 1993;**48**:1145–50.

184. Morgan AD, Peck DF, Buchanan DE, McHardy GJR. Effect of attitudes and beliefs on exercise tolerance in chronic bronchitis. *Br Med J* 1983;**286**:171–3.

185. Stubbing DG, Killian KJ, Campbell EJM. Weber's law and resistive load detection. *Am Rev Respir Dis* 1983;**127**:5–7.

186. Mador JM, Tobin MJ. Effect of alterations in mental activity on the breathing pattern in healthy subjects. *Am Rev Respir Dis* 1991;**144**:481–7.

187. Clark TJH, Cochrane GM. Effect of personality on alveolar ventilation in patients with chronic airways obstruction. *Br Med J* 1970;**1**:273–5.

188. Hudgel DW, Kinsman RA. Interactions among behavioural style, ventilatory drive and load recognition. *Am Rev Respir Dis* 1983;**128**:246–8.

189. Clague JE, Carter J, Pearson MG, Calverley PMA. Effort sensation, chemoreceptors and breathing pattern during inspiratory resistive loading. *J Appl Physiol* 1992;**73**:440–5.

190. Gottfried SB, Redline S, Altose MD. Respiratory sensation in chronic obstructive pulmonary disease. *Am Rev Respir Dis* 1985;**132**:954–9.

191. Oliven A, Kelsen SG, Deal EC, Cherniack NS. Respiratory pressure sensation. Relationship to changes in breathing pattern in patients with chronic obstructive lung disease. *Am Rev Respir Dis* 1985;**132**:1214–18.

192. Akiyama Y, Nishimura M, Kobayashi S, Yoshioka A, Yamamoyo K, Miyamoto K. Effects of naloxone on the sensation of dyspnea during acute respiratory loading in normal subjects. *J Appl Physiol* 1993;**74**:590–5.

193. Bardsley PA. Chronic respiratory failure in COPD: is there a place for a respiratory stimulant? *Thorax* 1993;**48**:781–4.

194. Moser KM, Luchsinger PC, Adamson JS, *et al.* Respiratory stimulation with intravenous doxapram in respiratory failure: a double-blind co-operative study. *N Engl J Med* 1973;**288**:427–31.

195. Calverley PMA, Robson RH, Wraith RH, Prescott LF, Flenley DC. The ventilatory effect of doxapram in normal man. *Clin Sci* 1983;**65**:65–9.

196. Powles AC, Tuxen DV, Mahood CB, Pugsley SO, Campbell EJM. The effect of intravenously administered almitrine, a peripheral chemoreceptor agonist, on patients with chronic air-flow obstruction. *Am Rev Respir Dis* 1983;**127**:284–9.

197. Connaughton JJ, Douglas NJ, Morgan AD, *et al.* Almitrine improves oxygenation when both awake and asleep in patients with hypoxia and carbon dioxide retention caused by chronic bronchitis and emphysema. *Am Rev Respir Dis* 1985;**132**:206–10.

198. MacNee W, Connaughton JJ, Rhind GB, *et al.* A comparison of the effects of almitrine or oxygen on pulmonary arterial pressure and right ventricular ejection fraction in hypoxic chronic bronchitis and emphysema. *Am Rev Respir Dis* 1986;**134**:559–65.

199. Watanabe S, Kanner RE, Cutiilo AG, *et al.* Long term effects of almitrene bismethylate in patients with hypoxic chronic obstructive pulmonary disease. *Am Rev Respir Dis* 1989;**140**:1269–73.

200. Bardsley PA, Howard P, De Backer W, *et al.* Two years' treatment with almitrine bismesylate in patients with hypoxic chronic obstructive pulmonary disease. *Eur Respir J* 1991;**4**:308–10.

201. Skatrud JB, Dempsey JA. Relative effectiveness of acetozolamide versus medroxyprogesterone acetate in the correction of chronic carbon dioxide retention. *Am Rev Respir Dis* 1983;**127**:405–12.

202. Petrof BJ, Calderini E, Gottfried SB. Effect of CPAP on respiratory effort and dyspnoea during exercise in severe COPD. *J Appl Physiol* 1990;**69**:179–88.

203. O'Donnell DE, Sanii R, Gresbrecht G, Younes M. Effect of continuous positive airway pressure on respiratory sensation in patients with chronic obstructive pulmonary disease during submaximal exercise. *Am Rev Respir Dis* 1988;**138**:1185–91.

204. Mitchell-Heggs P, Murphy K, Minty K, *et al.* Diazepam in the treatment of dyspnoea in the 'pink puffer' syndrome. *Q J Med* 1980;**193**:9–20.

205. Woodcock AA, Gross E, Geddes DM. Drug treatment of breathlessness: contrasting effects of diazepam and promethazine in pink puffers. *Br Med J* 1981;**283**:343–5.

206. Supinksi G, Dimarco A, Bark H, Chapman K, Clary S, Altose MD. Effect of codeine on the sensations elicited by loaded breathing. *Am Rev Respir Dis* 1990;**141**:1516–21.

207. Woodcock AA, Gross ER, Gellert A, *et al.* Effects of dihydrocodeine, alcohol and caffeine on breathlessness and exercise tolerance in patients with chronic obstructive lung disease and normal blood gases. *N Engl J Med* 1981;**305**:1611–16.

208. Johnson MA, Woodcock AA, Geddes DM. Dihydrocodeine for breathlessness in 'pink puffers'. *Br Med J* 1983;**276**:675–7.

209. Light RW, Muro JR, Sato RI, *et al.* Effects of oral morphine on breathlessness and exercise tolerance in patients with chronic obstructive pulmonary disease. *Am Rev Respir Dis* 1989;**139**:126–33.

210. Eiser N, Denman W, Luce P. Diamorphine in the treatment of dyspnoea in the 'pink puffer' syndrome of chronic airflow limitation. *Thorax* 1989;**44**:888P–9P.

211. Woodcock AA, Gross ER, Geddes DM. Oyxgen relieves breathlessness in 'pink puffers'. *Lancet* 1913;**i**:907–9.

212. Davidson AC, Leach R, George RJD, Geddes DM. Supplemental oxygen and exercise ability in chronic obstructive airways disease. *Thorax* 1988;**43**:965–71.

213. Leach RM, Davidson AC, Chinn S, Twort CHC, Cameron IR, Bateman NT. Portable liquid oxygen and exercise ability in severe respiratory disability. *Thorax* 1992;**47**:781–9.

214. O'Donnell DE, Bain DJ, Webb KA. Factors contributing to relief of exertional breathlessness during hyperoxia in chronic airflow limitation. *Am J Respir Crit Care Med* 1997;**155**:530–5.

215. Schwartzstein RM, Lahire K, Pope A, Weinberger SE, Weiss JW. Cold facial stimulation reduces breathlessness induced in normal subjects. *Am Rev Respir Dis* 1987;**136**:58–61.

216. Swinburn CR, Mould H, Stone TN, Corris PA, Gibson GJ. Symptomatic benefit of supplemental oxygen in hypoxemic patients with chronic lung disease. *Am Rev Respir Dis* 1991;**143**:913–15.

217. Killen JW, Corris PA. A pragmatic assessment of the placement of oxygen when given for exercise induced dyspnoea. *Thorax* 2000;**55**:544–6.

17

Pulmonary circulation

ROBERT NAEIJE AND WILLIAM MACNEE

INTRODUCTION

Although it had been known for many years that heart failure can complicate lung diseases, it was only in 1963 that a consensus conference sponsored by the World Health Organization pointed at the importance of 'pulmonary heart disease' or 'cor pulmonale' as a public health problem.[1] The report defined cor pulmonale as right ventricular hypertrophy resulting from diseases which affect the structure or function of the lungs. This purely pathologic definition proved impractical, so that cor pulmonale became better understood by clinicians as an alteration of right ventricular function, with right ventricular dilatation and hypertrophy, in response to increased pulmonary arterial pressures caused by pulmonary disease.[2–4] Pulmonary hypertension is a *sine qua non* for the development of cor pulmonale. The most common cause of cor pulmonale is COPD.

EPIDEMIOLOGY

The incidence of cor pulmonale in COPD is not exactly known, because there is no validated screening procedure. However, the condition is frequent in patients with COPD sick enough to be referred to specialized centers. Anatomical evidence of cor pulmonale can be found at autopsy in 10–40% of these patients, although most of these data are more than 20 years old.[5,6] The prevalence of clinical signs of cor pulmonale increases with worsening of airflow obstruction and deterioration of gas exchange: it is present in 40% of patients with a FEV_1 below 1 liter, and in 70% with a FEV_1 of 0.6 liter, and it is almost universal in patients with hypoxemia, hypercapnia and polycythemia.[7,8] Between 10 and 30% of hospital admissions for congestive heart failure are attributable to right heart failure secondary to hypoxemic chronic lung disease, that is most often COPD.[9,10] Pulmonary heart disease is considered to be the third most common cardiovascular condition, after left heart failure and systemic hypertension.[1–4]

PATHOPHYSIOLOGY

Pulmonary arterial hypertension

Pulmonary arterial hypertension has been defined as a mean pulmonary artery pressure greater than 25 mmHg at rest and 30 mmHg on exercise in a consensus statement for 'primary' pulmonary hypertension.[11] However, a mean resting pressure of greater than 20 mmHg at rest is considered in most studies to be abnormal.[12]

The normal pulmonary vasculature is both recruitable and distensible. A unilateral pulmonary artery occlusion (about 50% obstruction) increases mean pulmonary artery pressure to levels just above normal values (20 mmHg).

Higher levels of acute pulmonary vascular obstruction are associated with a hyperbolic increase in mean pulmonary artery pressure, which reaches 40 mmHg at a vascular obstruction of 80%.[13]

A decrease in the average cross-sectional area of the pulmonary resistive vessels can be caused by thrombotic obstruction, loss or obliteration because of inflammatory or destructive changes, or active vasoconstriction followed by remodeling.[14] The most potent pulmonary vasoconstricting stimulus is hypoxia. The reactivity of the pulmonary circulation to hypoxia varies in healthy subjects[15] and in patients with COPD.[16] However, the consequences of these variations in hypoxic vasoconstriction for the development of pulmonary hypertension are unknown. The biochemical mechanism of hypoxic pulmonary vasoconstriction remains incompletely understood. A current theory suggests that a decrease in P_{O_2} inhibits smooth muscle cell voltage-dependent potassium channels, resulting in membrane depolarization, influx of calcium and cell shortening.[17] Two such channels, $Kv_{2.1}$ and $Kv_{1.5}$, have been identified in rat pulmonary arteries.[18] However, the nature of the low P_{O_2} sensing mechanism remains elusive. A reduction in voltage-dependent potassium channel function has been reported in pulmonary artery smooth muscle cells of patients with primary pulmonary hypertension, and might thus be a universal pathway to enhanced pulmonary vascular reactivity and subsequent remodeling.[19] In addition to intrinsic smooth muscle cell reactivity to hypoxia, altered endothelium-mediated relaxation of pulmonary arteries,

particularly involving nitric oxide, might also play a role, as shown in experimental animals made chronically hypoxic[20] and in isolated pulmonary arteries from patients with COPD.[21] Hypoxic pulmonary vasoconstriction is enhanced by acidosis, while hypercapnia *per se* does not affect pulmonary vascular tone.[14] As indicated by the pulmonary vascular equation:

$$PVR = (Ppa - Pla)/Q$$

where PVR is pulmonary vascular resistance, Ppa mean pulmonary arterial pressure, Pla left atrial pressure and Q pulmonary blood flow. Pulmonary hypertension may be aggravated by a high pulmonary blood flow or an upstream transmission of increased pulmonary venous pressure.[14] An increased hematocrit further increases pulmonary vascular resistance.[14] Changes in lung volume may have profound effects on the pulmonary circulation: an increase in lung volume increases pulmonary vascular resistance by an increase in resistance of alveolar vessels, and a decrease in lung volume increases pulmonary vascular resistance by an increase in resistance of extraalveolar vessels.[22] Pulmonary vascular resistance is normally lowest at functional residual capacity.[22] Repeated stretching of resistive vessels in patients with obstructive lung diseases and hyperinflated chests may contribute to fixed structural changes.[23] As illustrated in Figure 17.1, all these mechanisms interact in patients with COPD to increase pulmonary artery pressures.

Pathological examination of the pulmonary circulation in COPD shows destruction of the capillaries,

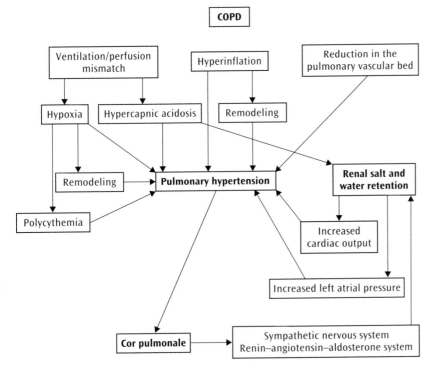

Figure 17.1 *Pathogenesis of pulmonary hypertension and cor pulmonale in COPD.*

muscularization of arterioles, and proliferation of longitudinal muscle in the intima of muscular arteries and larger arterioles.[23] The capillary destruction arises as part of the basic disease process. Muscularization of arterioles arises as a result of longstanding hypoxia, as seen in prolonged high-altitude hypoxia. Intimal longitudinal muscle results from recurrent stretching during breathing, with damage to the internal elastic lamina. Longitudinal muscle and associated fibrosis may completely obliterate vessel lumens. Prominent intimal proliferation may be related to inflammatory reaction to repeated stretching, and also to chronic cigarette smoke exposure.[24] These pathological aspects are illustrated in Plate 4. Although the vascular remodeling in the pulmonary circulation is thought to result mainly from chronic hypoxia, the ability of long-term oxygen therapy to reverse these changes remains controversial.[23,25]

Right ventricular function

The normal adult right ventricle has thin walls and a crescent shape, and is connected to a low-pressure vascular system, the pulmonary circulation. The left ventricle has thicker walls and an ovoid shape, and is connected to a high-pressure vascular system, the systemic circulation. The pumping action of the right ventricle has been compared to that of a bellows working in series with a low-resistance circuit, in contrast to the concentric contractions of the left ventricle. Small increments in pulmonary artery pressures result in a sharp decrease in right ventricular stroke volume, while the left ventricle is able to maintain stroke volume despite substantial increases in systemic artery pressures. Increases in filling pressures to the upper limit of normal, however, result in an increase in left ventricular stroke work that is five times that of right ventricular stroke work. The right ventricle therefore is generally said to be a 'flow generator' and the left ventricle a 'pressure generator'.[26] However, the function of both ventricles is qualitatively similar as described by a pressure–volume relationship.[27]

The normal right ventricle has been shown to fail, with acute dilatation and precipitous decline in cardiac output and systemic blood pressure, when mean Ppa is rapidly driven to about 40–50 mmHg, that is two to three times the upper limit of normal.[28] The level of pulmonary hypertension at which right ventricular failure occurs can be greatly increased by an increase in right coronary artery blood flow, which is critically dependent on systemic blood pressure. This observation is the basis of the treatment of acute right ventricular failure, or acute cor pulmonale, by systemic vasoconstrictors in the intensive care setting.[29] On the other hand, in response to chronic pressure load, the right ventricle dilates together with an increase in wall thickness and configuration,

making its aspect eventually similar to that of the left ventricle. The rate at which these changes occur in patients with pulmonary hypertension is not exactly known. However, right ventricular tolerance to mean pulmonary arterial pressure greater than 40–50 mmHg supports the view of a chronic rather than an acute pulmonary hypertensive process.

There has been discussion about the concept of cor pulmonale, with confusion regarding difficulties in clinical diagnosis and the concept itself of heart failure.[4] The debate may be clarified by the definition of heart failure proposed by Sagawa et al: 'as a state in which cardiac output cannot be maintained to meet peripheral systemic demand without an excessive use of physiologic compensatory mechanisms, mainly the increase in stroke volume associated with increased preload (Frank Starling mechanism)'.[27] This definition has the advantages of being physiologically sound, and of the integration of normal or even high cardiac output states as seen in patients with cor pulmonale.

Thus, in the presence of chronically increased pulmonary artery pressures, the right ventricle dilates with an increase in both end-diastolic and end-systolic volumes, a maintained stroke volume and a decreased ejection fraction. Secondary hypertrophy of the right ventricular wall decreases wall tension (or afterload). There is also an increase in contractility, as the autoregulation of ventricular function in response to increased afterload rapidly becomes homometric in addition to its initial heterometric adaptation classically described in Starling's law of the heart.[27] The increase in right ventricular end-diastolic volume, or preload, as an adaptation to increased afterload, is boosted by an increase in systemic venous return due to activation of sympathetic nervous and renin–angiotensin–aldosterone systems, and associated hypervolemia caused by renal salt and water retention (see below). Symptoms of right heart failure result from venous congestion secondary to upstream transmission of high right ventricular filling pressures and renal retention of salt and water in variable proportions. The pathogenesis of cor pulmonale in COPD is summarized in Figure 17.1.

PULMONARY HEMODYNAMICS IN COPD

At rest

Pulmonary hypertension in COPD is generally considered to be mild to moderate, based on reported hemodynamic profiles characterized by an increase in mean pulmonary arterial pressure to 20–35 mmHg, normal filling pressures of right and left ventricles, estimated by right atrial pressure and pulmonary artery occluded pressure, and a normal cardiac output.[16,30–39] This is very different from the pulmonary hypertension in left heart disease, congenital heart disease, thromboembolic disease and primary pulmonary hypertension where the mean pulmonary arterial pressures are greater than 40 mmHg. However, as illustrated in Table 17.1 and in Figure 17.2, there is considerable individual variability. Severe pulmonary hypertension, with a mean pulmonary arterial pressure higher than 40 mmHg, is not uncommon in patients who had at least one previous acute respiratory failure.[30] Pulmonary artery pressures in COPD have been repeatedly shown to correlate with the severity of hypoxemia and hypercapnia, but the correlation is not close (Figure 17.2). This is explained at least in part by intrinsic variability of the hypoxic pulmonary pressor response.[15,16]

Effects of pulmonary blood flow

In patients with COPD, the increase in pulmonary arterial pressure with blood flow is less than predicted by the pulmonary vascular resistance equation (Figure 17.3).

Table 17.1 *Hemodynamics and blood gases at rest in 74 patients with advanced COPD (From ref. 34 with permission from Elsevier Inc)*

Variables	COPD patients	Limits of normal
Pao_2 (mmHg)	43 ± 10	76–105
Sao_2 (%)	77 ± 11	94–1000
$Paco_2$ (mmHg)	51 ± 10	32–43
Q (L/min/m²)	3.8 ± 0.8	2.6–4.6
Pra (mmHg)	4 ± 4	2–9
Pla (mmHg)	6 ± 4	4–14
Ppa (mmHg)	35 ± 12	8–20
PVR (dyne/s/cm⁵/m²)	660 ± 284	40–200
RVSW (m/s)	17 ± 6	2–12

Values are shown as mean $\pm$ SD. Abbreviations: Pao_2: arterial Po_2; $Paco_2$: arterial Pco_2; Q: cardiac output; Pra: right atrial pressure; Pla: left atrial pressure (estimated by a pulmonary artery occluded pressure); Ppa: mean pulmonary artery pressure; PVR: pulmonary vascular resistance; RVSW: right ventricular stroke work.

Unilateral balloon occlusion studies have shown that the passive pulmonary arterial pressure–flow relationship in COPD is shifted to higher pressures, with a decreased slope and an increased extrapolated pressure intercept,[39–41] suggesting vascular closure.[40,41] An increase in pulmonary vascular closing pressure in COPD can be explained by increased lung volumes and gas trapping – inducing stretching of alveolar vessels[22] and dynamic hyperinflation-induced increased alveolar pressures.[42] Hypoxia-induced increase in tone and remodeling could also conceivably cause pulmonary vascular closure. A consequence of pulmonary artery pressure–flow relationship with decreased slope is that pulmonary vascular resistance becomes flow

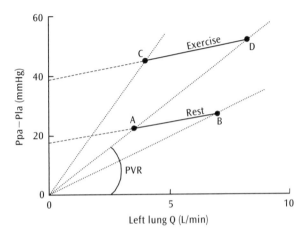

Figure 17.3 *Relationships between mean pulmonary artery pressure (Ppa) minus left atrial pressure (Pla) and left lung blood flow increased by contralateral pulmonary artery balloon occlusion in a representative patient with COPD at rest and at exercise. Pulmonary vascular resistance (PVR) is the slope of the (Ppa–Pla)/Q relationship. Passive increases in flow, from A to B and from C to D, increase pressure less than predicted by the PVR equation. Exercise, from A to C and from B to D, increases pressure more than predicted by the PVR equation. PVR is misleading for the evaluation of the functional state of the pulmonary circulation because it decreases from A to B and is unchanged from A to D. Q: cardiac output. (Adapted from ref. 34.)*

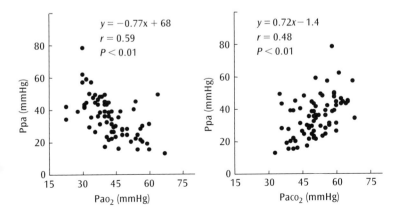

Figure 17.2 *Mean pulmonary artery pressures (Ppa) versus arterial Po_2 (Pao_2) and arterial Pco_2 ($Paco_2$) in 74 patients with advanced COPD. (From ref. 30.)*

dependent, making it unreliable for the estimation of changes in the functional state of pulmonary resistive vessels at variable flow (Figure 17.3).[14,40]

Effects of exercise

Exercise in COPD is associated with marked increases in mean pulmonary arterial pressure, especially in cases of severe disease with pre-existent pulmonary hypertension at rest.[31,32,39,43–47] As illustrated in Figure 17.3, the increase in pulmonary arterial pressure is more important than predicted by the pulmonary vascular resistance equation, indicating exercise-induced pulmonary vasoconstriction. This may be due to enhanced hypoxic pulmonary vasoconstriction by decreased mixed venous Po_2, increased sympathetic nervous system tone, and decreased arterial pH due to aggravated hypercapnia or lactic acidosis or both. Changes in intrathoracic pressures may also play a role. Exercise-induced increase in ventilation may aggravate dynamic hyperinflation, and thereby increase alveolar pressure at expiration. Increased ventilation in the presence of obstructed airways is associated with markedly negative inspiratory pleural pressures. Negative pleural pressures are associated with decreased ventricular pressures relative to alveolar pressure, and therefore correspond to an increase in right ventricular afterload.[48] This mechanism explains for example P pulmonale seen on the electrocardiogram of patients with status asthmaticus and normal (relative to atmosphere) pulmonary artery pressures.[49]

Effects of sleep

Sleep in COPD is associated with acute increases in pulmonary artery pressures.[50–52] Acute elevation of pulmonary arterial pressure is particularly observed during rapid eye movement sleep, when arterial oxygen saturation may decrease by 20–30%, and mean pulmonary arterial pressure may increase by 20–25 mmHg. In most patients there is a close relationship between the changes in Sao_2 and pulmonary arterial pressure during sleep.[51,52] Such increases in pulmonary hypertension during sleep are short lived, the pulmonary arterial pressure returning to its baseline level on waking in the morning.[52] Nocturnal oxygen desaturations in COPD have been shown to be due to relative hypoventilation and ventilation-perfusion mismatching.[53,54] Sleep apnea syndrome may occur co-incidentally in COPD patients and may aggravate nocturnal hypoxemia. Between 15 and 40% of subjects with sleep apnea syndrome have permanent pulmonary hypertension in the absence of intrinsic pulmonary or cardiac disease.[55,56]

Effects of acute respiratory failure

Worsening of hypoxemia and hypercapnia during episodes of acute respiratory failure are accompanied by

Table 17.2 *Hemodynamics and blood gases at rest in nine patients with COPD during acute respiratory failure and 1 month after recovery (From ref. 57)*

Variables	Acute respiratory failure	Recovery
Sao_2 (%)	62 ± 12	90 ± 5
$Paco_2$ (mmHg)	58 ± 6	43 ± 5
Q (L/min/m²)	4.7 ± 1.1	3.0 ± 0.7
Pra (mmHg)	16 ± 5	7 ± 3
Pla (mmHg)	15 ± 5	10 ± 4
Ppa (mmHg)	53 ± 11	30 ± 6

Values are shown as mean $\pm$ SD. Abbreviations: see Table 17.1.

marked increases in pulmonary arterial pressures.[57–59] Pulmonary arterial pressure may increase by up to 25–30 mmHg. Typical hemodynamics and blood gases in patients with COPD during acute respiratory failure and after recovery are shown in Table 17.2. The parallel improvements in arterial Po_2 and pulmonary hypertension during recovery are suggestive of an important role of hypoxic pulmonary vasoconstriction. However, hypervolemia may also be implicated, as suggested by frequently increased right and left atrial pressures during acute respiratory failure.[57–59] However, most patients return to their previous hemodynamic state within a few days after recovery.[36]

Longitudinal evolution

Studies on large series of patients followed over more than 10 years have shown that the spontaneous evolution of pulmonary hypertension secondary to COPD is slow, with an average yearly increase in mean pulmonary artery pressure of 0.5 mmHg.[34–37,60] However, in about one third of these patients, the aggravation of pulmonary hypertension follows a faster course.[60] These patients do not differ from the others at the onset, but are characterized by a progressive worsening of blood gases. Long-term oxygen therapy, at least 14–16 hours per day, may transiently prevent the progression of pulmonary hypertension in advanced COPD.[61–64] Follow-up studies of an average of 6 years duration show that oxygen therapy halts the progression of pulmonary hypertension even in patients with severe hypoxemia.[63,64]

RIGHT VENTRICULAR FUNCTION IN COPD

Volume and pressure measurements

Right ventricular function has been assessed by volume measurements using radionuclide angiocardiographic techniques, with focus on ejection fraction as an index of systolic function. Isotopic right ventricular ejection fraction is depressed, to less than 50%, in about half of unselected but advanced COPD patients.[65–67] This proportion increases on exercise.[68] Right ventricular ejection fraction is more frequently decreased in patients with a past history of clinical signs of right heart failure.[65–69] Technical improvement in the measurement of right ventricular ejection fraction by the use of krypton-81 m rather than technetium-99 m blood pool ventriculography decreases the percentage of low values at rest, confirms frequent absence of an increase on exercise in advanced COPD patients.[70]

Simultaneous hemodynamic and radionuclide measurements in patients with COPD show an inverse correlation between right ventricular ejection fraction and systolic pulmonary artery pressure or pulmonary vascular resistance in some,[69] but not all, studies,[71] but only a weak inverse correlation between right ventricular ejection fraction and end-diastolic right ventricular volume or right atrial pressure.[69] Right ventricular ejection fraction is also poorly correlated with cardiac index or with peak systolic pulmonary artery pressure divided by end-systolic volume as an index of contractility.[72] This is in keeping with the notion that ejection fraction is determined by a complex interplay between preload, afterload and contractility changes,[27] and that peak systolic ventricular pressure (isotonic conditions) cannot replace a measurement of end-systolic ventricular pressure (isometric condition) for the measurement of an end-systolic elastance.[27] Patients with COPD and similar pulmonary arterial pressures, right atrial pressure and pulmonary vascular resistance have a lower isotopic right ventricular ejection fraction in cases of clinical signs of right heart failure, which is explained by more important salt and water retention, increased venous return, and therefore more important increase in end-diastolic right ventricular volume.[72]

In spite of limitations of peak systolic pulmonary artery pressure versus end-systolic volume as an index of right ventricular contractility, its relatively elevated value[73] and further increase with minimal change in end-systolic right ventricular volumes at exercise[73] are suggestive of adaptative increase in right ventricular contractility in the face of increased afterload. This is in agreement with the increases in calculated right ventricular stroke work reported in exercising COPD patients.[73,74]

Effects of exercise

Patients with COPD have a lower maximum exercise capacity than normal controls, but no difference in slope of the oxygen consumption versus cardiac output relationship.[43] This has been taken as an indication that exercise limitation in advanced COPD is not of cardiovascular origin, but caused by ventilatory impairment and/ or muscular deconditioning. However, the argument is not convincing as oxygen consumption and cardiac output remain linearly related up to maximum oxygen consumption whatever the cause of limitation in exercise capacity.[75] Patients with advanced COPD frequently fail to increase, or even decrease, their right ventricular ejection fraction, which is rather in favor of a cardiac limitation to exercise capacity.[68,70] The fact that exercise in COPD increases peak systolic pulmonary arterial pressure at a given end-systolic right ventricular volume,[73] and right ventricular stroke work[74] does not prove that right ventricular adaptation is sufficient for an increase in systemic blood flow and oxygen transport that is matched to exercise-associated increase in oxygen consumption. As it stands, it is likely that exercise capacity is limited by altered right ventricular function in many patients with advanced COPD.

Effects on left ventricular function

Whether or not the left ventricle is abnormal in COPD patients with cor pulmonale has been discussed for many years. Autopsy studies have repeatedly shown an abnormally high incidence of left ventricular hypertrophy in patients with COPD.[76,77] However, the notion of abnormal left ventricle in COPD has been rejected on the basis of most hemodynamic studies showing normal left atrial pressures and left ventricular stroke work. But radionuclide angiocardiographic studies include a higher than normal proportion of COPD patients with lower left ventricular ejection fractions at rest and on exercise.[66,68] Depressed left ventricular ejection fractions appear to be most frequent in edematous COPD patients.[66] Whether or not a decreased left ventricular ejection fraction truly represents an altered left ventricular systolic function is particularly relevant to end-stage COPD patients considered for lung transplantation. In these patients, left ventricular dysfunction is a contraindication to lung transplantation. Recent studies show that the prevalence of decreased isotopic left ventricular ejection fraction in advanced COPD with a normal coronary angiogram is less than 5%.[78] In addition, low left ventricular ejection fractions in patients with advanced COPD return to normal after successful pulmonary transplantation.[78,79] This suggests that in most patients with advanced COPD, there is no intrinsic left ventricular dysfunction, and that altered left ventricular ejection fraction is related to a geometric distorsion caused by the overloaded right ventricle.[78,79] Accessory causes of abnormal left ventricular ejection fraction reported in a minority of patients may be negative inspiratory pressure swings, which increases left ventricular afterload, occult coronary heart disease and sometimes alcoholism.[79] Intrinsic effects of hypoxemia and acidosis of the severity generally seen in advanced COPD are very unlikely to affect left or right ventricular contractility.[79]

Edema formation

Many patients with advanced COPD present with ankle edema but normal right atrial pressures. It has long been recognized that edema in advanced COPD is related to hypercapnia rather than to raised jugular pressures.[80] Some authors have rejected the notion of right heart failure in COPD, based on the arguments of only mild pulmonary hypertension, normal or even high cardiac output, and edema without clear relation to right atrial or pulmonary artery pressures.[4,81] It is clear that some patients present with edema without hemodynamic signs of right heart failure or significant changes in pulmonary arterial pressure from baseline.[72,73] However, hemodynamic studies in patients with COPD who developed edema during exacerbations of their disease and who were studied again after recovery have shown a consistent pattern of abnormal increase in right ventricular diastolic pressures and markedly aggravated pulmonary hypertension together with hypoxemia and hypercapnia.[57,82,83] In cor pulmonale secondary to chronic respiratory insufficiency, hypoxemia and hypercapnia aggravate systemic congestion by a further activation of sympathetic nervous system, already stimulated by right atrial distension, leading to further decrease in renal plasma flow, activation of the renin–angiotensin–aldosterone system, and increased renal tubular reabsorption of bicarbonate, sodium and water. These effects are only temporarily and partially prevented by atrial natriuretic peptide released by distended atrial walls, and by an increase in renal output of dopamine. An increase in plasma vasopressin (by an as yet unclear mechanism) is observed in late-stage right heart failure, when patients become hyponatremic. Thus complex interactions between pulmonary hemodynamics, the renal effects of hypercapnia and reflex humoral activations (Figure 17.1) account for the edema in advanced COPD.

CLINICAL FINDINGS

Patients with COPD present with variable combinations of the 'blue bloater' or the 'pink puffer' clinical types. Blue bloaters are moderately to markedly overweight, present with chronic cough and sputum production, no or minimal dyspnea at rest, frequent bronchial infections, cyanosis, secondary erythrocytosis, edema and

mildly increased anteroposterior diameter of the thorax, which is moderately hyperresonant to percussion, with rales and ronchi at auscultation. Late clinical signs are confusion, flapping tremor, bounding pulse and peripheral vasodilatation due to hypercapnia, and eventually a positive hepatojugular reflux, hepatomegaly, ascites and aggravated edema due to right heart failure. Pink puffers are moderately underweight to wasted, present with little cough and sputum, unusual bronchial infections, marked dyspnea at rest, no cyanosis, no edema, no erythrocytosis, but an increased anteroposterior diameter of the thorax which is hyperresonant to percussion, with absent to depressed breath sounds at auscultation. Signs of hypercapnia or right heart failure are terminal in pink puffers.

It has been previously thought that the pink puffer type would be associated with relatively more emphysema, and the blue bloater type with relatively more airway inflammation and mucus gland hypertrophy.[8,84–86] However, the clinical prediction of emphysema or bronchial alterations has been shown to be quite unreliable by careful pathologic studies[87] and computed tomography (CT) densitometry measurements.[88] In addition, there has been no study showing a correlation between the amount of emphysema and the severity of pulmonary hypertension in COPD.[4] However it remains true that the blue bloater type is more constantly associated with pulmonary hypertension and cor pulmonale, in relation to more severe hypoxemia and earlier development of hypercapnia.[4]

The contribution of pulmonary hypertension per se to the clinical picture in COPD is difficult to assess because overlap of non-specific symptoms such as dyspnea, fatigue and chest pain, and problematical cardiac auscultation in patients with bronchial rales and inflated chests. Thus the typical auscultatory findings of pulmonary hypertension, with an ejection click or an increased pulmonary component of the second heart sound, a right ventricular third or a fourth heart sound, a high pitch early diastolic murmur of pulmonary insufficiency, and a pansystolic murmur of tricuspid regurgitation, are uncommon in COPD patients with cor pulmonale. The symptomatology of pulmonary hypertension with normal lung parenchyma is known from large series of patients with primary pulmonary hypertension.[89] These patients complain of dyspnea, fatigue and atypical chest pain on average during 2 years before diagnostic right heart catheterization, which then shows a mean pulmonary artery pressure around 60 mmHg, much higher than commonly found at rest in COPD patients. Patients with primary pulmonary hypertension start to present with exertional dyspnea and fatigue when mean pulmonary artery pressure increases to 30–40 mmHg at rest.[89] This severity of pulmonary hypertension is observed in advanced COPD.

SPECIAL STUDIES

Electrocardiogram

The sensitivity of the electrocardiogram for cor pulmonale is relatively low, the test being diagnostic in only 25–40% of patients with confirmed right ventricular hypertrophy.[26] Criteria of cor pulmonale include a mean QRS axis to the right of 120 degrees, an R/S amplitude ratio in V1 >1, an R/S amplitude ratio in V6 <1 (any of these first three criteria is sufficient to raise suspicion of right ventricular hypertrophy), a P-pulmonale pattern (right axis deviation and increased P-wave amplitude, $>0.25\,\mathrm{mV}$) in leads II, III and aVF, a S1Q3 or S1S2S3 pattern, and a normal voltage QRS. In COPD the electrocardiographic findings are affected by lung inflation. Electrocardiographic signs found in patients with pulmonary hypertension secondary to COPD also include low-voltage QRS and incomplete right bundle branch block, inverted, biphasic or flattened T waves in the right precordial leads, depressed ST segments in leads II, III, and aVF, and occasional large Q or Qs waves in the inferior or mid-precordial leads suggesting previous myocardial infarction. In general, electrocardiographic changes do not parallel the severity of underlying pulmonary hypertension.

Chest radiograph

The chest radiograph helps in the diagnosis of pulmonary hypertension as well as of the lung disease responsible for abnormal blood gases and cor pulmonale.[26] Signs of pulmonary hypertension are cardiomegaly due to an enlarged right ventricle, and enlarged pulmonary trunk and hilar vessels. Widening of the hilum is judged from the ratio of the distance between the start of divisions of the right and left main pulmonary arteries divided by the transverse diameter of the thorax. A ratio of more than 0.36 suggests pulmonary hypertension.[26] Another indicator is simple widening of the descending right pulmonary artery shadow (usually under $16\,\mathrm{mm}$) to over $20\,\mathrm{mm}$.[90] The enlarged right ventricle accounts for an increased cardiothoracic ratio above 0.5 together with encroachment of the retrosternal airspace on a lateral film. The vasculature in the peripheral lung fields may appear normal or decreased. A normal chest radiograph is against the diagnosis of pulmonary hypertension, but it should be noted that 6% of patients enroled in the National Institute of Health registry of primary pulmonary hypertension had a normal chest radiograph.[89]

Lung function tests

Lung function tests are necessary for the diagnosis of obstructive and restrictive lung diseases, or inadequate ventilatory drive, associated with pulmonary hypertension.[26] Arterial P_{O_2} and FEV_1 are the lung function tests that appear the most closely related to the severity of pulmonary hypertension in COPD.[4] Pulmonary hypertension has little effect *per se* on lung mechanics or gas exchange.[89]

Echocardiography

Echocardiography is the next indispensable diagnostic step in any patient suspected of cor pulmonale. The procedure is non-invasive, easily available in any cardiologic practice, and allows for the definite diagnosis of pulmonary hypertension and cor pulmonale,[91] in spite of technical difficulties that may be encountered by altered sound wave transmission through hyperinflated chests for some measurements.[92]

Typical signs are right ventricular and atrial enlargement with a normal or reduced left ventricular cavity, and eventually a reversal of the normal septal curvature. Transmitral Doppler studies may show an altered left ventricular compliance with redistribution of filling from early to late diastole. Doppler studies are also useful for the evaluation of the severity of pulmonary hypertension. The trans-tricuspid pressure gradient (ΔP) can be calculated from the maximum velocity of tricuspid regurgitant jets (v_{max}) and the simplified form of the Bernouilli equation: $\Delta P(mmHg) = v_{max}(m/s) \times 4$. An estimation of systolic right ventricular or pulmonary artery pressure is obtained by adding an estimate of right atrial pressure to ΔP. Another useful Doppler measurement is the pulmonary flow–velocity curve, which shows a shortening of the acceleration time (AT) in proportion to the severity of pulmonary hypertension, with a mid-systolic deceleration in the most severe cases. An AT of less than $100\,\mathrm{ms}$ or a ratio of AT to ejection time of less than 0.35 are very suggestive of pulmonary hypertension. Exemplary four-chamber views, and Doppler studies of tricuspid regurgitant and pulmonary arterial flow velocities are shown in Figure 17.4.

Echo Doppler evaluation can be particularly useful for the detection of early pulmonary hypertension, and for the monitoring of the severity of pulmonary hypertension and response to treatment. Echocardiography is also essential for the diagnosis of associated left heart disease. Transesophageal echocardiography has been more recently introduced for the precise assessment of intracardiac defects, sensitive detection of patent foramen ovale, and evaluation of pulmonary artery and venous flows. It may be a useful approach when the transthoracic is technically difficult, in obese or excessively hyperinflated patients.

Right heart catheterization

Right heart catheterization remains the gold standard for the diagnosis of pulmonary hypertension. The procedure

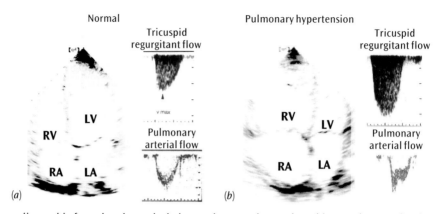

Figure 17.4 *Echocardiographic four-chamber apical view and concomitant tricuspid regurgitant and pulmonary arterial flows in a normal subject (a) and in a patient with severe pulmonary hypertension (b). Pulmonary hypertension is associated with an increase in right heart chambers and a leftward shift of the septum, an increase in velocity of tricuspid regurgitant flow, and a shortening of the acceleration time together with a mid-systolic deceleration of pulmonary arterial flow.*

allows a quantified evaluation of the contribution of increased pulmonary arterial pressures to the patient's symptoms at rest and at exercise, response to therapy and prognosis. Thermistance balloon-tipped catheters are used allowing for easy placement into the pulmonary arterial without fluoroscopic control, measurements of pulmonary artery pressures, occluded pulmonary artery pressure to estimate left atrial pressure, and cardiac output by thermodilution. Right heart catheterization is a safe procedure in expert hands, but, because of its invasive nature, it is preferably performed in a catheterization laboratory or an intensive care unit with adequate equipment for continuous monitoring and cardiopulmonary resuscitation. It is not routinely recommended in the assessment of patients with COPD.[93]

Polysomnography

Sleep studies are necessary for the diagnosis of sleep apnea syndrome, which will be suspected in COPD patients with obesity, snoring, daytime somnolence and fatigue, and hypercapnia out of proportion to lung function tests.

Cardiopulmonary exercise testing

Cardiopulmonary exercise testing, with measurements of heart rate, blood pressure and ventilatory variables at progressively increasing workload, for the determination of an anerobic threshold and a peak or a maximum oxygen consumption can be used to quantify the functional handicap in COPD patients.[75] A useful surrogate for cardiorespiratory exercise testing in clinical practice is the measurement of the distance walked in 6 minutes.[94] The 6-minute walk distance has been shown to be correlated

to pulmonary hemodynamics in patients with primary pulmonary hypertension,[89] but similar studies are not available in COPD patients. In COPD, an increase in the 6-minute walk distance by about 50 meters is associated with improved clinical state and quality of life.[94]

Ventilation-perfusion scintigraphy

Ventilation-perfusion scanning is used for the diagnosis of pulmonary embolism and thromboembolic pulmonary hypertension. However, markedly altered distributions of ventilation and perfusion in COPD make the identification of thromboembolic perfusion defects problematical.

Radionuclide angiography

This technique is usually performed using an intravenous injection of technetium-99 m-labeled erythrocytes or human serum albumin. A gamma camera is used to acquire a time–activity curve, either during the first pass of the radiolabeled tracer through the central circulation, or by gating counts from several points throughout the cardiac cycle once the radiotracer has equilibrated in the blood pool. Ejection fraction is calculated from the difference between end-diastolic and end-systolic counts, divided by end-diastolic counts. Krypton-81m may be a better isotope for right ventricular ejection fraction mesurement because of a short half-life and rapid escape from the lungs.[70] The normal right ventricular ejection fraction measured by this method ranges from 0.4 to 0.8. Right ventricular ejection fraction decreases in proportion to the severity of pulmonary hypertension, but is otherwise of limited help in the evaluation of cor pulmonale in clinical practice.[95]

Pulmonary angiography and spiral volumetric CT

Pulmonary angiography is indicated in cases of clinical suspicion of pulmonary embolism or chronic thromboembolic pulmonary hypertension. However, the procedure tends to be replaced by spiral volumetric computed tomography (CT) of the lungs. A spiral CT is easily completed by a thin-section CT, which is helpful for the differential diagnosis of dyspnea, and allows for the quantification of emphysema. Spiral CT has been shown to be as sensitive and specific as a pulmonary angiogram for the diagnosis of pulmonary emboli down to subsegmental pulmonary arteries.[96] More than 90% of acute embolic events occur upstream to subsegmental pulmonary arteries.[97] Surgically operable thromboembolic pulmonary hypertension also mainly concerns the most proximal portion of the pulmonary arterial tree.[98]

Magnetic resonance imaging

New generations of magnetic resonance imaging scanners with improved software offer great promise in the diagnosis of pulmonary hypertension and altered right ventricular structure and function. Their sensitivity is currently under evaluation.

MEDICAL TREATMENT

General measures

CORRECTION OF UNDERLYING CAUSE

Prevention of the development of pulmonary hypertension in COPD would be best achieved by preventing the decline in lung function which is characteristic of COPD. Present therapies have however failed to achieve this goal. Exacerbation of COPD may be reversed with the help of antibiotics, bronchodilators, chest physiotherapy and judicious use of corticosteroids.[2,3,99] Relief of hypoxemia, hypercapnic acidoses and hyperinflation will result in decreased pulmonary vascular resistance and strain on the right heart. Pulmonary hypertension may be relieved by nasal continuous positive airway pressure, tracheostomy or surgery for upper airway obstruction in patients with obstructive sleep apnea. Expanding surgical experience with thromboendarteriectomy and lung transplantation in recent years has shown that even the most advanced right heart failure secondary to severe pulmonary hypertension may be reversible.

CARDIAC GLYCOSIDES

There is little logic in the use of an inotropic drug as a first choice in the treatment of afterload-induced ventricular failure. It is therefore not surprising that cardiac glycosides have not shown to be useful in the treatment of cor pulmonale due to COPD. The risk of digitalis toxicity is enhanced by hypoxemia and by diuretic-induced hypokalemia. Digitalis may be given to slow the ventricular response to atrial flutter or fibrillation.[2,3,26]

DIURETICS

Diuretics have to be given with more care than usual, because of associated risks of aggravated metabolic alkalosis, leading to aggravated hypercapnia, excessive hypovolemia, compromising adequate filling of the afterloaded right ventricle, and increased blood viscosity by an increase in hematocrit in an already polycythemic patient.[2,3,26] Meticulous monitoring of plasma electrolytes is mandatory, and potassium and magnesium supplementation may be necessary. Therapy is instituted with low doses of loop diuretics, for example furosemide (frusemide), 20–40 mg/day, increased as needed and tolerated. Some patients with severe right heart failure may require huge doses of diuretics, for example furosemide up to 500 mg/day.

ANTICOAGULANT THERAPY

Severe pulmonary hypertension carries a risk of thromboembolism because of sedentary lifestyle, venous insufficiency, dilated right-sided heart chambers and sluggish pulmonary blood flow.[2,3] Thrombotic lesions are frequently found at autopsy in such patients. Anticoagulation has been shown to improve survival rate in primary pulmonary hypertension,[89] and is an undisputed therapy in thromboembolic pulmonary hypertension.[98] Until now, no study has proved anticoagulant therapy to be beneficial in cor pulmonale secondary to COPD. In these patients, it seems advisable to administer antiplatelet agents, and routine prophylaxis with low molecular weight heparin during periods of hospitalization or prolonged immobilization.[3]

Oxygen supplementation

Oxygen is the only treatment which has been shown to improve survival in patients with COPD, on the basis of two controlled studies reported in the early 1980s.[61,100] Current recommendation is to administer at least 15 hours/day of oxygen in patients with a PaO_2 below 55 mmHg, or a resting PaO_2 of 56–59 mmHg together with cor pulmonale or polycythemia (hematocrit above 55%).[101]

In patients with COPD, administration of high inspired oxygen concentrations carries a risk of aggravation of hypercapnic acidosis; however, slight increases in the fraction of inspired oxygen will most often increase arterial PO_2 above 60 mmHg, associated with a 90% saturation of hemoglobin. Therefore, oxygen has to be given in a controlled fashion (24–28%) in these patients.

Acute oxygen administration in patients with advanced COPD at rest has little effect on pulmonary hemodynamics[102,103] or right ventricular ejection fraction.[71,104] However, acute administration of oxygen at exercise often improves pulmonary hemodynamics[35,62] and right ventricular ejection fraction.[104]

Chronic supplemental oxygen improves pulmonary hemodynamics and right ventricular function in patients with COPD, with a slowing or even a reversal of the annual progression of pulmonary hypertension, and improved exercise pulmonary hemodynamics and right ventricular ejection fraction.[61–65] The best hemodynamic results have been in the studies with the highest daily duration of oxygen.[62,63] Attempts at prediction of pulmonary hemodynamic response to long-term oxygen therapy on the basis of short-term hemodynamic studies, exercise testing or change in right ventricular ejection fraction have been disappointing.

Vasodilators

Many vasodilators, including beta$_2$ stimulants, nitrates, calcium channel blockers, hydralazine, angiotensin converting enzyme inhibitors, phosphodiesterase inhibitors, alpha$_1$-receptor antagonists and hydralazine, have been repeatedly tried over the years for the treatment of cor pulmonale secondary to COPD.[4,30] In the search for the ideal drug, an optimal vasodilator response was defined as a decrease in pulmonary arterial pressure accompanied by an increase in cardiac output, no or minimal decrease in systemic arterial pressure and arterial oxygenation. In practice, the most common response has proved to be a relatively unchanged pulmonary arterial pressure, an increase in cardiac output, and mild to moderate decreases in systemic arterial pressure and arterial oxygenation.[4,30] There has been no randomized controlled trial showing benefit of long-term therapy with vasodilators in patients with cor pulmonale secondary to advanced COPD. This may be because sustained high pulmonary artery pressure and increased cardiac output lead to a decreased calculated pulmonary vascular resistance, but correspond in reality to an increased afterload of the right ventricle (increased wall tension because of increased preload in the presence of unchanged ejection pressure). Vasodilators in COPD also have many side effects, particularly worsening gas exchange. But the main reason for the clinical failure of most vasodilators in patients with pulmonary hypertension secondary to COPD may be the absence of effect on the progression of the remodeling of the pulmonary circulation.

At present, only two vasodilating treatments have been shown to improve clinical state and survival in pulmonary hypertension, and these results are restricted to patients with primary pulmonary hypertension.[89] The first is the oral administration of calcium-channel blockers at high doses, either nifedipine 30 to 240 mg/day, or diltiazem, 120–900 mg/day. Only 20–25% of patients respond by a decrease in both pulmonary artery pressures and resistance, and administration of the first dose carries a somewhat unpredictable risk of shock or sudden death by excessive systemic hypotension compromising right coronary perfusion pressure. The second is the continuous infusion of prostacyclin using a portable pump. About 70–80% of patients with primary pulmonary hypertension respond to this treatment, at least transiently. However, prostacyclin therapy is expensive, not without complications, and dose requirements tend to increase over time. Continuous infusion of prostacyclin is used as a bridge to transplantation for patients with severe pulmonary hypertension in several centers. Trials are currently under way to study the effects of inhaled or even oral prostacyclin analogue formulations. There are no trials of prostacycline in patients with COPD. There may be perspective in using inhaled nitric oxide, whose strong and specific pulmonary vasodilating effect[106] can be obtained with small pulses synchronized on the onset of each inspiration.[107,108] Chronic therapy with inhaled nitric oxide has been used to bridge patients to transplantation.[108] Inhaled, nitric oxide has been shown to improve pulmonary hemodynamics in COPD[109] but at the expense of worsening gas exchange.[110] Since vasodilators are less effective in COPD than in primary pulmonary hypertension, the associated side effects and the lack of a selective pulmonary vasodilator, long-term use of vasodilators is not recommended in COPD patients.

Phlebotomy

A decrease in hematocrit decreases pulmonary arterial pressures and resistance, increases resting right ventricular ejection fraction, and improves exercise tolerance in polycythemic patients with COPD.[32,111,112] The ideal hematocrit in hypoxemic COPD is not exactly known. Phlebotomy is recommended in polycythemic patients to maintain the hematocrit below 50–55%.

Transplantation

Single- or double-lung transplantation has been shown to be a suitable alternative for combined heart–lung transplantation in patients with end-stage lung disease.[113] Single-lung transplantation has been reported to normalize pulmonary hemodynamics in COPD.[114] Survival rates are reported as 60% at 1 year and 40% at 5 years, with most deaths resulting from infection, bronchiolitis obliterans and chronic rejection. Survival in patients with pulmonary vascular disease is in general not as good as in patients with parenchymal lung disease.

Lung volume reduction surgery (LVRS)

Selected patients with emphysema and lung overinflation may benefit from LVRS.[115,116] Patients with moderate to severe pulmonary hypertension (pulmonary arterial pressure = 35 mmHg) are not considered candidates for LVRS. Limited studies of pulmonary hemodynamics before and after LVRS[118–120] have shown conflicting results with increases in pulmonary arterial pressure post LVRS in some studies[117] but not in others.[118,119]

PROGNOSIS

At the same level of airflow obstruction, patients with COPD have a much greater longevity without than with pulmonary hypertension. A study on 175 patients with COPD showed a 7-year survival rate of 56% if the initial mean pulmonary arterial pressure was below 20 mmHg ($n = 113$), and of 29% if the initial mean pulmonary artery pressure was higher than 20 mmHg ($n = 62$).[38] Another study on 128 patients showed a 5-year survival rate of 85% with a mean pulmonary arterial pressure below 25 mmHg, and around 40% with a mean pulmonary arterial pressure between 30 and 45 mmHg.[120] As illustrated in Figure 17.5, survival in patients with a mean pulmonary arterial pressure of more than 40 mmHg

is similar to survival rates reported in patients with primary pulmonary hypertension.[89] The presence of clinical signs of right heart failure (edema) decreases the 5-year survival rate to only 27–33%.[4]

Pulmonary hypertension is still a good predictor of mortality in COPD patients treated with supplemental oxygen. In a series of 84 patients with advanced COPD treated with long-term oxygen, the 5-year survival rate was 62% in 44 patients with a mean pulmonary arterial pressure below 25 mmHg, and only 36% in 40 patients with a mean pulmonary arterial pressure higher than 25 mmHg.[121] It is of interest that in this large group of patients with advanced COPD, the level of pulmonary arterial pressure appeared to be a better prognostic factor than hypoxemia, hypercapnia or even airflow obstruction.

ACKNOWLEDGEMENT

The pathologic pictures were provided by Dr M. Wilkinson.

REFERENCES

1. World Health Organization. Chronic cor pulmonale. A report of the Expert Committee. *Circulation* 1993;**27**:594–8.
2. Fishman AP. Chronic cor pulmonale. *Am Rev Respir Dis* 1978;**114**:775–94.
3. Palevsky HL, Fishman AP. Chronic cor pulmonale. Etiology and management. *JAMA* 1990;**263**:2347–53.
4. MacNee W. Pathophysiology of cor pulmonale in chronic obstructive pulmonary disease. *Am J Respir Crit Care Med* 1994;**150**:833–52, 1158–68.
5. Heath D, Brewer D, Hicken P. Mechanisms and pathology. In: CC Thomas, ed. *Cor Pulmonale in Emphysema.* Thomas, Springfield, IL, 1968, pp 1–37.
6. Vogt P, Ruttner JR. Das cor pulmonale aus pathologisch-anatomischer sicht. *Schweiz Med Wochenschr* 1977;**107**: 549–53.
7. Renzetti AD Jr, McClement JH, Litt BD. The Veterans Administration cooperative study of pulmonary function. III: Mortality in relation to respiratory function in chronic obstructive pulmonary disease. *Am J Med* 1966;**41**:115–19.
8. Mitchell RS, Vincent TN, Filley GF. Chronic obstructive bronchopulmonary disease. IV. The clinical and physiological differential of chronic bronchitis and emphysema. *Am J Med Sci* 1964;**247**:513–17.
9. Stuart-Harris CH, Twiddle RHS, Clifton MA. Hospital study of congestive heart failure with special reference to cor pulmonale. *Br Med J* 1959;**2**:201.
10. Inter-Society Commission for Heart Disease Resources. Primary prevention of pulmonary heart disease. *Circulation* 1970;**41**:A-17.
11. Rubin LJ. ACCP Consensus Statement. *Chest* 1993;**104**:236–50.
12. Tartulier M, Bourret M, Deyreux F. Les pressions arterielles pulmonaires chez l'homme normal. Effects de l'age et de l'exercice musculaire. *Bull Physiopathol Respir* 1972;**8**: 1295–321.
13. Mélot C, Naeije R. Pulmonary vascular diseases. In: J Roca, R Rodriguez-Roisin, PD Wagner, eds. *Pulmonary and Peripheral*

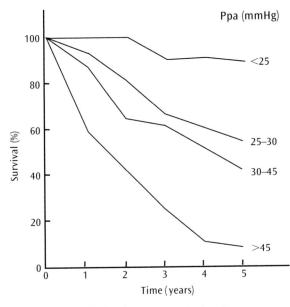

Figure 17.5 *Correlation between survival and mean pulmonary artery pressure in patients with COPD. (From ref. 105.)*

Gas Exchange in Health and Disease. Lung Biology in Health and Disease, vol 148. Marcel Dekker, New York, 2000, pp 285–302.

14. Fishman AP. Pulmonary circulation. In: Handbook of Physiology. The Respiratory System. Circulation and Nonrespiratory Functions, sect 3, vol 1. American Physiology Society, Bethesda, MD, 1985, pp 93–166.

15. Grover RF. Chronic hypoxic pulmonary hypertension. In: AP Fishman, ed. The Pulmonary Circulation: Normal and Abnormal. University of Pennsylvania, Philadelphia, 1990, pp 283–99.

16. Weitzenblum E, Schrijen F, Mohan-Kumar T, Colas des Francs V, Lockhart A. Variability of pulmonary vascular response to acute hypoxia in chronic bronchitis. Chest 1988;94:772–8.

17. Weir EK, Archer SL. The mechanism of acute hypoxic pulmonary vasoconstriction: the tale of two channels. FASEB J 1995;9:183–9.

18. Archer SL, Souil E, Dinh-Xuan AT, et al. Molecular identification of the role of voltage-gated K$^+$ channels, Kv1.5 and Kv2.1, in hypoxic pulmonary vasoconstriction and control of resting membrane potential in rat pulmonary artery myocytes. J Clin Invest 1998;101:2319–30.

19. Yuan XJ, Aldinger AM, Juhaszova M, et al. Dysfunctional voltage-gated K$^+$ channels in pulmonary artery smooth cells of patients with primary pulmonary hypertension. Circulation 1998;98:1400–6.

20. Adnot S, Raffestin B, Eddahibi S, Braquet P, Chabrier PE. Loss of endothelium-dependent relaxant activity in the pulmonary circulation of rats exposed to chronic hypoxia. J Clin Invest 1991;87:155–62.

21. Dinh-Xuan AT, Higenbottam TW, Clelland CA, et al. Impairment of endothelium-dependent pulmonary artery relaxation in chronic obstructive lung disease. N Engl J Med 1991;324:1539–47.

22. Howell JBL, Permutt S, Proctor DF, Riley RL. Effect of inflation of the lung on different parts of the pulmonary vascular bed. J Appl Physiol 1961;16:71–6.

23. Wilkinson M, Langhorn CA, Heath D, Barer GR, Howard P. A pathophysiological study of 10 cases of hypoxic cor pulmonale. Q J Med 1988;66:65–85.

24. Peinado VI, Barbera JA, Abate P, et al. Inflammatory reaction in pulmonary muscular arteries of patients with mild chronic obstructive pulmonary disease. Am J Respir Crit Care Med 1999;59:1605–11.

25. Calverley PM, Howatson R, Flenley DC, Lamb D. Clinicopathological correlations in cor pulmonale. Thorax 1992;47:494–8.

26. Wiedemann HP, Matthay RA. Cor pulmonale. In: E Braunwald, ed. Heart Disease. A Textbook of Cardiovascular Medicine, 5th edn. WB Saunders, Philadelphia, 1997, pp 1604–25.

27. Sagawa S, Maughan L, Suga H, Sunagawa K. Cardiac Contraction and the Pressure–Volume Relationship. Oxford University Press, New York, 1988.

28. Guyton AC, Lindsay AW, Gilluly J. The limits of right ventricular compensation following acute increase in pulmonary circulation resistance. Circ Res 1954;2:326–32.

29. Calvin JE Jr. Acute right heart failure: pathophysiology, recognition and pharmacological management. J Cardiothorac Vasc Anesth 1991;5:507–13.

30. Naeije R. Should pulmonary hypertension be treated in chronic obstructive pulmonary disease? In: EK Weir, SL Archer, JT Reeves, eds. The Diagnosis and Treatment of Pulmonary Hypertension. Futura Publishing, New York, 1992, pp 209–39.

31. Riley RL, Himmelstein A, Morley HL, Motley HL, Weiner HM, Cournand A. Studies on the pulmonary circulation at rest and during exercise in normal individuals and in patients with chronic pulmonary disease. Am J Physiol 1948;152:372–82.

32. Segel N, Bishop JM. The circulation in patients with chronic bronchitis and emphysema at rest and during exercise with special reference to the influence of changes in blood viscosity and blood volume on the pulmonary circulation. J Clin Invest 1966;45:1555–68.

33. Burrows B. Arterial oxygenation and pulmonary hemodynamics in patients with chronic airflow obstruction. Am Rev Respir Dis 1974;110:64–70.

34. Boushy SF, North LB. Hemodynamic changes in chronic obstructive pulmonary disease. Chest 1977;72:562–70.

35. Burrows B, Kettel LJ, Nielsen AH, Rabinowitz M, Diener CF. Patterns of cardiovascular dysfunction in chronic obstructive lung disease. N Engl J Med 1972;286:912–18.

36. Weitzenblum E, Loiseau A, Hirth C, Mirhom R, Rasaholinjanahary J. Course of pulmonary hemodynamics in patients with chronic obstructive pulmonary disease. Chest 1979;75:656–62.

37. Schrijen F, Uffholz H, Plu JM, Poincelot F. Pulmonary and systemic hemodynamic evolution in chronic bronchitis. Am Rev Respir Dise 1978;117:25–31.

38. Weitzenblum E, Hirth C, Duculone A, Mirhom R, Rasaholinjanahary J, Ehrhart M. Prognostic value of pulmonary artery pressure in chronic obstructive pulmonary disease. Thorax 1981;36:752–8.

39. Harris P, Segel N, Bishop JM. The relation between pressure and flow in the pulmonary circulation in normal subjects and in patients with chronic bronchitis and mitral stenosis. Cardiovasc Res 1968;2:73–83.

40. McGregor M, Sniderman A. On pulmonary vascular resistance: the need for more precise definition. Am J Cardiol 1985;55:217–21.

41. Even P, Duroux P, Ruff F, Caubarrere I, Brouet G, de Vernejoul P. The pressure–flow relationship of the pulmonary circulation in normal man and in chronic obstructive pulmonary disease: effects of muscular exercise. Scand J Respir Dis 1977; 77(suppl):72–6.

42. Ninane V, Yernault JC, De Troyer A. Intrinsic PEEP in patients with chronic obstructive pulmonary disease: role of expiratory muscles. Am Rev Respir Dis 1993;148:1037–42.

43. Shaw DR, Grover RF, Reeves JT, Blount G Jr. Pulmonary circulation in chronic bronchitis and emphysema. Br Heart J 1965;27:674–83.

44. Lockhart A, Nader F, Tzareva M, Schrijen F. Comparative effects of exercise and isocapnic voluntary hyperventilation on pulmonary haemodynamics in chronic bronchitis and emphysema. Eur J Clin Invest 1970;1:69–76.

45. Weitzenblum E, El-Gharbi T, Vandevenne A, Bieger A, Hirth C, Oudet P. Pulmonary hemodynamic changes during muscular exercise in non decompensated chronic bronchitis. Bull Eur Physiopathol Respir 1972;8:49–71.

46. Light RW, Mintz HM, Linden GS, Brown SE. Hemodynamics of patients with severe chronic obstructive pulmonary disease during progressive upright exercise. Am Rev Respir Dis 1984;130:391–5.

47. Mahler DA, Brent BN, Loke J, Zaret BL, Matthay RA. Right ventricular performance and central circulatory hemodynamics during upright exercise in patients with chronic obstructive pulmonary disease. Am Rev Respir Dis 1984;130:722–9.

48. Robotham JL. Cardiovascular disturbances in chronic respiratory insufficiency. Am J Cardiol 1981;47:941–9.

49. Gelb AF, Lyons HA, Fairshter RD, et al. P pulmonale in status asthmaticus. J Allergy Clin Immunol 1978;64:18–22.

50. Coccagna G, Lugaresi E. Arterial blood gases and pulmonary and systemic arterial pressure during sleep in chronic obstructive pulmonary disease. Sleep 1978;1:117–24.

51. Boysen PG, Block AJ, Wynne JW, Hunt LA, Flick MR. Nocturnal pulmonary hypertension in patients with chronic obstructive pulmonary disease. *Chest* 1979;**76**:536–42.

52. Weitzenblum E, Muzet A, Ehrhart M, Ehrhart J, Sautegeau A, Weber L. Variations nocturnes des gaz du sang et de la pression artérielle pulmonaire chez les bronchitiques chroniques insuffisants respiratoires. *Nouv Presse Med* 1982;**11**:1119–22.

53. Fletcher EC, Gray BA, Levin DC. Non-apneic mechanism of arterial oxygen desaturation during rapid-eye-movement sleep. *J Appl Physiol* 1983;**54**:632–9.

54. Hudgel DW, Martin RJ, Capehart M, Johnson B, Hill P. Contribution of hypoventilation to sleep oxygen desaturation in chronic obstructive pulmonary disease. *J Appl Physiol* 1983;**55**:669–77.

55. Weitzenblum E, Krieger J, Apprill M, *et al*. Daytime pulmonary hypertension in patients with obstructive sleep apnea syndrome. *Am Rev Respir Dis* 1988;**138**:345–9.

56. Sajkov D, Wang T, Saunders NA, Bune AJ, Neill AM, McEvoy RD. Daytime pulmonary hemodynamics in patients with obstructive sleep apnea without lung disease. *Am J Respir Crit Care Med* 1999;**159**:1518–26.

57. Lockhart A, Tzareva M, Schrijen F, Sadoul P. Etudes hémodynamiques des décompensations respiratoires aiguës des bronchopneumopathies chroniques. *Bull Physiopathol Respir* 1967;**3**:645–67.

58. Abraham AS, Cole RB, Green ID, Hedworth-Whitty RB, Clarke SW, Bishop JM. Factors contributing to the reversible pulmonary hypertension of patients with acute respiratory failure studied by serial observations during recovery. *Circ Res* 1969;**24**:51–60.

59. Weitzenblum E, Hirth C, Roeslin N, Vandevenne A, Oudet P. Les modifications hémodynamiques pulmonaires au cours de l'insuffisance respiratoire aiguë des bronchopneumopathies chroniques. *Respiration* 1971;**28**:539–54.

60. Weitzenblum E, Sautegeau A, Ehrhart M, Mammoser M, Hirth C, Roegel E. Long-term course of pulmonary artery pressure in chronic obstructive pulmonary disease. *Am Rev Respir Dis* 1984;**117**:25–31.

61. Medical Research Council Working Party. Long-term domiciliary oxygen therapy in chronic hypoxic cor pulmonale complicating chronic bronchitis and emphysema. *Lancet* 1981;**i**:681–6.

62. Timms RM, Khaja FU, Williams GW, and the Nocturnal Oxygen Therapy Trial Group. Hemodynamic response to oxygen therapy in chronic obstructive pulmonary disease. *Ann Intern Med* 1985;**102**:29–36.

63. Weitzenblum E, Sautegeau A, Ehrhart M, Mammosser M, Pelletier A. Long-term oxygen therapy can reverse the progression of pulmonary hypertension in patients withchronic obstructive pulmonary disease. *Am Rev Respir Dis* 1985;**131**:493–8.

64. Zielinski J, Tobiasz M, Hawrylkiewicz I, Sliwinski P, Palasiewicz G. Effects of long-term oxygen therapy on pulmonary hemodynamics in COPD patients: a 6-year prospective study. *Chest* 1998;**113**:65–70.

65. Ellis JH, Kirch D, Steele PP. Right ventricular ejection fraction in severe chronic airflow obstruction. *Chest* 1977; **71**(suppl):281–2.

66. MacNee W, Xue QF, Hannan WJ, Flenley DC, Adie CJ, Muir AL. Assessment by radionuclide angiography of right and left ventricular function in chronic bronchitis and emphysema. *Thorax* 1983;**38**:494–500.

67. Berger HJ, Matthay RA, Loke J, Marshal RC, Gottschalk A, Zaret BL. Cardiac performance with quantitative radionuclide angiocardiography: right ventricular ejection fraction with reference to findings in chronic obstructive pulmonary disease. *Am J Cardiol* 1978;**41**:897–905.

68. Matthay RA, Berger HJ, Davies RA, *et al*. Right and left ventricular exercise performance in chronic obstructive pulmonary disease. *Ann Intern Med* 1980;**93**:234–9.

69. Brent BN, Berger HJ, Matthay RA, Mahler D, Pytlik L, Zaret BL. Physiological correlates of right ventricular ejection fraction in chronic obstructive pulmonary disease. A combined radionuclide hemodynamic study. *Am J Cardiol* 1982;**50**:225–62.

70. Oliver RM, Fleming JS, Waller DG. Right ventricular function at rest and during exercise in chronic obstructive pulmonary disease. Comparison of two radionuclide techniques. *Chest* 1993;**103**:74–80.

71. Biernacki W, Flenley DC, Muir AL, MacNee W. Pulmonary hypertension and right ventricular function in COPD. *Chest* 1988;**94**:1169–75.

72. MacNee W, Wathen C, Flenley D, Muir AL. The effects of controlled oxygen therapy on ventricular function in acute and chronic respiratory failure. *Am Rev Respir Dis* 1988;**137**:1289–95.

73. MacNee W, Wathen CG, Hannan WJ, Flenley DC, Muir AL. Effect of pirbiterol and sodium nitroprusside on pulmonary hemodynamics in hypoxic cor pulmonale. *Br Med J* 1983;**287**:1169–72.

74. Khaja F, Parker JO. Right and left ventricular performance in chronic obstructive lung disease. *Am Heart J* 1971;**82**:319–27.

75. Wasserman K, Whipp BJ. Exercise physiology in health and disease. *Am Rev Respir Dis* 1975;**112**:219–49.

76. Kountz WB, Alexander HL, Prizmetal M. The heart in emphysema. *Am Heart J* 1936;**11**:163–72.

77. Kohama A, Tanouchi J, Masatsugu H, Kitabatake A, Kamada T. Pathologic involvement of the left ventricle in cor pulmonale. *Chest* 1990;**98**:794–800.

78. Vizza D, Lynch JP, Ochoa LL, Richardson G, Trulock EP. Right and left ventricular dysfunction in patients with severe pulmonary disease. *Chest* 1998;**113**:576–83.

79. Mal H, Levy A, Laperche T, *et al*. Limitations of radionuclide angiographic assessment of left ventricular systolic function before lung transplantation. *Am J Respir Crit Care Med* 1998;**158**:1396–402.

80. Campbell EJM, Short DS. The cause of oedema in 'cor pulmonale'. *Lancet* 1960;**i**:1184–6.

81. Bauduin SV. Oedema and cor pulmonale revisited. *Thorax* 1997;**52**:401–2.

82. Weitzenblum E, Apprill M, Oswald M, Chaouat A, Imbs JL. Pulmonary hemodynamics in patients with chronic obstructive pulmonary disease before and during an episode of peripheral edema. *Chest* 1994;**105**:1377–82.

83. Anand IS, Chandrasekhar Y, Ferrari R, *et al*. Pathogenesis of congestive state in chronic obstructive pulmonary disease. *Circulation* 1992;**86**:12–21.

84. Dornhorst A. Respiratory insufficiency. *Lancet* 1955;**i**:1185–7.

85. Burrows B, Fletcher CM, Heard BE, Jones NL, Woatliff JS. Emphysematous and bronchial types of chronic airways obstruction: clinicopathological study of patients in London and Chicago. *Lancet* 1966;**i**:830–5.

86. Filley GF. Emphysema and chronic bronchitis: clinical manifestations and their physiological significance. *Med Clin North Am* 1967;**51**:283–92.

87. Jamal K, Fleetham JA, Thurlbeck WM. Cor pulmonale: correlations with central airways lesions, peripheral airways lesions, emphysema, and control of breathing. *Am Rev Respir Dis* 1990;**141**:1172–7.

88. Biernacki W, Gould GA, Whyte KF, Flenley DC. Pulmonary hemodynamics, gas exchange, and the severity of emphysema as assessed by quantitative CT scan in chronic bronchitis and emphysema. *Am Rev Respir Dis* 1989;**139**: 1509–15.

89. Rubin LJ. Primary pulmonary hypertension. *N Engl J Med* 1997;**336**:111–17.

90. Matthay RA, Schwarz MI, Ellis JH, Steele PP, Seibert PE, Durrance JR, Levin DC. Pulmonary artery hypertension in chronic obstructive lung disease: determination by chest radiography. *Invest Radiol* 1981;**16**:95–100.

91. Naeije R, Torbicki A. More on the noninvasive diagnosis of pulmonary hypertension. Doppler echocardiography revisited. *Eur Respir J* 1995;**8**:1445–9.

92. Torbicki A, Skwarski K, Hawrylkiewicz I, Pasierski T, Miskiewicz Z, Zielinski J. Attempts of measuring pulmonary artery pressure by means of Doppler echocardiography in patients with chronic lung disease. *Eur Respir J* 1989;**2**: 856–60.

93. Pauwels RA, Buist AS, Calverley MA, Jenkins CR, Hurd SS, GOLD Scientific Committee. Global strategy for the diagnosis, management, and prevention of chronic obstructive pulmonary disease: National Heart, Lung, and Blood Institute and World Health Organization Global Initiative for Chronic Obstructive Lung Disease (GOLD): executive summary. *Resp Care* 2001;**46**:798–825.

94. Redelmeier DA, Bayoumi AM, Goldstein RS, Guyatt GH. Interpreting small differences in functional status: the six minute walk test in chronic lung disease patients. *Am J Respir Crit Care Med* 1997;**155**:1278–82.

95. Weitzenblum E, Chaouat A. Right ventricular function in COPD. Can it be assessed reliably by the measurement of right ventricular ejection fraction. *Chest* 1998;**113**:567–8.

96. Quanadli SD, El Hajjam M, Mesurolle B, *et al.* Pulmonary embolism: prospective evaluation of dual-section helical CT versus selective pulmonary arteriography in 157 patients. *Radiology* 2000;**217**:447–55.

97. Stein PD, Henry JW. Prevalence of acute pulmonary embolism in central and subsegmental pulmonary arteries and relation to probability interpretation of ventilation/ perfusion lung scan. *Chest* 1997;**111**:1246–8.

98. Moser KM, Auger WR, Fedullo PF, Jamieson SW. Chronic thromboembolic pulmonary hypertension: clinical picture and surgical treatment. *Eur Respir J* 1992;**5**:334–42.

99. Ferguson GT, Cherniack RM. Management of chronic obstructive pulmonary disease. *N Engl J Med* 1993;**328**: 1017–22.

100. Nocturnal Oxygen Therapy Trial Group. Continuous or nocturnal oxygen therapy in hypoxemic chronic obstructive lung disease: a clinical trial. *Ann Intern Med* 1980;**93**: 391–8.

101. Tarpy SP, Celli BR. Long-term oxygen therapy. *N Engl J Med* 1995;**333**:710–14.

102. Fishman AP, McClement J, Himmelstein A. Effects of acute anoxia on the circulation and respiration in patients with chronic pulmonary disease studied during the steady state. *J Clin Invest* 1952;**31**:770–81.

103. Degaute JP, Domenighetti G, Naeije R, Vincent JL, Treyvaud D, Perret C. Oxygen delivery in acute exacerbation of chronic obstructive pulmonary disease. Effects of controlled oxygen therapy. *Am Rev Respir Dis* 1981;**124**:26–30.

104. Olvey SK, Reduto LA, Stevens PM, Deaton WJ, Miller RR. First pass radionuclide assessment of right and left ventricular ejection fraction in chronic pulmonary disease. Effect of oxygen upon exercise response. *Chest* 1980;**78**:4–9.

105. Sliwinski P, Hawrylkiewicz I, Gorecka D, Zielinski J. Acute testing of oxygen on pulmonary arterial pressure does not predict survival on long-term oxygen therapy in patients with chronic obstructive pulmonary disease. *Am Rev Respir Dis* 1992;**146**:665–9.

106. Roger N, Barbera JA, Roca J, Rovira I, Gomez FP, Rodriguez-Roisin R. Nitric oxide inhalation during exercise in chronic obstructive pulmonary disease. *Am J Respir Crit Care Med* 1997;**156**:800–6.

107. Katayama Y, Higenbottam TW, Cremona G, *et al.* Minimizing the inhaled dose of NO with breath-by-breath delivery of spikes of concentrated gas. *Circulation* 1998;**98**:2429–32.

108. Channick RN, Newhart JW, Johnson FW, *et al.* Pulsed delivery of inhaled nitric oxide to patients with primary pulmonary hypertension: an ambulatory delivery system and initial clinical tests. *Chest* 1996;**109**:1545–9.

109. Adnot S, Kouyoumdjian C, Defouilloy C, *et al.* Hemodynamic and gas exchange responses to infusion of acetylcholine and inhalation of nitric oxide in patients with chronic obstructive lung disease and pulmonary hypertension. *Am Rev Respir Dis* 1993;**148**:310–16.

110. Katayama Y, Higenbottam TW, Diaz de Atauri MJ, *et al.* Inhaled nitric oxide and arterial oxygen tension in patients with chronic obstructive pulmonary disease and severe pulmonary hypertension. *Thorax* 1997;**52**:120–4.

111. Erickson AD, Golde WA, Claunch BC, Donat WE, Kaemmerlen JT. Acute effects of phlebotomy on right ventricular size and performance in polycythemic patients with chronic obstructive pulmonary disease. *Am J Cardiol* 1983;**52**:163–6.

112. Chetty KG, Brown SE, Light RW. Improved exercise tolerance in the polycythemic lung patient following phlebotomy. *Am J Med* 1983;**74**:415–20.

113. Corris PA. Lung transplantation. In: AJ Peacock, ed. *Pulmonary Circulation: A Handbook for Clinicians.* Chapman & Hall Medical, London, 1996, pp 348–58.

114. Bjortuft O, Simonsen S, Geiran OR, Fjeld JG, Skovlund E, Boe J. Pulmonary haemodynamics after single-lung transplantation for end-stage pulmonary parenchymal disease. *Eur Respir J* 1996;**9**:2007–11.

115. Cooper JD, Trulock EP, Triantafillou AN, *et al.* Bilateral pneumectomy (volume reduction) for chronic obstructive pulmonary disease. *J Thorac Cardiovasc Surg* 1995;**109**: 106–16.

116. Sciurba FC, Rogers RM, Keenan RJ, *et al.* Improvement in pulmonary function and elastic recoil after lung-reduction surgery for diffuse emphysema. *N Engl J Med* 1996;**334**: 1095–9.

117. Weg IL, Rossoff L, McKeon K, Michael GL, Scharf SM. Development of pulmonary hypertension after lung volume reduction surgery. *Am J Respir Crit Care Med* 1999;**159**: 552–6.

118. Oswald-Mammosser M, Kessler R, Massard G, Wihlm JM, Weitzenblum E, Lonsdorfer J. Effect of lung volume reduction surgery on gas exchange and pulmonary hemodynamics at rest and during exercise. *Am J Respir Crit Care Med* 1998;**158**:1020–5.

119. Kubo K, Koizumi T, Fujimoto K, *et al.* Effects of lung volume reduction surgery on exercise pulmonary hemodynamics in severe emphysema. *Chest* 1998;**114**:1575–82.

120. Bishop JM. Hypoxia and pulmonary hypertension in chronic bronchitis. *Prog Respir Dis* 1975;**9**:10–16.

121. Oswald-Mammoser M, Weitzenblum E, Quoix E, *et al.* Prognostic factors in COPD patients receiving long-term oxygen therapy. Importance of pulmonary artery pressure. *Chest* 1995;**107**:1193–8.

18

Exercise

DENIS E O'DONNELL AND KATHERINE A WEBB

INTRODUCTION

The inability to engage in the usual activities of daily living is one of the most distressing experiences of people afflicted with COPD. Exercise intolerance progresses relentlessly as the disease advances and can lead to virtual immobility and social isolation. A pervasive skepticism about the value of therapeutic interventions in this population has now given way to a general acceptance that comprehensive management strategies, that are based on a sound physiologic rationale, are clinically effective, even in advanced disease. Our understanding of the complex interface between physiological impairment and disability in COPD has increased considerably in recent years and is the main focus of this chapter. It has become clear that in COPD, exercise intolerance ultimately reflects integrated abnormalities of the ventilatory, cardiovascular, peripheral muscle and neurosensory systems. Ventilatory limitation is the dominant contributor to exercise curtailment in more advanced disease and will be considered in detail. Ventilatory responses to exercise in health will be reviewed so as to better understand the derangements of ventilatory mechanics peculiar to this disease, and how these can be therapeutically manipulated to improve exercise performance. Recent important research into the role of peripheral muscle dysfunction in exercise limitation will be reviewed, as well as emerging concepts on the pathophysiology of cardiopulmonary interactions in COPD.

VENTILATORY RESPONSE TO EXERCISE IN HEALTH

In health, the respiratory system admirably fulfils its task of ensuring adequate gas exchange to meet the challenge of increasing energy expenditure during exercise. Precise humoral and neuromechanical regulation ensures that alveolar ventilation rises linearly as a function of carbon dioxide output ($\dot{V}CO_2$) so that alveolar CO_2 and CO_2 and O_2, and thus arterial PO_2 and PCO_2 are maintained near resting values throughout exercise. The respiratory system is highly efficient during maximal exercise: young, untrained adults can accomplish very high ventilation levels (~120 L/min) while using only 5–7% of the total body oxygen uptake ($\dot{V}O_2$).[1]

During exercise in health, ventilatory work and the oxygen cost of breathing are minimized through several acute physiological adjustments. Progressive expiratory muscle recruitment reduces dynamic end-expiratory lung volume (EELV) below the relaxation volume of the respiratory system (Vr)[2–4] (Figure 18.1). The magnitude of EELV reduction varies with the type and intensity of exercise – average reductions between 0.3 and 1.0 L below Vr have been reported.[4–6] Expiratory muscle recruitment offers the following advantages in health. It allows tidal volume (VT) to expand to a maximum of 50 to 60% of the vital capacity (VC) by encroaching equally on the expiratory and inspiratory reserve volumes (ERV and IRV)[6] (Figure 18.1). This ensures that VT is positioned on the linear portion of the respiratory system's pressure–volume

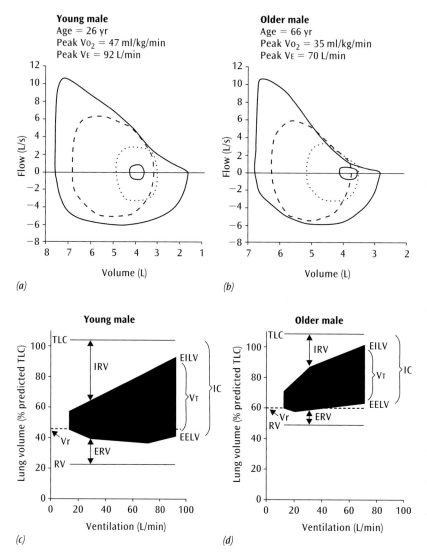

Figure 18.1 *Maximal and tidal flow–volume loops are shown at rest and during incremental cycle exercise in a healthy, younger (a) and older (b) male subjects. Tidal flow–volume loops are provided at rest (solid line), at a submaximal ventilation of approximately 30 L/min (dotted line), and at peak exercise (dashed line). Note expiratory flow limitation (tidal expiratory flow overlapping the maximal curve) and an increase in dynamic end-expiratory lung volume (EELV) during exercise in the older male. (c,d) In the same subjects, lung volumes are shown relative to ventilation during exercise. There are greater volume constraints on V_T expansion (solid area) during exercise in the older subject: i.e. increased RV and dynamic EELV, and a relatively reduced inspiratory reserve volume (i.e. IRV = TLC − EILV) at similar submaximal levels of ventilation. See text for definition of abbreviations.*

relationship (i.e. 20–80% of VC) throughout exercise, thus avoiding the alinear extremes where there is increased elastic loading[6] (Figures 18.1 and 18.2). The release of stored energy from the expiratory (abdominal) muscles also serves to assist the inspiratory muscles and the increased intra-abdominal pressure optimizes diaphragmatic length at the onset of the ensuing inspiration.[3] In young adults, the pressures generated by the expiratory muscles during exercise are generally well below the critical pressures associated with expiratory flow limitation.[7] Therefore, the avoidance of expiratory flow limitation and consequent dynamic airway compression contributes importantly to ventilatory efficiency in health.[7]

The resistive work of breathing is minimized during exercise despite large increases in respired flow rates by: (i) switching from nasal breathing to oronasal breathing; (ii) phasic activation of upper airway abductor muscles; and (iii) airway bronchodilatation as a result of increased circulating catecholamines.[8] In health, there is little difference between the total ventilation (V_E) and alveolar ventilation ($\dot{V}_A$) when both are expressed as a function of $\dot{V}_{O_2}$ or work rate.[9] This matching occurs because physiologic deadspace (V_D/V_T) progressively declines by approximately 30% of the baseline value at the end of exercise – in healthy young people deadspace ventilation represents only about 13% of the total ventilation at maximal exercise.[10]

Ventilatory responses in elderly, healthy individuals

Since COPD is primarily a disease of the elderly, the most appropriate 'control group' for the study of cardioventilatory responses to exercise is that of age-matched healthy subjects. In contrast to youth, these older individuals demonstrate significant ventilatory constraints, particularly under conditions of high ventilatory demand.[10–13] The oxygen cost of breathing required to maintain high ventilation levels in the elderly is higher than in youth for a number of reasons. Progressive structural changes in the connective tissue matrix of the lung parenchyma cause loss of the static lung elastic recoil pressures which drive expiratory flow.[14–17] Therefore, expiratory flow rates decline, particularly over the effort-independent portion of the maximal expiratory flow–volume curve, and flow limitation becomes evident[18] (Figure 18.1). Moreover, chest wall compliance is reduced due to decreased intervertebral disc spaces (mild kyphosis) and calcification of the costal cartilage.[18,19] These combined effects alter respiratory system mechanics such that functional residual capacity (FRC) and residual volume (RV) are increased with reciprocal decrease of inspiratory capacity (IC) and VC, respectively.[17,19] Total lung capacity (TLC) is generally preserved in the elderly.[19]

During strenuous exercise, the ability to reduce EELV below the resting relaxation volume of the respiratory system is diminished because of expiratory flow limitation (Figure 18.1). In fact, at high ventilation levels, increases in dynamic EELV occur as a result of reduced lung emptying and air trapping.[11–13] This is termed dynamic hyperinflation (DH). The propensity to develop DH is increased by the combination of flow limitation and increased ventilatory demand in the elderly (compared with youth). The latter reflects a higher physiologic deadspace, which is a result of greater ventilation-perfusion inequalities in the aged lung. V_D/V_T has been estimated to be as much as 30% of V_E in the elderly.[20] DH results in higher dynamic end-inspiratory lung volume (EILV) relative to TLC than in youth at a given submaximal ventilation[10,20] (Figure 18.1). Although DH optimizes expiratory flow rates by avoiding expiratory flow limitation at volumes near RV, it increases the elastic work on the inspiratory muscles.[11] As a result, the pressures generated by the inspiratory muscles during tidal breathing in the elderly represent a higher fraction of the maximal possible dynamic inspiratory force generating capacity than in youth for a given V_E and $\dot{V}_{O_2}$.[11,21] Consequently, the oxygen cost of breathing at maximal exercise represents approximately 13% of the total body $\dot{V}_{O_2}$, or almost 40% greater than in an untrained youth at a similar V_E.[10,11] Therefore, in many respects, the ventilatory response to exercise in the elderly is similar to that of mild COPD (see below).

However, in the elderly, metabolic demands and VC appear to fall in parallel with the passage of time, and it is only in highly fit individuals with high peak $\dot{V}_{O_2}$ and V_E that ventilatory constraints may actually curtail exercise performance.[10]

EXERCISE LIMITATION IN COPD

Exercise limitation is multifactorial in COPD. Recognized contributing factors include: (i) ventilatory limitation due to impaired respiratory system mechanics and ventilatory muscle dysfunction; (ii) metabolic and gas exchange abnormalities; (iii) peripheral muscle dysfunction; (iv) cardiac impairment; (v) intolerable exertional symptoms; and (vi) any combination of these interdependent factors. The predominant contributing factors to exercise limitation vary among patients with COPD or, indeed, in a given patient over time. The more advanced the disease, the more of these factors come into play in a complex integrative manner.

Ventilatory constraints on exercise performance in COPD

In patients with severe COPD, ventilatory limitation is often the predominant contributor to exercise intolerance. The patient is deemed to have ventilatory limitation if, at the breakpoint of exercise, he or she has reached estimated maximum ventilatory capacity (MVC), while at the same time cardiac and other physiologic functions are operating below maximal capacity.

In practice, it is difficult to precisely determine if ventilatory limitation is the proximate boundary to exercise performance in a given individual. Attendant respiratory discomfort may limit exercise before actual physiologic limitation occurs, and the relative importance of other non-ventilatory factors is impossible to quantify with precision. Our assessment of the MVC, as estimated from resting spirometry (i.e. $FEV_{1.0} \times 35$ or 40)[22,23] or from brief bursts of voluntary hyperventilation is inaccurate.[24] Prediction of the peak ventilation actually achieved during exercise from maximal voluntary ventilation at rest is problematic because the pattern of ventilatory muscle recruitment, the changes in intrathoracic pressures and in respired flows and volumes, and the extent of DH are often vastly different under the two conditions.[24] While an increased ratio (i.e. >90%) of peak exercise ventilation (V_E) to the estimated MVC strongly suggests limiting ventilatory constraints, a preserved peak V_E/MVC ratio (i.e. <75%) by no means excludes the possibility of significant ventilatory impairment during exercise.[25] Thus, simultaneous analysis of exercise flow–volume loops at the symptom-limited peak of exercise may show marked constraints on flow and volume generation in the presence of an apparently adequate ventilatory reserve as estimated from the peak V_E/MVC ratios.[25]

Ventilatory mechanics in COPD

COPD is a heterogeneous disorder characterized by dysfunction of the small and large airways and by parenchymal and vascular destruction, in highly variable combinations. Although the most obvious physiologic defect in COPD is expiratory flow limitation, due to

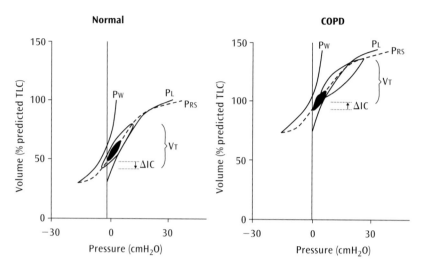

Figure 18.2 *Pressure–volume (P–V) relationships of the lung (PL), chest wall (PW) and total respiratory system (PRS) in health and in COPD. Tidal pressure–volume curves during rest (filled area) and exercise (open area) are provided. Note that in COPD, because of resting and dynamic hyperinflation (a further decreased IC), exercise VT encroaches on the upper alinear extreme of the respiratory system's P–V curve where there is increased elastic loading.*

combined reduced lung recoil (and airway tethering effects) as well as intrinsic airway narrowing, the most important mechanical consequence of this is a 'restrictive' ventilatory deficit due to DH[25–27] (Figure 18.2). When expiratory flow limitation reaches a critical level, lung emptying becomes incomplete during resting tidal breathing, and lung volume fails to decline to its natural equilibrium point (i.e. the relaxation volume of the respiratory system). EELV, therefore, becomes dynamically and not statically determined and represents a higher resting lung volume than in health[26] (Figure 18.2). In flow-limited patients, EELV is therefore, a continuous variable which fluctuates widely with rest and activity. When ventilation (VE) increases in flow-limited patients, as for example during exercise, increases in EELV (or DH) are inevitable (Figure 18.3). As already mentioned, DH (and its negative mechanical consequences) can occur in the healthy elderly, but at much higher VE and $\dot{V}_{O_2}$ levels than in COPD.[10]

The extent to which EELV exceeds the relaxation volume of the respiratory system depends on the magnitude of VT, expiratory time (TE), and the time constant (resistance × compliance) for emptying of the respiratory system as expressed in the equation:[28]

$$EELV - Vr = \frac{V_T}{e^{T_E/trs} - 1}$$

where Vr = relaxation volume, trs = time constant for emptying of the respiratory system, base e = 2.718282. As VT is increased during exercise, more time is required to allow volumes to decrease to Vr – an increase in VT at the same (or shorter TE) results in increased EELV. For practical purposes, the extent of DH during exercise depends on the extent of expiratory flow limitation, the level of baseline lung hyperinflation, the prevailing ventilatory demand and the breathing pattern for a given ventilation.[25] A possible compensatory strategy in the face of flow limitation is to increase TE, or reduce the inspiratory

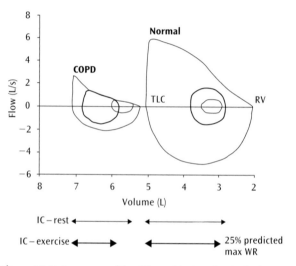

Figure 18.3 *In a normal healthy subject and a typical patient with COPD, tidal flow–volume loops at rest and during exercise (peak exercise in COPD compared with exercise at a comparable metabolic load in the age-matched person) are shown in relation to their respective maximal flow–volume loops. WR: work rate. (Adapted from ref. 184.)*

duty cycle (TI/TTOT). Given the markedly reduced maximal expiratory flow rates at lower lung volumes (i.e. 0.4 L/s near Vr), substantial prolongation of TE would be required to facilitate lung emptying. Such delays are not usually observed in COPD during exercise. Several studies have shown that in severe COPD, TI/TTOT remains relatively fixed from rest to peak exercise.[29–31] Moreover, a further reduction in TI/TTOT would require a corresponding increase in mean inspiratory flow rates (VT/TI) to preserve VT. This in turn would translate into increased velocity of shortening of the inspiratory muscles, with associated functional inspiratory muscle weakness, which would be expected to further hasten ventilatory limitation.[21]

Serial IC measurements have been used to track EELV during exercise for more than 30 years.[30-33] This approach is based on the reasonable assumption that TLC does not change appreciably during exercise in COPD and that reductions in dynamic IC must, therefore, reflect increases in EELV.[33] However, regardless of any possible changes in TLC with exercise, progressive reduction of an already diminished resting IC means that VT becomes positioned closer to the actual TLC and the upper, alinear extreme of the respiratory system's pressure–volume relationship, where there is increased elastic loading of the respiratory muscles (Figure 18.2). Reduction of IC as exercise progresses is likely a true reflection of shifts in EELV rather than simply the inability to generate maximal effort because of dyspnea or functional muscle weakness. In fact, several studies have established that dyspneic patients, even at the end of exhaustive exercise, are capable of generating maximal inspiratory efforts, as assessed by peak inspiratory esophageal pressures.[34,35] Moreover, we have recently shown that IC measurements during constant-load cycle exercise are both highly reproducible and responsive in patients with severe COPD, provided due attention is taken with their measurement.[36]

The extent and pattern of DH development in COPD patients during exercise is highly variable (Figure 18.4). Clearly, some patients do not increase EELV during exercise, whereas others show dramatic increases (i.e. >1 L).[30-36] We recently studied the pattern and magnitude of DH during incremental cycle exercise in 105 patients with COPD (FEV$_{1.0}$ = 37 ± 13% predicted; mean ± SD)[25] (Figures 18.4, 18.5). The majority of this sample (80%) demonstrated significant increases in EELV above resting values: dynamic IC decreased significantly by 0.37 ± 0.39 L (or 14 ± 15% predicted) from rest.[25] Similar levels of DH have recently been reported in COPD patients after completing a 6-minute walking test while breathing without an imposed mouthpiece.[37] For the same FEV$_{1.0}$, patients with a lower diffusion capacity (DLco < 50 % predicted), and presumably more emphysema, had faster rates of DH at lower exercise levels, earlier attainment of critical volume constraints (peak VT), greater exertional dyspnea and lower peak VE and V̇o$_2$ when compared with patients with a relatively preserved DLco.[25] In the latter group, the magnitude of rest to peak change in EELV was similar to that of the low DLco group, but air trapping increased at a relatively constant, slower rate up to a higher V̇o$_2$ and VE. Patients with predominant emphysema likely had faster rates of DH because of reduced elastic lung recoil (and airway tethering), and an increased propensity to expiratory flow limitation. In this group, DH is often further compounded by a greater ventilatory demand as a result of higher physiologic deadspace, reflecting greater ventilation-perfusion abnormalities.[38] The extent of DH during exercise is inversely correlated with the level of

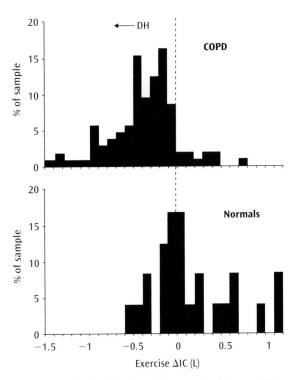

Figure 18.4 *The distribution of the extent of change (Δ) in IC during exercise is shown in COPD (n = 105) and in age-matched normal subjects (n = 25). A negative ΔIC reflects dynamic hyperinflation (DH) during exercise; each bar width corresponds to a ΔIC range of 0.10 L. In contrast to normals, the majority of patients with COPD experienced significant DH during exercise despite reaching a much lower peak ventilation, i.e. 33 versus 64 L/min in COPD and normals, respectively. (From ref. 25 with permission.)*

resting lung hyperinflation: patients who were severely hyperinflated at rest showed minimal further DH during exercise.[25]

Tidal volume restriction and exercise intolerance

An important mechanical consequence of DH is severe mechanical constraints on tidal volume expansion during exercise: VT is truncated from below by the increasing EELV and constrained from above by the TLC envelope and the relatively reduced IRV (Figure 18.5). Thus, compared with age-matched healthy individuals, COPD patients at comparable low work rates and VE showed substantially greater increases in dynamic EILV, a greater ratio of VT to IC, and marked reduction in the IRV (Figure 18.5). In 105 COPD patients, the EILV was found to be 94 ± 5% of TLC at a peak symptom-limited V̇o$_2$ of only 12.6 ± 5.0 ml/kg/min – this indicates that the diaphragm is maximally shortened at this volume and

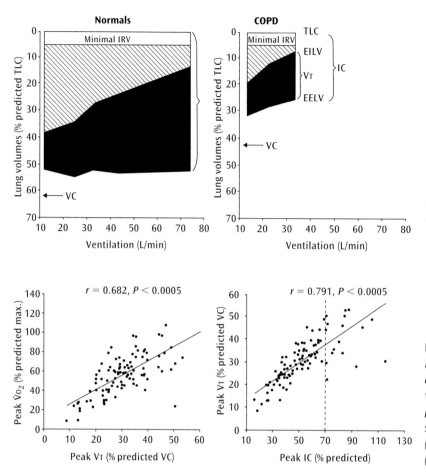

Figure 18.5 *Changes in operational lung volumes are shown as ventilation increases with exercise in COPD and in normal subjects. 'Restrictive' constraints on tidal volume (VT, solid area) expansion during exercise are significantly greater in the COPD group from both below (reduced IC) and above (minimal IRV, open area). (From ref. 25 with permission.)*

Figure 18.6 *In COPD (n = 105), the best correlate of peak oxygen consumption ($\dot{V}O_2$) was the peak tidal volume attained (VT standardized as % predicted vital capacity). In turn, the strongest correlate of peak VT was the (peak) inspiratory capacity (IC). (Adapted from ref. 25.)*

greatly compromised in its ability to generate greater inspiratory pressures.[25]

The resting IC and, in particular, the dynamic IC during exercise (and not the resting VC) represent the true operating limits for VT expansion in any given patient. Therefore, when VT approximates the peak dynamic IC during exercise or the dynamic EILV encroaches on the TLC envelope, further volume expansion is impossible, even in the face of increased central drive and electrical activation of the diaphragm.[39] In our study, using multiple regression analysis with symptom-limited peak $\dot{V}O_2$ as the dependent variable and several relevant physiological measurements as independent variables (including $FEV_{1.0}/FVC$ ratio and VE/MVC), peak VT (standardized as % predicted VC) emerged as the strongest contributory variable, explaining 47% of the variance[25] (Figure 18.6). Peak VT, in turn, correlated strongly with both the resting and peak dynamic IC (Figure 18.6). It is noteworthy that this correlation was particularly strong ($r = 0.9$) in approximately 80% of the sample, who had a diminished resting and peak dynamic IC (i.e. <70% predicted) (Figure 18.6). Studies by Tantucci *et al.*[40] have provided evidence that such patients with a diminished resting IC have demonstrable resting expiratory flow limitation by the negative expiratory pressure (NEP) technique.

Recent studies have confirmed that in patients with COPD, a reduced resting IC with evidence of resting expiratory flow limitation have poorer exercise performance when compared with those with a better preserved resting IC with no evidence of expiratory flow limitation at rest.[25,41,42]

Dynamic hyperinflation and inspiratory muscle dysfunction

While DH serves to maximize tidal expiratory flow rates during exercise, it has serious consequences with respect to dynamic ventilatory mechanics, inspiratory muscle function, perceived respiratory discomfort and, probably, cardiac function (Table 18.1). As already noted DH resulted in 'high-end' pressure–volume mechanics in contrast to health, where the relationship between pressure and volume is relatively constant throughout exercise (Figure 18.2). This results in increased elastic loading of muscles already burdened with increased resistive work. The combined elastic and resistive loads on the ventilatory muscles substantially increase the mechanical work and the oxygen cost of breathing at a given ventilation compared with health (Figure 18.7). It has been estimated

Table 18.1 *Negative effects of dynamic hyperinflation during exercise*

• ↑Elastic/threshold loads • Inspiratory muscle weakness	} ↑Pes/PImax 'effort'
• Reduced VT expansion → tachypnea	} ↓CLdyn ↑VD/VT ↑PaCO2

• Early ventilatory limitation to
  exercise
• ↑Exertional dyspnea
• ↓Cardiovascular function

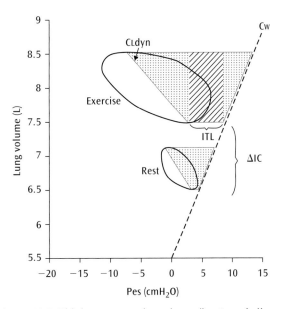

Figure 18.7 *Tidal pressure–volume loops (i.e. Campbell diagrams) during rest and exercise in a patient with COPD. Note the increased elastic (dotted area) and inspiratory threshold loads (hatched area) as a result of dynamic hyperinflation (ΔIC). CLdyn: dynamic lung compliance; Cw: chest wall compliance; Pes: esophageal pressure ITL: inspiratory threshold load.*

that at a peak exercise $\dot{V}_E$ of approximately 20 L/min, ventilatory work may approach 20 joules/min and respiratory muscle $\dot{V}_{O_2}$ may be as much as 300 ml/min in severe, mechanically compromised COPD patients.[43] In patients with poor exercise performance (peak symptom-limited $\dot{V}_{O_2} < 1$ L/min) this represents a much higher fraction (approximately one-third) of the total body $\dot{V}_{O_2}$ at this low ventilation compared with health.[43]

Another more recently recognized mechanical consequence of DH is inspiratory muscle threshold loading (ITL).[26,44] Since, in flow-limited patients, inspiration begins before tidal lung emptying is complete, the inspiratory muscles must first counterbalance the combined inward (expiratory) recoil at the lung and chest wall before inspiratory flow is initiated. This phenomenon (i.e. reduced lung emptying) is associated with positive intrapulmonary pressures at the end of quiet expiration (i.e. autoPEEP or intrinsic PEEP) and may have important implications for dyspnea causation.[45] The ITL, which is present throughout inspiration and which may occur at rest in flow-limited patients, further increases in conjunction with DH during exercise and can be substantial[35] (Figure 18.7).

DH alters the length–tension relationship of the inspiratory muscles, particularly the diaphragm, and compromises its ability to generate pressure. Sinderby et al.[39] have recently shown that DH during exercise greatly compromises the diaphragm's pressure-generating capacity; during progressive exercise, transdiaphragmatic pressures increased only modestly and plateaued at a relatively low $\dot{V}_{O_2}$ (Figure 18.8). However, simultaneous diaphragmatic electrical activity (relative to maximum) increased progressively; at end-exercise this was estimated to be as much as 81% of the maximal possible value[39] (Figure 18.8). These results indicated that central inhibition of respiratory drive, as a result of mechanical overloading, does not appear to occur during exercise in patients with severe COPD, and that severe neuromechanical dissociation is present (see below).

The tachypnea associated with an increased elastic load causes increased velocity of muscle shortening during

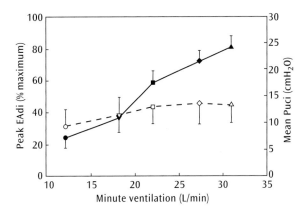

Figure 18.8 *Graph showing the group mean values of peak diaphragm electrical activity (EAdi: closed symbols, left y-axis) and mean transdiaphragmatic pressure (Puci: open symbols, right y-axis) plotted against minute ventilation (x-axis) during resting breathing (circles), as well as 0–3% (triangle with base up), 33–66% (squares), 66–99% (diamond) and 100% (triangle with base down) of exercise time. Values are mean ± SD. Solid line represents peak EAdi; dashed line represents mean PDi. (From ref. 39 with permission.)*

exercise and results in further functional inspiratory muscle weakness.[26] Exercise tachypnea also results in reduced dynamic lung compliance, which has an exaggerated frequency dependence in COPD.[26] Because of

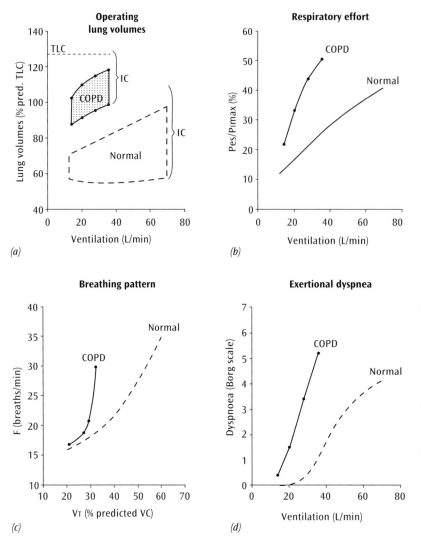

Figure 18.9 *Behavior of (a) operating lung volumes, (b) respiratory effort (Pes/Pimax) and (d) exertional dyspnea as ventilation increases throughout exercise in normals and COPD. In COPD, tidal volume (Vt) takes up a larger proportion of the reduced inspiratory capacity (IC), and the inspiratory reserve volume (IRV) is decreased at any given ventilation – these mechanical constraints on tidal volume expansion are further compounded because of dynamic hyperinflation during exercise. (c) Due to a truncated Vt response to exercise, patients with COPD must rely more on increasing breathing frequency (F) to generate increases in ventilation. (Adapted from ref. 35.)*

weakened inspiratory muscles, and the intrinsic mechanical loads already described, tidal inspiratory pressures represent a high fraction of their maximal force-generating capacity[21,46–48] (Figure 18.9). Moreover, DH results in a disproportionate increase in the end-expiratory rib cage volume, which probably decreases the effectiveness of sternocleidomastoid and scalene muscle activity.[30,32] Therefore, DH may alter the pattern of ventilatory muscle recruitment to a more inefficient pattern, with negative implications for muscle energetics.

The net effect of DH during exercise in COPD is, therefore, that the Vt response to increasing exercise is progressively constrained despite near maximal inspiratory efforts[35] (Figure 18.9). The ratio of tidal esophageal pressure relative to maximum (Pes/Pimax) to tidal volume Vt/VC or Vt/predicted IC is significantly higher at any given work rate or ventilation in COPD, compared with health (Figure 18.9).

Dynamic hyperinflation and dyspnea

Dyspnea intensity during exercise has been shown to correlate well with concomitant measures of dynamic lung hyperinflation[29,35] (Figure 18.10). In a multiple regression analysis with Borg ratings of dyspnea intensity as the dependent variable versus a number of independent physiologic variables, the change in EILV (expressed as % of TLC) during exercise emerged as the strongest independent correlate ($r = 0.63$, $P = 0.001$) in 23 patients with advanced COPD (average $FEV_{1.0}$, 36% predicted).[29] The change in EELV and change in Vt (components of EILV) emerged as significant contributors to exertional breathlessness and, together with increased breathing frequency, accounted for 61% of the variance in exercise Borg ratings.[29] A second study showed equally strong correlations between the intensity of perceived inspiratory difficulty during exercise and EILV/TLC

Inter-relationships at a standardized level of exercise

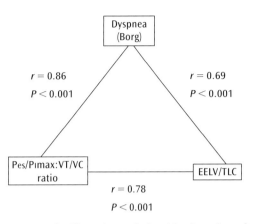

Figure 18.10 *Significant interrelationships have been found between dyspnea intensity, neuromechanical dissociation (Pes/Vt ratio) and the extent of DH (EELV) at a standardized level of exercise in COPD. (Adapted from ref. 35.)*

$(r = 0.69, P < 0.01)$.[35] Dyspnea intensity also correlates well with the ratio of effort (Pes/Pimax) to the tidal volume response (Vt/VC)[35] (Figure 18.10). This increased effort-displacement ratio in COPD ultimately reflects neuromechanical dissociation (or uncoupling) of the ventilatory pump.

We postulated that some of the distinct qualitative dimensions of exertional dyspnea in COPD may have their origin in this neuromechanical dissociation.[35] At the peak of symptom-limited exercise, both healthy individuals and COPD patients chose qualitative descriptors of dyspnea denoting increased work/effort of breathing. However, only COPD patients consistently selected descriptors denoting increased inspiratory difficulty (i.e. 67% selected 'my breath does not go in all the way') and 92% of the sample described unsatisfied inspiratory effort (i.e. 'can't get enough air in').[35] In health, during resting spontaneous breathing, there is harmonious neuromechanical coupling so that the level of ventilatory output is commensurate with the central medullary respiratory drive. This relationship between central motor command output and the anticipated ventilatory consequence (or the effort displacement ratio) is preserved during exercise in health (Figure 18.11). Although perceived effort of breathing increases, it remains appropriately rewarded and subjects do not describe inspiratory difficulty or unsatisfied inspiratory effort, even at peak exercise (Figure 18.11). By contrast, in patients with COPD, this relationship between effort and instantaneous respired volume (or flow) may be abnormal at rest, particularly if they are breathing above the relaxation volume of the respiratory system, and is further seriously disrupted during exercise because of increased intrinsic loading and a progressively restrictive mechanical response in the setting of increased ventilatory demand[35] (Figure 18.11). In this setting, patients experience incapacitating inspiratory difficulty, which encompasses the distressing sensation of unsatisfied inspiratory effort. A striking example of unsatisfied inspiration is the period of isometric tension development at the onset of each inspiration, when expended inspiratory effort is not rewarded until the ITL is counterbalanced[45] (Figure 18.11).

Current evidence suggests that breathlessness is not only a function of the amplitude of central motor output, but is also importantly modulated by peripheral feedback from a host of respiratory mechanoreceptors (for comprehensive reviews see refs 49–52). Thus, the psychophysical basis of neuromechanical dissociation likely resides in the complex central processing and integration of signals that mediate: (i) central motor command output;[53–55] and (ii) sensory feedback from various mechanoreceptors that provide precise instantaneous proprioceptive information about muscle displacement (muscle spindles and joint receptors), tension development (Golgi tendon organs) and change in respired volume or flow (lung and airway mechanoreceptors).[56–63] Awareness of the disparity between effort and ventilatory output may elicit patterned psychological and neurohumoral responses that culminate in respiratory distress, which is an important affective dimension of perceived inspiratory difficulty.[64,65]

Further indirect evidence of the importance of DH in contributing to exertional dyspnea in COPD has come from a number of studies that have shown that dyspnea was effectively ameliorated by interventions that reduced operating lung volumes (either pharmacologically or surgically), or that counterbalanced the negative effects of DH on the inspiratory muscles (i.e. continuous positive airway pressure).[66–73] Consistently strong correlations have been reported between reduced Borg ratings of dyspnea and reduced DH during exercise in a number of studies following various bronchodilators and lung volume reduction surgery [66–73] (Table 18.2).

It must be emphasized that DH represents only one stimulus for exertional dyspnea in COPD. Although the neurophysiological underpinnings of exertional dyspnea remain conjectural, our understanding of the integrated central and peripheral mechanisms involved continues to increase.[46–52] Increased central drive and attendant corollary discharge may be perceived as a sense of inspiratory muscle effort, which may have its origins in the central cortex.[53–55] Increased medullary drive secondary to chemical (hypoxia, hypercapnia) and neuromechanical (muscle loading ± weakness) stimuli, may be more relevant than increased voluntary muscle effort in mediating dyspnea. Altered vagal afferent activity, in response to lung overdistension and other mechanical perturbations (i.e. increased airways resistance) likely contribute to dyspnea or some of its qualitative dimensions.[49–63] Hypercapnia alone may directly give rise to unpleasant

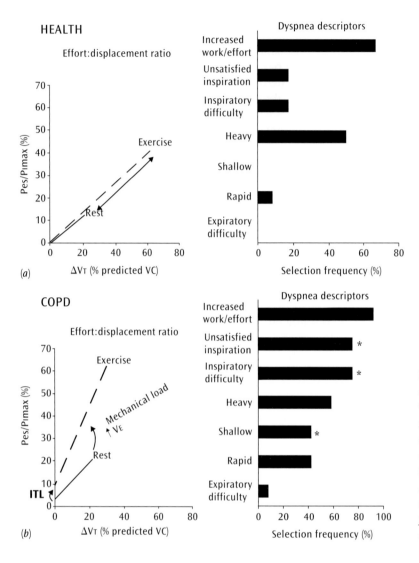

Figure 18.11 *The relationship between respiratory effort (Pes/Pimax) and tidal volume (Vt) at rest and peak exercise with simultaneous qualitative descriptors of exertional breathlessness in health (a) and in COPD (b). Note the inspiratory threshold load (ITL), the disparity between effort and Vt, and the different descriptor choices in COPD. (Adapted from ref. 35.) *P < 0.05 Significant difference between COPD and health.*

Table 18.2 *Correlates of change (Δ) in standardized Borg dyspnea ratings during exercise in COPD*

Author, year	Intervention	n	Independent variable	Significance
O'Donnell, 1999[69]	Ipratropium bromide	29	ΔIC% predicted at isotime exercise	$r = -0.33, P < 0.05$
Belman, 1996[66]	Albuterol	13	ΔEILV/TLC at isotime exercise	$r = 0.749, P < 0.01$
Martinez, 1997[70]	LVRS	12	ΔEELV/predicted TLC at isotime exercise	$r = 0.75, P < 0.01$
O'Donnell, 1996[72]	LVRS	8	ΔEELV/predicted TLC at isotime exercise	$r = 0.84, P < 0.05$

LVRS: lung volume reduction surgery; IC: inspiratory capacity; EELV: end-expiratory lung volume; EILV: end-inspiratory lung volumes; TLC: total lung capacity.

respiratory sensations independent of ventilatory muscle activity in some patients during exercise.[58]

Ventilatory limitation and gas exchange abnormalities in COPD

Arterial hypoxemia during exercise commonly occurs in patients with severe COPD as a result of the effect of a fall in mixed venous oxygen tension (Pv_{O_2}) on low ventilation–perfusion lung units, and shunting.[74] In severe COPD, both the ability to increase lung perfusion and to distribute inspired ventilation throughout the lungs during exercise is compromised.[74] Resting physiologic deadspace is often increased, reflecting ventilation-perfusion inequalities, and fails to decline further during exercise as is the case in health.[74,75] As we have seen, to maintain appropriate alveolar ventilation and blood gas homostasis in the face of increased physiologic

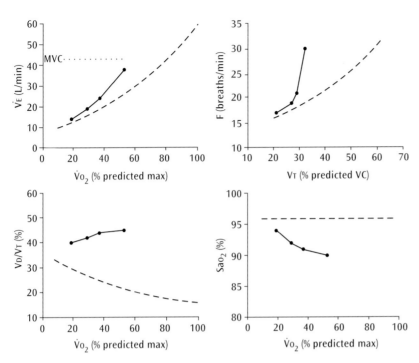

Figure 18.12 *Plots of ventilation (VE), physiological deadspace (VD/VT) and arterial oxygen saturation (Sao₂) versus Vo₂ and breathing pattern (F/VT) in COPD (solid lines) and in age-matched healthy subjects (dotted lines).*

deadspace, minute ventilation must increase. In this regard, several studies have confirmed high submaximal ventilation levels during exercise in COPD compared with health[38,76,77] (Figure 18.12).

In more advanced COPD, arterial hypoxemia during exercise occurs as a result of alveolar hypoventilation.[78,79] The reduced exercise ventilation relative to metabolic demand may reflect reduced output of the central controller ('won't breathe' hypothesis), or a preserved or amplified central respiratory drive in the presence of an impaired mechanical/ventilatory muscle response ('can't breathe' hypothesis).[80–82] It has further been postulated that CO_2 retention during exercise may result from the 'behavioral' adoption of a shallow breathing pattern, which would serve to minimize intrathoracic pressure perturbations, reduce respiratory discomfort, and possibly obviate the development of respiratory muscle fatigue ('wise fighter' hypothesis).[27]

The evidence that CO_2 retention during exercise is the result of reduced central or peripheral chemosensitivity is inconclusive. The resting ventilatory response to hypoxic or hypercapnic stimulation fails to predict exercise CO_2 retention in COPD.[83,84] Moreover, studies that have measured mouth occlusion pressure in the first 0.1 second of inspiration ($P_{0.1}$) during chemical stimulation tests have shown that this index of central drive is not different in patients who are hypercapnic compared with those who are eucapnic during exercise.[85,86]

Theoretically, the imbalance between inspiratory muscle load and capacity may predispose patients with COPD to inspiratory muscle fatigue or frank task failure and consequent CO_2 retention.[78] However, Montes de

Oca and Celli[87] have recently shown that maximal inspiratory pressure generation, the pattern of ventilatory muscle recruitment and breathing pattern were not different in those who maintained eucapnia and those who developed hypercapnia during exercise, thereby casting doubt on fatigue, or its avoidance, by the adoption of a rapid shallow breathing pattern as the explanation for CO_2 retention.

We recently reported that in a sample of 20 patients with advanced COPD (i.e. $FEV_{1.0}$ = 34% predicted), those who retained CO_2 following hyperoxic breathing at rest (i.e. 60% O_2 ⩾10 minutes) were more inclined to retain CO_2 during exercise: the change of arterial Pco_2 from rest to peak exercise correlated with the change of arterial Pco_2 following hyperoxia (r^2 = 0.62, P = <0.0005).[88] COPD patients with chronic hypoxemia demonstrate adaptations to preserve V_A, such as hypoxic pulmonary vasoconstriction (to reduce ventilation-perfusion mismatching) and increased peripheral chemoresponsiveness to hypoxia (to increase VE). Although these adaptations successfully maintain CO_2 homostasis at rest, they are quickly overwhelmed during exercise as Vco_2 increases and the mechanical constraints on ventilation reach their early critical limiting point.[88]

In our study, those who retained CO_2 during exercise could not be distinguished from non-retainers on the basis of resting $FEV_{1.0}$, resting lung volumes, resting $Paco_2$, or VD/VT. Similarly, breathing pattern responses and measured physiologic deadspace during exercise were not different between the two groups.[88] The rapid shallow breathing pattern, which is invariable in advanced COPD during exercise, is likely to be largely dictated by restrictive mechanics and the increased elastic load. However, CO_2 retainers showed greater DH and earlier attainment of their peak alveolar ventilation than non-CO_2 retainers. In the group as a whole, there was a good correlation between the EELV/TLC and the Pa_{CO_2} measured simultaneously during exercise ($r = 0.68$, $P < 0.005$).[88] We concluded that CO_2 retention occurred in part because of greater dynamic mechanical constraints in the setting of a fixed high physiologic deadspace during exercise.

Increased ventilatory demand during exercise in COPD

The effects of the above outlined mechanical derangements in COPD are often amplified by concomitantly increased ventilatory demand. A high physiologic deadspace that fails to decline with exercise is the primary stimulus for increased submaximal ventilation in this population (Figure 18.12). Other factors contributing to increased submaximal ventilation include early lactic acidosis, hypoxemia, high metabolic demands of breathing, low arterial CO_2 set points and other non-metabolic sources of ventilatory stimulation (i.e. anxiety). As we have seen, the extent of DH and its consequent negative sensory consequences in flow-limited patients will vary with ventilatory demand. There is abundant evidence that increased ventilatory demand contributes to dyspnea causation in COPD: dyspnea intensity during exercise had been shown to correlate strongly with the change in V_E or with V_E expressed as a fraction of maximal ventilatory capacity.[29] Flow-limited patients with the highest ventilation will develop limiting ventilatory constraints on flow and volume generation, and greater dyspnea early in exercise.[25] For a given $FEV_{1.0}$, patients who have greater ventilatory demands have been shown in one study to have more severe chronic activity-related dyspnea.[38] Moreover, exertional dyspnea relief and improved exercise endurance following interventions such as exercise training,[89] oxygen therapy[90] and opiates[91] has been shown to result, in part, from the attendant reduction in submaximal ventilation (see below).

Inspiratory muscle weakness during exercise in COPD

Reduced ventilatory capacity, due to reduced ventilatory muscle strength, could theoretically contribute to ventilatory limitation in patients with advanced COPD.[46–48] We have seen that DH during exercise can contribute to functional inspiratory muscle weakness by altering length–tension and force–velocity characteristics of the inspiratory muscles. Additionally, factors such as chronic

hypoxia and hypercapnia, steroid overusage, electrolytic disturbances and malnutrition could predispose to ventilatory muscle weakness in COPD. However, the evidence that a weakened ventilatory pump is a common contributor to exercise intolerance is inconclusive.[92–95] The prevalence of inspiratory muscle weakness in COPD patients has not been established and may not be as pervasive as previously thought. In fact, there is evidence that functional muscle strength is remarkably preserved in some patients with advanced chronic ventilatory insufficiency.[96] Biopsies of the diaphragm in patients with advanced COPD have shown several adaptations to chronic intrinsic mechanical loading. These include: (i) reduction of sarcomere length, which enhances the capacity of the muscles to generate pressure at high lung volumes;[97] (ii) increase in the proportion of Type I fibers, which are slow-twitch and fatigue resistant;[98] and (iii) increase in mitochondrial concentration, which improves oxidative capacity.[99]

To the extent that inspiratory muscle weakness contributes to exercise limitation in COPD, then targeted strengthening of these muscles should improve exercise performance. The results of studies on the effectiveness of specific inspiratory muscle training using a variety of techniques (i.e. voluntary isocapnic hyperventilation, inspiratory resistive loading and inspiratory threshold loading) have been inconsistent. A meta-analysis of 17 clinical studies concluded that there is insufficient evidence to recommend specific inspiratory muscle training for routine clinical purposes.[100]

Notwithstanding this negative meta-analysis, a few important controlled studies have shown that inspiratory muscle training using targeted resistive or inspiratory threshold loading, improved dyspnea and exercise endurance in patients with COPD, and that these improvements correlated with physiological improvements (i.e. increased static maximal inspiratory pressure (MIP)).[101–103] It would appear, therefore, that a subset of patients with COPD do have critical inspiratory muscle weakness which can contribute to exercise intolerance and dyspnea.

Inspiratory muscle fatigue in COPD

The imbalance between energy supply and demand could predispose to inspiratory muscle fatigue during exercise in COPD.[93] However, to date, the evidence that contractile fatigue contributes to exercise intolerance in COPD is not convincing. Bye et al.[92] demonstrated a change in the diaphragmatic electromyogram (EMG) power spectrum (i.e. a fall in the high/low ratio) during exercise in some COPD patients during exercise. EMG power spectrum analysis is often problematic at higher exercise levels because of possible changes in the relationship between the electrodes and underlying muscle during alterations in breathing pattern. Additionally, there is the potential for contamination of the EMG signal due to altered patterns of recruitment of different ventilatory muscles at the higher exercise levels. These authors proposed that a change in the EMG spectrum towards a less fatiguing pattern during added oxygen therapy could indicate that this intervention effectively delayed fatigue, and that this, in turn, contributed importantly to improved exercise endurance.[92] However, other explanations are equally plausible. Oxygen, for example, has been shown to reduce submaximal ventilation and, consequently, DH, which together delay the onset of critical ventilatory limitation.[90,104–106] These effects could collectively influence EMG signal recordings, independent of the existence of inspiratory muscle fatigue.

Kyroussis et al.[94,107] demonstrated a slowing of maximal sniff inspiratory muscle relaxation rates following exhaustive exercise in patients with COPD, and suggested that this may be an indicator of incipient inspiratory muscle fatigue. These authors showed a reduction of this slowing effect and improved exercise endurance following pressure support (PS = 15 cmH$_2$O) in six patients with severe COPD (FEV$_{1.0}$ = 22% predicted) compared with unassisted control.[107] These results indicate that PS successfully reduced the load on the inspiratory muscles and, therefore, we can conclude that this load, or its perception by the patient, contributed to exercise intolerance during unassisted walking. However, the extent to which inspiratory muscle fatigue was delayed by PS remains conjectural.

Mador et al.[108] measured twitch transdiaphragmatic pressures in patients with moderate to severe COPD during high intensity constant load cycle exercise to tolerance. The results of this study indicated that the majority of these patients showed no evidence of contractile fatigue of the diaphragm following symptom-limited exercise. In reality, many patients with COPD may stop exercise because of intolerable exertional symptoms well before fatigue or contractile failure actually develops. There is also increasing evidence that the diaphragm may adapt to chronic intrinsic loading by becoming more resistant to fatigue.[96–99]

Expiratory muscle activity during exercise in COPD

In the presence of expiratory flow limitation, tidal expiratory flow rates are independent of expiratory transpulmonary pressures beyond a critical level.[109] In fact, increasing expiratory effort beyond this level not only fails to increase expiratory flow, but also results in dynamic airway compression of airways downstream from the flow-limiting segment.[109] Expiratory muscle

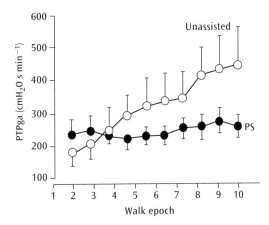

Figure 18.13 *Progression of pressure–time products of gastric pressure (PTPga) by 10% epoch of walk duration during free (open circle) and equidistant positive-pressure ventilation-assisted (closed circle) walking (six subjects) are presented. Results shown are mean ± SEM. PS: pressure support. (From ref. 107.)*

recruitment appears to be highly variable in COPD during exercise.[30–35,94,110,111] During constant-load exercise, some patients allow expiratory transpulmonary pressures to reach, but not exceed, the critical flow-limiting pressure, thus attenuating dynamic airway compression and its consequences.[111] However, other studies have shown marked expiratory muscle activity (i.e. expiratory pleural pressures >20 cmH$_2$O), particularly at high work rates in some COPD patients[31,107] (Figure 18.13). As previously discussed, expiratory muscle recruitment during exercise is advantageous in health, through optimization of diaphragmatic length and dynamic ventilatory mechanics. These important advantages are lost in COPD. Increased abdominal pressure generation (relative to expiratory intercostal activity) should increase diaphragmatic length at end expiration and, therefore, assist the inspiratory muscles. However, the extent to which this expiratory/inspiratory synergy exists in COPD has not been fully established.[27] Moreover, any increase in EILV (or V$_T$) as a result of inspiratory muscle activity augmented in this manner would be expected to have a net negative effect: an increase in the EILV at a fixed TE (not unusual in COPD) will result in further DH.

Aggravation of dynamic airway compression during forced expiratory efforts may have deleterious sensory consequences and/or may reflexly increase ventilation with attendant aggravation of DH.[112,113] Increased expiratory muscle action, in the setting of expiratory flow limitation, will reduce the velocity of shortening (V$_T$/T$_E$) of these muscles. The consequent amplified abdominal and intrathoracic pressure development throughout expiration will compromise cardiac output by reducing venous return and by increasing pulmonary vascular resistance through intrathoracic compression of alveolar vessels.

Kayser et al.[114] recently completed experiments where expiratory flow limitation and dyspnea were induced in young healthy individuals during exercise by means of a Starling resistor. Aliverti et al.[115] showed that this imposed load resulted in marked expiratory muscle activity, and caused what essentially was a prolonged Valsalva maneuver throughout expiration and early inspiration, with attendant measurable shifts of blood from the thorax to the extremities.

The importance of this mechanism in contributing to cardiac compromise and exercise intolerance in COPD patients remains to be established, particularly given the large intersubject variability of expiratory muscle activity. However, it would appear that the deleterious effects of vigorous expiratory muscle contraction on cardiac performance outweigh potential beneficial effects on inspiratory muscle function in many patients with COPD. Excessive expiratory activity is possibly maladaptive during exercise in COPD. It may represent a programed response to markedly increased central respiratory drive in these patients with compromised diaphragmatic function. In this regard, a recent interesting study by Kyroussis et al.[107] showed that effective mechanical unloading of the inspiratory muscles during exercise using PS was accompanied by consistent and marked reductions in the expiratory muscle pressure–time product, possibly due to reduced central respiratory drive (Figure 18.13).

Dynamic airway compression and dyspnea

There is evidence that dynamic airway distortion and collapse, induced in the laboratory by applying negative expiratory pressure (i.e. $-12\,cmH_2O$) to demonstrably flow-limited subjects, may give rise to unpleasant respiratory sensations.[112,113] The mechanisms of discomfort may include altered afferent information from airway mechanoreceptors or from ventilatory stimulation and tachypneic effects that may worsen lung hyperinflation in these mechanically compromised patients.[63] The contribution of dynamic compression (in isolation) to the intensity and quality of dyspnea, however, remains conjectural. The fact that COPD patients rarely complain of expiratory difficulty or unsatisfied expiration during exercise, and that interventions designed to attenuate dynamic collapse (such as positive expiratory pressure) have inconsistent effects on dyspnea intensity in flow-limited patients, does not support an important dyspnogenic role for dynamic compression during exercise.[45,113,116]

Clearly, the effects of dynamic compression and DH on dyspnea in COPD patients are inextricably linked; to the extent that avoidance of dynamic airway compression and the attendant unpleasant respiratory sensations is desirable, termination of expiration (and onset of neural inspiration) before expiratory flow is complete may determine the magnitude of DH and, ultimately, the intensity of exertional dyspnea.

PERIPHERAL MUSCLE DYSFUNCTION AND EXERCISE INTOLERANCE IN COPD

Recently, there has been heightened interest in the role of abnormalities of peripheral muscle structure and function in exercise limitation in COPD (for excellent comprehensive reviews see Gosker et al.[117] and Casaburi[118]). The importance of increased leg effort as an exercise-limiting symptom in COPD was first highlighted by Killian et al.[119] These authors studied the intensity of exercise-limiting symptoms during incremental cycle exercise in a sample of 97 patients with COPD ($FEV_{1.0}$ = 46.6% predicted). They found that 43% of the sample rated leg effort (by Borg scale) higher than dyspnea, 26% rated dyspnea intensity greater than leg effort, and the remainder (31%) noted the intensity of leg effort and dyspnea equally. The authors extended this study to show that the distribution of exercise-limiting symptoms in COPD was remarkably similar to that of healthy individuals and patients with congestive heart failure (CHF) at the end of incremental exercise.[120]

It must be remembered that these patients were asked to rate perceived leg 'effort', and not whether severe leg 'discomfort' was the primary exercise-limiting symptom per se. It is perhaps not surprising that inactive, deconditioned, elderly patients would experience a sense of heightened leg effort during unwonted incremental cycle exercise in the laboratory. In clinical practice, such patients rarely complain of leg discomfort during their daily activities – they are much more likely to complain of exertional dyspnea. We recently studied the distribution of exercise-limiting symptoms in 105 clinically stable patients ($FEV_{1.0}$ 37% predicted) with poor exercise performance, who were referred to respirology clinics at our institution.[25] Severe breathing discomfort was the primary symptom limiting incremental cycle exercise in 61% of this sample; combined dyspnea and leg discomfort limited exercise in 19%, and only 18% stopped primarily because of leg discomfort.[25] This frequency distribution of exercise-limiting symptoms was very similar to that found in a previous study in 125 patients entering a pulmonary rehabilitation program.[121] We demonstrated that patients who stopped exercise primarily because of dyspnea had greater levels of DH, greater ventilatory constraints and poorer exercise performance than the minority who stopped mainly because of leg discomfort.[25]

Peripheral muscle dysfunction is a potentially reversible cause of exercise curtailment in COPD and is currently the focus of intense study.[122–131] Abnormalities of peripheral muscle structure and function have now been extensively documented in COPD.[117,118,121] Many of these abnormalities ultimately represent the effects of reduced activity levels or immobility because of overwhelming dyspnea. These abnormalities include: loss of muscle mass and mitochrondrial (aerobic) potential and compromised oxidative phosphorylation which results in an exaggerated dependence on high energy phosphate transfer and anaerobic glycolysis.[122–127] Severe peripheral muscle weakness due in part to disuse atrophy has been reported in several studies.[122,124] In a number of studies, lactate thresholds (i.e. the $\dot{V}O_2$ at which lactate begins to increase) have been shown to be lower in COPD than in health. Casaburi[128] reported a mean lactate threshold in 33 COPD patients of 0.7 L/min, equivalent to a slow walking pace, as compared with 1.2 L/min in age-matched healthy individuals. $\dot{V}O_2$ kinetics at the peripheral muscle level have also been shown to be slower in COPD than in health.[129] Thus, in exercising COPD patients there is excessive accumulation of metabolic byproducts that impair contractility and increase the propensity to fatigue. The early metabolic acidosis (and increased CO_2 production through acid-buffering effects) may stimulate increased ventilation and hasten the onset of critical ventilatory limitation. Moreover, an acidic milieu, with an altered ionic status (e.g. increased potassium) of the active peripheral muscle, may also stimulate resident metaboreceptors, which may have important effects on ventilatory and sympathetic stimulation, as has been demonstrated in patients with CHF.[132]

Leg muscle biopsies in COPD have shown reduced capillarization with preserved or decreased capillary to fiber ratios.[125–127] These muscles show consistent reductions in Type I slow-twitch, high oxidative, low-tension, fatigue-resistant muscle fibers.[125–127] There is an increased preponderance of Type II fiber, which would be expected to be associated with an increased velocity of contraction, a reduced mechanical efficiency and increased fatigability.[133] General muscle wasting (cachexia) in COPD has

been associated with low circulating levels of anabolic steroids, growth hormone and altered circadian rhythms of leptin production in COPD.[134–137] It has recently been shown that exercise in COPD patients accelerated free radical formation.[138] If these are not scavenged by antioxidants, they can result in extensive damage to membranes and the cation cycling proteins.[139] Other well-recognized factors that contribute to peripheral muscle weakness in COPD, under certain circumstances, include: chronic oral steroid therapy, malnutrition, and the effects of hypoxia, hypercapnia and acidosis.

Improving peripheral muscle function in COPD

Exercise training has been shown to improve peripheral muscle function and perceived leg discomfort in both moderate and severe COPD[131,140,141] (Figure 18.14). Measurable improvements in peripheral muscle strength and endurance have been consistently reported.[77,89,143,144] Quadriceps muscle biopsies have confirmed increased aerobic enzyme concentrations and increased capillary density after supervised training.[141] $\dot{V}O_2$ kinetics are faster after training and blood lactate levels are lower at a standardized work.[131] Perceived leg discomfort is significantly less at any given work rate following exercise training and contributes to improved exercise endurance, particularly in patients where leg discomfort was the primary locus of sensory limitation prior to program entry[77,89] (Figure 18.14). The mechanisms of this improvement are unknown but may relate to improved peripheral muscle strength: less central motor command output (and therefore less perceived leg effort) is required for a given force generation in the newly strengthened muscle. Improvements in the local metabolic milieu of the active muscle after training may also alter afferent neural activity from this site, which by itself may modulate the sensory experience of leg discomfort. Ambulatory

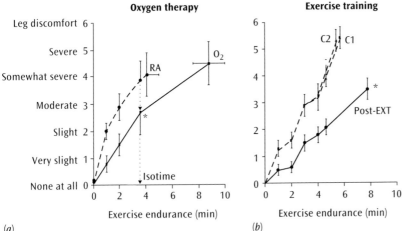

Figure 18.14 *Borg–time plots of leg discomfort during constant-load submaximal exercise in two groups of COPD patients following exercise training (b) and with supplemental oxygen (a). RA: room air; O_2: 60% oxygen; C1 and C2: before and after a control period prior to EXT; isotime: a standardized time near end-exercise; *P < 0.05 significant reduction in leg discomfort (b) and with supplemental oxygen. (Adapted from refs 88 and 89.)*

oxygen therapy has similarly been shown to consistently reduce perceived leg discomfort throughout exercise when compared with room air, presumably through similar mechanisms[90,104] (Figure 18.14).

Ventilatory–locomotor muscle competiton during exercise in COPD

The above outlined structural abnormalities of the peripheral muscle are not unique to COPD – identical abnormalities have been reported in CHF.[117] In addition to the metabolic abnormalities of the muscle, other factors may also contribute to locomotor dysfunction in COPD. Simon et al.[144] demonstrated that, at least in some patients (6/14) with COPD (FEV$_{1.0}$ = 35% predicted), leg $\dot{V}O_2$, leg blood flow and O_2 extraction plateau as exercise increases, despite progressive increases in total whole-body $\dot{V}O_2$ (Figure 18.15). This suggests a ventilatory

'steal' effect, at least in some patients, such that blood was diverted away from the competing locomotor muscles to the ventilatory muscles when cardiac output had reached its maximal level. Harms et al.[145] demonstrated this 'steal' phenomenon in highly trained athletes at the extremes of endurance, when maximal $\dot{V}O_2$ had plateaued. In these high-performance athletes, unloading of the ventilatory muscles using proportional assist ventilation (PAV) caused a significant increase in blood flow to the leg, with increased leg $\dot{V}O_2$.[145]

The concept of ventilatory–locomotor competition for a limited availability of energy supplies during exercise in COPD was bolstered by a recent study by Richardson et al.[146] These authors showed that in the absence of ventilatory competition, 'isolated' small muscle mass exercise resulted in a 2.2-fold greater muscle mass specific power output than during whole-body exercise, indicating substantial metabolic reserve. Improved power output occurred, presumably because of greater

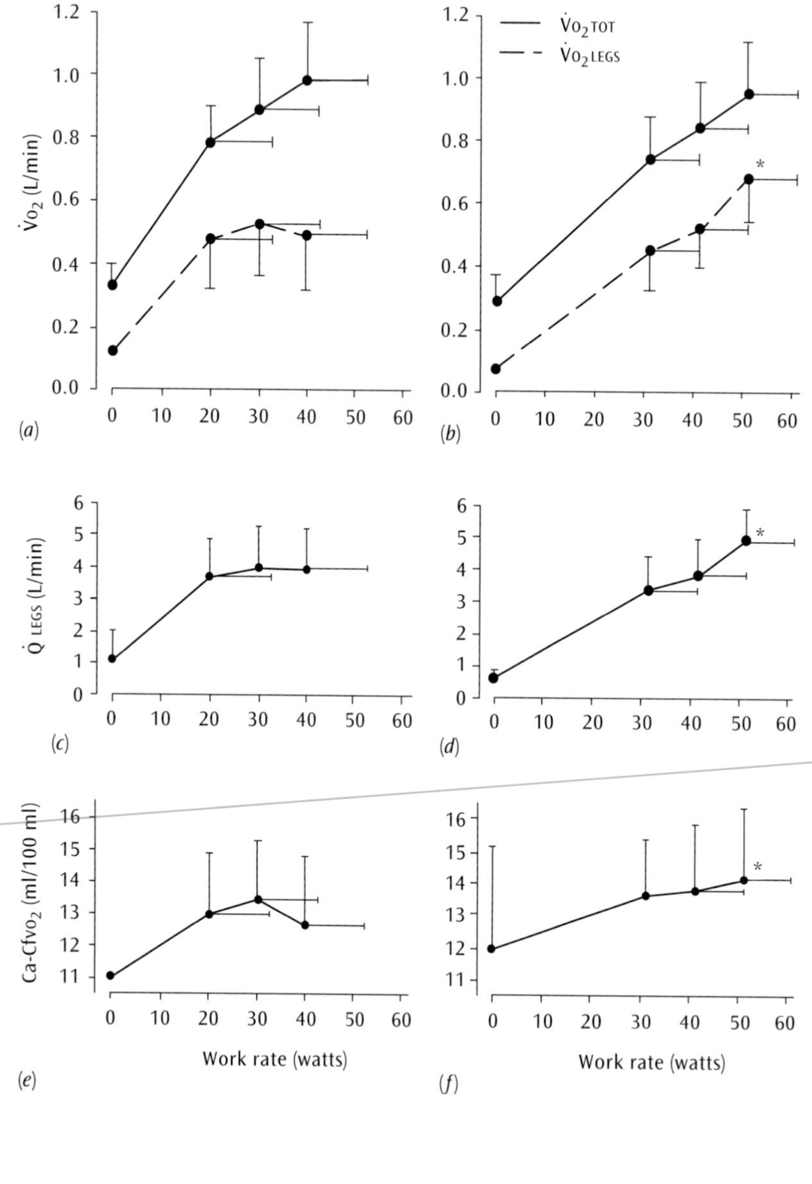

Figure 18.15 Total body $\dot{V}O_2$ ($\dot{V}O_2$TOT)–work rate and $\dot{V}O_2$LEGS–work rate (a,b), blood flow for both legs (QLEGS)–work rate (c,d), and arterial–femoral venous O_2 content difference (CaO_2 − CfvO_2)–work rate (e,f) relationships obtained in the group demonstrating (left) or not demonstrating (right) a plateau in $\dot{V}O_2$LEGS. CaO_2 − CfvO_2 is abbreviated as Ca-CfvO_2. In the non-plateau group, $\dot{V}O_2$LEGS, QLEGS and CaO_2 − CfvO_2 kept progressing while external work rate was increasing. In the other group, a plateau in $\dot{V}O_2$LEGS, QLEGS and CaO_2-CfvO_2 could be demonstrated despite the progression in $\dot{V}O_2$TOT and work rate. *P = 0.001 with the corresponding relationship in the plateau group. *P < 0.05: significant reduction in intensity of perceived exertional leg discomfort. Isotime: the highest equivalent exercise time (to the nearest whole minute) completed in both exercise tests. Results are expressed as mean ± SD. (Reproduced from ref. 144 with permission.)

blood perfusion and energy supplies to the small muscles, than during whole-body exercise where there was competition with the ventilatory muscles. Given the high oxygen cost of breathing at a given ventilation in severe COPD during exercise (see above), and compromised cardiac function (in part as a result of the effects of DH and excessive expiratory muscle recruitment), reduced blood flow to the exercising locomotor muscles may very well contribute to exercise intolerance.

In CHF patients in whom exercise was limited primarily by leg discomfort, we have recently shown that pressure support (PS) ventilation improved exercise endurance (by 40%), principally by reducing perceived leg discomfort.[147] Reduction of leg discomfort during exercise correlated well with the reduced total body $\dot{V}O_2$ during unloading, which in turn correlated with reduced inspiratory esophageal pressures.[147] We speculated that during PS there was reduced competition for a finite low cardiac output and that leg discomfort was reduced because of a consequently improved blood flow and/or oxygen delivery to the active muscle. In COPD, a preliminary study by Onorati et al.[148] found no evidence of increased blood flow to the leg or of increased leg $\dot{V}O_2$ following PAV in six patients with COPD ($FEV_{1.0}$ = 40% predicted) during high-level exercise. Further studies on the interaction between cardiopulmonary and peripheral muscle systems during ventilatory muscle unloading (using mechanical assistance and pharmacologic volume reduction) are required before any definitive conclusions can be reached concerning the importance of ventilatory–locomotor competition in exercising COPD patients.

Cardiovascular factors

The effect of COPD on cardiac performance during exercise is complex and multifactorial, and has received relatively little attention. Severe lung hyperinflation and excessive expiratory muscle recruitment can impair venous return and reduce right ventricular preload in COPD. Several studies have demonstrated increased pulmonary vascular resistance during exercise in COPD.[149–151] This results from emphysematous vascular destruction with reduced area, or compliance, of the pulmonary vascular bed and, in some cases, from critical hypoxemia as a result of alveolar hypoventilation.[152,153] Pulmonary artery pressures and right ventricular afterload are generally much higher than in health at a given cardiac output in COPD.[152,153] Right ventricular afterload during exercise is also increased because of the increased pulmonary vascular resistance associated with breathing at lung volumes close to TLC (i.e. DH).[151–154] Earlier studies have shown that right ventricular ejection fraction failed to increase despite a rise in right ventricular end-diastolic

pressure in COPD during exercise.[150] The left ventricular ejection fraction is generally preserved in COPD in the absence of concomitant ischemic heart disease or hypertension.[154,155] Left ventricular diastolic function may be impaired because of ventricular interdependence: increased tension or displacement of the right ventricle (because of increased pulmonary vascular resistance) may impede left diastolic filling.[154,155] Left ventricular afterload is increased during exercise because the left ventricular transmural pressure gradient is increased as a result of progressively negative intrathoracic pressure generation. Cardiac output has been found to increase normally with $\dot{V}O_2$ during submaximal exercise in COPD, despite the increased pulmonary vascular resistance, but peak cardiac output (and $\dot{V}O_2$) reaches a lower maximal value than in health.[149,156] Stroke volume is generally smaller and heart rate correspondingly higher, at a given $\dot{V}O_2$ in COPD compared with health.[149]

Cardiopulmonary interaction in COPD

Reduced peak cardiac output was shown to correlate well with the extent of prevailing expiratory flow limitation.[157,158] Morrison et al.[156] found that peak symptom-limited $\dot{V}O_2$ correlated strongly with reduced cardiac output in COPD: reduced cardiac output alone accounted for 63% of variance in exercise performance. Montes de Oca[159] showed a statistical correlation between oxygen pulse ($\dot{V}O_2$/heart rate), which is a crude measure of stroke volume, and the magnitude of pleural pressure swings during exercise. Oelberg et al.[160] showed that helium/oxygen breathing in COPD patients with low cardiac outputs during exercise resulted in an increase in VE by 32% and in peak $\dot{V}O_2$ by 16%, while causing no further increase in cardiac output. One possible explanation for this finding is that unloading of the ventilatory system in these patients may have reduced ventilatory 'steal', with the result that greater blood flow and oxygen uptake occurred in active peripheral locomotor muscles at a given cardiac output. These studies collectively attest to the importance of cardiopulmonary interactions during exercise in COPD and their potential contribution to poor exercise performance.

IMPROVING EXERCISE PEFORMANCE IN COPD

Quantitative flow–volume loop analysis during constant-load exercise testing (at approximately 60% of the achievable peak work rate or $\dot{V}O_2$) allows a non-invasive assessment of ventilatory mechanics in COPD.[36] Changes in dynamic IC correlate strongly with the elastic load and this measurement is, therefore, a useful surrogate for direct esophageal pressure measurements[35,66] (Figure 18.10). Furthermore, comparison of exercise flow–volume loops before and after therapeutic interventions at a standardized time, using a constant-load endurance protocol, provide valuable insights into the mechanisms of improved exercise performance and symptoms.[36] To improve exercise capacity in symptomatic COPD patients, therapeutic interventions must either increase ventilatory capacity (i.e. the maximal flow–volume envelope), delay the rate of DH (i.e. the shift of exercise tidal flow–volume loops towards TLC) or a combination of both. The effect of a few common therapeutic interventions on exercise performance in COPD is described below.

Bronchodilator therapy

Bronchodilator therapy is the first step in the management of patients with symptomatic COPD. All classes of bronchodilator therapy (i.e. inhaled beta$_2$-agonists, inhaled anticholinergics and oral theophyllines) have been shown to improve exertional dyspnea and increase exercise capacity in COPD patients when tested in placebo-controlled studies.[161–164] Constant-load endurance cycle exercise protocols have been shown to be more responsive to the effects of bronchodilators than incremental protocols or the 6-minute walk distance test.[165] The mechanisms of improved exercise endurance following bronchodilators are complex and not fully elucidated. From the available literature on the topic, it is clear that meaningful improvement in symptoms, activity levels and quality of life can occur in the presence of only modest changes in FEV$_{1.0}$ after bronchodilator therapy.[161–164]

Bronchodilators improve dynamic small airway function and lung emptying, and reduce the resistive and elastic loads on the respiratory muscles. Belman et al.,[66] in an elegant mechanical study, showed that relief of dyspnea following albuterol (salbutamol) therapy in advanced COPD correlated well with reduction in operating lung volumes as well as a reduction in inspiratory effort required for a given tidal volume, the latter an indication of improved neuromechanical coupling of the respiratory system. In that study, important reductions in lung volume occurred in the presence of only minimal changes in FEV$_{1.0}$.[66] This likely reflects the fact that FEV$_{1.0}$ provides, at best, a crude estimation of the extent of prevailing expiratory flow limitation, which is a primary determinant of DH. In severe COPD, improvement in lung volumes, which reflect increased conductance of the small airways, are likely to be more relevant measurements for the assessment of bronchodilator efficacy than traditional FEV$_{1.0}$ measurements.[166,167] Chrystyn et al.[67] showed that improvement in exercise endurance (i.e. the 6-minute walk distance) following incremental oral theophylline therapy was associated, in a dose–response

manner, with the reduction in resting plethysmographic FRC and trapped gas volume (plethysmographic versus helium-derived lung volumes). Again in this study, there was little change in the post-bronchodilator FEV$_{1.0}$.

We have shown[36] in a placebo-controlled study that relief of exertional dyspnea and improved exercise endurance following acute anticholinergic therapy (nebulized ipratropium bromide, 500 µg) in advanced COPD correlated best with improvement in dynamic IC measurements which reflect reductions in the EELV (Figure 18.16). IC-derived measures such as EILV, the IRV and the V$_T$/IC ratio, also correlated well with reduced exertional dyspnea measured by the Borg scale.[36] As a result of the bronchodilator-induced increase in expiratory flow rates over the tidal volume range, more effective lung emptying was achieved at rest (Figure 18.16). Patients, therefore, could maintain the same, or greater, ventilation while breathing at lower lung volumes, with a more efficient breathing pattern, and reduced exertional dyspnea. During bronchodilator therapy the IRV was significantly increased at submaximal levels of exercise and at peak exercise, despite a 32% increase in exercise endurance[36] (Figure 18.16). Because of this delay in ventilatory limitation, dyspnea was displaced by leg discomfort as the primary exercise-limiting symptom in many of the study patients.

Increased IC and IRV following bronchodilators meant that V$_T$ at end-exercise was positioned on a lower, more linear portion, of the respiratory system's pressure–volume relationship, where there is reduced elastic and inspiratory threshold loading of the inspiratory muscles (Figure 18.2). Therefore, less pressure is required by the inspiratory muscles for a greater V$_T$ response.[66] Evidence is accumulating that relatively small changes in resting IC (i.e. in the order of 0.3 to 0.4 L) or in plethysmographic lung volumes can translate into clinically important improvements in exercise endurance in severe COPD.[66,69] Similarly, close correlations between reduced operating lung volumes and dyspnea relief have been shown after surgical volume reduction[70,71] (Table 18.1).

Exercise training

Patients who, despite optimized combination pharmacotherapy, have persistent activity-related dyspnea and exercise curtailment, should be encouraged to undergo exercise training. The aim of exercise training is to break the vicious cycle of skeletal muscle deconditioning, progressive dyspnea and immobility, so as to improve symptoms and activity levels, and restore patients to the highest level of independent function. There is now abundant evidence for important symptom alleviation and increased exercise performance as a result of exercise training, at least in the short term.[168–174]

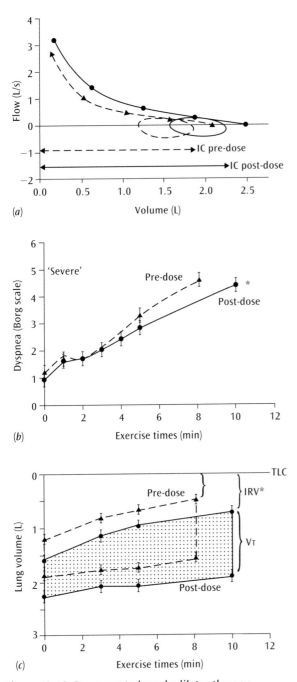

Figure 18.16 *Responses to bronchodilator therapy (nebulized ipratropium bromide, 500 μg) are shown. As post-dose maximal expiratory flow–volume relationships improved, tidal flow–volume curves at rest can shift to the right, i.e. lung hyperinflation is reduced as reflected by an increased IC (a). Exertional dyspnea decreased significantly (*P < 0.05) in response to bronchodilator therapy (b). Operating lung volumes improve in response to bronchodilator therapy, i.e. mechanical constraints on V_T expansion are reduced as IC and IRV are increased significantly (*P < 0.05) (c). Dashed lines: pre-dose data; solid lines: post-dose data. (Adapted from ref. 69.)*

The physiologic mechanisms of improved dyspnea and exercise performance following exercise training are not fully understood. Potential mechanisms include: (i) reduced ventilatory demands secondary to improved aerobic capacity or increased efficiency; (ii) increased inspiratory muscle strength and endurance; (iii) improved breathing pattern with a greater efficiency of CO_2 elimination; (iv) habituation to dyspnea or increased tolerance of dyspneogenic sensory perturbations; (v) improved peripheral muscle strength and endurance with reduced leg discomfort; and (vi) improved cardio-vascular function.

In patients with moderate disease (i.e. mean $FEV_{1.0}$ of 1.8 L, 56% predicted) and demonstrable lactic acidosis during incremental cycle testing, intensive exercise training targeted at a level above the patient's anaerobic threshold, has been shown to delay lactate accumulation with a concomitant reduction in ventilation (i.e. 1 mEq lactate reduction resulted in reduction in $\dot{V}_E$ by 2.5 L/ min).[139] Reduced ventilation at a given work rate or $\dot{V}_{O_2}$ should translate into delayed ventilatory limitation, reduced dyspnea and improved exercise capacity. In patients with more severe COPD with a symptom-limited peak $\dot{V}_{O_2}$ below 1 L/min (or approximately 60% predicted), anaerobic thresholds may not be discernible at baseline and, therefore, may not appreciably change following supervised exercise training. However, controlled studies have shown that, in patients with advanced COPD, submaximal $\dot{V}_E$ falls significantly by a range of 3 to 6 L/min after training[77,89] (Figure 18.17). This reduction in $\dot{V}_E$ usually reflects improved efficiency (i.e. reduced $\dot{V}_{CO_2}$ and $\dot{V}_{O_2}$ at any given submaximal work rate)[89] (Figure 18.17). In such patients, exercise ventilation falls predominantly as a result of reduced breathing frequency rather than change in V_T, which is relatively fixed in more advanced disease.[77,89]

Exercise training (EXT) has been shown not to improve gas exchange, and has only minor inconsistent effects on resting ventilatory mechanics.[172–174] In one study, resting IC improved significantly following exercise training by an average of 0.3 L compared with control (P < 0.003).[89] Dynamic ventilatory mechanics may improve as the result of reduced ventilation. Reduction in $\dot{V}_E/\dot{V}_{O_2}$ slopes was shown to be the predominant correlate of improved Borg ratings in a multiple regression analysis.[89] This study also showed that, at a given ventilation after training, dyspnea ratings fell significantly.[89] Possible explanations for this include altered mechanical loading due to decreased DH, improved inspiratory muscle strength or altered central perception of dyspneogenic stimuli. Increase in resting IC, together with increases in dynamic IC during exercise (because of reduced ventilation and air trapping), may reduce elastic/mechanical loading, provided the EILV does not increase. However, reduced mechanical loading as a

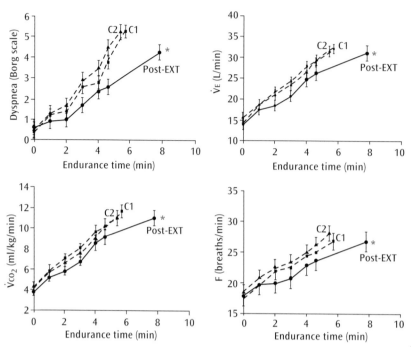

Figure 18.17 *Dyspnea, $\dot{V}_E$, $\dot{V}_{CO_2}$ and breathing frequency (F) versus endurance time during constant-load submaximal cycle exercise testing before (C1 and C2 control) and after exercise training (EXT). Note significant (*P < 0.05) reductions in dyspnea, $\dot{V}_E$, $\dot{V}_{CO_2}$ and F after training. (Adapted from ref. 89.)*

consequence of EXT remains a theoretical contributor to improved exercise performance, which requires further study.

EXT has been shown to significantly increase inspiratory (P_{Imax}) and expiratory (MEP) muscle strength in one study by 29% and 27% respectively, and resulted in a threefold increase in inspiratory muscle endurance.[77] These improvements are comparable to those achieved by specific inspiratory muscle training and occurred in response to the stimulus of sustained increases in ventilation for increasing periods of time during exercise training.[101] Thus, sustained targeted high ventilatory levels will result in functional adaptation of ventilatory muscles given their increased intrinsic mechanical loads. Increased inspiratory strength means that reduced neural activation or central motor command output is required for a given force generation by the muscles.[51,63] This should reduce the perceived respiratory discomfort.

Reduction in dyspnea at any given ventilation may also occur as a result of altered central perception of sensory stimuli. Prolonged supervised training, in a secure healthcare environment, may result in patients overcoming their fear of dyspnea-provoking activity, or may favorably alter the affective response to dyspnea provocation. This phenomenon of temporal adaptation or desensitization to dyspnea has been reported extensively, although its psychophysical basis remains obscure.[175] It is likely that in many patients with COPD, relatively small improvements in ventilatory demand, inspiratory muscle function and ventilatory mechanics, together with increased well being and motivation, all combine to ameliorate dyspnea and exercise capacity.

Oxygen therapy during exercise

The effects of ambulatory oxygen on dyspnea and exercise performance in any given individual with symptomatic COPD is unpredictable.[176–181] Furthermore, the mechanisms of improved exercise performance in those who do respond positively are multifactorial, and not fully understood. In advanced disease, the main mechanism appears to be that of a delay in reaching critical ventilatory limitation as a result of reduced ventilatory demand. Potential mechanisms of reduced ventilation include reduced central motor command output as a result of diminished hypoxic drive from peripheral chemoreceptors.[176–181] Alternatively, or in addition, reduced activity-generated metabolic acidosis as a result of improved oxygen delivery or utilization by the active locomotor muscles may reduce ventilatory requirements during added oxygen.[90,181] Additional contributors to improved exercise performance during oxygen therapy include: (i) reduced perceived respiratory discomfort; (ii) improved peripheral muscle function with reduced leg discomfort; and (iii) enhanced cardiac function.

The question of whether relief of dyspnea during oxygen therapy is solely a function of the attendant reduction of ventilation, or is independent of this effect, has not been conclusively answered. Some studies in normals and in patients with COPD during rest and exercise have shown that dyspnea relief can be independent of the reduction in ventilation,[176] while others have not.[90,177] Dyspnea amelioration at a given ventilation following oxygen therapy could be explained by: (i) concomitant reductions in DH due to altered

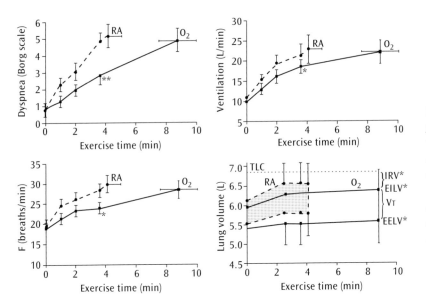

Figure 18.18 *Dyspnea, V_E, breathing frequency (F) and operating lung volumes plotted against exercise time in patients randomized to breathe either room air (RA) or 60% oxygen. While breathing oxygen, exercise endurance increased significantly in conjunction with significant decreases in dyspnea, V_E, F, EELV (i.e. increased IC) and EILV (i.e. increased IRV) at isotime during exercise (*P < 0.05, **P < 0.01). (Adapted from ref. 104.)*

breathing pattern (i.e. prolonged expiratory time)(see below); (ii) altered perception of dyspneogenic stimuli; and (iii) decreased afferent inputs from the pulmonary vasculature or right heart chambers secondary to acute decreases in pulmonary artery pressure.

Reduced peripheral chemoreceptor activity in response to oxygen has long been thought to be the primary mechanism of reduced dyspnea–ventilation slopes in COPD. However, mildly hypoxic patients, who would not be expected to rely on an increased hypoxic drive to breathe, also showed reduced submaximal ventilation with improvements in dyspnea and exercise endurance during added oxygen.[90,105] Studies conducted in patients with advanced disease, but with only mild exercise hypoxemia, have shown that reduction of standardized Borg ratings during added oxygen therapy (compared with control) was directly related to reduced submaximal ventilation which, in turn, correlated strongly with reduced metabolic acidosis (i.e. reduced blood lactate concentrations).[90,104]

Since the extent of DH during exercise in flow-limited patients depends on ventilation and breathing pattern for a given ventilation, it follows that therapeutic interventions, such as oxygen, that reduce submaximal ventilation by reducing breathing frequency (and increasing T_E), should delay the rate of DH and the onset of critical ventilatory constraints that limit exercise. In a recent placebo-controlled, crossover study, where patients with advanced COPD received either 60% oxygen or room air, we showed that hyperoxia more than doubled the time that it took to reach ventilatory limitation compared with breathing room air[105] (Figure 18.18). In this study the improvements in dyspnea and exercise endurance during hyperoxia were explained, in large measure, by the effects of reduced ventilatory demand and operating lung volumes. At a standardized submaximal work rate, V_E decreased by approximately 3 L/min and the IRV increased by 0.3 L during 60% oxygen compared with room air.[105]

Somfay *et al.*[182] recently confirmed the effects of supplemental oxygen on DH in a dose–response study to added oxygen in normoxic COPD. These authors demonstrated that with increasing levels of supplemental oxygen, correspondingly greater reductions of DH were achieved with maximal effects occurring at an added oxygen level of 50%. We have recently reported the results of a preliminary study which showed that in advanced Stage III COPD patients ($FEV_{1.0} < 35\%$ predicted), responses to supplemental oxygen (i.e. increased exercise endurance and reduced dyspnea) occurred independently of the baseline or exercise gas-exchange abnormalities.[105] Thus, small reductions in ventilation in the order of 4 L/min, in conjunction with reduced metabolic acidosis, caused concomitant reductions in dynamic operating lung volumes and translated into meaningful improvements in symptoms and exercise performance even in mildly hypoxemic patients with advanced disease.[105]

A comprehensive approach to exercise intolerance in COPD

To optimize exercise performance in advanced COPD, a step-by-step, integrated approach to management achieves best results. Combination bronchodilator therapy should be carefully optimized to achieve sustained 24-hour lung volume reduction. Oxygen therapy, in selected individuals, provides further performance enhancement. Positive responders to oxygen can easily be identified by a randomized case control study using a

Table 18.3 *Case example of a 73-year-old male with COPD (FEV$_{1.0}$ = 35% predicted) showing the magnitude of improvement after stepwise therapy*

Improvement	Magnitude
Changes in pulmonary function at rest:	
ΔFEV$_{1.0}$	+90 mL
ΔFRC	−400 mL
ΔMIP	+20 cmH$_2$O (30%)
ΔMEP	+24 cmH$_2$O (27%)
ΔInspiratory muscle endurance (breathing at 50% of MIP)	+3.5 min (230%)
Changes at a standardized level of exercise:	
ΔEELV (or IC)	−420 mL
ΔIRV	+350 mL
ΔVentilation	−5 L/min
ΔF	−6 breaths/min

Note: see text for definition of abbreviations.

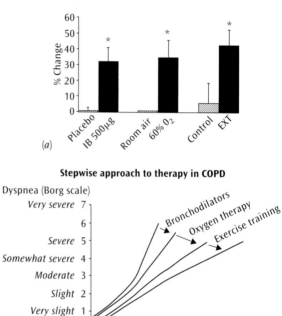

Figure 18.19 *(a) Exercise endurance increased significantly (*P < 0.05) in response to nebulized ipratropium bromide (IB, 500 μg),[36] 60% O$_2$[90] and exercise training (EXT)[89] in three groups of patients with severe COPD. No improvements were seen with placebo, room air or control, respectively. (b) Exertional dyspnea and exercise endurance progressively improves with a stepwise approach to therapy. (Adapted from ref. 183.)*

constant-load endurance protocol, where individuals are randomized to room air or oxygen (to maintain oxygen saturation >90%). Exercise endurance times, dyspnea intensity and leg discomfort (at a standardized time) are compared between the two conditions. Exercise training remains the pivotal intervention to maximize activity levels. These combined therapies cause a myriad of relatively small changes in a number of physiologic parameters (rarely measured in practice), which culminate in meaningful clinical improvement.

To illustrate this, we present the case of a 73-year-old male (FEV$_{1.0}$ = 35% predicted) with advanced COPD who participated in sequential studies in our laboratory on the effects of bronchodilators, oxygen therapy and exercise training (Table 18.3, Figure 18.19). Despite minimal changes in the FEV$_{1.0}$, this patient showed progressive increases in exercise endurance. These improvements were attributable to reduction in resting lung volumes, improvements in inspiratory muscle strength and endurance, reduction in dynamic lung volumes and ventilatory demand, with a more efficient breathing pattern during exercise, and reduced exertional dyspnea and leg discomfort. It is important to emphasize that the magnitude of the response to each of these therapeutic interventions will vary widely between individuals, but that additive or synergistic effects are to be expected with multiple interventions.

SUMMARY

On the basis of extensive studies in COPD patients, we can conclude that ventilatory limitation contributes importantly, and often predominantly, to exercise limitation. Expiratory flow limitation is the hallmark of this heterogeneous condition and its most important consequence is resting hyperinflation and further dynamic hyperinflation during exercise, which accelerates ventilatory limitation, respiratory discomfort and exercise termination. The recognition that DH is one factor contributing to reduced ventilatory capacity is potentially clinically important, since this is at least partially reversible and can, therefore, be manipulated for the patient's benefit. Interventions that improve airway function and lung emptying (i.e. bronchodilators) will reduce operating lung volumes during exercise and delay the occurrence of critical ventilatory constraints, thus improving exercise endurance and symptoms. Similarly, interventions that reduce ventilatory demand (i.e. oxygen therapy) will also delay the rate of DH and its deleterious consequences in selected patients.

Reduced activity levels, as a result of dyspnea and cardioventilatory impairment, eventually lead to alterations in the structure and function of the peripheral muscles, which further curtail exercise capacity in a vicious cycle.

Disuse atrophy, reduced oxygen delivery and/or blood perfusion to the active muscle, together with perceived leg discomfort, are all likely to be instrumental in contributing to exercise limitation. There is now good evidence that exercise reconditioning and strength training can partially reverse these abnormalities. Comprehensive management strategies that incorporate pharmacologic therapies and exercise training can maximize exercise capabilities and, thus, the health status of patients with advanced symptomatic disease.

REFERENCES

1. Aaron EA, Johnson BD, Seow KC, Dempsey JA. Oxygen cost of exercise hyperpnea: implications for performance. *J Appl Physiol* 1992;**72**:1818–25.
2. Henke KG, Sharratt M, Pegelow DF, Dempsey JA. Regulation of end-expiratory lung volume during exercise. *J Appl Physiol* 1988;**64**:135–46.
3. Druz WS, Sharp JT. Activity of respiratory muscles in upright and recumbent humans. *J Appl Physiol* 1981;**51**:1522–61.
4. Lind F, Hesser CM. Breathing pattern and lung volumes during exercise. *Acta Physiol Scand* 1984;**120**:123–19.
5. Linnarson D. Dynamics of pulmonary gas-exchange at start and end of exercise. *Acta Physiol Scand Suppl* 1974;**415**:1–68.
6. Younes M, Kivinen G. Respiratory mechanics and breathing pattern during and following maximal exercise. *J Appl Physiol* 1984;**57**:1773–82.
7. Olafsson S, Hyatt RE. Ventilatory mechanics and expiratory flow limitation during exercise in normal subjects. *J Clin Invest* 1969;**48**:564–73.
8. Warren JB, Jennings SJ, Clark TJH. Effect of adrenergic and vagal blockade on the normal human airway response to exercise. *Clin Sci* 1984;**66**:79–85.
9. Gledhill N, Froese A, Dempsey J. Ventilation to perfusion distribution during exercise in health. In: J Dempsey, C Reed, eds. *Muscular Exercise and the Lung*. University of Wisconsin Press, Madison, 1977, p 325.
10. Johnson BD, Badr MS, Dempsey JA. Impact of the aging pulmonary system on the response to exercise. In: IM Weisman, RJ Zeballos, eds. *Clinics in Chest Medicine*, vol 15. WB Saunders, Philadelphia, 1994, pp 229–46.
11. Johnson BD, Dempsey JA. Demand vs capacity in the aging pulmonary system. In: JO Holloszy, ed. *Exercise and Sports Science Reviews*. Williams & Wilkins, Baltimore, 1991, pp 171–210.
12. Johnson BD, Reddan DF, Pegelow KC, Seow KC, Dempsey JA. Flow limitation and regulation of functional residual capacity during exercise in a physically active aging population. *Am Rev Respir Dis* 1991;**143**:960–7.
13. Johnson BD, Reddan WG, Seow KC, Dempsey JA. Mechanical constraints on exercise hyperpnea in a fit aging population. *Am Rev Respir Dis* 1991;**143**:968–77.
14. Anthonisen NR, Danson J, Robertson PC, Ross WR. Airway closure as a function of age. *Respir Physiol* 1969;**8**:58–65.
15. Frank NR, Mead J, Ferris BG Jr. The mechanical behaviour of the lungs in healthy elderly persons. *J Clin Invest* 1957;**36**:1680.
16. D'Errico A, Scarani P, Colosimo E, Spina M, Grigioni WF, Mancini AM. Changes in the alveolar connective tissue of the aging lung. *Virch Arch A Pathol Anat* 1989;**415**:137–44.
17. Gibson GJ, Pride NB, O'Cain C, Quagliato R. Sex and age differences in pulmonary mechanics in normal non-smoking subjects. *J Appl Physiol* 1976;**41**:20–5.
18. Rizzato G, Marazzini L. Thoracoabdominal mechanics in elderly men. *J Appl Physiol* 1970;**28**:457–60.
19. Knudson RJ, Clark DF, Kennedy TC, Knudson DE. Effect of aging alone on mechanical properties of the normal adult human lung. *J Appl Physiol* 1977;**43**:1054–62.
20. Tenney SM, Miller RM. Dead space ventilation in old age. *J Appl Physiol* 1956;**9**:321.
21. Leblanc P, Summers E, Inman MD, Jones NL, Campbell EJ, Killian KJ. Inspiratory muscles during exercise: a problem of supply and demand. *J Appl Physiol* 1988;**64**:2482–9.
22. Gandevia B, Hugh-Jones P. Terminology of measurements of ventilatory capacity. *Thorax* 1957;**1**:290–3.
23. Dillard TA, Piantadosi S, Rajagopal KR. Determinants of maximum exercise capacity in patients with chronic airflow obstruction. *Chest* 1989;**96**:267–71.
24. Johnson BD, Weisman IM, Zeballos RJ, Beck KC. Emerging concepts in the evaluation of ventilatory limitation during exercise: the exercise tidal flow–volume loop. *Chest* 1999;**116**:488–503.
25. O'Donnell DE, Revill S, Webb KA. Dynamic hyperinflation and exercise intolerance in COPD. *Am J Respir Crit Care Med* 2001;**164**:770–7.
26. Pride NB, Macklem PT. Lung mechanics in disease. In: AP Fishman, ed. *Handbook of Physiology*, section 3, vol III, part 2: *The Respiratory System*. American Physiological Society, Bethesda, MD, 1986, pp 659–92.
27. Younes M. Determinants of thoracic excursions during exercise. In: BJ Whipp, K Wasserman, eds. *Lung Biology in Health and Disease*, vol 42: *Exercise, Pulmonary Physiology and Pathophysiology*. Marcel Dekker, New York, 1991, pp 1–65.
28. Vinegar A, Sinnett EE, Leith DE. Dynamic mechanisms determine functional residual capacity in mice. *J Appl Physiol* 1979;**46**:867–91.
29. O'Donnell DE, Webb KA. Exertional breathlessness in patients with chronic airflow limitation: the role of hyperinflation. *Am Rev Respir Dis* 1993;**148**:1351–7.
30. Grimby G, Bunn J, Mead J. Relative contribution of rib cage and abdomen to ventilation during exercise. *J Appl Physiol* 1968;**24**:159–66.
31. Potter WA, Olafsson S, Hyatt RE. Ventilatory mechanics and expiratory flow limitation during exercise in patients with obstructive lung disease. *J Clin Invest* 1971;**50**:910–19.
32. Dodd DS, Brancatisano T, Engel LA. Chest wall mechanics during exercise in patients with severe chronic airway obstruction. *Am Rev Respir Dis* 1984;**129**:33–8.
33. Stubbing DG, Pengelly LD, Morse JLC, Jones NL. Pulmonary mechanics during exercise in subjects with chronic airflow obstruction. *J Appl Physiol* 1980;**49**:511–15.
34. Yan S, Kaminski D, Sliwinski P. Reliability of inspiratory capacity for estimating end-expiratory lung volume changes during exercise in patients with chronic obstructive pulmonary disease. *Am J Respir Crit Care Med* 1997;**156**:55–9.
35. O'Donnell DE, Chau LKL, Bertley JC, Webb KA. Qualitative aspects of exertional breathlessness in chronic airflow limitation:pathophysiologic mechanisms. *Am J Respir Crit Care Med* 1997;**155**:109–15.
36. O'Donnell DE, Lam M, Webb KA. Measurement of symptoms, lung hyperinflation and endurance during exercise in chronic obstructive pulmonary disease. *Am J Respir Crit Care Med* 1998;**158**:1557–65.
37. Marin JM, Carrizo SJ, Gascon M, Sanchez A, Gallego BA, Celli BR. Inspiratory capacity, dynamic hyperinflation,

breathlessness and exercise performance during the 6-minute-walk test in chronic obstructive pulmonary disease. *Am J Respir Crit Care Med* 2001;**163**:1395–9.

38. O'Donnell DE, Webb KA. Breathlessness in patients with severe chronic airflow limitation: physiological correlates. *Chest* 1992;**102**:824–31.

39. Sinderby C, Spahija J, Beck J, *et al.* Diaphragm activation during exercise in chronic obstructive pulmonary disease. *Am J Respir Crit Care Med* 2001;**163**:1637–41.

40. Tantucci C, Duguet A, Similowski T, Zelter M, Derenne JP, Milic-Emili J. Effect of salbutamol on dynamic hyperinflation in chronic obstructive pulmonary disease patients. *Eur Respir J* 1998;**12**:799–804.

41. Diaz O, Villafranco C, Ghezzo H, *et al.* Exercise tolerance in COPD patients with and without tidal expiratory flow limitation at rest. *Eur Respir J* 2000;**16**:269–75.

42. Eltayara L, Becklake MR, Volta CA, Milic-Emili J. Relationship between chronic dyspnea and expiratory flow limitation in patients with chronic obstructive pulmonary disease. *Am J Respir Crit Care Med* 1996;**154**:1726–34.

43. Levison H, Cherniack RM. Ventilatory cost of exercise in chronic obstructive pulmonary disease. *J Appl Physiol* 1968;**25**:21–7.

44. Ninane V, Yernault JC, de Troyer A. Intrinsic PEEP in patients with chronic obstructive pulmonary disease. *Am Rev Respir Dis* 1993;**148**:1037–42.

45. Lougheed MD, Webb KA, O'Donnell DE. Breathlessness during induced lung hyperinflation in asthma:the role of the inspiratory threshold load. *Am J Respir Crit Care Med* 1995;**152**:911–20.

46. Rochester DF. The diaphragm in COPD:better than expected, but not good enough. *N Engl J Med* 1991;**325**:961–2.

47. Rochester DF, Braun NMT. Determinants of maximal inspiratory pressure in chronic obstructive pulmonary disease. *Am Rev Respir Dis* 1970;**132**:42–7.

48. Killian KJ, Jones NJ. Respiratory muscles and dyspnea. *Clin Chest Med* 1988;**9**:237–48.

49. Meek PM, Schwartzstein RMS, Adams L, *et al.* Dyspnea mechanisms, assessment and management: a consensus statement (American Thoracic Society). *Am J Respir Crit Care Med* 1999;**159**:321–40.

50. O'Donnell DE. Exertional breathlessness in chronic respiratory disease. In: DA Mahler, ed. *Lung Biology in Health and Disease*, vol III: *Dyspnea*. Marcel Dekker, New York, 1998, pp 97–147.

51. Killian KJ, Campbell EJM. Dyspnea. In: C Roussos, PT Macklem, eds. *Lung Biology in Health and Disease*, vol 29, part B: *The Thorax*. Marcel Dekker, New York, 1985, pp 787–828.

52. Altose M, Cherniack N, Fishman AP. Respiratory sensations and dyspnea: perspectives. *J Appl Physiol* 1985;**58**:1051–4.

53. Chen Z, Eldridge FL, Wagner PG. Respiratory associated rhythmic firing of midbrain neurones in cats: relation to level of respiratory drive. *J Appl Physiol* 1991;**437**:305–25.

54. Chen Z, Eldridge FL, Wagner PG. Respiratory-associated thalamic activity is related to level of respiratory drive. *Respir Physiol* 1992;**90**:99–113.

55. Davenport PW, Friedman WA, Thompson FJ, Franzen O. Respiratory-related cortical potentials evoked by inspiratory occlusion in humans. *J Appl Physiol* 1986;**60**:1843–8.

56. Gandevia SC, Macefield G. Projection of low threshold afferents from human intercostal muscles to the cerebral cortex. *Respir Physiol* 1989;**77**:203–14.

57. Homma I, Kanamara A, Sibuya M. Proprioceptive chest wall afferents and the effect on respiratory sensation. In: C Von Euler, M Katz-Salamon, eds. *Respiratory Psychophysiology*. Stockton Press, New York, 1988, pp 161–6.

58. Banzett RB, Lansing RW, Reid MB, Adams L, Brown R. 'Air hunger' arising from increased Pco_2 in mechanically ventilated quadriplegics. *Respir Physiol* 1989;**76**:53–68.

59. Altose MD, Syed I, Shoos L. Effects of chest wall vibration on the intensity of dyspnea during constrained breathing. *Proc Int Union Physiol Sci* 1989;**17**:288.

60. Matthews PBC. Where does Sherrington's 'muscular sense' originate: muscles, joints, corollary discharge? *Ann Rev Neurosci* 1982;**5**:189–218.

61. Roland PE, Ladegaard-Pederson HA. A quantitative analysis of sensation of tension and kinaesthesia in man. Evidence for peripherally originating muscular sense and a sense of effort. *Brain* 1977;**100**:671–92.

62. Noble MIM, Eisele JH, Trenchard D, Guz A. Effect of selective peripheral nerve blocks on respiratory sensations. In: R Porter, ed. *Breathing: Hering-Breyer Symposium*. Churchill, London, 1970, pp 233–46.

63. Zechman FR Jr, Wiley RL. Afferent inputs to breathing: respiratory sensation. In: AP Fishman, ed. *Handbook of Physiology*, section 3, vol II, part 2: *The Respiratory System*. American Physiology Society, Bethesda, MD, 1986, pp 449–74.

64. Banzett RB, Dempsey JA, O'Donnell DE, Wamboldt MZ. Symptom perception and respiratory sensation in asthma. *Am J Respir Crit Care Med* 2000;**162**:1178–82.

65. Kukorelli T, Namenyi J, Adam G. Visceral afferent projection areas in the cortex representation of the carotid sinus receptor area. *Acta Physiol Acad Sci* 1969;**36**:261–3.

66. Belman MJ, Botnick WC, Shin JW. Inhaled bronchodilators reduce dynamic hyperinflation during exercise in patients with chronic obstructive pulmonary disease. *Am J Respir Crit Care Med* 1996;**153**:967–75.

67. Chrystyn H, Mulley BA, Peake MD. Dose response relation to oral theophylline in severe chronic obstructive airways disease. *Br Med J* 1988;**297**:1506–10.

68. O'Donnell DE, Sanii R, Younes M. Improvements in exercise endurance in patients with chronic airflow limitation using CPAP. *Am Rev Respir Dis* 1988;**138**:1510–14.

69. O'Donnell DE, Lam M, Webb KA. Spirometric correlates of improvement in exercise performance after anticholinergic therapy in COPD. *Am J Respir Crit Care Med* 1999;**160**:524–49.

70. Martinez FJ, Montes de Oca M, Whyte RI, Stetz J, Gay SE, Celli BR. Lung-volume reduction improves dyspnea, dynamic hyperinflation and respiratory muscle function. *Am J Respir Crit Care Med* 1997;**155**:1984–90.

71. Laghi F, Jurban A, Topeli A, *et al.* Effect of lung volume reduction surgery on neuromechanical coupling of the diaphgram. *Am J Respir Crit Care Med* 1998;**157**:475–83.

72. O'Donnell DE, Bertley J, Webb KA, Conlan AA. Mechanisms of relief of exertional breathlessness following unilateral bullectomy and lung volume reduction surgery in advanced chronic airflow limitation. *Chest* 1996;**110**:18–27.

73. Petrof BJ, Calderini E, Gottfried SB. Effect of CPAP on respiratory effort and dyspnea during exercise in severe COPD. *J Appl Physiol* 1990;**69**:178–88.

74. Barbera JA, Roca J, Ramirez J, Wagner PD, Usetti P, Rodriquez-Roisin R. Gas exchange during exercise in mild chronic obstructive pulmonary disease: correlation with lung structure. *Am Rev Respir Dis* 1991;**144**:520–5.

75. Dantzker DR, D'Alonzo GE. The effect of exercise on pulmonary gas exchange in patients with severe chronic obstructive pulmonary disease. *Am Rev Respir Dis* 1986;**134**:1135–9.

76. Dillard TA, Piantadosi S, Rajagopal KR. Prediction of ventilation at maximal exercise in chronic airflow obstruction. *Am Rev Respir Dis* 1985;**132**:230–5.

77. O'Donnell DE, McGuire M, Samis L, Webb KA. Effects of general exercise training on ventilatory and peripheral muscle strength and endurance in chronic airflow limitation. *Am J Respir Crit Care Med* 1998;**157**:1489–97.

78. Begin P, Grassino A. Inspiratory muscle dysfunction and chronic hypercapnia in chronic obstructive pulmonary disease. *Am Rev Respir Dis* 1991;**143**:905–12.

79. Borrows B, Earle RH. Course and prognosis of chronic obstructive lung disease: a prospective study of 200 patients. *N Engl J Med* 1969;**280**:397–404.

80. Altose MD, McCauley WC, Kelsen SG, Cherniack NS. Effects of hypercapnia and inspiratory flow-resistive loading on respiratory activity in chronic airways obstruction. *J Clin Invest* 1977;**59**:500–7.

81. Light RW, Mahutte CK, Brown SE. Etiology of carbon dioxide retention at rest and during exercise in chronic airflow obstruction. *Chest* 1988;**94**:61–7.

82. DeTroyer A, Leeper JB, McKenzie D, Gandevia S. Neural drive to the diaphragm in patients with severe COPD. *Am J Respir Crit Care Med* 1997;**155**:1335–40.

83. Sorli J, Grassino A, Lorange G, Milic-Emili J. Control of breathing in patients with chronic obstructive lung disease. *Clin Sci Mol Med* 1978;**54**:296–304.

84. Moutain R, Zwillich C, Weil J. Hypoventilation in obstructive lung disease. The role of familial factors. *N Engl J Med* 1978;**298**:521–5.

85. Montes de Oca M, Celli BR. Mouth occlusion pressure, CO_2 response and hypercapnia in severe obstructive pulmonary disease. *Eur Respir J* 1998;**12**:666–71.

86. Scano G, Spinelli A, Duranti R, *et al.* Carbon dioxide responsiveness in COPD patients with and without hypercapnia. *Eur Respir J* 1995;**8**:78–85.

87. Montes de Oca M, Celli B. Respiratory muscle recruitment and exercise performance in eucapnic and hypercapnic severe chronic obstructive pulmonary disease. *Am J Respir Crit Care Med* 2000;**61**:880–5.

88. O'Donnell DE, D'Arsigny C, Webb KA. Mechanisms of exercise-induced hypercapnia in advanced COPD. *Am J Respir Crit Care Med* 2001;**63**:A21.

89. O'Donnell DE, McGuire M, Samis L, Webb KA. The impact of exercise reconditioning on breathlessness in severe chronic airflow limitation. *Am J Respir Crit Care Med* 1995;**152**:2005–13.

90. O'Donnell DE, Bain DJ, Webb KA. Factors contributing to relief of exertional breathlessness during hyperoxia in chronic airflow limitation. *Am J Respir Crit Care Med* 1997;**155**:530–5.

91. Light RW, Muro JR, Sato RI, Stansbury DW, Fischer CE, Brown SE. Effects of oral morphine on breathlessness and exercise tolerance in patients with chronic obstructive pulmonary disease. *Am Rev Respir Dis* 1989;**139**:126–33.

92. Bye PTP, Esau SA, Levy RO, *et al.* Ventilatory muscle function during exercise in air and oxygen in patients with chronic airflow limitation. *Am Rev Respir Dis* 1985;**32**:236–40.

93. Grassino A, Gross D, Macklem PT, Roussos C, Zagelbaum G. Inspiratory muscle fatigue as a factor limiting exercise. *Bull Eur Pathophysiol Respir* 1979;**15**:105–11.

94. Kyroussis D, Polkey MI, Keilty SEJ, *et al.* Exhaustive exercise slows inspiratory muscle relaxation rate in chronic obstructive pulmonary disease. *Am J Respir Crit Care Med* 1996;**153**:787–93.

95. Polkey MI, Kyroussis D, Mills GH, *et al.* Inspiratory pressure support reduces slowing of inspiratory muscle relaxation rate during exhaustive treadmill walking in severe COPD. *Am J Respir Crit Care Med* 1996;**154**:1146–50.

96. Similowski T, Yan S, Gauthier AP, Macklem PT, Bellemare F. Contractile properties of the human diaphragm during chronic hyperinflation. *N Engl J Med* 1991;**325**:917–23.

97. Orozco-Levi M, Gea J, Lloreta JL, *et al.* Subcellular adaptation of the human diaphragm in chronic obstructive pulmonary disease. *Eur Respir J* 1999;**13**:371–8.

98. Levine S, Kaiser L, Leferovich J, Tikunov B. Cellular adaptations in the diaphragm in chronic obstructive pulmonary disease. *N Engl J Med* 1997;**337**:1799–806.

99. Mercadier JJ, Schwartz K, Schiaffino S, *et al.* Myosin heavy chain gene expression changes in the diaphragm of patients with chronic lung hyperinflation. *Am J Physiol* 1998:**274**:L527–34.

100. Smith K, Cook D, Guyatt GH, Madhoven J, Oxman AD. Respiratory muscle training in chronic airflow obstruction. *Am Rev Respir Dis* 1992;**145**:533–9.

101. Harver A, Mahler DA, Daubenspeck JA. Targeted inspiratory muscle training improves respiratory muscle function and reduces dyspnea in chronic obstructive pulmonary disease. *Ann Intern Med* 1989;**111**:117–24.

102. Kim J, Larson J, Covey M, Vitalo C, Alex C, Patel M. Inspiratory muscle training in patients with chronic obstructive pulmonary disease. *Nurs Res* 1993;**42**:356–62.

103. Lisboa C, Munoz V, Beroiza T, Leiva A, Cruz E. Inspiratory muscle training in chronic airflow limitation: comparison of two different training loads with a threshold device. *Eur Respir J* 1994;**7**:1266–74.

104. O'Donnell DE, D'Arsigny C, Webb KA. Effects of hyperoxia on ventilatory limitation during exercise in advanced chronic obstructive pulmonary disease. *Am J Respir Crit Care Med* 2001;**163**:892–8.

105. Webb KA, D'Arsigny C, O'Donnell DE. Exercise response to added oxygen in patients with COPD and variable gas exchange abnormalities. *Am J Respir Crit Care Med* 2001;**163**:A169.

106. O'Donnell DE, D'Arsigny C, Fitzpatrick M, Webb KA. Exercise hypercapnia in advanced chronic obstructive pulmonary disease. *Am J Respir Crit Care Med* 2002;**166**:663–8.

107. Kyroussis D, Polkey MI, Hamnegard CH, Mills GH, Green M, Moxham J. Respiratory muscle activity in patients with COPD walking to exhaustion with and without pressure support. *Eur Respir J* 2000;**15**:649–55.

108. Mador MJ, Kufel TJ, Pineda LA, Sharma GK. Diaphragmatic fatigue and high intensity exercise in patients with chronic obstructive pulmonary disease. *Am J Respir Crit Care Med* 2000;**161**:118–23.

109. Hyatt RE. Expiratory flow limitation. *J Appl Physiol* 1983;**55**:1–8.

110. Roussos C, Macklem PT. The respiratory muscles. *N Engl J Med* 1982;**307**:786–97.

111. Leaver DG, Pride NB. Flow volume curves and expiratory pressures during exercise in patients with chronic airflow obstruction. *Scand J Respir Dis* 1971;**42**(suppl):23–7.

112. O'Donnell DE, Sanii R, Anthonisen NR, Younes M. Effect of dynamic airway compression on breathing pattern and respiratory sensation in severe chronic obstructive pulmonary disease. *Am Rev Respir Dis* 1987;**135**:912–18.

113. O'Donnell DE, Sanii R, Anthonisen NR, Younes M. Expiratory resistive loading in patients with severe chronic airflow limitation: an evaluation of ventilatory mechanics and compensatory responses. *Am Rev Respir Dis* 1987;**136**:102–7.

114. Kayser B, Sliwinski P, Yan S, Tobias M, Macklem PT. Respiratory effort sensation during exercise with induced expiratory flow limitation in healthy humans. *J Appl Physiol* 1997;**83**:936–47.

115. Aliverti A, Andelli I, Kayser B, *et al*. Pathophysiology of expiratory flow limitation (EFL): blood volume shifts. *Eur Respir J* 2000;**16**(suppl 31):190S.

116. O'Donnell DE, Sanii R, Giesbrecht G, Younes M. The effect of continuous positive airway pressure on respiratory sensation in patients with COPD during submaximal exercise. *Am Rev Respir Dis* 1988;**138**:1185–91.

117. Gosker HR, Wouters EF, Van der Vusse GJ, Schols AM. Skeletal muscle dysfunction in chronic obstructive pulmonary disease and chronic heart failure: underlying mechanisms and therapy perspectives. *Am J Clin Nutr* 2000;**71**:1033–47.

118. Casaburi R. Skeletal muscle dysfunction in chronic obstructive pulmonary disease. *Med Sci Sports Exerc* 2001;**33**(suppl 7):S662–70.

119. Killian KJ, Leblanc P, Martin DH, Summers E, Jones NL, Campbell EJM. Exercise capacity and ventilatory, circulatory and symptom limitation in patients with chronic airflow limitation. *Am Rev Respir Dis* 1992;**146**:935–40.

120. Hamilton AL, Killian KJ, Summers E, Jones NL. Symptom intensity and subjective limitation to exercise in patients with cardiorespiratory disorders. *Chest* 1996;**110**:1255–63.

121. O'Donnell DE, Webb KA. Exercise reconditioning in patients with chronic airflow limitation. In: Torg JS, Shepherd RJ, eds. *Current Therapy in Sports Medicine*, 3rd edn. Mosby Year Book, St Louis, MO, 1995, pp 678–84.

122. Bernard S, Leblanc P, Whittom F, *et al*. Peripheral muscle weakness in patients with chronic obstructive pulmonary disease. *Am J Respir Crit Care Med* 1998;**158**:629–34.

123. Wilson DO, Rogers RM, Wright EC, Anthonisen NR. Body weight in chronic obstructive pulmonary disease: the National Institutes of Health intermittent positive pressure breathing trial. *Am Rev Respir Dis* 1989;**139**:1435–8.

124. Gosselink R, Troosters T, Decramer M. Peripheral muscle weakness contributes to exercise limitation in COPD. *Am J Respir Crit Care Med* 1996;**153**:976–80.

125. Whittom F, Jobin J, Simard PM, *et al*. Histochemical and morphological characteristics of the vastus lateralis muscle in patients with chronic obstructive pulmonary disease. *Med Sci Sports Exerc* 1998;**30**:1467–74.

126. Jakobsson P, Jorfeldt L, Henriksson J. Metabolic enzyme activity in the quadriceps femoris muscle in patients with severe chronic obstructive pulmonary disease. *Am J Respir Crit Care Med* 1995;**151**:374–7.

127. Jobin J, Maltais F, Doyon JF, *et al*. Chronic obstructive pulmonary disease: capillarity and fiber-type characteristics of skeletal muscle. *J Cardiopul Rehab* 1998;**18**:432–7.

128. Casaburi R. Deconditioning. In: AP Fishman, ed. *Lung Biology in Health and Disease Series: Pulmonary Rehabilitation*. Marcel Dekker, New York, 1996, pp 213–30.

129. Casaburi R. Exercise training in chronic obstructive lung disease. In: R Casaburi, TL Petty, eds. *Principles and Practice of Pulmonary Rehabilitation*. WB Saunders, Philadelphia, 1993, pp 204–24.

130. Cooper CB. Determining the role of exercise in patients with chronic obstructive pulmonary disease. *Med Sci Sports Exerc* 1995;**27**:147–57.

131. Casaburi R, Porszasz J, Burns MR, Carithers ER, Chang RSY, Cooper CB. Physiologic benefits of exercise training in rehabilitation of patients with severe chronic obstructive pulmonary disease. *Am J Respir Crit Care Med* 1997;**155**:1541–51.

132. Wilson JR, Martin JL, Schwartz D, Ferraro N. Exercise intolerance in patients with chronic heart failure: role of impaired nutritive flow to skeletal muscle. *Circulation* 1984;**69**:1079–87.

133. Green HR. Myofibrillar composition and mechanical function in mammalian skeletal muscle. In: Shepard RJ, ed. *Sports Science Reviews*. Human Kinetic Publishers, Champaign, IL, 1992, pp 43–64.

134. Semple PD, Bestall GH, Watson WS, Hume R. Hypothalamic-pituitary dysfunction in respiratory hypoxia. *Thorax* 1981;**36**:605–9.

135. Semple PD, Bestall GH, Watson WS, Hume R. Serum testosterone depression associated with hypoxia in respiratory failure. *Clin Sci* 1989;**58**:105–6.

136. Semple PD, Watson WS, Bestall GH, Bethel MIF, Grant JK, Hume R. Diet, absorption, and hormone studies in relation to body weight in obstructive airways disease. *Thorax* 1979;**34**:783–8.

137. Takabatake N, Nakamura H, Mingmihaba O, *et al*. A novel pathophysiologic phenomenon in cachexic patients with chronic obstructive pulmonary disease. *Am J Respir Crit Car Med* 2001;**163**:1314–19.

138. Heunks KMA, Vina J, Van Herwaarden CLA, Folgering MTM, Gimeno A, Dekhuizen PNR. Xanthine oxidase is involved in exercise-induced oxidative stress in chronic obstructive pulmonary disease. *Am J Physiol* 1999;**277**:R1697–704.

139. Vina J, Severa E, Acensi M, *et al*. Exercise causes blood glutathione oxidation in chronic obstructive pulmonary disease and prevention by O_2 therapy. *J Appl Physiol* 1996;**81**:2198–202.

140. Casaburi R, Patessio A, Ioli F, Zanaboni S, Donner CF, Wasserman K. Reduction in exercise lactic acidosis and ventilation as a result of exercise training in obstructive lung disease. *Am Rev Respir Dis* 1991;**143**:9–18.

141. Maltais F, Leblanc P, Simard C, *et al*. Skeletal muscle adaptation to endurance training in patients with chronic obstructive pulmonary disease. *Am J Respir Crit Care Med* 1996;**154**:442–7.

142. Bernard S, Whittom F, Leblanc P, *et al*. Aerobic and strength training in patients with chronic obstructive pulmonary disease. *Am J Respir Crit Care Med* 1999;**159**:896–901.

143. Kochakian CD, Stettner CE. Effect of testosterone propionate and grown hormone on weight and composition of body and organs of the mouse. *Am J Physiol* 1948;**155**: 255–65.

144. Simon M, Leblanc P, Jobin J, Desmeules M, Sullivan MJ, Maltais F. Limitation of lower limb V_{O_2} during cycling exercise in COPD patients. *J Appl Physiol* 2001;**90**: 1013–19.

145. Harms GA, Babcock MA, McClaren SR, *et al*. Respiratory muscle work compromises leg blood flow during maximal exercise. *J Appl Physiol* 1997;**82**:1573–83.

146. Richardson RS, Sheldon J, Poole DC, Hopkins SR, Ries AL, Wagner PD. Evidence of skeletal muscle metabolic reserve during whole body exercise in patients with chronic obstructive pulmonary disease. *Am J Respir Crit Care Med* 1999;**159**:881–5.

147. O'Donnell DE, D'Arsigny C, Raj S, Abdollah H, Webb KA. Ventilatory assistance improves exercise endurance in stable congestive heart failure. *Am J Respir Crit Care Med* 1999;**60**:1804–11.

148. Onorati P, Rabinovich R, Mancini M, *et al*. Effects of proportional assist ventilation (PAV) on limb exercise in COPD. *Am J Respir Crit Care Med* 2000;**161**:A228.

149. Light RW, Mintz WM, Linden GS, Brown SE. Hemodynamics of patients with severe chronic obstructive pulmonary disease during progressive upright exercise. *Am Rev Respir Dis* 1984;**130**:391–5.

150. Mahler DA, Brent BN, Loke J, Zaret BL, Matthay RA. Right ventricular performance and central hemodynamics during

upright exercise in patients with chronic obstructive pulmonary disease. *Am Rev Respir Dis* 1984;**130**:722–9.

151. Oswald-Mammosser M, Apprill M, Bachez P, Ehrhart M, Weitzenblum E. Pulmonary hemodynamics in chronic obstructive pulmonary disease of the emphysematous type. *Respiration* 1991;**58**:304–10.

152. Magee F, Wright JL, Wiggs BR, Pare PD, Hogg JC. Pulmonary vascular structure and function in chronic obstructive pulmonary disease. *Thorax* 1988;**43**:183–9.

153. Agusti AGN, Barbera JA, Roca J, Wagner PD, Guitart R, Rodriguez-Roisin R. Hypoxic pulmonary vasoconstriction and gas exchange during exercise in chronic obstructive pulmonary disease. *Chest* 1990;**97**:268–75.

154. Matthay RA, Berger HJ, Davies RA, *et al.* Right and left ventricular exercise performance in chronic obstructive pulmonary disease: radionuclide assessment. *Ann Int Med* 1980;**93**:234–9.

155. Vizza CD, Lynch JP, Ochoa LL, Richardson G, Trulock EP. Right and left ventricular dysfunction in patients with severe pulmonary disease. *Chest* 1998;**113**:576–83.

156. Morrison DA, Adock K, Collins CM, Goldman S, Caldwell JH, Schwartz MI. Right ventricular dysfunction and the exercise limitation of chronic obstructive pulmonary disease. *J Am Coll Cardiol* 1987;**9**:1219–29.

157. Dimopoulou I, Tsintzas OK, Daganou M, Cokkinos DV, Tzelepis GE. Contribution of lung function to exercise capacity in patients with chronic heart failure. *Respiration* 1999;**66**:144–9.

158. Koskolou MD, Calbet JA, Radegran G, Roach RC. Hypoxia and the cardiovascular response to dynamic knee-extensor exercise. *Am J Physiol* 1997;**272**:H2655–63.

159. Montes de Oca M, Rassulo J, Celli BR. Respiratory muscle and cardiopulmonary function during exercise in very severe COPD. *Am J Respir Crit Care Med* 1996;**154**:1284–9.

160. Oelberg DA, Kacmarek RM, Pappagianopoulos PP, Grims LC, Systrom DM. Ventilatory and cardiovascular responses to inspired He-O_2 during exercise in chronic obstructive pulmonary disease. *Am J Respir Crit Care Med* 1998;**158**:1876–82.

161. Spence DPS, Hay JG, Pearson MG, Calverley PMA. Oxygen desaturation and breathlessness during corridor walking in chronic obstructive lung disease. Effect of oxitropium bromide. *Thorax* 1993;**48**:1145–50.

162. Hay JG, Stone P, Carter J, *et al.* Bronchodilator reversibility, exercise performance and breathlessness in stable chronic obstructive pulmonary disease. *Eur Respir J* 1992;**5**:659–64.

163. Mahler DA, Mathay RA, Synder PE, Wells CK, Loke J. Sustained release theophylline reduces dyspnea in non-reversible obstructive airways disease. *Am Rev Respir Dis* 1985;**131**:22–5.

164. Papiris S, Galavotti V, Sturani C. Effects of beta agonists on breathlessness and exercise tolerance in patients with chronic obstructive pulmonary disease. *Respiration* 1986;**49**:101–8.

165. Oga T, Nishimura K, Tsukino M, Hajiro T, Ideda A, Izumi T. The effects of oxitropium bromide on exercise performance in patients with stable chronic obstructive pulmonary disease. A comparison of three different exercise tests. *Am J Respir Crit Care Med* 2000;**161**:1897–901.

166. O'Donnell DE, Forkert L, Webb KA. Evaluation of bronchodilator responses in patients with 'irreversible' emphysema. *Eur Respir J* 2001;**18**:914–20.

167. O'Donnell DE. Assessment of bronchodilator efficacy in symptomatic COPD: is spirometry useful? *Chest* 2000;**117**:S42–57.

168. Ries AL, Kaplan RM, Limberg TM, Prewitt LM. Effects of pulmonary rehabilitation on physiologic and psychosocial outcomes in patients with chronic obstructive pulmonary disease. *Ann Intern Med* 1995;**122**:823–32.

169. Casaburi R. Exercise training in chronic obstructive lung disease. In: R Casaburi, TL Petty, eds. *Principles and Practice of Pulmonary Rehabilitation*. WB Saunders, Philadelphia, 1993, p 204.

170. Strijbos JW, Sluiter JH, Postma DS, Gimeno F, Koeter GH. Objective and subjective performance indicators in COPD. *Eur Respir J* 1989;**2**:666–9.

171. Reardon J, Awad E, Normandin E, Vale F, Clark B, Zu Wallack RL. The effect of comprehensive outpatient pulmonary rehabilitation on dyspnea. *Chest* 1994;**105**:1046–52.

172. Cockroft AE, Saunders MJ, Berry G. Randomized controlled trial of rehabilitation in chronic respiratory disability. *Thorax* 1981;**36**:200–3.

173. Goldstein RS, Gork EH, Stubbing D, Avendano MA, Guyatt GH. Randomized controlled trials of respiratory rehabilitation. *Lancet* 1994;**344**:1394–7.

174. Cambach W, Wagenaar RC, Koelman TW, van Keimpema ARJT, Kemper HCG. The long-term effects of pulmonary rehabilitation in patients with asthma and chronic obstructive pulmonary disease: a research synthesis. *Arch Phys Med Rehabil* 1999;**80**:103–11.

175. Belman MJ, Brooks LR, Ross DJ, Mohsenifar Z. Variability of breathlessness measurement in patients with chronic obstructive pulmonary disease. *Chest* 1991;**99**:566–71.

176. Chronos N, Adams L, Guz A. Effect of hyperoxia and hypoxia on exercise-induced breathlessness in normal subjects. *Clin Sci* 1988;**74**:531–7.

177. Lane R, Cockcroft A, Adams L, Guz A. Arterial oxygen saturation and breathlessness in patients with chronic obstructive airways disease. *Clin Sci* 1987;**72**:693–8.

178. Woodcock AA, Gross ER, Geddes DM. Oxygen relieves breathlessness in 'pink puffers'. *Lancet* 1981;**i**:907–9.

179. Stein DA, Bradley BL, Miller W. Mechanisms of oxygen effects on exercise in patients with chronic obstructive pulmonary disease. *Chest* 1982;**81**:6–10.

180. Libby DM, Briscoe WA, King TKC. Relief of hypoxia-related bronchoconstriction by breathing 30 percent oxygen. *Am Rev Respir Dis* 1981;**123**:171–5.

181. Dean NC, Brown JK, Himelman RB, Doherty JJ, Gold WM, Stuhlbarg MS. Oxygen may improve dyspnea and endurance in patients with chronic obstructive pulmonary disease and only mild hypoxemia. *Am Rev Respir Dis* 1992;**148**:941–5.

182. Somfay A, Porszasz J, Lee SM, Casaburi R. Dose-response effect of oxygen on hyperinflation and exercise endurance in non-hypoxemic COPD patients. *Eur Respir J* 2001;**18**:77–84.

183. O'Donnell DE. Ventilatory limitations in chronic obstructive pulmonary disease. *Med Sci Sports Exer* 2001;**33**:S647–55.

Sleep

NEIL J DOUGLAS

INTRODUCTION

In the 1950s, Robin and colleagues found that expired carbon dioxide tension rose by 10 mmHg during sleep in seven patients with 'emphysema and chronic hypercapnia' and that four of the seven had Cheyne Stokes respiration during sleep.[1,2] In the early 1960s, studies using an early ear oximeter showed that arterial oxygen saturation fell during sleep in all the COPD patients, and the authors noted that the lowest oxygen saturations during sleep were recorded in those whose saturations were also lowest when awake.[3] All this was reported before the sleep apnea syndrome was recognized[4] in 1966. However, the great interest in breathing during sleep stimulated by the sleep apnea syndrome has resulted in increased attention

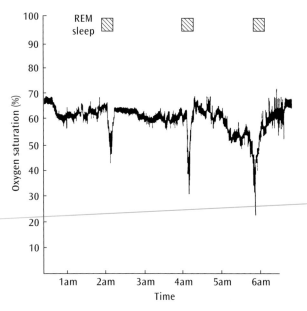

Figure 19.1 *Oxygen saturation throughout the night in a patient with COPD, the shaded areas representing rapid eye movement sleep.*

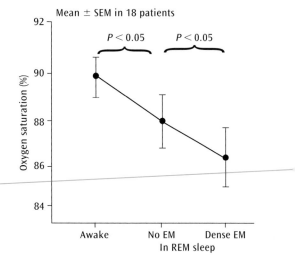

Figure 19.2 *The effect of sleep stage on oxygen saturation in 18 patients with COPD where rapid eye movement sleep is divided into periods with no eye movements (no EM) or periods with frequent eye movements (dense EM). (Data redrawn from ref. 15.)*

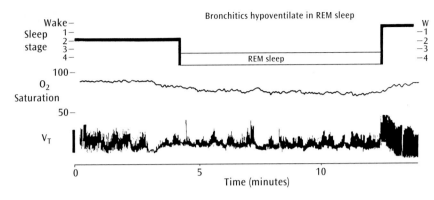

Figure 19.3 *Changes in oxygen saturation and 'tidal volume' measured by inductance plethysmography in a patient with COPD during an episode of rapid eye movement (REM) sleep. (Data redrawn from ref. 22.)*

being paid to breathing and oxygenation during sleep in patients with COPD.

Studies in which arterial blood gas tensions were monitored in sleeping patients with COPD demonstrated that the most severe hypoxemia and hypercapnia occurred during rapid eye movement (REM) sleep (Figure 19.1).[5–8] The development of accurate and progressively less obtrusive oximeters has allowed continuous measurement of arterial oxygenation in sleeping patients with COPD. Douglas *et al.*[9] reported that 23 of 28 episodes in which arterial oxygen saturation fell by more than 10% occurred during REM sleep (Figure 19.2) and that during such episodes arterial oxygen tension fell to as low as 26 mmHg, an observation confirmed by others.[10–14] The most severe hypoxemia occurs during episodes of REM sleep in which there are frequent eye movements (Figure 19.3).[15] During such hypoxemic episodes, arterial carbon dioxide tension also rises, but the nocturnal rise in measured transcutaneous carbon dioxide tension is usually relatively small.[16] Patients with COPD become more hypoxemic during sleep than during exercise.[17]

MECHANISMS OF HYPOXEMIA DURING SLEEP IN COPD

The major cause of REM hypoxemia in patients with COPD is hypoventilation but there are probably also contributions from a reduction in functional residual capacity and alterations in ventilation-perfusion matching.

Hypoventilation

Ventilation is lower during sleep than wakefulness in both normal subjects[18] and patients with COPD.[14] There is a relatively small decline in ventilation from wakefulness to non-REM sleep, but during REM sleep, there is intermittent marked hypoventilation[18] which is most severe during periods of intense eye movements.[19,20] This drop in ventilation is largely caused by a decrease in tidal volume. It is important to recognize that this hypoventilation is not associated with apneas.[20–22]

Although normal ventilation has not been accurately measured during sleep in patients with COPD, the thoracoabdominal movement during REM sleep is similar to that in normal subjects.[13] In normal subjects, it has been estimated that alveolar ventilation during REM sleep falls to around 60% of the level during wakefulness.[18,20] As patients with COPD have raised physiologic deadspace, the rapid shallow breathing during REM sleep may produce an even greater decrease in alveolar ventilation. It has been calculated that this could account for all of the REM hypoxemia observed in patients with COPD.[23] Ventilation has been measured during sleep in patients with COPD with 4 cmH$_2$O CPAP applied. This study found an 18% fall in ventilation from wakefulness to non-REM and a 35% fall from wakefulness to REM sleep, supporting the concept that hypoventilation is the major cause of REM hypoxemia.[24]

There are many factors which combine to produce hypoventilation during sleep. In normal subjects, ventilation falls during non-REM sleep, despite an increase in occlusion pressure.[25,26] This suggests that the increase in upper airways resistance which occurs during non-REM sleep[27,28] may contribute to the non-REM hypoventilation. This effect will be augmented because the ventilatory response to added resistance is impaired during non-REM sleep.[26,29] The increase in upper airways resistance is, however, unlikely to be a major factor in the additional hypoventilation and hypoxemia of REM sleep, because upper airways resistance is not greater in REM than non-REM sleep, at least in normal subjects.[28] Also, the 35% decrease in ventilation from wakefulness to REM sleep despite 4 cmH$_2$O of CPAP[24] strongly suggests upper airway obstruction is not a factor, as this would have been minimized by the CPAP. In addition, although few measurements have been made, the ventilatory response to added resistance appears to be similar between non-REM and REM sleep.[26,29] However, during REM sleep, there is marked alteration of brainstem function. In animals during REM sleep, there is phasic activity of respiratory neurones[30] and it seems probable that similar fluctuations in respiratory output may be a major determinant of the highly variable level of ventilation found during REM sleep in man.

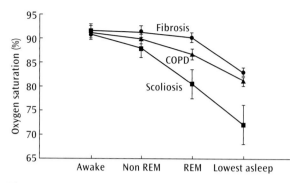

Figure 19.4 *Mean ± SEM oxygen saturation awake, during non-REM sleep, during REM sleep and at the lowest oxygen saturation recorded during sleep in patients with pulmonary fibrosis (filled circles), COPD (filled triangles) and kyphoscoliosis (filled squares). (Drawn from data in ref. 34.)*

Hypotonia of postural muscles during REM sleep[31] affects the intercostal muscles, resulting in a decreased ribcage contribution to ventilation.[21,32] In hyperinflated COPD patients, this ribcage flaccidity will result in grossly inefficient ventilation as the flattened diaphragms will then pull in the lower chest wall, further decreasing ventilation during REM sleep. In addition, the postural hypotonia during REM sleep also involves the accessory muscles of respiration,[33] which may be important in maintaining ventilation in patients with COPD. This may explain why hyperinflated patients with COPD tend to be more hypoxemic during REM sleep than are patients with fibrotic lung disease (Figure 19.4).[34]

The body's normal defense mechanism to hypoxemia would be to increase ventilation. However, during REM sleep there is marked reduction of the ventilatory responses both to hypoxia[35,36] and hypercapnia.[37,38] This, therefore, permits REM hypoxemia to occur.

Decrease in functional residual capacity

Functional residual capacity decreases during REM sleep in normal man.[28] Similar changes have been reported in patients with COPD[14] but this study used surface inductive plethysmography which may not be accurate during sleep.[39] A more recent study[40] using horizontal body plethysmography found no decrease in FRC during REM sleep in patients with COPD.

Ventilation/perfusion imbalance

The importance of the reported increase in ventilation/perfusion (V/Q) mismatching during REM sleep as a cause of REM hypoxemia in patients with COPD[6,7,22]

is difficult to assess. The data on which this assumption is based depend largely on the existence of a steady state of gas transfer which does not occur during REM hypoxemia in COPD.[23] However, the marked hypoventilation which occurs during REM sleep must result in alterations in V/Q matching. This conclusion is supported by the fact that cardiac output is maintained during the REM hypoventilation, indicating changes in overall V/Q matching.[22,23] However, current technology does not allow the relative importance of V/Q matching changes during this unsteady state to be adequately assessed.

COPD combined with the sleep apnea/hypopnea syndrome

Both COPD and the sleep apnea/hypopnea syndrome are relatively common conditions[41–43] and thus the two will coexist in some patients by chance alone. There is no doubt that the two conditions do coexist in some patients[44–46] but most studies performed in patients referred to respiratory clinics have not found an increased frequency of sleep apnea/hypopnea syndrome (SAHS) in patients with COPD compared to the normal population.[11–15] Looked at the other way round, one study has suggested that 10% of SAHS patients may have some degree of coexisting COPD.[47] However, an Australian study suggested that many patients with hypercapnic COPD have an increased frequency of hypopnoeas,[48] a finding at variance with the observations from ourselves and others in Europe and North America.[11–15] The same Australian study[48] indicated that hypercapnic patients with COPD have small upper airways.

Mechanisms of hypoxemia during sleep in COPD: conclusions

Hypoventilation is the main cause of hypoxemia during REM sleep in patients with COPD. In addition, however, there may be contributions from impairment of ventilation/perfusion matching and possibly also from a reduction in functional residual capacity. In a small minority of patients with COPD, there may also be coexisting obstructive sleep apnea/hypopnea syndrome.

CONSEQUENCES OF HYPOXEMIA DURING SLEEP IN COPD

REM sleep hypoxemia has significant cardiovascular and neurophysiologic sequelae in patients with COPD. In addition, REM hypoxemia may also have hematologic effects and may contribute to nocturnal death.

Cardiac dysrhythmias

Patients with COPD have an increased rate of ventricular ectopics during sleep.[49] However, no correlation could be found between ventricular ectopic frequency and oxygen saturation in a study of 42 patients with COPD, except in six of the 20 patients in whom oxygen saturation fell below 80%.[50] There was a non-significant trend for nocturnal oxygen therapy to reduce nocturnal ectopic frequency in COPD patients.[49] There is no evidence that such ventricular ectopics are of clinical importance.

Hemodynamics

Pulmonary arterial pressure rises during REM sleep in patients with COPD as oxygenation falls.[8,9,51] For example, in 12 patients with COPD, mean pulmonary arterial pressure rose from 37 to 55 mmHg as the mean arterial oxygen tension fell from 56 to 43 mmHg.[8] There is an inverse correlation between oxygen saturation and mean pulmonary arterial pressure with an average 1 mmHg rise in pulmonary arterial pressure per percent fall in SaO_2.[51] During these episodes of REM pulmonary hypertension, cardiac output increases little, if at all.[22,23]

The long-term significance of these episodes of REM sleep pulmonary hypertension is unknown. However, in rats, intermittent hypoxemia induced by breathing 12% oxygen for as little as 2 hours each day for 4 weeks led to a significant increase in right ventricular mass (Figure 19.5).[52] It thus seems probable that the intermittent REM hypoxemia seen in patients with COPD may have a similar effect on the human myocardium. Two studies have suggested that the short-term consequences of REM sleep hypoxemia on the myocardium in patients with COPD may be similar to those of maximal exercise when assessed either in terms of myocardial oxygen consumption[53] or left ventricular ejection.[54]

Pulmonary hemodynamics have been compared in patients with COPD who desaturate at night to at least 85% with more than 5 minutes spent below 90% in contrast to patients who did not desaturate in this way.[55] Those with such nocturnal desaturation had significantly higher daytime pulmonary arterial pressures and red cell masses than the non-desaturators. While the nocturnal hypoxemia may have produced these consequences, the nocturnal desaturators had significantly lower daytime oxygenation levels which could thus have contributed to the hemodynamic and haematological differences.

Polycythemia

Intermittent hypoxemia in rats results in elevation of red cell mass (Figure 19.5).[52] Thus, nocturnal desaturation in

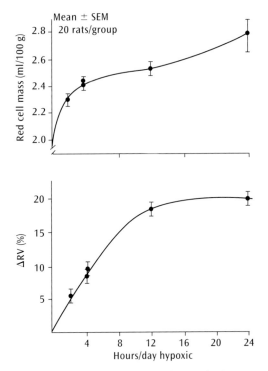

Figure 19.5 *Percentage change in right ventricular mass (ΔRV%) and changes in red cell mass in rats spending the number of hours per day indicated over a 28-day period breathing 12% oxygen. The two points at the 4-hour time point represent results obtained in rats spending a single 4-hour period and rats spending eight 30-minute periods per day breathing 12% oxygen, the latter to simulate transient sleep hypoxemia. (Data redrawn from ref. 52.)*

patients with COPD might also stimulate erythropiesis. Morning erythropietin levels have been found to be raised in some patients with COPD.[56–58] Patients whose oxygen saturations fall below 60% at night may have progressive rises in serum erythropietin during the night,[58] but more minor degrees of hypoxemia are not associated with measurable elevation of erythropietin levels.

Quality of sleep

Both symptomatic enquiry[59] and objective assessment with polysomnography[60–62] show that patients with COPD sleep poorly compared to normal subjects. Although COPD patients frequently arouse from sleep during episodes of desaturation,[61] the extent of sleep disruption appears to be at least as great in non-desaturating COPD patients;[62] thus, it may not be the desaturation *per se* which causes the sleep disruption. Despite the subjective and objective evidence of impaired sleep quality, there is no evidence of objective daytime sleepiness in patients with COPD when tested using the Multiple Sleep Latency Test.[63]

Death during sleep in COPD

Patients with COPD die more often at night than age-matched controls, and nocturnal death has been reported to be particularly common in COPD patients who are hypoxemic and hypercapnic.[64] In hypoxemic patients with COPD, nocturnal death is more common in those breathing air than in those receiving nocturnal oxygen therapy.[65] However, care must be taken not to equate nocturnal death with death during sleep.

Consequences of COPD combined with SAHS

Patients who have the combination of COPD and SAHS are more likely to develop pulmonary hypertension,[66] right heart failure[45,67] and carbon dioxide retention[68] than patients with either condition alone. This seems likely to be due to them having two separate causes for nocturnal hypoxemia, and thus they develop more severe nocturnal hypoxemia than would have occurred if they had had only one of these conditions.

Prediction of nocturnal oxygenation

For over 30 years, it has been known that the patients with COPD who are most hypoxic when awake were those who became the most hypoxemic during sleep.[3] This has since been widely confirmed by other workers[13,69,70] and several equations have been derived to predict the extent of nocturnal hypoxemia. Although each is statistically significant,[13,69,70] their clinical applicability is limited as there is marked scatter around the relationships, especially in the most hypoxemic patients (Figure 19.6). Such equations, however, do show that the extent of nocturnal hypoxemia is related not only to the level of daytime oxygenation, but also to daytime arterial carbon dioxide tension[69,70] and to the duration of REM sleep.[70] There has been considerable attention paid to the concept of 'nocturnal desaturators',[71] who have daytime arterial oxygen tensions of greater than 60 mmHg but who desaturate to some extent during sleep. Such patients have significantly lower daytime arterial oxygen tensions and higher arterial carbon dioxide tensions than those who do not desaturate, and thus from the above regression relationships[13,69,70] would be expected to desaturate more than the non-desaturators.

CLINICAL VALUE OF STUDIES OF BREATHING AND OXYGENATION DURING SLEEP IN PATIENTS WITH COPD

Overnight sleep studies could theoretically be of benefit in patients with COPD by detecting unsuspected cases of

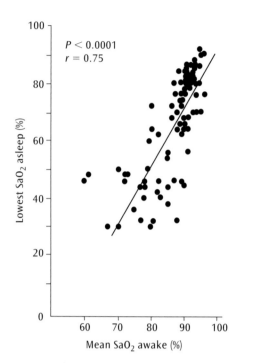

Figure 19.6 *Relationship between mean oxygen saturation during wakefulness and lowest nocturnal oxygenation during sleep in 97 patients with severe COPD. (Data redrawn from ref. 70.)*

the sleep apnea/hypopnea syndrome, by detecting clinically important excess hypoxemia during sleep in some patients, or by guiding selection of which patients might benefit from nocturnal oxygen therapy and/or what oxygen concentration such patients should inspire at night. These latter two roles will be discussed in the subsequent section on treatment.

Although no large studies have been carried out, there is as yet no convincing evidence that the prevalence of SAHS is increased in patients with COPD.[13] When SAHS coexists with COPD, the typical symptoms of SAHS[72,73] are present and current evidence suggests that sleep studies do not yield unsuspected cases of the sleep apnea/hypopnea syndrome,[70] provided an initial sleep history has been taken and hypersomnolence, snoring and witnessed apneas sought. Thus, the symptoms of SAHS should be sought in all patients with COPD, and if major symptoms exist, a clinical sleep study should be performed.

Oxygenation during sleep can be predicted from arterial blood gas tensions measured during wakefulness.[13,69,70] However, all such predictions leave considerable unexplained residual variance, but it is unclear whether this variance is of clinical importance. It has been claimed that measurements of nocturnal oxygenation in such patients can be a useful guide to treatment.[74] To establish the clinical importance of this variability between patients in the extent of sleep-related hypoxemia, Connaughton and colleagues[70] studied the relationship between nocturnal oxygen saturation and survival in 97 patients with COPD. Both mean nocturnal SaO_2 and the lowest SaO_2 during sleep were significantly related to survival, the patients with the lowest nocturnal oxygenation having the worst prognosis. However, neither nocturnal measure was a significantly better predictor of survival than the easier and cheaper measurements of oxygenation when awake or vital capacity.[70]

These investigators also studied the significance of the scatter around the regression relationship between measurements of oxygen saturation and PCO_2 when awake with oxygen saturation during sleep. Those patients who had excess nocturnal hypoxemia – the term used to describe those patients whose oxygen saturation during sleep was lower than that predicted from their oxygen saturation and arterial carbon dioxide tension during wakefulness – had similar survivals at a median of 70 months to those who became less hypoxemic at night relative to their awake oxygenation and $PaCO_2$ (Figure 19.7). A recent study found no significant relationship between the magnitude of nocturnal hypoxemia and the extent of daytime pulmonary hypertension,[75] again suggesting that the contribution of the additional hypoxemia during sleep to overall daytime pulmonary arterial pressure is relatively small.

Fletcher *et al.*[76] reported lower survival in 'desaturators' than non-desaturators. However, these groups were not matched for awake oxygenation which was significantly lower in the desaturators (67 vs. 75 mmHg; $P < 0.0001$).

Thus, it seems that there is no clinical value in performing routine polysomnography in patients with COPD. The only patients with COPD in whom I perform clinical sleep studies are those with symptoms of SAHS or, occasionally, those who have cor pulmonale or polycythemia but whose daytime arterial oxygen tension is more than 8 kPa. In this situation, it is imperative to perform full polysomnography as overnight oximetry is extremely difficult to interpret,[77] particularly in hypoxemic patients.

TREATMENT OF NOCTURNAL HYPOXEMIA IN COPD

Unsurprisingly, oxygen therapy improves oxygenation in sleeping patients with COPD,[9,61,78] although mild desaturation will still occur during REM sleep. The only firm evidence as to which patients benefit from domiciliary oxygen therapy remains the Nocturnal Oxygen Therapy Trial[79] and the Medical Research Council Study,[80] both of which showed that home oxygen therapy prolonged life in hypoxemic patients with COPD. However, in both studies the patient selection and choice of inspired oxygen concentration was entirely guided by daytime oxygenation. These studies were carried out on relatively hypoxemic patients who would be expected to become markedly hypoxemic at night. As the period of oxygen administration always included the night, it is tempting to conclude that at least some of the benefit of oxygen therapy was due to blunting the pulmonary arterial pressure rise during REM sleep.[81]

Two studies have attempted to answer the difficult question of whether measurement of nocturnal oxygenation should be used to guide oxygen therapy.[76,82] In a multicenter parallel group study, nocturnal oxygen therapy did not help survival in 'desaturators'.[76] Fletcher and colleagues[82] compared survival and physiologic measurements in a group of 38 patients with COPD who 'desaturated' at night. Unfortunately, only 16 patients completed the 3-year protocol, and only seven of these received nocturnal oxygen therapy. There was no significant effect of nocturnal oxygen therapy on survival, hospitalization or hematological variables, but the patients who received nocturnal oxygen therapy had a smaller rise in pulmonary arterial pressure than the controls. In a more recent study in 76 patients with a daytime PaO_2 greater than 7.3 kPa but nocturnal hypoxemia, nocturnal oxygen therapy did not affect survival nor pulmonary hemodynamics.[83] The clinical significance of this observation requires further assessment. Certainly, my policy is only to give oxygen therapy to patients with significant daytime hypoxemia.

Occasionally, patients will experience symptomatic carbon dioxide retention on nocturnal oxygen therapy, and this usually results in morning headaches. This seems to be particularly a problem in patients with coexisting

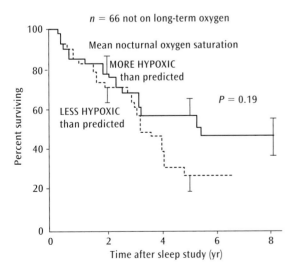

Figure 19.7 *Effect of nocturnal oxygenation on survival in 66 patients with COPD indicating the survival of those who were less hypoxic than predicted and those more hypoxic than predicted from the regression equation between oxygen saturation awake and mean nocturnal oxygen saturation. (From ref. 67 with permission.)*

sleep apnea/hypopnea syndrome[78] and I do perform polysomnography on patients who develop severe and intractable morning headaches on oxygen, although this is rare.

Some[60,78] but not all[61,84] studies have reported that correction of nocturnal hypoxemia improves sleep quality in patients with COPD. The inconsistency of this finding may result from differing severities of daytime hypoxemia and also from the lack of familiarization nights and of randomization in some studies.[61,78] It seems probable that severely hypoxemic patients with COPD do sleep better on nocturnal oxygen therapy, although this needs further testing.

Protriptyline

In an uncontrolled study, Series et al.[85] reported that protriptyline 20 mg daily improved nocturnal oxygenation in COPD by suppressing REM sleep. However, all patients experienced dryness of the mouth and six of the 11 patients also complained of dysuria. A subsequent non-randomized non-blinded trial[86] suggested that protriptyline may improve daytime arterial oxygen and carbon dioxide tension in patients with COPD, but again the side effects were common causing cessation of therapy within 10 weeks in four of 14 patients.

Medroxyprogesterone-acetate

Medroxyprogesterone-acetate (MPA) improved arterial oxygen tension and reduced arterial carbon dioxide tension during both wakefulness and non-REM sleep in five of 17 hypercapnic patients with COPD.[12] However, a double-blind controlled trial found no such beneficial effect.[87] Furthermore, MPA may cause troublesome side effects, including impotence in many patients.

Almitrine

Almitrine is an investigational drug which can raise arterial oxygen tension in patients with COPD. In a randomized double-blind study, 2 weeks of almitrine 50 mg twice daily improved oxygenation during sleep in patients with COPD without altering sleep quality.[88] This finding was subsequently confirmed by others.[89,90]

It was hoped that the combination of almitrine plus nocturnal oxygen therapy might produce greater improvements in oxygenation and right heart pressure than the use of either agent alone. However, this hope has not been fulfilled and there was no additional benefit in nocturnal oxygenation with the combination of the two therapies and there was a tendency for pulmonary arterial pressure to be higher in almitrine plus oxygen than when on oxygen alone.[91]

In addition, neither the dosage of almitrine[92] nor the importance of the peripheral neuropathy that has been associated with its use have as yet been established.

Acetazolamide

Acetazolamide improved both arterial oxygen tension when awake and asleep in five patients with COPD, but it did not alter arterial PCO_2 during sleep in two of the patients.[93] However, paresthesia, nephrolithiasis and acidosis may limit tolerance of this drug.

Beta-agonists

Oral sustained-release salbutamol had no effect on sleep, oxygenation or morning FEV_1 in 14 patients with moderately severe COPD.[94]

Theophylline

Oral theophyllines may improve overnight oxygen saturation and transcutaneous carbon dioxide levels[95,96] and morning peak flow rates[97] but may[96] or may not[95,97,98] improve sleep quality. Intravenous theophylline infusion did not improve overnight oxygenation in a study of 11 patients with COPD.[99]

Continuous positive airway pressure

Nocturnal continuous positive airway pressure has been reported to improve inspiratory muscle strength and 12-minute walking distances in eight patients with COPD[100] without altering nocturnal oxygenation or sleep quality. These data require confirmation.

Negative pressure ventilation

Negative pressure ventilation has been reported to reduce arterial carbon dioxide tension and increase respiratory muscle strength in some patients with COPD.[101,102] However, negative pressure ventilation results in increased upper airways obstruction and sleep disturbance[103] and thus has largely fallen out of use.

Intermittent positive pressure ventilation by nasal mask

Nocturnal intermittent positive pressure ventilation (NIPPV) via nasal mask was originally developed for use in patients with kyphoscoliosis or neuromuscular disorders.[104–107] However, some patients with COPD find this technique acceptable, and it also has the theoretical advantage over long-term oxygen therapy of reducing carbon dioxide tension. In those patients who can tolerate NIPPV, improvements in arterial blood gas tensions and sleep may be achieved[106,108] but nocturnal oxygenation is improved more by nocturnal oxygen therapy than by nocturnal IPPV alone.[109] Simultaneous nocturnal nasal IPPV and nocturnal oxygen therapy produced greater improvements in daytime arterial oxygen and carbon dioxide tensions and overnight arterial carbon dioxide tension, sleep quality and quality of life than oxygen therapy alone in a randomized control trial of 14 patients with COPD,[110] but long-term data, particularly data comparing the effect on survival of nasal IPPV with long-term oxygen therapy, is required before this promising technique can be widely advocated as first line therapy.

Hypnotics

Although hypnotics are often used to treat sleep disturbance in patients with COPD, they should not be used in hypercapnic patients in case ventilatory responses are further inhibited and acute on chronic ventilatory failure precipitated. Benzodiazepines have been reported to increase sleep duration in some[111–113] but not all[114] studies performed in eucapnic patients with COPD, but the frequency and severity of desaturation may increase.[111] Thus, even in eucapnic patients, hypnotics should only be used with great caution.

Alcohol

Alcohol ingestion before sleep may aggravate nocturnal hypoxemia[115] and increase ventricular ectopic frequency[116] in COPD patients. Heavy alcohol consumption by COPD patients may lead to hypercapnic respiratory failure[48] and right heart failure[117] and to more irregular breathing during sleep.[48] These data require confirmation and clarification, and in particular, it is not clear whether any effect of alcohol may be due to heavy drinkers being overweight. However, the two studies do suggest that alcohol consumption should be discouraged in COPD patients, and this may particularly apply to alcohol consumption in the evening which can contribute to the development of apneas and hypopneas during sleep.

TREATMENT OF COPD COMBINED WITH SAHS

There is relatively little evidence about how best to treat patients who have both COPD and the sleep apnea/hypopnea syndrome. A non-randomized study found

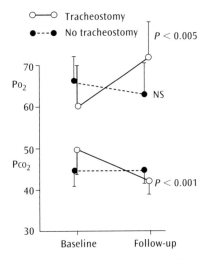

Figure 19.8 *Arterial oxygen and carbon dioxide tensions during the daytime in two groups of patients who had both COPD and the sleep apnea/hypopnea syndrome. In those who accepted tracheostomy, arterial blood gas tensions improved at follow-up, whereas there was no such change in those who declined tracheostomy. (Data redrawn from ref. 46.)*

that patients with both conditions improve their daytime arterial blood gas tensions and pulmonary arterial pressures only when their SAHS was adequately treated, the treatment used then being tracheostomy (Figure 19.8).[46] The patients who declined tracheostomy had no improvement in their blood gas tensions even although nine of the 10 received domiciliary oxygen therapy. Thus, it is reasonable to conclude that it is important to recognize coexisting sleep apnea/hypopnea syndrome in such patients and to treat it aggressively. These days, this would usually mean treatment with CPAP therapy with or without supplemental oxygen. Nocturnal nasal IPPV is an alternative.

BREATHING DURING SLEEP IN COPD: CONCLUSIONS

Patients with COPD become hypoxemic during sleep, especially during rapid eye movement sleep. There is no evidence that measurement of nocturnal hypoxemia or breathing patterns in individual patients provide prognostic information which adds significantly to the more simple measurements of oxygenation and lung function made during wakefulness. In a small minority of COPD patients, the sleep apnea/hypopnea syndrome may coexist and any COPD patient with a history suggestive of SAHS should have full polysomnography with those found to have SAHS having their SAHS treated aggressively. Domiciliary oxygen therapy is the current treatment of choice in COPD patients who are hypoxemic by day and night, although the roles of respiratory stimulants and of nocturnal intermittent positive pressure ventilation may grow.

REFERENCES

1. Robin ED, Whaley RD, Crump CH, *et al.* The nature of the respiratory acidosis of sleep and of the respiratory alkalosis of hepatic comas (abstract). *J Clin Invest* 1957;**36**:24.
2. Robin ED. Some interrelations between sleep and disease. *Arch Intern Med* 1958;**102**:669–75.
3. Trask CH, Cree EM. Oximeter studies on patients with chronic obstructive emphysema, awake and during sleep. *N Engl J Med* 1962;**266**:639–42.
4. Gastaut H, Tassinari CA, Duron B. Polygraphic study of the episodic diurnal and nocturnal (hypnic and respiratory) manifestations of the Pickwick syndrome. *Brain Res* 1966;**1**:167–86.
5. Pierce AK, Jarrett CE, Werkle G, *et al.* Respiratory function during sleep in patients with chronic obstructive lung disease. *J Clin Invest* 1966;**45**:631–6.
6. Koo KW, Sax DS, Snider GL. Arterial blood gases and pH during sleep in chronic obstructive pulmonary disease. *Am J Med* 1975;**58**:663–70.
7. Leitch AG, Clancy LJ, Leggett RJE, Tweeddale P, Dawson P, Evans JI. Arterial blood gas tensions, hydrogen ion, and electroencephalogram during sleep in patients with chronic ventilatory failure. *Thorax* 1976;**31**:730–5.
8. Coccagna G, Lugaresi E. Arterial blood gases and pulmonary and systemic arterial pressure during sleep in chronic obstructive pulmonary disease. *Sleep* 1978;**1**:117–24.
9. Douglas NJ, Calverley PMA, Leggett RJE, Brash HM, Flenley DC, Brezinova V. Transient hypoxemia during sleep in chronic bronchitis and emphysema. *Lancet* 1979;**i**:1–4.
10. Wynne JW, Block AJ, Hemenway J, *et al.* Disordered breathing and oxygen desaturation during sleep in patients with chronic obstructive lung disease (COLD). *Am J Med* 1979;**66**:573–9.
11. Fleetham JA, Mezon B, West P, *et al.* Chemical control of ventilation and sleep arterial oxygen desaturation in patients with COPD. *Am Rev Respir Dis* 1980;**122**:583–9.
12. Skatrud JB, Dempsey JA, Iber C, *et al.* Correction of CO_2 retention during sleep in patients with chronic obstructive pulmonary diseases. *Am Rev Respir Dis* 1981;**124**:260–8.
13. Catterall JR, Douglas NJ, Calverley PMA, *et al.* Transient hypoxemia during sleep in chronic obstructive pulmonary disease is not a sleep apnea syndrome. *Am Rev Respir Dis* 1983;**128**:24–9.
14. Hudgel DW, Martin RJ, Capehart M, *et al.* Contribution of hypoventilation to sleep oxygen desaturation in chronic obstructive pulmonary disease. *J Appl Physiol* 1983;**55**:669–77.
15. George CF, West P, Kryger MH. Oxygenation and breathing pattern during phasic and tonic REM in patients with chronic obstructive pulmonary disease. *Sleep* 1987;**10**:234–43.
16. Midgren B, Hansson L. Changes in transcutaneous Pco_2 with sleep in normal subjects and in patients with chronic respiratory diseases. *Eur J Respir Dis* 1987;**71**:384–7.
17. Mulloy E, McNicholas WT. Theophylline improves gas exchange during rest, exercise and sleep in severe chronic obstructive pulmonary disease. *Am Rev Respir Dis* 1993;**148**:1030–6.
18. Douglas NJ, White DP, Pickett CK, Weil JV, Zwillich CW. Respiration during sleep in normal man. *Thorax* 1982;**37**:840–4.
19. Aserinsky E. Periodic respiratory pattern occurring in conjunction with eye movements during sleep. *Science* 1965;**150**:763–6.
20. Gould GA, Gugger M, Molloy J, Tsara V, Shapiro CM, Douglas NJ. Breathing pattern and eye movement density during REM sleep in man. *Am Rev Respir Dis* 1988;**138**:874–7.
21. Millman RP, Knight H, Kline LR, *et al.* Changes in compartmental ventilation in association with eye movements during REM sleep. *J Appl Physiol* 1988;**65**:1196–202.
22. Fletcher EC, Gray BA, Levin DC. Non-apneic mechanisms of arterial oxygen desaturation during rapid-eye movement sleep. *J Appl Physiol* 1983;**54**:632–9.
23. Catterall JR, Calverley PMA, MacNee W, *et al.* Mechanism of transient nocturnal hypoxemia in hypoxic chronic bronchitis and emphysema. *J Appl Physiol* 1985;**59**:1698–703.
24. Becker HF, Piper AJ, Flynn WE, *et al.* Breathing during sleep in patients with nocturnal desaturation. *Am J Respir Crit Care Med* 1999;**159**:112–18.
25. White DP. Occlusion pressure and ventilation during sleep in normal humans. *J Appl Physiol* 1986;**61**:1279–87.
26. Gugger M, Molloy J, Gould GA, *et al.* Ventilatory and arousal responses to added inspiratory resistance during sleep. *Am Rev Respir Dis* 1989;**140**:1301–7.
27. Lopes JM, Tabachnik E, Muller NL, *et al.* Total airway resistance and respiratory muscle activity during sleep. *J Appl Physiol* 1983;**54**:773–7.
28. Hudgel DW, Martin RJ, Johnson B, *et al.* Mechanics of the respiratory system and breathing pattern during sleep in normal humans. *J Appl Physiol* 1984;**56**:133–7.
29. Wiegand L, Zwillich CW, White DP. Sleep and the ventilatory response to resistive loading in normal men. *J Appl Physiol* 1988;**64**:1186–95.
30. Orem J. Medullary respiratory neuron activity: relationship to tonic and phasic REM sleep. *J Appl Physiol* 1980;**48**:54–65.
31. Tabachnik E, Muller NL, Bryan AC, *et al.* Changes in ventilation and chest wall mechanics during sleep in normal adolescents. *J Appl Physiol* 1981;**51**:557–64.
32. White JES, Drinnan MJ, Smithson AJ, *et al.* Respiratory muscle activity during rapid eye movement (REM) sleep in patients with chronic obstructive pulmonary disease. *Thorax* 1995;**50**:376–82.
33. Johnson MW, Remmers JE. Accessory muscle activity during sleep in chronic obstructive pulmonary disease. *J Appl Physiol* 1984;**57**:1011–17.
34. Midgren B. Oxygen desaturation during sleep as a function of the underlying respiratory disease. *Am Rev Respir Dis* 1990;**141**:43–6.
35. Douglas NJ, White DP, Weil JV, *et al.* Hypoxic ventilatory response decreases during sleep in normal men. *Am Rev Respir Dis* 1982;**125**:286–9.
36. Berthon-Jones M, Sullivan CE. Ventilatory and arousal responses to hypoxia in sleeping humans. *Am Rev Respir Dis* 1982;**125**:632–9.
37. Douglas NJ, White DP, Weil JV, Pickett CK, Zwillich CW. Hypercapnic ventilatory response in sleeping adults. *Am Rev Respir Dis* 1982;**126**:758–62.
38. Berthon-Jones M, Sullivan CE. Ventilation and arousal responses to hypercapnia in normal sleeping adults. *J Appl Physiol* 1984;**57**:59–67.

39. Whyte KF, Gugger M, Gould GA, *et al.* Accuracy of the respiratory inductive plethysmograph in measuring tidal volume during sleep. *J Appl Physiol* 1991;**71**:1866–71.

40. Ballard RD, Clover CW, Suh BY. Influence of sleep on respiratory function in emphysema. *Am J Respir Crit Care Med* 1995;**151**:945–51.

41. Franceschi M, Zamproni P, Crippa D, *et al.* Excessive daytime sleepiness: a 1-year study in an unselected in-patient population. *Sleep* 1982;**5**:239–47.

42. Lavie P. Incidence of sleep apnea in a presumably healthy, working population: a significant relationship with excessive daytime sleepiness. *Sleep* 1983;**6**:312–18.

43. Stradling JR, Crosby JH. Predictors and prevalence of obstructive sleep apnoea and snoring in 1001 middle aged men. *Thorax* 1991;**46**:85–90.

44. Guilleminault C, Cummiskey J, Motta J. Chronic obstructive airflow disease and sleep studies. *Am Rev Respir Dis* 1980;**122**:397–406.

45. Bradley TD, Rutherford R, Grossman RF, *et al.* Role of daytime hypoxemia in the pathogenesis of right heart failure in the obstructive sleep apnea syndrome. *Am Rev Respir Dis* 1985;**131**:835–9.

46. Fletcher EC, Schaaf JW, Miller J, *et al.* Long-term cardiopulmonary sequelae in patients with sleep apnea and chronic lung disease. *Am Rev Respir Dis* 1987;**135**:525–33.

47. Chaouat A, Weitzenblum E, Krieger J, *et al.* Association of chronic-obstructive pulmonary disease and sleep apnoea syndrome. *Am J Respir Crit Care Med* 1995;**151**:82–6.

48. Chan CS, Bye PTP, Woolcock AJ, *et al.* Eucapnia and hypercapnia in patients with chronic airflow limitation: the role of the upper airway. *Am Rev Respir Dis* 1990;**141**:861–5.

49. Flick MR, Block AJ. Nocturnal versus diurnal cardiac arrhythmias in patients with chronic obstructive pulmonary disease. *Chest* 1979;**75**:8–11.

50. Shepard JW, Garrison MW, Grither DA, *et al.* Relationship of ventricular ectopy to nocturnal oxygen desaturation in patients with chronic obstructive pulmonary disease. *Am J Med* 1985;**78**:28–34.

51. Boysen PG, Block AJ, Wynne JW, *et al.* Nocturnal pulmonary hypertension in patients with chronic obstructive pulmonary disease. *Chest* 1979;**76**:536–42.

52. Moore-Gillon JC, Cameron IR. Right ventricular hypertrophy and polycythemia in rats after intermittent exposure to hypoxia. *Clin Sci* 1985;**69**:595–9.

53. Shepard JW, Schweitzer PK, Keller CA, *et al.* Myocardial stress: exercise versus sleep in patients with COPD. *Chest* 1984;**86**:366–74.

54. Levy PA, Guilleminault C, Fagret D, *et al.* Changes in left ventricular ejection fraction during REM sleep on exercise in chronic obstructive pulmonary disease in sleep apnoea syndrome. *Eur Respir J* 1991;**4**:347–52.

55. Fletcher EC, Luckett RA, Miller T, *et al.* Pulmonary vascular hemodynamics in chronic lung disease patients with and without oxyhemoglobin desaturation during sleep. *Chest* 1989;**95**:757–64.

56. Miller ME, Garcia JF, Cohen RA, *et al.* Diurnal levels of immunoreactive erythropoietin in normal subjects and subjects with chronic lung disease. *Br J Haematol* 1981;**49**:189–200.

57. Wedzicha JA, Cotes PM, Empey DW. Serum immuno-reactive erythropoietin and hypoxic lung disease with and without polycythemia. *Clin Sci* 1985;**69**:413–22.

58. Fitzpatrick MF, McMahon G, Whyte KF, *et al.* Does oxygen desaturation during sleep cause release of erythropoietin in patients with COPD? *Clin Sci* 1993;**84**:319–24.

59. Cormick W, Olsen LG, Hensley MJ, *et al.* Nocturnal hypoxemia and quality of sleep in patients with chronic obstructive lung disease. *Thorax* 1986;**41**:846–54.

60. Calverley PMA, Brezinova V, Douglas NJ, Catterall JR, Flenley DC. The effect of oxygenation on sleep quality in chronic bronchitis and emphysema. *Am Rev Respir Dis* 1982;**126**:206–10.

61. Fleetham J, West P, Mezon B, *et al.* Sleep, arousals and oxygen desaturation in chronic obstructive pulmonary disease. *Am Rev Respir Dis* 1982;**126**:429–33.

62. Brezinova V, Catterall JR, Douglas NJ, Calverley PMA, Flenley DC. Night sleep of patients with chronic ventilatory failure and age-matched controls. Number and duration of ECG episodes of intervening wakefulness and drowsiness. *Sleep* 1982;**5**:123–30.

63. Orr WC, Shamma-Othman Z, Levin D, *et al.* Persistent hypoxemia and excessive daytime sleepiness in chronic obstructive pulmonary disease. *Chest* 1990;**97**:583–5.

64. McNicholas WT, Fitzgerald MX. Nocturnal deaths in patients with chronic bronchitis and emphysema. *Br Med J* 1984;**289**:878.

65. Douglas NJ. Breathing during sleep in patients with respiratory disease. In: C Guilleminault, M Partinen, eds. *Obstructive Sleep Apnea Syndrome*. Raven Press, New York, 1990, pp 37–48.

66. Weitzenblum E, Krieger J, Apprill M, *et al.* Daytime pulmonary hypertension in patients with obstructive sleep apnea syndrome. *Am Rev Respir Dis* 1988;**138**:345–9.

67. Whyte KF, Douglas NJ. Peripheral edema in the sleep apnea/hypopnea syndrome. *Sleep* 1991;**14**:354–6.

68. Bradley TD, Rutherford R, Lue F, *et al.* Role of diffuse airway obstruction in the hypercapnia of obstructive sleep apnea. *Am Rev Respir Dis* 1986;**134**:920–4.

69. McKeon JL, Muree-Allan K, Saunders NA. Prediction of oxygenation during sleep in patients with chronic obstructive lung disease. *Thorax* 1988;**43**:312–17.

70. Connaughton JJ, Catterall JR, Elton RA, Stradling JR, Douglas NJ. Do sleep studies contribute to the management of patients with severe chronic obstructive pulmonary disease? *Am Rev Respir Dis* 1988;**138**:341–4.

71. Fletcher EC, Miller J, Devine GW, *et al.* Nocturnal oxyhemoglobin desaturation in COPD patients with arterial oxygen tensions above 60 mmHg. *Chest* 1987;**92**:604–8.

72. Guilleminault C, van den Hoed J, Mitler MM. Clinical overview of the sleep apnea syndromes. In: C Guilleminault, WC Dement, eds. *Sleep Apnea Syndromes*. Alan R Liss, New York, 1978, pp 1–12.

73. Whyte KF, Allen MB, Jeffrey AA, Gould GA, Douglas NJ. Clinical features of the sleep apnoea/hypopnoea syndrome. *Q J Med* 1989;**72**:659–66.

74. Phillipson EA, Remmers JE, Chairmen. Indications and standards for cardio-pulmonary sleep studies. *Am Rev Respir Dis* 1989;**139**:559–68.

75. Chaouat A, Weitzenblum E, Kessler R, *et al.* Sleep-related O$_2$ desaturation and daytime pulmonary haemodynamics in COPD patients with mild hypoxaemia. *Eur Respir J* 1997;**10**:1730–5.

76. Fletcher EC, Donner CF, Midgren B, *et al.* Survival in COPD patients with a daytime Pao$_2$ > 60 mmHg with and without nocturnal oxyhemoglobin desaturation. *Chest* 1992;**101**:649–55.

77. Douglas NJ, Thomas S, Jan MA. Clinical value of polysomnography. *Lancet* 1992;**339**:347–50.

78. Goldstein RS, Ramcharan V, Bowes G, *et al.* Effect of supplemental nocturnal oxygen on gas exchange in patients

with severe obstructive lung disease. *N Engl J Med* 1984;**310**:425–9.

79. Nocturnal Oxygen Therapy Trial Group: Continuous or nocturnal oxygen therapy in hypoxemic chronic obstructive lung disease: a clinical trial. *Ann Intern Med* 1980;**93**:391–8.

80. Medical Research Council Working Party Report. Long-term domiciliary oxygen therapy in chronic hypoxic cor pulmonale complicating chronic bronchitis and emphysema. *Lancet* 1981;**i**:681–6.

81. Fletcher EC, Levin DC. Cardiopulmonary hemodynamics during sleep in subjects with chronic obstructive pulmonary disease: the effect of short and long-term oxygen. *Chest* 1984;**85**:6–14.

82. Fletcher EC, Luckett R, Goodnight-White S, Miller CC, Qian W, Costarangos-Galarza C. A double-blind trial of nocturnal supplemental oxygen for sleep desaturation in patients with chronic obstructive pulmonary disease and a daytime Pao$_2$ above 60 mmHg. *Am Rev Respir Dis* 1992;**145**:1070–6.

83. Chaouat A, Weitzenblum E, Kessler R, *et al.* A randomized trial of nocturnal oxygen therapy in chronic obstructive pulmonary disease. *Eur Respir J* 1999;**14**:1002–8.

84. McKeon JL, Murree-Allen K, Saunders NA. Supplemental oxygen and quality of sleep in patients with chronic obstructive lung disease. *Thorax* 1989;**44**:184–8.

85. Series F, Cormier Y, La Forge J. Changes in day and in night time oxygenation with protriptyline in patients with chronic obstructive lung disease. *Thorax* 1989;**44**:275–9.

86. Series F, Cormier Y. Effects of protriptyline on diurnal and nocturnal oxygenation in patients with chronic obstructive pulmonary disease. *Ann Intern Med* 1990;**113**:507–11.

87. Dolly FR, Block AJ. Medroxyprogesterone acetate in COPD: effect on breathing and oxygenation in sleeping and awake patients. *Chest* 1983;**84**:394–8.

88. Connaughton JJ, Douglas NJ, Morgan AD, *et al.* Almitrine improves oxygenation when both awake and asleep in patients with hypoxia and carbon dioxide retention caused by chronic bronchitis and emphysema. *Am Rev Respir Dis* 1985;**132**:206–10.

89. Daskalopoulou E, Patakas D, Tsara V, *et al.* Comparison of almitrine bismesylate and medroxyprogesterone acetate on oxygenation during wakefulness and sleep in patients with chronic obstructive lung disease. *Thorax* 1990;**45**:666–9.

90. Gothe B, Cherniack NS, Bachandrt RT, *et al.* Long-term effects of almitrine bismesylate on oxygenation during wakefulness and sleep in chronic obstructive pulmonary disease. *Am J Med* 1988;**84**:436–43.

91. Ruhle KH, Kempf P, Mossinger B, *et al.* Einfluss von almitrin einem chemorezeptoren stimulator, auf die nachtliche hyperkapnie und dem pulmonarteriellen druck unter O$_2$ atmung bei chronisch obstruktiver lungenerkrankung. *Prax Clin Pneumol* 1988;**42**:411–14.

92. Howard P. Hypoxia, almitrine and peripheral neuropathy. *Thorax* 1989;**44**:247–50.

93. Skatrud JB, Dempsey JA. Relative effectiveness of acetazolamide versus medroxyprogesterone acetate in correction of carbon dioxide retention. *Am Rev Respir Dis* 1983;**127**:405–12.

94. Veale D, Cooper BG, Griffiths CJ, Corris PA, Gibson GJ. The effect of controlled-release salbutamol on sleep and nocturnal oxygenation in patients with asthma and chronic obstructive pulmonary disease. *Respir Med* 1994;**88**:121–4.

95. Berry RB, Desa MM, Branum JP, *et al.* Effect of theophylline on sleep and sleep-disordered breathing in patients with chronic obstructive pulmonary disease. *Am Rev Respir Dis* 1991;**143**:245–50.

96. Mulloy E, McNicholas WT. Theophylline improves gas exchange during rest, exercise and sleep in severe chronic obstructive pulmonary disease. *Am Rev Respir Dis* 1993;**148**:1030–6.

97. Man GCW, Chapman KR, Habib AS, *et al.* Sleep quality and nocturnal respiratory function with once-daily theophylline (Uniphyl) and inhaled salbutamol in patients with COPD. *Chest* 1996;**110**:648–53.

98. Martin RJ, Pak J. Overnight theophylline concentrations and effects on sleep and lung function in chronic obstructive pulmonary disease. *Am Rev Respir Dis* 1992;**145**:540–4.

99. Ebden P, Vathenen AS. Does aminophylline improve nocturnal hypoxia in patients with chronic airflow obstruction? *Eur J Respir Dis* 1987;**71**:384–7.

100. Mezzanotte WS, Tangel DJ, Fox AM, Ballard RD, White DP. Nocturnal nasal continuous positive airway pressure in patients with chronic obstructive pulmonary disease: influence on waking respiratory muscle function. *Chest* 1994;**106**:1100–8.

101. Brown NMT, Marino WD. Effective daily intermittent rest of respiratory muscles in patients with severe chronic airflow limitation. *Chest* 1984;**85**:59S–60S.

102. Crop AJ, Di Marco AF. Effects of intermittent negative pressure ventilation on respiratory muscle function in patients with severe chronic obstructive pulmonary disease. *Am Rev Respir Dis* 1987;**35**:1056–61.

103. Levy RD, Cosio MG, Gibbons L, Macklem PT, Martin JG. Induction of sleep apnoea with negative pressure ventilation in patients with chronic obstructive lung disease. *Thorax* 1992;**47**:612–15.

104. Ellis ER, Bye PTP, Bruderer JW, *et al.* Treatment of respiratory failure during sleep in patients with neuromuscular disease. *Am Rev Respir Dis* 1987;**135**:148–52.

105. Kerby GR, Mayer LS, Pringleton SK. Nocturnal positive pressure ventilation via nasal mask. *Am Rev Respir Dis* 1987;**135**:738–40.

106. Carroll N, Branthwaite MA. Control of nocturnal hypoventilation by nasal intermittent positive pressure ventilation. *Thorax* 1988;**43**:349–53.

107. Ellis ER, Grunstein RR, Chan S, *et al.* Noninvasive ventilatory support during sleep improves respiratory failure in kyphoscoliosis. *Chest* 1988;**94**:811–15.

108. Elliot MW, Simonds AK, Carroll MP, Wedzicha JA, Branthwaite MA. Domiciliary nocturnal nasal intermittent positive pressure ventilation in hypercapnic respiratory failure due to chronic obstructive lung disease: effects on sleep and quality of life. *Thorax* 1992;**47**:342–8.

109. Lin CC. Comparison between nocturnal nasal positive pressure ventilation combined with oxygen therapy and oxygen monotherapy in patients with severe COPD. *Am J Respir Crit Care Med* 1996;**154**:353–8.

110. Meecham Jones DJ, Paul EA, Jones PW, *et al.* Nasal pressure support ventilation plus oxygen compared with oxygen therapy alone in hypercapnic COPD. *Am J Respir Crit Care Med* 1995;**152**:538–44.

111. Block AJ, Dolly FR, Slayton PC. Does flurazepam ingestion affect breathing and oxygenation during sleep in patients with chronic obstructive lung disease? *Am Rev Respir Dis* 1984;**129**:230–3.

112. Wedzicha J, Wallis PJW, Ingram DA, *et al.* Effect of diazepam on sleep in patients with chronic airflow obstruction. *Thorax* 1988;**43**:729–30.

113. Midgren B, Hansson L, Skeidsvoll H, *et al.* The effects of nitrazepam and flunitrazepam on oxygen desaturation during sleep in stable hypoxemic non hypercapnic COPD. *Chest* 1989;**5**:765–8.

114. Cummiskey J, Guilleminault C, Rio GD, *et al*. The effects of flurazepam on sleep studies in patients with chronic obstructive pulmonary disease. *Chest* 1983;**84**:143–7.

115. Easton PA, West P, Meatherall RC, *et al*. The effect of excessive ethanol ingestion on sleep in severe chronic obstructive pulmonary disease. *Sleep* 1987;**10**:224–33.

116. Dolly FR, Block AJ. Increased ventricular ectopy and sleep apnea following ethanol ingestion in COPD patients. *Chest* 1983;**83**:469–72.

117. Jalleh R, Fitzpatrick MF, Jan MA, *et al*. Alcohol and cor pulmonale in chronic bronchitis and emphysema. *Br Med J* 1993;**306**:374.

20

Clinical and laboratory assessment

PETER MA CALVERLEY AND MG PEARSON

Although the definition of COPD in clinicopathologic terms presents continuing difficulties (see Chapter 1), the identification of symptomatic patients is more straightforward. The pathologic changes of inflammation, distortion of the small airways and patchy loss of the alveolar wall antedate the onset of symptoms, even those of mucus hypersecretion in regular smokers. The identification of these presymptomatic individuals is difficult but by the time the patient recognizes their symptoms, there is physiological evidence of airflow limitation and there may be abnormal physical signs. However, these signs may be undramatic, and are not always present. This chapter will review the clinical and laboratory findings which favor a diagnosis of COPD, consider some of its different clinical presentations and look at the practical aspects of achieving a diagnostic formulation on which treatment can be based.

SYMPTOMS IN COPD

The principal symptoms of which patients complain are breathlessness on exertion, wheeze and cough (usually with sputum).[1] Of these, breathlessness is the most important and disabling and the one most likely to lead the patients to seek medical help. However, it is not usually the first to appear, as a significant amount of ventilatory capacity has to be lost before respiratory disability is noticeable.[2] The clinical picture of COPD will vary both over time as the severity increases and with the ability of the patient to adapt to his or her limitations. Only some

of the features below will apply to individual patients at any one point in time. However respiratory symptoms are reported by a majority of patients with objective airflow limitation, even when their reduction in FEV_1 is quite modest.[3,4]

Cough

In 75% of COPD patients cough either precedes the onset of breathlessness or appears simultaneously with it.[5] Cough productive of sputum occurs in up to 50% of cigarette smokers[5,6] and may be present within 10 years of starting to smoke. In COPD the cough is usually worse in the morning but seldom disturbs the patient's sleep and is often dismissed as a 'smokers cough' of little importance. Its significance was recognized in early attempts to define COPD[7] and the MRC symptom questionnaire used cough and sputum production as the defining characteristics of clinical chronic bronchitis.[8] However, occupational studies have shown that cough relates to increases in inhaled dust burden rather than changes in lung function,[9] whilst most, but not all, longitudinal studies in COPD have found no association between mortality and symptoms of cough and/or sputum production.[2,10,11] When cigarette smokers stop smoking cough diminishes or disappears in 94% of cases[12,13] but abnormalities in lung function persist. Thus cough is a marker of the processes leading to disability but does not produce disabling symptoms in the early stage of the disease. This has led to its use in defining an 'at risk' population in the GOLD classification of

COPD.[14] This remains an operational approach to early disease intervention rather than a statement related to disease pathophysiology.

Whether cough in COPD is a normal physiologic response to increased mucus production or is itself pathologic remains controversial. Studies in asthma have demonstrated a consistently low cough threshold to inhaled capsaicin[15] possibly due to the release of inflammatory mediators.[16] Data in COPD are less consistent and appear to depend upon the technique and dosimeter used. Nonetheless, we have found similar reductions in the cough threshold in both chronic asthma and COPD (Figure 20.1),[17] a finding more marked in those receiving anticholinergic treatment. Subjective reports of coughing were only weakly related to these abnormalities, which also explains the poor relationship between reported cough and pathologic evidence of increased glandular hypertrophy.[13]

Sputum production is increased in COPD but mucociliary clearance (as assessed by radioisotope methods) is reduced[18] due to direct ciliotoxicity[19] and possibly increases in sputum viscosity. Interpretation of total sputum clearance is difficult without allowing for the variation in the frequency of cough. Thus Loudon and coworkers using objectively recorded cough counts detected an average of 120 coughs during 8 hours overnight recording compared with just 23 coughs per night in patients being treated for tuberculosis.[20] However, nocturnal cough frequency does not appear to be increased in stable COPD.[21] The variability in cough threshold, total sputum volume and the ability to swallow rather than expectorate sputum, between individual patients, make it hard to interpret sputum production objectively. Nonetheless, sputum purulence, as reflected in sputum color, is a reasonably reliable sign of endobronchial infection which merits antibiotic treatment.[22]

When severe airflow obstruction is present, recurrent coughing bouts can be severe enough to produce 'cough syncope'[23] and 'cough fractures' of the ribs.[24] These events probably share a common mechanism with high intrathoracic pressures being developed during coughing in patients whose relatively long mechanical time constants prevent adequate pulmonary deflation before the next cough begins.

Wheezing

This complaint is difficult to evaluate because of its intermittent nature and limitation in patient understanding. It is usually associated with wheeze audible on auscultation but this feature is not universal. Some patients can produce convincing wheeze from their larynx as do those with factitious asthma.[25] Whether this is a psychologic problem or is an attempt to modify expiratory airflow is unknown. Wheeze is not specific to COPD. It is due to turbulent airflow through larger airways narrowed from any cause, for example smooth muscle contraction, anatomic distortion or the presence of excess secretions. Although the Intermittent Positive Pressure Breathing (IPPB) trial found the presence of wheezing to be commoner in those patients showing a bronchodilator response the interpretation of these data is difficult[26] (see below). We could not confirm this relationship in our study of over 200 patients assessed with nebulized beta-agonists and oral corticosteroids. The presence of wheezing is believed to be a pointer against the diagnosis of COPD but we found that in our series of moderate to severe patients 83% reported that they wheezed on most days whilst wheeze on auscultation was present in 66% of patients.

Breathlessness

The physiologic basis of breathlessness is reviewed in Chapter 16. This is the symptom associated with the worst prognosis, greatest disability and largest loss of lung function over time.[10] In early COPD behavior can be modified to limit breathlessness, for example not talking when walking, using a car for short journeys. The gradual increase in background respiratory impedance over the years makes detection of further acute changes harder and patients may alter their breathing pattern to minimize the sensation of breathlessness. Thus a greater degree of inspiratory effort can be tolerated for the same level of discomfort.[27] How rapidly this adaptive behavior occurs is not known but many patients presenting to their physicians have substantially reduced ventilatory capacity, often less than 50% of predicted. By the time the FEV_1 has fallen to 30% or less predicted (equivalent to an FEV_1 of about 1.0 L) and the $\dot{V}O_{2max}$ is less than 15 ml/kg/min, the patient is breathless on minimal

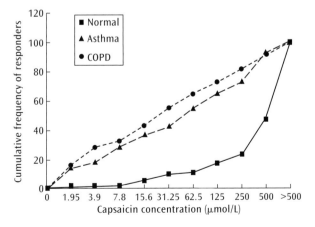

Figure 20.1 *Cumulative frequency plot of the dose of inhaled capsaicin required to induce 5 coughs in normal subjects and patients with chronic asthma or COPD. Note the similarity between asthma and COPD wth a significant reduction in cough threshold in both diseases.*

exertion.[28] However, it is difficult to accurately grade symptoms such as breathlessness from simple spirometric percentages, as hyperinflation which develops at a variable rate as FEV_1 declines and pulmonary hypertension, especially on exercise, will both affect exercise tolerance. The wide range of breathlessness intensity perceived at any given level of lung function is illustrated by data from Wolkove and colleagues using a 10-point Borg scale. They found that for any given level of lung function impairment there was a range of scoring of five or more points.[29] Moreover, mental state is a crucial determinant of the severity of perceived breathlessness in COPD.[30] For example, occupational medicolegal claimants have a significantly higher level of symptoms for each level of lung impairment than do patients with no claim to support.[31] Despite this, the impact of breathlessness on daily activity, as captured in a modified version of the MRC breathlessness scale, provides a useful surrogate for more detailed health status measurements.[32]

The terms used by patients to describe breathlessness vary widely. Specific clusters of symptoms have been reported in COPD and in asthma but may be modified by local experience. Thus in Liverpool, men complain of 'blowing for tugs' when describing their breathlessness, meaning 'wheezing as loudly as a ship's horn calling for tugs to help the ship into its docking berth'! The degree of breathlessness may be recorded by relating it to specific tasks, for example shopping or climbing stairs, or can be formally quantified using one of the several scales developed to assess breathlessness. The MRC scale is simple and has been extensively used as an epidemiologic tool. It is still a valuable way of describing population behavior but is relatively insensitive to small changes in symptoms produced by most medical treatment. Dramatic changes in symptoms after lung volume reduction surgery or intensive rehabilitation can change the reported MRC grade (see Chapters 30 and 32).

Short-term assessments with category scales such as the Borg scale or with visual analog scales are helpful in monitoring the progress of specific symptoms but a more global view is obtained by detailed questionnaire-based studies using the baseline and transitional dyspnea index.[33]

In severe COPD, orthopnea can occur reflecting the increased diaphragmatic activity required to maintain lung volume when supine[34] but some patients, especially those with marked increases in FRC, complain of breathlessness worse on leaning forward which is relieved by lying flat.[35] Again this reflects particular chest wall configurations and patterns of respiratory muscle activation.

Other symptoms

Chest pain is a common complaint in COPD but is not usually related to the disease itself. Ischemic heart disease is frequent in any population of heavy smokers and may be difficult to distinguish from symptoms of gastroesophageal reflux. Acid reflux occurs in up to 40% of COPD patients[36] presumably due to impairment of the pinch-cock mechanism at the esophageal hiatus secondary to hyperinflation and/or methylxanthine therapy.[37,38] COPD patients often complain of chest tightness during exacerbations which is not pleuritic and for which no cause is found. Possible explanations include intercostal muscle ischemia due to the increased work of respiration or trapped air under pressure in poorly ventilated peripheral areas of lung. Dull persistent pain, especially if accompanied by increasing breathlessness or fixed wheezing, raises the possibility of a central bronchial neoplasm, whilst acute pleurisy and dyspnea require that pulmonary embolism, pneumothorax or pneumonia be urgently excluded.

Ankle swelling may simply reflect immobility but if there is pitting edema and an elevated jugular venous pressure, cor pulmonale is a possibility. The difficulties associated with this commonly used term are reviewed in Chapter 17. A recent survey of acute exacerbation admissions showed that presenting with ankle swelling was one of three factors predictive of death within 3 months.[39] Hemoptysis, especially if it occurs as streaks of blood in purulent phlegm, may be due simply to airway inflammation.[40] However, this can never be assumed until bronchoscopy and a CT scan have excluded bronchial carcinoma or bronchiectasis.

Anorexia and weight loss often occurs in advanced disease and are markers of a worse prognosis.[41] Their cause is unclear but a reduction in calorie intake and hypermetabolism have been suggested.[42,43] Psychiatric morbidity is high in COPD reflecting the social isolation the disease produces, its chronicity and the neurological effects of hypoxemia.[44–46] Sleep quality is impaired in advanced disease, more so in the 'pink and puffing' than the 'blue and bloated' patients,[47] and this may contribute to impaired neuropsychiatric performance. Data in hypoxemic hypercapnic COPD patients suggest a specific pattern of cognitive deterioration characterized by an impaired verbal memory test, well-preserved visual attention and diffuse worsening of other functions. These changes cannot be explained by age or associated vascular dementia.[48]

SOCIAL HISTORY

Smoking remains the principal cause of COPD in developed economies (see Chapter 3) and the diagnosis should always be made with great caution in non-smokers even when the history and physiology appear to be typical. It is useful to assess lifetime smoking habits in terms of

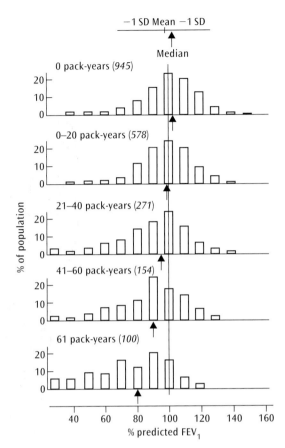

Figure 20.2 *The 'dose-related' effects of cigarette smoking in a population sample expressed as the percentage distribution of predicted FEV₁ for subjects divided by pack-years of smoking. Figures in brackets refer to the number in each sample and solid arrows to the median FEV₁ values. Mean and median FEV₁ fall as cigarette consumption increases but the individual change is still very variable and spirometry can be normal despite heavy tobacco exposure. (From ref. 49.)*

pack-years; one pack-year being equivalent to smoking 20 cigarettes per day for 1 year. This overcomes the problems of different durations and intensities of cigarette smoking but there is still considerable variation in the effects of apparently equivalent exposures on lung function, which is illustrated in Figure 20.2.[49] In general the greater the cumulative exposure, the worse the decline in FEV₁ but a very susceptible light smoker (1–20 pack-years) can have much worse lung function than a 'resistant' heavy smoker (61–80 pack-years). A similar spectrum of response is seen pathologically but patients can be assured that most smokers of 40 pack-years or more have pathological evidence of emphysema even if this is not yet affecting their pulmonary physiology![50] Some of this variability presumably reflects differences in puff size, cigarette type and the accuracy of the patient's own assessment of their

cigarette consumption but most represents the differences in susceptibility between individuals.

Although it is the most important factor leading to COPD, tobacco smoking is not the only cause and often interacts with other exposures in individuals with a family history of lung disease or reduction in lung function from other causes[51,52] (see Chapter 4). In some countries exposure to indoor pollution can be sufficient to produce a COPD-like illness[53,54] while exposure to coal dust underground may contribute to the annual decline in FEV₁ in a ratio of approximately 1:3.[55] Separating out the relative effects is difficult and controversial. However, the UK Industrial Injuries Advisory Committee concluded that coal miners with radiographic pneumoconiosis and airflow limitation should be compensated by the state for the airflow limitation irrespective of whether or not they have smoked cigarettes and the evidence supporting this has been presented.[56]

There is increasing evidence that COPD is commoner in certain families. This reflects the interplay of social and genetic factors and is reviewed in Chapter 4.

PHYSICAL SIGNS IN COPD

Unlike other respiratory diseases the most useful physical signs in COPD are those obtained by careful inspection rather than palpation or auscultation. They are qualitative rather than quantitative and support a diagnosis made from the history and investigations rather than being specific in their own right.

Many patients are distressed by minimal exertion and may appear tachypneic at rest. 'Nicotine-stained' fingers (a common misnomer since it is tar that stains) may belie the stated smoking habits while definite central cyanosis indicates significant hypoxemia. However, the assessment of cyanosis may be influenced both by the background lighting conditions and the presence of secondary polycythemia (see Chapter 17). Overall nutrition, especially limb muscle mass, may be reduced whilst a significant degree of finger clubbing suggests bronchiectasis or a pulmonary tumor.

It is important to observe the breathing pattern. Symptomatic patients will often have a prolonged expiratory phase and some will purse their lips in expiration. Patients adopting pursed lip breathing at rest usually have a severely reduced FEV₁ and pulmonary hyperinflation, i.e. an increase in resting FRC, but the physiologic basis of this sign is still obscure. Lip pursing may reduce expiratory airway collapse or slow the breathing frequency.[57] Pursed lip breathing when taught to patients as part of respiratory rehabilitation (see Chapter 30) is reported to improve oxygenation[58] but does not necessarily improve respiratory muscle function. Use of the accessory muscles, principally the sternomastoids, at rest suggests advanced disease and/or a clinical exacerbation. When the patient leans forward and supports themselves on a chair or handrail this fixes the shoulder girdle and allows the muscles such as the pectorals and latissimus dorsi to be used for increased ribcage movement.[59,60] Breathing frequency is usually more than 16/min even when rested and becomes rapid and shallow with exertion. Some patients can develop 'respiratory alternans' when they breathe alternately with predominantly diaphragmatic (abdominal) and ribcage movements. This is best documented in normal subjects during external-resistive breathing but may be seen in patients in the intensive care unit.[61,62]

Patients with advanced COPD develop progressive hyperinflation with an increased anteroposterior chest diameter, but the stage in the natural history when this changes starts is not well defined. Several mechanical consequences follow from these changes in lung volume. The ribs become more horizontal and since the trachea is fixed by the mediastinum it appears to be shortened, i.e. the distance between the cricoid cartilage and xiphisternal angle is less than three fingers' breadths, often less than one. Moreover the trachea appears to descend with each inspiration. The diaphragm becomes more horizontal and acts to pull in the lower ribs during inspiration – Hoover's sign. This is associated with a widened xiphisternal angle and apparent abdominal protuberance as the abdominal contents are displaced forwards. Some patients may be alarmed by this apparent 'weight gain' until it is explained to them. As the diaphragm descends the liver is displaced and may be palpable below the costal margin.

Low-frequency vesicular breath sounds are thought to originate from turbulent flow in the central airways attenuated by passage through the natural filters of the lung and chest wall.[63] These sounds are typically reduced in intensity in COPD producing the 'silent' chest found in advanced disease. This has been related to regional changes in ventilation and perfusion.[64] Breath sound intensity can be reproducibly recorded and when airflow is standardized there is no significant difference between COPD patients and observations in normal subjects.[65] Wheezes are often present but their clinical significance has not been systematically studied.[66] Similarly a few scanty crackles may be heard but can usually be easily distinguished from the coarse crackles of bronchiectasis and the persistent late inspiratory fine crackles of fibrosis or left heart failure.

Cardiovascular examination may reveal pitting edema, tricuspid regurgitation or elevation of the jugular venous pressure, all of which point to pulmonary hypertension. Although assessment of the jugular venous pressure can be difficult in patients with prominent accessory muscle activity, it remains one of the best clinical signs of right ventricular overload. When these signs are present, patients should be assessed with blood gases as potential candidates for long-term oxygen therapy (see Chapter 29).

CLINICAL SIGNIFICANCE OF SYMPTOMS AND SIGNS

Attempts to identify COPD patients on the basis of symptoms and signs alone have been disappointing. In a study examining the specificity of a range of markers of COPD, independent observers picked out a heavy smoking history and those already with a diagnosis of COPD, and the only additional diagnostic information came from the reduction in the intensity of breath sounds.[67] In a similar exercise Bohadana and colleagues found breath sound intensity during auscultation to be related to the FEV_1 and the specific airways conductance.[68] Both studies show the considerable variation in the criteria adopted for diagnosis even in skilled hands. When the diagnosis has been made, symptoms and signs have been suggested as potential predictors of response to bronchodilator therapy. Wardman and colleagues described a six-item combination with some predictive value but the work has not been replicated.[69] In our own study of 211 patients we could not identify any symptom or sign, either singly or in combination, that could predict the response to either bronchodilators or oral corticosteroids in the short or long term.

By contrast, spirometric screening of populations can identify significant numbers of pre-symptomatic COPD patients,[70,71] although the health economic case for this is yet to be established conclusively. An intermediate opportunistic approach has been reported by offering spirometry only in existing pulmonary centers where significant numbers of smokers and non-smokers alike have been identified when asymptomatic or with only mild symptoms.[72]

CLINICAL PRESENTATION

Patients reach their doctors by a variety of routes. Many with mild COPD will remain unidentified in the community, although some may be detected in a health screening program that includes spirometry. Most accept their cough and reduced exercise tolerance as part of being a smoker and have relatively advanced disease by the time they first seek attention. Since the lung damage takes time to develop, most patients are in their sixth decade or older at first presentation. In our own study of 211 COPD patients we found that although all complained of breathlessness and had spirometric airflow obstruction ($FEV_1/FVC < 60\%$), only 82% admitted to wheezing and 73% to having a cough. In spite of an average smoking history of 37 pack-years, only 64% fulfilled the MRC definition of chronic bronchitis which may in part reflect the fact that only 33% were still smoking by the time they presented to hospital for assessment. Patients described how their wheeze or their cough was worst at specific times of day but there was no discernible pattern to this and nor did it have bearing on their later response to bronchodilators or to an oral steroid trial.[73] Thus symptoms and history can suggest the diagnosis of COPD but cannot define either treatment or prognosis.

Whilst this is the usual pattern of patients seen in hospital outpatient clinics, two less common variants are worth noting. The first involves patients with advanced disease confirmed by markedly impaired spirometry who insist that they were fully active until the onset of a relatively recent intercurrent infection. It seems likely that such patients have been compensating well for their increasing airflow limitation until a final, relatively trivial, rise in respiratory impedance has been enough to provoke a host of symptoms. Whether these changes are psychological or physiological is not clear. Data from a large population survey of patients with a reported diagnosis of COPD or one of its synonyms[74] have recently confirmed that although patients are disabled in terms of their daily activities, they often understate the impact that this has on their lives. Secondly, some patients present with fluid retention, persistent hypoxemic hypercapnia and relatively well-preserved nutrition. The relationship of this presentation to abnormal ventilatory control, respiratory muscle function and the pulmonary circulation has already been touched on elsewhere (see Chapters 15, 16 and 17). Table 20.1 lists some typical features found in these patients, although the frequency of this particular presentation appears to be declining. Nonetheless they are important to identify as their mortality rate is approximately twice that of 'pink and puffing' patients with equivalent degrees of airflow obstruction.[75]

MEASUREMENTS

Diagnostic imaging

This topic is considered elsewhere (see Chapter 21). Good quality posteroanterior and lateral chest radiographs are essential to exclude other diagnoses, for example bronchial tumor, pneumothorax, heart failure and possibly bronchiectasis. Diagnostic features of COPD are rare but if large emphysematous bullae are identified occupying more than one-third of the hemithorax on a plain radiograph surgical resection should be considered (see Chapter 32).

High-resolution CT scanning provides a detailed assessment of the degree of macroscopic alveolar destruction, its distribution and likely pathologic type (see Chapter 21). It is essential in planning lung volume reduction surgery,[76] but until data about its relationship to the natural history of COPD are available, it cannot be recommended for routine evaluation of COPD. Ventilation–perfusion scanning is difficult to interpret in patients with severe airflow obstruction in whom ventilation–perfusion mismatching is part of the condition. It can lead to an erroneous diagnosis of pulmonary embolism.

Physiological assessment

The cardinal feature of COPD is obstruction to forced expiratory airflow.[14,77,78] The degree of airflow obstruction cannot be predicted on the basis of the symptoms or signs and therefore can only be quantified by making measurements. Despite this half of all physicians in a UK audit of patients admitted to hospital with an acute exacerbation managed the patient with no FEV_1 measure at any time before during or after the episode.[79] In primary care in the UK approximately half of all practices have no spirometer available to them. In a study that asked physicians to evaluate a hypothetical COPD case history a similar pattern emerged.[80] This may reflect what has

Table 20.1 Clinical and physiological features of 'pink and puffing' and 'blue and bloated' patients

	'Pink and puffing'	'Blue and bloated'
Synonym	Type A	Type B
Clinical	Dyspneic at rest	Less dyspneic
	Thin	Obese
	Hyperinflated	Edematous
Gas exchange		
K_{CO}	Low/normal	Normal
Pao_2 resting	>60 mmHg	<60 mmHg
$Paco_2$ resting	<50 mmHg	>50 mmHg, usually
Pao_2 exercise	Reduced	Variable
Total lung capacity	Moderate increase	Small increase
Static lung compliance	Normal/high	Normal
Pulmonary artery pressure	Normal	Modest elevation
Red cell mass	Normal–low	High

These represent extreme ends of a spectrum of disease with many patients lying between these extremes. In general, clinic spirometry is equally disturbed in both groups whilst argument persists about the amount of macroscopic emphysema present within their lungs. Classically this is more obvious in the 'pink and puffing' patients but not all studies support this view.

been custom but it also shows that some clinicians appear to find it difficult to relate their undergraduate physiology to the practical tests that are available. In this section we will consider what these tests are, how they should be performed, and what abnormalities are likely in COPD.

The earliest changes in COPD affect the alveolar walls and small airways and the consequent increase in peripheral airway resistance may be detectable by subtle modifications in lung mechanics and gas exchange, at least in the research setting. However these tests are difficult to perform, have high coefficients of variation and are only really valid when the pulmonary elastic recoil is normal and there is no proximal airway limitation, conditions that are seldom met even in mild COPD.

As the disease progresses, spirometric values begin to fall and end-expiratory volumes begin to rise. The work required of the inspiratory muscles increases and the breathing pattern changes, attempting to minimize respiratory discomfort. The reduced alveolar surface area is reflected in a reduced DLco (diffusing capacity for carbon monoxide) and changes in the pulmonary circulation coupled with ventilation–perfusion mismatching lead to hypoxemia. Finally in very severe disease the combination of ventilation–perfusion mismatching, circulatory changes and compromise of respiratory muscle function lead to daytime hypercapnia and sometimes clinical 'cor pulmonale'.

As COPD progresses the number of physiologic tests showing abnormality rises, but no single variable can characterize the whole process either in individuals or in a cohort. This general truism has been set out in tabular form in various publications of which the most recent is in the GOLD guideline[14] – a product of both clinical and epidemiologic viewpoints. We have set out an alternative purely clinical view in Table 20.2 which approximates the clinical presentation to the physiological abnormalities likely to be present. Tables 20.3 and 20.4 summarize the most commonly reported measures of pulmonary function, their physiologic basis and their derangement in COPD.

DYNAMIC TESTS OF LUNG FUNCTION – SPIROMETRY

Volumetric spirometers record volume by displacement and derive flow by differention of the volume signal. Since volume is recorded directly as the primary measurement, the accuracy of the volume is high and the device can never overestimate. The disadvantages of volume-based spirometers are a small resistance that has to be overcome in order to move the recording apparatus and their bulk. There are subtle but predictable differences between flow–volume loops generated on such machines as compared to the flow-based devices.[81] Clinically, the differences are too small to be important.

Flow-based spirometers (pneumotachygraphs, turbine spirometers and others) record pressure changes with time, assume that the relationship between pressure and time is linear and then integrate the flow/time signal to obtain volume. The method is highly dependent upon computing but the better systems are robust and can correct for the non-linearity between pressure and flow which is most marked at low flows. The devices have become small, cheap, portable and widely available.

Table 20.2 *Schematic relationship between disease progression, symptoms and physiologic test results*

Clinical state	Results of measurements
Stage 1 No symptoms No abnormal signs	Abnormalities reported on specialized tests, e.g. frequency dependence of compliance, closing volume and N_2 slope increased, volume of helium iso-flow increased, elastic recoil reduced Of limited value for practical patient management
Stage 2 'Smokers' cough' but no breathlessness No abnormal signs	Abnormalities as in stage 1 plus small reductions in FEV_1, FEV_1/VC ratio and other indice of expiratory airflow
Stage 3 Breathlessness (±wheeze) on exertion, cough (±sputum) and some abnormal signs	Reduction in FEV_1 often to less than 50% predicted Variable increases in FRC Reductions in DLco Some patients hypoxemic but normocapnic
Stage 4 Breathless on minimal exertion. Wheeze and cough prominent Clinical evidence of hyperinflation usual plus cyanosis and polycythemia in some	Severe airflow limitation ($FEV_1 < 30\%$ predicted) Marked hyperinflation (RV and FRC) Wide range of DLco Reduced maximum inspiratory pressures Hypoxemia usual and hypercapnia in some

There is one important caveat: calibration errors can be difficult to detect and they can be wrongly calibrated to yield either falsely low or high results.

Spirometry was introduced in the late 1950s but was not standardized until the American Thoracic Society's 'Snowbird' workshop produced technical guidelines for spirometers and made recommendations about how to perform the test.[82] These were revised by the ATS in 1987,[83] 1991[84] and 1994;[85] and it is to these standards that most equipment manufacturers produce spirometers. Separately, European guidelines on lung function were produced in 1983[86] and revised in 1993.[87] Good quality spirometry depends more on the care and training of the supervising technician than on any differences in equipment.[88]

All the guidance on spirometry including the most recent GOLD guideline[14] recommend that there should be a hardcopy output from the test that can be inspected. There should be:

- At least three technically satisfactory readings, i.e. volume/time curves should be smooth and free from irregularities that might indicate either variable submaximal effort or coughing.
- The recording has been continued until a volume plateau has been reached. This can take up to 15 or more seconds to achieve in severe COPD.
- Both FEV_1 and FVC should be the largest values from any of the three curves.
- The FEV_1 and FVC values should vary by not more than 100 ml or 5%, whichever is the greater.

Representative traces are shown in Figure 20.3.

The greatest errors arise from submaximal efforts, and are unlikely to be detected unless the actual traces are checked.[88] The FVC can be significantly underestimated if a full expiration is not performed.[89,90] Both ATS and European standards advocate that vital capacity should be measured either from a relaxed expiration or from an

Table 20.3 *Dynamic or spirometric tests*

Name	Test	Physiological basis	Results	Comment
FEV_1	Forced expiratory volume in first second from TLC	During a forced expiration the driving pressure is sufficient that at any given lung volume, the airflow is limited by the cross-sectional area of the flow limiting segment of the airways. Reproducible because depends more on airway dimensions than on test effort	Always ↓, often very low	Reproducible to ±200 ml, always abnormal in COPD so that COPD usually defined in terms of FEV_1/VC ratio
FVC	Forced expiratory volume from TLC to RV (see also VC)		Normal or ↓	Nearly as reproducible as FEV_1 but can be underestimated if expiration not continued for up to 15 seconds
PEF	Peak expiratory flow from TLC		Usually ↓	The most effort dependent of the three – may be relatively preserved compared to FEV_1. Less sensitive and less reproducible (±60 L/min) but easily repeated
Flow–volume loop	Maximum expiration from TLC, followed by maximum inspiration to TLC; usually preceded by a tidal breathing loop	As above for the expiratory phase. Inspiration more dependent on effort than airway dimensions	Characteristic shape of expiratory phase (Figure 20.3)	Many measurements can be calculated from the loop, but none have better predictive power than FEV_1 and FVC. Shape of loop may indicate airway collapsibility

These are the most important lung function measurements simple, quick, highly reproducible and surprisingly sensitive. Note that a reduced FEV_1/VC ratio is an important defining characteristic of airways obstruction.

Table 20.4 *Static lung volumes*

Name	Test	Physiologic basis	Results	Comment
TLC	Total lung capacity – lung volume at maximum inspiration	Depends on size and balance between maximum inspiratory pressure and elastic recoil of the respiratory system	Normal or ↑	Respiratory muscles adapt to a high TLC and work more efficiently. Reproducible ±5%
VC	Slow or relaxed vital capacity. Maximum volume of gas expired slowly from TLC to RV (or vice versa) (slow or relaxed vital capacity)	Depends on the different factors influencing the TLC and RV	Usually ↓	Can be preserved if both TLC and RV increase in parallel. Usually larger than FVC because less air trapping. Simple and reproducible. Relates well to self-paced walking distance
FRC	Functional residual capacity – lung volume at the end of tidal breath (elastic equilibrium volume) should be measured when relaxed – sensitive to changes in breathing pattern	Volume at which lung elastic recoil exactly balances outward chest wall recoil. Dynamic effects very important in COPD	Usually ↑	Affected by small reductions in lung elasticity. Limited reproducibility clinically (±10%), FRC may increase dynamically as respiratory rate increases
RV	Residual volume – volume of air remaining in lungs at end expiration	Depends on the balance of expiratory pressure and the outward recoil of the chest wall at low lung volumes and the collapsibility of the airways	Raised, often markedly	Reproducible to ±10%, a measure of hyperinflation due to early airway closure. Some airways may begin to close during tidal breathing in severe COPD. Raised by bronchospasm/pulmonary edema

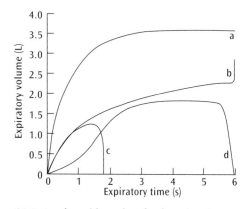

Figure 20.3 *A volume/time plot of a forced expiratory maneuver on a typical display which only shows 6 seconds on the x-axis. (a) Health with FEV$_1$ 2.7 L and FVC 3.6 L – the curve plateaus at 3.5 seconds. (b) A good sustained expiratory effort in COPD with an FEV$_1$ of 1.2 L. The trace stopped moving at 6 seconds, and the vertical line indicates a further 0.45 L were breathed out after this to make total FVC of 2.7 L. (c) Good initial effort in the same patient to give an FEV$_1$ of 1.15 L but stopping expiration at 1.5 seconds means no FVC can be recorded. (d) In the same COPD patient showing a poor effort, not sustained for even 6 seconds, resulting in falsely low volumes. To be acceptable, curves must be smooth and convex upwards throughout.*

inspiratory maneuver whenever possible. If this is not possible in clinical practice, the physician should be aware that FVC is a potential underestimate.

It has been suggested that the ATS criteria could be modified so that the maximum effort is made in the first part of the maneuver, and then a relaxed expiration encouraged after the airflow has fallen below 200 ml/s.[90] Quality control procedures developed in the original Lung Health Study[91] suggested that the patient should obtain reproducible peak expiratory flow values if the maneuver was to be classed as satisfactory. Unpublished data from the ISOLDE study[92] found that this criteria was hard to achieve in patients with a low FEV$_1$ but this did not compromise the reproducibility of the FEV$_1$ value. Some patients who did not sustain expiration for at least 12 seconds produced suboptimal FVC data which might influence their classification. This is in contrast to the large general population of patients more recently reported where FEV$_6$ was well correlated with FVC.[93] We recommend that care be taken to ensure repeatability of the FVC if the starting FEV$_1$ is <50% predicted.

The more recent guidelines recommend that the best FEV$_1$ and the best FVC should be reported from at least three acceptable tracings even if the values do not come from the same expiratory effort. However many computerized systems use the FEV_1 and FVC from the best loop, (defined as the loop with the largest sum of FEV_1 and FVC).

Individual values can be interpreted by comparison with a predicted value based on the subject's age, sex, height and race. Thus, for example, Negroes have lung volumes that are 13% less than Caucasians with Asians being in an intermediate range. European laboratories usually use the European Coal and Steel values which have been updated since their first publication in the early 1970s.[87] In North America each laboratory is encouraged to establish its own reference range. Using different published US equations can result in a 10% difference in the predicted value and hence a 10% variability in spirometry expressed as a percent predicted.[84,94]

For FEV_1 and FVC the lower limit of normal equates to about 80% of the predicted normal value. However the standard deviation from the predicted equation is the same at all ages and sizes and is not proportional to the FEV_1. Thus in older smaller people two standard deviations could equate to a value of 65% predicted. This has led to suggestions that results be expressed as the number of 'residual standard deviations' below the normal value.[95] Although statistically sound, clinicians do not seem to have found this appealing as a concept. There is an important distinction between the absolute level of FEV_1 and the ratio of FEV_1 to vital capacity whether expressed as FVC or VC. Airflow obstruction is defined in terms of an abnormal FEV_1/VC ratio,[14] while it is the absolute level of FEV_1 that correlates best with performance and has prognostic value. In the GOLD guideline, stage 1 is defined as an FEV_1 above 80% predicted and an FEV_1/FVC ratio below 70%. While these patients technically do have airflow limitation, the normal FEV_1 means that few if any will require medical attention. Moreover there are data that the FEV_1/FVC ratio declines with age in healthy non-smokers which could lead to some misclassification,[96] at least in epidemiologic studies. The GOLD approach is an empirical one designed to meet very different needs in different countries and this should be borne in mind when considering these borderline areas.

Although spirometry is recorded from a forced expiratory maneuver, the results obtained are largely independent of the effort used because the determining factors in the size of the FEV_1 include the dynamic cross-sectional area of the flow-limiting segments within the airways. These flow-limiting segments change during expiration with changing lung volume, elastic recoil pressure and the extent of airway disease. Thus the FEV_1 is in effect a proxy measurement of overall airway narrowing (see Chapter 13) and hence has proved to be the most robust general marker of pathology and prognosis in COPD. Alternatively results may be interpreted in terms of the FEV_1 alone (e.g. as per cent predicted) to

Table 20.5(a) *Disability and lung function (Data from ref. 83)*

Obstructive abnormality: the FEV_1/VC ratio must be below the normal range	
	FEV_1 expressed as % predicted
May be a physiologic variant	>101
Mild	70–100
Moderate	60–69
Moderately severe	50–59
Severe	35–49
Very severe	<35

Table 20.5(b) *(Data from ref. 84)*

Mean FEV_1		Dyspnea grade
L	% predicted	(0–4)
3.2	95	0
2.4	62	1
1.8	45	2
1.2	35	3
0.75	–	4

indicate how advanced the disease is, and by repeating the observations over time to assess progress. A rapid decline in FEV_1 indicates a worse prognosis.

Spirometry before and after bronchodilators may yield clinically useful information about some aspects of diagnosis but its importance in established COPD is more limited than initially believed (see below). FEV_1 data can be used to predict maximum ventilation during exercise. The conventional equation of $FEV_1 \times 35$ probably underestimates peak voluntary ventilation at least in moderate-severe COPD[97] and a better alternative is $(18.9 \times FEV_1) + 19.7$ L/min.[98] FEV_1 can be a guide to general disability and a general scheme is indicated in Table 20.5. As noted earlier, the relationship between impairment of FEV_1 and increase in symptoms is not a simple one and there are many other variables that influence that separately impact on the subjective effect of COPD – thus although the general trends are true, they must not be applied rigidly to the assessment of individual patients.

TESTS OF FLOW IN RELATION TO VOLUME

The graphic display of flow and volume provides a complementary approach to the usual volume/time plot and adds some information about lung mechanics in COPD especially when the tidal volume loop is considered in relation to the maximum flow–volume envelope. Figure 20.4 shows the flow–volume loop in severe COPD, illustrating the airway collapse which begins after the first 200–300 ml have been expelled from the trachea and main airways

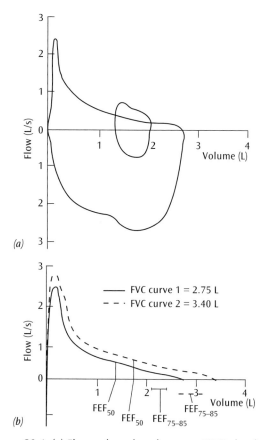

Figure 20.4 *(a) Flow–volume loop in severe COPD showing a relatively preserved PEF followed by a rapid diminution in flow as airways collapse. Inspiratory flows better preserved. Flow during tidal breathing (low effort) exceeds that during forced expiration. (b) Expiratory flow volume curve before (solid line) and after (dashed line) bronchodilator. TLC has been assumed constant for the purpose of illustration. Changed FVC leads to flow measurements being made at different absolute lung volumes.*

and continues throughout expiration. Quiet non-forced breathing such as tidal breathing often results in better flow rates at the same lung volume.

A number of measurements have been made from the flow–volume loop, including FEF_{50}, FEF_{75} and FEF_{75-85}. All have problems of reproducibility such that the values have to fall below 50% of predicted for them to be outside the normal range. Flows in the latter part of the expiratory curve were thought to be an indicator of small airway function, but at least one long-term study has shown that all the clinically useful information is provided by the FEV_1 and FVC.[99]

There are technical reasons why flow measurements made at iso-volume are so variable. Volume calculated from flows at the mouth makes no allowance for the effect of thoracic gas compression during expiration. Hence there are small but systematic differences between tests using a spirometer and those performed in a body

plethysmograph. More importantly if the FVC changes between two tests after an intervention (e.g. a bronchodilator) or because of too short a forced expiratory time, then the reported flow indices will have been derived at different lung absolute lung volumes. They will therefore relate to a different set of mechanical and geometric factors and will not be strictly comparable (Figure 20.4(b)).

Although most of the flow measurements from the flow–volume loop may be of limited value, there is useful information from the shape of the loop particularly for the detection of unsuspected conditions such as main airways obstruction by tumor or stricture, since though rare these conditions can be misdiagnosed for some time as COPD and appropriate treatment delayed.

Peak flow measurements

This can be read from the flow–volume loop or measured independently with a hand-held peakflow meter. These use a linear scale but are not in fact linear with respect to flow,[100] and so not directly comparable with levels of PEF in the laboratory. The value of the portable instruments lies in the ease with which measurements can be repeated at home. The importance of diurnal variability as a reliable defining characteristic of asthma is well established,[101,102] but the same is not true for COPD. Most patients show little change during the day and caution should be exercised when reporting the absolute values of PEF as a surrogate for FEV_1. During the first part of expiration air is rapidly expelled from the trachea and main airways before the more distal airways collapse limits further flow. The initial peak flow is less affected by this than is the FEV_1, which records all airflow in the first second. Thus relying on the PEF may overestimate airway caliber as assessed by the FEV_1. Moreover peak flow when recorded alone cannot differentiate whether a reduced value is due to restrictive disease or is the result of airway obstruction.

Single measurements of PEF are very variable and changes of 60 L/min are within the natural variability of the measurement.[103] Serial PEF values reduced the variability and can give information similar to the FEV_1.[104,105] However the role of these measurements in detecting a clinically important response to treatment is disputed and at present this approach is not recommended.

STATIC TESTS OF LUNG MECHANICS

The main determinants of TLC, RV and FRC are summarized in Table 20.4. These measures are indicators of the severity of hyperinflation, i.e. the progressive rise in FRC, and usually also in RV that results from the loss of pulmonary elastic recoil and airway collapse. In addition there is a dynamic component to the hyperinflation (see Chapter 18) such that it worsens during exercise. This cannot be predicted from data obtained during tidal breathing. Hyperinflation is a major determinant of symptoms such as breathlessness on exertions as it increases the elastic work of breathing and reduces inspiratory capacity. There are several methods for assessing static lung volumes:

- Helium dilution during rebreathing – this is long established and widely available, but in severe COPD poorly ventilated areas of lung (including bullae) do not have time to equilibrate properly with the inspired helium and so the measured residual volume (and hence total lung capacity) can be underestimated.
- Helium dilution during a single breath – this is calculated during the measurement of DLCO (see below) but is even more subject to underestimates than the above.
- Body plethysmography – this relies on the accurate measurement of small fluctuations in mouth and box pressure during gentle panting against a closed shutter and uses Boyle's law to calculate lung volumes. Computerized systems make it quick and practical to measure all the trapped air within the thorax including that in poorly ventilated areas and therefore produces a higher value than does helium dilution methods. However artefacts due to delayed equilibration of pressure between alveoli and mouth can lead to overestimation of volumes[106] and this can be made worse by an increased panting frequency[107] or the 'shunt compliance' of the upper airways. The latter problem can be reduced by supporting the cheeks with both hands.[108]
- X-ray planimetry – this apparently cheap and simple means of deriving an estimate of lung volume from a posteroanterior and lateral radiograph was made possible by computerization.[109] However standardization proved difficult and although there are reports suggesting that valid results can be obtained, we were unable to confirm them. In studies on normal and COPD subjects compared with helium dilution and body plethysmography methods we found 95% confidence intervals in individuals were up to 2 L of volume in either direction.[110]

Showing that FRC, residual volume and possibly TLC are raised supports the diagnosis of COPD and may help to explain why a patient with relatively modest spirometric abnormality, is particularly symptomatic. Changes in lung volumes after bronchodilators provide an alternative means of assessing response[111,112] but are more time consuming than simple spirometry. A potential refinement has been to look for changes in 'trapped gas volume', i.e. the difference between the volume measured with plethysmography and with helium dilution methods.[113] This corresponds to the 'slow ventilating' compartment described by the physiologists of the 1960s. Changes in trapped gas volume were claimed to be an indicator of response to bronchodilator and to relate to exercise performance. However the initial report has never been replicated and the methodologic problems of subtracting one inherently variable number from another make its routine use impractical.[110]

Maximum pressure generation

The measurement of maximum inspiratory and expiratory pressures has become more popular in recent years, mainly to monitor progress during pulmonary rehabilitation. Normal values have been defined[114] but these measurements are still not available in many laboratories. Their physiologic significance is reviewed elsewhere (see Chapter 15). The test equipment is now relatively inexpensive but several practical issues should be considered. Care is needed to ensure that the patient seals his or her lips around the mouthpiece and some practice is required to obtain reproducible results. Maximum efforts are normally reached within five attempts but the patient tires if the test is prolonged beyond this. The development of simple portable instruments has made this test more clinically valuable.[115]

Bronchodilator reversibility testing

Reversibility can be defined as an improvement in an index of airflow obstruction and/or relevant functional variable in response to an active treatment which is greater than that likely to have occurred by chance. Reversibility testing is usually recommended in the management of COPD,[14,77] usually as a means of differentiating from asthma. However, there is little agreement about which test should be used, what doses and types of drug to use and what a positive result signifies.[116] Reversibility can be assessed in terms of changes in symptoms (e.g. breathlessness) or exercise performance (e.g. self-paced walking tests) but is usually done using either FEV$_1$ or PEF. Several factors determine the outcome of reversibility testing.

LIMITATIONS OF THE MEASUREMENT

The coefficient of variation for FEV$_1$ is reported to be less than 5% in normal subjects.[117] In fact the variability is independent of baseline FEV$_1$ and is of similar absolute size whatever the FEV$_1$. Tweedale, Alexander and McHardy[118] found that the standard deviation of repeated measurements on the same day was 102 ml. This means that only if a change in FEV$_1$ exceeds 170 ml can it be considered to have arisen other than by chance. ATS,[85] European[87] and GOLD[14] guidelines recommend that changes should only be considered significant if they exceed an absolute volume of 200 ml. Our own data support this.[119,120]

RESPONSE CRITERIA

The commonest approach in the past has been to define a response in terms of the percentage change from the initial value, for example a rise of 15%. However, in subjects with a low FEV_1 a 20% rise may still be within the range of spontaneous variability of the measurement. To overcome this the British Thoracic Society (BTS) recommended that a response be defined as an increase in FEV_1, greater than both 15% of baseline and 200 ml,[87] an approach adopted in some physiologic studies.[119,121] The ATS and GOLD suggest a significant change of both 200 ml and a 12% change in the predicted normal FEV_1 value.[14,85] A third approach, adopted in Europe, is to express the change as a percentage of the potential possible change (i.e. a percentage of the predicted value).[103]

Criteria based on a percentage change from baseline alone are more likely to report patients as being reversible than those where an absolute change in FEV_1 is used (Figure 20.5).

CHANGE IN BASELINE AIRWAY CALIBER

If on the test day a patient has a relatively high level of airway smooth muscle tone and hence a lower initial FEV_1, there is a greater chance of observing a 200 ml (or greater) change in FEV_1 occurring than on another day when

resting tone happens to be lower and the initial FEV_1 higher. Thus about one-third of those who are graded responders on day 1 may be classed as non-responders on day 2 and vice versa.[23] In the ISOLDE study when patients were tested on three occasions over 2 months and classified as reversible or not by the ATS criteria only 52% remained within the same bronchodilator category on all three occasions. All these patients met the ERS criteria of being irreversible to one drug but when tested with two drugs over a third changed their responder status when retested. Again these changes were largely due to differences in the starting airway caliber between test days.

CHOICE OF DRUG AND DOSAGE

A small dose of bronchodilator from a metered dose inhaler (MDI) will cause fewer subjects to have a significant response than would repeated doses from the MDI or a larger dose by nebulizer.[122] Adding a second drug will further increase the FEV_1 and response rate of some patients.[123,124] Given the uncertainties above, it is difficult to make definitive statements about the relative efficacy of beta-agonist and anticholinergic agents.[120] The balance of evidence suggests that ipratropium is more likely to elicit a bronchodilator response than salbutamol (See Chapter 24). Beta-agonists have the advantage of a

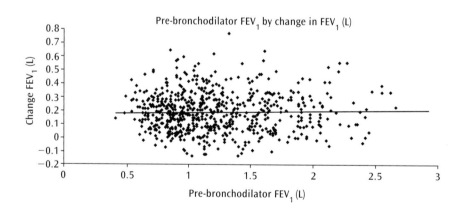

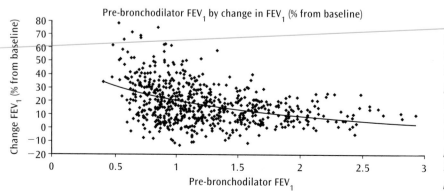

Figure 20.5 *Change in FEV$_1$ after inhaling 200 mcg salbutamol and 80 mcg ipratropium in 660 COPD patients. Upper panel presents the absolute change which is independent of baseline FEV$_1$. Lower panel plots the data as the percentage change from baseline, larger changes occurring at lower prebronchodilator FEV$_1$ values.*

quicker onset of action (15 min vs. 45 min), leading to a shorter test time. However, which single drug or combination should be used remains unclear because there are few data relating laboratory tests to treatment outcome. Timing is often decided more by convenience than the pharmacology, as seen in the Lung Health Study where testing took place only 15 minutes after isoproteronol.[125]

Corticosteroids

The role of corticosteroids in acute and stable disease is reviewed in Chapter 25.

Many clinicians give a short course of oral corticosteroids, in addition to the short-acting bronchodilator tests, to identify potentially responsive COPD patients. The commonest doses used have been 30 mg prednisolone or 0.6 mg/kg/day and the commonest trial period is 2 weeks. All the problems of defining a response described above apply to oral corticosteroid trials but there are no published studies of reproducibility. Our own data using 30 mg prednisolone for 2 weeks and defining a response as a 200 ml or greater rise in FEV_1, showed that 44/211 consecutive referrals were responsive (21%).[73] All but three also responded to bronchodilators. We were unable to identify either singly or in combination any part of clinical history, examination or laboratory tests that would predict the response and avoid the need for trial of steroids.

The time before a response to oral prednisolone occurs has not been examined in COPD but Weir et al. suggested that 6 weeks was required before a response could be expected if inhaled corticosteroids were used.[126] However these studies did use a mixture of end-points involving changes in FEV_1, FVC and PEF.[126,127] Patients with a positive response to beta-agonists, whether from a metered dose inhaler[128] or a nebulizer,[73] are more likely to subsequently respond to oral prednisolone. Nebulized anticholinergic drugs can identify a few additional cases.[120] In our series a small number of corticosteroid-responsive patients were not identified whichever bronchodilator was used, but the improvement in FEV_1 after oral corticosteroids in this group was small, normally being less than 250 ml. A response to oral steroids could not be predicted from the appearance of the flow–volume loop lung volumes, DL_{CO} or atopic status.[129]

In patients with limited responses to inhaled bronchodilators oral prednisolone produces a small but still statistically significant increase in FEV_1. The distribution of this response is normal (Figure 20.6) with no clear group of 'responsive' patients. Those who lie in the extremes of the distribution showed the greatest day-to-day variation in post-bronchodilator FEV_1. No factor predicted the magnitude of this response except smoking status. Ex-smokers had a significantly greater response than those who continued to smoke during the oral corticosteroid trial.[130]

CLINICAL SIGNIFICANCE

Very large changes in FEV_1 are likely to suggest either asthma or at least an asthmatic component that justifies treatment as for asthma. An FEV_1 that returns to the normal range or a response that is greater than 400 ml (more than twice the variability of the measurement) is highly suggestive that this is the case. Most COPD patients will have smaller responses and the usual hope is that the acute bronchodilator trial will identify patients likely to have the greatest reduction in symptoms and improvement in exercise tolerance after treatment. However there are now ample data showing that this is not the case with short-acting beta-agonists, anticholingerics,[131] or long-acting inhaled beta-agonists. Typical are the data of Hay et al. who found that 80 μg of oxitropium bromide increased exercise tolerance and reduced symptoms by approximately 13% in 32 patients with stable COPD.[119] Responses were similar, whether or not the patients had been shown before to be reversible to bronchodilator. Berger and Smith showed similar changes in self-paced walking distance after orciprenaline in patients with fixed airflow obstruction,[132] whilst both Corris et al.[133] and Spence et al.[134] found similar functional improvements even in patients unresponsive to oral corticosteroids. This is not surprising given that bronchodilators can reduce hyperinflation both at rest[135] and on exercise[136] with relatively little change in FEV_1.

The variability in response criteria and the normal distribution of response described above make separation of patients treated over longer periods particularly unreliable. Single-dose testing has not been shown to predict long-term response. Nor were bronchodilator responses or the responses to oral corticosteroids predictive of the subsequent decline in FEV_1, health status or the number of exacerbations in the ISOLDE study.

However, there are potential benefits in establishing the reversibility status. Data from the IPPB study suggested that those patients with the least bronchodilator response

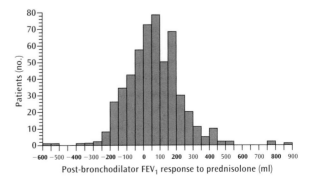

Figure 20.6 *Change in post-bronchodilator FEV_1 in 660 COPD patients receiving 30 mg prednisolone for 2 weeks. Note the normal distribution of the response.*

were most likely to lose lung function rapidly over time even allowing for other risk factors,[75] a finding supported by data from Holland.[137] We have found that patients with a positive corticosteroid trial have a more favorable outcome spirometrically and symptomatically over 1 year.[138]

Gas transfer factor

The diffusing capacity for carbon monoxide is a measure of the passive transfer of gas across the alveolar membrane and into the blood. Its size reflects the alveolar surface area but changes in the blood component must not be overlooked. Thus an increase in pulmonary capillary blood volume, for example during pulmonary edema, an increased pulmonary blood flow, for example on exercise or with a left to right cardiac shunt or a raised hemoglobin, for example polycythemia, will lead to higher values. Conversely, anemia or a high carboxyhemoglobin level will depress the measured DLco.

At present there are several different methods by which this measurement can be made, each yielding rather different answers in COPD patients. The method described by Ogilvie and colleagues in 1957 recorded the rate of carbon monoxide uptake during a 10-second breath-hold and related this to the alveolar volume derived by adding the inspired volume to the residual volume measured in a separate helium dilution test.[139] More widely used is the single-breath modification suggested by Mitchell and Renzetti who used helium to calculate alveolar volume.[140] This will underestimate alveolar volume in severe COPD and produce a lower value for the DLco measurement. Although this was accepted by the ATS and initial European guidelines, the most recent European revision[87] has advocated reversion to the original method especially in patients with COPD. The method of calculation can completely change the result for a given patient. Thus, for example, a man with bullous emphysema may have an inspiratory capacity of 3 liters during the single-breath maneuver and a residual volume of 2 liters from the single-breath helium dilution but 4.5 liters from the multiple-breath dilution. The alveolar volume in one method is 5 liters and in the other 7.5, which could represent a DLco of 60%, predicted against 90%. One way around this dilemma is to report diffusing capacity as the Krogh constant (Kco; i.e. DLco divided by alveolar volume), which effectively represents diffusion per unit lung volume. Although an attractive idea, the prediction equations are not well documented and the European statement[87] does not even recommend a standard prediction set. Confusion is likely to remain until the international standards are in agreement.

There is little doubt that the DLco values are below normal in many patients with COPD and this has been related to the presence of macroscopic emphysema[141,142]

and more recently to COPD on CT scan. However, the correlation between the severity of COPD and the reduction of DLco in the individual patients is relatively poor. Nonetheless, at least one study has reported a significant inverse relationship between DLco and 3-year survival.[143] Those patients with a Kco of less than 70% predicted have a mortality of over 80% compared with 30% of those with a Kco of more than 70% predicted. However, earlier studies did not observe this large effect,[144,145] whilst a more recent study reported a DLco rise even when the underlying disease was progressing,[146] possibly due to the subtle changes in ventilation–perfusion matching in the lungs of ex-smokers.

In summary a low DLco is suggestive of a significant degree of alveolar damage probably due to emphysema, but a normal DLco does not exclude the diagnosis of COPD.

Tests of gas exchange

The modern approach to gas exchange in COPD is discussed in Chapter 14. However, many clinicians find it difficult to apply logarthimic dispersions of ventilation and perfusion to bedside problems and still rely on the rather simpler concepts of the three-compartment model described by Riley and Cournand.[147] This considers the lung as three theoretical compartments; one in which there is 'ideal' ventilation but no perfusion (physiologic deadspace), a second with 'ideal' ventilation and perfusion and a third in which there is 'ideal' perfusion but no ventilation.

In practice the first compartment includes a contribution from units of above average V_A/Q dispersion and the anatomical deadspace. Within the physiologic deadspace (V_D) all the ventilation is wasted and the ventilation to perfusion ratio is infinity. The size of V_D can be calculated from the mixed expired (P_{ECO_2}) and arterial (Pa_{CO_2}) carbon dioxide tensions and the tidal volume. Thus:

$$V_D = V_T \left(1 - \left[\frac{P_{ECO_2}}{Pa_{CO_2}} \right] \right)$$

Physiologic deadspace is useful conceptually but is of less value clinically. The calculation of the deadspace to tidal volume ratio V_D/V_T is useful during exercise as a measure of the general effectiveness of ventilation and gas exchange. The concept can be used to understand what determines the level of arterial CO_2 in an individual. Thus:

$$Pa_{CO_2} = \frac{\dot{V}_{CO_2}}{\dot{V}_A} K$$

where $\dot{V}_A$ is the alveolar ventilation and K is a constant. Alveolar ventilation is $F \times (V_T - V_D)$ giving the revised equation:

$$Pa_{CO_2} = \frac{\dot{V}_{CO_2} \times K}{f \times (V_T - V_D)}$$

When metabolic CO_2 production is constant, for example at rest with no fever and no parenteral feeding, any reduction in breathing frequency or tidal volume (e.g. from ventilation-depressing drugs) or rise in physiologic deadspace (e.g. during exacerbations of COPD) will elevate the $Paco_2$. Most COPD patients maintain their CO_2 tension within the normal range, despite a large physiologic deadspace, until the airflow obstruction is severe (e.g. FEV_1 less than 1.2 L). An elevated $Paco_2$ without a mechanical explanation (i.e. low FEV_1) should prompt a search for an additional cause, for example sleep apnea or neuromuscular disease.

The third theoretical compartment has no ventilation, i.e. a $\dot{V}A/\dot{Q}$ ratio of zero. The partially saturated pulmonary arterial blood behaves as though it passes through this compartment unchanged. If the saturation of the systemic mixed venous blood and the arterial blood are known then the proportion of cardiac output passing though this theoretical compartment can be calculated (the venous admixture fraction). In practice the measurements and calculations necessary mean that formal shunt fraction assessment is confined to the research laboratory and to the intensive care unit where oxygen delivery must be optimized.

Since nitrogen plays no part in gas exchange, it follows that the non-nitrogen part of the inhaled gas mixture can be considered separately. CO_2 replaces some of the O_2 in the alveoli and a simple equation for use at the bedside can be derived relating the arterial blood gas tensions, the inspired oxygen concentration and the alveolar–arterial oxygen difference $((A - a)D)$: Thus:

$$FIO_2 = PO_2 + \frac{PCO_2}{0.8} + (A - a)D$$

where FIO_2 is the inspired O_2 tension, PO_2 and PCO_2 are the arterial blood gas tensions, $(A - a)D$ is the alveolar–arterial oxygen difference.

Since the percentage of oxygen in air is very close numerically to the partial pressure of oxygen in air expressed in kPa, the various factors can be related with simple mental arithmetic. For example the alveolar–arterial oxygen difference in a normal person breathing air could be:

$$21 = 13.3 + \frac{5.2}{0.8} + (A - a)D$$

so the $(A - a)D = 1.2\,kPa$
or in severe COPD, breathing 24% O_2:

$$24 = 7.3 + \frac{7.6}{0.8} + (A - a)D$$

so the $(A - a)D = 7.2\,kPa$.

Conversely by making an assumption of the likely high $(A-a)D$ in severe COPD patient, it is possible to back calculate the likely FIO_2 being administered – this

can be useful in detecting patients who have inadvertently been overprescribed oxygen, for example when given bronchodilators via an oxygen-powered nebulizer.

When the Pao_2 is above 8 kPa then a raised $(A-a)D$ is a surrogate measure of an increased venous admixture. When the Pao_2 is lower, small changes in PO_2 correspond to larger changes in oxygen fraction and this simple estimation will underestimate the true level of physiologic shunting.

ARTERIAL BLOOD GASES

The methodology of taking arterial blood for blood gases and some aspects of interpretation of the results are dealt with in Chapter 14. Arterial blood gas measurement is an essential part of the assessment of COPD to confirm the degree of hypoxia, assess if hypercapnia is present and, in the acutely ill patients, detect pH changes. These are dynamic measurements and values change rapidly in unstable patients. However, it may take 30 minutes for changes in inspired oxygen concentration to become fully apparent in the PO_2 because of the prolonged time constraints for alveolar gas equilibration. In the stable patient, resting hypoxemia is prognostically important, although the absolute oxygen tension is less important than the fact that it is below 7.5 kPa. By contrast, hypercapnia is a less predictive variable and survival is improved in patients receiving domiciliary oxygen despite a small increase in CO_2 tensions during treatment.[148]

Pulse oximetry and transcutaneous tensions

The relatively inexpensive and reliable non-invasive oximeters have aided the assessment of arterial oxygenation.[149] These devices measure oxygen saturation reliably down to approximately 75% but are sensitive to changes in the carboxyhemoglobin concentration, which may be elevated in chronic smokers.[149] They should not replace blood gases as the first measurement in a sick patient, but once the initial gas tensions are known pulse oximetry is a valuable tool with which to monitor progress during acute episodes, overnight or to screen potentially hypoxemic patients in the clinic.[150]

Oxygen saturation measurement takes no account of CO_2 tension, and during an acute exacerbation the saturation levels may be maintained (by additional oxygen being administered). This can lull the unwary into a false sense of security that results in deteriorating acid–base status. It is better to make repeated estimates of blood gas tensions, if necessary by inserting an arterial cannula, than to place undue reliance on saturation measurements in this setting. Measurements of transcutaneous oxygen and CO_2 tensions have still to find a useful place in adult practice as particular care is needed to obtain a stable and reliable signal. These devices require a biological calibration for each individual and tend to record CO_2 tensions, which are higher than the true arterial values although this can be allowed for. Since they operate at temperatures higher than 37°C there is always the risk of thermal injury if they are used for prolonged periods.

ACID–BASE STATUS

Arterial pH and bicarbonate measurements are normally reported at the same time as gas tensions and provide complementary information. Unfortunately acid–base physiology generates confusion easily but this has been lucidly reviewed in several texts.[151,152] A major problem is the logarithmic nature of the pH scale and most people (including ourselves) find the negative logarithm to the base 10 of the hydrogen ion concentration a difficult concept with which to grapple. It is much easier to think in terms of the modified Henderson equation:

$$\left[H^+\right] = k \times \frac{Pco_2}{HCO_3}$$

where H^+ is the concentration of hydrogen ions, k is a constant, HCO_3 bicarbonate concentration and Pco_2 is arterial CO_2 tensions.

Thus increases in CO_2 tension, which are usually rapid, can be compensated by renal conservation of bicarbonate, a relatively slow process. Once any two variables are known the third can be calculated. It is useful to think about, and with serial data plot out, the changes in H^+ concentration (pH) and Pco_2 on a non-logarithmic diagram (Figure 20.7). The version we use is that of Flenley[153] which incorporates data derived from carefully characterized patients with acute and chronic respiratory acidosis, the latter being compensated by increased levels of bicarbonate as well as data from patients with chronic stable metabolic acidosis and alkalosis. The position of the Pco_2/H^+ point within these boundaries indicates how much of any acid–base problems results from acute changes in CO_2 tension and how much from coexisting metabolic or chronic respiratory derangements. Many hypoxemic COPD patients have a normal pH despite their elevated $Paco_2$ due to chronic HCO_3 conservation and they lie within the chronic respiratory acidosis band. Although this is at best a semiquantitative approach it removes many of the problems found in the practical management of acid–base chemistry.

Exercise tests

Of all the more complex procedures exercise testing is the most frequently performed and potentially most informative. Several different protocols have been devised and the test chosen should be specific for the information desired. The relationship of exercise to respiratory muscle function and gas exchange have already been considered and the topic reviewed in detail in Chapter 18.

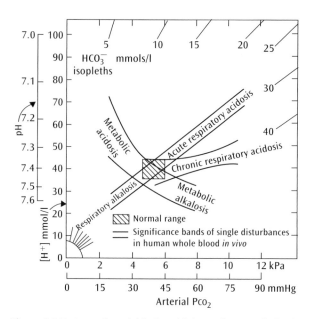

Figure 20.7 *A non-logarithimic acid–base diagram derived from the measured acid–base status of patients within the five abnormal bands illustrated and of normal subjects (hatched box). This plot of CO_2 tension against hydrogen ion concentration (pH) allows the likely acid–base disturbance calculated and the carbonate value (obtained from the relevant isopleth) to be rapidly determined whilst changes during treatment can be plotted serially for each patient. (Adapted from ref. 153.)*

Three forms of exercise testing are available and they are complementary rather than competitive in nature.

PROGRESSIVE SYMPTOM-LIMITED EXERCISE

Although the protocol employed, particularly the rate of workload increase, varies between laboratories and some investigators use treadmill rather than cycle ergometry, the overall objective is to assess cardiorespiratory performance as workload is increased in a steady ramp-like fashion. The patient is encouraged to maintain the exercise until symptoms terminate the test and symptom scoring of breathlessness during the test provides useful information along with the more conventional metabolic ventilatory and cardiac variables (Table 20.6). A number of criteria for defining a maximum test are available, the most commonly applied being a heart rate in excess of 85% predicted or ventilation greater than 90% predicted. Conventional oxygen desaturation criteria are hard to apply in patients who are already hypoxemic and particular caution is needed in interpreting end-tidal gas tensions in COPD patients. We have found that simultaneous automatic monitoring of ECG for ST segment depression and blood pressure to ensure an appropriate cardiovascular response greatly increases the usefulness of the test protocol.

At present data from cycle ergometry are largely of diagnostic rather than therapeutic or prognostic value.

Table 20.6 *Variables measured during cycle ergometry*

Term	Recording	COPD	Comment
Work (W)	Measured in watt or k pond meters per minute	Reduced	A common denominator in exercise tests, related to aerobic work capacity
Oxygen consumption ($\dot{V}O_2$) (ml/min)	Calculated from mixed expired oxygen content – needs correction if FIO_2 increased	Reduced	A common denominator of exercise capacity linearly related to ventilation below the anerobic threshold. $\dot{V}O_{2max}$ is recorded at the maximum workload achieved
Carbon dioxide production ($\dot{V}CO_2$) (ml/min)	Calculated from mixed expired CO_2 tension	Reduced	Related to ventilation at all workloads
Heart rate (beats/min)	Usually from chest leads of ECG	Normal for the $\dot{V}O_2$ achieved unless coexisting cardiac problem	Useful to monitor 12-lead ECG during exercise to detect occult cardiac ischemia
Oxygen pulse (ml/beat)	Amount of O_2 extracted per heartbeat	Usually normal	A surrogate for stroke volume provided SaO_2 normal
Minute ventilation ($\dot{V}E$) (L/min)	Usually expired ventilation ($\dot{V}E$) – may be measured cumulatively or averaged from 'instantaneous minute ventilation' of each breath	Reduced, often substantially	Often related to predicted values based on $FEV_1 \times 35$ – this does not allow for effects of $PImax$ (see text)
Tidal volume (V_T)	Volume of each breath – may be measured by pneumotachygraph or turbine spirometer	Normal or reduced	Rapid shallow breathing is common and may increase deadspace/tidal volume ratio
Respiratory frequency (f)	Derived from the timed ventilation	Often increased	Rapid shallow breathing is common and may increase deadspace/tidal volume ratio
Ventilatory equivalent ($\dot{V}E/\dot{V}O_2$)	Derived from ventilation $\dot{V}O_2$ at a specified level of ventilation or at $\dot{V}E_{max}$	Increased due to ventilation of high V/Q units	Values of 40 are seen – normal up to 30
Oxygen saturation (SaO_2)	Assessed non-invasively by pulse oximetry	Usually falls rapidly with exercise but some hypoxemic patients may maintain or increase SaO_2 with exercise	Cycle ergometry underestimates desaturation as compared to treadmill exercise. A hidden cause of polycythemia
Breathlessness	Assessed by visual analogue or Borg scales	Increased at every level of ventilation. Significant intersubject variability	Less reproducible in exercise than during CO_2 rebreathing. Limits exercise in 40% of cases

Results have good between-day reproducibility[154] and are invaluable in trying to determine how much functional limitation is due to coexisting cardiac or psychologic factors. Typical examples of the different types of test are given in Figure 20.8.

EXTERNALLY PACED WALKING TESTS

This type of test was developed as a simple 'field' test of maximum exercise capacity and involves the patients completing a 5-meter shuttle in response to a taped auditory prompt. The time between prompts is progressively reduced requiring the patient to walk more quickly until they are unable to continue. The heart rate and oxygen saturation can be measured during testing to confirm that the patient is not limited by cardiac disease or exercise desaturation. These tests relate well to maximum exercise capacity measured on a cycle ergometer,[155] are reproducible[156] and are responsive to treatments like

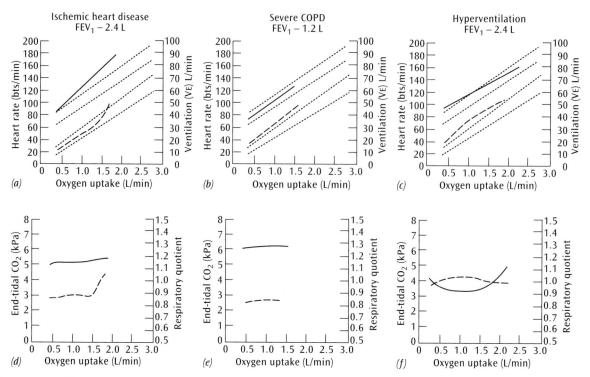

Figure 20.8 *Different responses to exercise in three different clinical situations. Solid lines refer to the left axis, dashed lines to the right. Dotted lines in upper panels refer to normal range for heart rate response (upper values) and ventilatory response (lower values) to exercise. In myocardial dysfunction (a, d), the heart rate is increased at each workload to compensate for its inability to increase stroke volume (lower O_2 pulse). The ECG showed ST segment depression of 2.1 mm at the end of the test which was terminated because the patient noted chest pain and maximum predicted heart rate was reached. Anaerobic threshold occurs early at a workload less than 70% predicted maximum. Arterial oxygen desaturation occurs above the anaerobic threshold as the vascular system fails to deliver enough oxygen to satisfy the demands of the skeletal musculature. Ventilatory responses at each workload are entirely normal.*

In COPD (b, e), the cardiac function may be entirely normal, but the minute ventilation ($\dot{V}E$) is disproportionately high at each workload. The test finished because of breathlessness at which point the patient was breathing at 51 L/min which is 123% of his predicted maximum ventilation (from $35 \times FEV_1$). The ventilatory equivalent is high reflecting the increased physiologic deadspace and the tidal volume never rises above 1.1 L reflecting the low resting FEV_1. Despite the increased ventilation at each workload the $Petco_2$ remains normal with a tendency to rise as the test progresses, indicating a relative alveolar hypoventilation, resulting in mild progressive oxygen desaturation. The RQ remains less than unity since the man fails to reach an anaerobic threshold.

In (c) and (f) are the results of a 55-year-old man who presented with breathlessness on 'any' exercise and chest tightness – sometimes at rest. The cardiac responses are normal. Ventilation (particularly respiratory frequency) increases rapidly as exercise commences, the ventilatory equivalent is high, the end-tidal CO_2 falls and the RQ is artificially high. As exercise progresses the relative alveolar hyperventilation becomes less marked. The patient reached 84% of his predicted maximum $\dot{V}o_2$ and stopped because of lightheadedness and tired legs. The ability to exercise to an acceptable workload without cardiac or respiratory limitation and without desaturation suggests that this man's problem is not cardiorespiratory structural damage but an inappropriate pattern of breathing.

pulmonary rehabilitation and bronchodilators.[156,157] They appear less sensitive to the number of trial attempts and self-paced tests (see below), although a warm up or initial test period is probably useful.

SELF-PACED EXERCISE TESTS

These are simple to perform and can yield information about more sustained exercise performance which itself may be more relevant to everyday life. Here the patient determines the intensity of exercise rather than having it imposed externally. McGavin and colleagues[158] advocated a 12-minute test in which patients were instructed to walk as far as they could along a measured distance in a hospital corridor. Stops were permitted if necessary, instructions to patients were standardized and the result recorded as the total distance in meters. The test was reasonably reproducible (coefficient of variation 8%)[159] but others have subsequently showed that a 6-minute walk is as reproducible and easier to perform.[160] Attempts to shorten this to 2 minutes have led to a loss of reproducibility.[161]

Apart from the lack of metabolic data there are two important limitations to these tests. Firstly, there is an effect of familiarization such that after the first one or two walks the patients will perform consistently better. One paper has suggested that as many as four walks on successive days are needed before a plateau is reached[161] but the protocol adopted was atypical and others have not found any significant change once two practice walks have been performed.[119] Secondly, the test is only applicable to patients with moderate to severe COPD (i.e. FEV_1 of less than 1.5 L), as milder patients would not be sufficiently stressed by walking and tend to plateau at around 600 meters in 6 minutes. There is a crude relationship between FEV_1 and walking distance[158,162] but if a more restricted population, for example FEV_1 less than 1 liter, is studied this disappears and other factors including the level of breathlessness,[163] severity of hyperinflation[164] and patient motivation[30] become dominant. Oxygen desaturation occurs frequently during corridor walking[165] and some have related this exercise-induced desaturation to the DLCO.[166] Walking distance also predicts survival, at least in patients who have undergone pulmonary rehabilitation,[167] and is responsive to interventions like bronchodilator drugs, rehabilitation and lung volume reduction surgery.[119,168,169]

Walking tests are a useful way of monitoring progress in a rehabilitation program. However, it is not clear whether practice walks are needed on every occasion once the patient has been familiarized with the test.

ENDURANCE EXERCISE TESTS

There is renewed interest in this type of exercise testing as it appears to be more sensitive to treatment interventions like oxygen[170] and bronchodilators[131] and is more likely to mimic the activities patients undertake themselves. If cycle or treadmill ergometry is used then setting the workload at 70% of peak oxygen consumption is useful in less disabled patients, though 50% is often more appropriate in severe disease where the anerobic threshold is reached much sooner.[171] Shuttle walking tests have been successfully adapted to an endurance format based on the walking speed when the heart rate reaches 70% of the peak value during a preliminary incremental test.[172] Again, this may be a useful monitor for treatment interventions.

Other complex tests

These involve more equipment, are more time consuming, may be more invasive and are needed to answer specific subsidiary questions rather than being part of the routine patient evaluation.

MEASUREMENT OF ESOPHAGEAL AND GASTRIC PRESSURE

This is readily done by swallowing an esophageal balloon catheter and is needed if the volume/pressure curve is to be measured and static lung compliance calculated. Catheter positioning and its response characteristics affect these results, as does the amount of esophageal pressure artefact, a common feature when the patient is supine. If a gastric balloon is also swallowed, the transdiaphragmatic pressure can be calculated by subtraction and this can be useful if symptoms are disproportionate to spirometric testing. Values for maximum transdiaphragmatic pressures vary with the technique employed,[173] especially the amount of abdominal activation.[174] Diaphragm function can be more simply assessed using the unoccluded sniff method, normal ranges for which are available.[175] The usefulness of electrical and magnetic nerve stimulation in assessing respiratory muscle function is considered in Chapter 16.

PULMONARY ARTERY CATHETERIZATION

This is used in the ITU to assess gas exchange, the degree of pulmonary hypertension and possibly the adequacy of left ventricular function as indicated by the wedge pressure (see Chapter 17). Although popular as a research tool in the investigation of the pulmonary vascular consequences of chronic hypoxemia and initially advocated as a guide to prognosis in long-term oxygen treatment,[176,177] more recent data suggest that acute trials of oxygen in chronically hypoxic COPD patients are of little value in predicting the long-term pulmonary vascular response or mortality experience.[178]

SLEEP STUDIES

As noted elsewhere there is no role at present for full polysomnography in the assessment of the typical COPD patients even if hypoxemic by day (see Chapter 19). Overnight oximetry is a useful way of assessing the adequacy of supplementary oxygen therapy but there is no data to show that this refinement improves the prognosis of these patients.

ASSESSMENTS OF OVERALL FUNCTION – HEALTH STATUS

This topic is discussed in detail in Chapter 31. There is a clearly a need to develop a readily administered and interpreted test that reliably evaluates health status in COPD. Present questionnaires are time consuming and only suited to research applications. Indeed the relationship of individual changes in health status as a marker of improvement is not well developed as current data address the effect of therapy on the notional average patient rather than the more complex issues involved in individual interpretation.

In COPD here is a good relationship between the MRC dyspnea grade and the total St George's score[32] and this remains the easiest assessment to make in practice.

Other non-physiological assessments

A range of other investigations can give useful additional information in COPD and are readily available.

Hematology

The important abnormality here is polycythemia. Since the advent of oxygen concentrators that can supply continuous oxygen sufficient to alleviate most of the nocturnal hypoxia, this has become a relatively rare complication of COPD.

It should be suspected when the hematocrit is elevated (greater than 52% in men, 47% in women) and/or the hemoglobin is raised (greater than 18 g/dl in men, 16 g/dl in women). However, some caution is needed since these values represent the combined effects of increases in red cell mass and plasma volume. Although changes in the latter parallel the former, plasma volume can be reduced by diuretics, dehydration and cigarette smoking thereby producing spurious polycythemia (Figure 20.9). Although desirable, routine measurement of red cell mass by radioisotopes is difficult and most treatment is guided by the simple indirect measurements. Red cell mass can be elevated as part of a myeloproliferative disorder or more commonly due to chronic hypoxia with or without cigarette smoking. Smoker's polycythemia was recognized by Smith and Landaw who described elevated red cell masses in 12 of 22 heavy smokers.[179] Variations in red cell mass were well correlated with mean carboxyhaemoglobin exposure in a large group of hypoxic COPD patents,[180] and along with chronic hypoxia, smoking was thought to explain the polycythemia via its effects on oxygen delivery to the kidney. Other important stimuli to polycythemia include nocturnal desaturation[181] and exercise,[166] which can add substantially to the overall hypoxic stimulus during the day. By contrast, intercurrent infection depresses red cell production. Given the many factors, which influence tissue oxygen delivery, it is not surprising that the relationship between polycythemia and chronic hypoxemia is a complex one.[182]

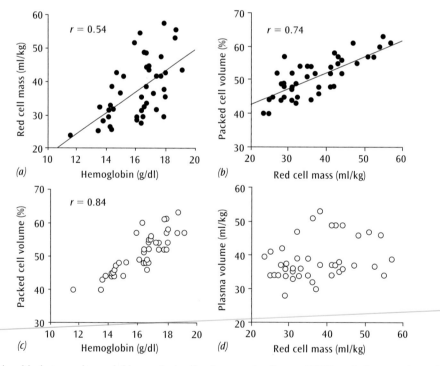

Figure 20.9 *Relationship between hemoglobin, packed cell volume, red cell mass (RCM) and plasma volume (PV) (measured radio-isotopically) in 43 patients with stable hypoxemic COPD (mean FEV$_1$ 0.92 L, Pao$_2$ less than 7.5 kPa). Although there is a relationship between hemoglobin and red cell mass (a) this is relatively weak and individuals with hemoglobin of 18 g/dl may have a normal to greatly increased RCM. Packed cell volume is a better guide, values of 50% or more indicating significant polycythemia (b). The variability of PCV and hemoglobin increases as hemoglobin rises (c). The discrepancy between RCM and hemoglobin is due to the variation in plasma volume which is unrelated to RCM and reflects other changes, e.g. diuretic therapy. Thus clinical decisions on venesection should be based on PCV, not hemoglobin, when no RCM data are available.*

Identifying polycythemia is important as increased blood viscosity predisposes to vascular events and there is some evidence that venesection improves exercise performance.[183,184] The best method for venesection is uncertain as is the time course of any resulting benefit. While erythropheresis and plasma replacement is elegant and safe,[185] most clinicians rely on the removal of the occasional unit of blood and its replacement with Dextran to try and limit rebound hyperviscocity. Generally this process is repeated over several days until the hematocrit falls below 60% although there are no data to support the choice of this particular level.

Other hematological changes are worth noting. Chronically hypoxemic patients often have raised MCV values. This cannot be accounted for by vitamin deficiencies or alcohol excess. Eosinophilia may be a marker of a potential response to oral corticosteroids, although this is an extremely infrequent finding in our hands. Nonetheless, patients with evidence of eosinophilia appear to follow a more benign course.[186] Finally there is evidence of enhanced platelet activity in hypoxemic COPD with a reduced survival time and increase in plasma and beta thromboglobulin.[187,188] The relevance of these changes to subsequent pulmonary and systemic vascular disease is presently obscure.

BIOCHEMISTRY

Hypoxemic COPD patients have reduced water clearance and an activate renin–angiotensin system (see Chapter 17). Moreover they receive diuretics to control peripheral edema and so reductions in serum sodium and potassium are relatively common. Whether chronic beta-agonist therapy produces sustained hypokalemia is more doubtful (see Chapter 24). Hypophosphatemia has been reported in 17% of COPD patients compared with 5% of non-respiratory patients,[189] presumably reflecting malnutrition and the effects of respiratory acidosis. This can have clinically important effects, at least in the ITU, as low phosphate impairs respiratory muscle function and prolongs ventilatory weaning.[190]

ALPHA-1-ANTITRYPSIN

This is discussed in full elsewhere (see Chapter 9).

ECG

The ECG is abnormal in up to 75% of advanced COPD patients (see Chapter 17) but the significance of these changes either for diagnosis or prognosis is dubious. Most of these reflect changes in cardiac configuration secondary to hyperinflation. Changes in the P wave are a better guide to right ventricular overload and are the most reliable pointer to increase in right ventricular mass, being abnormal in 50% of our cor pulmonale patients.[191] However, other abnormalities suggestive of cor pulmonale are disappointingly insensitive. These criteria were developed largely in patients with congenital heart disease and do not take account of the coexisting problems of hyperinflation in COPD.

DIFFERENTIAL DIAGNOSIS

Several other illnesses can be confused with or exist alongside COPD and their differential diagnosis is not always easy.

Heart failure

Many patients have pulmonary edema due to left ventricular dysfunction as well as chronic airways disease and the relative roles of each pathology may need cycle ergometry and echocardiography to resolve. However, the presence of dyspnea and angina does not mean that the latter causes the former and evidence of radiographic pulmonary edema or symptoms disproportionate to lung function should be sought before 'cardiac failure' is diagnosed. Peripheral edema and an elevated jugular venous pressure are not necessarily due to biventricular disease as previously noted.

Mitral valve disease

Abnormal spirometry has long been recognized in severe mitral stenosis. There is evidence of mild airflow limitation in some cases[192] but reductions in vital capacity and increases in residual volume are more frequent[192] and related to disease severity.[193] The signs of valvular heart disease may be difficult to elicit in an overinflated chest and echocardiography will be needed when the clinical suspicion is high.

Bronchiectasis

Less acute presentations are usually resolved by a mixture of investigations and clinical assessment. Bronchiectasis can be associated with progressively declining lung function, although this is far from universal. Large volumes of purulent sputum with or without a predisposing factor, for example past tuberculosis, cystic fibrosis, together with CT scanning makes this differential diagnosis relatively straightforward.

Bronchiolitis

This is a more taxing differential that can be very nonspecific in its presentation. Progressive airways obstruction especially in a relatively young person with a history of toxic fume exposure should always raise the possibility of this diagnosis. It has been reported in patients with rheumatoid arthritis and should always be considered when COPD develops without reason – as in a none or very light smoker. Imaging can be helpful with hypodense areas on an expiratory HRCT scan supporting the diagnosis as these reflect areas of local air trapping. Of more local interest are the unusual problems of panbronchiolitis, which have been described in Japan and are associated with a distinctive pathology and progressive airflow limitation.[194]

Asthma

The commonest and in may ways most difficult differential is that of bronchial asthma. As noted in Chapter 1 it can be very difficult and there is obviously an overlap between the features of asthma, bronchitis and emphysema, particularly when bronchial re-modeling has occurred in chronic asthma. Endobronchial biopsy data is probably the best solution but at present is still too experimental a technique for clinical purposes. One promising technique is the measurement of exhaled nitric oxide. This is elevated in bronchial asthma[195] but normal or low in COPD due to its conversion to peroxynitrite.[196] One group has reported that patients with high exhaled NO are more likely to respond to inhaled corticosteroids, a finding in keeping with a more 'asthmatic' pattern of response.[197] Irrespective of the diagnostic label this may prove useful but care is needed with the measurement which must be made in a standardized fashion if it is to be clinically helpful. The final terminology applied to the patient with chronic airflow obstruction will often depend upon an arbitrary decision about how large changes in FEV_1 after bronchodilator testing is really required to make the diagnosis of asthma.

Ultimately it is more important that the patients receive the correct treatment rather than the diagnostic label being modified to fit clinical preconceptions.

GENERAL ASSESSMENT OF COPD

This will always involve as detailed a history and clinical examination as the patient's condition permits. Most patients need at least one chest radiograph and ECG, full blood count and clinical chemistry but the selection of further investigations will vary with the clinical setting. The single most useful diagnostic test remains spirometry to first confirm that obstruction is present and second to demonstrate the severity of the disease. In patients with mild impairment and few symptoms, no further investigation may be required.

In the more severe but still ambulatory patients, as well as spirometry, preferably accompanied by a flow–volume loop, to confirm the diagnosis and assess severity, the measurement of lung volumes and DLCO is often helpful. There is a temptation to use pulse oximetry to identify the persistently hypoxemic patient but blood gas tensions are much more informative. This test is usually reserved for those patients with an $FEV_1 < 1.0$ L or with evidence of cyanosis. Nebulized bronchodilator testing with a combination of beta-agonists and anticholinergics is helpful in establishing the maximum bronchodilatation that can be achieved and relating subsequent therapy to this whilst those patients showing the largest absolute increase in FEV_1 are the ones in which some form of corticosteroid trial can be expected to yield benefits.

In general, corticosteroid trials are only worthwhile in patients with atypical features, for example low cigarette consumption, high DLCO and/or an unexpectedly large response to bronchodilator drugs which would normally be greater than 400 ml above baseline.

In the acute exacerbation requiring hospitalization, arterial blood gas tensions are probably the single most useful guide to severity. Acidosis, especially with a raised PCO2, requires active support. Once controlled then measurement of the arterial blood gases (with and without supplementary oxygen) gives the most useful and reliable guide to severity and prognosis. It is always worth trying to record baseline spirometry and repeating this as the patient's condition improves, while the patient is in hospital but more detailed assessment can usually be reserved for later outpatient clinic visits.

REFERENCES

1. Fletcher C, Peto R. The natural history of chronic airway obstruction. Br Med J 1977;**1**:1645–8.
2. Peto R, Speizer FE, Cochrane AL, et al. The relevance in adults of air-flow obstruction, but not of mucus hypersecretion, to mortality from chronic lung disease. Results from 20 years of prospective observation. Am Rev Respir Dis 1983;**128**:491–500.
3. Lofdahl CG, Postma DS, Laitinen LA, Ohlsson SV, Pauwels RA, Pride NB. The European Respiratory Society study on chronic obstructive pulmonary disease (EUROSCOP): recruitment methods and strategies. Respir Med 1998;**92**:467–72.
4. Anthonisen NR, Connett JE, Kiley JP, et al. Effects of smoking intervention and the use of an inhaled anticholinergic bronchodilator on the rate of decline of FEV_1. The Lung Health Study. JAMA 1994;**272**:1497–505.
5. Burrows B, Niden AH, Barclay WR, Kasik JE. Chronic obstructive lung disease II. Relationship of clinical and physiological findings to the severity of airway obstruction. Am Rev Respir Dis 1965;**91**:665–78.
6. Madison JM, Irwin RS. Chronic obstructive pulmonary disease. Lancet 1998;**352**:467–73.
7. CIBA Guest Symposium report. Terminology, definitions and classification of chronic pulmonary emphysema and related conditions. Thorax 1959;**14**:286–99.
8. Medical Research Council Committee on Research into Chronic Bronchitis. Instructions for the Use of the Questionnaire on Respiratory Symptoms. 1966. WJ Holman, Devon, UK.

9. Morgan WK. Bronchitis, airways obstruction and occupation. In: WR Parkes, ed. *Occupational Lung Disorders*. Butterworth-Heinemann, Oxford, 1993, pp 238–52.

10. Kerstjens HA, Brand PL, Postma DS. Risk factors for accelerated decline among patients with chronic obstructive pulmonary disease. *Am J Respir Crit Care Med* 1996;**154**: S266–72.

11. Vestbo J, Prescott E, Lange P. Association of chronic mucus hypersecretion with FEV_1 decline and chronic obstructive pulmonary disease morbidity. Copenhagen City Heart Study Group. *Am J Respir Crit Care Med* 1996;**153**:1530–5.

12. Brinkman GL, Block DL, Cress C. Effects of bronchitis and occupation on pulmonary ventilation over an 11-year period. *J Occup Med* 1972;**14**:615–20.

13. Jamal K, Cooney TP, Fleetham JA, Thurlbeck WM. Chronic bronchitis. Correlation of morphologic findings to sputum production and flow rates. *Am Rev Respir Dis* 1984;**129**: 719–22.

14. Pauwels RA, Buist AS, Calverley PMA, Jenkins CR, Hurd SS. Global strategy for the diagnosis,management and prevention of chronic obstructive pulmonary disease. *Am J Respir Crit Care Med* 2001;**163**:1256–76.

15. Fuller RW, Jackson DM. Physiology and treatment of cough. *Thorax* 1990;**45**:425–30.

16. Choudry NB, Fuller RW, Pride NB. Sensitivity of the human cough reflex: effect of inflammatory mediators prostaglandin E2, bradykinin, and histamine. *Am Rev Respir Dis* 1989;**140**: 137–41.

17. Doherty MJ, Mister R, Pearson MG, Calverley PM. Capsaicin responsiveness and cough in asthma and chronic obstructive pulmonary disease. *Thorax* 2000;**55**:643–9.

18. Goodman RM, Yergin BM, Landa JF, Golivanux MH, Sackner MA. Relationship of smoking history and pulmonary function tests to tracheal mucous velocity in nonsmokers, young smokers, ex-smokers, and patients with chronic bronchitis. *Am Rev Respir Dis* 1978;**117**:205–14.

19. Puchelle E, Zahm JM, Girard F, *et al*. Mucociliary transport *in vivo* and *in vitro*. Relations to sputum properties in chronic bronchitis. *Eur J Respir Dis* 1980;**61**:254–64.

20. Loudon RG, Brown LC. Cough frequency in patients with respiratory disease. *Am Rev Respir Dis* 1967;**96**:1137–43.

21. Power JT, Stewart IC, Connaughton JJ, *et al*. Nocturnal cough in patients with chronic bronchitis and emphysema. *Am Rev Respir Dis* 1984;**130**:999–1001.

22. Stockley RA, Bayley D, Hill SL, Hill AT, Crooks S, Campbell EJ. Assessment of airway neutrophils by sputum colour: correlation with airways inflammation. *Thorax* 2001;**56**:366–72.

23. Aaronson DW, Rovner RN, Patterson R. Cough syncope: case presentation and review. *J Allergy* 1970;**46**:359–63.

24. Irwin RS, Madison JM. The diagnosis and treatment of cough. *N Engl J Med* 2000;**343**:1715–21.

25. Rodenstein DO, Francis C, Stanescu DC. Emotional laryngeal wheezing:a new syndrome. *Am Rev Respir Dis* 1983;**127**: 354–6.

26. Anthonisen NR, Wright EC. Bronchodilator response in chronic obstructive pulmonary disease. *Am Rev Respir Dis* 1986;**133**:814–19.

27. Gottfried SB, Altose MD, Kelsen SG, Cherniack NS. Perception of changes in airflow resistance in obstructive pulmonary disorders. *Am Rev Respir Dis* 1981;**124**:566–70.

28. American Medical Association. *The Respiratory System. Guides to the Evaluation of Permanent Impairment*. Chicago, 1984, pp 85–107.

29. Wolkove N, Dajczman E, Colacone A, Kreisman H. The relationship between pulmonary function and dyspnea in obstructive lung disease. *Chest* 1989;**96**:1247–51.

30. Morgan AD, Peck DF, Buchanan DR, McHardy GJ. Effect of attitudes and beliefs on exercise tolerance in chronic bronchitis. *Br Med J* 1983;**286**:171–3.

31. Morgan WK. Disability or disinclination? Impairment or importuning? *Chest* 1979;**75**:712–15.

32. Bestall JC, Paul EA, Garrod R, Garnham R, Jones PW, Wedzicha JA. Usefulness of the Medical Research Council (MRC) dyspnoea scale as a measure of disability in patients with chronic obstructive pulmonary disease. *Thorax* 1999;**54**:581–6.

33. Mahler DA, Weinberg DH, Wells CK, Feinstein AR. The measurement of dyspnea. Contents, interobserver agreement, and physiologic correlates of two new clinical indexes. *Chest* 1984;**85**:751–8.

34. Druz WS, Sharp JT. Electrical and mechanical activity of the diaphragm accompanying body position in severe chronic obstructive pulmonary disease. *Am Rev Respir Dis* 1982; **125**:275–80.

35. Sharp JT, Drutz WS, Moisan T, Foster J, Machnach W. Postural relief of dyspnea in severe chronic obstructive pulmonary disease. *Am Rev Respir Dis* 1980;**122**:201–11.

36. David P, Denis P, Nouvet G, Pasquis P, Lefrancois R, Morere P. Lung function and gastroesophageal reflux during chronic bronchitis. *Bull Eur Physiopathol Respir* 1982;**18**:81–6.

37. Pellegrino R, Brusasco V. Lung hyperinflation and flow limitation in chronic airway obstruction. *Eur Respir J* 1997;**10**:543–9.

38. Berquist WE, Rachelefsky GS, Kadden M, *et al*. Effect of theophylline on gastroesophageal reflux in normal adults. *J Allergy Clin Immunol* 1981;**67**:407–11.

39. Roberts CM, Lowe D, Bucknall CE, Ryland I, Kelly Y, Pearson MG. Clinical audit indicators of outcome following admission to hospital with acute exacerbation of chronic obstructive pulmonary disease. *Thorax* 2002;**57**:137–41.

40. Poole G, Stradling P. Routine radiography for haemoptysis. *Br Med J* 1964;**1**:341–2.

41. Schols AM, Slangen J, Volovics L, Wouters EF. Weight loss is a reversible factor in the prognosis of chronic obstructive pulmonary disease. *Am J Respir Crit Care Med* 1998;**157**: 1791–7.

42. Baarends EM, Schols AM, Westerterp KR, Wouters EF. Total daily energy expenditure relative to resting energy expenditure in clinically stable patients with COPD. *Thorax* 1997;**52**:780–5.

43. Schols AM, Buurman WA, Staal van den Brekel AJ, Dentener MA, Wouters EF. Evidence for a relation between metabolic derangements and increased levels of inflammatory mediators in a subgroup of patients with chronic obstructive pulmonary disease. *Thorax* 1996;**51**:819–24.

44. Grant I, Heaton RK, McSweeny AJ, Adams KM, Timms RM. Neuropsychologic findings in hypoxemic chronic obstructive pulmonary disease. *Arch Intern Med* 1982;**142**: 1470–6.

45. McSweeny AJ, Grant I, Heaton RK, Adams KM, Timms RM. Life quality of patients with chronic obstructive pulmonary disease. *Arch Intern Med* 1982;**142**:473–8.

46. Calverley PM. Neuropsychological deficits in chronic obstructive pulmonary disease. *Monaldi Arch Chest Dis* 1996;**51**:5–6.

47. Calverley PM, Brezinova V, Douglas NJ, Catterall JR, Flenley DC. The effect of oxygenation on sleep quality in chronic bronchitis and emphysema. *Am Rev Respir Dis* 1982;**126**:206–10.

48. Incalzi RA, Chiappini F, Fuso L, Torrice MP, Gemma A, Pistelli R. Predicting cognitive decline in patients with hypoxaemic COPD. *Respir Med* 1998;**92**:527–33.

49. Burrows B, Knudson RJ, Cline MG, Lebowitz MD. Quantitative relationships between cigarette smoking and ventilatory function. *Am Rev Respir Dis* 1977;**115**:195–205.

50. Petty TL, Ryan SF, Mitchell RS. Cigarette smoking and the lungs. Relation to postmortem evidence of emphysema, chronic bronchitis, and black lung pigmentation. *Arch Environ Health* 1967;**14**:172–7.

51. Silverman EK, Chapman HA, Drazen JM, *et al.* Genetic epidemiology of severe, early-onset chronic obstructive pulmonary disease. Risk to relatives for airflow obstruction and chronic bronchitis. *Am J Respir Crit Care Med* 1998; **157**:1770–8.

52. McCloskey SC, Patel BD, Hinchliffe SJ, Reid ED, Wareham NJ, Lomas DA. Siblings of patients with severe chronic obstructive pulmonary disease have a significant risk of airflow obstruction. *Am J Respir Crit Care Med* 2001;**164**:1419–24.

53. Pandey MR, Regmi HN, Neupane RP, Gautam A, Bhandari DP. Domestic smoke pollution and respiratory function in rural Nepal. *Tokai J Exp Clin Med* 1985;**10**:471–81.

54. Pandey MR. Prevalence of chronic bronchitis in a rural community of the Hill Region of Nepal. *Thorax* 1984; **39**:331–6.

55. Love RG, Miller BG. Longitudinal study of lung function in coal-miners. *Thorax* 1982;**37**:193–7.

56. Newman-Taylor A, Coggon D. Industrial injuries benefits for coal miners with obstructive lung disease. *Thorax* 1999;**54**:282.

57. Ingram RH Jr, Schilder DP. Effect of pursed lips expiration on the pulmonary pressure–flow relationship in obstructive lung disease. *Am Rev Respir Dis* 1967;**96**:381–8.

58. Tiep BL, Burns M, Kas D, *et al.* Pursed lip breathing training using ear oximetry. *Chest* 1986;**90**:218–21.

59. Banzett RB, Topulos GP, Leith DE, Nations CS. Bracing arms increases the capacity for sustained hyperpnea. *Am Rev Respir Dis* 1988;**138**:106–9.

60. Celli BR, Rassulo J, Make BJ. Dyssynchronous breathing during arm but not leg exercise in patients with chronic airflow obstruction. *N Engl J Med* 1986;**314**:1485–90.

61. Tobin MJ, Perez W, Guenther SM, Lodato RF, Dantzker DR. Does rib cage-abdominal paradox signify respiratory muscle fatigue? *J Appl Physiol* 1987;**63**:851–60.

62. Cohen CA, Zagelbaum G, Gross D, Roussos C, Macklem PT. Clinical manifestations of inspiratory muscle fatigue. *Am J Med* 1982;**73**:308–16.

63. Loudon R, Murphy RL Jr. Lung sounds. *Am Rev Respir Dis* 1984;**130**:663–73.

64. Ploysongsang Y, Pare JA, Macklem PT. Correlation of regional breath sound with regional ventilation in emphysema. *Am Rev Respir Dis* 1982;**126**:526–9.

65. Schreur HJ, Sterk PJ, Vanderschoot J, van Klink HC, van Vollenhoven E, Dijkman JH. Lung sound intensity in patients with emphysema and in normal subjects at standardised airflows. *Thorax* 1992;**47**:674–9.

66. Marini JJ, Pierson DJ, Hudson LD, Lakshminarayan S. The significance of wheezing in chronic airflow obstruction. *Am Rev Respir Dis* 1979;**120**:1069–72.

67. Badgett RG, Tanaka DJ, Hunt DK, *et al.* Can moderate chronic obstructive pulmonary disease be diagnosed by historical and physical findings alone? *Am J Med* 1993;**94**:188–96.

68. Bohadana AB, Peslin R, Uffholtz H. Breath sounds in the clinical assessment of airflow obstruction. *Thorax* 1978;**33**:345–51.

69. Wardman AG, Binns V, Clayden AD, Cooke NJ. The diagnosis and treatment of adults with obstructive airways disease in general practice. *Br J Dis Chest* 1986;**80**:19–26.

70. Mannino DM, Gagnon RC, Petty TL, Lydick E. Obstructive lung disease and low lung function in adults in the United States: data from the National Health and Nutrition Examination Survey, 1988–1994. *Arch Intern Med* 2000; **160**:1683–9.

71. van den Boom G, Van Schayck CP, van Mollen MP, *et al.* Active detection of chronic obstructive pulmonary disease and asthma in the general population. Results and economic consequences of the DIMCA program. *Am J Respir Crit Care Med* 1998;**158**:1730–8.

72. Zielinski J, Bednarek M. Early detection of COPD in a high-risk population using spirometric screening. *Chest* 2001; **119**:731–6.

73. Nisar M, Walshaw M, Earis JE, Pearson MG, Calverley PM. Assessment of reversibility of airway obstruction in patients with chronic obstructive airways disease. *Thorax* 1990;**45**: 190–4.

74. Rennard SI, Decramer M, Calverley PMA, *et al.* The impact of COPD in North America and Europe: the patient's perspectiver of the Confronting COPD International survey. *Eur Respir J* 2002;**20**:1–7.

75. Anthonisen NR. Prognosis in chronic obstructive pulmonary disease: results from multicenter clinical trials. *Am Rev Respir Dis* 1989;**140**:S95–9.

76. National Emphysema Treatment Trial Research Group. Patients at high risk of death after lung-volume-reduction surgery. *N Engl J Med* 2001;**345**:1075–83.

77. American Thoracic Society. Standards for the diagnosis and care of patients with chronic obstructive pulmonary disease. *Am J Respir Crit Care Med* 1995;**152**:S77–120.

78. Fletcher CM, Pride NB. Definitions of emphysema, chronic bronchitis, asthma, and airflow obstruction: 25 years on from the Ciba symposium. *Thorax* 1984;**39**:81–5.

79. Roberts CM, Ryland I, Lowe D, Kelly Y, Bucknall CE, Pearson MG. Audit of acute admissions of COPD: standards of care and management in the hospital setting. *Eur Respir J* 2001;**17**:343–9.

80. Kesten S, Chapman KR. Physician perceptions and management of COPD. *Chest* 1993;**104**:254–8.

81. Ingram RH Jr, Schilder DP. Effect of gas compression on pulmonary pressure, flow, and volume relationship. *J Appl Physiol* 1966;**21**:1821–6.

82. American Thoracic Society. ATS Statement. Snowbird Workshop on Standardization of Spirometry. *Am Rev Respir Dis* 1979;**119**:831–8.

83. Standardization of spirometry – 1987 update. Statement of the American Thoracic Society. *Am Rev Respir Dis* 1987; **136**:1285–98.

84. American Thoracic Society Lung function testing: selection of reference values and interpretative strategies. *Am Rev Respir Dis* 1991; **144**:1202–28.

85. American Thoracic Society. ATS Standardization of Spirometry 1994 Update. *Am J Respir Crit Care Med* 1994;**152**: 1107–36.

86. Quanjer PH, ed. Standardised lung function testing. *Bull Eur Physiopathol Respir* 1983;**19**(suppl):1–95.

87. Quanjer PH, Tammeling GJ, Cotes JE, Pedersen OF, Peslin R, Yernault JC. Lung volumes and forced ventilatory flows. Report of Working Party Standardization of Lung Function Tests, European Community for Steel and Coal. Official Statement of the European Respiratory Society. *Eur Respir J* 1993;**16**(suppl):5–40.

88. Krowka MJ, Enright PL, Rodarte JR, Hyatt RE. Effect of effort on measurement of forced expiratory volume in one second. *Am Rev Respir Dis* 1987;**136**:829–33.

89. Hyatt RF, Okeson GC, Rodarte JR. Influence of expiratory flow limitation on the pattern of lung emptying in man. *J Appl Physiol* 1973;**35**:411–19.

90. Stoller JK, Basheda S, Laskowski D, Goormastic M, McCarthy K. Trial of standard versus modified expiration to achieve end-of-test spirometry criteria. *Am Rev Respir Dis* 1993;**148**:275–80.

91. Enright PL, Johnson LR, Connett JE, Voelker H, Buist AS. Spirometry in the Lung Health Study. 1. Methods and quality control. *Am Rev Respir Dis* 1991;**143**:1215–23.

92. Burge PS, Calverley PM, Jones PW, Spencer S, Anderson JA, Maslen TK. Randomised, double blind, placebo controlled study of fluticasone propionate in patients with moderate to severe chronic obstructive pulmonary disease: the ISOLDE trial. *Br Med J* 2000;**320**:1297–303.

93. Swanney MP, Jensen RL, Crichton DA, Beckert LE, Cardno LA, Crapo RO. FEV_6 is an acceptable surrogate for FVC in the spirometric diagnosis of airway obstruction and restriction. *Am J Respir Crit Care Med* 2000;**162**:917–19.

94. Hankinson JL, Bang KM. Acceptability and reproducibility criteria of the American Thoracic Society as observed in a sample of the general population. *Am Rev Respir Dis* 1991;**143**:516–21.

95. Miller MR, Pincock AC. Predicted values: how should we use them? *Thorax* 1988;**43**:265–7.

96. Enright PL, Crapo RO. Controversies in the use of spirometry for early recognition and diagnosis of chronic obstructive pulmonary disease in cigarette smokers. *Clin Chest Med* 2000;**21**:645–52.

97. Dillard TA, Hnatiuk OW, McCumber TR. Maximum voluntary ventilation: spirometric determinants in chronic obstructive pulmonary disease patients and normal subjects. *Am Rev Respir Dis* 1993;**147**:870–5.

98. Spiro SG, Hahn HL, Edwards RH, Pride NB. An analysis of the physiological strain of submaximal exercise in patients with chronic obstructive bronchitis. *Thorax* 1975;**30**:415–25.

99. Detels R, Tashkin DP, Simmons MS, *et al.* The UCLA population studies of chronic obstructive respiraory disease 5. Agreement and disagreement of tests in identifying abnormal lung function. *Chest* 1982;**82**:630–5.

100. Miller MR, Dickinson SA, Hitchings DJ. The accuracy of portable peak flow meters. *Thorax* 1992;**47**:904.

101. Higgins BG, Britton JR, Chinn S, Cooper S, Burney PG, Tattersfield AE. Comparison of bronchial reactivity and peak expiratory flow variability measurements for epidemiologic studies. *Am Rev Respir Dis* 1992;**145**:588–93.

102. Higgins BG, Britton JR, Chinn S, *et al.* The distribution of peak expiratory flow variability in a population sample. *Am Rev Respir Dis* 1989;**140**:1368–72.

103. Brand PL, Quanjer PH, Postma DS, *et al.* Interpretation of bronchodilator response in patients with obstructive airways disease. The Dutch Chronic Non-Specific Lung Disease (CNSLD) Study Group. *Thorax* 1992;**47**:429–36.

104. Mitchell DM, Gildeh P, Dimond AH, Collins JV. Value of serial peak expiratory flow measurements in assessing treatment response in chronic airflow limitation. *Thorax* 1986;**41**:606–10.

105. Hansen EF, Vestbo J, Phanareth K, Kok-Jensen A, Dirksen A. Peak flow as predictor of overall mortality in asthma and chronic obstructive pulmonary disease. *Am J Respir Crit Care Med* 2001;**163**:690–3.

106. Rodenstein DO, Stanescu D. The assessment of lung volumes and measurement by helium dilution and by body plethysmography in chronic airflow limitation. *Am Rev Respir Dis* 1982;**126**:1040–4.

107. Rodenstein DO, Stanescu DC, Francis C. Demonstration of failure of body plethysmography in airway obstruction. *J Appl Physiol* 1982;**52**:949–54

108. Liistro G, Stanescu D, Rodenstein D, Veriter C. Reassessment of the interruption technique for measuring flow resistance in humans. *J Appl Physiol* 1989;**67**:933–7.

109. Pierce RJ, Brown DJ, Holmes M, Cumming G, Denison DM. Estimation of lung volumes from chest radiographs using shape information. *Thorax* 1979;**34**:726–34.

110. Spence DP, Kelly YJ, Ahmed J, Calverley PM, Pearson MG. Critical evaluation of computerised x ray planimetry for the measurement of lung volumes. *Thorax* 1995;**50**:383–6.

111. Gross NJ. Role of the parasympathetic system in airways obstruction due to emphysema. *N Engl J Med* 1984;**311**:421–5.

112. Taylor DR, Buick B, Kinney C, Lowry RC, McDevitt DG. The efficacy of orally administered theophylline, inhaled salbutamol, and a combination of the two as chronic therapy in the management of chronic bronchitis with reversible airflow obstruction. *Am Rev Respir Dis* 1985;**131**:747–51.

113. Chrystyn H, Mulley BA, Peake MD. Dose response relation to oral theophylline in severe chronic obstructive airways disease. *Br Med J* 1988;**297**:1506–10.

114. Wilson SH, Cooke NT, Edwards RH, Spiro SG. Predicted normal values for maximal respiratory pressures in caucasian adults and children. *Thorax* 1984;**39**:535–8.

115. Carroll N, Clague JE, Pollard MH, Horan MA, Edwards RH, Calverley PM. Portable maximum respiratory pressure measurement – a comparison with laboratory techniques. *J Med Engineer Technol* 1992;**16**:82–6.

116. Eliasson O, Degraff AC Jr. The use of criteria for reversibility and obstruction to define patient groups for bronchodilator trials. Influence of clinical diagnosis, spirometric, and anthropometric variables. *Am Rev Respir Dis* 1985;**132**:858–64.

117. Meslier N, Racineux JL, Six P, Lockhart A. Diagnostic value of reversibility of chronic airway obstruction to separate asthma from chronic bronchitis:a statistical approach. *Eur Respir J* 1989;**2**:497–505.

118. Tweedale PM, Alexander F, McHardy GJ. Short term variability in FEV_1 and bronchodilator responsiveness in patients with obstructive ventilatory defects. *Thorax* 1987;**42**:487–90.

119. Hay JG, Stone P, Carter J, *et al.* Bronchodilator reversibility, exercise performance and breathlessness in stable chronic obstructive pulmonary disease. *Eur Respir J* 1992;**5**:659–64.

120. Nisar M, Earis JE, Pearson MG, Calverley PM. Acute bronchodilator trials in chronic obstructive pulmonary disease. *Am Rev Respir Dis* 1992;**146**:555–9.

121. Filuk RB, Easton PA, Anthonisen NR. Responses to large doses of salbutamol and theophylline in patients with chronic obstructive pulmonary disease. *Am Rev Respir Dis* 1985;**132**:871–4.

122. Gross NJ, Petty TL, Friedman M, Skorodin MS, Silvers GW, Donohue JF. Dose response to ipratropium as a nebulized solution in patients with chronic obstructive pulmonary disease. A three-center study. *Am Rev Respir Dis* 1989;**139**:1188–91.

123. Nishimura K, Koyama H, Ikeda A, Sugiura N, Kawakatsu K, Izumi T. The additive effect of theophylline on a high-dose combination of inhaled salbutamol and ipratropium bromide in stable COPD. *Chest* 1995;**107**:718–23.

124. Van Schayck CP, Folgering H, Harbers H, Maas KL, Van Weel C. Effects of allergy and age on responses to salbutamol and ipratropium bromide in moderate asthma and chronic bronchitis. *Thorax* 1991;**46**:355–9.

125. Enright PL, Connett JE, Kanner RE, Johnson LR, Lee WW. Spirometry in the Lung Health Study: II. Determinants of short-term intraindividual variability. *Am J Respir Crit Care Med* 1995;**151**:406–11.

126. Weir DC, Robertson AS, Gove RI, Burge PS. Time course of response to oral and inhaled corticosteroids in non-asthmatic chronic airflow obstruction. *Thorax* 1990;**45**:118–21.

127. Weir DC, Gove RI, Robertson AS, Burge PS. Corticosteroid trials in non-asthmatic chronic airflow obstruction:a comparison of oral prednisolone and inhaled beclomethasone dipropionate. *Thorax* 1990;**45**:112–17.

128. Mendella LA, Manfreda J, Warren CP, Anthonisen NR. Steroid response in stable chronic obstructive pulmonary disease. *Ann Intern Med* 1982;**96**:17–21.

129. Weir DC, Gove RI, Robertson AS, Burge PS. Response to corticosteroids in chronic airflow obstruction: relationship to emphysema and airways collapse. *Eur Respir J* 1991; **4**:1185–90.

130. Burge PS, Calverley PMA, Jones PW, Spencer S, Anderson JA. Prednisolone response in chronic obstructive pulmonary disease. *Thorax* 2003 (in press).

131. O'Donnell DE, Lam M, Webb KA. Spirometric correlates of improvement in exercise performance after anticholinergic therapy in chronic obstructive pulmonary disease. *Am J Respir Crit Care Med* 1999;**160**:542–9.

132. Berger R, Smith D. Effect of inhaled metaproterenol on exercise performance in patients with stable 'fixed' airway obstruction. *Am Rev Respir Dis* 1988;**138**:624–9.

133. Corris PA, Neville E, Nariman S, Gibson GJ. Dose–response study of inhaled salbutamol powder in chronic airflow obstruction. *Thorax* 1983;**38**:292–6.

134. Spence DP, Hay JG, Carter J, Pearson MG, Calverley PM. Oxygen desaturation and breathlessness during corridor walking in chronic obstructive pulmonary disease: effect of oxitropium bromide. *Thorax* 1993;**48**:1145–50.

135. Hadcroft J, Calverley PM. Alternative methods for assessing bronchodilator reversibility in chronic obstructive pulmonary disease. *Thorax* 2001;**56**:713–20.

136. O'Donnell DE, Lam M, Webb KA. Measurement of symptoms, lung hyperinflation, and endurance during exercise in chronic obstructive pulmonary disease. *Am J Respir Crit Care Med* 1998;**158**:1557–65.

137. Postma DS, Gimeno F, van der Weele LT, Sluiter HJ. Assessment of ventilatory variables in survival prediction of patients with chronic airflow obstruction: the importance of reversibility. *Eur J Respir Dis* 1985;**67**:360–8.

138. Davies L, Nisar M, Pearson MG, Costello RW, Earis JE, Calverley PMA. Oral corticosteroid trials in the management of stable chronic obstructive pulmonary disease. *Q J Med* 1999;**92**:395–400.

139. Ogilvie CM, Forster RE, Blakemore WS, Morton JW. A standardised breathholding technique for the clinical measurement of the diffusing capacity of the lung for carbon monoxide. *J Clin Invest* 1957;**36**:1–17.

140. Mitchell MM, Renzetti AD Jr. Application of the single-breath method of total lung capacity measurement to the calculation of the carbon monoxide diffusing capacity. *Am Rev Respir Dis* 1968;**97**:581–4.

141. McLean A, Warren PM, Gillooly M, MacNee W, Lamb D. Microscopic and macroscopic measurements of emphysema: relation to carbon monoxide gas transfer. *Thorax* 1992;**47**:144–9.

142. Gould GA, MacNee W, McLean A, Warren PM, Redpath A, Best JJ, *et al.* CT measurements of lung density in life can quantitate distal airspace enlargement – an essential defining feature of human emphysema. *Am Rev Respir Dis* 1988;**137**:380–92.

143. Dubois P, Machiels J, Smeets F, Delwiche JP, Lulling J. CO transfer capacity as a determining factor of survival for severe hypoxaemic COPD patients under long-term oxygen therapy. *Eur Respir J* 1990;**3**:1042–7.

144. Anthonisen NR, Wright EC, Hodgkin JE. Prognosis in chronic obstructive pulmonary disease. *Am Rev Respir Dis* 1986; **133**:14–20.

145. Burrows B. The course and prognosis of different types of chronic airflow limitation in a general population sample from Arizona: comparison with the Chicago 'COPD' series. *Am Rev Respir Dis* 1989;**140**:S92–4.

146. Watson A, Joyce H, Hopper L, Pride NB. Influence of smoking habits on change in carbon monoxide transfer factor over 10 years in middle aged men. *Thorax* 1993;**48**:119–24.

147. Riley RL, Cournand A. 'Ideal' alveolar air and the analysis of ventilation-perfusion relationships in the lungs. *J Appl Physiol* 1949;**1**:825–47.

148. Baudouin SV, Waterhouse JC, Tahtamouni T, Smith JA, Baxter J, Howard P. Long term domiciliary oxygen treatment for chronic respiratory failure reviewed. *Thorax* 1990;**45**: 195–8.

149. Douglas NJ, Brash HM, Wraith PK, *et al.* Accuracy sensitivity to carboxyhemoglobin, and speed of response of the Hewlett-Packard 47201A ear oximeter. *Am Rev Respir Dis* 1979;**119**:311–13.

150. Roberts CM, Bugler JR, Melchor R, Hetzel MR, Spiro SG. Value of pulse oximetry in screening for long-term oxygen therapy requirement. *Eur Respir J* 1993;**6**:559–62.

151. Effros RM. Acid base balance. In: JF Murray, JA Nadel, eds. *Textbook of Respiratory Medicine.* WB Saunders, Philadelphia, 1988, pp 129–48.

152. Gibson GJ. Carbon dioxide carriage in the blood. In: GJ Gibson, ed. *Clinical Tests of Respiratory Function.* Macmillan, London, 1984, pp 87–99.

153. Flenley DC. Another non-logarithmic acid–base diagram? *Lancet* 1971;**i**:961–5.

154. Brown SE, Fischer CE, Stansbury DW, Light RW. Reproducibility of Vo_{2max} in patients with chronic air-flow obstruction. *Am Rev Respir Dis* 1985;**131**:435–8.

155. Singh SJ, Morgan MD, Scott S, Walters D, Hardman AE. Development of a shuttle walking test of disability in patients with chronic airways obstruction. *Thorax* 1992;**47**:1019–24.

156. Dyer CA, Singh SJ, Stockley RA, Sinclair AJ, Hill SL. The incremental shuttle walking test in elderly people with chronic airflow limitation. *Thorax* 2002;**57**:34–8.

157. Griffiths TL, Burr ML, Campbell IA, *et al.* Results at 1 year of out-patient multidisciplinary pulmonary rehabilitation. *Lancet* 2000;**355**:362–8.

158. McGavin CR, Gupta SP, McHardy GJ. Twelve-minute walking test for assessing disability in chronic bronchitis. *Br Med J* 1976;**1**:822–3.

159. Mungall IP, Hainsworth R. Assessment of respiratory function in patients with chronic obstructive airways disease. *Thorax* 1979;**34**:254–8.

160. Butland RJA, Gross ER, Pang J, Woodcock AA, Geddes DM. Two, six and twelve minute walking tests in respiratory diseases. *Br Med J* 1982;**284**:1607–8.

161. Knox AJ, Morrison JF, Muers MF. Reproducibility of walking test results in chronic obstructive airways disease. *Thorax* 1988;**43**:388–92.

162. Swinburn CR, Wakefield JM, Jones PW. Performance, ventilation, and oxygen consumption in three different types of exercise test in patients with chronic obstructive lung disease. *Thorax* 1985;**40**:581–6.

163. O'Donnell DE, Webb KA. Exertional breathlessness in patients with chronic airflow limitation. The role of lung hyperinflation. *Am Rev Respir Dis* 1993;**148**:1351–7.

164. O'Donnell DE, Revill SM, Webb KA. Dynamic hyperinflation and exercise intolerance in chronic obstructive pulmonary disease. *Am J Respir Crit Care Med* 2001;**164**:770–7.

165. Mak VH, Bugler JR, Roberts CM, Spiro SG. Effect of arterial oxygen desaturation on six minute walk distance, perceived effort, and perceived breathlessness in patients with airflow limitation. *Thorax* 1993;**48**:33–8.

166. Owens GR, Rogers RM, Pennock BE, Levin D. The diffusing capacity as a predictor of arterial oxygen desaturation during exercise in patients with chronic obstructive pulmonary disease. *N Engl J Med* 1984;**310**:1218–21.

167. Bowen JB, Votto JJ, Thrall RS, *et al.* Functional status and survival following pulmonary rehabilitation. *Chest* 2000;**118**:697–703.

168. Lacasse Y, Wong E, Guyatt GH, King D, Cook DJ, Goldstein RS. Meta-analysis of respiratory rehabilitation in chronic obstructive pulmonary disease. *Lancet* 1996;**348**:1115–19.

169. Geddes D, Davies M, Koyama H, *et al.* Effect of lung-volume-reduction surgery in patients with severe emphysema. *N Engl J Med* 2000;**343**:239–45.

170. O'Donnell DE, Bain DJ, Webb KA. Factors contributing to relief of exertional breathlessness during hyperoxia in chronic airflow limitation. *Am J Respir Crit Care Med* 1997;**155**:530–5.

171. Maltais F, LeBlanc P, Jobin J, *et al.* Intensity of training and physiologic adaptation in patients with chronic obstructive pulmonary disease. *Am J Respir Crit Care Med* 1997;**155**: 555–61.

172. Revill SM, Morgan MDL, Singh SJ, Williams J, Hardman AE. The endurance shuttle walk: a new field test for the assessment of endurance capacity in chronic obstructive pulmonary disease. *Thorax* 1999;**54**:213–22.

173. Laporta D, Grassino A. Assessment of transdiaphragmatic pressure in humans. *J Appl Physiol* 1985;**58**:1469–76.

174. Hillman DR, Markos J, Finucane KE. Effect of abdominal compression on maximum transdiaphragmatic pressure. *J Appl Physiol* 1990;**68**:2296–304.

175. Laroche CM, Mier AK, Moxham J, Green M. The value of sniff esophageal pressures in the assessment of global inspiratory muscle strength. *Am Rev Respir Dis* 1988;**138**:598–603.

176. Ashutosh K, Mead G, Dunsky M. Early effects of oxygen administration and prognosis in chronic obstructive pulmonary disease and cor pulmonale. *Am Rev Respir Dis* 1983;**127**:399–404.

177. Timms RM, Khaja FU, Williams GW. Hemodynamic response to oxygen therapy in chronic obstructive pulmonary disease. *Ann Intern Med* 1985;**102**:29–36.

178. Sliwinski P, Hawrylkiewicz I, Gorecka D, Zielinski J. Acute effect of oxygen on pulmonary arterial pressure does not predict survival on long-term oxygen therapy in patients with chronic obstructive pulmonary disease. *Am Rev Respir Dis* 1992;**146**:665–9.

179. Smith JR, Landaw SA. Smokers' polycythemia. *N Engl J Med* 1978;**298**:6–10.

180. Calverley PM, Leggett RJ, McElderry L, Flenley DC. Cigarette smoking and secondary polycythemia in hypoxic cor pulmonale. *Am Rev Respir Dis* 1982;**125**:507–10.

181. Wedzicha JA, Cotes PM, Empey DW, Newland AC, Royston JP, Tam RC. Serum immunoreactive erythropoietin in hypoxic lung disease with and without polycythaemia. *Clin Sci (Lond)* 1985;**69**:413–22.

182. Stradling JR, Lane DJ. Development of secondary polycythaemia in chronic airways obstruction. *Thorax* 1981;**36**:321–5.

183. Harrison BD, Davis J, Madgwick RG, Evans M. The effects of therapeutic decrease in packed cell volume on the responses to exercise of patients with polycythaemia secondary to lung disease. *Clin Sci Mol Med* 1973;**45**:833–47.

184. Chetty KG, Brown SE, Light RW. Improved exercise tolerance of the polycythemic lung patient following phlebotomy. *Am J Med* 1983;**74**:415–20.

185. Wedzicha JA, Cotter FE, Rudd RM, Apps MC, Newland AC, Empey DW. Erythropheresis compared with placebo apheresis in patients with polycythaemia secondary to hypoxic lung disease. *Eur J Respir Dis* 1984;**65**:579–85.

186. Burrows B, Bloom JW, Traver GA, Cline MG. The course and prognosis of different forms of chronic airways obstruction in a sample from the general population. *N Engl J Med* 1987;**317**:1309–14.

187. Steele P, Ellis JH Jr, Weily HS, Genton E. Platelet survival time in patients with hypoxemia and pulmonary hypertension. *Circulation* 1977;**55**:660–1.

188. Cordova C, Musca A, Violi F, Alessandri C, Perrone A, Balsano F. Platelet hyperfunction in patients with chronic airways obstruction. *Eur J Respir Dis* 1985;**66**:9–12.

189. Fisher J, Magid N, Kallman C, *et al.* Respiratory illness and hypophosphatemia. *Chest* 1983;**83**:504–8.

190. Aubier M, Murciano D, Lecocguic Y, *et al.* Effect of hypophosphatemia on diaphragmatic contractility in patients with acute respiratory failure. *N Engl J Med* 1985;**313**:420–4.

191. Calverley PM, Howatson R, Flenley DC, Lamb D. Clinicopathological correlations in cor pulmonale. *Thorax* 1992;**47**:494–8.

192. Rhodes KM, Evemy K, Nariman S, Gibson GJ. Effects of mitral valve surgery on static lung function and exercise performance. *Thorax* 1985;**40**:107–12.

193. Wood TE, McLeod P, Anthonisen NR, Macklem PT. Mechanics of breathing in mitral stenosis. *Am Rev Respir Dis* 1971;**104**:52–60.

194. Kitaichi M, Nishimura K, Izumi T. Diffuse panbronchiolitis. In: OP Sharma, ed. *Lung Disease in the Tropics.* Marcel Dekker, New York, 1991, pp 479–510.

195. Kharitonov SA, Barnes PJ. Exhaled markers of pulmonary disease. *Am J Respir Crit Care Med* 2001;**163**:1693–722 [review].

196. Maziak W, Loukides S, Culpitt S, Sullivan P, Kharitonov SA, Barnes PJ. Exhaled nitric oxide in chronic obstructive pulmonary disease. *Am J Respir Crit Care Med* 1998;**157**:998–1002.

197. Papi A, Romagnoli M, Baraldo S, *et al.* Partial reversibility of airflow limitation and increased exhaled NO and sputum eosinophilia in chronic obstructive pulmonary disease. *Am J Respir Crit Care Med* 2000;**162**:1773–7.

21

Imaging

KAREN-LISBETH DIRKSEN AND ASGER DIRKSEN

Imaging plays an important role in the assessment of patients with COPD, although the two components of the disease, chronic bronchitis and emphysema, do not lend themselves equally well to imaging. Chronic bronchitis is defined clinically as cough and mucus production, and this definition does not provide insight on the abnormalities that may be of significance for imaging.[1] However, emphysema is defined anatomically as enlargement of the airspaces distal to the terminal bronchiole, with destruction of alveolar structures which can be detected by imaging such as plain radiography and particularly by high-resolution computed tomography (HRCT).

PLAIN RADIOGRAPHIC (CHEST X-RAY) FINDINGS IN COPD

Emphysema implies loss of elastic recoil producing airway collapse and gas trapping, resulting in hyperinflation which is a useful but non-specific feature on chest X-ray (CXR), whereas loss of lung tissue and alterations in the pulmonary vasculature can only be accurately assessed by computed tomography (CT), especially with high-resolution technique (HRCT).

The plain chest film (CXR) is usually not helpful in the diagnosis of chronic bronchitis, and most patients with pure chronic bronchitis will show a normal CXR.[2] The main purpose of CXR in this condition is to exclude other diseases which may mimic chronic bronchitis and to suggest concomitant emphysema.

Chest X-ray findings in emphysema

Several early studies have compared roentgenological features of emphysema with necropsy-assessed disease.[3–9] These papers were mainly descriptive and emphasize different imaging aspects of emphysema, and a general consensus was never reached. Nevertheless, the papers contain important information. Features of hyperinflation on CXR include increase in the retrosternal space and depression of the diaphragm, i.e. location of the right hemidiaphragm at or below the anterior end of the 7th rib.[10] Nicklaus *et al.*[6] found that diaphragmatic flattening (or even concavity) in the lateral projection was the most accurate sign of overinflation (Figure 21.1). In

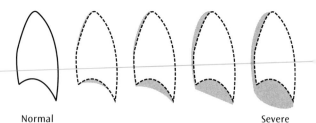

Normal   Severe

Figure 21.1 *The contour of the diaphragm on the lateral chest radiograph – from left to right changes with progressive hyperinflation. On the left the convexity of the normal diaphragm, in the middle flattening of the contour and concurrent increase in the retrosternal space, and on the right eventually concavity of the diaphragm, which is seen in very severe emphysema, only. (Adapted from ref. 140.)*

the posteroanterior view the contour of the diaphragm is more important in the diagnosis of overinflation than its position based on rib level.[5,11] However, population-based studies of imaging in COPD do not exist, which means that published frequencies and correlations must be interpreted with caution.

When a straight line is drawn from the costophrenic junction to the sternophrenic junction on the film of the lateral view, the height of the arc should be greater than 2.5 cm; measurements less than this correlate well with functionally important airflow obstruction.[12] Another useful index of this change is the presence of a 90-degree or larger sternodiaphragmatic angle. In most patients with emphysema, this junction is more readily seen than in subjects with normal chests.[13] Diaphragmatic changes are more reliable and sensitive indicators of hyperinflation than an increase in the retrosternal space, defined horizontally as greater than 2.5 cm from the posterior sternum to the most anterior margin of the ascending aorta.[7,13,14]

Alterations in the pulmonary vessel size and course were originally described by Simon,[2] and he concluded that focal or generalized oligemia or arterial depletion correlates significantly with emphysema at necropsy[14] and abnormal gas exchange,[15,16] but poorly with airflow obstruction.[10,17] Alterations in lung vessels include a reduction in the caliber and number of peripheral vessels[3] and widened branching angles with loss of side branches.[18] Emphysema has a patchy distribution, and due to compensatory engorgement the more normal areas of lung may show prominent vessels, termed 'marker vessels' by Simon,[15] and vascular marginal blurring.[19]

Although detecting alterations in lung vessels is more subjective and less reproducible than detecting overinflation, the information provided by the vascular pattern is supplementary[15] and can help in diagnosis when overinflation is not obvious.[6] Pulmonary vessels must be seen directly to evaluate subtle vascular changes, and generally increased lucency or 'transradiancy' of the lung should be disregarded because it is highly dependent on the radiographic technique. Superimposed conditions, such as the development of left heart failure, may mask emphysema by increasing the number of peripheral markings.[1,20]

On CXR bullae appear as totally avascular round or oval areas demarcated by a distinct hair-line density of lobular septae and atelectasis of surrounding lung tissue. The presence of one or more bullae on CXR cannot be considered diagnostic of emphysema, but their presence in association with other signs of emphysema usually indicates gross widespread disease and a poorer prognosis.[20]

Bullae are more commonly seen on CT, and even a large bulla may not be visible on CXR if peripheral or surrounded by normal lung parenchyma. In a study of patients referred for bullectomy, two-thirds of the patients' CT scans showed more extensive disease or bilateral disease where only unilateral was suspected from posteroanterior

and lateral chest radiographs.[21] Furthermore, CT makes it easier to distinguish between generalized emphysema, which is locally worse in the area of the suspected bulla, and well-defined bullae, which are potentially amenable to surgery.[22]

Idiopathic giant bullous emphysema, also known as vanishing lung syndrome, occurs in both smokers and non-smokers. The usual patient is a young male. The bullae are paraseptal on HRCT and occupy at least one-third of a hemithorax (Figure 21.2).[23]

Chest X-ray findings in chronic bronchitis

Most patients considered to have chronic bronchitis have a normal CXR, and the abnormalities which may be seen are usually subtle and non-specific. The term increased lung markings or 'dirty chest' refers to ill-defined linear densities in the lungs fields. In chronic bronchitis multiple minor insults from mucus plugging of small airways and repeated or chronic infection will result in scarring and minor areas of fibrosis. However, the relationship of chronic bronchitis to the 'dirty chest' is only presumptive, and knowledge of the variety of pathologic conditions that can produce the 'dirty chest' is still incomplete.[24]

Other radiographic abnormalities associated with cigarette smoking include bronchial wall thickening. Thickening of bronchial walls causes ring shadows[25] and parallel linear shadows, also known as tubular shadows or slightly tapering line shadows outside the boundaries of the pulmonary hila. However, the radiologic diagnosis of bronchial disease is more subjective and variable than that of emphysema, and an increase in the thickness of bronchial walls probably does not occur in chronic bronchitis.[1,10,20]

In COPD, destruction of the capillary bed and reflex vasoconstriction secondary to hypoxemia may cause elevation of pulmonary vascular resistance and pulmonary arterial hypertension. The principal radiographic sign of pulmonary hypertension is enlargement of central pulmonary arteries. In the posteroanterior view, the diameter of the right descending pulmonary artery should not exceed 16 mm, and the descending left pulmonary artery should not exceed 18 mm.[26] However, only a weak correlation was found between the caliber of the central arteries and the pulmonary artery pressure, and CT[27,28] and especially magnetic resonance imaging (MRI)[29,30] are probably more accurate in diagnosing pulmonary arterial hypertension.

Chest radiography plays a role in detecting other causes of worsening dyspnea in patients with chronic bronchitis such as pneumonia, pneumothorax, cancer and congestive heart failure, but the routine use of CXR in acute exacerbations of chronic bronchitis has little impact on patient management. In 242 patients hospitalized

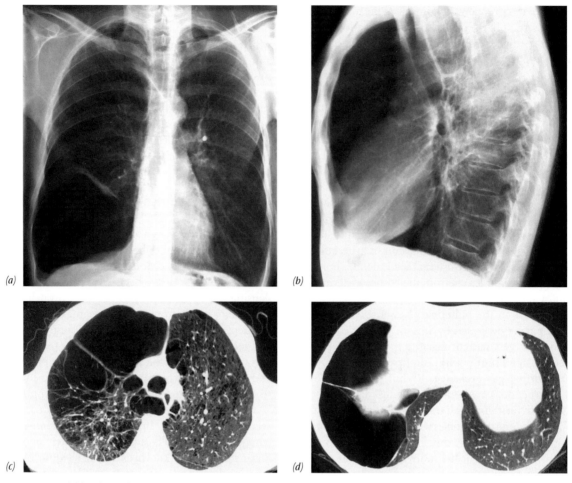

Figure 21.2 *Vanishing lung. (a,b) The CXR raised suspicion of a right-sided basal pneumothorax. CT scans above (c) and below (d) the carinal level showed that the abnormal radiolucency was due to severe destruction of the right lung, whereas the left lung seemed to be less involved.*

with an exacerbation of COPD, Sherman *et al.*[31] found that CXR resulted in management changes in only 11 cases (4.5%). In another study[32] Tsai *et al.* concluded that patients with acute exacerbations of obstructive airway disease who are otherwise uncomplicated do not benefit from routine admission CXR. However, in this study COPD, as defined by the American Thoracic Society, was the most common reason for classification of a patient as complicated, and management was altered by the chest radiography in 26 out of 84 complicated patients.

In severe emphysema, pneumonia may have an unusual appearance. Organisms that typically cause dense consolidation, such as pneumococci, may cause inhomogeneous consolidation or even a coarse interstitial pattern, reflecting the presence of aerated emphysematous spaces within consolidated parenchyma.[33]

COPD accounts for about half of the cases of secondary pneumothorax. The distinction between pneumothorax and a large bulla may be difficult, and occasionally CT may be necessary to make the distinction (Figure 21.2).[34]

Tracheal deformities in COPD

Tracheal deformities have been related to COPD. The cross-sectional shape of the trachea can be described by the tracheal index, which is the ratio between the coronal and sagittal diameters of the trachea. A 'saber-sheath' trachea is defined as a tracheal index less than 0.6 measured at a level 1 cm above the upper margin of the aortic arch.

In children, a near circular tracheal shape prevails, and women retain a tracheal index approaching one. With advancing age men reconfigure their trachea to show an increase in sagittal diameter and a decrease in coronal diameter, and on chest radiographs, a saber-sheath trachea can be identified in 5% of elderly men.[35]

A possible cause of the saber-sheath deformity may be air-trapping in the upper lobes related to centrilobular emphysema (Figure 21.3). In a study of 60 patients with saber-sheath trachea Greene found that 57 had clinical evidence of COPD, as compared with 11 of 60 control patients with normal tracheal index.[36] Of those with clinical evidence of COPD almost half had no other

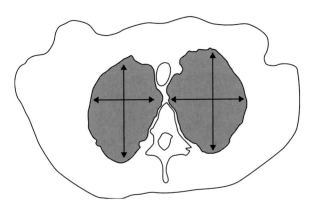

Figure 21.3 *Illustration of the mechanical stress exercised on the trachea by chest hyperinflation. (Produced by Karina Bjerregaard, Tegnestuen, Gentofte Hospital, Copenhagen.)*

conventional radiographic evidence of COPD other than the saber-sheath deformity.

Another tracheal deformity is tracheobronchomegaly, which is relatively rare, and its association with COPD has not been as well established as that of saber-sheath trachea in spite of the fact that a higher incidence of COPD can be expected in patients with dilatation of the central airways.[37]

BRONCHOGRAPHY FINDINGS IN COPD

Although bronchography has now been replaced by CT, previous bronchographic studies have given considerable insight into marked structural and functional changes in COPD.

Bronchography findings in emphysema

Bronchographic features of emphysema relate to peripheral lung structures.[2,38–41] The smaller bronchi may show an increase in their dividing angle. Contrast material penetrates the lungs poorly, and this may result in a 'leafless-tree' appearance, with no alveolar filling and incomplete filling of small bronchi. In centrilobular emphysema contrast material may enter enlarged peripheral airspaces and appear as smooth-walled opacities 2–5 mm in diameter ('peripheral pools'), irregular opacities 5–10 mm in diameter with lateral projections ('spiders') or larger, irregular opacities measuring 5–20 mm in diameter ('flowers').[42,43] The extent of emphysematous changes correlated positively with the severity of fixed airflow obstruction, and negatively with the bronchodilator response.[44]

Bronchography findings in chronic bronchitis

Bronchographic features of chronic bronchitis are distinctive, possibly even diagnostic, and relate to the airways. The bronchographic abnormalities are closely related to

the clinical severity of the disease.[45] A minor degree of irregularity of medium-sized bronchi or a mild generalized increase in the caliber of the airways are subtle changes of early bronchitis.[2,41] In advanced disease irregularity or 'beading' and excessive variation in caliber with ventilation (reflecting flaccidity of the wall) can be seen in airways of all sizes from large bronchi to bronchioles, and the changes may be so severe as to make the differentiation from bronchiectasis arbitrary.[20] However, bronchiectasis is a more localized disease, whereas the changes in bronchitis, although they may be patchy, involve most lobes.

Increased mucus production is associated with opacification of the ducts of enlarged mucous glands by contrast material, especially in the major bronchi. The ducts appear as multiple small projections from the bronchial lumen, mainly on their inferior surface (bronchial diverticulosis). These findings, which are not pathognomonic of chronic bronchitis, are visible in about half of patients suffering from this condition.[2]

The most commonly seen bronchographic abnormality in chronic bronchitis is an abrupt or tapered termination of smaller bronchi or bronchioles and an associated absence of peripheral filling in these regions.[40,41,46]

COMPUTED TOMOGRAPHY FINDINGS IN COPD

Whereas little has been written about CT findings in chronic bronchitis, the literature on CT findings in emphysema is extensive.

CT findings in emphysema

The clinical features of emphysema such as insidious onset of exertional dyspnea may only be recognized late in the course of the disease and are imprecise in the diagnosis of this condition. The radiologic signs of emphysema on CXR, such as hyperinflation and reduced vascularity, are no more precise than the clinical features in diagnosing this condition, and the hope that tests of pulmonary function would be sensitive and specific enough to detect emphysema has also not been realized. However, major advance in the *in vivo* diagnosis and quantification of emphysema has come from CT.[47–49]

In the 1970s when Hounsfield developed CT for clinical use, he envisaged the scanner as a measuring device, because it provides precise information on the density of tissues derived from the attenuation of X-rays. Furthermore, the pathologic correlate of emphysema is loss of lung tissue, and therefore it is logical that CT has greatly improved the diagnosis and especially the quantification of emphysema.

Emphysema was first described by CT in the late 1970s and early 1980s.[50,51] Since that time, several studies

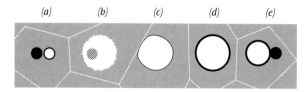

Figure 21.4 *Conditions characterized by decreased lung density. (a) Normal lung: bronchiolar and pulmonary artery branches of equal diameter lay together in the center of the pulmonary lobule surrounded by alveolar tissue and connective tissue interlobular septae that contain pulmonary veins (not shown) and lymphatic branches (not shown). (b) Emphysema: destructive lesions usually without visible walls, and sometimes with a persistent vessel (hatched) in the center of the lesion. (c) Bulla: a sharply demarcated area of emphysema, measuring 1 cm or more in diameter, and possessing a wall less than 1 mm in thickness. (d) Cyst: as opposed to bulla, the term cyst has no relation to emphysema and refers to a circumscribed, air- (or fluid-) containing lesion, 1 cm or more in diameter with a thin wall (usually less than 3 mm). (e) Bronchiectasis can sometimes be hard to differentiate from cysts, but in bronchiectasis an adjacent pulmonary artery can usually be identified (signet-ring sign). (Produced by Karina Bjerregaard, Tegnestuen, Gentofte Hospital, Copenhagen.)*

have compared CT and pathologic findings, and with improved resolution, faster scan times, and thinner collimation, the correlation of CT scores and pathologic grading has improved. Because of its tomographic nature and improved contrast resolution, CT is superior to plain radiography in detection,[52,53] characterization and grading of emphysema,[54] and at present CT is the imaging method of choice to diagnose emphysema in living patients.[55,56]

The CT diagnosis of emphysema is morphological[57] and based on visual inspection for low attenuation areas (LAA), i.e. regions of parenchymal destruction. The density of emphysematous lung as measured by the pixel attenuation values (in HU = Hounsfield units) is decreased as compared with normal lung, and the severity of the disease can be assessed by quantitative analyses of the CT density of the lung.

CT MORPHOLOGY OF EMPHYSEMA

Emphysema is characterized by focal areas of abnormally low attenuation usually without visible walls, and sometimes with a persistent vessel in the center of the lesion (Figure 21.4). An appropriately low window setting (-600 to -900 HU) is essential for diagnosing emphysema.[58]

CT has a high specificity,[59-63] but low sensitivity. CT misses very small areas of emphysema, and using 10 mm collimation only half of those patients with mild to moderate levels of parenchymal destruction are detected.[64-66] As a result of decreased volume averaging and higher spatial resolution, HRCT offers a clear advantage over 10-mm collimation in identification of small areas of emphysema.[66-68]

Preliminary observations indicate that high-quality, diagnostic images of the lung can be obtained with a very low radiation dose,[69,70] which opens up a potential use of HRCT as a screen for emphysema. Wider use of CT for investigation of relatively asymptomatic smokers may allow early diagnosis of emphysema and provide more information on the natural history of this disease.[52]

Based on the distribution of emphysema within the secondary lobule and with respect to fissures and exterior pleural surfaces, it is possible on HRCT to separate various subtypes of emphysema (Figures 21.5–21.7):[58]

- Centrilobular emphysema: multiple, small, centrilobular lucencies, patchy in central parts of lobes and predominantly upper lobe distribution (Figure 21.5).
- Panlobular emphysema: uniform destruction of lobules, extensive, predominant lower lobe distribution (Figure 21.6).
- Paraseptal emphysema: subpleural and perihilar bullae and cysts, visible walls. This form of emphysema is associated with spontaneous pneumothorax (Figure 21.7).[71,72]
- Irregular airspace enlargement: irregular areas of decreased opacity in regions of fibrosis (Figure 21.7).

Centrilobular emphysema with upper lobe predominance is the most common type of emphysema in smokers,[9] whereas the lung disease associated with alpha-1-antitrypsin deficiency is usually panlobular emphysema with lower lobe predominance.[9,73-76] The distribution pattern, such as homogeneous diffuse versus heterogeneous lobe predominance, is associated with outcome after lung volume reduction surgery, the latter being associated with a better outcome.[77-80]

Dependent ground-glass opacities in emphysematous lung is probably due to relaxation atelectasis. Because emphysema is often patchy in distribution, some lobules preserve more elastic recoil than others, allowing them to collapse partially and thereby increase their attenuation. Unlike the ground-glass opacities seen in interstitial lung disease, dependent atelectasis reaerates and loses its ground-glass appearance when the patient changes position (e.g. turns from supine to prone).

The walls of paraseptal emphysematous spaces are often thicker than those of other emphysematous spaces, and it may be difficult to distinguish paraseptal emphysema from scarring and honeycomb cysts in lung fibrosis. In paraseptal emphysema the spaces are usually larger than in honeycomb lung, and it may be useful to look for vessels or strands of residual lung tissue or vessels within the spaces, which may be present in emphysematous spaces or bullae, but not in honeycomb cysts. Another distinguishing feature is that honeycomb cysts

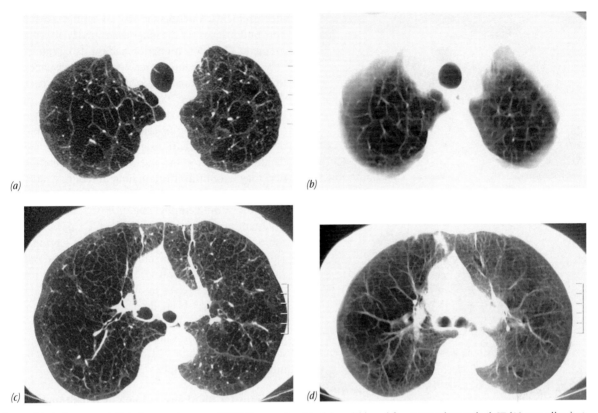

Figure 21.5 *Severe centrilobular emphysema. HRCT (1-mm slices) in (a) and (c) and for comparison spiral CT (10-mm slices) at same level (b) and (d). Low attenuation areas (LAA), i.e. regions of parenchymal destruction, are more conspicuous on HRCT.*

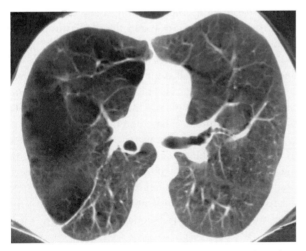

Figure 21.6 *Panlobular emphysema in alpha-1-antitrypsin deficient (type PI*ZZ) patient. Vascular distortion and pruning is more predominant than parenchymal destruction.*

are arranged in multiple rows along the visceral pleura, whereas the emphysematous spaces of paraseptal emphysema are typically confined to a single row.[56]

OTHER CT CHARACTERISTICS OF EMPHYSEMA

Because of the uniform nature of the process in panlobular emphysema, non-peripheral low-attenuation areas are

less easily appreciated than with centrilobular emphysema, and vascular distortion and pruning become more predominant CT features.[9]

As a result of overinflation the right and left lung may approach each other closely in the retrosternal region to form an anterior junction line. In the CT section at the carinal level, an anterior junction line of more than 3 cm and a sterno-aortic distance of more than 4 cm corresponds to an increase in the retrosternal space on CXR[81] and to airflow limitation.[82] In the region inferior to the aortic arch other lines and stripes have been described with a similar connotation,[83] and intercostal lung bulging where the pleura takes a wavy configuration has also been associated with airways obstruction.[82]

Due to its cross-sectional nature, a diagnosis of saber-sheath trachea is easy by CT. A small tracheal index correlates with an increase in FRC and sterno-spinal distance, and thus it was concluded that saber-sheath trachea is basically a sign of overinflation.[84] A small tracheal index also correlates with airflow limitation.[82] Apart from the tracheal deformities, overinflation is less conspicuous on CT than on CXR because the changes in ribcage dimensions are rather complex in the cross-sectional view.[82,85,86]

Emphysema is associated with loss of elastic recoil which is the physiologic basis for permanent enlargement of airspaces,[87] and CT scans taken at full expiration

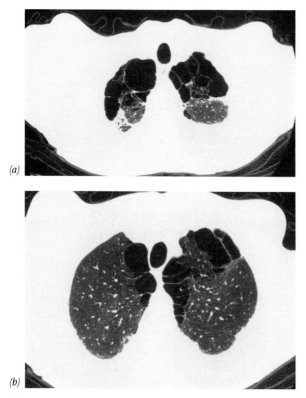

(a)

(b)

Figure 21.7 *(a,b) Paraseptal emphysema. Subpleural and perihilar bullae with visible walls. In the apical regions, emphysema is often accompanied by some scarring (irregular emphysema). From a radiologic point of view it is not always easy to distinguish between benign scarring and an apical neoplasm (Pancoast tumor).*

can effectively reveal the abnormal enlargement of airspaces which defines emphysema.[88] Although emphysema scored on expiratory scans correlated better with functional assessment of airway obstruction (FEV₁),[89,90] scans obtained in exhalation appeared to underestimate the severity of emphysema,[68] and inspiratory CT was more accurate than expiratory CT for quantifying emphysema.[90] In other words, expiratory CT reflects airway obstruction and air trapping (see below) more than it does emphysema.[65] Furthermore, CT volumetric assessments of abnormally low attenuation of the lung at inspiration and expiration had a high correlation, suggesting that a dedicated expiratory examination is not needed.[91]

CT QUANTITATION OF EMPHYSEMA

More than 20 years ago it was noted that the CT density of emphysematous lung was decreased as compared with normal lung.[50,51] Several studies have correlated the quantitative assessment of emphysema by CT with pathologic findings[9,52,64,66,67,90,92–108] and pulmonary function and exercise tests.[51–54,64,68,87–91,96,98,99,101,104–107,109–132] In patients with bullous disease, the extent of bullous emphysema correlated poorly with respiratory function

measurements, but the severity of emphysema in the non-bullous parts of the lungs correlated well with measurements of airflow limitation and diffusing capacity.[133]

CT grading of emphysema, whether by visual estimation or computer analysis, correlates best with decreased diffusing capacity[98,99,110] and less well with airflow obstruction (e.g. FEV₁)[51–53,60,68,87–90,96,101,104–107,109,111–113,115–118,120–124,126,129–132] In centrilobular emphysema, lung destruction is concentrated in the upper lobes, where little gas exchange occurs and where even severe destruction may have little effect on lung function,[114] and CT is more sensitive than pulmonary function testing in the diagnosis of mild emphysema.[52,64,92,100,121]

Quantitation of emphysema by CT can be based on subjective (visual) or objective (computer) scoring. Visual scoring is both time consuming and subject to observer variability.[97,108,124] Because of their digital nature, CT images lend themselves to objective computer analysis, and software has been developed for semi-automatic calculation of so-called densitometric parameters from the pixel attenuation values of the CT images. At present such software (Figure 21.8) is available on a limited number of scanners only.

CT quantitation of emphysema by densitometric parameters

Quantitative analysis of CT lung density begins with the delineation of lung in the images. At a given threshold for the soft tissue–lung interface, lung tissue can be separated from the thoracic wall and the mediastinum by a semi-automatic contour tracing algorithm.[134,135] From the pixel attenuation values (HU) within the lung, a frequency distribution called the CT lung density histogram is generated (Figure 21.9). This histogram is usually unimodal, but in bullous disease the histogram may show a bimodal distribution.[101] Based on the histogram various types of densitometric parameters can be calculated. Due to low reproducibility, simple parameters such as the mean, median and mode of the histogram, have not been used much for the quantitation of emphysema,[126,136–138] whereas two more sophisticated parameters, the pixel percentile and the pixel index, have proven more useful.[111,113,130]

The percentile method was introduced by the Edinburgh group.[96] The pixel percentile is the cut-off point in the histogram that defines a given percentile of the histogram. For example, the 10th pixel percentile is extracted from the histogram as the density value (HU) at which 10% of the pixels have lower densities.

The 'density mask' method leads to the pixel index that is presumed to indicate the percentage of lung volume affected by emphysema. The pixel index is defined as the relative volume of lung for which pixel attenuation values fall below a given threshold. Originally the Vancouver group used a threshold of −910 HU,[97] and later

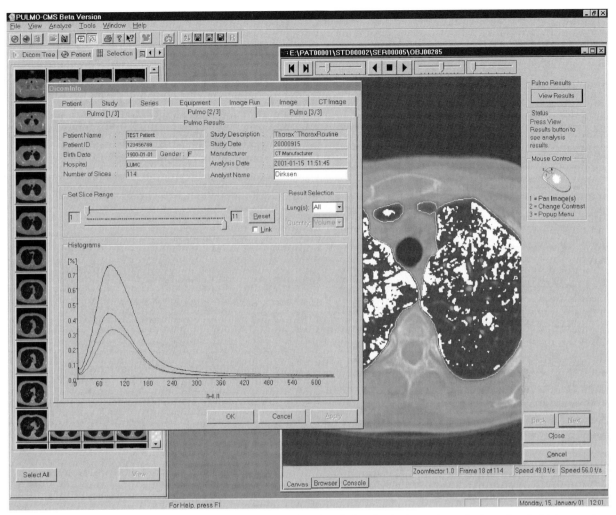

Figure 21.8 *Sample of software for analyzing CT lung density. The window in the front shows the lung density histogram for the whole lung and for the left and right lungs, separately (x-axis, pixel density values in grams per liter (g/L); y-axis, percentage of pixels). The modal values are around 100 g/L (corresponding to −900 HU), and the curves have a tail to the right mainly because of the higher density of vascular structures and partial volume effects along the border of the lung. The window in the back shows a 'density-mask' analysis where emphysematous (low attenuation) areas are highlighted (white). This software package called* PULMO-CMS *detects the lungs in CT scans and automatically analyzes the density distribution of the lungs. From the CT lung density histograms several parameters can be saved (for further analysis) such as: the total lung volume, mean lung density, the lung weight (which is equal to the product of volume and density), and various pixel percentiles and pixel indexes.* PULMO-CMS *has been developed for a standard PC and runs under the Windows-NT and Windows-2000 operating system. It is able to read CT images obtained with scanners from different manufacturers through the image standards ACR-NEMA 1.0, ACR-NEMA 2.0 and DICOM 3.0. (*PULMO-CMS *has been developed by the image processing division (Dutch abbreviation: LKEB) of the Radiology Department of the Leiden University Medical Center in The Netherlands in collaboration with a medical imaging company MEDIS. For further information contact:* b.c.stoel@lumc.nl.)

Gevenois found a better correlation with both microscopic and macroscopic emphysema at a threshold of −950 HU.[90,103,105]

Using the density mask method it is possible to highlight areas of attenuation below a given threshold, thus making it easy to identify and visualize (even three-dimensionally) the emphysematous regions (Figure 21.8). Several studies have found a close relationship between the pixel index and the extent of improvement after lung volume reduction surgery.[79,124,139] However, adequate amounts of normal or near-normal lung need to be present for optimal results.[79,140]

CT monitoring of the progress of emphysema

Measurements of lung density or tissue mass by CT are based on an approximately linear relationship between attenuation of the X-ray beam and the mass density of materials such as air, blood and lung tissue. Attenuation

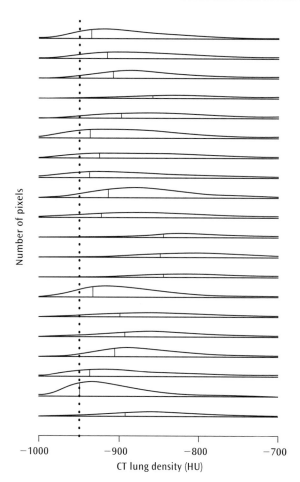

Number of pixels

CT lung density (HU)

Figure 21.9 *CT lung density histograms of 20 patients with moderate to severe emphysema and alpha-1-antitrypsin deficiency (type PI*Z).[153] The areas under the curves correspond to total lung volumes. The vertical dotted line indicates a threshold of −950 HU for calculating the pixel index, whereas the solid vertical line in each histogram indicates the 20th pixel percentile. As emphysema progresses the histograms move to the left. Both pixel index and pixel percentile vary much between patients. Intuitively it can be inferred from the figure that the absolute change over time is less dependent on the baseline value for the pixel percentile than for the pixel index, which gives the pixel percentile an advantage as an indicator of progression of emphysema.*

is expressed in terms of the HU scale in which water is 0 HU and air is −1000 HU. Hounsfield units can be converted to tissue density by adding 1000 to the HU value. Thus, an attenuation value of −950 HU corresponds to a tissue density of 50 g/L.

Estimates of lung density based on CT have been shown to correspond closely to gravimetric estimates within a margin of 4%,[141] and dependence on the reconstruction filter was negligible.[142,143] Variability is inversely related to slice thickness.[69,143] There was some variability in HU between different CT scanners.[144] Furthermore, pixel

attenuation values fluctuated with the position in the thorax and change with aging of the X-ray tube.[145]

The principal source of variation of lung density measurements is the depth of inspiration. Ranging from full inspiration to full expiration, lung densities more than double.[146,147] The volume of air in the lung can be derived from the CT images, i.e. the CT lung density histogram.[111,127,148] Half of the lung density is composed of blood in the microvascular circulation,[149] and when taking a deep breath not only the volume of air increases, but also blood is sucked into the lung, which makes the relation between inspiratory level and lung density more complicated.

Some investigators[89,134,150–152] have tried to standardize the amount of air in the lung by spirometrically controlled CT, i.e. by having the patients breathe through a spirometer during the examination. As soon as a preselected inspiration level is reached, the CT scan is initiated during breath holding. Using this technique, CT lung density measurements were most reproducible at inspiration as compared to expiration,[151] but patients with COPD were less able to reproduce the levels of full expiration and inspiration required for standardizing the level of inspiration in successive examinations.[150,152]

Recently analysis of repeated CT scans at various levels of inspiration has revealed the relationship within an individual between lung density and volume. Based on this relationship, densitometric parameters can be standardized by log-transformed lung volume, which corrects for differences in lung volume between scans and eliminates the need for spirometrically controlled CT.[153]

CT quantitation of emphysema by densitometric parameters seems to be a more sensitive measure of the progress of emphysema as compared to pulmonary function tests (e.g. FEV_1).[154–156] Inspiratory CT was superior to expiratory CT for longitudinal estimation of structural abnormalities caused by aging and smoking,[156] and the pixel percentile was more robust than the pixel index for monitoring the progress of emphysema (Figure 21.9).[153]

It has been shown that CT lung density is influenced by age, and normal CT attenuation values for the lung by age should be established.[113,141,147,156,157]

Of serious consideration when using CT for monitoring the progress of emphysema is the inherent radiation exposure. A reduction of the electrical current (mA) to levels ten times below standard settings has little influence on lung density measurements.[144]

CT findings in chronic bronchitis

Specific findings have proven difficult to define. The following abnormalities may occur: bronchial wall thickening and interlobular septal thickening;[158,159] mucous plugging of bronchioles resembling a branching tree in the lung periphery ('tree-in-bud');[160] air-trapping manifested as a lack of expected increase in lung opacity on exhalation scans; central arterial dilatation reflecting pulmonary arterial hypertension; and modest mediastinal lymphadenopathy reflecting chronic, low-grade infection.

CT findings in small airways disease

The major CT sign of small airways disease is regional decreased attenuation of the lung parenchyma.[161] Reduction of lung volume on expiratory CT scans usually results in a uniform increase in attenuation. In small airways disease increased resistance to airflow results in air trapping on expiration leading to decreased attenuation and less volume loss than normal lung.[162] Small airways disease is usually patchy in distribution, and expiratory scans accentuate subtle differences between normal and abnormal lung.[161]

Because low attenuation areas are also the main characteristic of emphysema, small airways disease may be mistaken for emphysema. The introduction of multislice CT scanners may solve this confusion. Small detectors arranged in large matrices and image reconstruction with isotropic pixels will make it possible to track airways three dimensionally down to a diameter of only a few millimeters, and that may revolutionize our understanding of disorders of these small airways in the near future.

Small airways disease is seen to a variable extent in a wide range of diffuse pulmonary diseases, and it is one of the abnormalities that leads to airway obstruction in COPD.[40] The poor correlation between CT emphysema scores and airflow limitation, found in some studies, may be explained by small airways inflammation of varying extent.[106,113,115,163] Therefore, in the evaluation of COPD, CT measurement of emphysema and airway dimensions may both be useful and complementary.[164] However, the role and contribution of emphysema and small airways disease in causing expiratory airflow limitation in COPD is still controversial.[104]

A window level of −500 HU and a width of 1500 HU is optimal for the study of lung parenchyma and airway lumen and wall dimensions.[165] The bronchiole and the branch of the pulmonary artery supplying the pulmonary lobule have equal diameter and are located in the center of the lobule, whereas branches of the pulmonary veins are located peripherally within the interlobular septa (Figure 21.10). This accounts for the characteristic centrilobular distribution of bronchiolar abnormalities on HRCT.[166]

In healthy adult cigarette smokers, apart from destructive lesions, HRCT may also reveal inflammatory changes such as ill-defined 2- to 3-mm centrilobular micronodules and patchy ground-glass opacities.[158,159,167] These abnormalities indicate small airways disease and it

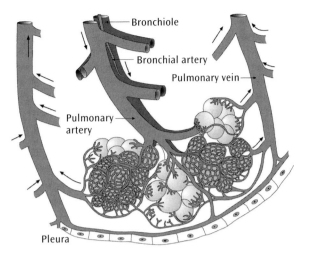

Figure 21.10 *The bronchiole and the branch of the pulmonary artery supplying the pulmonary lobule have equal diameter and are located in the center of the lobule, whereas branches of the pulmonary veins are located peripherally within the interlobular septa.*

is hypothesized that it may progress to respiratory bronchiolitis interstitial lung disease (RBILD).[24,168,169] If smoking is stopped, the changes show no further progression or resolve slowly.

Expiratory air trapping can be detected in most patients with airway obstruction. In COPD, pulmonary function (FEV_1 and $DLCO$) was negatively correlated to both an air trapping score[170–173] and a reduction score.[123,171,172] The air trapping score was defined as the ratio of the cross-sectional air trapping area versus the total cross-sectional lung area on expiratory CT, and the reduction score was defined as the change in cross-sectional lung area or mean lung attenuation at inspiration and expiration.

However, limited or focal air trapping is seen in normal subjects,[172] particularly in the superior segment of the lower lobe,[173] and the frequency of air trapping increases with age, and its severity increases with age and smoking in asymptomatic subjects.[174] Furthermore, diffuse air trapping without intervening areas of normal lung may be difficult to appreciate, even on expiratory scans.[175]

In many diseases resulting in small airways abnormalities, large airway abnormalities such as bronchiectasis are also visible. Although bronchiectasis by definition is a disease separate from COPD, in patients with bronchiectasis there is a high prevalence of emphysema, which on HRCT is mainly localized in the bronchiectatic lobes,[122] and the severity and extent of bronchiectasis correlates with severity of airways obstruction.[176,177] In bronchiectasis the airflow obstruction is primarily linked to evidence of small airways disease, such as the extent of decreased attenuation on the expiratory CT, and not so much to bronchiectatic abnormalities in large airways, emphysema or retained endobronchial secretions.[178]

Is COPD associated with CT evidence of bronchiectasis?

In a recent study HRCT evidence of predominantly tubular bronchiectasis was noted in 29% of 110 patients who presented to primary care with a diagnosis of an acute exacerbation of COPD.[179]

Whereas the association between alpha-1-antitrypsin deficiency and the development of premature emphysema has long been recognized, only a limited number of studies have assessed the association between alpha-1-antitrypsin deficiency and bronchiectasis. In Eriksson's original patients, bronchiectasis was reported in two of 23 patients.[180] Guest observed bronchial wall thickening and/or dilatation in seven out of 17 patients with alpha-1-antitrypsin deficiency,[76] and King found evidence of bronchiectasis in six of 14 patients with alpha-1-antitrypsin deficiency.[181] However, the frequency of alpha-1-antitrypsin alleles was not increased among patients with bronchiectasis.[182]

OTHER IMAGING TECHNIQUES IN COPD

Magnetic resonance imaging (MRI) has the advantage of being a radiation-free modality. It has a large potential, although it cannot yet match the resolution of CT in most thoracic applications. Dynamic gradient fast spin echo sequences are extremely effective at showing diaphragm and chest wall motion in the sagittal and coronal plane.[140,183] Axial MRI has also been used to assess the change in total lung volume following lung volume reduction surgery, although spiral CT can be used just as effectively for this purpose.[184,185]

MRI with polarized noble gases such as helium-3 and xenon-129 is a promising new modality for the assessment of pulmonary ventilation and its abnormalities in COPD, but it needs additional studies to determine its potential clinical role.[186,187]

Several types of scintigraphs have been used to assess emphysema.[125] In mild to moderate COPD with a normal CXR, multiple small matched defects may be found on ventilation-perfusion scans,[188] but the spatial resolution of CT is superior to scintigraphy, and usually there is a strong correlation between lung perfusion assessed by HRCT and lung perfusion on scintigraphy.[189] Ventilation scintigraphy may be useful for diagnostic assessment of panlobular emphysema, which is difficult to distinguish from normal lung by CT.[190]

The most important selection criteria for lung volume reduction surgery is the presence of a bilateral upper lobe heterogeneity both with regard to pattern of emphysema on CT[77–80] and lung perfusion scanning.[191] Heterogeneity on CT was better for the prediction of improvement after lung volume reduction surgery than was heterogeneity on lung perfusion scans. However, perfusion scintigraphy may be helpful to identify target areas for resection in candidates for lung volume reduction surgery with homogeneous CT morphology.[192] Since CT is an anatomic technique and perfusion scanning is a functional technique, the two techniques provide complementary information,[193] and perfusion scintigraphy may be useful in selecting patients with successful outcomes after lung volume reduction surgery.[194]

CONCLUSIONS

Chronic bronchitis is virtually invisible by diagnostic imaging, and the role for plain radiography is to exclude other disorders such as cancer or bronchiectasis and detect complications such as pneumonia, pneumothorax and pulmonary hypertension. Reliable CT findings have not been established in chronic bronchitis.

On the contrary, emphysema has a characteristic and pleomorphic appearance. Hyperinflation is the most useful feature on CXR, whereas on CT the parenchymal destruction is directly visible. Thus, CT is superior to both plain radiography and pulmonary function tests in determining the type, distribution and severity of emphysema, and *in vivo*, HRCT is the most accurate method for detecting emphysema. The principal finding on CT is focal areas of abnormally low attenuation usually without visible walls.

As surgical and medical treatment of emphysema advances, it will be necessary to grade emphysema in an objective and reproducible manner. Preliminary data indicate that lung density measurements based on CT may be more sensitive and specific than pulmonary function tests for monitoring the progress of emphysema. Provided low-dose techniques can be applied without loss of precision and measurements can be automated and standardized, CT may replace pulmonary function measurements (FEV_1) as the gold standard for assessing the response to treatment in clinical trials of emphysema.

There are many important epidemiologic questions regarding the natural history of emphysema and its importance in COPD that can only be answered by using CT. But first, the lung community must do the same painstaking work of standardizing and validating CT that it did for spirometry.

REFERENCES

1. Sanders C. The radiographic diagnosis of emphysema. *Radiol Clin North Am* 1991;**29**:1019–30.
2. Simon G, Galbraith H-JB. *Radiology* of chronic bronchitis. *Lancet* 1953;**2**(6791):850–2.

3. Laws JW, Heard BE. Emphysema and the chest film: a retrospective radiological and pathological study. *Br J Radiol* 1962;**35**:750–61.

4. Reid L, Millard FJC. Correlation between radiological diagnosis and structural lung changes in emphysema. *Clin Radiol* 1964;**15**:307–11.

5. Suitinen S, Christoforidis AJ, Klugh GA, Pratt PC. Roentgenologic criteria for the recognition of nonsymptomatic pulmonary emphysema. Correlation between roentgenologic findings and pulmonary pathology. *Am Rev Respir Dis* 1965;**91**:69–76.

6. Nicklaus TM, Stowell DW, Christiansen WR, Renzetti AD Jr. The accuracy of the roentgenologic diagnosis of chronic pulmonary emphysema. *Am Rev Respir Dis* 1966;**93**:889–99.

7. Katsura S, Martin CJ. The roentgenologic diagnosis of anatomic emphysema. *Am Rev Respir Dis* 1967;**96**:700–6.

8. Thurlbeck WM, Henderson JA, Fraser RG, Bates DV. Chronic obstructive lung disease. A comparison between clinical, roentgenologic, functional and morphologic criteria in chronic bronchitis, emphysema, asthma and bronchiectasis. *Medicine* 1970;**49**:81–145.

9. Foster WL Jr, Gimenez EI, Roubidoux MA *et al.* The emphysemas: radiologic–pathologic correlations. *Radiographics* 1993;**13**:311–28.

10. Burki NK, Krumpelman JL. Correlation of pulmonary function with the chest roentgenogram in chronic airway obstruction. *Am Rev Respir Dis* 1980;**121**:217–23.

11. Rothpearl A, Varma AO, Goodman K. Radiographic measures of hyperinflation in clinical emphysema. Discrimination of patients from controls and relationship to physiologic and mechanical lung function. *Chest* 1988;**94**:907–13.

12. Reich SB, Weinshelbaum A, Yee J. Correlation of radiographic measurements and pulmonary function tests in chronic obstructive pulmonary disease. *AJR* 1985;**144**:695–9.

13. Pratt PC. Role of conventional chest radiography in diagnosis and exclusion of emphysema. *Am J Med* 1987;**82**:998–1006.

14. Thurlbeck WM, Simon G. Radiographic appearance of the chest in emphysema. *AJR* 1978;**130**:429–40.

15. Simon G, Pride NB, Jones NL, Raimondi AC. Relation between abnormalities in the chest radiograph and changes in pulmonary function in chronic bronchitis and emphysema. *Thorax* 1973;**28**:15–23.

16. Musk AW. Relation of pulmonary vessel size to transfer factor in subjects with airflow obstruction. *AJR* 1983;**141**:915–18.

17. Colp C, Park SS, Williams MH Jr. Emphysema with little airway obstruction. *Am Rev Respir Dis* 1970;**101**:615–19.

18. Stein PD, Leu JD, Welch MH, Guenter CA. Pathophysiology of the pulmonary circulation in emphysema associated with alpha antitrypsin deficiency. *Circulation* 1971;**43**:227–39.

19. Milne EN, Bass H. The roentgenologic diagnosis of early chronic obstructive pulmonary disease. *J Can Assoc Radiol* 1969;**20**:3–15.

20. Gamsu G, Nadel JA. The roentgenologic manifestations of emphysema and chronic bronchitis. *Med Clin North Am* 1973;**57**:719–33.

21. Carr DH, Pride NB. Computed tomography in pre-operative assessment of bullous emphysema. *Clin Radiol* 1984;**35**:43–5.

22. Morgan MD, Denison DM, Strickland B. Value of computed tomography for selecting patients with bullous lung disease for surgery. *Thorax* 1986;**41**:855–62.

23. Stern EJ, Webb WR, Weinacker A, Müller NL. Idiopathic giant bullous emphysema (vanishing lung syndrome): imaging findings in nine patients. *AJR* 1994;**162**:279–82.

24. Guckel C, Hansell DM. Imaging the 'dirty lung' – has high resolution computed tomography cleared the smoke? *Clin Radiol* 1998;**53**:717–22.

25. Fraser RG, Fraser RS, Renner JW, Bernard C, Fitzgerald PJ. The roentgenologic diagnosis of chronic bronchitis: a reassessment with emphasis on parahilar bronchi seen end-on. *Radiology* 1976;**120**:1–9.

26. Matthay RA, Schwarz MI, Ellis JH Jr, *et al.* Pulmonary artery hypertension in chronic obstructive pulmonary disease: determination by chest radiography. *Invest Radiol* 1981;**16**:95–100.

27. Kuriyama K, Gamsu G, Stern RG, Cann CE, Herfkens RJ, Brundage BH. CT-determined pulmonary artery diameters in predicting pulmonary hypertension. *Invest Radiol* 1984;**19**:16–22.

28. Tan RT, Kuzo R, Goodman LR, Siegel R, Haasler GB, Presberg KW. Utility of CT scan evaluation for predicting pulmonary hypertension in patients with parenchymal lung disease. *Chest* 1998;**113**:1250–6.

29. Gefter WB, Hatabu H, Dinsmore BJ, *et al.* Pulmonary vascular cine MR imaging: a noninvasive approach to dynamic imaging of the pulmonary circulation. *Radiology* 1990;**176**:761–70.

30. Kondo C, Caputo GR, Masui T, *et al.* Pulmonary hypertension: pulmonary flow quantification and flow profile analysis with velocity-encoded cine MR imaging. *Radiology* 1992;**183**:751–8.

31. Sherman S, Skoney JA, Ravikrishnan KP. Routine chest radiographs in exacerbations of chronic obstructive pulmonary disease. Diagnostic value. *Arch Intern Med* 1989;**149**:2493–6.

32. Tsai TW, Gallagher EJ, Lombardi G, Gennis P, Carter W. Guidelines for the selective ordering of admission chest radiography in adult obstructive airway disease. *Ann Emerg Med* 1993;**22**:1854–8.

33. Ziskind MM, Schwarz MI, George RB, *et al.* Incomplete consolidation in pneumococcal lobar pneumonia complicating pulmonary emphysema. *Ann Intern Med* 1970;**72**:835–9.

34. Bourgouin P, Cousineau G, Lemire P, Hebert G. Computed tomography used to exclude pneumothorax in bullous lung disease. *J Can Assoc Radiol* 1985;**36**:341–2.

35. Greene R, Lechner GL. 'Saber-Sheath' trachea: a clinical and functional study of coronal narrowing of the intrathoracic trachea. *Radiology* 1975;**115**:265–8.

36. Greene R. 'Saber-sheath' trachea: relation to chronic obstructive pulmonary disease. *AJR* 1978;**130**:441–5.

37. Stark P, Norbash A. Imaging of the trachea and upper airways in patients with chronic obstructive airway disease. *Radiol Clin North Am* 1998;**36**:91–105 [review].

38. Reid LM. Correlation of certain bronchographic abnormalities seen in chronic bronchitis with the pathological changes. *Thorax* 1955;**10**:199–204.

39. Freimanis AK, Molnar W. Chronic bronchitis and emphysema at bronchography. Survey of diagnostic features obtained by reviewing 2000 bronchograms. *Radiology* 1960;**74**:194–205.

40. Hogg JC, Macklem PT, Thurlbeck WM. Site and nature of airway obstruction in chronic obstructive lung disease. *N Engl J Med* 1968;**278**:1355–60.

41. Gregg I, Trapnell DH. The bronchographic appearances of early chronic bronchitis. *Br J Radiol* 1969;**42**:132–9.

42. Leopold JG, Seal RM. The bronchographic appearance of 'peripheral pooling' attributed to the filling of centrilobular emphysematous spaces. *Thorax* 1961;**16**:70–7.

43. Duinker NW, Huizinga E. The 'flowers' in bronchography. *Thorax* 1962;**17**:175–8.

44. Koyama H, Nishimura K, Mio T, Izumi T. Emphysematous changes assessed by selective alveolobronchography and

bronchodilator response in chronic airflow obstruction. *Lung* 1994;**172**:103–12.

45. Ogilvie AG. Bronchography in chronic bronchitis. *Thorax* 1975;**30**:631–5.

46. Friedman PJ. Radiology of the airways with emphasis on the small airways. *J Thorac Imaging* 1986;**1**:7–22 [review].

47. Flenley DC. Diagnosis and follow-up of emphysema. *Eur Respir J* 1990;**9**(suppl):5s–8s.

48. Webb WR. High-resolution computed tomography of obstructive lung disease. *Radiol Clin North Am* 1994; **32**:745–57 [review].

49. Stern EJ, Song JK, Frank MS. CT of the lungs in patients with pulmonary emphysema. *Semin Ultrasound CT MR* 1995; **16**:345–52 [review].

50. Rosenblum LJ, Mauceri RA, Wellenstein DE, Bassano DA, Cohen WN, Heitzman ER. Computed tomography of the lung. *Radiology* 1978;**129**:521–4.

51. Goddard PR, Nicholson EM, Laszlo G, Watt I. Computed tomography in pulmonary emphysema. *Clin Radiol* 1982;**33**:379–87.

52. Sanders C, Nath PH, Bailey WC. Detection of emphysema with computed tomography. Correlation with pulmonary function tests and chest radiography. *Invest Radiol* 1988;**23**:262–6.

53. Klein JS, Gamsu G, Webb WR, Golden JA, Müller NL. High-resolution CT diagnosis of emphysema in symptomatic patients with normal chest radiographs and isolated low diffusing capacity. *Radiology* 1992;**182**:817–21.

54. Miniati M, Filippi E, Falaschi F, *et al.* Radiologic evaluation of emphysema in patients with chronic obstructive pulmonary disease. Chest radiography versus high resolution computed tomography. *Am J Respir Crit Care Med* 1995;**151**: 1359–67.

55. Thurlbeck WM, Müller NL. Emphysema: definition, imaging, and quantification. *AJR* 1994;**163**:1017–25 [review].

56. Takasugi JE, Godwin JD. Radiology of chronic obstructive pulmonary disease. *Radiol Clin North Am* 1998;**36**:29–55 [review].

57. Bonelli FS, Hartman TE, Swensen SJ, Sherrick A. Accuracy of high-resolution CT in diagnosing lung diseases. *AJR* 1998; **170**:1507–12.

58. Webb WR, Müller NL, Naidich DP. *High Resolution CT of the Lung*, 3rd edn. Lippincott Williams & Wilkins, New York, 2000.

59. Kinsella M, Müller NL, Staples C, Vedal S, Chan Yeung M. Hyperinflation in asthma and emphysema. Assessment by pulmonary function testing and computed tomography. *Chest* 1988;**94**:286–9.

60. Kondoh Y, Taniguchi H, Yokoyama S, Taki F, Takagi K, Satake T. Emphysematous change in chronic asthma in relation to cigarette smoking. Assessment by computed tomography. *Chest* 1990;**97**:845–9.

61. Paganin F, Seneterre E, Chanez P, *et al.* Computed tomography of the lungs in asthma: influence of disease severity and etiology. *Am J Respir Crit Care Med* 1996;**153**: 110–14.

62. Biernacki W, Redpath AT, Best JJ, MacNee W. Measurement of CT lung density in patients with chronic asthma. *Eur Respir J* 1997;**10**:2455–9.

63. Mochizuki T, Nakajima H, Kokubu F, Kushihashi T, Adachi M. Evaluation of emphysema in patients with reversible airway obstruction using high-resolution CT. *Chest* 1997;**112**: 1522–6.

64. Bergin C, Muller N, Nichols DM, *et al.* The diagnosis of emphysema. A computed tomographic–pathologic correlation. *Am Rev Respir Dis* 1986;**133**:541–6.

65. Müller NL, Thurlbeck WM. Thin-section CT, emphysema, air trapping, and airway obstruction. *Radiology* 1996;**199**:621–2.

66. Miller RR, Müller NL, Vedal S, Morrison NJ, Staples CA. Limitations of computed tomography in the assessment of emphysema. *Am Rev Respir Dis* 1989;**139**:980–3.

67. Spouge D, Cardoso W, Müller NL. Panacinar emphysema: CT and pathologic findings. *J Comput Assist Tomogr* 1993;**17**: 710–13.

68. Nishimura K, Murata K, Yamagishi M, *et al.* Comparison of different computed tomography scanning methods for quantifying emphysema. *J Thorac Imaging* 1998;**13**:193–8.

69. Naidich DP, Shall CH, Gribbin C, Arams RS, McCauley DI. Low-dose CT of the lungs: preliminary observations. *Radiology* 1990;**175**:729–31.

70. Zwirewich CV, Müller NL. Low-dose high-resolution CT of lung parenchyma. *Radiology* 1991;**180**:413–17.

71. Lesur O, Delorme N, Fromaget JM, Bernadac P, Polu JM. Computed tomography in the etiologic assessment of idiopathic spontaneous pneumothorax. *Chest* 1990; **98**:341–7.

72. Bense L, Lewander R, Eklund G, Hedenstierna G, Wiman LG. Nonsmoking, non-alpha-1-antitrypsin deficiency-induced emphysema in nonsmokers with healed spontaneous pneumothorax, identified by computed tomography of the lungs. *Chest* 1993;**103**:433–8.

73. Guenter CA, Welch MH, Russell TR, Hyde RM, Hammarsten JF. The pattern of lung disease associated with alpha-1-antitrypsin deficiency. *Arch Intern Med* 1968;**122**:254–7.

74. Gishen P, Saunders AJ, Tobin MJ, Hutchison DC. Alpha-1-antitrypsin deficiency: the radiological features of pulmonary emphysema in subjects of Pi type Z and Pi type SZ: a survey by the British Thoracic Association. *Clin Radiol* 1982;**33**:371–7.

75. Brantly ML, Paul LD, Miller BH, Falk RT, Wu M, Crystal RG. Clinical features and history of the destructive lung disease associated with alpha-1-antitrypsin deficiency of adults with pulmonary symptoms. *Am Rev Respir Dis* 1988;**138**:327–36.

76. Guest PJ, Hansell DM. High resolution computed tomography (HRCT) in emphysema associated with alpha-1-antitrypsin deficiency. *Clin Radiol* 1992;**45**:260–6.

77. Weder W, Thurnheer R, Stammberger U, Burge M, Russi EW, Bloch KE. Radiologic emphysema morphology is associated with outcome after surgical lung volume reduction. *Ann Thorac Surg* 1997;**64**:313–19;discussion 319–20.

78. Slone RM, Pilgram TK, Gierada DS, *et al.* Lung volume reduction surgery: comparison of preoperative radiologic features and clinical outcome. *Radiology* 1997;**204**: 685–93.

79. Gierada DS, Slone RM, Bae KT, Yusen RD, Lefrak SS, Cooper JD. Pulmonary emphysema: comparison of preoperative quantitative CT and physiologic index values with clinical outcome after lung-volume reduction surgery. *Radiology* 1997;**205**:235–42.

80. Wisser W, Klepetko W, Kontrus M, *et al.* Morphologic grading of the emphysematous lung and its relation to improvement after lung volume reduction surgery. *Ann Thorac Surg* 1998;**65**:793–9.

81. Hagen G, Kolbenstvedt A. CT measurement of mediastinal anterior junction line in emphysema patients. *Acta Radiol* 1993;**34**:194–5.

82. Arakawa H, Kurihara Y, Nakajima Y, Niimi H, Ishikawa T, Tokuda M. Computed tomography measurements of overinflation in chronic obstructive pulmonary disease: evaluation of various radiographic signs. *J Thorac Imaging* 1998;**13**:188–92.

83. Curtis BR, Fisher MS. Posterior inferior junction line and left pleuroesophageal stripe: their association with emphysema. *J Thorac Imaging* 1998;**13**:184–7.

84. Trigaux JP, Hermes G, Dubois P, Van Beers B, Delaunois L, Jamart J. CT of saber-sheath trachea. Correlation with clinical, chest radiographic and functional findings. *Acta Radiol* 1994;**35**:247–50.

85. Kilburn KH, Asmundsson T. Anteroposterior chest diameter in emphysema. *Arch Intern Med* 1969;**123**:379–82.

86. Cassart M, Gevenois PA, Estenne M. Rib cage dimensions in hyperinflated patients with severe chronic obstructive pulmonary disease. *Am J Respir Crit Care Med* 1996;**154**:800–5.

87. Gugger M, Gould G, Sudlow MF, Wraith PK, MacNee W. Extent of pulmonary emphysema in man and its relation to the loss of elastic recoil. *Clin Sci* 1991;**80**:353–8.

88. Knudson RJ, Standen JR, Kaltenborn WT, *et al.* Expiratory computed tomography for assessment of suspected pulmonary emphysema. *Chest* 1991;**99**:1357–66.

89. Lamers RJ, Thelissen GR, Kessels AG, Wouters EF, van Engelshoven JM. Chronic obstructive pulmonary disease: evaluation with spirometrically controlled CT lung densitometry. *Radiology* 1994;**193**:109–13.

90. Gevenois PA, De Vuyst P, Sy M, *et al.* Pulmonary emphysema: quantitative CT during expiration. *Radiology* 1996;**199**:825–9.

91. Mergo PJ, Williams WF, Gonzalez Rothi R, *et al.* Three-dimensional volumetric assessment of abnormally low attenuation of the lung from routine helical CT: inspiratory and expiratory quantification. *AJR* 1998;**170**:1355–60.

92. Hayhurst MD, MacNee W, Flenley DC, *et al.* Diagnosis of pulmonary emphysema by computerised tomography. *Lancet* 1984;**ii**(8398):320–2.

93. Foster WL Jr, Pratt PC, Roggli VL, Godwin JD, Halvorsen RA Jr, Putman CE. Centrilobular emphysema: CT–pathologic correlation. *Radiology* 1986;**159**:27–32.

94. Murata K, Itoh H, Todo G, *et al.* Centrilobular lesions of the lung: demonstration by high-resolution CT and pathologic correlation. *Radiology* 1986;**161**:641–5.

95. Hruban RH, Meziane MA, Zerhouni EA, *et al.* High resolution computed tomography of inflation-fixed lungs. Pathologic–radiologic correlation of centrilobular emphysema. *Am Rev Respir Dis* 1987;**136**:935–40.

96. Gould GA, MacNee W, McLean A, *et al.* CT measurements of lung density in life can quantitate distal airspace enlargement – an essential defining feature of human emphysema. *Am Rev Respir Dis* 1988;**137**:380–92.

97. Müller NL, Staples CA, Miller RR, Abboud RT. 'Density mask'. An objective method to quantitate emphysema using computed tomography. *Chest* 1988;**94**:782–7.

98. Morrison NJ, Abboud RT, Ramadan F, *et al.* Comparison of single breath carbon monoxide diffusing capacity and pressure–volume curves in detecting emphysema. *Am Rev Respir Dis* 1989;**139**:1179–87.

99. Morrison NJ, Abboud RT, Müller NL, *et al.* Pulmonary capillary blood volume in emphysema. *Am Rev Respir Dis* 1990;**141**:53–61.

100. Kuwano K, Matsuba K, Ikeda T, *et al.* The diagnosis of mild emphysema. Correlation of computed tomography and pathology scores. *Am Rev Respir Dis* 1990;**141**:169–78.

101. MacNee W, Gould G, Lamb D. Quantifying emphysema by CT scanning. Clinicopathologic correlates. *Ann NY Acad Sci* 1991;**624**:179–94 [review].

102. Hamada T, Sasaguri T, Hisaoka M, *et al.* Mild emphysema: a novel method using formalin-fixed lungs for computed tomography and pathological analyses. *Virchows Arch* 1995;**426**:597–602.

103. Gevenois PA, de Maertelaer V, De Vuyst P, Zanen J, Yernault JC. Comparison of computed density and macroscopic morphometry in pulmonary emphysema. *Am J Respir Crit Care Med* 1995;**152**:653–7.

104. Gelb AF, Hogg JC, Müller NL, *et al.* Contribution of emphysema and small airways in COPD. *Chest* 1996;**109**:353–9.

105. Gevenois PA, De Vuyst P, de Maertelaer V, *et al.* Comparison of computed density and microscopic morphometry in pulmonary emphysema. *Am J Respir Crit Care Med* 1996;**154**:187–92.

106. Gelb AF, Zamel N, Hogg JC, Müller NL, Schein MJ. Pseudophysiologic emphysema resulting from severe small-airways disease. *Am J Respir Crit Care Med* 1998;**158**:815–19.

107. Coxson HO, Rogers RM, Whittall KP, D'yachkova Y, Pare PD, Sciurba FC, Hogg JC. A quantification of the lung surface area in emphysema using computed tomography. *Am J Respir Crit Care Med* 1999;**159**:851–6.

108. Bankier AA, De Maertelaer V, Keyzer C, Gevenois PA. Pulmonary emphysema: subjective visual grading versus objective quantification with macroscopic morphometry and thin-section CT densitometry. *Radiology* 1999;**211**:851–8.

109. Sakai F, Gamsu G, Im JG, Ray CS. Pulmonary function abnormalities in patients with CT-determined emphysema. *J Comput Assist Tomogr* 1987;**11**:963–8.

110. Biernacki W, Gould GA, Whyte KF, Flenley DC. Pulmonary hemodynamics, gas exchange, and the severity of emphysema as assessed by quantitative CT scan in chronic bronchitis and emphysema. *Am Rev Respir Dis* 1989;**139**:1509–15.

111. Kinsella M, Müller NL, Abboud RT, Morrison NJ, DyBuncio A. Quantitation of emphysema by computed tomography using a 'density mask' program and correlation with pulmonary function tests. *Chest* 1990;**97**:315–21.

112. Fujita J, Nelson NL, Daughton DM, *et al.* Evaluation of elastase and antielastase balance in patients with chronic bronchitis and pulmonary emphysema. *Am Rev Respir Dis* 1990;**142**:57–62.

113. Gould GA, Redpath AT, Ryan M, *et al.* Lung CT density correlates with measurements of airflow limitation and the diffusing capacity. *Eur Respir J* 1991;**4**:141–6.

114. Gurney JW, Jones KK, Robbins RA, *et al.* Regional distribution of emphysema: correlation of high-resolution CT with pulmonary function tests in unselected smokers. *Radiology* 1992;**183**:457–63.

115. Gelb AF, Schein M, Kuei J, *et al.* Limited contribution of emphysema in advanced chronic obstructive pulmonary disease. *Am Rev Respir Dis* 1993;**147**:1157–61.

116. Wakayama K, Kurihara N, Fujimoto S, Hata M, Takeda T. Relationship between exercise capacity and the severity of emphysema as determined by high resolution CT. *Eur Respir J* 1993;**6**:1362–7.

117. Watanuki Y, Suzuki S, Nishikawa M, Miyashita A, Okubo T. Correlation of quantitative CT with selective alveolobronchogram and pulmonary function tests in emphysema. *Chest* 1994;**106**:806–13.

118. Sakai N, Mishima M, Nishimura K, Itoh H, Kuno K. An automated method to assess the distribution of low attenuation areas on chest CT scans in chronic pulmonary emphysema patients. *Chest* 1994;**106**:1319–25.

119. Crausman RS, Ferguson G, Irvin CG, Make B, Newell JD Jr. Quantitative chest computed tomography as a means of predicting exercise performance in severe emphysema. *Acad Radiol* 1995;**2**:463–9.

120. Beinert T, Brand P, Behr J, Vogelmeier C, Heyder J. Peripheral airspace dimensions in patients with COPD. *Chest* 1995;**108**:998–1003.

121. Betsuyaku T, Yoshioka A, Nishimura M, Miyamoto K, Kawakami Y. Pulmonary function is diminished in older asymptomatic smokers and ex-smokers with low attenuation areas on high-resolution computed tomography. *Respiration* 1996;**63**:333–8.

122. Loubeyre P, Paret M, Revel D, Wiesendanger T, Brune J. Thin-section CT detection of emphysema associated with bronchiectasis and correlation with pulmonary function tests. *Chest* 1996;**109**:360–5.

123. Eda S, Kubo K, Fujimoto K, Matsuzawa Y, Sekiguchi M, Sakai F. The relations between expiratory chest CT using helical CT and pulmonary function tests in emphysema. *Am J Respir Crit Care Med* 1997;**155**:1290–4.

124. Bae KT, Slone RM, Gierada DS, Yusen RD, Cooper JD. Patients with emphysema: quantitative CT analysis before and after lung volume reduction surgery. *Radiology* 1997;**203**:705–14.

125. Satoh K, Nakano S, Tanabe M, *et al.* A clinical comparison between Technegas SPECT, CT, and pulmonary function tests in patients with emphysema. *Radiation Med* 1997;**15**:277–82.

126. Haraguchi M, Shimura S, Hida W, Shirato K. Pulmonary function and regional distribution of emphysema as determined by high-resolution computed tomography. *Respiration* 1998;**65**:125–9.

127. Kauczor HU, Heussel CP, Fischer B, Klamm R, Mildenberger P, Thelen M. Assessment of lung volumes using helical CT at inspiration and expiration: comparison with pulmonary function tests. *AJR* 1998;**171**:1091–5.

128. Schwaiblmair M, Beinert T, Seemann M, Behr J, Reiser M, Vogelmeier C. Relations between cardiopulmonary exercise testing and quantitative high-resolution computed tomography associated in patients with alpha-1-antitrypsin deficiency. *Eur J Med Res* 1998;**3**:527–32.

129. Nakano Y, Sakai H, Muro S, *et al.* Comparison of low attenuation areas on computed tomographic scans between inner and outer segments of the lung in patients with chronic obstructive pulmonary disease: incidence and contribution to lung function. *Thorax* 1999;**54**:384–9.

130. Park KJ, Bergin CJ, Clausen JL. Quantitation of emphysema with three-dimensional CT densitometry: comparison with two-dimensional analysis, visual emphysema scores, and pulmonary function test results. *Radiology* 1999;**211**:541–7.

131. Mishima M, Hirai T, Itoh H, *et al.* Complexity of terminal airspace geometry assessed by lung computed tomography in normal subjects and patients with chronic obstructive pulmonary disease. *Proc Natl Acad Sci USA* 1999;**96**:8829–34.

132. Wilson JS, Galvin JR. Normal diffusing capacity in patients with PiZ alpha-antitrypsin deficiency, severe airflow obstruction, and significant radiographic emphysema. *Chest* 2000;**118**:867–71.

133. Gould GA, Redpath AT, Ryan M, *et al.* Parenchymal emphysema measured by CT lung density correlates with lung function in patients with bullous disease. *Eur Respir J* 1993;**6**:698–704.

134. Kalender WA, Fichte H, Bautz W, Skalej M. Semiautomatic evaluation procedures for quantitative CT of the lung. *J Comput Assist Tomogr* 1991;**15**:248–55.

135. Zagers R, Vrooman HA, Aarts NJ, *et al.* Quantitative analysis of computed tomography scans of the lungs for the diagnosis of pulmonary emphysema. A validation study of a semiautomated contour detection technique. *Invest Radiol* 1995;**30**:552–62.

136. Guenard H, Diallo MH, Laurent F, Vergeret J. Lung density and lung mass in emphysema. *Chest* 1992;**102**:198–203.

137. Heremans A, Verschakelen JA, Van Fraeyenhoven L, Demedts M. Measurement of lung density by means of quantitative CT scanning. A study of correlations with pulmonary function tests. *Chest* 1992;**102**:805–11.

138. Zagers H, Vrooman HA, Aarts NJ, *et al.* Assessment of the progression of emphysema by quantitative analysis of spirometrically gated computed tomography images. *Invest Radiol* 1996;**31**:761–7.

139. Rogers RM, Coxson HO, Sciurba FC, Keenan RJ, Whittall KP, Hogg JC. Preoperative severity of emphysema predictive of improvement after lung volume reduction surgery: use of CT morphometry. *Chest* 2000;**118**:1240–7.

140. Slone RM, Gierada DS. Radiology of pulmonary emphysema and lung volume reduction surgery. *Semin Thorac Cardiovasc Surg* 1996;**8**:61–82.

141. Hedlund LW, Vock P, Effmann EL. Computed tomography of the lung. Densitometric studies. *Radiol Clin North Am* 1983;**21**:775–88.

142. Kemerink GJ, Lamers RJ, Thelissen GR, van Engelshoven JM. CT densitometry of the lungs: scanner performance. *J Comput Assist Tomogr* 1996;**20**:24–33.

143. Kemerink GJ, Kruize HH, Lamers RJ, van Engelshoven JM. CT lung densitometry: dependence of CT number histograms on sample volume and consequences for scan protocol comparability. *J Comput Assist Tomogr* 1997;**21**:948–54.

144. Mishima M, Hirai T, Jin Z, *et al.* Standardization of low attenuation area versus total lung area in chest X-ray CT as an indicator of chronic pulmonary emphysema. *Front Med Biol Eng* 1997;**8**:79–86.

145. Stoel BC, Vrooman HA, Stolk J, Reiber JH. Sources of error in lung densitometry with CT. *Invest Radiol* 1999;**34**:303–9.

146. Robinson PJ, Kreel L. Pulmonary tissue attenuation with computed tomography: comparison of inspiration and expiration scans. *J Comput Assist Tomogr* 1979;**3**:740–8.

147. Rosenblum LJ, Mauceri RA, Wellenstein DE, *et al.* Density patterns in the normal lung as determined by computed tomography. *Radiology* 1980;**137**:409–16.

148. Perhomaa M, Jauhiainen J, Lahde S, Ojala A, Suramo I. CT lung densitometry in assessing intralobular air content. An experimental and clinical study. *Acta Radiol* 2000;**41**:242–8.

149. Levant MN, Bass H, Anthonisen N, Fraser RG. Microvascular circulation of the lungs in emphysema: correlation of results obtained with roentgenologic and radioactive-isotope techniques. *J Can Assoc Radiol* 1968;**19**:130–4.

150. Kalender WA, Rienmuller R, Seissler W, Behr J, Welke M, Fichte H. Measurement of pulmonary parenchymal attenuation: use of spirometric gating with quantitative CT. *Radiology* 1990;**175**:265–8.

151. Lamers RJ, Kemerink GJ, Drent M, van Engelshoven JM. Reproducibility of spirometrically controlled CT lung densitometry in a clinical setting. *Eur Respir J* 1998;**11**:942–5.

152. Kohz P, Stabler A, Beinert T, *et al.* Reproducibility of quantitative, spirometrically controlled CT. *Radiology* 1995;**197**:539–42.

153. Dirksen A, Friis M, Olesen KP, Skovgaard LT, Sorensen K. Progress of emphysema in severe alpha-1-antitrypsin deficiency as assessed by annual CT. *Acta Radiol* 1997;**38**:826–32.

154. Biernacki W, Ryan M, MacNee W, Flenley DC. Can the quantitative CT scan detect progression of emphysema. *Am Rev Respir Dis* 1989;**139**(suppl):A120.

155. Dirksen A, Dijkman JH, Madsen F, *et al.* A randomized clinical trial of alpha-1-antitrypsin augmentation therapy. *Am J Respir Crit Care Med* 1999;**160**:1468–72.

156. Soejima K, Yamaguchi K, Kohda E, *et al.* Longitudinal follow-up study of smoking-induced lung density changes by high-resolution computed tomography. *Am J Respir Crit Care Med* 2000;**161**:1264–73.

157. Gevenois PA, Scillia P, de Maertelaer V, Michils A, De Vuyst P, Yernault JC. The effects of age, sex, lung size, and hyperinflation on CT lung densitometry. *AJR* 1996;**167**: 1169–73.

158. Remy-Jardin M, Remy J, Boulenguez C, Sobaszek A, Edme JL, Furon D. Morphologic effects of cigarette smoking on airways and pulmonary parenchyma in healthy adult volunteers: CT evaluation and correlation with pulmonary function tests. *Radiology* 1993;**186**: 107–15.

159. Remy-Jardin M, Remy J, Gosselin B, Becette V, Edme JL. Lung parenchymal changes secondary to cigarette smoking: pathologic-CT correlations. *Radiology* 1993;**186**:643–51.

160. Collins J, Blankenbaker D, Stern EJ. CT patterns of bronchiolar disease: what is 'tree-in-bud'? *AJR* 1998; **171**:365–70.

161. Ng CS, Desai SR, Rubens MB, Padley SP, Wells AU, Hansell DM. Visual quantitation and observer variation of signs of small airways disease at inspiratory and expiratory CT. *J Thorac Imaging* 1999;**14**:279–85.

162. Sutherland GR, Hume R, James WB, Davison M, Kennedy J. Correlation of regional densitometry patterns, radiological appearances, and pulmonary function tests in chronic bronchitis and emphysema. *Thorax* 1971;**26**:716–20.

163. Snider GL. CT and COPD. *Am J Respir Crit Care Med* 1994; **149**:552–3.

164. Nakano Y, Muro S, Sakai H, *et al.* Computed tomographic measurements of airway dimensions and emphysema in smokers. Correlation with lung function. *Am J Respir Crit Care Med* 2000;**162**:1102–8.

165. King GG, Müller NL, Pare PD. Evaluation of airways in obstructive pulmonary disease using high-resolution computed tomography. *Am J Respir Crit Care Med* 1999; **159**:992–1004.

166. Worthy SA, Müller NL. Small airway diseases. *Radiol Clin North Am* 1998;**36**:163–73 [review].

167. Moon J, du Bois RM, Colby TV, Hansell DM, Nicholson AG. Clinical significance of respiratory bronchiolitis on open lung biopsy and its relationship to smoking related interstitial lung disease. *Thorax* 1999;**54**:1009–14.

168. Holt RM, Schmidt RA, Godwin JD, Raghu G. High resolution CT in respiratory bronchiolitis-associated interstitial lung disease. *J Comput Assist Tomogr* 1993;**17**:46–50.

169. Heyneman LE, Ward S, Lynch DA, Remy Jardin M, Johkoh T, Müller NL. Respiratory bronchiolitis, respiratory bronchiolitis-associated interstitial lung disease, and desquamative interstitial pneumonia: different entities or part of the spectrum of the same disease process? *AJR* 1999;**173**:1617–22.

170. Stern EJ, Webb WR, Gamsu G. Dynamic quantitative computed tomography. A predictor of pulmonary function in obstructive lung diseases. *Invest Radiol* 1994;**29**:564–9.

171. Lucidarme O, Coche E, Cluzel P, Mourey Gerosa I, Howarth N, Grenier P. Expiratory CT scans for chronic airway disease: correlation with pulmonary function test results. *AJR* 1998;**170**:301–7.

172. Chen D, Webb WR, Storto ML, Lee KN. Assessment of air trapping using postexpiratory high-resolution computed tomography. *J Thorac Imaging* 1998;**13**:135–43.

173. Verschakelen JA, Scheinbaum K, Bogaert J, Demedts M, Lacquet LL, Baert AL. Expiratory CT in cigarette smokers: correlation between areas of decreased lung attenuation, pulmonary function tests and smoking history. *Eur Radiol* 1998;**8**:1391–9.

174. Lee KW, Chung SY, Yang I, Lee Y, Ko EY, Park MJ. Correlation of aging and smoking with air trapping at thin-section CT of the lung in asymptomatic subjects. *Radiology* 2000;**214**: 831–6.

175. Stern EJ, Frank MS. Small-airway diseases of the lungs: findings at expiratory CT. *AJR* 1994;**163**:37–41.

176. Wong You Cheong JJ, Leahy BC, Taylor PM, Church SE. Airways obstruction and bronchiectasis: correlation with duration of symptoms and extent of bronchiectasis on computed tomography. *Clin Radiol* 1992;**45**: 256–9.

177. Lynch DA, Newell J, Hale V, *et al.* Correlation of CT findings with clinical evaluations in 261 patients with symptomatic bronchiectasis. *AJR* 1999;**173**:53–8.

178. Roberts HR, Wells AU, Milne DG, *et al.* Airflow obstruction in bronchiectasis: correlation between computed tomography features and pulmonary function tests. *Thorax* 2000;**55**:198–204.

179. O'Brien C, Guest PJ, Hill SL, Stockley RA. Physiological and radiological characterisation of patients diagnosed with chronic obstructive pulmonary disease in primary care. *Thorax* 2000;**55**:635–42.

180. Eriksson S. Studies in alpha-1 antitrypsin deficiency. *Acta Med Scand* 1965;**177**:1–85.

181. King MA, Stone JA, Diaz PT, Mueller CF, Becker WJ, Gadek JE. Alpha-1-antitrypsin deficiency: evaluation of bronchiectasis with CT. *Radiology* 1996;**199**:137–41.

182. Cuvelier A, Muir JF, Hellot MF, *et al.* Distribution of alpha-antitrypsin alleles in patients with bronchiectasis. *Chest* 2000;**117**:415–19.

183. Suga K, Tsukuda T, Awaya H, *et al.* Impaired respiratory mechanics in pulmonary emphysema: evaluation with dynamic breathing MRI. *J Magn Reson Imaging* 1999;**10**: 510–20.

184. Gierada DS, Hakimian S, Slone RM, Yusen RD. MR analysis of lung volume and thoracic dimensions in patients with emphysema before and after lung volume reduction surgery. *AJR* 1998;**170**:707–14.

185. Cleverley JR, Hansell DM. Imaging of patients with severe emphysema considered for lung volume reduction surgery. *Br J Radiol* 1999;**72**:227–35.

186. Kauczor HU, Ebert M, Kreitner KF, *et al.* Imaging of the lungs using ^{3}He MRI: preliminary clinical experience in 18 patients with and without lung disease. *J Magn Reson Imaging* 1997;**7**:538–43.

187. de Lange EE, Mugler JP 3rd, Brookeman JR, *et al.* Lung air spaces: MR imaging evaluation with hyperpolarized ^{3}He gas. *Radiology* 1999;**210**:851–7.

188. Alderson PO, Secker Walker RH, Forrest JV. Detection of obstructive pulmonary disease. Relative sensitivity of ventilation-perfusion studies and chest radiography. *Radiology* 1974;**112**:643–8.

189. Cleverley JR, Desai SR, Wells AU, *et al.* Evaluation of patients undergoing lung volume reduction

surgery: ancillary information available from computed tomography. *Clin Radiol* 2000;**55**:45–50.

190. Satoh K, Takahashi K, Kobayashi T, Yamamoto Y, Nishiyama Y, Tanabe M. The usefulness of [99 m]Tc-Technegas scintigraphy for diagnosing pulmonary impairment caused by pulmonary emphysema. *Acta Med Okayama* 1998;**52**:97–103.

191. McKenna RJ Jr, Brenner M, Fischel RJ, *et al.* Patient selection criteria for lung volume reduction surgery. *J Thorac Cardiovasc Surg* 1997;**114**:957–64;discussion 964–7.

192. Thurnheer R, Engel H, Weder W, *et al.* Role of lung perfusion scintigraphy in relation to chest computed tomography and pulmonary function in the evaluation of candidates for lung volume reduction surgery. *Am J Respir Crit Care Med* 1999;**159**:301–10.

193. Salzman SH. Can CT measurement of emphysema severity aid patient selection for lung volume reduction surgery? *Chest* 2000;**118**:1231–2.

194. Jamadar DA, Kazerooni EA, Tinez FJ, Wahl RL. Semi-quantitative ventilation/perfusion scintigraphy and single-photon emission tomography for evaluation of lung volume reduction surgery candidates: description and prediction of clinical outcome. *Eur J Nucl Med* 1999;**26**: 734–42.

22

Smoking cessation

STEPHEN I RENNARD AND DAVID M DAUGHTON

INTRODUCTION

While not the only risk factor for the development of COPD, cigarette smoking is far and away the most important risk factor.[1–3] Between 80 and 90% of US patients with COPD are current or former smokers.[4] In addition, passive smoke exposure may contribute to the development of COPD in the 10–20% of non-smokers who develop COPD.[5] Other factors clearly play a role. There is, moreover, marked individual susceptibility to the effects of cigarette smoke. The 10–15% of smokers who are most susceptible were traditionally regarded as those who developed COPD.[1] It is clear, however, that on average most smokers will show evidence of lung damage and physiologic compromise.[6] While often undiagnosed, these patients have increased mortality[7] and may be more symptomatic than traditionally believed. Eliminating cigarette smoking, therefore, is the most important intervention for the prevention of COPD and for the slowing of its progression.

The traditional view that cigarette smoking represents a 'lifestyle choice' has been replaced with the concept that cigarette smoking should be regarded as a primary disease.[8] In this context, COPD can be regarded as one of the many secondary complications of the primary disorder: cigarette smoking. The best results in dealing with this disease are currently obtained with a multifaceted, multidisciplinary approach including sociopolitical strategies, public health interventions and behavioral and pharmacologic treatments. The individual smoker, moreover, should be regarded as having a chronic relapsing disorder, and each smoking cessation attempt should be regarded as an attempt to induce a long-term remission. Currently available strategies to treat smoking cessation can have a major impact in facilitating cessation with a corresponding impact on the many diseases including the COPD from which many smokers will suffer.

SMOKING AS AN ADDICTION

Cigarette smoke contains more than 6000 chemical moieties and its composition varies with the type of cigarette and how it is smoked.[9,10] The most important addicting substance in cigarette smoke is nicotine,[11] although other psychoactive compounds are also present and may contribute to cigarette smoking. When a cigarette is smoked, air is inhaled through the burning tobacco at the end of the cigarette.[12] This heats the air so that as it passes over the unburned tobacco more proximally in the cigarette rod it causes the nicotine present to volatilize. As the airstream cools, this nicotine vapour condenses on the particles of smoke generated in the burning process. This results in a nicotine-containing aerosol of very small particle size which delivers nicotine with considerable efficiency to the alveolar space. Nicotine is lipid soluble and, as a result, rapidly diffuses across the alveolar wall into the pulmonary capillary blood. It is then transported through the arterial circulation and to the body. Upon reaching the brain, nicotine can interact with nicotinic receptors and can induce a variety of physiologic responses. Cigarette smoking, because it delivers nicotine as a bolus, is particularly potent from an addiction perspective.[13,14] Specifically, the euphoria induced by addicting drugs and the biological alterations thought to underlie addiction are believed to depend on both the amount of drug that reaches the relevant receptors in the brain and on the pharmacokinetics of delivery. Boluses with rapid rises are believed to be much more potent than are similar amounts of drug delivered gradually.[15] These aspects of nicotine pharmacokinetics are relevant when considering nicotine replacement as a form of treatment for nicotine addiction (see below).

Nicotine exerts a number of psychoactive effects. It causes a sensation of euphoria which, in a blinded controlled trial, was similar in magnitude to the euphoria experienced when drug-experienced volunteers received cocaine or morphine.[14] Nicotine also has a modest antidepressant effect.[16,17] Other components present in cigarette smoke may contribute to altered mood in smokers. At least one substance that is not nicotine, which is contained in cigarette smoke, has been demonstrated to have monoamine oxidase inhibitory activity.[18] Nicotine can, in addition, have an effect on cognitive function. Nicotine improves performance of tasks requiring attention to detail in relatively unstimulating situations.[19,20] Nicotine may also partially ameliorate some of the cognitive disturbances present in schizophrenics.[21,22] Cigarette smoking, likely involving more than nicotine alone, can also affect appetite and result in a modest weight loss.[23] Smokers vary in their reasons for smoking, but many or all of these psychoactive effects may contribute.

Neurones present in the mesolimbic system with projections into the nucleus accumbens are believed to play a particularly important role in the addiction process.[24–26] These neurones utilize dopamine as a neurotransmitter. Nicotinic receptors on the axons of these neurons are capable of modulating dopamine release, an action that is similar to the effects of opiates. Interestingly, cocaine and norepinephrine (noradrenaline) are also able to modulate dopaminergic transmission by displacing dopamine from its storage vesicles or by inhibiting its reuptake.[27] It is believed that all these drugs of addiction co-opt similar neuropathways involved in learning complex behaviors.[24–26] Like other addicting drugs, nicotine alters the expression of its own receptors.[28,29] These effects can be exceedingly long lasting. In animal models, fetal exposures result in alterations in brain nicotinic receptors that persist well after birth.[30,31] Similarly, smokers have altered nicotinic receptor expression, and these persist for long periods following cessation.[32]

Most smokers begin smoking before reaching adulthood. Some begin smoking before adolescence. In the USA, peak smoking initiation rates occur between the ages of 13 and 18.[33,34] A number of factors can influence smoking initiation. These include the availability of cigarettes, the images associated with smoking,[35,36] the

number of smokers at home and smoking behavior among peers.[37,38] All of these may be amenable to interventions, and efforts to control advertising[35,39] and to restrict access[40] may be of benefit, though there is some controversy about the latter.[41,42] That social factors can have a major effect is demonstrated by Utah, a state with a large population of Latter Day Saints who eschew smoking. This state has the lowest smoking initiation and smoking prevalence rates in the USA.[34] Efforts at decreasing cigarette availability through restricted access and through increased price can also have an impact.[43] While smoking is clearly an addiction, increasing cigarette prices decreases cigarette usage. This may be associated with more efficient smoking of the remaining cigarettes. However, in Canada, increasing the cigarette price nearly threefold resulted in a reduction of approximately 60% in the number of adolescents smoking (Figure 22.1).[43]

In the USA, approximately three-quarters of adolescents will experiment with cigarettes.[34,44] Less than half will become regular smokers. While studies vary, about half of the variance in smoking behavior is believed to be on a social and environmental basis and about half of the variance is due to genetic factors.[45–48] Evidence supporting a genetic basis for cigarette smoking derives from twin studies,[45–48] from association studies with candidate genes, although there remains no clear consensus on the role of any gene as yet,[27,49–55] and from animal studies.[56,57] Twin studies support a genetic effect on both smoking initiation and on smoking maintenance.[45–48] Several candidate genes have been associated with cigarette smoking behavior,[27] including several involved in dopamine metabolism. Specifically, polymorphisms in the D2, D4 and D5 dopamine receptors and in the dopamine transporter have been associated with smoking. The polymorphism in the mixed function oxidase CYP2A6 has also been associated with smoking.[53]

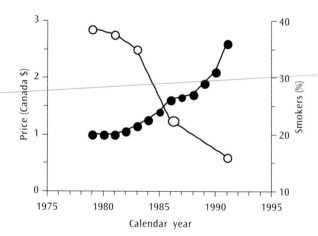

Figure 22.1 *Effect of price increase on smoking prevalence in Canadian children age 15–19. (Adapted from ref. 43.)*

CYP2A6 is the major enzyme that catabolizes nicotine into cotinine. Individuals with a null mutation for this gene metabolize nicotine more slowly and are less likely to become smokers. It is believed that these slower metabolizers are more likely to become nicotine toxic and, therefore, it is more difficult for them to 'learn' how to smoke. If such individuals do become smokers, interestingly, they smoke significantly fewer cigarettes than individuals with higher rates of CYP2A6 expression, and smoke those cigarettes less completely.[58] As a result, they may be at less risk to develop smoke-induced disease.[59] The genetic bases which underlie cigarette smoking are as yet incompletely defined.[53,60] It is estimated that as many 50 genes may contribute to the 50% of smoking behavior variance which appears to be accounted for in a genetic basis based on twin studies.[61,62] It is unlikely that any single gene, however, will account for more than 3–5% of this variance.

A significant minority, approximately 10–15%, of smokers in the USA, do not appear to be addicted.[63,64] These individuals smoke cigarettes in social situations, but may not smoke every day. On days on which they do not smoke, they do not experience withdrawal symptoms. The majority of smokers, however, among the other reasons for which they might smoke, are addicted to nicotine. Upon withdrawal, they experience a well-defined syndrome with recognizable symptoms (Table 22.1).[65] These symptoms are often most intense beginning the day after cessation and begin to ebb after a week or two. Some symptoms, particularly craving to smoke, can recur, often long after quitting and after other withdrawal symptoms have resolved. These urges have been described as resembling grief responses. That is, a smoker, particularly in situations where cues previously associated with smoking are present, will experience intense urges and cravings to smoke. The intensity of these sensations does not decrease as much with time as the frequency does. Smoking, of course, relieves these cravings, though they will also resolve in the absence of smoking. Cravings, as might be expected, are strongly associated with relapse.[66]

While the majority of smokers are addicted, many smokers smoke for reasons in addition to nicotine addiction.[67] As well as the physiological effects described above, which may be perceived as benefits by some smokers, the taste of cigarettes is also important. This and a variety of other factors, including advertising, contribute to brand preference.[68–71] This is well recognized by tobacco manufacturers who use advertising to create brand loyalty with a variety of images. Smokers, however, tend to show a modest ability to distinguish their cigarette from other brands,[72] and this likely contributes, in part, to brand loyalty. If nicotine addiction were the only reason driving smoking, such issues would be relatively unimportant in brand choice.

Just as smoking initiation rates peak in adolescence and decline in adulthood, smoking cessation rates increase with increasing age throughout adulthood.[73–75] Whether this reflects varying levels of commitment and motivation which are changing with age or reflects a biological basis is unknown. It is of interest, however, that expression of the dopaminergic receptors peaks in adolescence and then declines with increasing age, suggesting possible age-related mechanisms for susceptibility to smoking and to cessation.[76–78]

A clinician faced with a patient who is smoking, therefore, needs to recognize that smoking is a very complex disorder. Individuals vary in their susceptibility to the psychoactive and addicting effects of cigarette smoking. They differ in their psychosocial attitudes toward smoking and in their motivation to quit. By recognizing the complex factors which interact in driving smoking behavior, the clinician can be most effective in attempting to eliminate smoking and the associated risks to health.

METHODS FOR SMOKING CESSATION

General approach

As noted above, cigarette smoking should be regarded as the primary disorder. Recommendations from the Department of Health and Human Services in the USA suggest that cigarette smoking should be regarded as a 'vital sign' (Figure 22.2)[8,79] and that every smoker's

Table 22.1 *Nicotine withdrawal symptoms*

Dysphoric or depressed mood
Insomnia
Irritability, frustration or anger
Anxiety
Difficulty concentrating
Restlessness
Decreased heart rate
Increased appetite or weight gain

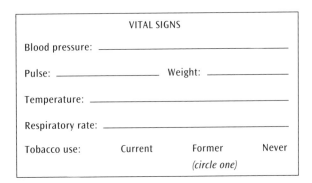

Figure 22.2 *Smoking as a vital sign. (Reproduced from ref. 8 with permission.)*

Table 22.2 *Classes of patients requiring special considerations*

Class of patient	Considerations
Gender and race	Approaches should be similar for men and women and for various races
Pregnancy	The pregnant smoker should be encouraged to quit. Behavioral approaches are recommended. Pharmacologic support can be offered if the benefits are felt to outweigh the risks. (Level of evidence* = C)
Hospitalized smokers	Smoking cessation can be offered in the hospital where it can be effective. (Level of evidence = B)
Adolescents	Similar approaches to those used in adults are recommended. However, evidence that they are effective is limited. (Level of evidence = C)
Older smokers	Smoking cessation is of benefit in the elderly. Such smokers should be offered interventions with demonstrated efficacy. (Level of evidence = A)
Patients with cardiac disease	Concurrent smoking and use of nicotine replacement was not found to be associated with increased incidence of acute myocardial events[156,157] and may improve performance.[158] Cardiac disease is not, therefore, a contraindication to use of pharmacologic support for smoking cessation.

Levels of evidence:
A: Multiple well-designed randomized clinical trials, directly relevant to the recommendation, yielded a consistent pattern of findings;
B: Some evidence from randomized clinical trials supported the recommendation, but the scientific support was not optimal.
For instance, few randomized trials existed, the trials that did exist were somewhat inconsistent, or the trials were not directly relevant to the recommendation; C: Reserved for important clinical situations where the panel achieved consensus on the recommendation in the absence of relevant randomized controlled trials.
*As assessed in the DHHS guideline.[8]

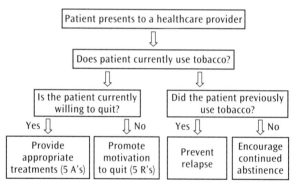

Figure 22.3 *Flow chart for a 'systems' approach to smoking. For an explanation of the 5 R's and 5 A's see Tables 22.3 and 22.4 respectively. (Reproduced from ref. 8 with permission.)*

Table 22.3 *The 5 R's: to motivate smokers unwilling to make a quit attempt at the present time*

Relevance	Tailor advice and discussion to each smoker
Risks	Outline risks of continued smoking
Rewards	Outline the benefits of quitting
Roadblocks	Identify barriers to quitting
Repetition	Reinforce the motivational message at every visit

smoking status should be assessed at every visit. An individualized approach to smoking should then be undertaken at every visit. As with all medical interventions, there are classes of patients for whom special considerations exist (Table 22.2). Appropriate interaction on the part of the physician can be accomplished in a very brief interval, often less than 1 minute. It is currently believed that continued repetition of messages related to smoking cessation is essential in obtaining best results. Integration of a proactive program to identify, classify and provide appropriate support for smoking control efforts should be a part of all healthcare delivery systems. A suggested paradigm is indicated in Figure 22.3.

Smokers are categorized as 'current', 'former' or 'lifelong non-smokers'.

Non-smokers are encouraged to remain abstinent. Some individuals, particularly adolescents, with an appropriate history of risks, for example, the presence of smokers in the household, smoking peers, etc. may offer the opportunity for smoking-initiation prophylaxis.

For individuals who are former smokers but have quit, continued abstinence should be encouraged. Support to prevent relapse should be provided (see below).

Individuals currently smoking should be categorized as those willing to make a quit attempt and those unwilling to do so.

Those unready to make a quit attempt should be offered encouragement. The 5 R's (Table 22.3) can serve as a guide to help motivate smokers toward making a quit attempt. As noted above, it is believed that a smoker's decision to

Table 22.4 *The 5 A's: for smokers willing to quit*

Ask	about tobacco use
Advise	to quit
Assess	willingness to make a quit attempt
Assist	in quit attempt
Arrange	for follow-up

make a quit attempt develops incrementally over time, and continued repetition of an anti-smoking message is important. In addition, it is likely that motivation to quit smoking varies with other health-related events. Intercurrent illness, for example, may be an important motivating factor,[80,81] and the astute clinician can exploit these windows of opportunity to help facilitate smoking cessation.

For smokers willing to make a quit attempt, several specific interventions should be offered. Current guidelines recommend a strategy that will optimize success from each serious quit attempt. To this end, behavioral support, pharmacologic treatment and follow-up have all been documented to improve quit rates, and all should, ideally, be offered.

Treatment of the smoker willing to quit

BEHAVIORAL SUPPORT

Even modest forms of behavioral support can greatly increase quit rates.[8] While the effect is small, simple physician recommendation to quit can more than double quit rates from the spontaneous rate of 2% to 4–6% and should always be offered.[8,82–85] Encouragement and support of cessation efforts from other healthcare providers and from members of the general community also aid in quit attempts.[8] Simple behavioral support recommendations, termed the 5 A's, have been developed by the National Cancer Institute in the USA and are currently recommended by the DHHS guidelines and endorsed by the British Thoracic Society (Table 22.4). These simple interventions should be integrated into other smoking cessation efforts. In particular, follow-up of all individuals making a serious quit attempt is highly recommended and has been shown to improve quit rates.[8]

A number of studies have evaluated the role of more intense behavioral interventions. A series of meta-analyses provides support for increasing effectiveness of more intense programs.[86] All smokers should therefore be offered participation in more intense behavioral programs. Those willing to consider such interventions should be encouraged to do so. Such programs can achieve quit rates of up to 20% among those who attend, and quit rates can be increased with the use of pharmacologic support.[84,87] The majority of smokers making a

quit attempt, however, will decline participation in such programs and will be dependent on the behavioral interventions offered by the healthcare provider. Support from both physician and non-physician providers is clearly beneficial. Training a range of personnel involved in patient contact in smoking cessation methods is recommended.[8]

Key features which can help individual smokers with quit attempts include:

- Set a target quit day within a 30-day period. Remind the smoker that quitting smoking is not a 1-day event. Use a calendar to guide the smoker to select a target quit day that is not followed by a major social or stress event for a 3-week period.
- Encourage the smoker to enlist support by enroling in a stop smoking programme or by contacting a friend.
- Review prior stop smoking attempts. Use the information to guide coping strategies and to evaluate whether the smoker would most likely benefit from a pharmaceutical aid to quitting smoking.
- Emphasize that total cessation is essential. Tobacco withdrawal symptoms are temporary for smokers who quit and who do not smoke a single puff.
- Prepare the smoker for the quit day and for the first weeks of quitting. Advise them to:
  - Discard all cigarettes, lighters and ash trays from the home, workplace and car prior to arising on the target quit day.
  - Keep cigarette substitutes handy: gum, candy, straws, carrot sticks, etc.
  - Avoid situations where people smoke and avoid or limit alcohol use until urges have greatly diminished.
  - Plan on using the five D's (Delay, Deep breathing, Drink water, Do something else, Distract yourself) when the urge to smoke is intolerable. Emphasize that the urge will remit whether they smoke or not.
  - Quit one day at a time. Some smokers become overwhelmed by the prospect of quitting for the rest of their lives. Quitting day by day is a realistic and achievable goal.
  - Schedule a follow-up contact within 1 week of the quit day.

Free telephone counseling to help smokers quit is now provided in many locations. Several studies support the efficacy of this type of intervention.[88,89] Follow-up of smokers by mail may also improve quit rates.[90] The general principle seems to be that the more involved the healthcare provider, and the more active the contact, the greater the success, particularly in preventing relapse.[91]

Tapering versus 'cold turkey'

Current recommendations suggest that abrupt smoking cessation is most effective. A number of smokers will, however, prefer to reduce the amount of smoking prior to making a quit attempt. Some data exist that support such an approach.[92,93] Abrupt abstinence, however, is the method that has been used in the development of pharmacologic support for smoking cessation (see below).

Other behavioral approaches

A range of techniques have been offered as aids to smoking cessation.[8,84,94] These include aversive therapies, hypnosis, acupuncture and a large number of other modalities. No data supporting their effectiveness beyond that of behavioral support exist. Obviously the goal is to quit smoking. Individuals who achieve abstinence with any modality should be encouraged to remain abstinent.

Psychiatric co-morbidity

As noted above, nicotine and other components in cigarette smoke have a number of potent psychoactive effects. Individuals with severe depression have a very high prevalence of cigarette smoking.[95] It is thought that many may smoke, at least in part, as an attempt to self-medicate their dysphoric mood. Similarly, schizophrenics have a very high smoking prevalence.[96] Nicotine, in this context, may have effects that affect disordered thought patterns.[21,22] Recognition of proper diagnosis and initiation of appropriate treatment of psychiatric co-morbidities may be essential prior to making an attempt at smoking cessation.

PHARMACOLOGIC SUPPORT

Nicotine replacement

Symptoms of nicotine withdrawal are believed to develop when nicotine levels fall below threshold level. Nicotine replacement as an aid to smoking cessation is based on the concept of providing steady-state nicotine levels to mitigate the symptoms of withdrawal. A smoker can, therefore, become abstinent and deal with the various psychological effects of becoming a non-smoker. Often this will require adoption of specific behavioral strategies for situations of high risk. Nicotine replacement formulations do not provide nicotine with the same bolus effect as does a cigarette. As a result, it is believed that nicotine replacement may not support the cellular and biochemical effects that maintain the addicted state as efficiently.

Five formulations of nicotine replacement have been approved, and several others are under development. These differ in their mode of administration and in their pharmacokinetics. All forms of nicotine replacement have similar efficacy in clinical trials.[8] All approximately double quit rates when compared to a placebo. Placebo quit rates, however, vary among studies. This likely reflects both patient selection, with some studies including patients who are less motivated to quit, as well as the intensity of the accompanying behavioral program.

The availability of multiple modalities creates several opportunities for the clinician. First, some individuals may prefer one form of nicotine administration.[97] Second, for individuals who fail or who relapse with one formulation, a second formulation can be tried. Third, the transdermal nicotine patch administers nicotine continuously. This may be of advantage for selected individuals. Alternatively, the other formulations administer nicotine upon dosing. This allows some degree of individual control both of the total dose and of the time of delivery. This may also offer advantages for selected individuals. Finally, it is possible to combine various nicotine formulations.[98] Combinations of transdermal nicotine systems with a nicotine inhaler, with nicotine nasal spray and with nicotine gum have been reported to be associated with improved quit rates.[99–101] Use of such combinations in individually tailored programs is often used by clinicians with experience in these medications, although these combinations have not been approved by drug registration agencies. Their use is recognized by guidelines, however.

Transdermal nicotine systems

The transdermal nicotine system or 'patch' is applied to the skin in a non-hairy area of the torso or proximal area of the extremities. Each device contains an adhesive, a reservoir which contains nicotine and an impermeant backing. Nicotine diffuses from the reservoir through the skin and is absorbed in the capillary blood of the skin. Absorption is continuous and relatively slow. Several formulations are available.[102] Some devices were approved for continuous usage with a new patch being applied every day. One system was evaluated with daytime use, being removed each night. The patch delivers nicotine very slowly. The high-dose patches (21 mg delivered per 24 hours) results in blood levels of approximately 20 ng/ml, roughly half that during steady state in a 30-cigarette per day smoker.[103] Transdermal nicotine reduces the intensity, but does not eliminate withdrawal symptoms.[104] Administration throughout the night provides for a morning blood level of nicotine, a feature of no other nicotine replacement formulation. This may help reduce early-morning cravings. Administration throughout the night, however, is also associated with vivid dreams. While not a problem for many individuals, these may require discontinuation of nocturnal administration. Other adverse affects associated with the transdermal nicotine systems are related to local irritation from the device (which should be rotated) and to allergic reactions. After use, the transdermal nicotine system still contains a considerable amount of nicotine. It should, therefore, be removed, as application of a second device can result in overdose.

Treatment with nicotine patches is generally recommended at 'full dose' for 4–6 weeks. This is often followed by a tapering regimen for several additional weeks. Use of the patch for longer periods of time, for example 22 weeks, has not demonstrated improved quit rates, although there may be benefits of use for longer intervals than tested in clinical trial, at least in selected individuals.[105] Use of higher-dose patches or patches in combination was not found to be effective in clinical trials, but has been recommended in selected individuals by some experts and may benefit some individuals.[106] Because of the ease of application, transdermal nicotine systems may be more effective in primary practice settings than is nicotine 'polacrilex'.

Chronic use of transdermal nicotine systems has not been reported.

Nicotine polacrilex

Nicotine polacrilex (gum) contains nicotine bound to a polacrilex resin together with a buffering agent. Chewing releases the nicotine from the polacrilex. Varying the rate of chewing varies the rate of nicotine release. Once released, nicotine is present in the saliva and is absorbed across the buccal mucosa. Low oral pH causes nicotine base to ionize, and the charged form is absorbed much more slowly. Acidic foods and beverages, therefore, should be avoided when using the gum. In addition, following chewing, the saliva must be allowed to remain in the mouth so that nicotine can be absorbed through the buccal mucosa. If swallowed, nicotine can cause gastric discomfort and hiccups. Nicotine will be absorbed from the gastro-intestinal tract, but first-pass metabolism in the liver prevents effective absorption into the systemic circulation. Nicotine polacrilex is also associated with other local side effects. The gum can traumatize dental appliances, and the chewing can be a problem for individuals with temporomandibular joint problems. Two-milligram and 4-mg gum formulations are available.[107,108] Heavier smokers who are highly dependent may benefit from the higher-dose formulation.

Two chewing regimens have been recommended.[8] Scheduled chewing of at least 10 gums per day may be associated with higher quit rates. Many smokers, however, will chew the gum on an as-needed basis. This can also be effective. Gum use is usually recommended for 3–6 months. Some individuals remain abstinent from smoking but continue to use gum over extended periods of time. Clearly nicotine gum can sustain the addiction in these individuals. Some individuals may use the gum to provide nicotine when in a smoke-free environment.[109] Hazards of such use are not defined. It is unlikely, however, that such use will lead to cessation.

Nicotine inhaler

The nicotine inhaler consists of a mouthpiece and a nicotine-containing cartridge.[110,111] Nicotine is released when air is inhaled through the device. Most of the nicotine is deposited in the mouth and absorbed through the buccal mucosa. The device should not, therefore, be inhaled like a cigarette as very little nicotine will reach the lower respiratory tract. Because the nicotine is absorbed through the buccal mucosa, absorption is into the venous circulation. The device contains about 10 mg of nicotine of which about 1 mg is released with approximately 100 inhalations. As a result, nicotine absorption is relatively slow. Ad lib. use of the nicotine inhaler results in blood levels approximately one-third those of average smokers consuming 30 cigarettes daily. Local irritation in the mouth and throat is common, particularly during early stages of use.

Nicotine nasal spray

The nicotine nasal spray consists of an aqueous solution of nicotine. It is delivered by direct spray to the nasal mucosa.[112,113] One spray in each nostril delivers 1 mg of nicotine. The nicotine is absorbed into the venous blood in the nasal mucosa. Absorption, however, is relatively rapid with peak levels being achieved in approximately 10 minutes. This comes closest to that observed with smoking. As a result, the nicotine nasal spray has increased potential for prolonging nicotine dependence as compared to other nicotine-replacement therapies. Local irritation is exceedingly common and can be severe, although most individuals are able to adjust to the local effects with continued use. Asthma exacerbation has been associated with nicotine nasal spray use and caution should be used when prescribing it to asthmatics.[114]

Nicotine lozenges

The most recently approved formulation of nicotine as an aid for smoking cessation is the nicotine lozenge.[115] It is approved for over-the-counter use in the USA and is available in 2- and 4-mg nicotine doses. The smoker is allowed to select the dose based on the time from awakening to the first cigarette, a measure of intensity of addiction. Those who use a cigarette within 30 minutes of awakening are advised to use the 4-mg nicotine dose. Dosing is recommended at 9 lozenges per day, one every 1–2 hours for up to 6 weeks followed by tapering of daily use with discontinuation after 6 months.

Bupropion

Bupropion is the only non-nicotine medication currently approved for use as an aid in smoking cessation. Bupropion has been used as an antidepressant since 1989. Its mechanism of action is believed to be through enhancing central nervous system dopaminergic and noradrenergic signaling. Following the empirical observation that depressed patients treated with bupropion lost their craving for cigarettes, it was tested and found to be efficacious as an aid to smoking cessation.[116,117] The slow-release formulation of bupropion is generally used for smoking cessation. The medication is started at 150 mg daily for 5 days and, if tolerated, is increased to 150 mg twice daily. After 1 week of treatment, the smoker should quit. Treatment is then continued for several months. Long-term treatment with bupropion may be associated with reduced relapse rates and with reduced weight gain following smoking cessation. Bupropion may also have advantages in treating smokers with a history of depression.[118] These individuals are often refractory to behavioral interventions and, in one study, were less benefited by nicotine replacement than by bupropion. Bupropion can be combined with nicotine replacement therapy,[117] and this can result in an improved rate of abstinence. Adverse effects include dry mouth and insomnia. Bupropion lowers seizure threshold and should not be used in individuals who are at increased risk for seizures, who have a pre-existing seizure disorder, anorexia or bulimia. In some countries, bupropion is available under two tradenames. Individuals concurrently treated with bupropion for depression should not receive additional bupropion for smoking cessation as overdose is possible.

Other pharmacologic therapies

Clonidine Clonidine is a hypotensive drug that acts on central nervous system noradrenergic pathways. Several controlled clinical trials have been performed following initial reports of its utility in smoking cessation. A meta-analysis of these trials has suggested efficacy.[119] It is recommended as a second-line option (off label) in the DHHS guidelines. The most common adverse effects include drowsiness, fatigue, dry mouth and postural hypotension.

Antidepressants A number of antidepressants have been assessed as aids in smoking cessation.[8,120] This should be distinguished from treating concurrent depression which may be important in selected individuals as a therapeutic goal in and of itself. When assessed specifically to aid smoking cessation, only nortriptyline,[121,122] a tricyclic antidepressant, has consistently been reported to be of benefit. Interestingly, two MAO inhibitors, moclobamide[123] and laxabemide,[124] have also been reported to be of benefit. Data relating to these agents, however, are limited, and neither is approved or recommended for use in smoking cessation. The DHHS guidelines suggest nortriptyline may be considered as a second-line treatment. Anxiolytic drugs have not shown dramatic effects.[120] A number of trials have been conducted with buspirone and while some have shown potential short-term benefits, these have been inconsistent. Such agents may be considered for individuals who experience considerable anxiety as part of their withdrawal syndrome.

Naloxone and naltrexone, opiate antagonists, have not been of benefit. Amphetamines may increase smoking behavior.[125]

Agents in evaluation

Clinical trials with novel smoking cessation modalities are currently in progress. One strategy is to utilize nicotine antagonists such as mecamylamine.[126,127] The concept is that the nicotine antagonist will block the effect of nicotine and thus prevent a smoker from becoming re-addicted when tempted during a potential relapse. The same strategy underlies the potential use of nicotine vaccines.[128,129] Agents acting on other receptors in the central nervous system are also being evaluated.[130] Whether any of these agents will prove safe and effective remains to be determined. It is likely, however, that there will be additional types of pharmacologic support for smoking cessation in the future.

HAZARDS OF SMOKING CESSATION

Smoking cessation is not without its hazards. As noted above, symptoms of withdrawal are common. In addition, smoking cessation can be associated with exacerbations of underlying depression, with exacerbations of ulcerative colitis[131] and with weight gain.

The depression associated with smoking cessation as a withdrawal symptom is usually mild. At times, however, it can be sufficiently severe that antidepressant therapy and even hospitalization is required. One study of 76 smokers with a prior history of major depression found that smoking cessation was associated with a significant risk of a major depressive episode.[132] Therefore, recognition of significant depression among smokers who quit, with initiation of appropriate therapy, should be an important part of every clinician's routine.

As noted above, cigarette smoking affects appetite and results in a several kilogram weight loss. Smoking cessation is generally associated with a 1–2 kilogram weight gain in the first few weeks followed by an additional 2–3 kilogram weight gain over the next several months. Some individuals, however, may gain substantially more weight than this.[133] This weight gain can compromise lung function by reducing the vital capacity.[134] Combining dietary interventions with a smoking cessation program has reported some success in limiting weight gain.[135] Bupropion may also be of benefit in controlling weight gain, at least as long as the medication is taken.[117]

COST EFFECTIVENESS OF SMOKING CESSATION

Compared to other medical interventions, smoking cessation is highly cost effective. When gauged as quality-adjusted life years gained, smoking cessation interventions are far more effective than are many medical interventions. One study, for example, estimated the cost per year of life gained from smoking cessation to be US$7000. This compares with $24 000 for year of life gained for treating mild hypertension.[136] One issue with respect to cost effectiveness in smoking cessation is the so-called 'moral hazard'. This concept has often been used to deny coverage of smoking cessation services by insurers. The idea is that highly motivated individuals will seek smoking cessation without provision of coverage. Providing coverage of services will encourage less motivated individuals to use the service. These individuals, however, because of their lower motivation, will not be successful. As a result, provision of the service would lead to increased utilization, but decreased quit rates and a 'waste' of potential resources.

This issue was evaluated in a large health maintenance organization where a variety of service coverages were provided.[137] The provision of increasing levels of service did increase utilization. Increased utilization, however, was not associated with substantial reductions in success in quitting. As a result, increasing the services available resulted in substantially increasing the number of successful quits. Another economic analysis, evaluating the treatments recommended by the DHHS guidelines, suggests the most aggressive treatments are the most cost effective.[138]

Smoking cessation interventions, therefore, should be regarded as among the most cost-effective healthcare interventions available. Smoking cessation services of the highest degree of effectiveness including both behavioral and pharmacologic support should be included in any comprehensive healthcare program.

RELAPSE PREVENTION

Smoking cessation interventions can frequently induce short-term cessation. Over time, however, many smokers will relapse. Efforts designed to prevent relapse, therefore, can greatly improve overall abstinence rates.[139,140] In this context, many smokers will relapse at times of stress or in situations with behaviors in social settings previously associated with smoking. Alcohol use, in particular, is associated with relapse. This is likely because smoking and drinking are often associated and with the fact that alcohol can reduce a smoker's resolve to maintain abstinence. Forewarning the newly quit smoker about high-risk situations can potentially prevent some relapses.[139]

Bupropion has been suggested to help prevent relapse by decreasing cravings.[141] One prospective trial evaluated newly abstinent smokers who quit with the aid of bupropion.[142] These individuals were then randomly assigned to receive year-long therapy with either placebo or bupropion. The long-term bupropion-treated group had significantly greater continuous abstinence after 24 weeks, although quit rates were similar after 1 year. Behavioral approaches designed to prevent relapse have had limited success.[143] Anticipatory interventions among women who quit smoking during pregnancy, for example, reduced relapse rates postpartum from 21 to 18.5%, a difference which was not statistically significant.[144] Contacting recent ex-smokers with repeated mailings, however, has been suggested to be of benefit.[91]

The smoker who relapses should not be regarded as a failure.[8] Rather, such individuals should be encouraged to make another quit attempt. In general, each quit attempt should be viewed as a step toward success, and the experience gained in each quit attempt should be used to inform subsequent efforts. Pharmacologic and behavioral support, for example, can be modified based on what was helpful and what needs were unmet. The majority of smokers do not achieve long-term abstinence on their first attempt.

HARM REDUCTION

Despite the best available interventions, some smokers are unable to quit. In addition, some smokers do not wish to quit. Options for such individuals are limited. The ultimate goal should be to patiently encourage continued attempts at smoking cessation hoping that these will eventually be successful. An alternative strategy, termed 'harm reduction' is to attempt to reduce the health hazards experienced by continued smokers.[145]

One strategy to achieve this is to replace some of the nicotine required by addicted smokers with nicotine derived from nicotine-replacement formulations.[146] Such strategies may reduce exposure to many of the toxins contained in cigarette smoke. Such strategies may also be associated with reductions in lower respiratory tract inflammation.[147]

An alternative strategy is to vary the materials smoked. The burning tobacco at the distal end of the cigarette serves as a heat source, but also produces the majority of the toxic species contained in cigarette smoke. Devices that do not burn tobacco but generate heat by an alternate mechanism have the potential for reducing toxin exposure.[142] Two such products are currently available.[148,149] The health effects of such devices are under investigation.

Another strategy is to modify the tobacco leaf so that carcinogens are reduced. Again products reported to have dramatically reduced nitrosamines in promotional materials are available, although the health consequences associated with the use of such products are unknown. A modification of this approach is the substitution of moist snuff for smoking.[150] Moist snuff (snus) is a product widely used in Sweden.[151] It differs from other oral tobacco products and may be associated with less local adverse effects.[152] Its use may be associated with a significant reduction in smoking-associated lung cancer among Swedish men, but cause and effect remains to be demonstrated.[153]

The harm-reduction strategy was the subject of a recent review by the Institute of Medicine.[145] While harm-reduction approaches should be considered as part of any comprehensive strategy to approach the health burden caused by cigarette smoking, they pose a number of practical and theoretical problems. First, assessing health benefits of harm reduction products will be difficult. Second, the availability of such products may discourage some smokers from making an active quit attempt. Moreover, such products may encourage smoking initiation either directly because products assumed to be 'safer' may be available or indirectly by eroding public opinion against smoking. Finally, products such as low-tar, low-nicotine cigarettes that clearly do not have any health benefits were promoted by the tobacco industry to health-conscious consumers as improved products.[154,155] These products were widely adopted based on poor information and misperceptions. How to regulate the promotion and public information required for harm-reduction products, therefore, remains problematical.

At present, while harm reduction remains an interesting and potentially important approach, available data are insufficient to recommend this strategy from a health perspective.

SUMMARY RECOMMENDATIONS

- Smoking should be regarded as a primary disorder. The majority of smokers are addicted to nicotine. This process has a clear biological and cellular basis.
- Smoking cessation approaches should be multidisciplinary and multifactorial. Public health measures can help prevent smoking initiation and can help facilitate smoking cessation. Social attitudes toward smoking are crucial in both.
- Healthcare systems should provide a system-based approach to the problem of tobacco use. Smoking status should be assessed at all visits. Non-smokers should be encouraged to remain abstinent. Ex-smokers should be congratulated, and attempts should be made to prevent relapse. Current smokers should be assessed regarding their willingness to quit. Those unwilling to make a quit attempt should be systematically encouraged to do so. Smokers willing to make a quit attempt should be offered the best possible chances for success. This includes behavioral support combined with pharmacologic treatment.

REFERENCES

1. Fletcher C, Peto R, Tinker C, Speizer FE. *The Natural History of Chronic Bronchitis and Emphysema.* Oxford University Press, New York, 1976, pp 1–272.
2. Buist AS, Vollmer WM. Smoking and other risk factors. In: JF Murray, Nadel, eds. *Textbook of Respiratory Medicine.* WB Saunders, Philadelphia, 1994, pp 1259–87.
3. Mossberg B, Strandberg K, Philipson K, Camner P. Tracheobronchial clearance in bronchial asthma: response to beta-adrenoceptor stimulation. *J Respir Dis* 1976;**57:** 119–28.
4. Mannino DM, Gagnon RC, Petty TL, Lydick E. Obstructive lung disease and low lung function in adults in the United States: data from the National Health and Nutrition Examination Survey, 1988–1994. *Arch Intern Med* 2000;**160:**1683–9.
5. Leuenberger P, Schwartz J, Ackermann-Liebrich U, *et al.* Passive smoking exposure in adults and chronic respiratory symptoms (SAPALDIA Study). *Am J Respir Crit Care Med* 1994;**150:**1222–8.
6. Burrows B, Knudson RJ, Cline MG, Lebowitz MD. Quantitative relationships between cigarette smoking and ventilatory function. *Am Rev Respir Dis* 1977;**115:**195–205.
7. Ashley F, Kannel WB, Sorlie PD, Masson R. Pulmonary function: relation to aging, cigarette habit, and mortality. *Ann Intern Med* 1975;**82:**739–45.
8. Fiore MC. US public health service clinical practice guideline: treating tobacco use and dependence. *Respir Care* 2000;**45:**1200–62.
9. Rodgman A, Smith CJ, Perfelli TA. The composition of cigarette smoke: a retrospective, with emphasis on polycyclic components. *Hum Exp Toxicol* 2000;**19:**573–95.
10. Hoffmann D, Djordjevic MV, Hoffmann I. The changing cigarette. *Prev Med* 1997;**26:**427–34.
11. Benowitz NL. Nicotine addiction. *Prim Care* 1999;**26:** 611–31.
12. RJ Reynolds Tobacco Company. *New Cigarette Prototypes that Heat Instead of Burn Tobacco.* RJ Reynolds Tobacco Company, Winston-Salem, NC, 1988, p 744.
13. Benowitz NL. Pharmacokinetic considerations in understanding nicotine dependence. *Ciba Found Symp* 1990;**152:**186–200.
14. Henningfield JE, Miyasato K, Jasinski DR. Abuse liability and pharmacodynamic characteristics of intravenous and inhaled nicotine. *J Pharmacol Exp Ther* 1985;**234:**1–12.
15. Henningfield JE, Keenan RM. Nicotine delivery kinetics and abuse liability. *J Consulting Clin Psychol* 1993;**61:**743–50.
16. Salin-Pascual RJ. Relationship between mood improvement and sleep changes with acute nicotine administration in non-smoking major depressed patients. *Rev Invest Clin* 2002;**54:**36–40.
17. Salin-Pascual RJ, Rosas M, Jimenez-Genchi A, Rivera-Meza BL, Delgado-Parr V. Antidepressant effect of transdermal nicotine patches in nonsmoking patients with major depression. *J Clin Psychiatry* 1996;**57:**387–9.
18. Fowler JS, Volkow ND, Wang G-J, *et al.* Brain monoamine oxidase A inhibition in cigarette smokers. *Proc Natl Acad Sci USA* 1996;**93:**14065–9.
19. Sherwood N. Effects of cigarette smoking on performance in a simulated driving task. *Neuropsychobiology* 1995;**32:**161–5.
20. Mumenthaler MS, Taylor JL, O'Hara R, Yesavage JA. Influence of nicotine on simulator flight performance in non-smokers. *Psychopharmacology (Berl)* 1998;**140:**38–41.

21. Smith RC, Singh A, Infante M, Khandat A, Kloos A. Effects of cigarette smoking and nicotine nasal spray on psychiatric symptoms and cognition in schizophrenia. *Neuropsychopharmacology* 2002;**27**:479–97.

22. Freedman R, Adler LE, Bickford P, *et al*. Schizophrenia and nicotinic receptors. *Harv Rev Psychiatry* 1994;**2**:179–92.

23. Jo YH, Talmage DA, Role LW. Nicotinic receptor-mediated effects on appetite and food intake. *J Neurobiol* 2002; **53**:618–32.

24. Dackis CA, O'Brien CP. Cocaine dependence: a disease of the brain's reward centers. *J Subst Abuse Treat* 2001;**21**:111–17.

25. Martin-Solch C, Magyar S, Kunig G, Missimer J, Schultz W, Leenders KL. Changes in brain activation associated with reward processing in smokers and nonsmokers. A positron emission tomography study. *Exp Brain Res* 2001;**139**: 278–86.

26. Thomas MJ, Malenka RC, Bonci A. Modulation of long-term depression by dopamine in the mesolimbic system. *J Neurosci* 2000;**20**:5581–6.

27. Rossing MA. Genetic influences on smoking: candidate genes. *Environ Health Perspect* 1998;**106**:231–8.

28. Ridley DL, Rogers A, Wonnacott S. Differential effects of chronic drug treatment on alpha3* and alpha7 nicotinic receptor binding sites, in hippocampal neurones and SH-SY5Y cells. *Br J Pharmacol* 2001;**133**:1286–95.

29. Hellstrom-Lindahl E, Seiger A, Kjaeldgaard A, Nordberg A. Nicotine-induced alterations in the expression of nicotinic receptors in primary cultures from human prenatal brain. *Neuroscience* 2001;**105**:527–34.

30. Van de Kamp JL, Collins AC. Prenatal nicotine alters nicotinic receptor development in the mouse brain. *Pharmacol Biochem Behav* 1994;**47**:889–900.

31. Tizabi Y, Perry DC. Prenatal nicotine exposure is associated with an increase in [125I]epibatidine binding in discrete cortical regions in rats. *Pharmacol Biochem Behav* 2000;**67**:319–23.

32. Lebargy F, Benhammou K, Morin D, *et al*. Tobacco smoking induces expression of very high affinity nicotine binding sites on blood polymorphonuclear cells. *Am J Respir Crit Care Med* 1996;**153**:1056–63.

33. Escobedo LG, Anda RF, Smith PF, Remington PL, Mast EE. Sociodemographic characteristics of cigarette smoking initiation in the United States. *JAMA* 1990;**264**:1550–5.

34. Youth tobacco surveillance – United States, 2000. *MMWR CDC Surveill Summ* 2001;**50**:1–84.

35. Evans N, Farkas A, Gilpin E, Berry C, Pierce JP. Influence of tobacco marketing and exposure to smokers on adolescent susceptibility to smoking. *J Natl Cancer Inst* 1995;**87**: 1538–45.

36. Headen SW, Bauman KE, Deane GD, Koch GG. Are the correlates of cigarette smoking initiation different for black and white adolescents? *Am J Pub Health* 1991;**81**:854–8.

37. Santi S, Best JA, Brown KS, Cargo M. Social environment and smoking initiation. *Intl J Addiction* 1991;**25**:881–903.

38. Flay BR, Hu FB, Siddiqui O, *et al*. Differential influence of parental smoking and friends' smoking on adolescent initiation and escalation of smoking. *J Health Soc Behav* 1994;**35**:248–65.

39. Gilpin EA, Pierce JP. Trends in adolescent smoking initiation in the United States: is tobacco marketing an influence? *Tob Control* 1997;**6**:122–7.

40. Jason LA. Active enforcement of cigarette control laws in the prevention of cigarette sales to minors. *JAMA* 1991; **266**:3159–61.

41. Rigotti NA, DiFranza JR, Chang Y, Tisdale T, Kemp B, Singer DE. The effect of enforcing tobacco-sales law on adolescents' access to tobacco and smoking behavior. *N Engl J Med* 1997;**337**:1044–51.

42. Siegel M, Biener L, Rigotti NA. The effect of local tobacco sales laws on adolescent smoking initiation. *Prev Med* 1999;**29**:334–42.

43. Sweanor DT, Martial LR, Dossetor JB. *The Canadian Tobacco Tax Experience: A Case Study*. 1993. The Non-Smokers' Rights Association (Canada) and The Smoking and Health Action Foundation (Canada).

44. Flay BR, Phil D, Hu FB, Richardson J. Psychosocial predictors of different stages of cigarette smoking among high school students. *Prev Med* 1998;**27**(5 Pt 3):A9–18.

45. Kendler KS, Thornton LM, Pedersen NL. Tobacco consumption in Swedish twins reared apart and reared together. *Arch Gen Psychiatry* 2000;**57**:886–92.

46. Gynther LM, Hewitt JK, Heath AC, Eaves LJ. Phenotypic and genetic factors in motives for smoking. *Behav Genet* 1999; **29**:291–302.

47. Carmeli D, Swan G, Robinette D, Fabsitz R. Genetic influence on smoking – a study of male twins. *N Engl J Med* 1992;**327**:829–33.

48. True WR, Heath AC, Scherrer JF, *et al*. Genetic and environmental contributions to smoking. *Addiction* 1997;**92**:1277–87.

49. Noble EP, St Jeor ST, Ritchie T, *et al*. D2 dopamine receptor gene and cigarette smoking: a reward gene? *Med Hypotheses* 1994;**42**:257–60.

50. Vandenbergh DJ, Bennett CJ, Grant MD, *et al*. Smoking status and the human dopamine transporter variable number of tandem repeats (VNTR) polymorphism: failure to replicate and finding that never-smokers may be different. *Nicotine Tob Res* 2002;**4**:333–40.

51. Lerman C, Shields PG, Audrain J, *et al*. The role of serotonin transporter gene in cigarette smoking. *Cancer Epidem, Biomarkers & Prev* 1998;**7**:253–5.

52. Sullivan PF, Neale MC, Silverman MA, *et al*. An association study of DRD5 with smoking initiation and progression to nicotine dependence. *Am J Med Genet* 2001;**105**:259–65.

53. Pianezza ML, Sellers EM, Tyndale RF. Nicotine metabolism defect reduces smoking. *Nature* 1998;**393**:750.

54. Shields PG, Lerman C, Audrain J, *et al*. Dopamine D4 receptors and the risk of cigarette smoking in african-americans and caucasians. *Cancer Epidemiol Biomarkers Prev* 1998;**7**:453–8.

55. Lerman C, Audrain J, Main D, *et al*. Evidence suggesting the role of specific genetic factors in cigarette smoking. *Health Psychology* 1999;**18**:14–20.

56. Pomerleau OF. Individual differences in sensitivity to nicotine: Implications for genetic research on nicotine dependence. *Behav Genet* 1995;**25**:161–77.

57. Collins AC. Genetic influences on tobacco use: a review of human and animal studies. *Intl J Addict* 1990;**25**: 35–55.

58. Tyndale RF, Sellers EM. Genetic variation in CYP2A6-mediated nicotine metabolism alters smoking behavior. *Ther Drug Monit* 2002;**24**:163–71.

59. Ariyoshi N, Miyamoto M, Umetsu Y, *et al*. Genetic polymorphism of CYP2A6 gene and tobacco-induced lung cancer risk in male smokers. *Cancer Epidemiol Biomarkers Prev* 2002;**11**:890–4.

60. Lerman C, Niaura R. Applying genetic approaches to the treatment of nicotine dependence. *Oncogene* 2002;**21**: 7412–20.

61. Heath AC, Martin NG. Genetic models for the natural history of smoking: evidence for a genetic influence on smoking persistence. *Addictive Behav* 1993;**18**:19–34.

62. Sullivan PF, Kendler KS. The genetic epidemiology of smoking. *Nicotine Tob Res* 1999;**1**(suppl 2):S51–7; discussion S69–70.

63. Shiffman S. Tobacco 'chippers' – individual differences in tobacco dependence. *Psychopharmacology* 1989;**97**:539–47.

64. Shiffman S, Paty JA, Gnys M, Kassel JD, Elash C. Nicotine withdrawal in chippers and regular smokers: subjective and cognitive effects. *Health Psychol* 1995;**14**:301–9.

65. *Diagnostic and Statistical Manual of Mental Disorders*, vol. 3. American Psychiatric Association, Washington, DC, 1987.

66. Killen JD, Fortmann SP. Craving is associated with smoking relapse: findings from three prospective studies. *Exp Clin Psychopharmacol* 1997;**5**:137–42.

67. Woodson PP, Griffiths RR. Control of cigarette smoking topography: smoke filtration and draw resistance. *Behav Pharmacol* 1992;**3**:99–111.

68. Herskovic JE, Rose JE, Jarvik ME. Cigarette desirability and nicotine preference in smokers. *Pharmacol Biochem Behav* 1986;**24**:171–5.

69. Boren JJ, Stitzer ML, Henningfield JE. Preference among research cigarettes with varying nicotine yields. *Pharmacol Biochem Behav* 1990;**36**:191–3.

70. Volk RJ, Edwards DW, Lewis RA, Schulenberg J. Smoking and preference for brand of cigarette among adolescents. *J Subst Abuse* 1996;**8**:347–59.

71. DiFranza JR, Richards JW, Paulman PM, *et al.* RJR Nabisco's cartoon camel promotes Camel cigarettes to children. *JAMA* 1991;**266**:3149–53.

72. Jaffe AJ, Glaros AG. Taste dimensions in cigarette discrimination: a multidimensional scaling approach. *Addict Behav* 1986;**11**:407–13.

73. Brigham J, Henningfield JE, Stitzer ML. Smoking relapse: a review. *Int J Addict* 1990;**25**:1239–55.

74. Giovino GA, Shelton DM, Schooley MW. Trends in cigarette smoking cessation in the United States. *Tob Control* 1993;**2**:S3–16.

75. Ockene JK, Emmons KM, Mermelstein RJ, *et al.* Relapse and maintenance issues for smoking cessation. *Health Psychol* 2000;**19**(1 suppl):17–31.

76. Meng SZ, Ozawa Y, Itoh M, Takashima S. Developmental and age-related changes of dopamine transporter, and dopamine D1 and D2 receptors in human basal ganglia. *Brain Res* 1999;**843**:136–44.

77. Tohgi H, Utsugisawa K, Yoshimura M, Nagane Y, Mihara M. Age-related changes in D1 and D2 receptor mRNA expression in postmortem human putamen with and without multiple small infarcts. *Neurosci Lett* 1998; **243**:37–40.

78. Wang Y, Chan GL, Holden JE, *et al.* Age-dependent decline of dopamine D1 receptors in human brain: a PET study. *Synapse* 1998;**30**:56–61.

79. Fiore MC, Jorenby DE, Schensky AE, Smith SS, Bauer RR, Baker TB. Smoking status as the new vital sign: eon assessment and intervention in patients who smoke. *Mayo Clinic Proc* 1995;**70**:209–13.

80. Daughton DM, Susman J, Sitorius M, *et al.* Transdermal nicotine therapy and primary care: importance of counseling, demographic and patient selection factors on one-year quit rates. *Arch Fam Med* 1998; **7**:425–30.

81. Ockene JK, Kristeller JL, Goldberg R. Smoking cessation and severity of disease: The Coronary Artery Smoking Intervention Study. *Health Psychol* 1992;**11**:119–26.

82. Gilpin EA, Pierce JP, Johnson M, Bal D. Physician advice to quit smoking: results from the 1990 California Tobacco Survey. *J Gen Intern Med* 1993;**8**:549–53.

83. Silagy C, Stead LF. Physician advice for smoking cessation. *Cochrane Database Syst Rev* 2001;CD000165.

84. Schwartz JL. *Review and Evaluation of Smoking Cessation Methods: the United States and Canada, 1978–1985.* National Cancer Institute, Bethesda, MD, 1987.

85. Russell MAH, Wilson C, Taylor C, Baker CD. Effect of general practitioners' advice against smoking. *Br Med J* 1979;**2**: 231–5.

86. Fiore MC, Bailey WC, Cohen SJ. *Smoking Cessation. Guideline Technical Report No. 18.* Publication No. AHCPR 97-No 4. US Department of Health and Human Services, Public Health Service, Agency for Health Care Policy and Research, Rockville, MD, 1997.

87. Fiore MC, Smith SS, Jorenby DE, Baker TB. The effectiveness of the nicotine patch for smoking cessation. *JAMA* 1994; **271**:1940–7.

88. Miguez MC, Vazquez FL, Becona E. Effectiveness of telephone contact as an adjunct to a self-help program for smoking cessation: a randomized controlled trial in Spanish smokers. *Addict Behav* 2002;**27**:139–44.

89. Zhu SH, Anderson CM, Tedeschi GJ, *et al.* Evidence of real-world effectiveness of a telephone quitline for smokers. *N Engl J Med* 2002;**347**:1087–93.

90. Humerfelt S, Eide GE, Kvale G. Effectiveness of postal smoking cessation advice. A randomized controlled trial in young men with reduced FEV_1 and asbestos exposure. *Eur Respir J* 1998;**11**:284.

91. Brandon TH, Collins BN, Juliano LM, Lazev AB. Preventing relapse among former smokers: a comparison of minimal interventions through telephone and mail. *J Consult Clin Psychol* 2000;**68**:103–13.

92. Cinciripini PM, Lapitsky L, Seay S, Wallfisch A, Kitchens K, Vunakis H. Effects of smoking schedules on cessation outcome: can we improve on common methods of gradual and abrupt nicotine withdrawal. *J Consult Clin Psychol* **1995**: 388–99.

93. Cinciripini PM, Wetter DW, McClure JB. Scheduled reduced smoking: effects on smoking abstinence and potential mechanisms of action. *Addict Behav* 1997;**22**:759–67.

94. Schwartz JL. Methods for smoking cessation. *Clin Chest Med* 1991;**12**:737–53.

95. Covey LS, Glassman AH, Stetner F. Cigarette smoking and major depression. *J Addict Dis* 1998;**17**:35–46.

96. Lohr JB, Flynn K. Smoking and schizophrenia. *Schizophr Res* 1992;**8**:93–102.

97. West R, Hajek P, Nilsson F, Foulds J, May S, Meadows A. Individual differences in preferences for and responses to four nicotine replacement products. *Psychopharmacology (Berl)* 2001;**153**:225–30.

98. Sweeney CT, Fant RV, Fagerstrom KO, McGovern JF, Henningfield JE. Combination nicotine replacement therapy for smoking cessation: rationale, efficacy and tolerability. *CNS Drugs* 2001;**15**:453–67.

99. Bohadana A, Nilsson F, Rasmussen T, Martinet Y. Nicotine inhaler and nicotine patch as a combination therapy for smoking cessation: a randomized, double-blind, placebo-controlled trial. *Arch Intern Med* 2000;**160**: 3128–34.

100. Blondal T, Gudmundsson LJ, Olafsdottir I, Gustavsson G, Westin A. Nicotine nasal spray with nicotine patch for smoking cessation: randomised trial with six year follow up. *Br Med J* 1999;**318**:285–9.

101. Kornitzer M, Boutsen M, Dramaix M, Thijs J, Gustavsson G. Combined use of nicotine patch and gum in smoking cessaton: a placebo-controlled clinical trial. *Prevent Med* 1995;**24**:41–7.

102. Fiore MC, Jorenby DE, Baker TB, Kenford SL. Tobacco dependence and the nicotine patch. *JAMA* 1992;**268**: 2687–9.

103. Palmer KJ, Buckley MM, Faulds D. Transdermal nicotine: a review of its pharmacodynamic and pharmacokinetic properties, and therapeutic efficacy as an aid to smoking cessation. *Drugs* 1992;**44**:498–529.

104. Fiore MC, Jorenby DE, Baker TB. Tobacco dependence and the nicotine patch. Clinical guidelines for effective use. *JAMA* 1992;**268**:2687–94.

105. Shiffman S, Khayrallah M, Nowak R. Efficacy of the nicotine patch for relief of craving and withdrawal 7–10 weeks after cessation. *Nicotine Tob Res* 2000;**2**:371–8.

106. Tonnesen P, Paoletti P, Gustavsson G, *et al.* Higher dosage nicotine patches increase one-year smoking cessation rates: results from the European CEASE trial. Collaborative European Anti-Smoking Evaluation. European Respiratory Society. *Eur Respir J* 1999;**13**:238–46.

107. Blondal T. Contolled trial of nicotine polacrilex gum with supportive measures. *Arch Intern Med* 1989;**149**:1818–21.

108. Glover ED, Sachs DPL, Stitzer ML, *et al.* Smoking cessation in highly dependent smokers with 4 mg nicotine polacrilex. *Am J Health Behav* 1996;**20**:319–32.

109. Daughton DM, Thompson AB, Hatlelid K, Rennard SI. Smoke-free environments and nicotine polacrilex. *Am J Med* 1992;**92**:340–1.

110. Schneider NG, Olmstead RE, Franzon MA, Lunell E. The nicotine inhaler: clinical pharmacokinetics and comparison with other nicotine treatments. *Clin Pharmacokinet* 2001;**40**:661–84.

111. Schneider NG, Olmstead R, Nilsson F, Mody FV, Franzon M, Doan K. Efficacy of a nicotine inhaler in smoking cessation: a double-blind, placebo-controlled trial. *Addiction* 1996; **91**:1293–306.

112. Hurt RD, Dale LC, Croghan GA, Croghan IT, Gomez-Dahl LC, Offord KP. Nicotine nasal spray for smoking cessation: pattern of use, side effects, relief of withdrawal symptoms, and cotinine levels. *Mayo Clin Proc* 1998;**73**:118–25.

113. Blondal T, Franzon M, Westin A. A double-blind randomized trial of nicotine nasal spray as an aid in smoking cessation. *Eur Respir J* 1997;**10**:1585–90.

114. Roth MT, Westman EC. Asthma exacerbation after administration of nicotine nasal spray for smoking cessation. *Pharmacotherapy* 2002;**22**:779–82.

115. Shiffman S, Dresler CM, Hajek P, Gilburt SJ, Targett DA, Strahs KR. Efficacy of a nicotine lozenge for smoking cessation. *Arch Intern Med* 2002;**162**:1267–76.

116. Hurt RD, Sachs DP, Glover ED, *et al.* A comparison of sustained-release bupropion and placebo for smoking cessation. *N Engl J Med* 1997;**337**:1195–202.

117. Jorenby DE, Leischow SJ, Nides MA, *et al.* A controlled trial of sustained-release bupropion, a nicotine patch, or both for smoking cessation. *N Engl J Med* 1999;**340**: 685–91.

118. Hayford KE, Patten CA, Rummans TA, *et al.* Efficacy of bupropion for smoking cessation in smokers with a former history of major depression or alcoholism. *Br J Psychiatry* 1999;**174**:173–8.

119. Gourlay SG, Stead LF, Benowitz NL. Clonidine for smoking cessation. *Cochrane Database Syst Rev* 2000;2.

120. Hughes JR, Stead LF, Lancaster T. Anxiolytics and antidepressants for smoking cessation. *Cochrane Database Syst Rev* 2000;2.

121. Hall SM, Reus VI, Munoz RF, *et al.* Nortriptyline and cognitive-behavioral therapy in the treatment of cigarette smoking. *Arch Gen Psychiatry* 1998;**55**:683–90.

122. Prochazka AV, Weaver MJ, Keller RT, Fryer GE, Licari PA, Lofaso D. A randomized trial of nortriptyline for smoking cessation. *Arch Intern Med* 1998;**158**:2035–9.

123. Berlin I, Said S, Spreux-Varoquaux O, *et al.* A reversible monoamine oxidase A inhibitor (moclobemide) facilitates smoking cessation and abstinence in heavy, dependent smokers. *Clin Pharmacol Ther* 1995;**58**:444–52.

124. Berlin I, Aubin HJ, Pedarriosse AM, Rames A, Lancrenon S, Lagrue G. Lazabemide, a selective, reversible monoamine oxidase B inhibitor, as an aid to smoking cessation. *Addiction* 2002;**97**:1347–54.

125. Center for Disease Control, US Department of Health and Human Services, Public Health Service, Center for Health Promotion and Education, Office on Smoking and Health. *The Health Consequences of Smoking, Nicotine Addiction. A Report of the Surgeon General.* US Government Printing Office, Rockville, MD, 1988.

126. Rose JE, Behm FM, Westman EC, Levin ED, Stein RM, Ripka GV. Mecamylamine combined with nicotine skin patch facilitates smoking cessation beyond nicotine patch treatment alone. *Clin Pharmacol Ther* 1994;**56**:86–99.

127. Lancaster T, Stead LF. Mecamylamine (a nicotine antagonist) for smoking cessation. *Cochrane Database Syst Rev* 2000;CD001009.

128. Pentel P, Malin D. A vaccine for nicotine dependence: targeting the drug rather than the brain. *Respiration* 2002;**69**:193–7.

129. Pentel PR, Malin DH, Ennifar S, *et al.* A nicotine conjugate vaccine reduces nicotine distribution to brain and attenuates its behavioral and cardiovascular effects in rats. *Pharmacol Biochem Behav* 2000;**65**:191–8.

130. Cohen C, Perrault G, Voltz C, Steinberg R, Soubrie P. SR141716, a central cannabinoid (CB) receptor antagonist, blocks the motivational and dopamine-releasing effects of nicotine in rats. *Behav Pharmacol* 2002;**13**:451–63.

131. Motley RJ, Rhodes J, Ford GA, *et al.* Time relationships between cessation of smoking and onset of ulcerative colitis. *Digestion* 1987;**37**:125–7.

132. Glassman AH, Covey LS, Stetner F, Rivelli S. Smoking cessation and the course of major depression: a follow-up study. *Lancet* 2001;**357**:1929–32.

133. O'Hara P, Connett JE, Lee WW, Nides M, Murray R, Wise R. Early and late weight gain following smoking cessation in the Lung Health Study. *Am J Epidemiol* 1998;**148**:821–30.

134. Wise RA, Enright PL, Connett JE, *et al.* Effect of weight gain on pulmonary function after smoking cessation in the Lung Health Study. *Am J Respir Crit Care Med* 1998;**157**:866–72.

135. Danielsson T, Rossner S, Westin A. Open randomised trial of intermittent very low energy diet together with nicotine gum for stopping smoking in women who gained weight in previous attempts to quit. *Br Med J* 1999;**319**:490–3; discussion 494.

136. Croghan IT, Offord KP, Evans RW, *et al.* Cost-effectiveness of treating nicotine dependence: The Mayo Clinic Experience. *Mayo Clin Proc* 1997;**72**:917–24.

137. Curry SJ, Grothaus LC, McAfee T, Painiak C. Use and cost effectiveness of smoking cessation services under four insurance plans in a health maintenance organization. *N Engl J Med* 1998;**339**:673–9.

138. Cromwell J, Bartosch WJ, Barendregt JJ, Bonneux L. AHCPR guidelines on smoking cessation found cost-effective – more intensive interventions cost less per quitter. *Am J Health Syst Pharm* 1998;**55**:211–12.

139. Irvin JE, Bowers CA, Dunn ME, Wang MC. Efficacy of relapse prevention: a meta-analytic review. *J Consult Clin Psychol* 1999;**67**:563–70.

140. Kenford SL, Smith SS, Wetter DW, Jorenby DE, Fiore MC, Baker TB. Predicting relapse back to smoking: contrasting affective and physical models of dependence. *J Consult Clin Psychol* 2002;**70**:216–27.

141. Durcan MJ, Deener G, White J, *et al.* The effect of bupropion sustained-release on cigarette craving after smoking cessation. *Clin Ther* 2002;**24**:540–51.

142. Hays JT, Hurt RD, Rigotti NA, *et al.* Sustained-release bupropion for pharmacologic relapse prevention after smoking cessation. A randomized, controlled trial. *Ann Intern Med* 2001;**135**:423–33.

143. Smith SS, Jorenby DE, Fiore MC, *et al.* Strike while the iron is hot: can stepped-care treatments resurrect relapsing smokers? *J Consult Clin Psychol* 2001;**69**:429–39.

144. Ratner PA, Johnson JL, Bottorff JL, Dahinten S, Hall W. Twelve-month follow-up of a smoking relapse prevention intervention for postpartum women. *Addict Behav* 2000;**25**:81–92.

145. Stratton K, Shetty P, Wallace R, Bondurant S, eds. *Clearing the Smoke*. National Academy Press, Washington, DC, 2001.

146. Russell MAH, Wilson C, Feyerabend C, Cole PV. Effect of nicotine chewing gum on smoking behaviour and as an aid to cigarette withdrawal. *Br Med J* 1976;**2**:391–3.

147. Rennard SI, Daughton D, Fujita J, *et al.* Short-term smoking reduction is associated with reduction in measures of lower respiratory tract inflammation in heavy smokers. *Eur Respir J* 1990;**3**:752–9.

148. Stapleton JA, Russell MAH, Sutherland G, Feyerabend C. Nicotine availabity from Eclipse tobacco-heating cigarette. *Psychopharmacology* 1998;**139**:288–90.

149. Buchhalter AR, Eissenberg T. Preliminary evaluation of a novel smoking system: effects on subjective and physiological measures and on smoking behavior. *Nicotine Tob Res* 2000;**2**:39–43.

150. Andersson G, Axell T, Curvall M. Reduction in nicotine intake and oral mucosal changes among users of Swedish oral moist snuff after switching to a low-nicotine product. *J Oral Pathol Med* 1995;**24**:244–50.

151. Henningfield JE, Fagerstrom KO. Swedish Match Company, Swedish snus and public health: a harm reduction experiment in progress? *Tob Control* 2001;**10**:253–7.

152. Idris AM, Ibrahim SO, Vasstrand EN, *et al.* The Swedish snus and the Sudanese toombak: are they different? *Oral Oncol* 1998;**34**:558–66.

153. Wramner B, Zatonski W, Pellmer K. Premature mortality in lung cancer as an indicator of effectiveness of tobacco use prevention in a gender perspective – a comparison between Poland and Sweden. *Cent Eur J Public Health* 2001;**9**:69–73.

154. Kozlowski LT, Goldberg ME, Yost BA, White EL, Sweeney CT, Pillitteri JL. Smokers' misperceptions of light and ultra-light cigarettes may keep them smoking. *Am J Prev Med* 1998;**15**:9–16.

155. Pollay RW, Dewhirst T. The dark side of marketing seemingly 'Light' cigarettes: successful images and failed fact. *Tob Control* 2002;**11**(suppl 1):118–31.

156. Joseph AM. Nicotine replacement therapy for cardiac patients. *Am J Health Behav* 1996;**20**:261–9.

157. Working Group for the Study of Transdermal Nicotine in Patients with Coronary Artery Disease. Nicotine replacement therapy for patients with coronary artery disease. *Arch Intern Med* 1994;**154**:989–95.

158. Mahmarian JJ, Moye LA, Nasser GA. Nicotine patch therapy in smoking cessation reduces the extent of exercise-induced myocardial ischemia. *J Am Coll Cardiol* 1997;**30**:125–30.

23

Pharmacology

RICHARD COSTELLO

Pharmacologic therapy for patients with COPD is aimed at both achieving relief of symptoms and altering the progression of the disease. Since the principal symptom of COPD is breathlessness, symptomatic management is aimed at controlling this symptom and involves the use of a wide variety of bronchodilator drugs. The mechanism of action, chemical properties and rationale for use of these medications will be discussed in this chapter. Several pharmacologic strategies have been developed with the aim of inhibiting the progression of the disease. Unfortunately to date the results of these studies have largely been disappointing and so the pharmacology of these agents is not discussed in detail. In addition to these broad classes of agents other therapies such as oxygen, antibiotics and nutritional agents are also widely used in the management of patients with COPD; the rationale for the use of these agents is discussed elsewhere in this book.

ANTICHOLINERGIC DRUGS

Administration of acetylcholine or stimulation of the parasympathetic nerves in the vagus causes the airway smooth muscle to contract,[1] the glandular tissue to secrete mucus[2,3] and the bronchial circulation to dilate.[4,5] As both airflow obstruction and increased mucus production are among the dominant symptoms in patients with COPD, it follows that inhibiting parasympathetic nerves is likely to be of benefit in this condition. In support of this observation is the fact that anticholinergic

agents are often recommended as the first-line therapeutic agents in patients with COPD.

Distribution of parasympathetic nerves and muscarinic receptors in the lungs

The axons of the parasympathetic vagus nerves that innervate the lungs extend from cell bodies in the medulla through the neck to the thorax.[6,7] Branches of the vagi enter the lungs at the cardiac plexus, in the mediastinum and extend through the trachea and major bronchi where they relay at cholinergic ganglia. Short postganglionic fibers extend from these cell bodies to the airway smooth muscle and glands. The hilum is the site of the densest collection of ganglia and the greatest influence of vagally mediated bronchoconstriction is at this site and at points of branching of the major bronchi. From the hilum down, the ganglia decrease in density, as do the numbers of both postganglionic fibers and muscarinic receptors. Functional studies cannot demonstrate an effect of stimulation of the vagus nerves on the respiratory bronchioles and alveoli. That there is a paucity of cholinergic nerves in the small airways is of relevance for the treatment of patients with COPD because exercise-induced dyspnea in COPD appears to result from dynamic hyperinflation due to narrowing of smaller airways.[8,9] Under normal circumstances the vagus nerves maintain a constant tonic control over the caliber of the airways and so even in normal individuals inhibiting the vagus leads to some degree of bronchodilatation.[10–12] Thus, even in the absence of stimuli that may activate the

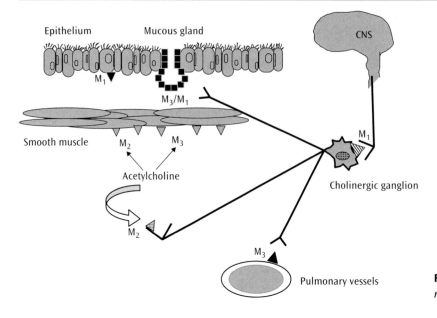

Figure 23.1 *Distribution of muscarinic receptors in the lungs.*

cholinergic nerves there is a constant vagal tonic contraction of the airway smooth muscle which can be overcome with anticholinergic agents.

Muscarinic receptors

The parasympathetic nerves release acetylcholine onto nicotinic receptors on the cholinergic ganglia and onto muscarinic receptors. Muscarinic receptors are found on many structures in the lung, most of these being directly innervated by branches from the parasympathetic nerves. Based on genetic and functional studies with antagonists it has been identified that acetylcholine binds to five subtypes of muscarinic receptors.[13–15] Autoradiographic imaging and ligand-binding studies have established that M_1, M_2 and M_3 muscarinic receptors are found in the airways of all species studied including man.[16–20]

Muscarinic receptors share the common characteristics of being seven transmembrane domain G-protein-linked receptors.[13] There are considerable structural similarities between the five receptors, in particular their transmembrane folding structure. Each muscarinic receptor has a glycosylated extracellular NH_2 terminal. The seven transmembrane regions are all arranged in a similar manner, with each arranged as a parallel stacks of cylinders. Amino acid interactions determine the spacing of these cylinders. Agonist binding affinity and specificity for each receptor is determined by both the arrangement of amino acids that project into the spaces between the cylinders and by carbohydrate side chains on the extracellular domains of the receptor. The third intracellular loop of each receptor has a uniquely different arrangement of amino acids and the least homology between receptors is found within this region. Site-directed mutagenesis experiments have shown

that each of the different muscarinic receptors is linked to different G-proteins and thus different intracellular signal transduction systems at this site.[21–24] Binding of an agonist leads to phosphorylation of the third intracellular loop and COOH terminal tail which leads to homologous desensitization of these receptors.

MUSCARINIC RECEPTORS IN THE AIRWAYS

The distribution and function of each of these three muscarinic receptor subtypes will be discussed below and are shown in Figure 23.1. M_1 muscarinic receptors are coupled to the phospholipase enzyme via the G-protein $G_{q/11}$ and so stimulation of these receptors leads to the production of inositol phosphate, the intracellular second messenger system (Figure 23.2). M_1 muscarinic receptors comprise more than 50% of all muscarinic receptors found in human airways although most of them do not appear to be innervated by parasympathetic nerves.[25] The function of these non-innervated receptors is not yet established. M_1 muscarinic receptors which are innervated by parasympathetic nerves are found on pulmonary veins, epithelial cells and cholinergic ganglia. Under normal circumstances the function of M_1 muscarinic receptors within cholinergic ganglia is to play a role in facilitating neurotransmission.[26] Stimulation of submucosal glandular cell M_1 muscarinic receptors in the airways leads to the release of neutrophil and monocyte chemoattractants.[27–30]

M_2 muscarinic receptors are found on postganglionic parasympathetic nerves and on airway smooth muscle cells. M_2 muscarinic receptors are coupled to the pertussis toxin-sensitive G-protein, Gi. Stimulation of M_2 muscarinic receptors leads to a Gi-mediated inhibition of the adenylate cyclase enzyme.[13,22] Neuronal M_2 muscarinic receptors control the release of acetylcholine from

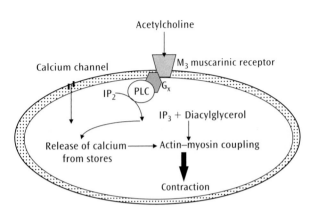

Figure 23.2 *Mechanism of the action of M_3 muscarinic receptor. Binding of acetylcholine to this G-protein coupled receptor leads to an activation of G_x which leads to activation of the enzyme diacylglycerol and the formation of inositol tri-phosphate. PLC = phospholipase C; IP_2 = inositol diphosphate, G_x = alpha subunit of the G-protein; IP_3 = inositol triphosphate.*

cholinergic nerves.[31,32] Stimulation of these receptors with a muscarinic receptor agonist such as pilocarpine inhibits the release of acetylcholine from these nerves. Thus, the function of neuronal M_2 muscarinic receptors is to inhibit the magnitude of vagally induced bronchoconstriction and mucus production induced by the parasympathetic nerves.[31-34] M_2 muscarinic receptors are also located on airway smooth muscle cells. Stimulation of these receptors leads to an inhibition of adenylate cyclase and so in effect these receptors inhibit beta$_2$-adrenoreceptor mediated smooth muscle relaxation.[35,36]

Muscarinic M_3 receptors are located on the airway smooth muscle, pulmonary endothelial vessels and on goblet and mucous glands. These receptors are coupled to the G-protein Gq; stimulation of these receptors leads to stimulation of the phospholipase enzyme. Functionally, stimulation of M_3 muscarinic receptors leads to smooth muscle contraction, relaxation of contracted pulmonary endothelial vessels, enhanced secretion of mucous and promotion of ciliary beat frequency.[34,37]

RELEVANCE OF MUSCARINIC RECEPTORS TO THE PATHOPHYSIOLOGY AND TREATMENT OF PATIENTS WITH COPD

As outlined above the vagus nerves maintain a constant tonic contraction of human airway smooth muscle, by the release of acetylcholine onto M_1 and M_3 receptors in the airways. Thus inhibiting these in subjects leads to bronchodilatation. By contrast, blockade of neuronal M_2 receptors leads to potentiation of vagally induced bronchoconstriction as has been demonstrated in animal studies.[38] Recently, it has been shown that pulmonary neuronal M_2 muscarinic receptors are functional in

patients with stable COPD. This suggests that inhibition of neuronal M_2 muscarinic receptors with the currently available non-selective antagonists may limit the effectiveness of these bronchodilators.[39]

In animal models, studies have shown that after exposure to parainfluenza virus, or the pollutant ozone, or following exposure of sensitized animals to antigen there is dysfunction of M_2 muscarinic receptors.[40-52] This dysfunction leads to an increase in both direct vagally mediated and reflex bronchoconstriction.[42] In patients with COPD this may occur during exacerbations since anticholinergic agents are of particular value at these times.

Another mechanism where anticholinergic agents may exert a beneficial effect is via inhibition of M_1 muscarinic receptors on cholinergic ganglia. As discussed above these receptors play a role in controlling neurotransmission, and administration of the M_1 muscarinic receptor antagonist pirenzipine causes bronchodilatation in humans.[53,54] M_1 muscarinic receptors release epithelial neutrophil and monocyte chemoattractants and the anti-inflammatory agent secretary leucocyte protease inhibitor from submucosal glandular tissue.[55] Although not established, *in vivo*, it seems possible that stimulation of M_1 muscarinic receptors contributes to the airway inflammation of neutrophils and macrophages seen in patients with COPD. Thus, inhibition of these receptors is likely to lead to an improvement in some of the features of COPD.

M_1 and M_3 muscarinic receptors play a role in mediating another characteristic feature of COPD, increased sputum production. Stimulation of M_3 muscarinic receptors causes mucus production and so it may be expected that anticholinergic agents would inhibit sputum production. Treatment of patients with either chronic bronchitis or diffuse panbronchiolitis with the anticholinergic medication oxitropium decreases sputum volume by about one-third, but increases the concentration of protein in the sputum by a third.[56] Thus, anticholinergic agents inhibit water secretion and so may make sputum more tenacious. Airway secretions are moved up through the airways by the beating action of cilia on the epithelial cells. The function of cilia activity is mediated in part by the action of M_1 and M_3 muscarinic receptors in epithelial cells.[29,30] Inhibition of this cilia-mediated clearance of mucus clearance is decreased by atropine, but not by ipratropium.[57]

In the pulmonary vasculature muscarinic M_3 receptors on the smooth muscle mediate contraction while M_3 receptors on pulmonary endothelial vessels mediate relaxation of contracted vessels. The role of these receptors in the development of chronic pulmonary hypertension and cor pulmonale in patients with COPD is not established. The very limited systemic absorption of inhaled anticholinergic agents means that these vascular muscarinic receptors are not likely to be influenced by anticholinergic therapy. This lack of effect on vascular muscarinic receptors may explain why there is no apparent worsening of ventilation or perfusion matching, as occurs following beta-adrenoreceptor agonists when these drugs are administered to subjects during an exacerbation of COPD.

Anticholinergic agents

Anticholinergic agents are composed of a trophane ring on which is located a nitrogen atom. In naturally occurring antagonists, such as atropine, this nitrogen atom is three-valent, and so these compounds are termed tertiary anticholinergics. Tertiary anticholinergic compounds are water soluble and so are readily absorbed when applied topically. Since systemic absorption is associated with several important side effects, outlined below, this limits their clinical usefulness. Quaternary ammonium anticholinergic compounds were designed by rational pharmacologic methods to overcome this problem.[58,59] Quaternary anticholinergic agents retain the trophane ring nitrogen, which is required for functional activity but they have been modified so that they exist in an ionized state (Figure 23.3). This modification has led to the development of compounds that are considerably less soluble in organic solvents compared to water and so have much less systemic absorption than do the tertiary compounds.

IPRATROPIUM BROMIDE AND OXITROPIUM BROMIDE

At present the most widely used anticholinergic agents in the management of dyspnea in COPD are the quaternary compounds ipratropium bromide, oxitropium bromide and tiotropium bromide (Figure 23.3). Both drugs

are non-selective antagonists at muscarinic receptors for example, the K_d for ipratropium at the M_{1-3} receptors is 1.23 ± 0.36, 3.54 ± 1.27 and 0.64 ± 0.07 nM respectively. Ipratropium bromide is available in both the USA and in Europe in both nebulized and metered dose preparations. A dose of 36 µg ipratropium bromide administered by metered dose results in a bronchodilatation that is equivalent to 100 µg delivered by a nebulizer. Studies using radiolabeled tracer suggest that <5% of the drug is absorbed when administered by the inhaled route. This limited absorption is due to the quaternary structure of the compound. Following oral aerosol inhalation of ipratropium, bronchodilatation starts after 15 minutes and reaches its peak effect 1–2 hours after administration. The duration of bronchodilatation induced by ipra-tropium bromide is approximately 4–6 hours. In dose– response studies in patients with COPD it has been demonstrated that the optimal dose of ipratropium when administered by aerosol is 36–72 µg and 400 µg when administered by nebulizer. The structure and peripheral action of oxitropium bromide is similar to that of ipratropium bromide, although a dose of 200 µg which achieves a similar degree of bronchodilatation as 36 µg of ipratropium lasts between 6 and 8 hours. Tracer studies have demonstrated that between 15 and 24% of ipratropium is excreted as the intact molecule in the urine, a further 40–60% in the feces. The trophane ring of ipratropium bromide is metabolized by hydrolysis which accounts for the rest of the drug metabolism.

The results of the large prospective multicenter 5-year study indicate that there is little evidence of tolerance to anticholinergic agents even after five years of regular use.[60] This lack of tolerance may be because the drug is an antagonist and there is no evidence of constitual activity of these receptors.

The naturally occurring tertiary ammonium agents such as atropine are associated with significant side effects including blurring of vision, tachycardia, dry eyes and mouth, urinary retention as well as irritability and confusion. These significant side effects of these inhaled agents is noteworthy since the systemic side effects of tertiary anticholinergic agents, in particular worsening of bladder outflow obstruction, confusion, postural hypotension and blurring of vision are more likely to occur in older subjects such as those with COPD. By contrast, the inhaled quaternary anticholinergic agents are poorly absorbed and so are associated with few systemic adverse effects. The quaternary anticholinergic agents do not inhibit mucociliary clearance, do not worsen narrow angle glaucoma or bladder outflow obstructive symptoms.[58,59,61] In particular, the drugs are well tolerated in subjects with COPD. For example, in the Lung Health Study the most important side effect was a dry mouth which occurred in less than 5% of subjects.[60] In contrast

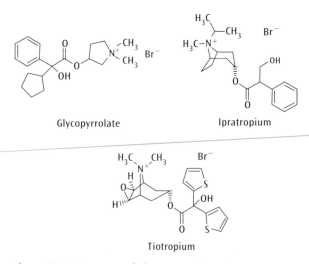

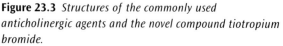

Figure 23.3 *Structures of the commonly used anticholinergic agents and the novel compound tiotropium bromide.*

to subjects with asthma paradoxical bronchoconstriction, worsening of symptoms after treatment with an inhaled anticholinergic agent due to a reaction to the solvent has not been reported to occur in patients with COPD.[62] To date there has been little investigation on the possible pharmacogenetics of muscarinic receptors. However, it is clear that there is a variability in the clinical response to these compounds suggesting that there is may be a genetic variability in muscarinic receptors or in the metabolism of these compounds.

In addition to these compounds several long-acting, functionally selective, anticholinergic compounds are being developed for clinical use, of these tiotropium bromide has recently become available.

TIOTROPIUM BROMIDE

Tiotropium is a positively charged compound with quaternary structure; as such it is similar in structure to ipratropium bromide but has, in addition, a thiophene group (Figure 23.3). The binding affinity for tiotropium at human muscarinic receptors is high and essentially the same for all three muscarinic receptors in the lungs (K_d 0.21 ± 0.06, 0.021 ± 0.06 and 0.014 ± 0.02 nM for M_1, M_2 and M_3 respectively.[63] Interestingly, however, tiotropium disassociates 100-fold more slowly than ipratropium bromide from M_1 and M_3 muscarinic receptors (dissociation half-life = 14.6, 3.6 and 34.7 hours, for M_1, M_2 and M_3 receptors, respectively). This unique feature of apparent kinetic selectivity for tiotropium bromide (the time constants for ipratropium bromide are in minutes rather than hours) means that although tiotropium bromide is not a selective muscarinic receptor antagonist, it selectively inhibits M_1 and M_3 muscarinic receptors. Functional studies on isolated airways show that tiotropium bromide inhibits methacholine-induced contraction with greater potency than the effect of either atropine or ipratropium bromide.[64] Tiotropium bromide also enhances electrical field-stimulated acetylcholine release due to M_2 receptor blockade. However, this enhancement is lost within 2 hours of washout of the drug at a time when M_3 muscarinic receptors are still blocked. This finding shows functional selectivity of tiotropium bromide for M_3 muscarinic receptors over M_2 muscarinic receptors. Although such artificial experiments demonstrate the pharmacologic selectivity of blockade of M_3 receptor by tiotropium bromide, it must be questioned as to whether this effect occurs *in vivo* since, unlike the situation in binding studies, the drug will potentially be able to rebind to M_2 muscarinic receptors *in vivo*.

In humans, *in vivo*, single dosing studies have established an effective dose that is not associated with systemic effects, consistent with a quaternary structured anticholinergic agent. In addition, tiotropium causes a sustained increase in FEV_1 of about 10% over baseline which is sustained for more than 24 hours.[65] In these studies, tiotropium was effective in inhibiting methacholine-induced bronchoconstriction; in other words it inhibited M_3 receptor stimulation. It remains to be seen if tiotropium bromide is any more effective against vagally mediated reflex bronchoconstriction. The results of studies using tiotropium in patients with COPD, using both single and multiple dosing studies, show it to be a safe, well-tolerated drug that causes a sustained bronchodilatation.[66–70] These studies have also shown tiotropium to be more effective than ipratropium bromide and tiotropium has the advantage of being taken once daily. In addition, it has been shown to increase quality of life scores, reduce the severity and duration of COPD exacerbations and increase exercise capacity.

GLYCOPYRROLATE

Glycopyrrolate is a quaternary ammonium anticholinergic agent, widely used in anesthesia and in veterinary medicine. It has not been used widely in the management of COPD, although placebo-controlled studies have shown that when given as a metered dose, glycopyrrolate is an effective long-acting bronchodilator in asthma. Recent work has shown glycopyrrolate to be threefold more potent than ipratropium bromide in inhibiting vagally induced bronchoconstriction.[71] In these studies, the duration of action of glycopyrrolate was significantly more prolonged compared to ipratropium bromide. There was no selectivity in its binding to rat M_1, M_2 and M_3 receptors, although kinetic studies have shown that glycopyrrolate dissociated significantly more slowly from human smooth muscle muscarinic receptors compared to ipratropium bromide. Thus, although there is little clinical data on the effectiveness of glycopyrrolate in COPD, it has many of the advantages of tiotropium bromide.

BETA-ADRENORECEPTOR AGONISTS

Studies by Oliver in the 1890s identified that adrenal gland extracts stimulated a rise in blood pressure.[72] The compound responsible for this action is adrenaline (epinephrine) isolated by Takamine while noradrenaline (norepinephrine), which has different systemic effects was identified by van Euler in 1947.[73] Studies by Ahlquist identified that the differences in the systemic activity of adrenaline and noradrenaline were due to their effects on different receptors which were termed adrenoreceptors.[74] Further studies identified that certain adrenoreceptor agonists preferentially bind to subgroups of adrenoreceptors, termed alpha$_{1-2}$ and beta$_{1-3}$.

Adrenoreceptors mediate the responses to sympathetic nerves

In humans, submucosal blood vessels, in particular in the upper airway, are well innervated with noradrenergic nerves.[75–77] Stimulation of these nerves constricts these blood vessels which in turn leads to changes in airflow and the heat exchange functions of the nose. Bronchial submucosal gland cells contain alpha- and beta-adrenoreceptors and stimulation of these receptors leads to mucus production. Thus, in theory, adrenoreceptor agonists which are widely used in the management of obstructive airways diseases such as asthma may therefore lead to mucus plugging of the airways. In practice, however, this effect is overshadowed by the effect of both alpha$_2$- and beta$_2$-adrenoreceptors located on postsynaptic nerve terminals. Stimulation of these postsynaptic adrenoreceptors prevents the release of acetylcholine from cholinergic nerves and of noradrenaline (norepinephrine) from noradrenergic nerves. These inhibitory effects on neurotransmitter release appear to be the dominant effect of adrenoreceptors in the airways.[78,79] Airway and vascular smooth muscle contains an abundance of beta$_2$-adrenoreceptors and a relatively small number of stimulatory alpha$_1$-adrenoreceptors.[80–85] The function of airway smooth muscle associated beta$_2$-adrenoreceptors is bronchodilatation. These receptors represent the principal pharmacologic site of interest in modulating the action of the sympathetic nervous system.

Chemical properties of beta-adrenoreceptor agonists

The chemical formulation of adrenaline (epinephrine) is shown in Figure 23.4; the compound contains a benzene ring and an ethylamine side chain. Substitutions on the benzene ring, either of the two side chain carbon molecules or the terminal amine group, leads to changes in the nature of the sympathetic activity. Increasing the size of the alkyl substituent of the amine group increases beta-adrenoreceptor activity. Molecular studies have shown that serine residues at position 207 and 204 interact with hydroxyl groups on position three and five of the aromatic ring.[86] Thus, a compound with OH-groups in these positions has greater selectivity for the beta-adrenoreceptor. Using these principals several beta-adrenoreceptors have been designed and introduced for the management of airways diseases.

THE BETA$_2$-ADRENORECEPTOR

The beta-adrenoreceptor is a seven transmembrane spanning G-protein as shown in Figure 23.4.[87] It consists of two disulfide bonds on the extracellular surface and

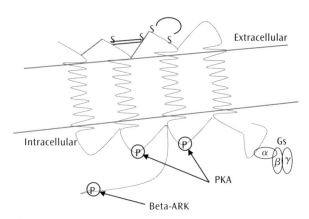

Figure 23.4 *The structure of the β$_2$-adrenoreceptor. The β$_2$-adrenoreceptor is a G-protein with intracellular and extracellular domains. The extracellular domain is maintained by two disulfide bonds and in addition to activating adenylate cyclase the receptor is both homologously and heterologously desensitized by phosphorylation at the sites shown on the intracellular domains by the letter P. PKA = protein kinase A; Beta-ARK = β-adrenoreceptor kinase.*

two sites for N-linked glycosylation. Stimulation of the beta-adrenoreceptor stimulates the Gs domain to activate the enzyme adenylate cyclase leading to the production of cAMP and the activation of intracellular kinase protein kinase A (PKA).[88] The intracellular domain contains sites for phosphorylation by the action of the cAMP dependent enzyme PKA, heterologous desensitization and a phosphorylation site at the C-terminus which is activated by beta-adrenoreceptor kinase (beta-ARK) which results in homologous desensitization of the receptor (Figure 23.5).[89]

SALBUTAMOL AND TERBUTALINE

The synthetic sympathomimetic amines most commonly used in the management of patients with COPD are terbutaline and salbutamol. The chemical formulations of these agents is shown in Figure 23.6. Both compounds have a high affinity for beta-adrenoreceptors with a pK$_a$ of 9.3 and 10.3; in contrast, neither compound has any significant affinity for alpha-adrenoreceptors.[90,91] Both compounds have greater selectivity for beta$_2$- compared to beta$_1$-adrenoreceptors and thus exert an effect on both airway smooth muscle cells and peripheral vascular blood vessels in preference to beta$_1$-adrenoreceptors which are found in particular on cardiac muscle cells.

Both salbutamol and terbutaline exist in two stereoisomeric forms referred to as (−) and (+) enantiomers. Most formulations consist of the compounds in both enantiomeric forms. Data from *in vitro* ligand-binding studies and functional studies in animals indicate

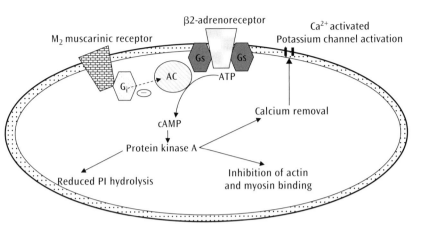

Figure 23.5 *Mechanism of action of the β$_2$- and M$_2$ muscarinic receptors in airway smooth muscle. Following activation of the β$_2$-adrenoreceptor by an agonist, Gs subunit is phosphorylated and activates the adenylate cyclase enzyme leading to the generation of cAMP.*

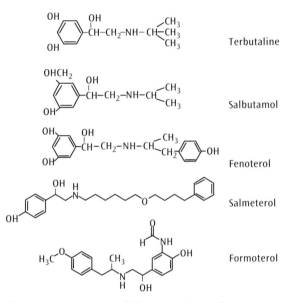

Figure 23.6 *Structures of the commonly used sympathomimetic agents.*

that the (+) enantiomer has as much as a 100-fold greater affinity for the beta$_2$-adrenoreceptor than the (−) enantiomer. By contrast, the (−) enantiomer may not be associated with any significant bronchodilatation and may in fact inhibit the functional effect of the (+) form.[92] Further, *in vivo*, studies in patients with obstructive airways diseases will need to be performed to establish the functional consequences of these *in vitro* observations.

Both salbutamol and terbutaline are highly water soluble and so both are readily absorbed from the respiratory tract. The peak blood levels of salbutamol after a nebulized dose of 3 mg is 2.1 ng/ml, which occurs approximately 50 minutes after administration. Bronchodilatation typically occurs 5–10 minutes after topical oral administration of either drug, peaks approximately after 1 hour and lasts 3–4 hours. The (+) enantiomer has

a shorter half-life and a lower bioavailability than the (−) enantiomer. Both salbutamol and terbutaline are metabolized in the liver by sulphate conjugation. Neither drug is metabolized by the enzyme C-OMT and neither is a substrate for catecholamine cellular uptake processes and so they can be used in conjunction with monoamine oxidase inhibitor (MAOI) antidepressant medications. After topical oral administration approximately 70% of the drug or its metabolites are excreted in the urine within 24 hours.

The beta$_2$-adrenoreceptor agonists are associated with the predictable side effects of all the sympathomimetic agents such as tachycardia, mild agitation, headaches and peripheral vasodilatation. In keeping with the presence of beta$_2$-adrenoreceptors on skeletal smooth cells these agonists can also cause fine motor tremor, cramps and occasionally with higher doses hypokalemia and hyperglycemia.[93]

Chronic agonist binding, including to beta-adrenoreceptors, leads to both homologous and heterologous desensitization of the receptor and downregulation of the receptor. In theory this should mean that repeated use of these agents leads to less efficacy or an increase in the dose of the drug required to induce the same degree of bronchodilatation. In practice, this does not appear to happen *in vivo* in most individuals with other airways diseases such as asthma.[94,95] However, there is some evidence that there are certain common polymorphic variations in the structure of beta$_2$-adrenoreceptors. These polymorphisms appear to alter the behavior of the receptor following agonist exposure and include Arg-Gly16, Glu-Gln27, and Thr-lle164. The Gly16 receptor downregulates to a greater extent and is associated with increased airway hyperreactivity, nocturnal symptoms and more severe asthma. The Glu27 form appears to protect against downregulation, is associated with less reactive airways and a greater tendency to desensitization.[96–98] To date studies examining whether this also occurs in subjects with COPD have not been reported.

SALMETEROL AND FORMOTEROL

Currently, there are two long-acting beta-adrenoreceptor agonists available for use in patients with COPD, salmeterol and formoterol. Formoterol was initially one of a group of phenyethanolamines that were being systematically analyzed for beta$_2$-adrenoreceptor potency.[99,100] By chance it was found that formoterol had an extended duration of action when delivered by an inhaled route and so the compound was further developed and brought into clinical trials in the mid 1990s. Subsequent studies have shown that the extended spectrum of activity of formoterol is due to its hydrophobic nature. Salmeterol was based on chemical principles, it was designed specifically to be a longer acting beta-adrenoreceptor.[100–102] The rationale for the design of salmeterol was that it would retain the COMT-resistant catechol nucleus of salbutamol but the N-subunits were extended to make them more hydrophobic and resistant to metabolism. The hydrophobic nature of both of these compounds explains the extended duration of action. Both drugs associate within the cell membrane lipid bilayers and diffuse from this to the beta$_2$-adrenoreceptor. *In vivo*, and, *in vitro*, studies have shown that these agents relax airway smooth muscle for considerably longer periods than short-acting beta$_2$-adrenoreceptor agonists. Differences in the lipid solubility of the two drugs explains the observed differences in the duration of their action. For example, after washing off a solution of 1×10^{-9} M formoterol results in a return of 50% relaxation capability of airway smooth muscle at 4 hours, in the same type of experiment 50% relaxation of airway smooth muscle occurs 24 hours after application of 1×10^{-7} M salmeterol.[103] *In vivo*, in humans a single dose of 50 µg of salmeterol or 24 µg of formoterol results in a sustained bronchodilatation for a period of 12 hours. There are some differences in the pharmacology of formoterol and salmeterol. For example, formoterol has a faster onset of action, i.e. 2–3 minutes compared to 10 minutes for salmeterol, and indeed the maximum bronchodilatation achieved by this agent takes several hours. Once again these differences reflect the different chemical nature of the two compounds. The efficacy of formoterol, i.e. its ability to relax airway smooth muscle relative to an agonist such as adrenaline (epinephrine), is substantially higher than that of either salbutamol or salmeterol.[103–105] The low intrinsic efficacy of salmeterol may be of clinical relevance, since this means that salmeterol is less likely to bind to and exert an effect in tissue where there are relatively small numbers of beta$_2$-adrenoreceptors compared with an equal dose of an agent with higher intrinsic efficacy, such as formoterol. The low intrinsic efficacy of salmeterol reduces its side effects in non-target organs where beta$_2$-adrenoreceptors are expressed in relatively low numbers, such as the heart. A second advantage of this partial efficacy is that less homologous desensitization occurs with partial agonists such as salmeterol. This is likely to result in less desensitization to the bronchodilator effects of short-acting beta$_2$-adrenoreceptor agonists when these drugs are administered in association with formoterol on a regular basis. In practice it is not clear whether either of these differences are relevant to patients with COPD.

Systemic absorption of inhaled salmeterol and formoterol occurs after topical application. There is an initial increase in the blood following administration due to absorption from the oropharynx and also approximately 45 minutes after delivery of the drug, a second increase in systemic levels occurs due to the effect of swallowing and absorption from the gastrointestinal tract. The levels of either drug in the blood do not correlate with the drug's functional activity since it is carried in the blood attached to proteins and in any case for both drugs the blood levels are relatively small. The drugs are extensively metabolized in the liver by hydroxylation or glucuronidation and eliminated in the feces. The side effects of long-acting beta$_2$-adrenoreceptor agonists are tachycardia, tremor, hypokalemia, hyperglycemia and an increase in Q-Tc intervals.[106]

THEOPHYLLINES

More than 150 years ago it was reported that the ingestion of strong infusions of tea or coffee were effective in the relief of breathlessness in patients with obstructive airways diseases.[107] It was later identified that the active bronchodilator substance in these beverages is a methylxanthine. Theophylline, a chemically synthesized methylxanthine, has been used for the treatment of dyspnea in patients with COPD for over 50 years. Notwithstanding the length of clinical experience with theophylline the exact mechanism of its action and its role in the management of patients with COPD still remains uncertain. This is because theophyllines have a narrow therapeutic window, i.e. at low doses they are only relatively weak bronchodilators while at higher doses they are associated with significant side effects. Consequently, the use of theophylline drugs in the management of dyspnea in patients with COPD has diminished in particular with the introduction of other long-lasting bronchodilator agents such as the long-acting beta-agonists.

Chemistry of theophyllines

Theophylline is a methylxanthine (Figure 23.7). It is sparingly soluble in water although its solubility is enhanced with increases in the pH of the solution. Derivatives of theophyllines including aminophylline, dyphylline and oxtriphylline have been synthesized to increase solubility.

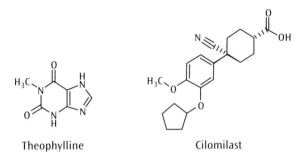

Figure 23.7 *Structures of the theophylline and cilomilast.*

Each of these compounds exert their effects by competitively inhibiting the action of the phosphodiesterase enzymes.[108] The phosphodiesterase enzymes are a superfamily of enzymes, found in almost all cells, whose function is the metabolism of the cyclic nucleotides, cyclic AMP and cyclic GMP. Thus, by inhibiting phosphodiesterases theophyllines lead to an increase in the cellular content of cyclic neucleotides. In airway smooth muscle cells the increased cyclic AMP levels induced by theophylline lead to the phosphorylation of protein kinase (PKA) and the opening of outwardly rectifying calcium channels and the relaxation of airway smooth muscle cells. It is reasonable to suppose that if this were the drug's principal mechanism of action then this would have a synergistic effect with beta$_2$-adrenoreceptor agonists, which increase cyclic AMP levels in smooth muscle cells. In practice, such synergism is not seen when theophylline is administered in the doses that are used in clinical practice. Alternative explanations for the effect of theophyllines in obstructive airways diseases include the hypothesis that they inhibit airway wall edema induced by activated sensory nerves or they inhibit the activation of certain populations of T cells or eosinophils.[109–120] In all of these studies the anti-inflammatory effects of theophylline is relatively weak. Another proposed explanation for the action of theophylline in COPD, in particular during acute exacerbations, is that they increase the force of contraction of the diaphragm.[121,122] However, this too is of uncertain clinical significance since there is little evidence that diaphragmatic fatigue occurs, *in vivo*, even during exacerbations of COPD. Thus, the mechanism of action of theophylline in patients with COPD has yet to be established.

Metabolism of theophyllines

Theophylline is absorbed from the gastrointestinal system. However, the rate of absorption depends on the nature of the preparation, in particular there is a considerable degree of variability in the rate of absorption of long-acting and enteric-coated preparations. Theophylline is not administered in an inhaled formulation since the clinical benefits are related to the serum concentrations of the drug. Theophylline is bound to protein in the serum and is metabolized by the liver's microsomal cytochrome P450/P448 system and excreted as 3-methylxanthine and dimethyluric acid into the urine. Thus, since the compound is carried protein bound in the systemic circulation and metabolized in the liver through the cytochrome P450 system it is not surprising that theophylline is associated with several important pharmacokinetic interactions. Therapeutically, there is a narrow window of blood levels between clinical effectiveness and side effects. It is well established that when the serum concentrations of theophylline are less than 5–10 μg/ml there is little clinical benefit while serum levels in excess of 20 μg/ml are associated with toxicity.

There is a marked variability in the rate of metabolism of the compound, for example in steady-state dosing schedule studies serum concentrations vary among patients by as much as sixfold and serum half-lives exhibit a wide variation due to variability in the rates of clearance. The serum half-life is quite constant for an individual, however it may be increased in patients with cor pulmonale, heart failure, liver disease, in cigarette smokers or following the ingestion of certain drugs.[123–125]

Side effects of theophyllines

There are two important types of side effects associated with theophyllines, systemic side effects and drug interactions. The systemic effects of theophyllines are mediated by the inhibition of phosphodiesterase enzymes that are not involved in its proposed therapeutic benefit. The common side effects of theophylline include nausea and vomiting, palpitations, tachycardia, arrhythmia, tremor, headaches, dizziness, seizures and electrolyte disturbances.[126]

Drug side effects of theophyllines are common since these drugs are metabolized by the hepatic microsomal system that is used by a number of other drugs and body products. A number of drugs or conditions associated with COPD including cigarette smoke, alcohol intake and viral infections as well as medications such as macrolide antibiotics, ciprofloxacin, cimetidine, phenytoin and phenobarbitone can alter the metabolism of theophyllines. Thus, the use of these drugs or the presence of these conditions can result in either accumulation of the drugs or altered clinical ineffectiveness.

PHOSPHODIESTERASE TYPE 4 INHIBITORS

As indicated above the phosphodiesterases comprise a superfamily of proteins with 10 individual families (PDE 1–10) whose function is to metabolize the intracellular messengers, the cyclic nucleotides cAMP and cGMP.[127–130] The individual families have different sites of distribution in the body, different substrate preferences and different activities. For example, PDE3 and PDE4 are found in the airway smooth muscle of the trachea and bronchi.[131–133] By contrast, in the smaller airways the PDE4 isoform appears to mediate smooth muscle relaxation and is also widely distributed in inflammatory cells such as macrophages, neutrophils and eosinophils.[115,134–138] This may be of relevance as these are the inflammatory cells implicated in the pathogenesis of COPD. Dilation of the small airways may be of greater importance in COPD and furthermore studies have shown that the PDE3 isoform mediates the cardiovascular effects of phosphodiesterase inhibition. Since the clinical effectiveness of theophylline is limited by side effects mediated by inhibition of phosphodiesterase enzymes not involved in its therapeutic benefit and PDE4 has a number of potentially beneficial effects selective PDE4 antagonists have been developed.

The PDE4 enzyme family are encoded for by four different genes termed A–D, each gene product may undergo alternative splicing thus leading to long and short forms of the enzyme. The initial PDE inhibitor rolipram, which was introduced as a potential antidepressant was limited in its use by the significant incidence of nausea and vomiting. Thus, two broad strategies have been used to develop novel PDE4 inhibitors.[139–141] For example, each subtype of PDE4 exists in either a low- or a high-affinity conformation which means that although an inhibitor may bind the same enzyme from different sites within the body with equal affinity, this may not be reflected in its ability to inhibit enzymatic function (different K_i). Studies have shown that in the brain and in particular within the emesis center the PDE4 enzyme is in the high-affinity conformation while in the lung the target PDE4 is in the low-affinity conformation state.[142] Thus, new PDE4 inhibitors have been designed with selective activity for one or other of the conformations. The other strategy used to develop a PDE4 inhibitor with the maximal clinical efficacy without side effects has been to selectively inhibit one of the four genetically different PDE4 enzymes.[140,141] This strategy is based on the fact that PDE4D protein expression is highest in the brainstem, while the A–C gene products are more widely expressed by inflammatory cells. However, before this strategy can be used clinically more information on the exact distribution of the PDE4 products in the lungs and brain as well as possible changes in their expression in diseases such as COPD and the mechanism of regulation of expression are all required.

There is relatively limited published information on the pharmacology of many of the new compounds that are in clinical development. Rolipram was the first PDE4 inhibitor and was initially brought into clinical trials as a potential antidepressant based on its ability to increase neurotransmission. In these clinical trials it was reported that these agents were not associated with any cardiac or circulatory side effects but that nausea and vomiting were important side effects, which occurred in approximately 20% of subjects.[143,144] This appears to be an effect of the compound on the central emesis center rather than a local irritant effect, since studies using analogs of rolipram that are not taken up into the central nervous system are associated with significantly less emesis. The second generation PDE4 inhibitors, CDP840 and SB 207499 (cilomilast), have been reported in clinical trials to be associated with significantly less emesis than rolipram, indeed the incidence of this symptom in clin-ical trials in patients with both compounds was similar to placebo.

Corticosteroids

Although corticosteroids are widely used in an attempt to control airway inflammation in asthma they have not been convincingly demonstrated to be of value in the majority of patients with COPD. Notwithstanding this limitation they are used in the management of some patients as discussed in a separate section of this book. The possible mechanism of action of these powerful anti-inflammatory agents in the airways is summarized in Figure 23.8. The most commonly used corticosteroids are beclomethasone and budesonide (dose in asthma 50–2400 μg/day) and fluticasone (dose in asthma 50–1000 μg/day). All contain a central steroid ring; fluticasone is a trifluorinated corticosteroid that is synthesized from a 19-carbon androsterone ring. Beclomethasone and budesonide are 21-carbon steroid molecules and are structurally related to hydrocortisone. They are readily absorbed from the gastrointestinal and respiratory tracts, all are metabolized in the liver and excreted in the urine. Local side effects, in particular oropharyngeal candidiasis, are common, cataracts, adrenal suppression and disturbance of glucose and bone turnover may occasionally be seen with very high doses of inhaled steroids.

Smoking cessation medications
(see also Chapter 22)

Nicotine replacement patches have been used in conjunction with smoking cessation counseling for some years.[145–147] Nicotine is a pyridine alkaloid and is available for administration as nicotine polacrilex, a sugar-free chewing gum (dose 2–4 mg), as a nasal or oral inhaler (delivers approximately 15 ng per activation) and in a transdermal absorbable form (dose ranges from 30 to 130 μg/cm^2/h, which results in an equivalent of 21 mg/day). Nicotine is an agonist at cholinergic ganglion receptors at peripheral ganglia, within the adrenal

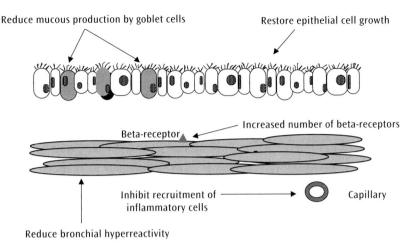

Reduce mucous production by goblet cells

Restore epithelial cell growth

Increased number of beta-receptors

Beta-receptor

Inhibit recruitment of inflammatory cells

Capillary

Reduce bronchial hyperreactivity

Figure 23.8 *Mechanism of action of glucocorticoids. These compounds exert a wide variety of potentially useful effects in the airways of subjects with COPD.*

medulla, at neuromuscular junctions and in the central nervous system. Initially the compound may induce agonist effects although later tolerance to chronically administered nicotine develops. Following administration of a dose of nicotine a number of effects are seen due to the stimulation of nicotinic receptors which lead to an increase in heart rate, blood pressure, stimulation of the gastrointestinal tract, and in the central nervous system stimulation of alertness and cognitive performance.[148,149] Absorption of nicotine is most rapid when administered as a topical spray (plasma level in 15 minutes), while the plasma level following chewing the nicotine gum is 25 minutes and following transdermal administration the drug is absorbed at a slower rate, the peak plasma level is seen at 2 hours.[150,151] Thus, the inhaled form is useful acutely as a cigarette substitute while the patch is useful for chronic avoidance. The half-life of nicotine in the plasma is 3 hours and 12 hours following the removal of a nicotine patch the plasma levels of nicotine are undetectable. Aside from local effects due to topical administration adverse effects of nicotine replacement are usually mild and transient and are due to the local effects of the nicotine. However such side effects can be sufficient to discourage poorly motivated smokers. In large doses there can be cardiovascular side effects, including worsening of angina and limb claudication, arrhythmias and hypertension, since these conditions often associated with COPD mean that nicotine replacement may not be tolerated by some patients.

Bupropion is a tricyclic antidepressant which has recently been licensed for use as an adjunct for smoking cessation.[152] The mechanism of action is not established but may in part be due to inhibition of nicotine withdrawal symptoms and prevention of decline in mood associated with nicotine by dopaminergic and noradrenergic effects.[153] Prospective, randomized clinical trials have established that bupropion is more effective than

standard therapeutic approaches using nicotine replacement and supportive counseling.[154–157] Other, less expensive tricyclic antidepressant agents such as nortriptyline have also been shown to be of benefit in achieving effective smoking cessation.

Bupropion is an aminoketone derivative that is structurally unrelated to any other antidepressant agent and so is not associated with some of the usual side effects of the other antidepressants. The drug is administered as an oral preparation, a dose of 150–300 mg per day has been shown to be more effective than placebo in achieving smoking cessation. It is absorbed from the gastrointestinal tract in 2–3 hours, the half-life is between 8–24 hours and is metabolized in the liver by hydroxylation. The mechanism of action is uncertain, although wholebody turnover of noradrenaline (norepinephrine) is reduced.[158–160] Buproprion has a relatively safe side effect even in patients with COPD. For example, in a recent study of 204 subjects with COPD, 6% of participants reported side effects of anxiety and insomnia.[161] Thus, this may be an effective and safe medication for use as an aid in smoking cessation, still the only proven diseasemodifying intervention in COPD.

CONCLUSIONS

A large number of compounds are available for use in the symptomatic management of patients with COPD. Several of these compounds have been the subject of intensive research and development to improve their clinical effectiveness and limit their side effects. Further developments in the development of agents with an ability to inhibit the tissue destruction and inflammation caused by cigarettes and relief of symptoms such as cough and mucus production would be useful new agents to have in clinical practice.

REFERENCES

1. Olsen C, Colebatch H, Mebel P, Nadel J, Staub N. Motor control of pulmonary airways studied by nerve stimulation. *J Appl Physiol* 1965;**20**:202–8.

2. Brody JS, Klempfner G, Staum MM, Vidyasagas D, Kuhl DE, Waldhausen JA. Mucociliary clearence after lung denervation and bronchial transection. *J Appl Physiol* 1972;**32**:160–4.

3. Gallagher JT, Kent PW, Passatore M, Phipps RJ, Richardson PS. The composition of tracheal mucus and the nervous control of its secretion in the cat. *Proc R Soc Lond* 1976;**192**:49–76.

4. McCormack DG, Mak JC, Minette P, Barnes PJ. Muscarinic receptor subtypes mediating vasodilation in the pulmonary artery. *Eur J Pharmacol* 1988;**158**:293–7.

5. Coleridge HM, Coleridge JC. Neural regulation of bronchial blood flow. *Respir Physiol* 1994;**98**:1–13.

6. Mann SP. The innervation of mammalian bronchial smooth muscle: the localization of catecholamines and cholinesterases. *Histochemistry* 1971;**3**:319–31.

7. Richardson JB. Nerve supply to the lungs. *Am Rev Respir* 1979;**119**:785–802.

8. O'Donnell DE, Lam M, Webb KA. Spirometric correlates of improvement in exercise performance after anticholinergic therapy in chronic obstructive pulmonary disease. *Am J Respir Crit Care Med* 1999;**160**:542–9.

9. O'Donnell DE, Lam M, Webb KA. Measurement of symptoms, lung hyperinflation, and endurance during exercise in chronic obstructive pulmonary disease. *Am J Respir Crit Care Med* 1998;**158**:1557–65.

10. Severinghaus JW, Stupfel M. Respiratory dead space increases following atropine in man and atropine, vagal or ganglionic blockade and hypothermia in dogs. *J Appl Physiol* 1955;**8**:81–6.

11. Douglas NJ, Sudlow MF, Flenley DC. Effect of an inhaled atropinelike agent on normal airway function. *J Appl Physiol* 1979;**46**:256–62.

12. Gross NJ, Co E, Skorodin MS. Cholinergic bronchomotor tone in COPD. Estimates of its amount in comparison with that in normal subjects. *Chest* 1989;**96**:984–7.

13. Hulme EC, Kurtenbach E, Curtis CA. Muscarinic acetylcholine receptors: structure and function. *Biochem Soc Trans* 1991;**19**:133–8.

14. Lechleiter J, Peralta E, Clapham D. Diverse functions of muscarinic acetylcholine receptor subtypes. *Trends Pharmacol Sci* 1989;(suppl):34–8.

15. Ramachandran J, Peralta EG, Ashkenazi A, Winslow JW, Capon DJ. The structural and functional interrelationships of muscarinic acetylcholine receptor subtypes. *Bioessays* 1989;**10**:54–7.

16. Mak JC, Barnes PJ. Muscarinic receptor subtypes in human and guinea pig lung. *Eur J Pharmacol* 1989;**164**:223–30.

17. Mak JC, Barnes PJ. Autoradiographic visualization of muscarinic receptor subtypes in human and guinea pig lung. *Am Rev Respir Dis* 1990;**141**:1559–68.

18. Mak JC, Baraniuk JN, Barnes PJ. Localization of muscarinic receptor subtype mRNAs in human lung. *Am J Respir Cell Mol Biol* 1992;**7**:344–8.

19. Haddad EB, Mak JC, Hislop A, Haworth SG, Barnes PJ. Characterization of muscarinic receptor subtypes in pig airways: radioligand binding and northern blotting studies. *Am J Physiol* 1994;**266**:L642–8.

20. Haddad EB, Mak JC, Belvisi MG, Nishikawa M, Rousell J, Barnes PJ. Muscarinic and beta-adrenergic receptor expression in peripheral lung from normal and asthmatic patients. *Am J Physiol* 1996;**270**:L947–53.

21. Buckley NJ, Bonner TI, Buckley CM, Brann MR. Antagonist binding properties of five cloned muscarinic receptors expressed in CHO-K1 cells. *Mol Pharmacol* 1989;**35**:469–76.

22. Wess J, Blin N, Mutschler E, Bluml K. Muscarinic acetylcholine receptors: structural basis of ligand binding and G protein coupling. *Life Sci* 1995;**56**:915–22.

23. Wess J. Molecular basis of receptor/G-protein-coupling selectivity. *Pharmacol Ther* 1998;**80**:231–64.

24. Wess J, Liu J, Blin N, Yun J, Lerche C, Kostenis E. Structural basis of receptor/G protein coupling selectivity studied with muscarinic receptors as model systems. *Life Sci* 1997;**60**:1007–14.

25. Casale TB, Ecklund P. Characterization of muscarinic receptor subtypes on human peripheral lung. *J Appl Physiol* 1988;**65**:594–600.

26. Myers AC, Undem BJ, Weinreich D. Electrophysiological properties of neurons in guinea pig bronchial parasympathetic ganglia. *Am J Physiol* 1990;**259**:L403–9.

27. Koyama S, Rennard SI, Robbins RA. Acetylcholine stimulates bronchial epithelial cells to release neutrophil and monocyte chemotactic activity. *Am J Physiol* 1992;**262**:L466–71.

28. Ueda F, Ban K, Ishima T. Irsogladine activates gap-junctional intercellular communication through M1 muscarinic acetylcholine receptor. *J Pharmacol Exp Ther* 1995;**274**:815–19.

29. Yang B, McCaffrey TV. The roles of muscarinic receptor subtypes in modulation of nasal ciliary action. *Rhinology* 1996;**34**:136–9.

30. Yang B, Schlosser RJ, McCaffrey TV. Signal transduction pathways in modulation of ciliary beat frequency by methacholine. *Ann Otol Rhinol Laryngol* 1997;**106**:230–6.

31. Fryer AD, Maclagan J. Muscarinic inhibitory receptors in pulmonary parasympathetic nerves in the guinea-pig. *Br J Pharmacol* 1984;**83**:973–8.

32. Blaber LC, Fryer AD, Maclagan J. Neuronal muscarinic receptors attenuate vagally-induced contraction of feline bronchial smooth muscle. *Br J Pharmacol* 1985;**86**:723–8.

33. Patel HJ, Barnes PJ, Takahashi T, Tadjkarimi S, Yacoub MH, Belvisi MG. Evidence for prejunctional muscarinic autoreceptors in human and guinea pig trachea. *Am J Respir Crit Care Med* 1995;**152**:872–8.

34. Ramnarine SI, Haddad EB, Khawaja AM, Mak JC, Rogers DF. On muscarinic control of neurogenic mucus secretion in ferret trachea. *J Physiol* 1996;**494**:577–86.

35. Sankary RM, Jones CA, Madison JM, Brown JK. Muscarinic cholinergic inhibition of cyclic AMP accumulation in airway smooth muscle. Role of a pertussis toxin-sensitive protein. *Am Rev Respir Dis* 1988;**138**:145–50.

36. Fernandes LB, Fryer AD, Hirshman CA. M2 muscarinic receptors inhibit isoproterenol-induced relaxation of canine airway smooth muscle. *J Pharmacol Exp Ther* 1992;**262**:119–26.

37. Roffel AF, Elzinga CRS, Zaagsma J. Muscarinic M₃ receptors mediate contraction of human central and peripheral airway smooth muscle. *Pulmonary Pharm* 1990;**3**:47–51.

38. Fryer AD, Maclagan J. Ipratropium bromide potentiates bronchoconstriction induced by vagal nerve stimulation in the guinea-pig. *Eur J Pharmacol* 1987;**139**:187–91.

39. On LS, Boonyongsunchai P, Webb S, Davies L, Calverley PM, Costello RW. Function of pulmonary neuronal M2 muscarinic receptors in stable chronic obstructive pulmonary disease. *Am J Respir Crit Care Med* 2001;**163**:1320–5.

40. Evans CM, Belmonte KE, Costello RW, Jacoby DB, Gleich GJ, Fryer AD. Substance P-induced airway hyperreactivity is mediated by neuronal M2 receptor dysfunction. *Am J Physiol Lung Cell Mol Physiol* 2000;**279**:L477–86.

41. Adamko DJ, Yost BL, Gleich GJ, Fryer AD, Jacoby DB. Ovalbumin sensitization changes the inflammatory response to subsequent parainfluenza infection. Eosinophils mediate airway hyperresponsiveness, m^2 muscarinic receptor dysfunction, and antiviral effects. *J Exp Med* 1999;**190**: 1465–78.

42. Costello RW, Evans CM, Yost BL, *et al.* Antigen-induced hyperreactivity to histamine: role of the vagus nerves and eosinophils. *Am J Physiol* 1999;**276**:L709–14.

43. Jacoby DB, Xiao HQ, Lee NH, Chan-Li Y, Fryer AD. Virus- and interferon-induced loss of inhibitory M2 muscarinic receptor function and gene expression in cultured airway parasympathetic neurons. *J Clin Invest* 1998;**102**:242–8.

44. Evans CM, Fryer AD, Jacoby DB, Gleich GJ, Costello RW. Pretreatment with antibody to eosinophil major basic protein prevents hyperresponsiveness by protecting neuronal M2 muscarinic receptors in antigen-challenged guinea pigs. *J Clin Invest* 1997;**100**:2254–62.

45. Costello RW, Schofield BH, Kephart GM, Gleich GJ, Jacoby DB, Fryer AD. Localization of eosinophils to airway nerves and effect on neuronal M2 muscarinic receptor function. *Am J Physiol* 1997;**273**:L93–103.

46. Kahn RM, Okanlami OA, Jacoby DB, Fryer AD. Viral infection induces dependence of neuronal M2 muscarinic receptors on cyclooxygenase in guinea pig lung. *J Clin Invest* 1996; **98**:299–307.

47. Elbon CL, Jacoby DB, Fryer AD. Pretreatment with an antibody to interleukin-5 prevents loss of pulmonary M2 muscarinic receptor function in antigen-challenged guinea pigs. *Am J Respir Cell Mol Biol* 1995;**12**:320–8.

48. Fryer AD, Yarkony KA, Jacoby DB. The effect of leukocyte depletion on pulmonary M2 muscarinic receptor function in parainfluenza virus-infected guinea-pigs. *Br J Pharmacol* 1994;**112**:588–94.

49. Jacoby DB, Gleich GJ, Fryer AD. Human eosinophil major basic protein is an endogenous allosteric antagonist at the inhibitory muscarinic M2 receptor. *J Clin Invest* 1993; **91**:1314–18.

50. Fryer AD, Jacoby DB. Function of pulmonary M2 muscarinic receptors in antigen-challenged guinea pigs is restored by heparin and poly-L-glutamate. *J Clin Invest* 1992;**90**:2292–8.

51. Jacoby DB, Fryer AD. Virus-induced airway hyperresponsiveness – possible involvement of neural mechanisms. *Am Rev Respir Dis* 1991;**144**:1422–3.

52. Fryer AD, Jacoby DB. Parainfluenza virus infection damages inhibitory M2 muscarinic receptors on pulmonary parasympathetic nerves in the guinea-pig. *Br J Pharmacol* 1991;**102**:267–71.

53. Lammers JW, Barnes PJ, Chung KF. Nonadrenergic, noncholinergic airway inhibitory nerves. *Eur Respir J* 1992; **5**:239–46.

54. Cazzola M, Matera MG, Liccardi G, Sacerdoti G, D'Amato G, Rossi F. Effect of telenzepine, an M1-selective muscarinic receptor antagonist, in patients with nocturnal asthma. *Pulm Pharmacol* 1994;**7**:91–7.

55. Saitoh H, Masuda T, Shimura S, Fushimi T, Shirato K. Secretion and gene expression of secretory leukocyte protease inhibitor by human airway submucosal glands. *Am J Physiol Lung Cell Mol Physiol* 2001;**280**:L79–87.

56. Tamaoki J, Chiyotani A, Tagaya E, Sakai N, Konno K. Effect of long term treatment with oxitropium bromide on airway secretion in chronic bronchitis and diffuse panbronchiolitis. *Thorax* 1994;**49**:545–8.

57. Wanner A. Effect of ipratropium bromide on airway mucociliary function. *Am J Med* 1986;**81**:23–7.

58. Cugell DW. Clinical pharmacology and toxicology of ipratropium bromide. *Am J Med* 1986;**81**:18–22.

59. Pakes GE, Brogden RN, Heel RC, Speight TM, Avery GS. Ipratropium bromide: a review of its pharmacological properties and therapeutic efficacy in asthma and chronic bronchitis. *Drugs* 1980;**20**:237–66.

60. Anthonisen NR, Connett JE, Kiley JP, *et al.* Effects of smoking intervention and the use of an inhaled anticholinergic bronchodilator on the rate of decline of FEV_1. The Lung Health Study. *JAMA* 1994;**272**:1497–505.

61. Anderson WM. Hemodynamic and non-bronchial effects of ipratropium bromide. *Am J Med* 1986;**81**:45–53.

62. Beasley CR, Rafferty P, Holgate ST. Bronchoconstrictor properties of preservatives in ipratropium bromide (Atrovent) nebuliser solution. *Br Med J (Clin Res Ed)* 1987;**294**:1197–8.

63. Haddad EB, Mak JC, Barnes PJ. Characterization of [^{3}H]Ba 679 BR, a slowly dissociating muscarinic antagonist, in human lung: radioligand binding and autoradiographic mapping. *Mol Pharmacol* 1994;**45**:899–907.

64. Takahashi T, Belvisi MG, Patel H, *et al.* Effect of Ba 679 BR, a novel long-acting anticholinergic agent, noncholinergic neurotransmission in guinea pig and human airways. *Am J Respir Crit Care Med* 1994;**150**:1640–5.

65. O'Connor BJ, Towse LJ, Barnes PJ. Prolonged effect of tiotropium bromide on methacholine-induced bronchoconstriction in asthma. *Am J Respir Crit Care Med* 1996;**154**:876–80.

66. Littner MR, Ilowite JS, Tashkin DP, *et al.* Long-acting bronchodilation with once-daily dosing of tiotropium (Spiriva) in stable chronic obstructive pulmonary disease. *Am J Respir Crit Care Med* 2000;**161**:1136–42.

67. van Noord JA, Bantje TA, Eland ME, Korducki L, Cornelissen PJ. A randomised controlled comparison of tiotropium and ipratropium in the treatment of chronic obstructive pulmonary disease. The Dutch Tiotropium Study Group. *Thorax* 2000;**55**:289–94.

68. Calverley PM. The future for tiotropium. *Chest* 2000;**117**:67S-9S.

69. Barnes PJ. The pharmacological properties of tiotropium. *Chest* 2000;**117**:63S-6S.

70. Maesen FP, Smeets JJ, Sledsens TJ, Wald FD, Cornelissen PJ. Tiotropium bromide, a new long-acting antimuscarinic bronchodilator: a pharmacodynamic study in patients with chronic obstructive pulmonary disease (COPD). Dutch Study Group. *Eur Respir J* 1995;**8**:1506–13.

71. Haddad EB, Patel H, Keeling JE, Yacoub MH, Barnes PJ, Belvisi MG. Pharmacological characterization of the muscarinic receptor antagonist, glycopyrrolate, in human and guinea-pig airways. *Br J Pharmacol* 1999;**127**:413–20.

72. Oliver G, Schafer EA. The physiological effects of extracts of the suprarenal capsules. *J Physiol* 1895;**18**:270–6.

73. Davenport HW. Early history of the concept of chemical transmission of the nerve impulse. *The Physiologist* 1991; **34**:129–90.

74. Ahlquist RPA. A study of the adrenotropic receptors. *Am J Physiol* 1948;**153**:586–600.

75. Baraniuk JN, Kowalski ML, Kaliner MA. Relationships between permeable vessels, nerves, and mast cells in rat cutaneous neurogenic inflammation. *J Appl Physiol* 1990;**68**:2305–11.

76. Baraniuk JN. Neural control of human nasal secretion. *Pulm Pharmacol* 1991;**4**:20–31.

77. Chen Y, Getchell TV, Sparks DL, Getchell ML. Patterns of adrenergic and peptidergic innervation in human olfactory mucosa: age-related trends. *J Comp Neurol* 1993;**334**:104–16.

78. Bergendal A, Linden A, Lotvall J, Skoogh BE, Lofdahl CG. Different effects of salmeterol, formoterol and

salbutamol on cholinergic responses in the ferret trachea. *Br J Pharmacol* 1995;**114**:1478–82.

79. Skoogh BE, Ullman A. Modulation of cholinergic neurotransmission to the airways. *Am Rev Respir Dis* 1991; **143**:1427–8.

80. Xue QF, Maurer R, Engel G. Selective distribution of beta- and alpha 1-adrenoceptors in rat lung visualized by autoradiography. *Arch Int Pharmacodyn Ther* 1983; **266**:308–14.

81. Carstairs JR, Nimmo AJ, Barnes PJ. Autoradiographic localisation of beta-adrenoceptors in human lung. *Eur J Pharmacol* 1984;**103**:189–90.

82. Carstairs JR, Nimmo AJ, Barnes PJ. Autoradiographic visualization of beta-adrenoceptor subtypes in human lung. *Am Rev Respir Dis* 1985;**132**:541–7.

83. Spina D, Rigby PJ, Paterson JW, Goldie RG. Autoradiographic localization of beta-adrenoceptors in asthmatic human lung. *Am Rev Respir Dis* 1989;**140**:1410–15.

84. Spina D, Rigby PJ, Paterson JW, Goldie RG. Alpha 1-adrenoceptor function and autoradiographic distribution in human asthmatic lung. *Br J Pharmacol* 1989;**97**:701–8.

85. Henry PJ, Rigby PJ, Goldie RG. Distribution of beta 1- and beta 2-adrenoceptors in mouse trachea and lung: a quantitative autoradiographic study. *Br J Pharmacol* 1990; **99**:136–44.

86. Strader CD, Sigal IS, Dixon RA. Mapping the functional domains of the beta-adrenergic receptor. *Am J Respir Cell Mol Biol* 1989;**1**:81–6.

87. Johnson M. The beta-adrenoceptor. *Am J Respir Crit Care Med* 1998;**158**:S146–53.

88. Collins S, Caron MG, Lefkowitz RJ. From ligand binding to gene expression: new insights into the regulation of G-protein-coupled receptors. *Trends Biochem Sci* 1992;**17**: 37–9.

89. Hausdorff WP, Caron MG, Lefkowitz RJ. Turning off the signal: desensitization of beta-adrenergic receptor function. *Faseb J* 1990;**4**:2881–9.

90. Svedmyr N. Fenoterol: a beta2-adrenergic agonist for use in asthma. Pharmacology, pharmacokinetics, clinical efficacy and adverse effects. *Pharmacotherapy* 1985;**5**:109–26.

91. Heel RC, Brogden RN, Speight TM, Avery GS. Fenoterol: a review of its pharmacological properties and therapeutic efficacy in asthma. *Drugs* 1978;**15**:3–32.

92. Brittain RT, Farmer JB, Marshall RJ. Some observations on the adrenoceptor agonist properties of the isomers of salbutamol. *Br J Pharmacol* 1973;**48**:144–7.

93. Lulich KM, Goldie RG, Ryan G, Paterson JW. Adverse reactions to beta 2-agonist bronchodilators. *Med Toxicol* 1986; **1**:286–99.

94. Israel E, Drazen JM, Liggett SB, Boushey HA, Cherniack RM, Chinchilli VM, *et al.* The effect of polymorphisms of the beta$_2$-adrenergic receptor on the response to regular use of albuterol in asthma. *Am J Respir Crit Care Med* 2000;**162**:75–80.

95. Drazen JM, Israel E, Boushey HA, Chinchilli VM, Fahy JV, Fish JE, *et al.* Comparison of regularly scheduled with as-needed use of albuterol in mild asthma. Asthma Clinical Research Network. *N Engl J Med* 1996;**335**:841–7.

96. Lipworth BJ, Hall IP, Aziz I, Tan KS, Wheatley A. Beta$_2$-adrenoceptor polymorphism and bronchoprotective sensitivity with regular short- and long-acting beta$_2$-agonist therapy. *Clin Sci (Colch)* 1999;**96**:253–9.

97. Aziz I, Tan KS, Hall IP, Devlin MM, Lipworth BJ. Subsensitivity to bronchoprotection against adenosine monophosphate challenge following regular once-daily formoterol. *Eur Respir J* 1998;**12**:580–4.

98. Tan S, Hall IP, Dewar J, Dow E, Lipworth B. Association between beta 2-adrenoceptor polymorphism and susceptibility to bronchodilator desensitisation in moderately severe stable asthmatics. *Lancet* 1997;**350**:995–9.

99. Anderson GP. Formoterol: pharmacology, molecular basis of agonism, and mechanism of long duration of a highly potent and selective beta 2-adrenoceptor agonist bronchodilator. *Life Sci* 1993;**52**:2145–60.

100. Lofdahl CG. Basic pharmacology of new long-acting sympathomimetics. *Lung* 1990;**168**:18–21.

101. Johnson M. Salmeterol: a novel drug for the treatment of asthma. *Agents Actions Suppl* 1991;**34**:79–95.

102. Johnson M. The pharmacology of salmeterol. *Lung* 1990;**168**: 115–19.

103. Moore RH, Khan A, Dickey BF. Long-acting inhaled beta$_2$-agonists in asthma therapy. *Chest* 1998;**113**:1095–108.

104. Linden A, Rabe KF, Lofdahl CG. Pharmacological basis for duration of effect: formoterol and salmeterol versus short-acting beta 2-adrenoceptor agonists. *Lung* 1996; **174**:1–22.

105. Waldeck B. Some pharmacodynamic aspects on long-acting beta-adrenoceptor agonists. *Gen Pharmacol* 1996;**27**: 575–80.

106. Boyd G, Morice AH, Pounsford JC, Siebert M, Peslis N, Crawford C. An evaluation of salmeterol in the treatment of chronic obstructive pulmonary disease (COPD). *Eur Respir J* 1997;**10**:815–21.

107. Salter H. On some points in the treatment and clinical history of asthma. *Edin Med J* 1859;**4**:1109–15.

108. Butcher RW, Sutherland EW. Adenosine 3′5′-phosphate in biological materials. *J Biol Chem* 1962;**237**:1244–50.

109. Yasui K, Hu B, Nakazawa T, Agematsu K, Komiyama A. Theophylline accelerates human granulocyte apoptosis not via phosphodiesterase inhibition. *J Clin Invest* 1997;**100**: 1677–84.

110. Okubo Y, Hossain M, Horie S, *et al.* Inhibitory effects of theophylline and procaterol on eosinophil function. *Intern Med* 1997;**36**:276–82.

111. Adachi T, Motojima S, Hirata A, *et al.* Eosinophil apoptosis caused by theophylline, glucocorticoids, and macrolides after stimulation with IL-5. *J Allergy Clin Immunol* 1996;**98**:S207–15.

112. Namovic MT, Walsh RE, Goodfellow C, Harris RR, Carter GW, Bell RL. Pharmacological modulation of eosinophil influx into the lungs of Brown Norway rats. *Eur J Pharmacol* 1996;**315**:81–8.

113. Cohan VL, Showell HJ, Fisher DA, *et al.* In vitro pharmacology of the novel phosphodiesterase type four inhibitor, CP-80633. *J Pharmacol Exp Ther* 1996;**278**: 1356–61.

114. Turner CR, Cohan VL, Cheng JB, Showell HJ, Pazoles CJ, Watson JW. The *in vivo* pharmacology of CP-80, 633, a selective inhibitor of phosphodiesterase 4. *J Pharmacol Exp Ther* 1996;**278**:1349–55.

115. Tenor H, Hatzelmann A, Church MK, Schudt C, Shute JK. Effects of theophylline and rolipram on leukotriene C4 (LTC4) synthesis and chemotaxis of human eosinophils from normal and atopic subjects. *Br J Pharmacol* 1996;**118**: 1727–35.

116. Sagara H, Fukuda T, Okada T, Ishikawa A, Makino S. Theophylline at therapeutic concentration suppresses PAF-induced upregulation of Mac-1 on human eosinophils. *Clin Exp Allergy* 1996;**26**:16–21.

117. Horiguchi T, Tachikawa S, Kasahara J, *et al.* Suppression of airway inflammation by theophylline in adult bronchial asthma. *Respiration* 1999;**66**:124–7.

118. Momose T, Okubo Y, Horie S, Suzuki J, Isobe M, Sekiguchi M. Effects of intracellular cyclic AMP modulators on human eosinophil survival, degranulation and CD11b expression. *Int Arch Allergy Immunol* 1998;**117**:138–45.

119. Spoelstra FM, Berends C, Dijkhuizen B, de Monchy JG, Kauffman HF. Effect of theophylline on CD11b and L-selectin expression and density of eosinophils and neutrophils *in vitro*. *Eur Respir J* 1998;**12**:585–91.

120. Peleman RA, Kips JC, Pauwels RA. Therapeutic activities of theophylline in chronic obstructive pulmonary disease. *Clin Exp Allergy* 1998;**28**:53–6.

121. Belman MJ. Effects of aminophylline on diaphragmatic fatigue during acute respiratory failure. *Am Rev Respir Dis* 1984;**130**:695.

122. Vires N, Aubier M, Murciano D, Fleury B, Talamo C, Pariente R. Effects of aminophylline on diaphragmatic fatigue during acute respiratory failure. *Am Rev Respir Dis* 1984;**129**:396–402.

123. Cooling DS. Theophylline toxicity. *J Emerg Med* 1993;**11**:415–25.

124. Sessler CN. Theophylline toxicity: clinical features of 116 consecutive cases. *Am J Med* 1990;**88**:567–76.

125. Tsiu SJ, Self TH, Burns R. Theophylline toxicity: update. *Ann Allergy* 1990;**64**:241–57.

126. Hardman JG, Goodman Gilman A, Limbird LE. *The Pharmacological Basis of Therapeutics*, 9th edn. McGraw-Hill, New York, 1996.

127. Houslay MD, Milligan G. Tailoring cAMP-signalling responses through isoform multiplicity. *Trends Biochem Sci* 1997;**22**:217–24.

128. Weishaar RE, Cain MH, Bristol JA. A new generation of phosphodiesterase inhibitors: multiple molecular forms of phosphodiesterase and the potential for drug selectivity. *J Med Chem* 1985;**28**:537–45.

129. Thompson WJ, Appleman MM. Characterization of cyclic nucleotide phosphodiesterases of rat tissues. *J Biol Chem* 1971;**246**:3145–50.

130. Thompson WJ, Appleman MM. Multiple cyclic nucleotide phosphodiesterase activities from rat brain. *Biochemistry* 1971;**10**:311–16.

131. Bernareggi MM, Belvisi MG, Patel H, Barnes PJ, Giembycz MA. Anti-spasmogenic activity of isoenzyme-selective phosphodiesterase inhibitors in guinea-pig trachealis. *Br J Pharmacol* 1999;**128**:327–36.

132. Challiss RA, Adams D, Mistry R, Nicholson CD. Modulation of spasmogen-stimulated Ins(1,4,5)P3 generation and functional responses by selective inhibitors of types three and four phosphodiesterase in airways smooth muscle. *Br J Pharmacol* 1998;**124**:47–54.

133. Spina D, Ferlenga P, Biasini I, *et al.* The effect duration of selective phosphodiesterase inhibitors in the guinea pig. *Life Sci* 1998;**62**:953–65.

134. Ezeamuzie CI. Involvement of A3 receptors in the potentiation by adenosine of the inhibitory effect of theophylline on human eosinophil degranulation: possible novel mechanism of the anti-inflammatory action of theophylline[1]. *Biochem Pharmacol* 2001;**61**:1551–9.

135. Hatzelmann A, Schudt C. Anti-inflammatory and immunomodulatory potential of the novel PDE4 inhibitor roflumilast *in vitro*. *J Pharmacol Exp Ther* 2001;**297**:267–79.

136. Cooper N, Teixeira MM, Warneck J, *et al.* A comparison of the inhibitory activity of PDE4 inhibitors on leukocyte PDE4 activity *in vitro* and eosinophil trafficking *in vivo*. *Br J Pharmacol* 1999;**126**:1863–71.

137. Blease K, Burke-Gaffney A, Hellewell PG. Modulation of cell adhesion molecule expression and function on human lung microvascular endothelial cells by inhibition of phosphodiesterases three and four. *Br J Pharmacol* 1998;**124**:229–37.

138. Gantner F, Tenor H, Gekeler V, Schudt C, Wendel A, Hatzelmann A. Phosphodiesterase profiles of highly purified human peripheral blood leukocyte populations from normal and atopic individuals: a comparative study. *J Allergy Clin Immunol* 1997;**100**:527–35.

139. Torphy TJ, Page C. Phosphodiesterases: the journey towards therapeutics. *Trends Pharmacol Sci* 2000;**21**:157–9.

140. Barnette MS, Underwood DC. New phosphodiesterase inhibitors as therapeutics for the treatment of chronic lung disease. *Curr Opin Pulm Med* 2000;**6**:164–9.

141. Barnette MS. Phosphodiesterase four (PDE4) inhibitors in asthma and chronic obstructive pulmonary disease (COPD). *Prog Drug Res* 1999;**53**:193–229.

142. Jacobitz S, McLaughlin MM, Livi GP, Burman M, Torphy TJ. Mapping the functional domains of human recombinant phosphodiesterase 4A: structural requirements for catalytic activity and rolipram binding. *Mol Pharmacol* 1996;**50**:891–9.

143. Zeller E, Stief HJ, Pflug B, Sastre-y-Hernandez M. Results of a phase II study of the antidepressant effect of rolipram. *Pharmacopsychiatry* 1984;**17**:188–90.

144. Wachtel H. Potential antidepressant activity of rolipram and other selective cyclic adenosine 3′,5′-monophosphate phosphodiesterase inhibitors. *Neuropharmacology* 1983;**22**:267–72.

145. Glover ED, Glover PN. Pharmacologic treatments for the nicotine dependent smoker. *Am J Health Behav* 2001;**25**:179–82.

146. Panchagnula R, Jain AK, Pillai O, Jaiswal J. Nicotine transdermal systems: pharmaceutical and clinical aspects. *Methods Find Exp Clin Pharmacol* 2000;**22**:299–308.

147. Silagy C, Mant D, Fowler G, Lancaster T. Nicotine replacement therapy for smoking cessation. *Cochrane Database Syst Rev* 2000;CD000146.

148. Benowitz NL, Gourlay SG. Cardiovascular toxicity of nicotine: implications for nicotine replacement therapy. *J Am Coll Cardiol* 1997;**29**:1422–31.

149. Pomerleau OF. Nicotine and the central nervous system: biobehavioral effects of cigarette smoking. *Am J Med* 1992;**93**:2S–7S.

150. Schneider NG, Lunell E, Olmstead RE, Fagerstrom KO. Clinical pharmacokinetics of nasal nicotine delivery. A review and comparison to other nicotine systems. *Clin Pharmacokinet* 1996;**31**:65–80.

151. Tonnesen P. Smoking cessation: nicotine replacement, gums and patches. *Monaldi Arch Chest Dis* 1999;**54**:489–94.

152. Prochazka AV. New developments in smoking cessation. *Chest* 2000;**117**:169S–75S.

153. Lief HI. Bupropion treatment of depression to assist smoking cessation. *Am J Psychiatry* 1996;**153**:442.

154. Hurt RD, Sachs DP, Glover ED, *et al.* A comparison of sustained-release bupropion and placebo for smoking cessation. *N Engl J Med* 1997;**337**:1195–202.

155. Hayford KE, Patten CA, Rummans TA, *et al.* Efficacy of bupropion for smoking cessation in smokers with a former history of major depression or alcoholism. *Br J Psychiatry* 1999;**174**:173–8.

156. Jorenby DE, Leischow SJ, Nides MA, *et al.* A controlled trial of sustained-release bupropion, a nicotine patch, or both for smoking cessation. *N Engl J Med* 1999;**340**:685–91.

157. Pasternak M. Sustained-release bupropion for smoking cessation. *N Engl J Med* 1998;**338**:619–20.

158. Ferris RM, Beaman OJ. Bupropion: a new antidepressant drug, the mechanism of action of which is not associated with down-regulation of postsynaptic beta-adrenergic, serotonergic (5-HT2), alpha 2-adrenergic, imipramine and dopaminergic receptors in brain. *Neuropharmacology* 1983;**22**:1257–67.

159. Ferris RM, Cooper BR, Maxwell RA. Studies of bupropion's mechanism of antidepressant activity. *J Clin Psychiatry* 1983;**44**:74–8.

160. Cooper BR, Hester TJ, Maxwell RA. Behavioral and biochemical effects of the antidepressant bupropion (Wellbutrin): evidence for selective blockade of dopamine uptake *in vivo. J Pharmacol Exp Ther* 1980;**215**:127–34.

161. Tashkin D, Kanner R, Bailey W, *et al.* Smoking cessation in patients with chronic obstructive pulmonary disease: a double-blind, placebo-controlled, randomised trial. *Lancet* 2001;**357**:1571–5.

24

Symptomatic bronchodilator treatment

PETER MA CALVERLEY

The use of bronchodilator drugs to reduce the symptoms and increase the exercise tolerance of patients with COPD is a cornerstone of management in these patients. The basic pharmacology of these drugs has already been reviewed (see Chapter 23) and this chapter focuses on the physiologic consequences of bronchodilator action as well as considering the evidence for their efficacy and the problems of treatment selection. Although 'functional' end-points such as reductions in breathlessness and increases in self-paced waking distance are important to patients, it is only relatively recently that simpler and reliable methods of assessing these variables have been developed. Surrogate end-points such as changes in FEV_1 or PEF after active bronchodilator have been reported in most clinical trials, usually over quite short periods of time, and these may underestimate the potential benefit of treatment. Unlike bronchial asthma where drug treatment can restore normal pulmonary function in most mild to moderate cases, the structural changes in COPD (see Chapter 2) preclude this and few studies have considered how effective a dose of bronchodilator is in relation to the maximum attainable bronchodilatation for that subject.[1,2] Moreover, clinically relevant changes in FEV_1 may be so small in severe COPD patients that they fall within the day-to-day reproducibility of the measurement (see Chapter 20). Problems such as these hamper interpretation of clinical studies of bronchodilator action and lead to an unduly pessimistic view of the benefit of treatment.[3]

Before considering the three principal groups of symptomatic bronchodilator, beta-agonist, anticholinergic and theophylline derivatives, it is useful to review how they might modify the pathophysiology of the COPD patient.

PHYSIOLOGIC BASIS OF BRONCHODILATOR ACTION

Although the most important effects of bronchodilators appear to be related to relaxation of the airway smooth muscle, a range of other actions with potential or actual clinical benefit have been reported (Table 24.1).

Changes in airway caliber

Central and peripheral airways resistance is increased in stable COPD at rest and falls after bronchodilator treatment,[4,5] presumably due to airway smooth muscle relaxation. The consequent rise in FEV_1 results from a combination of several factors including the distribution of the aerosol bolus, the degree of inhomogeneous airway pathology and the degree of resting cholinergic muscle tone. A range of secondary physiologic changes occur (see below) which are probably of greater importance than the modest improvement in FEV_1.

Reduction in pulmonary hyperinflation

This has been documented in several studies and is discussed in detail in Chapter 18. Dynamic increases in end

Table 24.1 *Potential beneficial effects of bronchodilator drugs in COPD*

1 Change in airway caliber	Central and/or peripheral Reduces inspiratory/expiratory airways resistance Reduces respiratory system time constants Mainly 'neural', i.e. abolishes airway smooth muscle tone
2 Reduction of pulmonary hyperinflation	Reduces the work of breathing Reduces passive and dynamic FRC Reduces threshold load due to PEEP Parallels the change in FEV_1 but not proportionately Changes in PIF/FIV_1 may be a useful guide Most evident during exercise
3 Changes in mucociliary clearance	A long-term benefit Clinical significance unclear
4 Improved respiratory muscle strength/endurance	Shown in animal studies with several drugs Hard to separate from changes in 1 and 2
5 Anti-inflammatory activity	Remains of speculative importance only as yet – although experimental evidence is accumulating to support this

expiratory lung volume due to an inadequate time for lung emptying occur but static increases in residual volume are also relevant and both can change after bronchodilator treatment. Changes in end-expiratory lung volume are rather greater than those in FEV_1 and are accompanied by an increased tidal volume.[6] There is no clear relationship between these effects and the change in tidal airflow limitation, but when end-inspiratory lung volume decreases there is a reduction in the degree of breathlessness.[6–9] Pulmonary elastic recoil is an important determinant of airway caliber but changes in this variable principally reflect those occurring in lung volume.

Changes in mucociliary clearance

This is impaired in most forms of COPD[10] reflecting structural damage to the cilia and the ciliotoxic effects of cigarette smoke.[11,12] Beta-agonists can increase ciliary beat frequency and accelerate mucociliary clearance whilst anticholinergic drugs might impair this, although clinical studies suggest this is not the case (see below). There are no good clinical studies of the effects of long-term bronchodilators on mucociliary clearance which control for the effects of changes in cigarette smoking or of cough. This latter is a major mechanism of particulate clearance and is reduced by bronchodilator drugs. Clinically these effects appear to be insignificant.

Improving respiratory muscle function

The debate about the ability of theophyllines to increase respiratory muscle endurance and strength continues and much of the evidence for this is reviewed in Chapter 15.

It is difficult to believe that there is significant effect in spontaneously breathing patients at the accepted therapeutic levels of theophylline since the respiratory muscles appear to cope surprisingly well with their increased loading given their geometric disadvantage[13] (see Chapter 15).

Anti-inflammatory actions

This is a rather unsatisfactory term used to describe changes in mediators or cellular elements produced by drugs normally thought of as working by their effect on airway caliber. There is no evidence that anticholinergic drugs modulate any process other than muscarinic receptor activation in airway smooth muscle and at the nerve endings. By contrast, short-acting beta-agonists and low doses of theophylline in asthmatics have been thought to have some anti-inflammatory action,[14] though data in COPD are scanty. Much the most studied drug has been salmeterol which has a number of non-bronchodilator properties reviewed elsewhere.[15] *In vitro* this drug shows a dose-dependent suppression of superoxide production from stimulated neutrophils,[16] reduces their adherence to bronchial epithelium and promotes neutrophil apoptosis. There is limited clinical evidence that neutrophil numbers can be decreased by salmeterol treatment. *In vitro* studies of the number of ciliated epithelial cells in the airway show that salmeterol protects against damage produced by *Haemophilus influenzae* and *Pseudomonas*[17,18] and rather surprisingly the number of patients reporting bronchitic symptoms is significantly fewer in salmeterol-treated patients.[19]

Table 24.2 *Commonly used formulations of bronchodilator drugs (Data derived from refs 137, 138)*

Drug	Parental	Metered dose inhaler (μg)	Nebulizer (mg)	Oral (mg)	Duration of action (h)
Isoprenaline sulphate (isoproterenol)	–	200–400	0.8–4.0	–	1–2
Orciprenaline, (metaproterenol)	–	750–1500	–	20	3–4
Salbutamol (albuterol)	3–20 μg/min	100–200	2.5–5.0	4	4–6
Terbutaline	1.5–5 μg/min	250–500	5–10	5	4–6
Fenoterol*	–	100–200	–	–	4–6
Salmeterol	–	50–100	–	–	12+
Formoterol	–	12–24	–	–	12+
Ipratropium bromide	–	40–80	0.25–0.5	–	6–8
Oxitropium bromide[†]	–	200	–	–	7–9
Tiotropium[†]	–	36	–	–	24+
Theophylline	–	–	–	100–400	Variable, up to 12
Aminophylline	500 μg/kg/h	–	–	225–450	Variable, up to 12

Names in parentheses refer to North American generic terms where different from the UK.
Total daily dose quoted
Short-acting drugs are given up to four times daily (see text) whilst long-acting inhaled beta-agonists are given twice daily and in the case of tiotropium once daily.
Theophyllines require dose titration depending on side effects and plasma theophylline (see text).
*Not available in USA – caution redosage in view of concerns raised in asthmatic patients.
[†]Not available in USA.

Although these non-bronchodilator effects are of scientific interest the similarities in action between the anticholinergic and the other drugs listed above make changes in airways caliber as a consequence of these agents much the most likely explanation of their overall effect.

Most actions of bronchodilator drugs can be explained by the abolition of the normal resting cholinergically mediated smooth muscle tone, a reduction in pathologically increased smooth muscle tone or a decrease in airway wall thickness either from anti-inflammatory or vascular effects. There is evidence for tonic airway smooth muscle contraction as a minor degree of bronchodilatation occurs after inhaled atropine and ipratropium.[20] Studies in normal subjects and COPD suggest that day-to-day variations in airway caliber are due to fluctuations in this smooth muscle tone.[21,22] (Figure 24.1) This is supported by the observation in bronchodilator studies that a bronchodilator response is more likely when the baseline airway caliber is lower on a particular test day. Whether the degree of cholinergic tone is truly 'pathologic' or simply reflects normal fluctuations in smooth muscle activity in an airway of reduced baseline caliber, is much more debatable.[23]

Non-specific bronchial reactivity in response to either histamine or methacholine is increased in COPD[24,25] but this is usually attributed to geometric factors since even a small change in airway caliber will increase resistance dramatically when the resting airway diameter is reduced. A more elaborate analysis has been reported by Wiggs *et al.*[26] Using data derived from directly measured

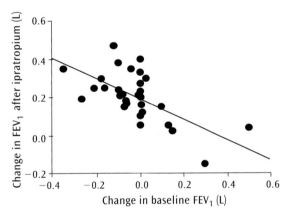

Figure 24.1 *Relationship between the change in baseline airway caliber and the response to 50 μg nebulized ipratropium bromide in 33 stable COPD patients. Patients attended on two days and received ipratropium or salbutamol in randomized order. On days when baseline airway caliber had increased, there was little or no further bronchodilatation with ipratropium and vice versa. This suggests that airway tone may be cholinergically mediated since anticholinergic blockade on days when airway tone was relatively low, i.e. FEV_1 had risen, was ineffective. (From ref. 22 with permission.)*

airway wall thickness in asthmatic and COPD patients and applying a series of reasonable physiological assumptions, they have developed a model for bronchial reactivity which emphasizes the role of airway wall thickness as the cause of increases in reactivity in both conditions.

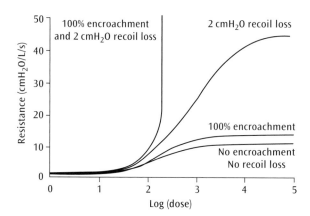

Figure 24.2 *Theoretical model predictions of changes in resistance with increasing dose of an agonist drug derived using actual measurements of airway wall thickness.[23] When there is no encroachment on the lumen and no loss of recoil a plateau of increasing resistance is reached after three log doses. With the addition of a 2 cm H_2O loss of elastic recoil the airway resistance for a given change in agonists increases dramatically, even with normal wall thickness. The in vivo situation is likely to lie in between this relationship and that when there was 100% increase in encroachment and a loss of recoil, and this could contribute to closure of critically narrowed airways subtending specific lung units. This model takes no account of dynamic compensatory responses, which might modify the behavior of the respiratory system in vivo. (From ref. 26 with permission.)*

Moreover, these effects are greatly exaggerated by even modest changes in pulmonary elastic recoil (Figure 24.2). Although they now believe that much of these results in asthmatics can be explained by smooth muscle hypertrophy, a comparable analysis for reactivity in COPD has not been developed.

The consequences of bronchodilatation are complex. As well as improving the FEV_1 and PEF, bronchodilators can promote a slower, deeper breathing pattern, which favors more complete lung emptying. Whether this is due to some local reflex action or, more likely, simply to the reduction in inspiratory impedance associated with changes in airway caliber and lung volume is not clear. Not only do these changes reduce the work of breathing due to hyperinflation, but also they reduce the hidden threshold load of intrinsic PEEP (see Chapter 13) and increase the previously diminished inspiratory force reserve.[27] A fall in airways resistance shortens the time constant of the respiratory system. These show marked frequency dependence in COPD (see Chapter 13) and by reducing this effect the bronchodilator not only increases maximum ventilation but allows this to be reached with a smaller degree of pulmonary hyperinflation. The relationships between tidal and maximum flows and the influence of resting lung volume are shown schematically in Figure 24.3 and are similar to those reported in

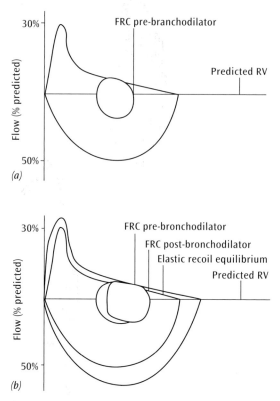

(a)

(b)

Figure 24.3 *Schematic flow volume before (a) and after an active bronchodilator drug. In (b), the changes are superimposed upon baseline results for comparison. Inspiratory flows are downwards and expiratory flows are upwards. (a) Residual volume is increased and there is an additional increase in dynamic FRC due to the breathing pattern adopted. Forced expiratory flow is flow limited at most lung volumes including those during tidal breathing. Expiratory flows can only be increased by a further increase in dynamic FRC (dynamic hyperinflation). After the bronchodilator (b) there is a fall in the dynamic FRC as well as in the residual volume. There are modest increases in mid and late maximum expiratory flows (FEF_{50} and FEF_{75}) as well as an increase in peak expiratory flow and peak inspiratory flow. Tidal expiratory flow is still flow limited but the increase in peak inspiratory flow means that it is possible to increase tidal inspiratory flow at the same lung volume without the same cost in terms of the respiratory muscle energetics. These predictions have been confirmed by direct observation.[8]*

patients tested for bronchodilator responsiveness.[28] A further result in a transient mismatch in ventilation and perfusion can lead to a fall in PaO_2 at rest[29,30] (see Chapter 14), although whether this is significant during exercise remains more questionable.[31]

From this it is clear that relatively modest changes in airway dimension can have major effects on respiratory mechanics and hence symptoms as well as on maximum exercise capacity and, perhaps more relevantly, the amount of exercise that can be undertaken before further dynamic hyperinflation occurs. This analysis suggests a number of end-points, for example FEV_1, FVC, PEF, lung volume, symptoms and exercise tolerance that might demonstrate the benefits of a bronchodilator drug. However, not all of these variables will change to the same degree at the same time. In general, the effectiveness of a bronchodilator in COPD will depend upon:

1 Its potency and the dose used.
2 Its duration of action which itself can be influenced by (1) above.
3 Speed of onset of action – generally anti-inflammatory effects take weeks to months to be apparent whilst bronchodilators change airway caliber in minutes.
4 The clinical state of the patient – especially baseline FEV_1 which remains the simplest global measure of severity.

These features taken together with the side effect profile and the simplicity of use of the drug itself, determine the acceptability of treatment to these patients.

BETA-AGONISTS

These are available in a range of formulations and dosage schedules, representative examples of which are given in Table 24.2. Oral beta-agonists can be effective bronchodilators[32,33] but have lost favor even in older COPD patients as their simplicity of administration is marred by their higher side effect profile and slow onset of bronchodilatation. This is clearly demonstrated in an acute study of 17 patients where conventional doses of 5 mg oral terbutaline and 400 mg aminophylline were compared with 270 µg of inhaled salbutamol given from a metered dose inhaler (MDI). Oral therapy was marginally less effective (mean change in FEV_1 post-salbutamol 0.3 L vs. 0.21 L after oral therapy). Tremor, anxiety and nausea were reported by nine patients after oral treatment but by none after the inhaled drug.[34]

Oral and intravenous beta-agonists can act as pulmonary vasodilators at rest and may further reduce pulmonary artery pressure by lowering airways resistance.[35,36] The clinical significance of these effects remain dubious.

Episodic reports of bronchodilatation after beta-agonists inhalation in patients with 'emphysema' have been published for many years but the Intermittent Positive Pressure Breathing (IPPB) Trial group were the first to study this systematically. They examined the response to 250 µg of inhaled isoprenaline in 965 COPD patients repeatedly over 3 years.[37] The majority showed a significant degree of bronchodilatation to beta-agonists

however, expressed at one or more visits in this trial. Responders were more likely to complain of wheezing or reduced exercise capacity or to have shown a fall in baseline FEV_1 during the trial. There is an impression that conventional doses of salbutamol are more effective than orciprenaline (meta-proterenol). Direct comparisons are lacking in COPD patients but data for each drug compared against the same dose of ipratropium supports this view.[38] Three useful dose–response studies have examined the effects of salbutamol on spirometry in incompletely reversible or 'irreversible' COPD patients.[39–41] There appears to be a shallow but definite dose–response relationship best seen with FEV_1. The time to peak response may be slower than that reported in asthmatics but the time to 80% of the peak value is quite rapid. The duration of bronchodilatation and incidence of cardiac and metabolic side effects increases with the dose used[40] (Figure 24.4) and there seems to be little benefit in giving more than 1 mg salbutamol. Although salbutamol increases oxygen consumption acutely in healthy volunteers,[42] this effect wanes with regular treatment, unlike the bronchodilator effects.[43] How completely bronchodilatation protects against non-specific inhaled stimuli and is influenced by baseline airway reactivity has not been assessed in COPD, although data in asthmatic patients suggest that bronchoprotection against inhaled agonists is more short term.[44]

In unselected patient populations those who subsequently respond to corticosteroids often have the largest bronchodilator responses to beta-agonists.[45] However, there is still evidence of dose–response effect with inhaled beta-agonists even in patients with a previously negative corticosteroid trial.[28,41] Whether these short-acting agents should be given regularly remains uncertain and one randomized controlled trial has assessed this in COPD. In this study 53 patients were advised to use short-acting salbutamol in addition to regular ipratropium four times daily and received either active drug or placebo. Surprisingly, they used twice as much of the active drug when on regular treatment than they did when the medication was simply used as rescue therapy.[46] Given the data with long-acting inhaled beta-agonists where rescue medication use falls it may be that this is a consequence of the drug regime rather than stimulation of the beta-receptor.

Patients who do not show significant spirometric improvement can still benefit from beta-agonist treatment (Table 24.3). Changes in 12-minute corridor walking distance do not relate well to changes in simple spirometry after beta-agonists[47] (see Chapter 18), but 12-minute walking distance increased by 62 (15 meters) after 200 µg of inhaled salbutamol in one study of 24 severe COPD patients (mean FEV_1 0.83 L). Even patients who show 'no bronchodilator response' can still show significant improvement in mean (SD) treadmill and corridor

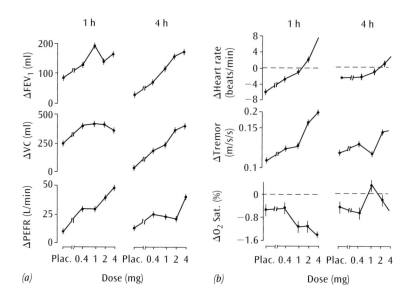

Figure 24.4 *(a) The changes in FEV$_1$, vital capacity and peak expiratory flow after placebo, and increasing doses of inhaled salbutamol given on different days in a group of 30 COPD patients (mean FEV$_1$ 0.9 (0.261)). This demonstrates the dose–response relationships with beta-agonists and the preservation of the bronchodilator effect over a 4-hour period. (b) Side effects noted at each dose increment. There was, again, a dose-related increase in heart rate, tremor and fall in oxygen saturation with the cardiovascular effects persisting more clearly at 4 hours than is the case with a change in saturation. The clinical significance of these effects for the group as a whole is likely to be small although individuals show marked idiosyncratic responses, at least in terms of tremor and heart rate. (Adapted from ref. 40 with permission.)*

Table 24.3 *Effect of short-acting beta-agonists on exercise capacity in COPD*

Study	No	Dose	Baseline FEV$_1$ (L/s)	FEV (L)	FVC (L)	Δ6MD (m)	Comment
Mohammed[33]	30	8 mg oral salb	1.03	0.09	0.17	30	6 weeks treatment NS compared to placebo
Corris[41]	8	400 µg 1600 µg inh salb	0.72 0.71	0.07 0.13	0.20 0.44	35* 38*	Patients corticosteroid irreversible; change in PIF a useful predictor
Vathenen[40]	30	400 µg 4 mg inh salb	0.09 0.9	0.12 0.16	0.36 0.42	20* 16*	Randomized study of multiple doses, no dose-related walking effect
Berger[48]	10	5 puffs orciprenaline	1.48	0.11	0.14	42*	Patients chosen to be 'irreversible'
Leitch[47]	24	200 µg inh salb	0.82	0.15	0.41	31*	Combination with anticholinergic beneficial

Δ6MD: change in 6-minute walking distance in meters – data converted to this from 12-minute walking by simple division; inh: inhaled; terb: terbutaline; salb: salbutamol.
*Significantly better than placebo.

walking times 112 (56 meters) and 82 (46 meters) respectively after supranormal doses of orciprenaline.[48] A scientifically more rigorous investigation was conducted in 13 COPD patients who received either inhaled salbutamol or an identical placebo and in whom measurements of intrathoracic pressures and lung volumes were made during exercise. In these patients there was a significant

reduction in breathlessness assessed by Borg score (4.5 to 3.1) and the change in breathlessness related to the change in end-inspiratory lung volumes standardized for total lung capacity. There was evidence of improved neuroventilatory coupling and this together with the changes in dynamic hyperinflation were thought to explain the improved exercise capacity.[9] Studies in a general practice

Table 24.4 *Effects of inhaled anticholinergic and oral theophyllines on exercise capacity in COPD*

Study	Patients (no.)	Dose	Baseline FEV$_1$ (L/s)	ΔFEV (L)	ΔFVC (L)	Δ6MD (m)	Comment
Leitch et al.[47]	24	40 µg ipra	0.85	0.15	0.44	22	?Type II error or dose effect
Hay et al.[69]	32	200 µg oxi	0.70	0.18	0.41	27*	Spirometric reversibility did not predict improvement in breathless scores following active drugs
Spence et al.[31]	32	200 µg oxi	0.77	0.18	0.42	20*	All patients unresponsive to a corticosteroid trial
Mahler et al.[85]	12	15 µg/ml theo	1.36	0.11	0.14	9.2	Improved overall dyspnea rating over 4 weeks therapy
Chrystyn et al.[83]	33	12.0 µg/ml 18.3 µg/ml theo	1.00	0.08 0.13	0.19 0.32	26* 56*	Dose-related reductions in 'trapped gas volume'; 8 weeks therapy
McKay et al.[89]	15	9.1 µg/ml 16.8 µg/ml theo	0.92	0.10 0.13	0.11 0.17	65 80*	Not a true 6MD but a treadmill walk; improved quality of lifescores on active drug? Selection bias; 7 weeks therapy
Guyatt et al.[88]	19	10 µg/ml theo	N/A	N/A	N/A	40*	Changes equivalent to inhaled salbutamol; 2 weeks therapy

ipra: ipratropium bromide; oxi: oxitropium bromide; theo: theophylline expressed as a mean serum theophylline concentration.
Note the variable confidence intervals for significant changes in the longer-term oral theophyllines studies reflecting the wider between day coefficient of variation in walking distance.
*Significantly different from placebo.

population of COPD patients in Holland studied found those who received regular beta-agonists appeared to have a more rapid disease progression than those on intermittent therapies (see discussion above), but this was not confirmed during a longer follow-up.[49,50]

Long-acting inhaled beta-agonists

The use of long-acting inhaled beta-agonists in COPD has been proven to be of significant clinical benefit and the key studies are presented in Table 24.5. Both salmeterol and formoterol are administered twice daily and produce a sustained improvement of FEV$_1$ and FVC over 24 hours in a wide range of COPD.[51,52] Treatment over 4 months is not associated with tachyphylaxis in these bronchodilator actions. Health status improves significantly compared to placebo in those receiving lower but not the higher dose of long-acting drug, possibly reflecting the effects of increased tremor and sleep disturbance which are more evident at these higher doses.[19,52] The similarity in the health status effects between salmeterol and formoterol as compared with placebo and their superiority to ipratropium when assessed using the same health status questionnaire is illustrated in Figure 24.5. More sensitive health status questionnaires such as the

Chronic Respiratory Disease questionnaire did not distinguish between the beneficial effects of four times daily ipratropium and regular salmeterol, a finding seen in two studies.[53,54] The effect of these drugs on exercise capacity, at least as assessed by corridor walking distance, remains disappointing. These studies also found a delay in the time to the next exacerbation in those patients treated with the active drug, a finding supported by large studies with formoterol that are currently awaiting publication. These changes appear to be a class effect and the drugs themselves seem equivalent in most respects.[55] However there are data to confirm that formoterol does have a more rapid onset of action in COPD,[56] which may have some benefits in exacerbation control. Whether this proves an important advantage in the long term remains to be seen.[57]

ANTICHOLINERGICS

Although smoking the leaves of *Datura stramonium* was one of the earliest herbal remedies for airflow limitation of all kinds,[58] treatment with anticholinergic drugs fell from favor due to their systemic atropine-like effects. Therapeutic interest revived in the 1970s with the development of the poorly absorbed inhaled quaternary ammonium compound, ipratropium bromide. The closely

Table 24.5 *Comparative effects of long-acting beta-agonists and regular short-acting anticholinergic drugs*

Study	Patients (no.)	Duration (weeks)	Dose	Baseline FEV_1 (L)	ΔFEV_1 (L)	ΔHealth status	Comment
Jones et al.[19,51]	674	16	Placebo	1.31	−0.03	1.4*	Ref 19 is a subset of 51
			salm 50 µg bd	1.31	0.08	6.8	No effect on walking distance
			Salm 100 µg bd	1.23	0.07	2.3	Higher dose had less beneficial effect on health status
Mahler et al.[53]	411	12	Placebo	1.31	0.000	–	salm had a longer action
			ipra 40 µg qds	1.18	0.25	6.8†	and delayed the time to
			salm 50 µg bd	1.36	0.25	7.1	next exacerbation – ipra was intermediate in this
Rennard et al.[54]	403	12	Placebo	1.30	0.05	6†	Similar data to ref. 53
			ipra 40 µg qds	1.22	0.25	9	above
			salm 50 µg bd	1.28	0.25	10	Significant trial effect on health status
Dahl et al.[52]	935	12	Placebo	1.29	0.00	1.5*	form was superior in
			ipra 40 µg qds	1.29	0.15	2.7	duration of effect and
			form 12 µg bd	1.31	0.35	6.6	reduced the number of
			form 24 µg bd	1.31	0.30	4.8	'bad' days. Higher doses were less effective

salm: salmeterol; form: formoterol; ipra: ipratropium.

*Total St George's Respiratory Questionnaire score, converted so that positive change reflects improved health status. Clinically significant change is 4 units.

†Summed Chronic Respiratory Disease Questionnaire score, clinically significant changes is 10 units.

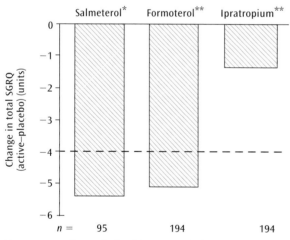

Figure 24.5 *Change in health status relative to placebo in patients treated with salmeterol, formoterol and ipratropium. Data are combined from two clinical trials (*ref. 19; **ref. 52) which use the same health status measurements, Total St George's Respiratory Questionnaire Score (SGRQ), and adopted a similar protocol with 3 months of treatment. The changes in health status after the lower dose of long-acting inhaled beta-agonists is identical in each group and significantly greater than those after regular short-acting anticholinergics. The largest changes in health status were seen at the lower dose of the beta-agonists in both trials.*

related derivative oxitropium bromide has been investigated but is only available in Europe and Japan and not North America. Detailed reviews of the clinical pharmacology of both are available.[59,60] Inhaled anticholinergics affect both central and peripheral airways[55] and produce significant falls in resting FRC[5,61] (Figure 24.6). When compared to beta-agonists, anticholinergics have a somewhat slower time to peak effect, usually between 30 and 60 minutes in most COPD patients, but are effective for rather longer than simple bronchodilators (approx. 6–10 hours).[62] Dose–response studies with both ipratropium and oxitropium[63–65] suggest optimal bronchodilation from a metered dose inhaler usually occurs with either 80 µg ipratropium or 200 µg oxitropium. Oxitropium bromide 200 µg appears to be equivalent to ipratropium 80 µg in terms of bronchodilatation and duration of action.[66]

The effect of inhaled anticholinergics on exercise performance, whether assessed by progressive cycle ergometry,[31,67] steady-state endurance exercise[8] or self-paced corridor walking tests[67] appears to be reasonably consistent (Table 24.4). Despite initial doubts about the effectiveness of ipratropium,[47] observations using oxitropium in a larger group of patients demonstrated that walking distance was increased and both resting and end-exercise breathlessness were reduced by active therapy.[68] These changes occurred irrespective of the magnitude of spirometric response. More detailed physiologic studies have shown that inhaled anticholinergics reduce FRC at rest

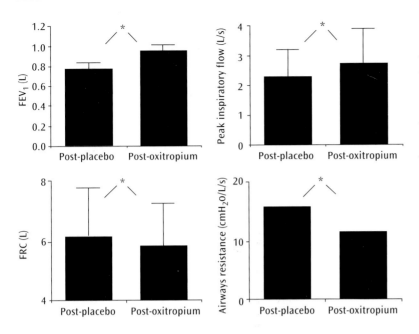

Figure 24.6 *Lung mechanics, in a group of 32 stable COPD patients (mean FEV$_1$ 0.81) recorded after 200 µg oxitropium bromide via a metered dose inhaler or after an identical placebo. There are significant increases in FEV$_1$, peak inspiratory flow and falls in both functional residual capacity and in airways resistance. These are paralleled by small but significant increases in corridor walking distance and reductions in perceived breathlessness at the end of exercise. Changes in FEV$_1$ were not proportional to changes in either walking distance or perceived breathlessness. Changes in intensity of breathlessness at the end of exercise were best related to changes in PIF (r = 0.57).*

and delay the onset of dynamic hyperinflation during exercise.[8] The resulting increase in exercise duration is most evident in steady-state studies. This is accompanied by falls in resting and end-exercise breathlessness as occurred in the self-paced studies. The magnitude of the changes in lung volume reported were similar to those seen with short-acting beta-agonists and are reviewed in detail in Chapter 18.

Anticholinergic drugs vary in their speed of onset of action and not only show dose-dependent increases in lung function but also in the accompanying side effects.[63] There is no evidence of tachyphylaxis in the spirometric response to these agents.[64] This is illustrated by data in the first Lung Health Study where one treatment limb studied the combination of anticholinergic drugs with smoking cessation. There was a small but sustained improvement in lung function over the 5 years of the trial in participants treated in this way.[69] Unfortunately, there was no evidence that the rate of disease progression, assessed by decline in FEV$_1$, was affected by the anticholinergic, either positively or negatively.[49] Unlike beta-agonists there is no suggestion of a loss of responsiveness to inhaled anticholinergics with age.

Long-acting inhaled anticholinergics

The latest inhaled anticholinergic to be developed is tiotropium bromide and should be available in Europe from 2002 onwards and North America subsequently. This is an exceptionally long-acting drug with unique pharmacokinetics (see Chapter 23). Its selective dissociation from muscarinic M2 receptor may be of more than theoretical interest since these receptors are now known

to be active even in patients with well-established COPD[70] (see Chapter 23). It has a rather slow onset of action over 1–2 hours and multiple dosing studies have shown that bronchodilatation is well maintained by a single daily dose over periods from 3 to 12 months[71,72] and it provides more sustained bronchodilitation than in the case of regular ipratropium.[73] It is able to block effects of methacholine challenge in asthmatic subjects[74] in the now conventional dose of 18 µg per day which is given via a dry powdered inhaler. The dose–response relationship appears to be relatively flat,[75] although it is possible that there is systemic absorption at higher doses which are not recommended. The timing of the dose does not modify the bronchodilator effect, which persists throughout the 24-hour day. There is still evidence of a normal circadian variation in airway caliber despite this peripheral anticholinergic blockade (Figure 24.7), suggesting that centrally mediated increases in airway smooth muscle tone are responsible for this effect.[76] Studies comparing tiotropium to placebo and regular ipratropium have a very consistent pattern of response with an increase in the morning FEV$_1$ which is well maintained throughout the follow-up period. It is accompanied by similar but proportionately more modest improvements in FVC and rather larger changes in peak expiratory flow.[72] Further comparative studies following a similar pattern over 12 months confirmed these earlier observations as well as indicating improved effectiveness compared with both placebo and regular anticholinergic treatment with shorter-acting drugs. Tiotropium produces significant improvements in total St George's Respiratory Questionnaire score as well as reductions in both the rate of exacerbation and hospitalization.[77,78] Tiotropium produces these effects with little

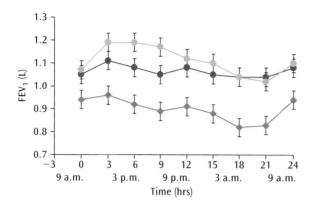

Figure 24.7 *The effect of a single dose of inhaled tiotropium on FEV$_1$ measured serially throughout the 24-hour day, in three groups of subjects receiving treatment in the evening (upper data points), morning (middle data points) or placebo (lower data points). All had a similar initial pattern of circadian variation in airway caliber before treatment and this was unchanged after the placebo drug. The bronchodilator increases lung function throughout the day without abolishing the nocturnal fall in FEV$_1$. Placebo significantly (P < 0.01) less than both a.m. and p.m. treatment values.*

in the way of anticholinergic toxicity and no sleep disturbance.[76] The most frequently reported side effect is a dry mouth. Although data on exercise capacity are awaited, there is evidence of a significant clinical improvement in the transitional dyspnea index in those patients studied for 1 year.

THEOPHYLLINE

Despite the drawbacks of a substantial and erratic side effect profile and limited efficacy as a bronchodilator, theophylline preparations are still widely prescribed among COPD patients although their popularity is declining. Theophyllines are available orally and rectally, although the latter route of administration is now seldom used. This limits their role as acute symptom relievers and explains their propensity for systemic side effects, particularly CNS and gastrointestinal ones. On the positive side they can potentially achieve similar concentrations throughout the airways, which may not be true of inhaled therapy. Earlier preparations were bedevilled by erratic absorption, which may explain their lack of clinical effectiveness.[79,80] These problems have now been overcome, aided by the development of simpler readily available laboratory theophylline assays, and more reliable long-acting formulations with a half-life of 12–18 hours are available.[81,82] Even when care is taken to ensure a stable plasma concentration, the bronchodilator action

is limited in stable COPD patients (Table 24.5), changes in FEV$_1$ ranging from 0 to 20%. There is evidence of a modest dose–response effect[83] but the confidence intervals of these changes are wide and like many other studies this report does not indicate how many patients had to enter the study to achieve the study population reported.

Some patients do report subjective improvement after theophyllines in the face of trivial spirometric changes and this may explain why formal assessments of breathlessness and exercise tolerance have been performed more often with this drug than with any other. Representative clinical trials data are summarized in Table 24.6. There are over a dozen reports of the effects of theophylline on exercise capacity in COPD. However these studies tend to be small and the use of coexisting rescue or regular therapies is seldom standardized. Some studies report no change in corridor walking distance[84,85] or improvement in the duration of cycle exercise.[86] Other studies report equivocal findings with responses in one variable but not another, for example improvement in walking distance after beta-agonist and theophylline combined but not either alone.[87] In the remaining studies there is a small but clear improvement in corridor and treadmill walking after theophylline, although whether this differs from beta-agonist is less clear.[83,88–90] There appears to be a dose–response relationship,[83,89] with clinically significant benefits only being seen at the higher dose levels. Quality of life assessments made after longer periods of treatment showed improvements in breathlessness during everyday activities and reductions in perceived fatigue on higher (i.e. >17 μg/ml) doses of theophylline, but whether these changes are greater than those seen after salbutamol is debatable.[88,89]

The slow onset of action and the difficulties in achieving stable plasma levels mean that most studies occur after 2–6 weeks rather than a few hours as is the case with inhaled therapy. In these periods tachyphylaxis to theophyllines is not apparent but extended follow-up beyond 12 weeks in COPD patients has not been reported, at least for the functional end-points which seem to be clinically most important.

The reasons for this functional improvement are still being investigated but are likely to be similar to those now established after inhaled bronchodilators. *In vitro* studies and observations in normal volunteers led to the suggestion that theophyllines protected against respiratory muscle fatigue and increased respiratory muscle strength.[91] In one particularly impressive placebo-controlled study in 60 patients with severe COPD there was a fall in FRC, an increase in inspiratory muscle strength and a lower tidal pleural pressure/maximum pleural pressure ratio after active therapy.[92]

However, even during acute fatiguing inspiratory loads oral theophyllines did not reduce dyspnea in COPD patients.[86] Decreases in dynamic hyperinflation

Table 24.6 *Effects of bronchodilator agents on spirometry and lung volumes in stable COPD*

	Gross and Skorodin[1]	Spence et al.[82]	Chrystyn et al.[83]	Murciano et al.[92]	Taylor et al.[98]
No drug	10/salb	32/oxi	33/theo	60/theo	12/theo
Dose	720 µg (atr) 3.0 mg (salb)	200 µg	12.1 µg/ml 18.3 µg/ml	14.8 µg/ml	12.0 µg/ml
FEV$_1$					
Baseline	1.12 1.19	0.77	1.00 1.00	31.5% p	1.14
Post-drug	1.42 1.51	0.95	1.08 1.13	35.7% p	1.27
% Change	27 27	24	8 13	13	11
FVC					
Baseline	– –	1.91	2.46 2.46	60.1% p	2.55
Post-drug	– –	2.33	2.65 2.78	63.2% p	2.69
% Change	–	22	8 13	5	5
FRC					
Baseline	217% p 220% p	5.28	6.76 6.76	161% p	5.01
Post-drug	195% p 188% p	4.93	6.28 6.24	157% p	4.9
% Change	10 14.5	7	7 7	2	2
RV					
Baseline	242% p 247% p	– –	4.24	4.23 4.23	4.12
Post-drug	197% p 180% p	– –	3.93	3.32 3.06	3.8
% Change	18.6 27	– –	7	22 28	8

Data expressed as absolute volumes (liters) or as % predicted (% p) depending on study.
atr: atropine methonitrite; salb: salbutamol; oxi: oxitropium bromide; theo: theophylline.

after theophylline remain the most likely explanation for the improvements seen in both symptoms and exercise tolerance. Thus Jenne and colleagues found that the work of breathing was reduced in 10 patients at modest theophylline levels (mean 10.3 µg/ml) whilst maximum exercise ventilation increased.[93] This is similar to data after an inhaled anticholinergic drug during cycle exercise where exercise desaturation and dyspnea were also reduced.[31] These findings make it unlikely that the beneficial effects of theophylline are occurring for reasons other than simple bronchodilatation.

SINGLE AGENT OR COMBINATION THERAPY?

The problem of suboptimal dosing when comparing different routes of administration makes interpretation of comparisons between agents very difficult. Most data rely on spirometric end-points and rather surprisingly there are no functional comparisons between high doses of beta-agonists and high doses of inhaled anticholinergics in COPD. The problems of the existing data are illustrated by the one study to compare walking distance after both drugs in the same patients.[47] As already noted, salbutamol but not 40 µg ipratropium improved exercise performance in these patients. However, combining the two drugs did produce a further significant functional improvement (changes in 12-minute distance post-salbutamol 62(SEM 15) meters), suggesting that one or both of the other drugs were being given in suboptimal doses.

There is convincing evidence that beta-agonists are more effective bronchodilators in asthmatics than are anticholinergics[94] but this is not true in COPD. Thus one reviewer found that 36 of 38 studies reported that anticholinergics were equivalent with or superior to beta-agonists in COPD patients.[95] An earlier well-conducted dose–response study suggested that inhaled atropine methonitrate could achieve more of the potentially available bronchodilatation than could salbutamol.[96] However, this finding is not universal. Among milder COPD patients who were assessed by short-term responses to 80 μg ipratropium and 400 μg salbutamol respectively, more patients responded to the former and achieved most of their maximal bronchodilation with ipratropium alone, a reverse of the situation in a parallel group of asthmatics.[96] Combining beta-agonists and anticholinergics in high doses produces a greater improvement in resting lung mechanics than either agent alone, leads to a further fall in end-expiratory and end-inspiratory lung volume and a reduction in resting breathlessness irrespective of the degree of tidal airflow limitation.[6] This is true in severe patients which may explain why some benefit from nebulized bronchodilators (see below). Even here more data about the effect on exercise capacity would be welcome.

Several studies have compared the effects of short-acting inhaled drugs with oral theophylline. Technically, this is more demanding because of the need to establish appropriate serum theophylline concentrations. Most of these studies have involved fairly small numbers of patients and relied on spirometric outcomes. When salbutamol and intravenous theophylline were compared, it was clear that the theophylline alone was not as effective a bronchodilator as the beta-agonist, irrespective of the order of administration. In a more complex study, Guyatt and colleagues compared inhaled salbutamol and oral aminophylline in high doses singly and in combination.[88] They chose a 4-week treatment period and assessed health status using the Chronic Respiratory Questionnaire. Although 612 were screened only 29 entered and 19 completed the study, which illustrates something of the atypical nature of data and trials such as this. The authors concluded that the combination treatment was more effective, although whether this would have been the case had a higher dose of salbutamol been used is less clear. However, studies of both pulmonary function and exercise capacity using either anticholinergics alone or a combination of anticholinergics and beta-agonists have shown significant further benefits when these are added to maintenance theophylline treatment.[96–99]

Studies comparing long- and short-acting inhaled bronchodilators are now beginning to be reported. A large trial conducted by van Noord and colleagues used a parallel group design to compare patients treated with placebo and salmeterol or salmeterol plus regular ipratropium.[100] The combination therapy was significantly better than its components and importantly the number of exacerbations during the 3-month study was lowest in those patients who received combined treatments.

A further large US study has shown the additive effects on spirometry of salmeterol and theophylline in combination which was clearly superior to either component alone.[101]

Italian investigators reported 80 well-controlled COPD patients who were randomized to 3 months treatment with either 50 μg of salmeterol twice daily, the same dose of salmeterol and either to 250 μg or 500 μg of fluticasone (an inhaled corticosteroid) of a high-dose corticosteroid beta-agonist regime and titrated theophyllines.[102] They showed clear benefit from the use of the inhaled corticosteroid and the long-acting beta-agonists, with a further additional improvement in lung function when theophylline treatment was added. A higher dose of the inhaled steroid appeared to be more effective in producing these more effects.[103] Significant improvements in dyspnea score and lung function disease have been seen with long-acting beta-agonist–inhaled steroid combination treatment in COPD, whilst a 1-year study has shown this produced the greatest change and health status, with the fewest number of study withdrawals, the largest reductions in rescue therapy and symptoms.[104]

Comparative trials using tiotropium have largely compared it to ipratropium (see above) where it is clearly superior over 3 and 12 months of use. Direct comparison with salmeterol showed that tiotropium was a more effective bronchodilator over six months use but there were no statistically significant differences between the drugs in the number of exacerbations reported, both being superior to placebo. As yet no trials of the combination of this drug and other agents have been published.

SIDE EFFECTS

Each of the three major bronchodilator groups exhibits dose-dependent side effects, which limit their usefulness but vary widely in severity between different patients. Although current beta-agonists drugs are relatively bronchoselective, oral therapy increases heart rate probably by peripheral vasodilatation, and promotes muscle tremor irrespective of the drug chosen. Larger doses given by MDI, i.e. above 1 mg, increase the heart rate and objectively reported somatic tremor as well as the patients perception of side effects[40] (see Figure 17.4). Despite these changes in resting heart rate, there is no excess of arrhythmia in COPD patients without coexisting cardiac disease,[105] but patients with ischemic heart disease do have more ventricular ectopic beats, the clinical significance of which remains unclear.[106] Detailed hemodynamic studies show that oral beta-agonists can reduce pulmonary vascular resistance and increase cardiac output, which may explain the patient's complaint of a more forceful heartbeat.[35] However, these favorable effects on tissue oxygen delivery are offset by falls in arterial saturation due to worsening ventilation–perfusion mismatching and the overall benefit or improvement in these hemodynamic variables is very difficult to predict (see Chapter 17).

Similar falls in oxygen saturation have been reported after high-dose short- and long-acting inhaled beta-agonists but these may not be relevant to everyday exercise as studies during self-paced corridor walking for 15 minutes and 2 hours after nebulized salbutamol show that the exercise-induced desaturation that normally occurs in these patients is not worsened by pre-treatment with a beta-agonist but their exercise-induced tolerance is increased. Like all sympathomimetic drugs, beta-agonists produce hypokalemia at least transiently, after their administration. COPD patients are older, may have occult ischemic disease and are often transiently or permanently hypoxemic and often receive other treatment, for example thiazide diuretics which worsen beta-agonist-induced hypokalemia.[107] Again, the lack of evidence of significant rhythm disturbances in these patients is reassuring, probably reflecting tachyphylaxis of these metabolic effects.[43] Nonetheless, it is worth monitoring serum potassium during high-dose nebulizer treatment of an acute exacerbation (see Chapter 26).

Inhaled anticholinergic drugs are relatively free from side effects although many patients complain of a slightly metallic taste, which they dislike. The lack of systemic absorption even at high doses protects against gastrointestinal and urinary problems, although the occasional patient can develop acute glaucoma if they inadvertently allow the nebulized aerosol to enter their eyes.[108] Early reports of paradoxical bronchoconstriction were confined to asthmatic patients and seem to have resolved after the benzalkonium chloride preservative was removed from the nebulizer formulation. Likewise, concerns about reduced mucociliary clearance have proven unfounded.[109] Unlike beta-agonists anticholinergics do not affect resting oxygen tensions[30] and improve exercise performance without changing the degree of exercise-induced desaturations.[31] The side effect profile of inhaled tiotropium appears to be similar to that of shorter-acting inhaled anticholinergic drugs with no evidence of impaired mucociliary clearance or prostatic symptoms. However dry mouth is reported more frequently with this drug, possibly because of its longer duration of action.

Theophylline therapy has a deservedly bad reputation for side effects among COPD patients. In one large study of patients attending an emergency department 10% of 5557 patients in whom theophylline levels were measured had values greater than 20 µg/ml and 116 cases exceeded 30 µg/ml.[110] Most of this toxicity was chronic and 6% of this group died of drug-related effects. Relatively minor problems include insomnia, headaches, nausea and gastrointestinal reflux symptoms (reflecting increased gastric acid production). However, serious cardiac rhythm disturbances can occur, especially multifocal atrial tachycardia and ventricular tachyarrhythmias.[111] Some patients develop grand mal seizures. This may result from theophylline toxicity which can induce significant falls in cerebral blood flow[112] and increase brain hypoxia.[113] It is tempting to suggest that the ventilatory stimulant effects of theophylline, if they exist,[114] are due to these mechanisms rather than its impact on CNS adenosine concentrations. COPD patients often have coexisting vascular disease and acid reflux disorders due to their smoking which may explain why side effects seem to occur at levels within the therapeutic range. Moreover, additional intravenous theophylline on a background of high-normal theophylline levels during an exacerbation is particularly hazardous and requires careful monitoring (Chapter 26).

Unlike other symptomatic treatments, oral theophylline needs considerable attention to detail if its modest benefits in terms of symptom reduction and improved exercise tolerance (which requires the highest tolerable theophylline levels) are not to provoke significant side effects (which requires the lowest practical serum levels). Theophylline is metabolized by the cytochrome P450 mixed function oxidize system and metabolizers may be fast or slow.[115] Theophylline clearance decreases with age[116] and is influenced by a host of other variables (Table 24.7).

Long-acting readily absorbed theophylline preparations have greatly improved the pharmacokinetic profile of these drugs which may account for the success in treating overnight peak flow changes in asthmatics. However, the once or twice daily recommended dose may be insufficient to give therapeutic serum theophylline levels in rapid metabolizers.[117] Slow-release theophyllines are still affected by the timing of the dose in relation to meals. When taken after a meal, absorption is slow and fluctuations in the theophylline level are

Table 24.7 *Theophylline metabolism in COPD*

Increased	Decreased
Cigarette smoking**	Arterial hypoxemia (<6.0 kPa)**
Anticonvulsant drugs	Respiratory acidosis*
Rifampicin	Congestive cardiac failure*
	Liver cirrhosis
	Erythromycin**
	Ciprofloxacin (not ofloxacin)
	Cimetidine (not ranitidine)
	Viral infections
	Old age*

Many factors influence theophylline metabolism and those posing particular problems in COPD are indicated by asterisks, the number depending upon the likely hazards.

reduced. If taken with food, especially if the fat content is high, then 'dose dumping' occurs and potentially toxic levels can develop due to enhanced absorption.[118] Given this multiplicity of problems, it is not surprising that routine theophylline treatment is so difficult, even when monitoring of serum levels is readily available.

DELIVERY DEVICES

Whatever its other problems oral therapy has the advantage of simplicity in use, which is not shared by inhaled bronchodilators. Studies of patients compliance with inhaled treatment in the Lung Health Study make depressing reading with an overall compliance with prescribed therapy of 65% and significant overreporting of inhaler use by patients keen to please their physician.[119] A clinical trial in mild-disease may not reflect more normal treatment patterns and patients with more severe disease and persistent symptoms appear to be more adherent with medical therapy. Thus 85% of participants in the ISOLDE study of inhaled corticosteroids took more than 70% of the prescribed doses over the 3-year period. More recent studies examining particle deposition suggest that patients with airflow obstruction and particularly COPD are more likely to have central drug deposition. This has some advantages in limiting absorption through the alveoli, although clearly this does occur as was seen from the changes in serum cortisol in patients treated with inhaled corticosteroids.[120]

Conventional MDIs pose particular problems especially for elderly patients.[121] The physics of aerosol generation and its deposition within the lungs have been studied in detail.[122] Key factors are the particle size, usually expressed as the mass median diameter, the hygroscopicity of the drug and the inspiratory flow rate. In general, particles between two and five microns mass median diameters (MMD) are deposited in the airway rather than the alveoli or mouth. Particles tend to absorb moisture and increase their MMD the further along the airway they travel. High initial inspiratory flows promote impaction in the pharynx and increase the dose swallowed. An ideal MDI technique has been suggested,[123] the principal features of which are summarized in Table 24.8 together with the particular problems for the older COPD patient. Incoordination of inspiratory effort and activation and breath-holding due to the 'cold freon' effect when the aerosol vaporizes appear to be particularly common.[124]

Many attempts have been made to overcome this. Dry powder formulations need less patient cooperation but require a higher inspiratory flow rate to ensure optimal lung deposition. Devices based on dry powder capsule, foil disks or miconized pure drug in a dry powder reservoir

Table 24.8 *Inhaler technique in COPD*

Ideal method	Difficulties in COPD
1 Remove cap	Occasionally forgotten
2 Shake inhaler	Occasionally forgotten
3 Hold inhaler upright	Often forgotten
4 Tilt head back 10–55 degrees	Often forgotten
5 Hold inhaler in front of open mouth	Advice often confused about this
6 Begin to inspire and activate inhaler	Coordination problems
7 Breathe in slowly and deeply	Difficult if hyperinflated already
8 Breath-hold for 10–15 seconds	Breath-hold time reduced
9 Breathe out slowly through the nose	High respiratory rate makes this harder
10 Use one puff at a time – wait 3–5 minutes between puffs	Often use multiple puffs in a single inspiration

are competing for this lucrative market. Radioactive tracer studies suggest that most of the inhaled drug from an MDI activation ends up in the stomach with only 10% reaching the lungs.[122] By introducing a space between the inhaler and the oropharynx, the aerosol forms a cloud, which can be inhaled. Large-volume 'spacer' devices utilize these effects. They involve less coordination and the larger particles deposit in the spacer before inhalation reducing the total drug dosage, although the amount reaching the lung is probably not very different. Although hard to assess directly at present with short-term bronchodilator drugs, studies with high-dose inhaled corticosteroids suggest that less drug is absorbed when spacers are used.[124] However, COPD patients may only be able to achieve low inspiratory flow rates. Usually the one-way plastic valve used in these devices opens even at flow rates of 40 L/min or less but it may stick if the spacer is not kept clean. Tube spacers represent an attempt to make these devices more portable but are generally less effective, at least in drug deposition terms.[125]

The deposition patterns of nebulized drugs are similar to those of the spacer, with larger particles being deposited within the facemask and tubing. They involve even less patient cooperation and yield a higher absolute dosage of the drug, which may explain some of their popularity with patients (see below).

Despite the enthusiasm for better devices, there are surprisingly few data about the benefits of improved delivery systems or even modifications of inhaler technique in COPD patients. Most deposition studies examine whole-lung differences resulting from change in delivery. Indeed, the poor 'clinical signal:noise ratio' in COPD makes practical clinical trials extremely difficult. However, a change in airway caliber will influence the deposition pattern[126] and favor more peripheral drug deposition.

DOMICILIARY NEBULIZER THERAPY

The continuing debate about efficacy and appropriateness of domiciliary nebulized bronchodilators in COPD illustrates many of the problems inherent in studies of bronchodilator action in these patients. There is a genuine concern that in some countries at least, the prescription of nebulizer solutions of bronchodilators from a portable compressor has increased unnecessarily.[127] The initial belief that a complex IPPB machine is better than a compressor has not been borne out,[128] although it would be interesting to know what effect IPPB and bronchodilator together have on intrinsic PEEP as either continuous or intermittent positive airways pressure (CPAP or IPAP) can reduce this in some circumstances.[129] A potent practical attraction of this therapy in the USA is the fact that it is fully reimbursable by the health insurers, unlike inhaled therapy given in other ways.

Using spirometric end-points and corridor walking exercise, nebulized salbutamol seems to be no more effective than lower doses of the same drug given through a spacer device.[39] However, these comparisons were relatively brief and studies of up to 1 year suggest that most (27 of 32) of a group of predominant COPD patients found nebulized treatment better than their previous inhaled therapy and also demonstrated an increase in home PEF of 40 L/min.[130] Several factors may explain these changes.

First, the total dose of drug delivered to the airways is large and although the dose–response effects of beta-agonists and anticholinergics are not impressive, a small change in FEV_1 is likely to produce a disproportionately large improvement in effort tolerance (see above). Second, the higher the initial FEV_1 the longer is the duration of action. This is clearly seen in a multidose study of ipratropium where the mean FEV_1 after 0.6 mg was significantly higher than that after 40 μg through a metered dose inhaler and remained 33% higher at 8 hours.[63] Finally, facial cooling that occurs when the nebulizer solution condenses within the mask can, itself, reduce dyspnea independent of any effect on airway caliber.[131]

Attempts at evaluating successful treatment have been restricted by the lack of suitable end-points, although a mixture of patient preference, home PEF and symptom scoring has been used.[132,133] Routine bronchodilator testing can separate relatively good responders but was less useful in long-term studies.[134] In this last report changes in specific airways conductance in the laboratory did seem a promising means of selecting 'good responders'. At present prescribing nebulizer treatment is

Table 24.9 *Key points in the assessment of wet-nebulizer treatment for COPD. (Modified from ref. 138.)*

1 Treatment is normally only indicated in patients with an $FEV_1 < 50\%$ predicted
2 An appropriate trial of alternative medications including a check on compliance and device preference should be conducted before considering regular nebulized bronchodilators
3 There is no clear agreement on what constitutes a 'positive' response. A subjective report of benefit following regular treatment is at least as valid as any objective assessment
4 A treatment trial should continue for at least 2 weeks
5 A positive response would be considered as a subjective change of 'definitely better or much better' and/or an increase in PEF by at least 10 and preferably 20% of the mean value recorded during the week before the trial began

more likely to be influenced by the enthusiasm (or lack of it) of the physician together with the anxiety of both patients and family that every form of treatment should be used to reduce distress. There is obviously a need for further large-scale systematic investigation to provide a firmer basis for the current recommendations. Until that time, the advice offered in the European Respiratory Society Nebuliser Guidelines remains a reasonable approach (Table 24.9).[33]

CLINICAL STRATEGIES OF BRONCHODILATOR USE

The increased number of studies about the multiple actions of bronchodilator drugs has led to a reasonable consensus about how and when they should be used,[135] although not necessarily about which treatment is most appropriate. Much depends upon the clinical setting, when the patient presents, local availability of pharmaceuticals and, more particularly, the healthcare system in which the physician operates. Thus in the UK if a patient attended a family physician with early symptoms suggestive of COPD, then establishing the diagnosis firmly and making some form of assessment of its severity preferably by spirometry, with encouragement to stop smoking should be the primary goal. Monotherapy with either beta-agonists or anticholinergics to provide adequate symptom control particularly during exacerbations is often all that is required.

Once symptoms and particularly breathlessness become persistent then maintenance bronchodilator therapy is required. At present there is more experience with long-acting beta-agonists but newer agents such as tiotropium may be equally effective as monotherapy. This should be combined with a short-acting bronchodilator as a 'rescue' therapy and most data suggest the relatively faster onset of beta-agonists is to be preferred. Whether rapid-onset long-acting drugs such as formoterol are a good or a bad thing will depend on the total dose of drug used and hence the risk of subsequent side effects. These are still to be appropriately tested in COPD. An alternative approach would be to use a regular short-acting beta-agonist–anticholinergic combination but this is less reliable since most patients are not as adherent with the four times a day treatment that is significantly more inconvenient. These considerations are true, whether the patient is managed in primary care or is attending hospital. In either case, assessing the maximum dilatation that can be achieved is a useful benchmark for judging subsequent progress.

The persistence of symptoms makes a trial of additional inhaled therapy appropriate. The aim should be to find a regimen which maximizes bronchodilatation, reduces symptoms and does so without increasing side effects. It is generally better to choose drugs at the mid-point of their dose–response relationship and combine them to minimize side effects, making a combination of an inhaled long-acting beta-agonist and anticholinergic an attractive, if untested, possibility. Whether this remains true with inhaled corticosteroids as a further supplementary therapy is not clear, as the majority of studies using lower doses of inhaled corticosteroids have been less successful at potentiating the effects of long-acting inhaled beta-agonists.

If the patient remains symptomatic despite these measurements, the introduction of a carefully monitored dose of theophylline is worthwhile, starting with a low dose, slowly increasing the dose to the upper limit of the therapeutic range over 2–4 weeks. The trend to give subtherapeutic doses, by analogy with the anti-inflammatory effects reported in asthma, has not been supported by good data in COPD. The assessment of inhaler technique and an early change to a simpler delivery system such as spacers or dry powder devices will often give the patient more confidence and save time in the long run. This is an important consideration whatever the stage of disease management.

A realistic explanation of the potential benefits and possible side effects, particularly when taking theophyllines, will help the patient to cope with their disability better. Whether such simple traditional medical attention is more effective than active bronchodilator therapy alone has not been assessed. Nebulized bronchodilator assessment is best reserved for patients with very severe symptoms where all other therapies have been judged inappropriate or have failed to provide adequate control. This form of treatment, like short-burst oxygen therapy, appears to be most appropriate for those having greatest difficulty in the community and who become 'revolving-door patients' with frequent hospitalizations. In these circumstances, nebulizer therapy is likely to have a powerful placebo effect, which may nonetheless be worthwhile for the patient.

FUTURE PROSPECTS

The last 5 years have seen important changes in the bronchodilator drugs available for treating COPD.[136,137] There is a better understanding of the value of non-spirometric end-points like breathlessness, exercise capacity, health status and the number of exacerbations in deciding the worth of these therapies. The greatest benefits have been seen with long-acting inhaled bronchodilators. These are being used more widely and their simple dosage regimen and acceptable side effect profile suggest that they will become the new standard therapy in countries where the costs inherent in their prescription can be met. Earlier concerns about problems with a change to CFC-free inhalers have proven groundless and these have now become the standard means of delivery of bronchodilator drugs.[138] The practical problems of an aging population in using these devices means that there is still much to be gained by developing more 'user-friendly' systems which can take advantage of the simpler dosing regimens now possible.

Clearly studies examining the effects of long-acting beta-agonists and tiotropium combinations will be undertaken and it is reasonable to predict that a useful additional benefit will be found. Similarly, combining these agents with inhaled corticosteroids, as has been done successfully in bronchial asthma, appears to offer benefits which the conventional pharmacologic explanations would not predict. There is still much to be done to determine whether it is possible to identify those patients who will show the greatest benefit from particular combinations of treatment and so 'customize' patient care.

The prospects for an acceptable oral bronchodilator with a more acceptable side effect pattern remain distant. Initial hopes have focused on the PDE IV inhibitors like ciliomilast which appear to achieve this in the short term. However this class offers more promise as an anti-inflammatory therapy and is considered elsewhere (see Chapter 25). For the foreseeable future we must concentrate on using our existing drugs more wisely rather than expecting major new breakthroughs in this area.

REFERENCES

1. Gross NJ. Role of the parasympathetic system in airways obstruction due to emphysema. *New Engl J Med* 1984;**311**:421–425.
2. Chaib J, Belcher N, Rees PJ. Maximum achievable bronchodilation in asthma. *Respir Med* 1989;**83**:497–502.

3. Rebuck AS, Galko BM. Bronchodilators in the treatment of bronchitis and emphysema. In: NS Cherniack, ed. *Chronic Obstructive Pulmonary Disease*. WB Saunders, Philadelphia, 1991, pp 487–9.

4. Yanai M, Sekizawa K, Ohrui T, Saski H, Takishima T. Site of airways obstruction in pulmonary disease: direct measurement of intrabronchial pressure. *J Appl Physiol* 1992;**72**:1016–23.

5. Takishma T, Sekizawa K, Tamura G, Inoue H. Anticholinergics in the treatment of COPD – site of bronchodilation. *Res Clin Forum* 1990;**13**:49–59.

6. Hadcroft J, Calverley PM. Alternative methods for assessing bronchodilator reversibility in chronic obstructive pulmonary disease. *Thorax* 2001;**56**:713–20.

7. O'Donnell DE, Lam M, Webb KA. Measurement of symptoms, lung hyperinflation, and endurance during exercise in chronic obstructive pulmonary disease. *Am J Respir Criti Care Med* 1998;**158**:1557–65.

8. O'Donnell DE, Lam M, Webb KA. Spirometric correlates of improvement in exercise performance after anticholinergic therapy in chronic obstructive pulmonary disease. *Am J Respir Crit Care Med* 1999;**160**:542–9.

9. Belman MJ, Botnick WC, Shin JW. Inhaled bronchodilators reduce dynamic hyperinflation during exercise in patients with chronic obstructive pulmonary disease. *Am J Respir Crit Care Med* 1996;**153**:967–75.

10. Puchelle E, Zahn JM, Girard R, *et al.* Mucociliary transport *in vivo* and *in vitro*. Relations to sputum properties in chronic bronchitis. *Eur J Respir Dis* 1980;**61**:254–64.

11. Barton AD, Weiss SGT, Lourenco RV, *et al.* Mucous glycoprotein content of chronic bronchitis sputum. *Proc Soc Exp Biol Med* 1977;**156**:8–13.

12. Lourenco RV, Klimek MF, Borouski CJ. Deposition and clearance of 2 µm particles in the tracheobronchial tree of normal subjects – smokers and non-smokers. *J Clin Invest* 1971;**50**:1411–20.

13. Similowski T, Yan S, Gauthier AP, Macklem PT. Contractile properties of the human diaphragm during chronic hyperinflation. *New Engl J Med* 1991;**325**:917–23.

14. Barnes PJ. Novel approaches and targets for treatment of chronic obstructive pulmonary disease. *Am J Resp Crit Care Med* 1999;**160**:S72–9.

15. Johnson M, Rennard S. Alternative mechanisms of long-acting beta 2-agonists in COPD. *Chest* 2001;**120**:258–70.

16. Ottonello L, Morone P, Dapino P, *et al.* Inhibitory effect of salmeterol on the respiratory burst of adherent human neutrophils. *Clin Exp Immumol* 1996;**106**:97–102.

17. Dowling RB, Rayner CF, Rutman A, *et al.* Effect of salmeterol on *Psuedomonas aeroginosa* infection of the respiratory mucosa. *Am J Respir Crit Care Med* 1997;**155**:327–36.

18. Dowling RB, Johnson M, Cole PJ, *et al.* Effect of salmeterol on *Haemophilus influenzae* infection of respiratory mucosa *in vitro*. *Eur Respir J* 1998;**11**:86–90.

19. Jones PW, Bosh TK. Quality of life changes in COPD patients treated with salmeterol. *Am J Respir Crit Care Med* 1997;**155**:1283–9.

20. De Troyer A, Yernault J-C, Rodenstein D. Effects of vagal blockade on lung mechanics in normal man. *J Appl Physiol* 1979;**46**:217–26.

21. Gross NJ, Co E, Skorodin MS. Cholinergic bronchomotor tone in COPD. *Chest* 1989;**96**:984–7.

22. Nisar M, Earis JE, Pearson MG, Calverley PM. Acute bronchodilator trials in chronic obstructive pulmonary disease. *Am Rev Respir Dis* 1992;**146**:555–9.

23. Bosken CH, Wiggs BR, Pare PD, Hogg JC. Small airway dimensions in smokers with obstruction of airflow. *Am Rev Respir Dis* 1990;**142**:563–70.

24. Ramsdell JW, Nachtwey FJ, Moser KM. Bronchial hyperreactivity in chronic obstructive bronchitis. *Am Rev Respir Dis* 1982;**126**:829–32.

25. Woolcock AJ, Anderson SD, Peat JK, *et al.* Characteristics of bronchial hyperresponsiveness in chronic obstructive pulmonary disease and in asthma. *Am Rev Respir Dis* 1991;**143**:1438–43.

26. Wiggs BR, Bosken CH, Pare PD, James A, Hogg JC. A model of airway narrowing in asthma and in chronic obstructive pulmonary disease. *Am Rev Respir Dis* 1992;**145**:1251–8.

27. Bellemare F, Grassino A. Force reserve of the diaphragm in patients with chronic obstructive pulmonary disease. *J Appl Physiol* 1983;**55**:8–15.

28. Burge PS, Calverley PMA, Jones PA, Spencer S, Anderson JA. Prednisolone response in patients with chronic obstructive pulmonary disease; results from the ISOLDE study. *Thorax* 2003 (in press).

29. Gross NJ, Bankwala Z. Effects of an anticholinergic bronchodilator on arterial blood gases of hypoxaemic patients with chronic obstructive pulmonary disease: comparison with an adrenergic agent. *Am Rev Respir Dis* 1987;**136**:1091–4.

30. Khoukaz G, Gross NJ. Effects of salmeterol on arterial blood gases in patients with stable chronic obstructive pulmonary disease. Comparison with albuterol and ipratropium. *Am J Respir Crit Care Med* 1999;**160**:1028–30.

31. Spence DP, Hay JG, Carter J, Pearson MG, Calverley PM. Oxygen desaturation and breathlessness during corridor walking in chronic obstructive pulmonary disease: effect of oxitropium bromide. *Thorax* 1993;**48**:1145–50.

32. Marvin PM, Baker BJ, Dutt AK, *et al.* Physiologic effects of oral bronchodilators during rest and exercise in chronic obstructive pulmonary disease. *Chest* 1983;**84**:684–9.

33. Mohammed AF, Anderson K, Matusiewicz SP, Boyd G, Greening AP, Thomson NC. Effect of controlled-release salbutamol in predominantly non-reversible chronic airflow obstruction. *Respir Med* 1991;**85**:495–500.

34. Shim CS, Williams MH. Bronchodilator response to oral aminophylline and terbutaline versus aerosol albuterol in patients with chronic obstructive pulmonary disease. *Am J Med* 1983;**75**:697–701.

35. Peacock A, Busset C, Dawkins K, Denison D. Response of pulmonary circulation to oral pirbuterol in chronic airflow obstruction. *Br Med J* 1983;**287**:1178–80.

36. Teule GJJ, Majid PA. Haemodynamic effects of terbutaline in chronic obstructive airways disease. *Thorax* 1980;**35**:536–42.

37. Anthonisen NR, Wright EC. Bronchodilator response in chronic obstructive pulmonary disease. *Am Rev Respir Dis* 1986;**133**:814–19.

38. Tashkin DP, Ashutosh K, Bleecker ER, *et al.* Comparison of the anticholinergic bronchodilator ipratropium bromide with metaproterenol in chronic obstructive pulmonary disease. A 90-day multi-center study. *Am J Med* 1986;**81**:81–90.

39. Jenkins SC, Moxham J. High dose salbutamol in chronic bronchitis: comparison of 400 µg, 1 mg, 1.6 mg, 2 mg and placebo delivered by rotahaler. *Br J Dis Chest* 1987;**81**:242–7.

40. Vathenen AS, Britton JR, Ebden P, Cookson JB, Wharrad HJ, Tattersfield AE. High-dose inhaled albuterol in severe chronic airflow limitation. *Am Rev Respir Dis* 1988;**138**:850–5.

41. Corris PA, Neville E, Nariman S, Gibson GJ. Dose–response study of inhaled salbutamol powder in chronic airflow obstruction. *Thorax* 1983;**38**:292–6.

42. Amoroso P, Wilson SR, Moxham J, Ponte J. Acute effects of inhaled salbutamol on the metabolic rate of normal subjects. *Thorax* 1993;**48**:882–5.

43. Wilson SR, Amoroso P, Moxham J, Ponte J. Modification of the thermogenic effect of acutely inhaled salbutamol by chronic inhalation in normal subjects. *Thorax* 1993; **48**:886–9.

44. Cheung D, Timmers MC, Zwinderman AH, Bel EH, Dijkman JH, Sterk PJ. Long term effects of a long acting beta-2-adrenoreceptor agonist, salmeterol, on airway hyperresponsiveness in patients with mild asthma. *N Engl J Med* 1992;**327**:1198–203.

45. Mendella LA, Manfreda J, Warren CP, Anthonisen NR. Steroid response in stable chronic obstructive pulmonary disease. *Ann Intern Med* 1982;**96**:17–21.

46. Cook D, Guyatt G, Wong E, *et al.* Regular versus as-needed short-acting inhaled beta-agonist therapy for chronic obstructive pulmonary disease. *Am J Respir Crit Care Med* 2001;**163**:85–90.

47. Leitch AG, Hopkin JM, Ellis DA, Merchant S, McHardy GJR. The effect of aerosol ipratropium bromide and salbutamol on exercise tolerance in chronic bronchitis. *Thorax* 1978; **33**:711–13.

48. Berger R, Smith D. Effect of inhaled metaproterenol on exercise performance in patients with stable 'fixed' airway obstruction. *Am Rev Respir Dis* 1988;**138**:624–9.

49. Van Schayck CP, Dompeling E, Van Herwaarden CL, *et al.* Bronchodilator treatment in moderate asthma or chronic bronchitis:continuous or on demand? A randomised controlled study. *Br Med J* 1991;**303**:1426–31 [see comments].

50. Van Schayck CP, Dompeling E, Van Herwaarden CL, *et al.* Continuous and on demand use of bronchodilators in patients with non-steroid dependent asthma and chronic bronchitis: four-year follow-up randomized controlled study. *Br J Gen Pract* 1995;**45**:239–44.

51. Boyd G, Morice AH, Pounsford JC, Siebert M, Peslis N, Crawford C. An evaluation of salmeterol in the treatment of chronic obstructive pulmonary disease (COPD). *Eur Respir J* 1997;**10**:815–21 [published erratum appears in *Eur Respir J* 1997;**10**:1696].

52. Dahl R, Greefhorst LA, Nowak D, *et al.* Inhaled formoterol dry powder versus ipratropium bromide in chronic obstructive pulmonary disease. *Am J Respir Crit Care Med* 2001; **164**:778–84.

53. Mahler DA, Donohue JF, Barbee RA, *et al.* Efficacy of salmeterol xinafoate in the treatment of COPD. *Chest* 1999;**115**:957–65.

54. Rennard SI, Anderson W, Wallack R, *et al.* Use of a long-acting inhaled beta-2-adrenergic agonist, salmeterol xinafoate, in patients with chronic obstructive pulmonary disease. *Am J Respir Crit Care Med* 2001;**163**:1087–92.

55. Celik G, Kayacan O, Beder S, Durmaz G. Formoterol and salmeterol in partially reversible chronic obstructive pulmonary disease: a crossover, placebo-controlled comparison of onset and duration of action. *Respiration* 1999;**66**:434–9.

56. Benhamou D, Cuvelier A, Muir JF, *et al.* Rapid onset of bronchodilation in COPD: a placebo-controlled study comparing formoterol (Foradil Aerolizer) with salbutamol (Ventodisk). *Respir Med* 2001;**95**:817–21.

57. Cazzola M, Di Perna F, D'Amato M, Califano C, Matera MG, D'Amato G. Formoterol Turbuhaler for as-needed therapy in patients with mild acute exacerbations of COPD. *Respir Med* 2001;**95**:917–21.

58. Gandevia B. Historical view of the use of parasympatholytic agents in the treatment of respiratory disorders. *Postgrad Med J* 1975;S1(suppl 7):13–20.

59. Gross NJ. Ipratropium bromide. *N Engl J Med* 1988;**319**: 486–94.

60. Calverley PMA. The clinical efficacy of oxitropium bromide. *Rev Contemp Pharmacother* 1992;**3**:189–96.

61. Poppius H, Salorinne Y. Comparative trial of a new anticholinergic bronchodilator Sch 1000 and salbutamol in chronic bronchitis. *Br Med J* 1973;**4**:134–6.

62. Gross NJ, Petty TL, Friedman M, Skorodin MS, Silvers GW, Donohue JF. Dose response to ipratropium as a nebulized solution in patients with chronic obstructive pulmonary disease. A three-center study. *Am Rev Respir Dis* 1989; **139**:1188–91.

63. Ikeda A, Nishimura K, Koyama H, Izumi T. Comparative dose–response study of three anticholinergic agents and fenoterol using a metered dose inhaler in patients with chronic obstructive pulmonary disease. *Thorax* 1995;**50**:62–6.

64. Rennard SI, Serby CW, Ghafouri M, Johnson PA, Friedman M. Extended therapy with ipratropium is associated with improved lung function in patients with COPD. A retrospective analysis of data from seven clinical trials. *Chest* 1996;**110**:62–70.

65. Allen CJ, Campbell AH. Dose response of ipratropium bromide assessed by two methods. *Thorax* 1980;**35**:137–9.

66. Peel ET, Anderson G. A dose–response study of oxitropium bromide in chronic bronchitis. *Thorax* 1984;**39**:453–6.

67. Ikeda A, Nishimura K, Koyama H, Sugiura, Izumi T. Oxitropium bromide improves exercise performance in patients with COPD. *Chest* 1994;**106**:1740–5.

68. Hay JG, Stone P, Carter J, *et al.* Bronchodilator reversibility, exercise performance and breathlessness in stable chronic obstructive pulmonary disease. *Eur Respir J* 1992;**5**:659–64.

69. Anthonisen NR, Connett JE, Kiley JP, *et al.* Effects of smoking intervention and the use of an inhaled anticholinergic bronchodilator on the rate of decline of FEV_1. The Lung Health Study. *JAMA* 1994;**272**:1497–505.

70. On LS, Boonyongsunchai P, Webb S, Davies L, Calverley PMA, Costello RW. Function of pulmonary neuronal M2 muscarinic receptors in stable chronic obstructive pulmonary disease. *Am J Respir Crit Care Med* 2001;**163**:1320–5.

71. Casaburi R, Briggs DDJ, Donohue JF, Serby CW, Menjoge SS, Witek TJ, Jr. The spirometric efficacy of once-daily dosing with tiotropium in stable COPD: a 13-week multicenter trial. The US Tiotropium Study Group. *Chest* 2000;**118**:1294–302.

72. Littner MR, Ilowite JS, Tashkin DP, *et al.* Long-acting bronchodilation with once-daily dosing of tiotropium (Spiriva) in stable chronic obstructive pulmonary disease. *Am J Respir Crit Care Med* 2000;**161**:1136–42.

73. Van Noord JA, Bantje TA, Eland ME, Korducki L, Cornelissen PJ. A randomised controlled comparison of tiotropium and ipratropium in the treatment of chronic obstructive pulmonary disease. The Dutch Tiotropium Study Group. *Thorax* 2000;**55**:289–94.

74. O'Connor BJ, Towse LJ, Barnes PJ. Prolonged effect of tiotropium bromide on methacholine-induced bronchoconstriction in asthma. *Am J Respir Crit Care Med* 1996;**154**:876–80.

75. Maesen FP, Smeets JJ, Sledsens TJ, Wald FD, Cornelissen PJ. Tiotropium bromide, a new long-acting antimuscarinic bronchodilator: a pharmacodynamic study in patients with chronic obstructive pulmonary disease (COPD). Dutch Study Group. *Eur Respir J* 1995;**8**:1506–13.

76. Calverley PMA, Lee A, Towse L, Witek TJ, Kesten S. The effect of tiotropium bromide on the circadian variation in airflow limitation in chronic obstructive pulmonary disease. *Thorax* 2003 (submitted).

77. Wincken W, van Noord JA, Greefhorst APM, *et al.* Improved health outcomes in patients with COPD during 1 years treatment with tiotropium. *Eur Respir J* 2002;**19**:209–16.

78. Casaburi R, Mahler DA, Jones PW, *et al.* A long term evaluation of once-daily inhaled tiotropium in chronic obstructive pulmonary disease. *Eur Respir J* 2002;**19**: 217–24.

79. Rogers RM, Owens GR, Pennock BE. The pendulum swings again toward a rationale use of theophylline. *Chest* 1985;**87**:280–2.

80. Alexander MR, Dull WL, Kasik JE. Treatment of chronic obstructive pulmonary disease with orally administered theophylline. *JAMA* 1980;**244**:2286–90.

81. Jenkins PF, White JP, Jariwalla AJ, Anderson G, Campbell IA. A controlled study of slow-release theophylline and aminophylline in patients with chronic bronchitis. *Br J Dis Chest* 1982;**76**:57–60.

82. Greening AP, Baillie E, Gubben HR, Pride NB. Sustained release oral aminophylline in patients with airflow obstruction. *Thorax* 1981;**36**:303–7.

83. Chrystyn H, Mulley BA, Peake MD. Dose response relation to oral theophylline in severe chronic obstructive airways disease. *Br Med J* 1988;**297**:1506–10.

84. Evans WV. Plasma theophylline concentrations, six minute walking distances and breathlessness in patients with chronic airflow obstruction. *Br Med J* 1984;**289**:1649–51.

85. Mahler DA, Malthay RA, Snyder PE, Wells CK, Loke J. Sustained release theophylline reduces dyspnea in non-reversible obstructive airways disease. *Am Rev Respir Dis* 1985;**131**:22–5.

86. Kongragunta WR, Druz WS, Sharp JL. Dyspnea and diaphragmatic fatigue in patients with chronic obstructive pulmonary disease. *Am Rev Respir Dis* 1988;**137**:662–7.

87. Dullinger D, Kronenberg R, Niewohner DE. Efficacy of inhaled metaproterenol and orally administered theophylline in patients with chronic airflow obstruction. *Chest* 1986;**89**:171–3.

88. Guyatt GH, Townsend M, Pugsley SO, *et al.* Bronchodilators in chronic airflow limitation. Effects on airway function, exercise capacity and quality of life. *Am Rev Respir Dis* 1987;**135**:1069–74.

89. McKay SE, Howie CA, Thomson AH, Whiting B, Addis GJ. Value of theophylline treatment in patients handicapped by chronic obstructive lung disease. *Thorax* 1993;**48**:227–32.

90. Leitch AG, Morgan A, Ellis DA, Bell G, Haslett C, McHardy GJR. Effect of oral salbutamol and slow-release theophylline on exercise tolerance in chronic bronchitis. *Thorax* 1981; **36**:787–.

91. Aubier M. Pharmacology of respiratory muscles. *Clin Chest Med* 1988;**9**:311–14.

92. Murciano D, Auclair M-H, Pariente R, Aubier M. A randomized, controlled trial of theophylline in patients with severe chronic obstructive pulmonary disease. *N Engl J Med* 1989;**320**:1521–5.

93. Jenne JW, Siever JR, Druz WS, Solano JV, Cohen SM, Sharp JT. The effect of maintenance theophylline therapy on lung work in severe chronic obstructive pulmonary disease while standing and walking. *Am Rev Respir Dis* 1984;**130**: 600–5.

94. Lefcoe NM, Toogood JH, Blenner Lassett G, Baskerville J, Patterson NAM. The addition of an aerosol anticholinergic to an oral beta agonist plus theophylline in asthma and bronchitis. *Chest* 1982;**82**:300–5.

95. Chapman KR. The role of anticholinergic bronchodilators in adult asthma and COPD. *Lung* 1990;**168**(suppl):295–303.

96. van Schayck CP, Folgering H, Harbers H, Maas KL, van Weel C. Effects of allergy and age on responses to salbutamol and ipratropium bromide in moderate asthma and chronic bronchitis. *Thorax* 1991;**46**:355–9.

97. Nishimura K, Koyama H, Ikeda A, Sugiura N, Kawakatsu K, Izumi T. The additive effect of theophylline on a high-dose combination of inhaled salbutamol and ipratropium bromide in stable COPD. *Chest* 1995;**107**:718–23.

98. Taylor DR, Buick B, Kinney C, Lowry RC, McDevitt DG. The efficacy of orally administered theophylline, inhaled salbutamol, and a combination of the two as chronic therapy in the management of chronic bronchitis and reversible airflow obstruction. *Am Rev Respir Dis* 1985; **131**:747–51.

99. Filuk RB, Easton PA, Anthonisen NR. Responses to large doses of salbutamol and theophylline in patients with chronic obstructive pulmonary disease. *Am Rev Respir Dis* 1985;**132**:871–4.

100. Van Noord JA, de Munck DR, Bantje TA, Hop WC, Akveld ML, Bommer AM. Long-term treatment of chronic obstructive pulmonary disease with salmeterol and the additive effect of ipratropium. *Eur Respir J* 2000;**15**:878–85.

101. Zuwallack RL, Mahler DA, Reilly D, *et al.* Salmeterol plus theophylline combination therapy in the treatment of COPD. *Chest* 2001;**119**:1661–70.

102. Cazzola M, Di Lorenzo G, Di Perna F, Calderaro F, Testi R, Centanni S. Additive effects of salmeterol and fluticasone or theophylline in COPD. *Chest* 2000;**118**:1576–81.

103. Hanania NA, Ramsdell J, Payne K, *et al.* Improvements in airflow and dyspnea in COPD patients following 26 weeks treatment with salmeterol 50 μg and fluticasone propionate 250 μg alone or in combination. *Am J Respir Crit Care Med* 2001;**163**:A279

104. Calverley PMA, Pauwels R, Vestbo J, *et al.* Combining salmeterol and fluticasone in the treatment of chronic obstructive pulmonary disease. *Lancet* 2003;**361**: 449–56.

105. Conradson TB, Eklundh G, Olofsson B, *et al.* Cardiac arrhythmias in patients with mild to moderate obstructive lung disease. *Chest* 1985;**88**:537–42.

106. Conradson TB, Eklundh G, Olofsson B, *et al.* Arrhythmogenicity from combined bronchodilator therapy in patients with obstructive lung disease and concomitant ischaemic heart disease. *Chest* 1987;**91**:5–9.

107. Lipworth BJ, McDevitt DG, Strathers AD. Electrocardiographic changes induced by inhaled salbutamol after treatment with bendrofluazide:effects of replacement therapy with potassium, magnesium and triamterene. *Clin Sci* 1990; **78**:255–9.

108. Patel KR, Tullett WM. Bronchoconstriction in response to ipratropium bromide. *Br Med J* 1983;**286**:1318.

109. Pavia D, Bateman JRM, Sheahan NF, Clarke SW. Effect of ipratropium bromide on mucociliary clearance and pulmonary function in reversible airways obstruction. *Thorax* 1979;**34**:501–7.

110. Sessler CN. Theophylline toxicity : clinical features of 116 consecutive cases. *Am J Med* 1990;**88**:567–76.

111. Levine JH, Michael JR, Guarnieri T. Multifocal atrial tachycardia: a toxic effect of theophylline. *Lancet* 1985;**i**:12–14.

112. Bowton DL, Alford PT, McLees BD, Prough DS, Stump DA. The effects of aminophylline on cerebral blood flow in patients with chronic obstructive pulmonary disease. *Chest* 1987;**91**:874–7.

113. Nishimura N, Suzuki A, Yoshioka A, *et al.* Effect of aminophylline on brain tissue oxygen tension in patients with chronic obstructive lung disease. *Thorax* 1992;**47**: 1025–9.

114. Swaminathan S, Paton JY, Davidson-Ward SL, Sargent CW, Keens TG. Theophylline does not increase ventilatory

responses to hypercapnia or hypoxia. *Am Rev Respir Dis* 1992;**146**:1398–401.

115. Miller CA, Shisher LB, Vesell ES. Polymorphism of theophylline metabolism in man. *J Clin Invest* 1985; **75**:1415–25.

116. Randolph WC, Seaman JJ, Dickson B, *et al.* The effect of age on theophylline clearance in normal subjects. *Br J Clin Pharmacol* 1986;**22**:603–5.

117. Weinberger M, Hendeles L. Slow-release theophylline: rationale and basis for product selection. *N Engl J Med* 1983;**308**:760–4.

118. Hendeles L, Weinberger M, Milavetz G, *et al.* Food-induced 'dose dumping' from a once-a-day theophylline product as a cause of theophylline toxicity. *Chest* 1985;**87**:758–65.

119. Rand CS, Wise RA, Nides M, *et al.* Metered-dose inhaler adherance in a clinical trial. *Am Rev Respir Dis* 1992; **146**:1559–64.

120. Burge PS, Calverley PM, Jones PW, Spencer S, Anderson JA, Maslen TK. Randomised, double blind, placebo controlled study of fluticasone propionate in patients with moderate to severe chronic obstructive pulmonary disease:the ISOLDE trial. *Br Med J* 2000;**320**:1297–303.

121. Crompton GK. Problems patients have using pressurised aerosol inhalers. *Eur J Respir Dis* 1982;**63**(suppl 119):101–4.

122. Newman SP, Pavia D, Moren F, Sheahan NF, Clarke SW. Deposition of pressurized aerosols in the human respiratory tract. *Thorax* 1981;**36**:52–5.

123. Dolovich MB, Ruffig RE, Roberts R, Newhouse MT. Optimal delivery of aerosols from metered-dose inhalers. *Chest* 1981;**80**(suppl):911–15.

124. Brown PH, Greening AP, Crompton GK. Large volume spacer devices and the influence of high dose beclomethasone dipropionate on hypothalamo–pituitary–adrenal axis function. *Thorax* 1993;**48**:233–8.

125. Godden DJ, Crompton GK. An objective assessment of the tube spacer in patients unable to use a conventional pressurized aerosol effectively. *Br J Dis Chest* 1981;**75**: 165–8.

126. Pavia D, Thomson ML, Clarke SW, Shannon HS. Effect of lung function and mode of inhalation on penetration of aerosol into the human lung. *Thorax* 1977;**32**:194–7.

127. Editorial. The nebuliser epidemic. *Lancet* 1984;**ii**:789–90.

128. Intermittent Positive Pressure Breathing Trial Group. Intermittent positive pressure breathing therapy of chronic obstructive pulmonary disease: a clinical trial. *Ann Intern Med* 1983;**99**:612–20.

129. Petrof BJ, Calderini E, Gottfried SB. Effect of CPAP on respiratory effort and dyspnoea during exercise in severe COPD. *J Appl Physiol* 1990;**69**:179–88.

130. O'Driscoll BR, Kay EA, Taylor RJ, Weatherby H, Chetty MCP, Bernstein A. A long-term prospective assessment of home nebulizer treatment. *Respir Med* 1992;**86**:317–25.

131. Spence DP, Graham DR, Ahmed J, Rees K, Pearson MG, Calverley PM. Does cold air affect exercise capacity and dyspnea in stable chronic obstructive pulmonary disease? *Chest* 1993;**103**:693–6.

132. O'Driscoll BR, Pearson MG, Muers MF. Nebulizers in severe stable chronic obstructive pulmonary disease. *Eur Respir Rev* 2001;**10**:516–22.

133. Hosker HS, Teale C, Greenstone MA, Muers MF. Assessment and provision of home nebulizers for chronic obstructive pulmonary disease (COPD) in the Yorkshire region of the UK. *Respir Med* 1995;**89**:47–52.

134. Teale CMF. Reversibility tests in chronic obstructive airways disease: their predictive value with reference to benefit from domiciliary nebuliser therapy. *Respir Med* 1991;**85**:281–4.

135. Pauwels RA, Buist AS, Calverley PMA, Jenkins CR, Hurd SS. Global strategy for the diagnosis, management and prevention of chronic obstructive pulmonary disease. *Am J Respir Crit Care Med* 2001;**163**:1256–76.

136. American Thoracic Society. Standard for the diagnosis and care of patients with chronic obstructive pulmonary disease and asthma. *Am Rev Respir Dis* 2001;**136**:225–44.

137. *British National Formulary*, 41. British Medical Association/ Royal Pharmaceutical Society of Great Britain, 2001.

138. Boe J, Dennis JH, O'Driscoll BR. European Respiratory Society Nebuliser Guidelines: clinical aspects. *Eur Respir Rev* 2000;**10**:516–22.

25

Anti-inflammatory therapy

PETER MA CALVERLEY AND DIRKJE S POSTMA

Since COPD is now defined, in part, by the presence of persistent inflammatory changes within the lung,[1] it is no surprise that suppression or elimination of these changes has been extensively studied. Any therapy, which leads to the removal of or reduction in exposure to a pro-inflammatory stimulus, could be considered to be an 'anti-inflammatory'. Thus smoking cessation, however induced, would meet this criterion although inflammation does persist even when this is done, at least in COPD patients with established physiological abnormalities.[2] In practice, most attention has focused on the suppression of chronic inflammation and whether corticosteroids administered either orally or by inhalation can achieve this.

The reasons for this are threefold. Firstly, these drugs have proven to be outstandingly successful in improving symptoms, lung function and patient well being in bronchial asthma,[3] the prototype of airway inflammatory disorders. Secondly, empirical studies over the last 40 years have noted that some patients who were thought to have COPD nonetheless showed surprisingly large improvements in lung function, usually after treatment with oral corticosteroids.[4] Moreover, two retrospective studies have shown that oral corticosteroids, at least in a dose of 7.5 mg per day or higher, reduced lung function decline in COPD patients with little reversibility of airflow limitation.[5,6] When oral corticosteroids were withdrawn due to substantial side effects, lung function deteriorated again.[6] This suggested that studies with corticosteroids with less side effects were needed to determine whether anti-inflammatory treatment could abate the relentless progression of the disease. Finally, these

agents have been widely used by chest physicians who are very familiar with their side effect profile. Although these effects are significant, especially during long-term use[7] they are believed to be more acceptable than those of immunosuppressive agents like cyclophosphamide or aziothioprine used in other pulmonary inflammatory disorders. This proposition, both with regards to effectiveness and tolerability, has yet to be tested in COPD.

The bulk of this chapter addresses the role of corticosteroids and especially inhaled corticosteroids in the management of stable COPD. The use of corticosteroids as a diagnostic tool to identify subtypes of COPD is considered in Chapter 20. A substantial body of data is now available on which to base treatment recommendations, and some conflicting data about the effects of corticosteroids in experimental situations has been published more recently. It is worth remembering that most studies of corticosteroids and COPD were designed and executed before experimental data evaluating their anti-inflammatory action in COPD were available which may explain the disappointing findings in a number of clinical trials.

RELEVANT PHARMACOLOGIC CONSIDERATIONS

The glucocorticosteroids used therapeutically are synthetic compounds based on the naturally occurring cortisone molecule. The most commonly used preparations are listed in Table 25.1. Oral preparations have good

Table 25.1 *Most commonly used corticosteroid preparations*

Drug	Route of administration	Daily dose	Regimen
Prednisolone	Oral	2.5–5 mg 30–40 mg daily in exacerbation	Once daily
Methylprednisone	IV	500 mg in exacerbation	6 hourly
Beclomethasone dipropionate	Inhaled – MDI, DPI	400–2000 mg	12 hourly
Budesonide	Inhaled – MDI, DPI, NEB	400–1600 mg 2000 mg in exacerbation	12 hourly
Fluticasone propionate	Inhaled – MDI, DPI	200–1000 mg	12 hourly
Triamcinolone acetonide	Inhaled – MDI, DPI	400–1200 mg	12 hourly

MDI: metered dose inhaler; DPI: dry powder inhaler; NEB: wet nebulizer.

bioavailability and a long half-life. Thus once daily dosing is sufficient to achieve a stable therapeutic effect. Inhaled preparations are usually given twice daily and similar considerations apply to their effective delivery as for bronchodilator drugs (see Chapter 24). A range of formulations is available and although triamcinolone has been given as six puffs twice daily to COPD patients,[8] the other commonly used corticosteroids require only two actuations twice a day to deliver an adequate dose. The time of onset of action varies with the end-point chosen and good studies of this phenomenon are lacking in COPD. Since anti-inflammatory therapy is usually chronic rather than acute this is not a significant drawback. Nonetheless when used in treating exacerbations of COPD where lung function is the outcome, changes in FEV_1 occur within 24 hours of the first dose[9] and possibly earlier, at least when pre-bronchodilator FEV_1 is the end-point.[10] Drug metabolism occurs in the liver and its rapidity varies with the drug used, being most complete with fluticasone propionate. However, this does not prevent some drug being available to systemic circulation since direct absorption after alveolar deposition can occur. This explains the significant short-term adrenal suppression seen with fluticasone in normal volunteers.[11] However when drug particle deposition is more central as occurs in both asthma and COPD,[12] the effect of fluticasone is proportionately less.[13,14] The main pharmacologically predictable side effects of corticosteroids are listed in Table 25.2. These are most obvious when oral corticosteroids are used either as maintenance treatment or when frequent courses are administered because of exacerbations, a common problem in severe COPD. The deleterious effects of oral corticosteroids on muscle function have now been clearly demonstrated in COPD patients. Thus higher doses of oral maintenance therapy (>4 mg per day) are associated with significant reductions in quadriceps force, increased health costs[15] and a higher mortality, a finding related to total oral corticosteroid use[16] (Figure 25.1). Using oral corticosteroids in this way in COPD patients is now no longer acceptable.[1]

Table 25.2 *Side effects of corticosteroids*

Central obesity, moon-face, 'buffalo hump'
Striae, thinning of skin
Spontaneous bruising
Glucose intolerance, diabetes mellitus
Osteoporosis
Avascular necrosis
Fluid retention
Peptic ulceration, gastrointestinal bleeding
Cataracts
Peripheral muscle myopathy
Adrenal suppression
Pharyngeal candidiasis*
Dysphonia*

*Only with inhaled form.

Selecting an appropriate dose of inhaled treatment for use in COPD remains difficult. The doses of inhaled corticosteroids conventionally used have tended towards the upper limit of the dosing range largely by extrapolating the results of retrospective data using oral corticosteroids (see below). There are limited data currently in abstract form looking at lower and higher doses of corticosteroids with and without salmeterol, which suggest that the higher doses were associated with greater symptomatic benefit. However similar studies have been conducted using modest doses of budesonide (total 800 µg per day) in more severe COPD and demonstrating reductions in exacerbations comparable to that seen with higher doses of fluticasone.[17] Thus the high doses so far studied may not always be needed.

MECHANISMS OF ACTION

Significant changes have occurred in our understanding of the mode of action of corticosteroids during the last five years. Initial assumptions that the effect of these drugs

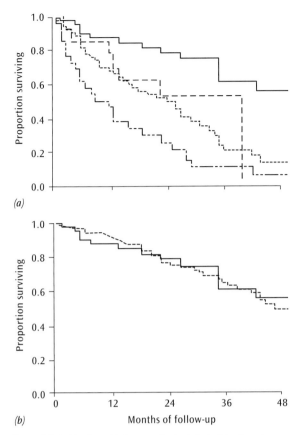

(a)

(b)

Months of follow-up

Figure 25.1 *Kaplan–Meier survival plots (a,b) of oral glucocorticoid users compared to similar patients not receiving maintenance therapy (solid line). There is a dose relationship with worse survival in those receiving 15 mg prednisolone daily (dash and dots) compared to 10 mg daily (dotted line) who are worse than the 5 mg daily group (dashed line). Survival was uninfluenced by regular inhaled corticosteroid use (in (b) dotted line is the inhaled steroid users). (From ref. 16.)*

required interaction with nuclear DNA and subsequent protein transcription have not been borne out and this helps explain why the onset of action of corticosteroids is rather more rapid than had previously been believed.

Three important steps occur.[18] Firstly, the glucocorticoid molecule combines with a soluble receptor causing it to shed the heat shock proteins, which 'chaperone' this molecule and prevent it from combining with the nucleus. Secondly, this molecular complex combines with specific areas within the DNA leading to upregulation of the number of beta-receptors and the production of lipocortin which is responsible for much of the systemic effects of these drugs. This positive action has been attributed to the 'glucocorticoid-responsive elements' within the DNA but the suppresser functions of these drugs have also been postulated to involve other more distant areas of the DNA and a nuclear sequence for this has been described. This was originally believed to be the

principal site of action for the anti-inflammatory effects of these drugs. However, there is a third step, which is increasingly recognized as being important, and which occurs before gene transcription and nuclear binding. Other transcription factors, particularly AP-1 and NF-κB, are known to be important regulators of cytokine production and their activity is increased in many inflammatory processes. There is evidence for intranuclear and cytoplasmic binding of the glucocorticoid receptor complex with these transcription factors, thereby directly reducing the production of pro-inflammatory products.

Access to the nuclear chromatin and hence to DNA transcription is regulated by the degree of coiling of the chromatin. This is in turn controlled by the extent of histone acetylation of the chromatin. When the corticosteroid receptor complex interacts with the nucleus histone deacetylase is activated, increasing the degree of DNA uncoiling and allowing the specific corticosteroid receptor to interact with the relevant nucleotides. However, this is less likely to occur in COPD patients, at least according to studies from the National Heart and Lung Institute (NHLI) in London.[19] This may explain the relative absence of anti-inflammatory effects of corticosteroids in COPD. It may also be influenced by the local oxidant– antioxidant balance, a finding supported by the clinical observation that the spirometric response to corticosteroids is smaller in patients who smoke than in those who do not.[20] These intriguing observations clearly require further study.

Experimental models of inflammation in COPD are limited by the uncertainty about which inflammatory marker best predicts future disease progression. No study has yet related phenotypic features of emphysema or directly measured airway pathology to the effects of short-term corticosteroid exposure. The resulting data using different end-points remain confusing. Thomson *et al.* treated 21 patients with COPD, mean FEV_1 50.6% predicted for 6 weeks with either beclometasone propionate or placebo and observed modest improvements in pulmonary function and a relative reduction in epithelial lining fluid albumen[21] (Figure 25.2). Llewellyn-Jones and colleagues examined sputum from 17 patients (mean FEV_1 0.71 L) with COPD before and after 8 weeks of 1.5 mg fluticasone propionate daily or placebo. They noted significant reductions in chemotactic activity and an increase in the neutrophil elastase inhibitory capacity of sputum in those patients treated with the corticosteroid.[22] Confalonieri and colleagues using induced sputum observed a fall in the total number of cells and the percentage that were neutrophils in COPD patients treated with 1.5 mg beclometasone for 2 months but not in patients randomized to control observation.[23] By contrast, a series of studies using similar methodology with patients with asthma acting as a reference group has been published from the NHLI that suggest quite a different

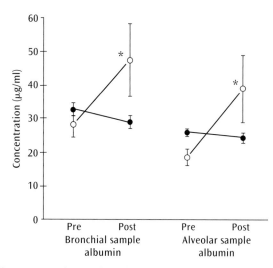

Figure 25.2 *Changes in estimated epithelial lining fluid albumen concentration after treatment with beclometasone (closed circles) or placebo (open circles). (Reproduced from ref. 21 with permission.)*

pattern. Although interleukin-8 (IL-8) and tumor necrosis factor alpha (TNF-α) were elevated in induced sputum,[24] treatment with corticosteroids did not change their levels nor did it modify the concentrations of matrix metalloproteinases.[25,26] Surprisingly there was no change in the sputum eosinophil count after corticosteroids. This differs from the findings of two other groups where the initial eosinophil count was higher and it was found that 2 weeks of treatment with corticosteroids produced a significant reduction in the number in this subset of patients.[27,28]

It is clear that no simple and consistent effect of corticosteroid therapy is present in any of these models. Worryingly, differences in experimental design, assay technique, patient selection and treatment duration contribute to these confusing data. Establishing a consensus about the most appropriate techniques to use, standardizing their measurement and confirming their robustness in different COPD populations is essential if a clear answer about the mechanism of corticosteroid action in this disease is ever to emerge. This has equally important implications in the assessment of new therapies now being developed.

One further possibility should be considered. Although corticosteroids have anti-inflammatory properties in a number of diseases, their effects are not confined to modifying the intensity of cellular inflammation. The standard method of classifying corticosteroid potency is the McKenzie skin blanching assay, a response which some have related to corticosteroid resistance in asthma.[29] Administering fluticasone to asthmatics reduces bronchial wall blood flow.[30] How persistent these effects are is not known but COPD airways treated with beclometasone appear less hyperemic than those

receiving placebo inhalations.[21] COPD patients have increased protein leakage into their airways[31] and, as noted above, this can be reduced with regular inhaled corticosteroids. Thus there are a range of 'non-inflammatory' effects of corticosteroid treatment which might produce small but physiologically important changes in airway wall thickness and hence modify the degree of pulmonary hyperinflation in more severe disease. Such an effect would certainly be more evident when baseline airway function was reduced and may prove more important in explaining the beneficial action of these drugs than changes in any of the currently reported inflammatory markers.

CORTICOSTEROIDS IN ACUTE EXACERBATIONS

Although short courses of oral corticosteroids have been used for the treatment of exacerbations of COPD for many years, clear evidence to support this practice has only been obtained recently. Albert *et al.* noted a significant increase in pre-bronchodilator FEV_1 measured over the first 6 hours of admission in patients treated with corticosteroids compared to placebo, although the post-bronchodilator FEV_1 effect was much smaller.[32] In a carefully conducted but small ($n = 17$) study of outpatients with COPD, those whose exacerbations were treated with a tapering dose of oral prednisone (total dose 360 mg) had a significantly higher FEV_1 and PaO_2 at days 3 and 10 compared with the placebo-treated patients. Although symptomatic improvement appeared to be more rapid in the active treatment group this was not statistically significant for the whole admission.[10] Two larger studies of patients admitted to hospital with exacerbations have supported these findings. Niewoehner and colleagues studied 271 patients using a treatment failure end-point (death, ventilation, readmission or treatment intensification) and found that those who received oral corticosteroids were less likely to relapse than those given placebo. However, there was no difference between 2 weeks and 2 months of this intensive treatment[33] (Figure 25.3). Post-bronchodilator FEV_1 increased more rapidly and hospital stay was shorter in the 56 patients studied by Davies *et al.*[9] (Figure 25.4). Although the change in FEV_1 was relatively modest, further analysis of the North American data showed that patients with the greatest FEV_1 improvement in the early stages of an exacerbation were less likely to relapse subsequently and confirmed the UK finding that this was more likely to be the case in the corticosteroid-treated individuals.[34] The total dose of oral corticosteroids (30 mg prednisolone daily for two weeks) in the UK study was significantly less than the cumulative doses

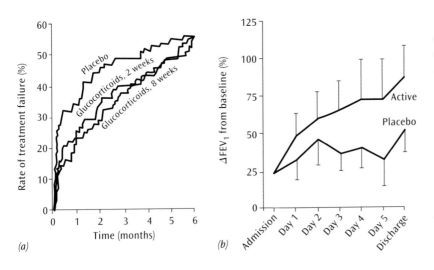

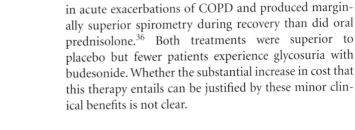

Figure 25.3 *COPD patients whose exacerbations are treated with oral corticosteroids are less likely to be treatment failures in the next 6 months of follow-up (a). This is mainly due to acute treatment with these drugs and can be achieved with lower doses as was seen in data in (b). In this study post-bronchodilator FEV$_1$ values improve significantly faster in patients receiving 30 mg oral prednisolone for 10 days than those getting placebo. ((a) Reproduced from ref. 34; (b) from ref. 9 with permission.)*

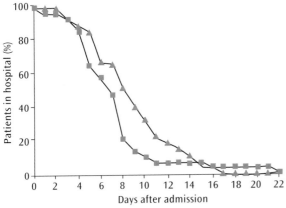

Figure 25.4 *Time to discharge from hospital is significantly shorter in patients treated with oral corticosteroids for their non-acidotic exacerbation of COPD. Treated patients: squares; placebo: triangles. (Reproduced from ref. 9 with permission.)*

in acute exacerbations of COPD and produced marginally superior spirometry during recovery than did oral prednisolone.[36] Both treatments were superior to placebo but fewer patients experience glycosuria with budesonide. Whether the substantial increase in cost that this therapy entails can be justified by these minor clinical benefits is not clear.

INHALED CORTICOSTEROIDS IN STABLE DISEASE

Given the unfavorable side effect profile of oral corticosteroids it is not surprising that attention has turned to the role of inhaled corticosteroids in chronic disease management. Retrospective studies of oral corticosteroids in COPD patients in general[37] and in those without clinical evidence of allergy[6] suggested that patients who received 10 mg or more of prednisolone daily showed significant FEV$_1$ improvement over time. Changes in FEV$_1$ took 6–24 months to appear, unlike the situation in bronchial asthma. Data of this type are essentially observational but it would be an oversimplification to suggest that any benefit that occurred was entirely due to a population of undiagnosed asthmatics, as is sometimes suggested.[38] This form of circular logic is unhelpful as it implies that any patient with COPD who shows improvement in lung function after treatment must actually have had asthma since COPD cannot be treated!

In normal clinical practice a group of patients exist who show improvement in FEV$_1$ after short-term treatment with oral corticosteroids[4,39] (Figure 25.5(a)). This effect is more evident in patients with a lower FEV$_1$[40] and these are the patients who are most likely to improve with inhaled corticosteroids during the next year of treatment[41] (Figure 25.5(b)). However, not all patients initially classified as responders to oral corticosteroids

used in the North American trial, but there was no clear difference in the magnitude of benefit. Whether it is the dose or duration of treatment that produces these effects remains unclear. An underpowered Turkish study has suggested that the benefits are greater if corticosteroids are given for 10 rather than 3 days;[35] larger trials will be needed to confirm this. Six of the UK patients developed transient glycosuria while hyperglycemia sufficient to require therapy was seen in 15% of glucocorticoid-treated patients. There is clearly a risk from repeated therapy with oral corticosteroids as noted above. Nonetheless, this is likely to remain the standard approach to treating more severe exacerbations, as increasing the dose of inhaled corticosteroids has not yet been shown to improve exacerbation control.

The role of nebulized corticosteroids has remained contentious but a large Canadian study has shown that high doses of nebulized budesonide were well tolerated

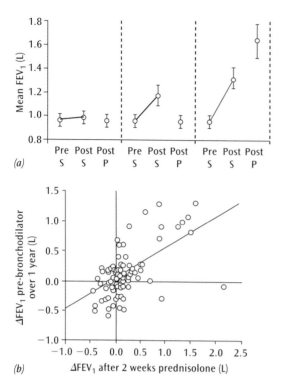

(a)

(b)

Figure 25.5 *Panel (a): In a population of stable patients with moderate to severe COPD defined spirometrically approximately 20% will show a 'significant' increase in FEV$_1$ after 2 weeks treatment with 30 mg oral prednisolone. Panel (b): Over the next year approximately half of these 'responder' patients will show a sustained improvement in FEV$_1$ when treated with inhaled corticosteroids (b), a finding not seen in those without such a large initial spirometric response. None of these patients had clinical, physiological or immunologic features suggestive of bronchial asthma. S: salbutamol; P: prednisolone. (Data from: (a) ref. 39; (b) ref. 41.)*

benefit spirometrically during follow-up. This is most obvious when the change in FEV$_1$ lies within the day-to-day reproducibility of the measurement, i.e. approximately 200 ml.[42] Those patients with a relatively large spirometric response after corticosteroids are more likely to show significant short-term increase in FEV$_1$ after an inhaled bronchodilator.[39] However, their identification is important practically, whatever the nomenclature adopted for their apparent 'reversibility'.

To avoid confusion with any coexisting 'asthmatic element' or 'overlap syndrome' recent treatment trials have gone to considerable lengths to exclude those patients with more labile airflow limitation who were included in earlier studies. Some regulatory groups now believe that COPD is defined by the absence of any significant improvement in FEV$_1$ after an inhaled bronchodilator, a feature not included in any current disease

definition. Nonetheless, it is this group of patients who form the core of subsequent investigations and who might be expected to show least spirometric benefit from treatment.

SHORT-TERM TREATMENT WITHIN INHALED CORTICOSTEROIDS

Between 1989 and 1992, seven studies of short-term (2–12 weeks) treatment of either beclomethasone or budesonide in doses of 800–600 μg per day were reported. They spanned a wide range of FEV$_1$ (mean values 97–44% predicted) and all together 238 patients were studied. In only two studies comprising 40 patients[21,43] did FEV$_1$ improve significantly (10 and 7.5% baseline respectively). This limited short-term responsiveness helps explain why brief periods of corticosteroid treatment, whether given orally or by inhalation, relate so poorly to subsequent disease progression.[20] Moreover emphasis on spirometric end-points may not be the best way of judging the effectiveness of anti-inflammatory treatment in this group of patients. However, studies investigating the effect on airway hyperresponsiveness, a COPD phenotype that is related to subsequent lung function decline,[44] also do not show an improvement with inhaled steroids. This is true both for direct measures of airways hyperresponsiveness[45] and for indirect challenges, for example adenosine-5-monophosphate.[46]

There have now been several long-term randomized, placebo-controlled studies published[8,14,47–54] assessing the long-term effect of inhaled corticosteroids in COPD. Tables 25.3–25.5 show the clinical characteristics of the patients included and the doses and types of inhaled corticosteroids used in the particular studies. The first studies were either in small groups of patients[47–49] or had a relatively short duration of observation.[50,51]

The relatively short-term studies with 6 months of follow-up obtained conflicting results.[50,51] The Canadian data did not show an effect of 800 μg of inhaled budesonide in 40 patients who did not respond to 2 weeks treatment with oral prednisone, when effects were compared with those 40 COPD patients who received placebo.[51] Assessments of other outcome parameters – including daily symptoms, exercise capacity and quality of life – led to the same conclusion. There were many dropouts making the power of the study too small to provide sufficient evidence that there was no effect. Numbers of withdrawals and reasons for withdrawal were comparable in both treatment arms. However, these data are compatible with the Copenhagen City Study,[53] in which individuals were included who did not respond to oral corticosteroids (to exclude asthmatics as far as possible). In this study also no significant effect on lung

Table 25.3 *Overview of results on inhaled corticosteroids in COPD*

	Study					
	Copen[53]	Euro[54]	Isolde[14]	Renk[49]	Gruns[52]	LHS[8]
Symptoms	−	−	+	+	nt	+
Exacerbations	−	−	+	−	−	+
FEV$_1$ 3–6 months	−	+	+	−	+	+?
FEV$_1$ years	−	−	−	−	high dose	−
PC$_{20}$	nt	nt	−	−	nt	+
QoL	nt	nt	+	nt	nt	+

nt: not tested; +: positive treatment effect; −: negative treatment effect; PC$_{20}$: bronchial responsiveness to histamine; QoL: quality of life.

Table 25.4 *Doses of inhaled steroid used in long-term treatment (>1 year follow-up) studies in COPD*

	Copen[53]	Euro[54]	Isolde[14]	Renk[49]	Gruns[52]	LHS[8]
Dose ICS (μg) first 6 months	1200 B	800 B	1000 F Oral CS	1600 B	1500 BDP 800 BDP 1600 B	1200 T
Dose ICS (μg) rest study	800 B	800 B	1000 F	1600 B	same	1200 T

ICS: inhaled corticosteroid; B: budesonide; F: fluticasone; BDP: beclomethasone dipropionate; T: triamcinolone; CS: corticosteroids.

Table 25.5 *Clinical characteristics of participants in long-term studies (>1 year follow-up) investigating treatment with inhaled corticosteroids*

	Copen[53]	Euro[54]	Isolde[14]	Renk[49]	Gruns[52]	LHS[8]
Number	290	1277	751	58	183	1116
Age (yr)	59	52	63	56	61	56
Male (%)	60	73	63	100	80	63
Atopy (%)	?	18	25	0	?	?
Pack-years	?	39	44	25	41	?
Current smoking (%)	76	100	77	44	37	90
FEV$_1$ (pb%pred)	86	80	50	68	45	68
ΔFEV$_1$ (%pred)	8*	3	4	6	3	7

*Derived from data in the paper.
pb = post-bronchodilator.

function (FEV$_1$) was observed within the first 6 months treatment with 1200 μg budesonide.

Paggiaro *et al.*[50] compared inhaled fluticasone 500 μg twice daily with placebo in current or ex-smokers with COPD (139 patients in the placebo group and 142 in the fluticasone group). They concluded that fluticasone might be of clinical benefit to patients with COPD, since PEF, FEV$_1$ and FVC values improved significantly more with fluticasone. When analyzing individual characteristics of responders, the patients' age, sex, baseline FEV$_1$ and bronchodilator response, smoking habit and serum cortisol did not predict who would respond. An interesting observation in a subanalysis was that individuals who had COPD for more than 10 years duration had a better response than those with recent presentation of disease. Since baseline FEV$_1$ values were comparable in the two groups, either these patients perceived their airway obstruction earlier, or they had, as the authors suggest, asthma that had developed already into an irreversible state at the time they were included in the study.

One study has looked at the effect of inhaled corticosteroids in COPD patients with an established rapid decline (mean 160 ml/yr) in FEV$_1$ over 2 years follow-up without using inhaled corticosteroids.[55] At the end of the 2 years follow-up, patients served as their own controls when 800 μg of inhaled beclomethasone was instituted. After institution of beclomethasone, patients with COPD improved their pre-bronchodilator FEV$_1$ significantly by

160 ml in the first 6 months of treatment, but the FEV_1 fell by 70 ml in the next 6 months, which was not significantly different from the decline in FEV_1 during the first 2 years. This study thus suggests that the observation of Paggiaro and coworkers cannot be extended over long periods of follow-up. This initial improvement in FEV_1, followed by the 'normal' course of disease, i.e. a slow but ongoing deterioration, has been shown now in other studies as well. It is comparable with the findings in post-bronchodilator FEV_1 in the Euroscop study in smoking individuals with early disease[54] and the ISOLDE study in patients with advanced disease.[14] The results of the Lung Health Study in 1116 persons with COPD whose FEV_1 ranged from 30 to 90% predicted also suggests a trend toward improvement in the first months treatment with triamcinolone, though it was not formally tested.[8]

By contrast, a study in a small group of COPD patients (without allergy) with a 2-year double-blind follow-up did not show this initial increase in FEV_1.[43] One individual in the inhaled corticosteroid group was responsive to a course of oral corticosteroids, otherwise all 38 patients in the inhaled corticosteroid and placebo group were non-responsive. This study did not find a different slope in FEV_1 between those treated with 1600 µg budesonide daily (median value 30 ml/yr) and placebo (median value 60 ml/yr). Airway hyperresponsiveness did not change with either corticosteroid treatment. Beneficial effects in this study were limited to symptoms and withdrawal rate due to pulmonary problems.

All studies assessing the influence of inhaled steroids over a long time of follow-up overall refute the hypothesis that corticosteroids might change the course of the disease, as assessed with FEV_1. Even when some beneficial effects can be seen in the first 6 months, an observation probably due to reduction of airway wall edema, the further downhill course of FEV_1 is not reversed, or even attenuated.

Effects on exacerbations and symptoms

There are some indications that the number and/or severity of exacerbations may be reduced by inhaled corticosteroids. The number of exacerbations per patient was lower in the fluticasone group in the study of Paggiaro et al.,[50] but not significantly so ($P = 0.067$). Nevertheless significantly fewer patients in the fluticasone group had severe and moderately severe exacerbations compared with placebo treatment. Furthermore, symptom scores and walking distance improved next to the improvement in lung function. In the study of Renkema et al.,[49] five patients dropped out in the placebo group due to pulmonary problems, whereas none dropped out in the inhaled steroid group. Moreover, symptoms improved significantly more in the group treated with inhaled corticosteroids. The number of exacerbations was the same in the

years without and with inhaled corticosteroids in the Dompeling et al. study[47] (a mean of 1.8 exacerbations per year in both periods) and in the placebo and inhaled corticosteroid arm in the Renkema et al. study,[49] i.e. 1 and 2, respectively 2 and 2.5 exacerbations per year in the first and second year of follow-up. Finally, the number of exacerbations were reported not to decrease in the Euroscop study,[54] but participants hardly had an exacerbation given the mild nature of their disease. Thus differences between the patients treated with corticosteroids and those with placebo could not be expected. The ISOLDE study[14] found a significant reduction in the number of exacerbations with corticosteroid treatment in patients with severe COPD, and the LHS found a lower rate of healthcare visits in the triamcinolone-treated group (1.2 per 100 person-years vs. 2.1 per 100 person-years, $P = 0.03$).[8] Moreover, there was less dyspnea and fewer new or worsening respiratory symptoms in those treated with triamcinolone. Further data supporting an effect of inhaled corticosteroids comes from two large studies comparing one year of placebo and inhaled fluticasone (500 µg bd) or placebo and inhaled budesonide (400 µg bd).[17,56] These show clearly that exacerbation frequency is reduced by approximately 25%, a change most evident in those patients whose FEV_1 was less than 50% predicted.

Effects on quality of life (health status)

The ISOLDE study and the Lung Health Study were the first investigations to assess the long-term effects of inhaled steroids on health status. The ISOLDE study[14] showed that health status deteriorated more slowly in those receiving inhaled corticosteroids, despite the fact that lung function did not further improve after the first 6 months and even deteriorated again.[57] Possible mechanisms contributing to this change are discussed in Chapter 31. The Lung Health Study found that none of the eight quality-of-life aspects showed changes associated with treatment assignment except the score on the mental health subscale. This scale was slightly worse at 36 months in the tramcinolone group (decrease from baseline, 2.3 + 0.6 vs. 0.1 + 0.7 on a scale of 100, $P = 0.03$). These findings require further study as to which aspects of inhaled corticosteroids would induce these changes. The recent 1-year studies show similar changes in health status to that seen in the ISOLDE study, although these investigations were not long enough for rate of change of health status to be reliably calculated.

GENERAL CONSIDERATIONS

Short-term studies are disappointing with regard to response to inhaled corticosteroids in COPD, both expressed as lung function, hyperresponsiveness and symptoms. Studies with a somewhat longer time of follow-up (i.e. a half-year treatment) have provided conflicting data. However, negative results were obtained in a study evaluating non-responders to oral corticosteroids[51] and a positive response in a study that did not assess the oral corticosteroid response.[50] Follow-up for many years shows that inhaled corticosteroids may provide a beneficial effect on FEV_1 in the initial months, but if it has this beneficial effect it wanes off during longer treatment.

However, other interpretations are also possible. The beneficial effects are presented in studies including patients with and without atopy. Thus differences in results might have been explained by the presence or absence of atopy. However, atopy did not present itself as a prognostic sign for better treatment response in the Euroscop study or in the ISOLDE data. The prevalence of smokers was different in the various studies mentioned as well. This can also not fully explain a lack of response or even a better response to treatment, since there existed an initial response in the Euroscop study[54] with 100% smokers and the ISOLDE study[14] which included 48% smokers, and no response in the study of Bourbeau and coworkers[51] with 39% smokers. One explanation might be that the pack-years of smoking is an important aspect of response to inhaled corticosteroids. The Euroscop study showed that individuals with less than 36 pack-years smoking had a more extensive response to the effects of inhaled steroids on lung function decline (Figure 25.6), suggesting that there might be a non-reversible phase in the disease. Data on pack-years have not been provided in the Lung Health Study and the Copenhagen study.

However, if this was applicable to all patients with COPD, one would have anticipated that the small study of Renkema and coworkers, with a mean number of pack-years of 25 would have provided better results.

The dose of the inhaled corticosteroid might have an effect on the outcome of the studies as well. This remains a matter that is open to debate, since the studies were performed with different types of drugs, i.e. beclomethasone, budesonide, fluticasone propionate and triamcinolone. With a daily dose of 800 μg of beclomethasone or budesonide a positive initial response occurred in the study of Dompeling et al.[47] and in the Euroscop study, yet no effect in the study of Bourbeau and coworkers.[51] Moreover, the Copenhagen study and Lung Health Study, in which higher doses of corticosteroids was used, i.e. 1200 μg of budesonide and triamcinolone respectively, did not have a positive effect either.

Results might be different due to a class effect, but positive effects were found with the inhalation of fluticasone,[14,50] with budesonide[54] and with beclomethasone[47] and negative effects as well with budesonide.[3] The severity of airflow limitation cannot explain the results either since positive and negative responses have been shown in patients with advanced as well as in patients with mild airflow limitation.

FUTURE PERSPECTIVES

It would be extremely attractive to assess which factors determine the response to treatment with inhaled corticosteroids in patients with COPD. This will need a large

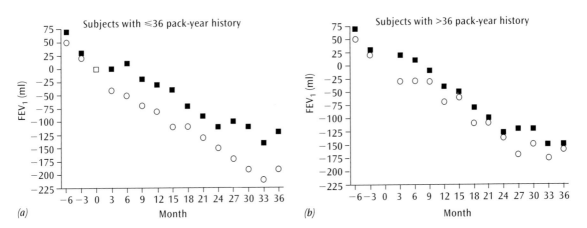

Figure 25.6 *Rate of decline of lung function over 3 years in the Euroscop trial of mild–moderate COPD patients. Data are separated into those with a smoking history below (a) or above (b) the median value of 36 pack-years. In this post hoc analysis the rate of decline of lung function was less during corticosteroid treatment in those with the lower tobacco exposure, a finding that would require further prospective study to validate. Budesonide-treated patients: squares; control subjects: circles. (From ref. 54 © 200 × Massachusetts Medical Society. All rights reserved.)*

cohort with variability in the parameters under study. So far, the Euroscop study suggested that administering inhaled steroids to COPD patients with a lower number of pack-years would reveal the beneficial effects of these drugs. However, this has not been evaluated in the other prospective large studies. The Lung Health Study reported that neither the severity of airway hyperresponsiveness, nor the severity of wheezing and presence or absence of a diagnosis of asthma, could identify any group that benefited in terms of decline in the FEV_1. Finally, one has to investigate why the spirometric response to treatment seems to be confined to the first 6 months. The effects of inhaled corticosteroids on airway wall and tissue remodeling have not been investigated in COPD so far. This is of prime interest, since this may explain the observed effects in the long-term studies. If corticosteroids first improve airway wall inflammation, but at the same time suppress airway remodeling, the positive effects of this drug may wane off with longer treatment. Therefore, focus on causes and consequences of airway and lung tissue remodeling in patients with mild to severe COPD is of great importance.

NEDOCROMIL SODIUM

One study has investigated short-term effects of inhaled nedocromil in patients with COPD.[58] Treatment with 4×8 mg nedocromil sodium for 10 weeks did not significantly change hyperresponsiveness to adenosine monophosphate, as was shown to be the case in asthmatic individuals. Moreover, it did not change lung function and symptoms. One finding is of interest, as it provides a different view on treatment with anti-inflammatory drugs. The number of study withdrawals due to exacerbations was largest in the placebo group. Again, as for other studies with inhaled corticosteroids, the data suggest that withdrawal of inhaled corticosteroids may lead to exacerbations and furthermore that institution of anti-inflammatory drugs may prevent it.

COMBINATION TREATMENT WITH BRONCHODILATOR DRUGS

The improvement in post-bronchodilator FEV_1 seen with some inhaled corticosteroids suggests a potential for synergy with inhaled corticosteroids. Experimental data have shown that corticosteroids increase the number of beta-receptors expressed on the cell surface[59] and this could translate into more potent airway smooth muscle relaxation and hence a greater improvement in lung

function. Whether this occurs in COPD is debatable, and the only currently published data[43] failed to show a statistically significant increase in bronchodilator effectiveness after treatment with inhaled beclomethasone. This was a relatively small study using a short-term inhaled bronchodilator and now larger scale investigations combining inhaled corticosteroids with the long-acting beta-agonist salmeterol have been reported. These studies involve more severe patients (mean FEV_1 36–44 predicted) who were randomly allocated to treatment with salmeterol 50 µg bd, fluticasone 500 µg bd; these doses in combination are an identical placebo in the case of the TRISTAN study[56] and 9 µg bd formoterol and/or 400 µg bd budesonide in a similar four-limb trial by Szfranski et al.[17] Over 2000 patients participated in these two trials and were followed for 12 months with similar outcome measures being used in each. In both studies statistically significant increases in FEV_1 were seen in the combination group compared with either component and in all three compared with placebo. More important clinically were the improvements in health status that only reached clinical significance in the combination therapy. In general long-acting beta-agonists improved health status more and inhaled corticosteroids had most effect on exacerbation frequency. The onset of lung function effect as assessed from daily PEF chart was seen within the first few days of treatment and was associated with less night waking and rescue therapy use. A further study from the USA has found that dyspnea assessed by the transitional dyspnea index, improves substantially in COPD patients treated for 6 months with combination therapy and this was significantly greater than the symptom change with either component.[60] Whether further benefits would occur were these treatments also combined with a long-acting inhaled anticholinergic blocker such as tiotropium remains to be determined.

NEWER ANTI-INFLAMMATORY AGENTS

However optimistically the data are viewed, corticosteroid therapy in COPD cannot be considered to be as effective as in bronchial asthma. In that disease, inhaled corticosteroids produce significant improvements in airway histology, but in COPD patients the effects are much more marginal. Changes in the pharmacokinetic properties of these drugs may reduce their propensity to produce side effects while combining them with long-acting beta-agonists may produce greater symptomatic benefit, but alternative approaches to controlling inflammation in COPD are needed.

A wide range of potential candidates are available to achieve this and these have been reviewed in detail.[61]

Most have not reached phase two clinical trials and some, like neutrophil elastase and matrix metalloproteinase inhibitors, have proven too toxic for use, at least in their current formulations. Nonetheless, several drugs are being considered for further study and have progressed to patient-based clinical trials.

Although there is no good evidence for a role of cysteinyl leukotrienes in COPD, a significant number of patients especially in the USA receive treatment with leukotriene-modifying drugs. There is a stronger theoretical case for involvement of leukotriene B_4 (LTB_4) in patients with COPD. This mediator is a potent neutrophil attractant and is present in increased concentration in the sputum of COPD patients.[62] A number of LTB_4 antagonists have been developed and are being studied in the treatment of disease exacerbations and in stable patients. It is too early as yet to confirm the effectiveness of this approach.

For many years, so-called 'mucolytic' agents have been widely used in the management of COPD especially in Central and Southern Europe. Objective assessments of conventional physiological end-points such as spirometry or exercise capacity have been disappointing but recently there has been renewed interest in the effects of these drugs in preventing exacerbations. Meta-analysis and systematic review of the available data provides a strong case that these drugs reduce the number of exacerbations of chronic bronchitis to a degree comparable to that reported with inhaled corticosteroids.[63,64] These data are heavily influenced by the large number of studies that used N-acetyl cysteine, which is more appropriately considered to be an orally active anti-oxidant (see Chapter 10). The ability of this drug to attain adequate tissue concentrations in the lung probably limits its effectiveness but a large multicenter prospective randomized study is now underway to test whether it reduces exacerbations and improves health status.[65] The development of newer antioxidant molecules remains an attractive approach to controlling pulmonary inflammation in COPD.

The most promising new anti-inflammatory agents are the PDE IV inhibitors. These drugs increase cyclic AMP in neutrophils, reduce the chemotactic activity, degranulation and adhesion of these cells and inhibit macrophage and CD8– T-lymphocytes[66] as well as promoting airway smooth muscle relaxation. This is a particularly attractive combination of properties for patients with COPD and the absence of PDE III inhibition removes the risk of the dangerous cardiac and neurologic side effects seen with oral theophyllines. The best studied compound so far is ciliomilast which produces significant increases in FEV_1, FVC and peak flow as well as a 3.9-unit improvement in total St George's Respiratory Questionnaire (SGRQ) during 6 weeks of treatment of 107 COPD patients (mean FEV_1 1.43 L).

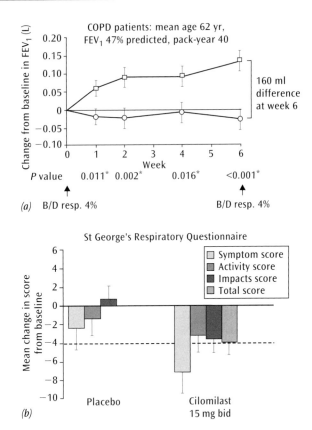

Figure 25.7 *The effect of 6 weeks' treatment with ciliomilast, a PDE IV inhibitor, on spirometry (a) and health status (b) in patients with stable COPD. The spirometric change persists after bronchodilator treatment while the health status change is mainly driven by a reduction in symptoms. ((a) * Significantly different from placebo. Placebo: open circle; ciliomilast 15 mg bid: open squares.) (Reproduced from ref. 67 with permission.)*

This was achieved without significant side effects but was only seen at the higher dose of 50 mg twice daily[67] (Figure 25.7). Nausea is reported in the early stages of treatment in a significant number of patients but seems to settle with treatment. The results of further long-term studies are awaited with interest, as are the effects of combining this drug with a long-acting beta-agonist, which should further increase the concentration of intracellular cyclic AMP.

The availability of each of these newer agents, some of which seem to have generally similar effects to existing drugs, is likely to complicate the therapeutic choices available in COPD management. It is to be hoped that drugs operating through different mechanisms will prove at least additive in their effectiveness, thereby increasing patient well being and perhaps ultimately achieving the reduction in decline in FEV_1 which remains the gold standard for the effectiveness of anti-inflammatory treatment in this condition.

REFERENCES

1. Pauwels RA, Buist AS, Calverley PMA, Jenkins CR, Hurd SS. Global strategy for the diagnosis, management and prevention of chronic obstructive pulmonary disease. *Am J Respir Crit Care Med* 2001;**163**:1256–76.

2. Turato G, Di Stefano A, Maestrelli P, *et al.* Effect of smoking cessation on airway inflammation in chronic bronchitis. *Am J Respir Crit Care Med* 1995;**152**:1262–7.

3. Barnes PJ. Efficacy of inhaled corticosteroids in asthma. *J Allergy Clin Immunol* 1998;**102**:531–8.

4. Nisar M, Earis JE, Pearson MG, Calverley PM. Acute bronchodilator trials in chronic obstructive pulmonary disease. *Am Rev Respir Dis* 1992;**146**:555–9.

5. Postma DS, Steenhuis EJ, van der Weele LT, Sluiter HJ. Severe chronic airflow obstruction: can corticosteroids slow down progression? *Eur J Respir Dis* 1985;**67**:56–64.

6. Postma DS, Peters I, Steenhuis EJ, Sluiter HJ. Moderately severe chronic airflow obstruction. Can corticosteroids slow down obstruction? *Eur Respir J* 1988;**1**:26.

7. Decramer M, Lacquet LM, Fagard R, Rogiers P. Corticosteroids contribute to muscle weakness in chronic airflow obstruction. *Am J Respir Crit Care Med* 1994;**150**:11–16.

8. The Lung Health Study Research Group. Effect of inhaled triamcinolone on the decline in pulmonary function in chronic obstructive pulmonary disease. *N Engl J Med* 2000; **343**:1902–9.

9. Davies L, Angus RM, Calverley PMA. Oral corticosteroids in patients admitted to hospital with exacerbations of chronic obstructive pulmonary disease: a prospective randomised controlled trial. *Lancet* 1999;**354**:456–60.

10. Thompson WH, Nielson CP, Carvalho P, Charan NB, Crowley, JJ. Controlled trial of oral prednisone in outpatients with acute COPD exacerbation. *Am J Respir Crit Care Med* 1996;**154**:407–12.

11. Wilson AM, Clark DJ, McFarlane L, Lipworth BJ. Adrenal suppression with high doses of inhaled fluticasone propionate and triamcinolone acetonide in healthy volunteers. *Eur J Clin Pharmacol* 1997;**53**:33–7.

12. Kim CS, Kang TC. Comparative measurement of lung deposition of inhaled fine particles in normal subjects and patients with obstructive airway disease. *Am J Respir Crit Care Med* 1997;**155**:899–905.

13. Nelson HS, Busse WW, DeBoisblanc BP, *et al.* Fluticasone propionate powder: oral corticosteroid-sparing effect and improved lung function and quality of life in patients with severe chronic asthma. *J Allergy Clin Immunol* 1999;**103**: 267–75.

14. Burge PS, Calverley PM, Jones PW, Spencer S, Anderson JA, Maslen TK. Randomised, double blind, placebo controlled study of fluticasone propionate in patients with moderate to severe chronic obstructive pulmonary disease: the ISOLDE trial. *Br Med J* 2000;**320**:1297–303.

15. Decramer M, Gosselink R, Troosters T, Verschueren M, Evers G. Muscle weakness is related to utilization of health care resources in COPD patients. *Eur Respir J* 1997;**10**:417–23.

16. Schols AM, Wesseling G, Kester AD, *et al.* Dose dependent increased mortality risk in COPD patients treated with oral glucocorticoids. *Eur Respir J* 2001;**17**:337–42.

17. Szafranski W, Cukier A, Ramirez A, *et al.* Efficacy and safety of budesonide/formoterol in the management of chronic obstructive pulmonary disease. *Eur Respir J* 2003;**21**:74–81.

18. Barnes PJ. Anti-inflammatory actions of glucocorticoids: molecular mechanisms. *Clin Sci* 1998;**94**:557–72 [review].

19. Ito K, Jazrawi E, Cosio B, Barnes PJ, Adcock IM. p65-activated histone acetyltransferase activity is repressed by glucocorticoids: mifepristone fails to recruit HDAC2 to the p65-HAT complex. *J Biol Chem* 2001;**276**:30208–15.

20. Burge PS, Calverley PMA, Jones PW, Spencer S, Anderson JA. Prednisolone response in chronic obstructive pulmonary disease. *Thorax* 2003 (in press).

21. Thompson AB, Mueller MB, Heires AJ, *et al.* Aerosolized beclomethasone in chronic bronchitis. Improved pulmonary function and diminished airway inflammation. *Am Rev Respir Dis* 1992;**146**:389–95.

22. Llewellyn-Jones CG, Harris TAJ, Stockley RA. Effect of fluticasone propionate on sputum of patients with chronic bronchitis and emphysema. *Am J Respir Crit Care Med* 1996;**153**:616–21.

23. Confalonieri M, Mainardi E, Della PR, *et al.* Inhaled corticosteroids reduce neutrophilic bronchial inflammation in patients with chronic obstructive pulmonary disease. *Thorax* 1998;**53**:583–5.

24. Keatings VM, Collins PD, Scott DM, Barnes PJ. Differences in interleukin-8 and tumor necrosis factor-alpha in induced sputum from patients with chronic obstructive pulmonary disease or asthma. *Am J Respir Crit Care Med* 1996;**153**:530–4.

25. Keatings VM, Jatakanon A, Worsdell YM, Barnes PJ. Effects of inhaled and oral glucocorticoids on inflammatory indices in asthma and COPD. *Am J Respir Crit Care Med* 1997;**155**:542–8.

26. Culpitt SV, Maziak W, Loukidis S, *et al.* Effect of high dose inhaled steroid on cells, cytokines, and proteases in induced sputum in chronic obstructive pulmonary disease. *Am J Respir Crit Care Med* 1999;**160**:1635–9.

27. Pizzichini E, Pizzichini MMM, Gibson P, *et al.* Sputum eosinophilia predicts benefit from prednisone in smokers with chronic obstructive bronchitis. *Am J Respir Crit Care Med* 1998; **158**:1511–17.

28. Brightling CE, Monteiro W, Ward R, *et al.* Sputum eosinophilia and short-term response to prednisolone in chronic obstructive pulmonary disease: a randomised controlled trial. *Lancet* 2000;**356**:1480–5.

29. Brown PH, Teelucksingh S, Matusiewicz SP, Greening AP, Crompton GK, Edwards CRW. Cutaneous vasoconstrictor response to glucocorticoids in asthma. *Lancet* 1991;**337**:576–80.

30. Kumar SD, Brieva JL, Danta I, Wanner A. Transient effect of inhaled fluticasone on airway mucosal blood flow in subjects with and without asthma. *Am J Respir Crit Care Med* 2000;**161**:918–21.

31. Hill AT, Bayley D, Stockley RA. The interrelationship of sputum inflammatory markers in patients with chronic bronchitis. *Am J Respir Crit Care Med* 1999;**160**:893–8.

32. Albert RK, Martin TR, Lewis SW. Controlled clinical trial of methylprednisolone in patients with chronic bronchitis and acute respiratory insufficiency. *Ann Intern Med* 1980;**92**:753–8.

33. Niewoehner DE, Erbland ML, Deupree RH, *et al.* Effect of systemic glucocorticoids on exacerbations of chronic obstructive pulmonary disease. *N Engl J Med* 1999;**340**:1941–7.

34. Niewoehner DE, Collins D, Erbland ML. Relation of FEV to clinical outcomes during exacerbations of chronic obstructive pulmonary disease. Department of Veterans Affairs Cooperative Study Group. *Am J Respir Crit Care Med* 2000;**161**:1201–5.

35. Sayiner A, Aytemur ZA, Cirit M, Unsal I. Systemic glucocorticoids in severe exacerbations of COPD. *Chest* 2001;**119**:726–30.

36. Maltais F, Ostinelli J, Bourbeau J, *et al.* Comparison of nebulized budesonide and oral prednisolone with placebo in the treatment of acute exacerbations of chronic obstructive pulmonary disease: a randomized controlled trial. *Am J Respir Crit Care Med* 2002;**165**:698–703.

37. Postma DS, Kerstjens HA. Are inhaled glucocorticosteroids effective in chronic obstructive pulmonary disease? *Am J Respir Crit Care Med* 1999;**160**:S66–71.

38. Barnes PJ. Inhaled corticosteroids are not beneficial in chronic obstructive pulmonary disease. *Am J Respir Crit Care Med* 2000;**161**:342–4.

39. Nisar M, Walshaw M, Earis JE, Pearson MG, Calverley PM. Assessment of reversibility of airway obstruction in patients with chronic obstructive airways disease. *Thorax* 1990;**45**:190–4.

40. Eliasson O, Hoffman J, Trueb D, Frederick D, McCormick JR. Corticosteroids in COPD. A clinical trial and reassessment of the literature. *Chest* 1986;**89**:484–90.

41. Davies L, Nisar M, Pearson MG, Costello RW, Earis JE, Calverley PMA. Oral corticosteroid trials in the management of stable chronic obstructive pulmonary disease. *Q J Med* 1999;**92**:395–400.

42. Tweeddale PM, Alexander F, McHardy GJ. Short term variability in FEV_1 and bronchodilator responsiveness in patients with obstructive ventilatory defects. *Thorax* 1987;**42**:487–90.

43. Wempe JB, Postma DS, Breederveld N, Kort E, van der Mark TW, Koeter GH. Effects of corticosteroids on bronchodilator action in chronic obstructive lung disease. *Thorax* 1992;**47**:616–21.

44. Hospers JJ, Postma DS, Rijcken B, Weiss ST, Schouten JP. Histamine airway hyper-responsiveness and mortality in chronic obstructive pulmonary disease. *Lancet* 2000;**356**:1313–17.

45. Auffarth B, Postma DS, de Monchy JG, van der Mark TW, Boorsma M, Koeter GH. Effects of inhaled budesonide on spirometric values, reversibility, airway responsiveness, and cough threshold in smokers with chronic obstructive lung disease. *Thorax* 1991;**46**:372–7.

46. Rutgers SR, Koeter GH, van der Mark TW, Postma DS. Short-term treatment with budesonide does not improve hyperresponsiveness to adenosine 5'-monophosphate in COPD. *Am J Respir Crit Care Med* 1998;**157**:880–6.

47. Dompeling E, Van Schayck CP, Molema J, Folgering H, Van Grunsven PM, Van Weel C. Inhaled beclomethasone improves the course of asthma and COPD. *Eur Respir J* 1992;**5**:945–52.

48. Van Schayck CP, Dompeling E, Van Herwaarden CL, *et al.* Bronchodilator treatment in moderate asthma or chronic bronchitis:continuous or on demand? A randomised controlled study. *Br Med J* 1991;**303**:1426–31.

49. Renkema TE, Schouten JP, Koeter GH, Postma DS. Effects of long-term treatment with corticosteroids in COPD. *Chest* 1996;**109**:1156–62.

50. Paggiaro PL, Dahle R, Bakran I, Frith L, Hollingworth K, Efthimiou J. Multicentre randomised placebo-controlled trial of inhaled fluticasone propionate in patients with chronic obstructive pulmonary disease. International COPD Study Group. *Lancet* 1998;**351**:773–80 (published erratum appears in *Lancet* 1998;**351**:1968).

51. Bourbeau J, Rouleau MY, Boucher S. Randomised controlled trial of inhaled corticosteroids in patients with chronic obstructive pulmonary disease. *Thorax* 1998;**53**:477–82.

52. Van Grunsven PM, Van Schayck CP, Derenne JP, *et al.* Long term effects of inhaled corticosteroids in chronic obstructive pulmonary disease: a meta-analysis. *Thorax* 1999;**54**:7–14.

53. Vestbo J, Sorensen T, Lange P, Brix A, Torre P, Viskum K. Long-term effect of inhaled budesonide in mild and moderate chronic obstructive pulmonary disease: a randomised controlled trial. *Lancet* 1999;**353**:1819–23.

54. Pauwels RA, Lofdahl C-G, Laitinen LA, *et al.* Long-term treatment with inhaled budesonide in persons with mild chronic obstructive pulmonary disease who continue smoking. *N Engl J Med* 1999;**340**:1948–53.

55. Dompeling E, Van Schayck CP, Van Grunsven PM, *et al.* Slowing the deterioration of asthma and chronic obstructive pulmonary disease observed during bronchodilator therapy by adding inhaled corticosteroids. A 4-year prospective study. *Ann Intern Med* 1993;**118**:770–8.

56. Calverley P, Pauwels R, Vestbo J, *et al.* Combined salmeterol and fluticasone in the treatment of chronic obstructive pulmonary disease: a randomised controlled trial. *Lancet* 2003;**361**:449–56.

57. Spencer S, Calverley PMA, Burge PS, Jones PW. Health status deterioration in patients with chronic obstructive pulmonary disease. *Am J Respir Crit Care Med* 1901;**163**:122–8.

58. De Jong PW, Postma DS, van der Mark TW, Koeter GH. Effect of nedocromil sodium in the treatment of non-allergic subjects with chronic obstructive pulmonary disease. *Thorax* 1994;**49**:1022–4.

59. Holgate ST, Baldwin CJ, Tatterfield AE. Beta-adrenergic agonist resistance in normal human airways. *Lancet* 1977;**ii**:375–6.

60. Mahler DA, Wire P, Horstmann D, *et al.* Effectiveness of fluticasone propionate and salmeterol combination delivered via the Diskus device in the treatment of chronic obstructive pulmonary disease. *Am J Respir Crit Care Med* 2002;**166**:1084–91.

61. Barnes PJ. Novel approaches and targets for treatment of chronic obstructive pulmonary disease. *Am J Respir Crit Care Med* 1999;**160**:S72–9.

62. Gompertz S, O'Brien C, Bayley DL, Hill SL, Stockley RA. Changes in bronchial inflammation during acute exacerbations of chronic bronchitis. *Eur Respir J* 2001;**17**:1112–19.

63. Poole PJ, Black PN. Mucolytic agents for chronic bronchitis or chronic obstructive pulmonary disease. *Cochrane Database System Rev* 2000;CD001287.

64. Poole P, Black P. Oral mucolytic drugs for exacerbations of chronic obstructive pulmonary disease: systematic review. *Br Med J* 2001;**322**:1271.

65. Decramer M, Dekhuijzen PN, Troosters T, *et al.* The Bronchitis Randomized On NAC Cost–Utility Study (BRONCUS): hypothesis and design. BRONCUS-trial Committee. *Eur Respir J* 2001;**17**:329–36.

66. Torphy TJ. Phosphodiesterase isozymes: molecular targets for novel antiasthma agents. *Am J Respir Crit Care Med* 1998;**157**:351–70.

67. Compton CH, Gubb J, Nieman R, *et al.* Cilomilast, a selective phosphodiesterase-4 inhibitor for treatment of patients with chronic obstructive pulmonary disease: a randomised, dose-ranging study. *Lancet* 2001;**358**:265–70.

26

Exacerbations

JADWIGA A WEDZICHA

INTRODUCTION

There is now considerable interest in the causes of and mechanisms underlying exacerbations of COPD as they are now recognized to be an important cause of the considerable morbidity and mortality found in COPD.[1] Some patients are prone to frequent exacerbations that are an important cause of hospital admission and readmission and these frequent episides may have considerable impact on quality of life and activities of daily living.[2] COPD exacerbations are also associated with considerable physiologic deterioration and increased airway inflammatory changes[3] that are caused by a variety of factors such as viruses, bacteria and common pollutants (Figure 26.1). COPD exacerbations are commoner in the winter months and there may be important interactions between cold temperatures and exacerbations caused by viruses or pollutants.[4]

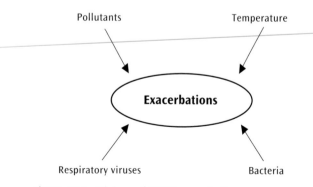

Figure 26.1 *Etiology of COPD exacerbations.*

DEFINITION OF A COPD EXACERBATION

Although there is no standardized definition of a COPD exacerbation, an exacerbation is often described as an acute worsening of respiratory symptoms. However some symptoms are more important in the description of an exacerbation than others and Anthonisen and colleagues some years ago defined exacerbations as Type 1 if they had all the major symptoms of increased dyspnea, sputum volume and sputum purulence, Type 2 exacerbations with two of the above symptoms and Type 3 when one of the symptoms was combined with cough, wheeze or symptoms of an upper respiratory tract infection.[5] Definitions based on symptoms have been used in other studies, though this definition depends on careful monitoring and changes in daily symptoms.[2-4] However definitions of exacerbations have also been proposed based on healthcare utilization, for example unscheduled physician visits, changes or increases in medication, use of oral steroids at exacerbation and hospital admission, or using the combination of worsening of symptoms and healthcare utilization.[6] However healthcare utilization in COPD varies from country to country and thus there may be considerable difficulty standardizing such a definition. Many exacerbations are not reported to healthcare professionals and this would bias any definition based on access to health care.[2]

EPIDEMIOLOGY OF COPD EXACERBATIONS

Earlier descriptions of COPD exacerbations have concentrated mainly on studies of hospital admission, although

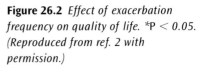

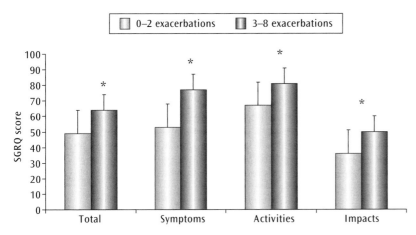

Figure 26.2 *Effect of exacerbation frequency on quality of life. *P < 0.05. (Reproduced from ref. 2 with permission.)*

most COPD exacerbations are treated in the community and not associated with hospital admission. A cohort of moderate to severe COPD patients, followed in East London, UK (East London COPD Study) with daily diary cards and peak flow readings, were asked to report exacerbations as soon as possible after symptomatic onset.[2] The diagnosis of COPD exacerbation was based on criteria modified from those described by Anthonisen and colleagues[5] that require two symptoms for diagnosis, one of which must be a major symptom of increased dyspnea, sputum volume or sputum purulence. Minor exacerbation symptoms included cough, wheeze, sore throat, nasal discharge or fever. The study found that about 50% of exacerbations were unreported to the research team, despite considerable encouragement to do so and were only diagnosed from diary cards.[2] Patients with COPD are accustomed to frequent symptom changes and this may explain their tendency to under report exacerbations to physicians. These patients have high levels of anxiety and depression and may accept their situation.[7,8] The tendency of patients to under report exacerbations may explain the higher total rate of exacerbation in this study at 2.7 per patient per year, which is higher than previously reported by Anthonisen and coworkers at 1.1 per patient per year.[5] However in the latter study, exacerbations were diagnosed from patients' recall of symptoms and daily monitoring of symptoms to detect exacerbation was not carried out.

Using the median number of exacerbations as a cut-off point, COPD patients in the East London Study were classified as frequent and infrequent exacerbators. Quality of life scores measured using a validated disease specific scale – the St George's Respiratory Questionnaire (SGRQ) – was significantly worse in all of its three component scores (symptoms, activities and impacts) in the frequent compared to the infrequent exacerbators (Figure 26.2). This suggests that exacerbation frequency is an important determinant of health status in COPD and is thus one of the important outcome measures in COPD. Factors

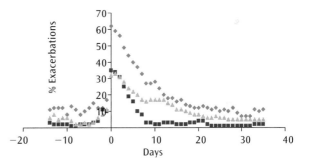

Figure 26.3 *Time course of a COPD exacerbation. Days −7 to −1, p < 0.05. Filled diamond: SOB; filled square: colds; filled triangle: cough. (Reproduced from ref. 10 with permission.)*

predictive of frequent exacerbations included daily cough and sputum and frequent exacerbations in the previous year. A previous study of acute infective exacerbations of chronic bronchitis found that one of the factors predicting exacerbation was also the number of exacerbations in the previous year,[9] though this study was limited to exacerbations presenting with purulent sputum and no physiologic data was available during the study.

In a further prospective analysis of 504 exacerbations, where daily monitoring was performed, there was some deterioration in symptoms, though no significant peak flow changes.[10] Falls in peak flow and FEV_1 at exacerbation were generally small and not useful in predicting exacerbations, but larger falls in peak flow were associated with symptoms of dyspnea, presence of colds and related to longer recovery time from exacerbations (Figure 26.3). Symptoms of dyspnea, common colds, sore throat and cough increased significantly during the prodromal phase suggesting that respiratory viruses may be important triggers of exacerbations. The median time to recovery of peak flow was 6 days and 7 days for symptoms, but at 35 days peak flow had returned to normal in only 75% of exacerbations, while at 91 days, 7.1% of exacerbations had not returned to baseline lung function. Recovery was longer in the presence of increased dyspnea or symptoms of a common cold at exacerbation. The changes observed in lung function at exacerbation were smaller than those observed at asthmatic exacerbations, though the average duration of an asthmatic exacerbation was longer at 9.6 days.[11,12]

The combination of the symptoms of increased dyspnea and of the common cold at exacerbation with a prolonged exacerbation recovery suggests that viral infections may lead to more prolonged exacerbations. As colds are associated with longer exacerbations, COPD patients who develop a cold may be prone to more severe exacerbations and should be considered for therapy early at onset of symptoms.

The reasons for the incomplete recovery of symptoms and lung function are not clear, but may involve inadequate treatment or persistence of the causative agent. The incomplete physiologic recovery after an exacerbation could contribute to the decline in lung function with time in patients with COPD. To date there is no evidence that patients with incomplete recovery of their exacerbation have a greater decline in lung function. However one recent study has suggested that in patients who are smokers exacerbations are associated with more lung function decline.[13] In another study, patients with a history of frequent exacerbations had a faster decline of FEV_1 compared to patients with a history of infrequent exacerbations.[14] Further long-term studies are required to evaluate the effect of exacerbations on disease progression in COPD.

AIRWAY INFLAMMATION AT EXACERBATION

Although it has been assumed that exacerbations are associated with increased airway inflammation there has been little information available on the nature of inflammatory markers, especially when studied close to an exacerbation, as performing bronchial biopsies at exacerbation is difficult in patients with moderate to severe COPD. The relation of any airway inflammatory changes to symptoms and physiologic changes at exacerbations of COPD is also an important factor to consider.

In one study, where biopsies were performed at exacerbation in patients with chronic bronchitis, increased airway eosinophilia was found, though the patients studied had only mild COPD.[15] At exacerbation, there were more modest increases observed in neutrophils, T-lymphocytes (CD3) and tumor necrosis factor alpha (TNF-α) positive cells, while there were no changes in CD4 or CD8 T cells, macrophages or mast cells. However the technique of sputum induction allows study of these patients at exacerbation and it has been shown that it is a safe and

well-tolerated technique in COPD patients.[16] Levels of inflammatory cytokines have been shown to be elevated in induced sputum in COPD patients when stable, though changes at exacerbation had not been previously studied.[17]

In a prospectively followed cohort of patients from the East London COPD Study inflammatory markers in induced sputum were related to symptoms and physiologic parameters both at baseline and at exacerbation.[3] There was a relationship between exacerbation frequency and sputum cytokines, in that there was increased sputum interleukin 6 (IL-6) and IL-8 found in patients at baseline when stable with frequent exacerbations compared to those with infrequent exacerbations (Figure 26.4), although there was no relationship between cytokines and baseline lung function. Sputum cell counts were not increased at baseline in patients with more frequent exacerbations suggesting that the increased cytokine production comes from the bronchial epithelium in COPD. As discussed below, exacerbations are triggered by viral infections, especially by rhinovirus that is the cause of the

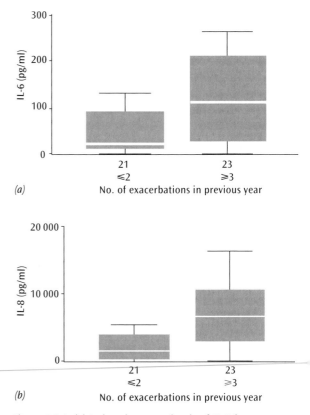

(a)

(b)

Figure 26.4 (a) Induced sputum levels of IL-6 in patients at baseline who are categorized as frequent exacerbators (≥ 3 exacerbations in the previous year) and those who are infrequent exacerbators (≤ 2 exacerbations in previous year). Data are expressed as medians (IQR). (From ref. 3.) (b) Induced sputum levels of IL-8 in patients with frequent exacerbations and infrequent exacerbations. Data are expressed as medians (IQR). (From ref. 3.)

common cold. Rhinovirus has been shown to increase cytokine production in an epithelial cell line[18] and thus repeated viral infection may lead to upregulation of cytokine airway expression.

At exacerbation increases were found in induced sputum IL-6 levels and the levels of IL-6 were higher when exacerbations were associated with symptoms of the common cold (Figure 26.5). Experimental rhinovirus infection has been shown to increase sputum IL-6 in normal subjects and asthmatics.[19–21] However increases in cell counts and IL-8 were more variable with exacerbation and not reaching statistical significance, suggesting marked heterogeneity in the degree of the inflammatory response at exacerbation or lack of reproducibility of the assay. The exacerbation of IL-8 levels was related to sputum neutrophil and total cell counts, indicating that neutrophil recruitment is the major source of airway IL-8 at exacerbation. Lower airway IL-8 has been shown to increase with experimental rhinovirus infection in normal and asthmatic patients in some studies,[20] but not in others.[21] However COPD patients already have upregulated airway IL-8 levels when stable due to their high sputum neutrophil load[17] and further increases in IL-8 would be unlikely. COPD exacerbations are associated with a less pronounced airway inflammatory response than asthmatic exacerbations,[22] and this may explain the relatively reduced response to steroids seen at exacerbation in COPD patients relative to asthma.[23–29]

In the study performed by Bhowmik and colleagues, there was no increase seen in the eosinophil count in induced sputum at exacerbation, even though the patients in that study were sampled early at exacerbation with onset of symptoms.[3] Compared to the study by Saetta and colleagues, where patients had mild COPD,[15] the patients had more severe and irreversible airflow obstruction with an FEV_1 at 39% predicted. Thus it is possible that the inflammatory response at exacerbation is different in nature in patients with moderate to severe COPD than in patients with milder COPD.

Patients were followed with daily diary cards in the study by Bhowmik and colleagues and thus the inflammatory response could be related to exacerbation recovery. There was no relation between the degree of inflammatory cell response during exacerbations and duration of symptoms and lung function changes. Induced sputum markers taken 3–6 weeks after exacerbation showed no relation to exacerbation changes. Thus levels of induced sputum markers at exacerbation do not predict the subsequent course of the exacerbation and did not appear to be useful in the prediction of exacerbation severity.

ETIOLOGY OF COPD EXACERBATION

COPD exacerbations have been associated with a number of etiological factors, including infection and pollution episodes (Table 26.1) (see Chapter 8). COPD exacerbations are frequently triggered by upper respiratory tract infections and these are commoner in the winter months, when there are more respiratory viral infections in the community. Patients may also be more prone to exacerbations in the winter months as lung function in COPD patients shows small but significant falls with reduction in outdoor temperature during the winter months.[4] COPD patients have been found to have increased hospital admissions, suggesting increased exacerbations when increasing environmental pollution occurs. During the December 1991 pollution episode in the UK, COPD mortality was increased together with an increase in hospital admission in elderly COPD patients.[30] However common pollutants especially oxides of nitrogen and particulates may interact with viral infection in asthma to precipitate exacerbation rather than acting alone and a similar mechanism may occur in COPD.[31]

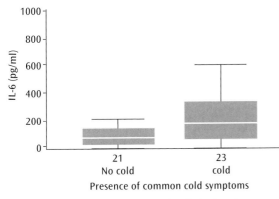

Figure 26.5 *Induced sputum IL-6 levels in the absence and presence of a natural cold. Data are expressed as medians (IQR). (From ref. 3.)*

Table 26.1 *Causes of COPD exacerbations*

Viruses	Bacteria	Common pollutants
Rhinovirus (common cold)	*Haemophilus influenzae*	Nitrogen dioxide
Influenza	*Streptococcus pneumoniae*	Particulates
Parainfluenza		Sulfur dioxide
Coronavirus	*Branhamella cattarhalis*	Ozone
Adenovirus		
RSV	*Staphylococcus aureus*	
Chlamydia pneumoniae	*Pseudomonas aeruginosa*	

Viral infections

Viral infections are an important trigger for COPD exacerbations. Studies in childhood asthma have shown that viruses, especially rhinovirus (the cause of the common cold), can be detected by the polymerase chain reaction (PCR) from a large number of these exacerbations.[32] Rhinovirus has not hitherto been considered to be of much significance during exacerbations of COPD as earlier studies have not used PCR techniques. In one of these studies of 44 chronic bronchitics over 2 years, Stott and colleagues found rhinovirus in 13 (14.9%) of 87 exacerbations of chronic bronchitis.[33] In a more detailed study of 25 chronic bronchitics with 116 exacerbations over 4 years, Gump et al. found that only 3.4% of exacerbations could be attributed to rhinoviruses.[34] In a more recent study of 35 episodes of COPD exacerbation using serological methods and nasal samples for viral culture, little evidence was found for a rhinovirus etiology of COPD exacerbation.[35]

Recent studies have shown that around half of COPD exacerbations were associated with viral infections, and that the majority of these were due to rhinovirus.[36–38] Viral exacerbations were associated with symptomatic colds and prolonged recovery.[9] However Seemungal and colleagues showed that rhinovirus can be recovered from induced sputum more frequently than from nasal aspirates at exacerbation, suggesting that wild-type rhinovirus can infect the lower airway and contribute to inflammatory changes at exacerbation.[37] They also found that exacerbations associated with the presence of rhinovirus in induced sputum had larger increases in airway IL-6 levels,[37] suggesting that viruses increase the severity of airway inflammation at exacerbation. This finding is in agreement with the data that respiratory viruses produce longer and more severe exacerbations and have a major impact on healthcare utilization.[10,36] Other viruses may trigger COPD exacerbation, though coronavirus was associated with only a small proportion of asthmatic exacerbations and is unlikely to play a major role in COPD.[32,39]

Bacterial infection (see also Chapter 8)

Airway bacterial colonization has been found in approximately 30% of COPD patients, and this colonization has been shown to be related to the degree of airflow obstruction and current cigarette smoking status.[40] Although bacteria such as *Haemophilus influenzae* and *Streptococcus pneumoniae* have been associated with COPD exacerbation, some studies have shown increasing bacterial counts during exacerbation, while others have not confirmed these findings.[41,42] Soler and colleagues showed that the presence of potentially pathogenic organisms in bronchoalveolar lavage from COPD

patients at bronchoscopy was associated with a greater degree of neutrophilia and higher TNF-α levels.[43] Hill and colleagues in a larger study showed that the airway bacterial load was related to inflammatory markers.[44] They also found that the bacterial species was related to the degree of inflammation, with *Pseudomonas aeruginosa* colonization showing greater myeloperoxidase activity (an indirect measure of neutrophil activation). Recently a study has suggested that isolation of a new bacterial strain was associated with an increased risk of an exacerbation, though this does not conclusively prove that bacteria are direct causes of exacerbations.[45]

Thus bacterial colonization in COPD may be an important determinant of airway inflammation and thus further long-term studies are required to determine whether bacterial colonization predisposes to decline in lung function, characteristic of COPD. There is now evidence that patients with frequent exacerbations have increased sputum bacterial colonization and this explains the higher cytokine levels observed in the frequent exacerbator patient group.[3,14] However it is also possible that there may be interactions between viral and bacterial infection at COPD exacerbation. Other organisms such as *Chlamydia pneumoniae* which have been associated with asthmatic exacerbation, may also play a role in COPD exacerbation.

PATHOPHYSIOLOGIC CHANGES AT COPD EXACERBATION

Relatively little information is available on pathologic changes in the airway during COPD exacerbation. In patients with moderate and severe COPD, the mechanical performance of the respiratory muscles is reduced (see Chapter 13). The airflow obstruction leads to hyperinflation, with the respiratory muscles acting at a mechanical disadvantage and generating reduced inspiratory pressures. The load on the respiratory muscles is also increased in patients with airflow obstruction by the presence of intrinsic positive end-expiratory pressure (PEEP). With an exacerbation of COPD, the increase in airflow obstruction will further increase the load on the respiratory muscles and increase the work of breathing, precipitating respiratory failure in more severe cases. Minute ventilation may be normal, but the respiratory pattern will be irregular with increased frequency and decreased tidal volume. The resultant hypercapnia and acidosis will then reduce inspiratory muscle function, contributing to further deterioration of the respiratory failure.

Hypoxemia in COPD usually occurs due to a combination of ventilation–perfusion mismatch and hypoventilation, although arteriovenous shunting can also contribute in the acute setting. This causes increase in pulmonary artery pressure, which can lead to salt and water retention and the development of edema. The degree of the ventilation–perfusion abnormalities increases during acute exacerbations and then resolves over the following few weeks. Acidosis is an important prognostic factor in survival from respiratory failure during a COPD exacerbation and thus early correction of acidosis is an essential goal of therapy.

TREATMENT

Inhaled bronchodilator therapy

Beta$_2$-agonists and anticholinergic agents are the inhaled bronchodilators most frequently used in the treatment of acute exacerbations of COPD. In patients with stable COPD, symptomatic benefit can be obtained with bronchodilator therapy in COPD, even without significant changes in spirometry. This is probably due to a reduction in dynamic hyperinflation that is characteristic of COPD and hence leads to a decrease in the sensation of dyspnea especially during exertion.[46] In stable COPD greater bronchodilatation has been demonstrated with anticholinergic agents than with beta$_2$-agonists, which may be due to the excessive cholinergic neuronal bronchoconstrictor tone.[47] However, studies investigating bronchodilator responses in acute exacerbations of COPD have shown no differences between agents used and no significant additive effect of the combination therapy, even though combination of an anticholinergic and bronchodilator has benefits in the stable state.[48,49] This difference in effect between the acute and stable states may be due to the fact that the larger doses of drug delivered in the acute setting produce maximal bronchodilatation, whereas the smaller doses administered in the stable condition may be having a submaximal effect.

Methylxanthines such as theophylline are sometimes used in the management of acute exacerbations of COPD. There is some evidence that theophyllines are useful in COPD, though the main limiting factor is the frequency of toxic side effects. The therapeutic action of theophylline is thought to be due to its inhibition of phosphodiesterase which breaks down cyclic AMP, an intracellular messenger, thus facilitating bronchodilatation, though further studies are required. However studies of intravenous aminophylline therapy in acute exacerbations of COPD have shown no significant beneficial effect over and above conventional therapy.[50]

Corticosteroids (see Chapter 25)

Only about 10–15% of patients with stable COPD show a spirometric response to oral corticosteroids[51] and, unlike the situation in asthma, steroids have variable effect on airway inflammatory markers in patients with COPD.[52,53] Although corticosteroids have traditionally been used in the management of acute exacerbations of COPD, there is only recently evidence of their beneficial role in the acute situation.[23–29]

A number of early studies have investigated the effects of corticosteroid therapy at COPD exacerbation. In an early controlled trial in patients with COPD exacerbations and acute respiratory failure, Albert and coworkers found that there were larger improvements in pre- and post-bronchodilator FEV$_1$ when patients were treated for the first 3 days of the hospital admission with intravenous methylprednisolone over those treated with placebo.[23] Another trial found that a single dose of methylprednisolone given within 30 minutes of arrival in the accident and emergency department produced no improvement after 5 hours in spirometry, and also had no effect on hospital admission, though another study reduced readmission.[24,25] A retrospective study comparing patients treated with steroids at exacerbation compared to those not treated showed that the steroid group had a reduced chance of relapse after therapy.[26]

Thompson and colleagues gave a 9-day course of prednisolone or placebo in a randomized manner to outpatients presenting with acute exacerbations of COPD.[27] Unlike the previous studies, these patients were either recruited from outpatients or from a group that were pre-enrolled and self reported the exacerbation to the study team. In this study patients with exacerbations associated with acidosis or pneumonia were excluded, so exacerbations of moderate severity were generally included. Patients in the steroid-treated group showed a more rapid improvement in Pa$_{O_2}$, alveolar–arterial oxygen gradient, FEV$_1$, peak expiratory flow rate and a trend towards a more rapid improvement in dyspnea in the steroid-treated group.

In a recent cohort study by Seemungal and colleagues, the effect of therapy with prednisolone on COPD exacerbations diagnosed and treated in the community was studied, though this particular study did not set out to evaluate the role of steroids in exacerbations and the evaluation was not controlled.[10] Exacerbations treated with steroids were more severe and associated with larger falls in peak flow rate. The treated exacerbations also had a longer recovery time to baseline for symptoms and peak flow rate. However, the rate of peak flow rate recovery was faster in the prednisolone-treated group, though not the rate of symptom score recovery. An interesting finding in this study was that steroids significantly prolonged the median time from the day of onset of the initial exacerbation to the next exacerbation from 60 days in the group not treated with prednisolone to 84 days in the patients treated with prednisolone. By contrast, antibiotic therapy had no effect on the time to the next exacerbation. If short course oral steroid therapy at exacerbation does prolong the time to the next exacerbation, then this could be an important way to reduce exacerbation frequency in COPD patients, which is an important determinant of health status.[2]

Davies and colleagues randomized patients admitted to hospital with COPD exacerbations to prednisolone or placebo.[28] In the prednisolone group, the FEV_1 rose faster until day 5, when a plateau was observed in the steroid-treated group. Changes in the pre-bronchodilator and post-bronchodilator FEV_1 were similar, suggesting that this is not just an effect on bronchomotor tone, but involves faster resolution of airway inflammatory changes or airway wall edema with exacerbation. Length of hospital stay analysis showed that patients treated with prednisolone had a significantly shorter length of stay. Six weeks later, there were no differences in spirometry between the patient groups and health status was similar to that measured at 5 days after admission. Thus the benefits of steroid therapy at exacerbation are most obvious in the early course of the exacerbation. A similar proportion of the patients, approximately 32% in both study groups, required further treatment for exacerbations within 6 weeks of follow-up, emphasizing the high exacerbation relapse rate in these patients.

Niewoehner and colleagues performed a randomized controlled trial of either a 2-week or 8-week intravenous methyl prednisolone course at exacerbation compared to placebo, in addition to other exacerbation therapy.[29] The primary end-point was a first treatment failure, including death, need for intubation, readmission or intensification of therapy. There was no difference in the results using the 2- or 8-week treatment protocol. The rates of treatment failure were higher in the placebo group at 30 days, compared to the combined 2- and 8-week prednisolone groups. As in the study by Davies and colleagues, the FEV_1 improved faster in the prednisolone-treated group, though there were no differences by 2 weeks. By contrast, Niewoehner and colleagues performed a detailed evaluation of steroid complications and found considerable evidence of hyperglycemia in the steroid-treated patients, which it is likely was due to the higher steroid doses used. Thus steroids should be used at COPD exacerbation in short courses of no more than 2 weeks' duration to avoid risk of complications.

Antibiotics

Acute exacerbations of COPD often present with increased sputum purulence and volume and antibiotics have traditionally been used as first line therapy in such exacerbations. However, viral infections may be the triggers in a significant proportion of acute infective exacerbations in COPD and antibiotics used for the consequences of secondary infection. A study investigating the benefit of antibiotics in over 300 acute exacerbations demonstrated a greater treatment success rate in patients treated with antibiotics, especially if their initial presentation was with the symptoms of increased dyspnea, sputum volume and purulence.[5] Patients with mild COPD obtained less benefit from antibiotic therapy. A randomized placebo-controlled study investigating the value of antibiotics in patients with mild obstructive lung disease in the community concluded that antibiotic therapy did not accelerate recovery or reduce the number of relapses.[54] A meta-analysis of trials of antibiotic therapy in COPD identified only nine studies of significant duration and concluded that antibiotic therapy offered a small but significant benefit in outcome in acute exacerbations.[55]

Management of respiratory failure

Hypoxemia occurs with more severe exacerbations and usually requires hospital admission. Caution should always be taken in providing supplemental oxygen to patients with COPD, particularly during acute exacerbations, when respiratory drive and muscle strength can be impaired leading to significant increases in carbon dioxide tension at relatively modest oxygen flow rates. However, in the vast majority of cases, the administration of supplemental oxygen increases arterial oxygen tension sufficiently without clinically significant rises in carbon dioxide. It is suggested that supplemental oxygen is delivered at an initial flow rate of 1–2 L/min via nasal cannulae or 24–28% inspired oxygen via Venturi mask, with repeat blood gas analysis after 30–45 minutes of oxygen therapy.

Hypercapnia during COPD exacerbations may be managed initially with the use of respiratory stimulants. The most commonly used is doxapram, which acts centrally to increase respiratory drive and respiratory muscle activity. The effect is probably only appreciable for 24–48 hours; the main factor limiting use being side effects which can lead to agitation and are often not tolerated by the patient. There are only a few studies of the clinical efficacy of doxapram and short-term investigations suggest that improvements in acidosis and arterial carbon dioxide tension can be attained.[56] A small study comparing doxapram with non-invasive positive pressure ventilation (NPPV) in acute exacerbations of COPD, suggested that NPPV was superior with regard to correction of blood gases during the initial treatment phase.[57] Increases in pulmonary artery pressure during acute exacerbations of COPD can result in right-sided cardiac dysfunction and development of peripheral edema. Diuretic therapy may thus be necessary if there is edema or a rise in jugular venous pressure.

Ventilatory support

NON-INVASIVE VENTILATION (see Chapter 27)

The introduction of NPPV using nasal or face masks has had a major impact on the management of acute exacerbations and has enabled acidosis to be corrected at an early stage. Studies have shown that NPPV can produce improvements in arterial blood gases, reduction in intubation and reduction of mortality.[58–61]

Studies have shown that NPPV can be successfully implemented in up to 80% of cases.[62,63] NPPV is less successful in patients who have worse blood gases at baseline before ventilation, are underweight, have a higher incidence of pneumonia, have a greater level of neurologic deterioration and where compliance with the ventilation is poor.[62] Moretti and colleagues have recently shown that 'late treatment failure' (after an initial 48 hours of therapy with NPPV) is up to 20% and that patients with late failure were more likely to have severe functional and clinical disease with more complications at the time of admission.[64] Identification of patients with a potentially poor outcome is important as delay in intubation can have serious consequences for the patient.

INDICATIONS FOR INVASIVE VENTILATION
(see Chapter 28)

If NPPV fails, or is unavailable in the hospital, invasive ventilation may be required in the presence of increasing acidosis. It may be considered when the pH falls below 7.26. Decisions to ventilate these patients may be difficult, though with improved modes of invasive ventilatory support and better weaning techniques, the outlook for the COPD patient is better. Patients will be suitable for tracheal intubation if this is the first presentation of COPD exacerbation or respiratory failure, or there is a treatable cause of respiratory failure, such as pneumonia. Information will be required on the past history and quality of life, especially the ability to perform daily activities. Patients with severe disabling and progressive COPD may be less suitable, but it is important that adequate and appropriate therapy has been used in these patients, with documented disease progression. The patient's wishes and those of any close relatives should be considered in any decision to institute or withhold life-supporting therapy.

Supported discharge

Many hospital admissions are related to exacerbations of COPD and thus reductions of admissions especially during the winter months when they are most frequent is particularly desirable. Over the last few years a number of different models of supported discharge have been developed and some evaluated.[65–68] Patients have been discharged early with an appropriate package of care organized, including domiciliary visits made to these patients after discharge by trained respiratory nurses.

Cotton and colleagues randomized patients to discharge on the next day or usual management and found that there were no differences in mortality or readmission rates between the two groups.[66] There was a reduction in hospital stay from a mean of 6.1 days to 3.2 days. In another larger study by Skwarska and colleagues, patients were randomized to discharge on the day of assessment or conventional management.[67] Again there were no differences in readmission rates, though these were high at around 30% of the study populations at 3 months. There were no differences in visits to primary care physicians and health status measured 8 weeks after discharge was similar in the two groups. The authors also demonstrated that there were significant cost savings of around 50% for the home support group, compared to the admitted group. Similar results were found by Davies and colleagues with no differences in mortality or readmission rate between the home and hospital treated group.[68] However only about 25% of patients presenting for hospital admission with a COPD exacerbation are suitable for home therapy and thus selection is required.[67,68] Other considerations need to be taken into account in organizing an assisted discharge service, in that resources have to be released for the nurses to follow the patients and the benefits may be seasonal, as COPD admissions are a particular problem in the winter months. Further work is required on the different models of supported discharge available and the cost effectiveness of these various programs.

PREVENTION OF COPD EXACERBATION

There has been relatively little attention paid to aspects of prevention of exacerbations in patients with COPD, though any therapy that can prevent exacerbations will have important health economic benefits and improve health status. As upper respiratory tract infections are common factors in causing exacerbation, influenza and pneumococcal vaccinations are recommended for all patients with significant COPD. A study that reviewed the outcome of influenza vaccination in a cohort of elderly patients with chronic lung disease found that influenza vaccination is associated with significant health benefits with fewer outpatient visits, fewer hospitalizations and a reduced mortality.[69] Long-term antibiotic therapy has been used in patients with very frequent exacerbations, though there is little evidence of effectiveness. Recently there has been a report of the effects of an immunostimulatory agent in patients with COPD exacerbations, with reduction in severe complications and hospital admissions in the actively treated group.[70] Further studies on the effects of these agents in the prevention of COPD exacerbation are required.

Mucolytic agents have also been prescribed in COPD though their use worldwide is very variable with little use in the UK and Australia and more prescriptions in Europe. A recent meta-analysis was published that assessed the effects of oral mucolytics in COPD.[71] A total of 23 randomized controlled trials was identified and the main outcome was that there was a 29% reduction in exacerbations with mucolytic therapy. The number of patients who had no exacerbations was greater in the mucolytic group and day of illness was also reduced, though mucolytics had no effect on lung function. The drug that contributed most to the beneficial results in the review was *N*-acetylcysteine, though the mechanism of action of *N*-acetylcysteine is not entirely clear and may be a combination of mucolytic and antioxidative effects. Further large studies on the effects of mucolytics are in progress and the results will be available in the next few years.

In the recent ISOLDE study of long-term inhaled steroids in patients with moderate to severe COPD, a reduction in exacerbation frequency of around 25% was shown. However the overall exacerbation frequency was relatively low in that study and this was probably due to a retrospective assessment of exacerbation.[72] The effect of inhaled steroids was greater in patients with more impaired lung function, suggesting that this is the group to target with long-term inhaled steroids therapy. Another earlier study suggested that the severity of exacerbations may be reduced with inhaled steroid therapy.[73] An observational study showed that exacerbations were increased following withdrawal of inhaled steroids, though this study was not placebo controlled.[74] Two recent studies have also shown that small reductions in exacerbations can be achieved with bronchodilator therapy, though both studies involved relatively short periods of therapy at 12 weeks.[75,76] Mahler and colleagues found that the time to the first exacerbation was longer with therapy with the long-acting beta-agonist, salmeterol, though the overall number of exacerbations during the study was relatively small.[75] Van Noord and colleagues in a similar study suggested that the combination of salmeterol and ipratropium was most effective in reduction of exacerbation.[76] Recently the new long-acting anticholinergic agent tiotropium has been shown to reduce exacerbations by 24% when studied over a 1-year period.[77] Longer term studies of the effects of bronchodilators on COPD exacerbation are now required.

Exacerbation frequency increases with progressive airflow obstruction and thus patients with chronic respiratory failure are particularly susceptible to exacerbation. Following the early experience of domiciliary long-term NPPV in patients with chest wall and neuromuscular disease, NPPV has also been evaluated in patients with hypercapnic COPD. An early observation on the effect of NPPV came from a randomized crossover study where NPPV given at home over a 3-month period had a significant beneficial effect on health status measured with the St George's Respiratory Questionnaire, though exacerbations were not measured in that study.[78] As health status is such an important determinant of exacerbation frequency,[2] it is possible that the improvement in health status is due to a reduction of exacerbation frequency. Two open studies have shown that use of NPPV in patients with hypercapnic COPD is associated with a reduction in hospitalization,[79,80] and thus larger controlled studies are now required to evaluate the effect of NPPV on exacerbation in these patients.

CONCLUSIONS

COPD exacerbations are an important cause of morbidity and mortality in COPD and have significant health economic consequences. There is a need for increased patient education about the detection and treatment of exacerbations early in the natural history. More specific written treatment plans for COPD patients at risk may be useful, as are those produced for asthmatics, though such an approach requires formal testing. Following an exacerbation, the condition of the patient with COPD should be reviewed and attention given to risk factors and compliance with therapy. Strategies to reduce exacerbation frequency need to be urgently developed and evaluated in randomized controlled trials. We will then be in a better position to reduce significantly the morbidity associated with COPD exacerbation and improve the health-related quality of life of our patients in this disabling condition.

REFERENCES

1. Fletcher CM, Peto R, Tinker CM, Speizer FE. *Natural History of Chronic Bronchitis and Emphysema*. Oxford University Press, Oxford, 1976.
2. Seemungal TAR, Donaldson GC, Paul EA, Bestall JC, Jeffries DJ, Wedzicha JA. Effect of exacerbation on quality of life in patients with chronic obstructive pulmonary disease. *Am J Respir Crit Care Med* 1998;**151**:1418–22.
3. Bhowmik A, Seemungal TAR, Sapsford RJ, Wedzicha JA. Relation of sputum inflammatory markers to symptoms and physiological changes at COPD exacerbations. *Thorax* 2000;**55**:114–200.
4. Donaldson GC, Seemungal T, Jeffries DJ, Wedzicha JA. Effect of environmental temperature on symptoms, lung function and mortality in COPD patients. *Eur Respir J* 1999;**13**:844–9.

5. Anthonisen NR, Manfreda J, Warren CPW, Hershfield ES, Harding GKM, Nelson NA. Antibiotic therapy in exacerbations of chronic obstructive pulmonary disease. *Ann Intern Med* 1987;**106**:196–20.

6. Rodriguez-Roisin R. Towards a consensus definition for COPD exacerbations. *Chest* 2000;**117**:398S–401S.

7. Okubadejo AA, Jones PW, Wedzicha JA. Quality of life in patients with COPD and severe hypoxaemia. *Thorax* 1996;**51**:44–47.

8. Okubadejo AA, O'Shea L, Jones PW, Wedzicha JA. Home assessment of activities of daily living in patients with severe chronic obstructive pulmonary disease on long term oxygen therapy. *Eur Respir J* 1997;**10**:1572–5.

9. Ball P, Harris JM, Lowson D, Tillotson G, Wilson R. Acute infective exacerbations of chronic bronchitis. *Q J Med* 1995;**88**:61–8.

10. Seemungal TAR, Donaldson GC, Bhowmik A, Jeffries DJ, Wedzicha JA. Time course and recovery of exacerbations in patients with chronic obstructive pulmonary disease. *Am J Respir Crit Care Med* 2000;**161**:1608–13.

11. Reddel HS, Ware S, Marks G, Salome C, Jenkins C, Woolcock A. Differences between asthma exacerbations and poor asthma control. *Lancet* 1999;**353**:364–9.

12. Tattersfield AE, Postma DS, Barnes PJ, *et al.* Exacerbations of asthma. *Am J Respir Crit Care Med* 1999;**160**:594–9.

13. Kanner RE, Anthonisen NR, Connett JE. Lower respiratory illnesses promote FEV_1 decline in current smokers but not ex-smokers with mild chronic obstructive lung disease: results from the Lung Health Study. *Am J Respir Crit Care Med* 2001;**164**:358–64.

14. Donaldson GC, Seemungal TAR, Bhowmik A, Wedzicha JA. The relationship between exacerbation frequency and lung function decline in chronic obstructive pulmonary disease. *Thorax* 2002 (in press).

15. Saetta M, Di Stefano A, Maestrelli P, *et al.* Airway eosinophilia in chronic bronchitis during exacerbations. *Am J Respir Crit Care Med* 1994;**150**:1646–52.

16. Bhowmik A, Seemungal TAR, Sapsford RJ, Devalia JL, Wedzicha JA. Comparison of spontaneous and induced sputum for investigation of airway inflammation in chronic obstructive pulmonary disease. *Thorax* 1998;**53**:953–6.

17. Keatings VM, Collins PD, Scott DM, *et al.* Differences in Interleukin-8 and Tumour Necrosis Factor in induced sputum from patients with chronic obstructive pulmonary disease and asthma. *Am J Respir Crit Care Med* 1996;**153**:530–4.

18. Subauste MC, Jacoby DB, Richards SM, Proud D. Infection of a human respiratory epithelial cell line with rhinovirus. *J Clin Invest* 1995;**96**:549–57.

19. Fraenkel DJ, Bardin PG, Sanderson G, *et al.* Lower airways inflammation during rhinovirus colds in normal and in asthmatic subjects. *Am J Respir Crit Care Med* 1995;**151**:879–86.

20. Grunberg K, Smits HH, Timmers MC, *et al.* Experimental rhinovirus 16 infection: effects on cell differentials and soluble markers in sputum of asthmatic subjects. *Am J Respir Crit Care Med* 1997;**156**:609–16.

21. Fleming HE, Little EF, Schnurr D, *et al.* Rhinovirus-16 colds in healthy and asthmatic subjects. *Am J Respir Crit Care Med* 1999;**160**:100–8.

22. Pizzicini MMM, Pizzichini E, Clelland L, *et al.* Sputum in severe exacerbations of asthma:kinetics of inflammatory indices after prednisone treatment. *Am J Respir Crit Care Med* 1997;**155**:1501–8.

23. Albert RK, Martin TR, Lewis SW. Controlled clinical trial of methylprednisolone in patients with chronic bronchitis and acute respiratory insufficiency. *Ann Intern Med* 1980;**92**:753–8.

24. Emerman CL, Connors AF, Lukens TW, May ME, Effron D. A randomized controlled trial of methylprednisolone in the emergency treatment of acute exacerbations of chronic obstructive pulmonary disease. *Chest* 1989;**95**:563–7.

25. Bullard MJ, Liaw SJ, Tsai YH, Min HP. Early corticosteroid use in acute exacerbations of chronic airflow limitation. *Am J Emerg Med* 1996;**14**:139–43.

26. Murata GH, Gorby MS, Chick TW, Halperin AK. Intravenous and oral corticosteroids for the prevention of relapse after treatment of decompensated COPD. *Chest* 1990;**98**:845–9.

27. Thompson WH, Nielson CP, Carvalho P, *et al.* Controlled trial of oral prednisolone in outpatients with acute COPD exacerbation. *Am J Respir Crit Care Med* 1996;**154**:407–12.

28. Davies L, Angus RM, Calverley PMA. Oral corticosteroids in patients admitted to hospital with exacerbations of chronic obstructive pulmonary disease: a prospective randomized controlled trial. *Lancet* 1999;**354**:456–60.

29. Niewoehner DE, Erbland ML, Deupree RH, *et al.* Effect of systemic glucocorticoids on exacerbations of chronic obstructive pulmonary disease. *N Engl J Med* 1999;**340**:1941–7.

30. Anderson HR, Limb ES, Bland JM, Ponce de Leon A, Strachan DP, Bower JS. Health effects of an air pollution episode in London, December 1991. *Thorax* 1995;**50**:1188–93.

31. Linaker CH, Coggon D, Holgate ST, *et al.* Personal exposure to nitrogen dioxide and risk of airflow obstruction in asthmatic children with upper respiratory infection. *Thorax* 2000;**55**:930–3.

32. Johnston SL, Pattemore PK, Sanderson G, *et al.* Community study of the role of viral infections in exacerbations of asthma in 9–11 year old children. *Br Med J* 1995;**310**:1225–9.

33. Stott EJ, Grist NR, Eadie MB. Rhinovirus infections in chronic bronchitis:isolation of eight possible new rhinovirus serotypes. *J Med Microbiol* 1968;**109**:117.

34. Gump DW, Phillips CA, Forsyth BR. Role of infection in chronic bronchitis. *Am Rev Respir Dis* 1976;**113**:465–73.

35. Philit F, Etienne J, Calvet A, *et al.* Infectious agents associated with exacerbations of chronic obstructive pulmonary disease and attacks of asthma. *Rev Mal Respir* 1992;**9**:191–6.

36. Greenberg SB, Allen M, Wilson J, Atmar RL. Respiratory viral infections in adults with and without chronic obstructive pulmonary disease. *Am J Respir Crit Care Med* 2000;**162**:167–73.

37. Seemungal TAR, Harper-Owen R, Bhowmik A, Jeffries DJ, Wedzicha JA. Detection of rhinovirus in induced sputum at exacerbation of chronic obstructive pulmonary disease. *Eur Respir J* 2000;**16**:67–83.

38. Seemungal TAR, Harper-Owen R, Bhowmik A, *et al.* Respiratory viruses, symptoms and inflammatory markers in acute exacerbations and stable chronic obstructive pulmonary disease. *Am J Respir Crit Care Med* 2001;**164**:1618–23.

39. Nicholson KG, Kent J, Ireland DC. Respiratory viruses and exacerbations of asthma in adults. *Br Med J* 1993;**307**:982–6.

40. Zalacain R, Sobradillo V, Amilibia J, *et al.* Predisposing factors to bacterial colonization in chronic obstructive pulmonary disease. *Eur Respir J* 1999;**13**:343–8.

41. Monso E, Rosell A, Bonet G, *et al.* Risk factors for lower airway bacterial colonization in chronic bronchitis. *Eur Respir J* 1999;**13**:338–42.

42. Wilson R. Bacterial infection and chronic obstructive pulmonary disease. *Eur Respir J* 1999;**13**:233–5.

43. Soler N, Ewig S, Torres A, Filella X, Gonzalez J, Zaubet A. Airway inflammation and bronchial microbial patterns in patients with stable chronic obstructive pulmonary disease. *Eur Respir J* 1999;**14**:1015–22.

44. Hill AT, Campbell EJ, Hill SL, Bayley DL, Stockley RA. Association between airway bacterial load and markers of airway inflammation in patients with chronic bronchitis. *Am J Med* 2000;**109**:288–95.

45. Sethi S, Evans N, Grant BJB, Murphy TF. New strains of bacteria and exacerbations of chronic obstructive pulmonary disease. *N Engl J Med* 2002;**347**:465–71.

46. Belman MJ, Botnick WC, Shin JW. Inhaled bronchodilators reduce dynamic hyperinflation during exercise in patients with chronic obstructive pulmonary disease. *Am J Respir Crit Care Med* 1996;**153**:967–75.

47. Braun SR, McKenzie WN, Copeland C, Knight L, Ellersieck M. A comparison of the effect of ipratropium and albuterol in the treatment of chronic obstructive airway disease. *Arch Intern Med* 1989;**149**:544–7.

48. Combivent Inhalation Aerosol Study Group. In chronic obstructive pulmonary disease, a combination of ipratropium and albuterol is more effective than either agent alone. *Chest* 1994;**105**:1411–19.

49. Rebuck AS, Chapman KR, Abboud R, *et al.* Nebulized anticholinergic and sympathomimetic treatment of asthma and chronic obstructive airways disease in the emergency room. *Am J Med* 1987;**82**:59–64.

50. Rice KL, Leatherman JW, Duane PG, *et al.* Aminophylline for acute exacerbations of chronic obstructive pulmonary disease. A controlled trial. *Ann Intern Med* 1987;**107**:305–9.

51. Callahan CM, Cittus RS, Katz BP. Oral corticosteroid therapy for patients with stable chronic obstructive pulmonary disease:a meta-analysis. *Ann Intern Med* 1991;**114**:216–23.

52. Keatings VM, Jatakanon A, Worsdell Y, Barnes PJ. Effects of inhaled and oral glucocorticoids on inflammatory indices in asthma and COPD. *Am J Respir Crit Care Med* 1997;**155**:542–8.

53. Culpitt SV, Maziak W, Loukidis S, *et al.* Effects of high dose inhaled steroids on cells, cytokines and proteases in induced sputum in chronic obstructive pulmonary disease. *Am J Respir Crit Care Med* 1999;**160**:1635–9.

54. Sachs APE, Koeter GH, Groenier KH, Van der Waaij D, Schiphuis J, Meyboom-de Jong B. Changes in symptoms, peak expiratory flow and sputum flora during treatment with antibiotics of exacerbations in patients with chronic obstructive pulmonary disease in general practice. *Thorax* 1995;**50**:758–63.

55. Saint S, Bent S, Vittinghoff E, Grady D. Antibiotics in chronic obstructive pulmonary disease exacerbations. A meta-analysis. *JAMA* 1995;**273**:957–60.

56. Moser KM, Luchsinger PC, Adamson JS, *et al.* Respiratory stimulation with intravenous doxapram in respiratory failure. *N Engl J Med* 1973;**288**:427–31.

57. Angus RM, Ahmed AA, Fenwick LJ, Peacock AJ. Comparison of the acute effects on gas exchange of nasal ventilation and doxapram in exacerbations of chronic obstructive pulmonary disease. *Thorax* 1996;**51**:1048–50.

58. Bott J, Carroll MP, Conway JH, *et al.* Randomized controlled trial of nasal ventilation in acute ventilatory failure due to chronic obstructive airways disease. *Lancet* 1993;**341**:1555–7.

60. Brochard L, Mancebo J, Wysocki M, *et al.* Noninvasive ventilation for acute exacerbations of chronic obstructive pulmonary disease. *N Engl J Med* 1995;**333**:817–22.

60. Kramer N, Meyer TJ, Meharg J, Cece RD, Hill NS. Randomized prospective trial of noninvasive positive pressure ventilation in acute respiratory failure. *Am J Respir Crit Care Med* 1995;**151**:1799–806.

61. Plant PK, Owen JL, Elliott MW. A multicentre randomized controlled trial of the early use of non-invasive ventilation for acute exacerbations of chronic obstructive pulmonary disease on general respiratory wards. *Lancet* 2000;**355**:1931–5.

62. Ambrosino N, Foglio K, Rubini F, Clini E, Nava S, Vitacca M. Non-invasive mechanical ventilation in acute respiratory failure due to chronic obstructive pulmonary disease: correlates for success. *Thorax* 1995;**50**:755–7.

63. Brown JS, Meecham Jones DJ, Mikelsons C, Paul EA, Wedzicha JA. Outcome of nasal intermittent positive pressure ventilation when used for acute-on-chronic respiratory failure on a general respiratory ward. *J R Coll Physicians Lond* 1998;**32**:219–24.

64. Morretti M, Cilione C, Tampieri A, *et al.* Incidence and causes of non-invasive mechanical ventilation failure after initial success. *Thorax* 2000;**55**:819–25.

65. Gravil JH, Al-Rawas OA, Cotton MM, *et al.* Home treatment of exacerbations of COPD by an acute respiratory assessment service. *Lancet* 1998;**351**:1853–5.

66. Cotton MM, Bucknall CE, Dagg KD, *et al.* Early discharge for patients with exacerbations of COPD: a randomized controlled trial. *Thorax* 2000;**55**:902–6.

67. Skwarska E, Cohen G, Skwarski KM, *et al.* A randomized controlled trial of supported discharge in patients with exacerbations of COPD. *Thorax* 2000;**55**:907–12.

68. Davies L, Wilkinson M, Bonner S, Calverley PMA, Angus RM. Hospital at home versus hospital care in patients with exacerbations of chronic obstructive pulmonary disease: prospective randomized controlled trial. *Br Med J* 2000;**321**:1265–8.

69. Nichol KL, Baken L, Nelson A. Relation between influenza vaccination and out patient visits, hospitalization and mortality in elderly patients with chronic lung disease. *Ann Intern Med* 1999;**130**:397–403.

70. Collet JP, Shapiro S, Ernst P, *et al.* Effect of an immunostimulating agent on acute exacerbations and hospitalization in COPD patients. *Am J Respir Crit Care Med* 1997;**156**:1719–24.

71. Poole PJ, Black PN. Oral mucolytic drugs for exacerbations of chronic obstructive pulmonary disease: systematic review. *Br Med J* 2001;**322**:1271–4.

72. Burge PS, Calverley PMA, Jones PW, *et al.* Randomized, double blind, placebo controlled study of fluticasone propionate in patients with moderate to severe chronic obstructive pulmonary disease:the ISOLDE trial. *Br Med J* 2000;**320**:1297–303.

73. Paggiaro PL, Dahle R, Bakran I, Frith L, Hollingworth K, Efthimiou J. Multicentre randomized placebo-controlled trial of inhaled fluticasone propionate in patients with chronic obstructive pulmonary disease. *Lancet* 1998;**351**:773–80.

74. Jarad N, Wedzicha JA, Burge PS, Calverley PMA. An observational study of inhaled corticosteroid withdrawal in patients with stable chronic obstructive pulmonary disease. *Respir Med* 1999;**93**:161–6.

75. Mahler DA, Donohue JF, Barbee RA, *et al.* Efficacy of salmeterol xinafoate in the treatment of COPD. *Chest* 1999;**115**:957–65.

76. Van Noord JA, de Munck DRAJ, Bantje ThA, *et al.* Long-term treatment of chronic obstructive pulmonary disease with salmeterol and the additive effect of ipratropium. *Eur Respir J* 2000;**15**:878–85.

77. Vincken W, van Noord JA, Greefhorst APM. Improved health outcomes in patients with COPD during 1 year's treatment with tiotropium. *Eur Respir J* 2002;**19**:209–16.

78. Meecham Jones DJ, Paul EA, Jones PW, Wedzicha JA. Nasal pressure support ventilation plus oxygen compared with oxygen therapy alone in hypercapnic COPD: a randomized controlled study. *Am J Respir Crit Care Med* 1995;**152**:538–44.

79. Leger P, Bedicam JM, Cornette A, *et al.* Nasal intermittent positive pressure ventilation. Longterm follow-up in patients with severe chronic respiratory insufficiency. *Chest* 1994; **105**:100–5.

80. Jones S, Packham S, Hebden M, Smith AP. Domiciliary nocturnal intermittent positive pressure ventilation in patients with respiratory failure due to severe COPD: long term follow up and effect on survival. *Thorax* 1998; **53**:495–8.

27

Non-invasive ventilation

MARK W ELLIOTT

INTRODUCTION

Non-invasive ventilation (NIV) has been one of the major advances in respiratory medicine in the last decade. In particular it has found widespread application in the management of patients with COPD. There is a robust evidence base for its use in acute exacerbations of COPD. The evidence that it is effective in chronic COPD is much less strong but despite this COPD is one of the major reasons for long-term home mechanical ventilation. This chapter focuses mainly on non-invasive ventilation in acute exacerbations of COPD, but also reviews the evidence in chronic ventilatory failure due to COPD.

PATHOPHYSIOLOGY OF ACUTE VENTILATORY FAILURE (See Chapter 13)

For ventilation to be effective the respiratory muscle pump must have the capacity to sustain ventilation against a given load, with sufficient drive from the central nervous system. In patients with COPD the primary abnormality leading to the development of ventilatory failure is that of increased load, due to airways obstruction. However the capacity of the respiratory muscle pump may also be reduced, either because the respiratory muscles are working at a mechanical disadvantage as a consequence of hyperinflation[1] or because of intrinsic

weakness due to malnutrition[2] or steroid therapy.[3] Drive may be chronically reduced by nocturnal hypoventilation; and abnormalities of breathing during sleep are well recognized in patients with COPD.[4,5] An excessive rise in $PaCO_2$ causes a transient acidosis, which results in a compensatory renal retention of bicarbonate and as a result chemosensitivity to CO_2, which is mediated by changes in pH, is reduced. Drive can also be reduced by sedative drugs and injudicious oxygen therapy, if it causes severe carbon dioxide retention.[6] Figure 27.1 shows schematically how derangement of any one of these parameters may precipitate a deterioration in others. For example the patient with severe COPD may be able to maintain adequate, though not normal, blood gas tensions until in acute exacerbation load is increased by bronchospasm or secretion retention. They then develop a rapid shallow pattern of breathing in an attempt to protect the respiratory muscles against fatigue.[7] There is insufficient time for emptying of lung units with long time constants, leading to dynamic hyperinflation and intrinsic positive end-expiratory pressure (PEEPi). Hyperinflation places the respiratory muscle at a worse mechanical advantage and in addition PEEPi, acting as an inspiratory threshold load, further increases the work of breathing. The already loaded system is now working with reduced capacity and against an even greater load. Capacity may be reduced further by deterioration in arterial gas tensions, with an abnormal pH reducing respiratory muscle strength.[8] If $PaCO_2$ rises excessively

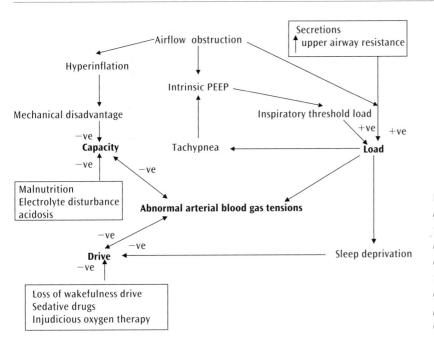

Figure 27.1 *The pathophysiology of acute ventilatory failure in patients with an exacerbation of COPD. There are a number of self-perpetuating cycles which if left untreated lead to worsening respiratory failure. By contrast, reversal of a particular process may lead to a virtuous cycle of improvement.*

narcosis may develop with a consequent reduction in the central drive to breathe. As can be seen from Figure 27.1 a number of potential vicious cycles are initiated, culminating in a downward spiral of arterial blood gas tensions.

RATIONALE FOR USE OF ASSISTED VENTILATION IN ACUTE EXACERBATIONS OF COPD

The aim of assisted ventilation is to restore the patient to how they were before the onset of acute on chronic ventilatory failure. Treatment of the precipitating cause is key and is often sufficient, however in some patients assisted ventilation is also required to offload the respiratory muscles and increase alveolar ventilation. This requires either that the work of ventilation is completely subsumed by the ventilator or more commonly that spontaneous breaths are augmented by machine-delivered breaths, triggered in response to patient effort. This requires that the patient and ventilator be in synchrony, with machine breaths coinciding with patient efforts. Asynchrony may be uncomfortable for the patient and does not reduce the work of breathing to the same extent as well-synchronized ventilation, because respiratory efforts are wasted.[9] Assisted ventilation is usually seen as a means of buying time for other therapies to work. However it may be a therapy in its own right, by breaking some of the above vicious cycles (Figure 27.1). For instance a slight improvement in arterial blood gas tensions and offloading of the respiratory muscles allows some recovery of respiratory muscle function, which in turn facilitates the return to the *status quo ante*.

PHYSIOLOGIC EFFECTS OF NIV

Physiologically NIV is little different to invasive mechanical ventilation; positive pressure is delivered to the lungs, but because of difficulties in getting a perfect seal with the mask it is theoretically less efficient than invasive ventilation. On the other hand the fact that NIV is relatively less efficient may be to its advantage. Barotrauma such as pneumothorax is not uncommon with ventilation after intubation but it has not been reported in any of the major studies of NIV, perhaps due to the lack of a perfect seal acting as a safety valve preventing high pressures being transmitted to the lungs. NIV decreases inspiratory muscle effort and respiratory rate and increases tidal volumes and oxygen saturation in stable COPD patients[10,11] and during an acute exacerbation.[12] A greater reduction in the sensation of dyspnea, measured by a visual analog scale, in NIV-treated patients compared to the conventionally treated patients,[13] also suggests significant unloading of the respiratory muscles by NIV. NIV increases PaO_2 and decreases $PaCO_2$.[14,15] For the same FIO_2 the alveolar-arterial oxygen difference ($AaDO_2$) increases due to a rise in clearance of CO_2 and hence increased respiratory exchange ratio, but there appears to be no improvement in VA/Q ratio with NIV.[15]

Airway obstruction may cause the development of PEEPi because alveolar emptying is incomplete by the end of expiration. Gas flow into the alveoli occurs only when the pressure within them falls below the pressure at the mouth and nose. In the presence of PEEPi, there is an inspiratory threshold load and the first part of each inspiratory effort is wasted because gas decompression occurs without airflow. This increases the work of breathing and decreases ventilatory efficiency. It may also increase patient–ventilator asynchrony because inspiratory efforts are not sufficient to trigger the ventilator during assisted modes of ventilation.[9,16] The addition of extrinsic PEEP (PEEPe or EPAP) to counterbalance intrinsic PEEP results in a greater reduction in the work of breathing for the same level of pressure support.[17] The addition of PEEPe may also have other important beneficial effects. It lavages CO_2 from the mask[18] and helps to stabilize the upper airway in patients who develop obstruction during sleep.

NIV may have potentially deleterious effects upon cardiac function in some patients. In contrast to mechanical ventilation via endotracheal tube however, hemodynamic collapse is rarely seen during NIV for acute ventilatory failure. This probably relates to the fact that anesthetic agents are not needed and positive pressure changes within the thorax are less marked. Ambrosino et al.[19] demonstrated a small reduction in cardiac output and oxygen delivery with pressure support ventilation via nasal mask when PEEP was added; in some patients this fact may be critical in determining the success or otherwise of the technique.

EVIDENCE BASE FOR NIV IN ACUTE EXACERBATIONS OF COPD (Table 27.1)

Severe exacerbations (mean pH < 7.30)

Case series of the use of NIV in acute exacerbations of COPD were followed by a number of prospective randomized controlled trials. Brochard et al.[20] showed that NIV for patients with exacerbations of COPD in the ICU reduced the intubation and mortality rates compared to conventional medical therapy. NIV also improved pH, PaO_2, respiratory rate and encephalopathy score at 1 hour and was associated with a shorter hospital stay (23 days vs. 35 days, $P = 0.005$) and a lower complication rate (16% vs. 48%, $P = 0.001$). Most of the excess mortality and complications, particularly pneumonia, were attributed to endotracheal intubation (ETI). On the face of it these data suggest that NIV may be superior to intermittent mandatory ventilation, but importantly this was a highly selected group of patients with the majority (70%) of potentially eligible patients excluded from the study.

In a smaller study ($n = 31$) in two North American ICUs Kramer et al.[21] showed a marked reduction in intubation rate, particularly in the subgroup with COPD. However mortality, hospital stay and charges were unaffected. Those enroled had a severe exacerbation, as evidenced by a mean pH of 7.28. In a further ICU study Celikel et al.[22] showed a more rapid improvement in various physiologic parameters, but there was no difference in intubation rate or survival. However some patients randomized to standard therapy subsequently received NIV and there was a significant reduction in treatment failure rate, defined as the need for ventilatory support; at the time of failure all patients had a decrement in pH.

Martin et al.[23] in a prospective randomized controlled trial comparing NIV with usual medical care in 61 patients, including 23 with COPD showed, in common with other studies, that there was a significant reduction

Table 27.1 Prospective randomized controlled trials of NIV in acute exacerbations of COPD

	Disease (n)	Setting	Baseline data pH or PaO_2/FIO_2	ETI or 'surrogate'	Mortality
Severe exacerbations					
Brochard et al.[20]	COPD[85]	ICU	7.28 vs. 7.27	**11/43 vs. 31/42**	**4/43 vs. 12/42**
Kramer et al.[21]	Mixed COPD[23]	ICU	7.28 vs. 7.27	**31% vs. 73%**	1/16 vs. 2/15
			7.29 vs. 7.27	**9% vs. 67%**	
Celikel et al.[22]	COPD[30]	ICU	7.27 vs. 7.28	**1/16 vs. 6/15**	0/15 vs. 1/15
Martin et al.[23]	COPD[23]	ICU	7.27 vs. 7.28	**6.4 vs. 21.3/100**	2.4 vs. 4.27/100
	Non COPD[38]		103 vs. 110	ICU days	ICU days
Moderately severe exacerbations					
Bott et al.[13]	COPD[60]	Ward	7.35	0/30 vs. 5/30	3/30 vs. 9/30
Barbe et al.[32]	COPD[24]	ER and ward	7.33	0/12 vs. 0/12	0/12 vs. 0/12
Angus et al.[29]	COPD[17]	Ward	7.31 vs. 7.30	0/9 vs. 5/8	0/9 vs. 3/8
Wood et al.[34]	Mixed[27] COPD[6]	ER	7.35 vs. 7.34	7/16 vs. 5/11	4/16 vs. 0/11
Bardi et al.[30]	COPD[30]	Ward	7.36 vs. 7.39	1/15 vs. 2/15	0/15 vs. 1/15
Plant et al.[31]	COPD[236]	Ward	7.32 vs. 7.31	**15% vs. 27%**	**10% vs. 20%**

ER: emergency room; ICU: intensive care unit; **Bold** text indicates $p < 0.05$.

in intubation rate (6.4 vs. 21.3 intubations per 100 ICU days, $p = 0.002$). However there was no difference in mortality (2.4 vs. 4.3 deaths per 100 ICU days, $p = 0.21$). Although the intubation rate was lower in the COPD subgroup (5.3 vs. 15.6 intubations per 100 ICU days, $p = 0.12$) this did not reach statistical significance; this may simply reflect the small sample size. Three patients in the NIV group and one in the control group required ETI to maximize the safety of other procedures (e.g. bronchoscopy) and two patients in the NIV group required ETI because of hemodynamic compromise related to massive gastrointestinal bleeding. All other patients required ETI because of progressive ventilatory failure; in other words only four of the intubations in the NIV group were because of a failure to control respiratory failure compared with 16 in the control group.

It is important to note that there is no direct comparison between intermittent mandatory ventilation and NIV and the two techniques should be viewed as complementary, with NIV considered a means of obviating the need for ETI rather than as a direct alternative. These studies, performed on ICUs show that NIV is possible and that the prevention of ETI is advantageous. A reduction in the incidence of nosocomial infection is a consistent and important advantage of NIV compared with intermittent mandatory ventilation.[24,25] In intubated patients there is a 1% risk per day of developing nosocomial pneumonia.[26] This complication of invasive ventilation is associated with a longer ICU stay, increased costs and a worse outcome.[27] The reduction in nosocomial infections is probably the most important advantage of avoiding ETI using NIV.

Moderately severe exacerbations (mean pH 7.30–7.35)

It has been suggested that NIV should be introduced when the pH falls below 7.35[28] and the evidence for the effectiveness of NIV in these less severely affected patients is now reviewed. Bott et al.[13] randomized 60 patients with COPD to either conventional treatment or NIV on a general ward. NIV initiation, by research staff, took 90 minutes on average (range 15 mins to 4 hrs) and it led to a more rapid correction of pH and $PaCO_2$. On an intention to treat analysis there was no significant benefit from NIV, but when those unable to tolerate NIV were excluded a significant survival benefit was seen (9/30 vs. 1/26, $p = 0.014$). The high mortality rate (30%) in the control group was surprising considering that the mean pH was only 7.34. In addition the low intubation rate, while probably reflecting UK practice, has been criticized.

Angus et al.[29] compared NIV and doxapram in patients with COPD and type II respiratory failure in a small randomized trial on a general ward. NIV resulted in a significant improvement in both PaO_2 and $PaCO_2$ at 4 hours. By contrast, no fall in $PaCO_2$ occurred in those patients treated with doxapram and an initial improvement in PaO_2 was not sustained at 4 hours. At both 1 and 4 hours pH was significantly better in the NIV group as compared with the doxapram group. All the patients in the NIV group were discharged home, although one required doxapram in addition to NIV during their acute illness. Three out of eight patients in the doxapram group died and a further two received NIV. This small study suggests that NIV is more effective than doxapram in the treatment of respiratory failure associated with COPD. However no comparisons were made of nursing workload, patient tolerance or complication rates between the two groups.

Bardi et al.[30] found no significant differences in hospital outcome between NIV and conventional therapy in a study of 30 patients with COPD, with the majority of patients in both groups recovering without the need for invasive ventilation. Because they did not have an ICU on site NIV was started early and given the fact the mean pH in the two groups were 7.36 and 7.39 and no patient in either group had a pH less than 7.30 these results are not surprising. However a surprising finding was that the outcome in the patients who had received NIV was better than in those who had not at 3, 6 and 12 months. Although at admission there was no difference between the two groups in FEV_1, at discharge that in the NIV treated group was 49.4% predicted and in the standard therapy group 40.5%; it seems unlikely that this increase in FEV_1 was an effect of NIV and more probably that these patients had less severe chronic disease. Furthermore a number of the patients who died had significant coexistent disease.

A multicenter randomized controlled trial of NIV in acute exacerbations of COPD ($n = 236$) on general respiratory wards in 13 centers has recently been reported.[31] NIV was applied by the usual ward staff, using a bilevel device in spontaneous mode according to a simple protocol. NIV led to a fall in respiratory rate and a more rapid improvement in pH associated with a statistically non-significant fall in $PaCO_2$. 'Treatment failure', defined by a priori criteria, a surrogate for the need for intubation, was reduced from 27 to 15% by NIV ($p < 0.05$). In-hospital mortality was also reduced from 20 to 10% ($p < 0.05$). Subgroup analysis suggested that the outcome in patients with pH less than 7.30 after initial treatment was inferior to that in the studies performed in the ICU. NIV led to a more rapid relief of breathlessness. The median time to relief of breathlessness was 4 days in the NIV group and 7 days in the standard group. However NIV neither delayed nor expedited patient mobility or nutritional intake. NIV led to a modest increase in nursing workload in the first 8 hours of the admission, equating to 26 minutes. No difference was identified after

8 hours. The median length of stay was the same for both groups at 10 days (range standard group 2–119, NIV group 4–137, $p = 0.269$). No statistically significant differences were identified in discharge blood gases on air or spirometry. This study suggests that, with adequate staff training, NIV can be applied with benefit outside the ICU by the usual ward staff and that the early introduction of NIV on a general ward results in a better outcome than providing no ventilatory support for acidotic patients outside the ICU.

Barbe et al.[32] initiated NIV in the emergency department in patients presenting with an acute exacerbation of COPD and continued it on a general ward. To ease some of the problems of workload and compliance NIV was administered for 3 hours twice a day. In this small study ($n = 24$) there were no intubations nor deaths in either group and arterial blood gas tensions improved equally in both the NIV group and in the controls. However the mean pH at entry in each group was 7.33 and at this level of acidosis significant mortality is not expected; in other words it was unlikely that such a small study would show an improved outcome when recovery would be expected anyway.[33]

Wood et al.[34] randomized 27 patients with acute respiratory distress, due to a variety of different conditions, to conventional treatment or NIV in the emergency department. Intubation rates were similar (7/16 vs. 5/11) but there was a non-significant trend towards increased mortality in those given NIV (4/16 vs. 0/11, $p = 0.123$). The authors attributed the excess mortality to delay in intubation as conventional patients requiring invasive ventilation were intubated after a mean of 4.8 hours compared to 26 hours in those on NIV ($p = 0.055$). It is difficult to draw many conclusions from this study given its small size, the fact that the numbers of patients in each group were different and that the patients were not matched for etiology of respiratory failure. Another possible reason why these studies in which NIV was initiated in the emergency room[32,34] both failed to show any advantage to NIV over conventional therapy includes the fact that patients are usually admitted to ICU when other therapies have failed whereas most of those presenting to the emergency room have not received any treatment. A proportion are going to improve after initiation of standard medical therapy. In a 1-year period prevalence study[35] of patients with acute exacerbations of COPD of 954 patients admitted through the emergency rooms in Leeds, 20% were acidotic on arrival in the department and of these 25% had completely corrected their pH by the time of arrival on the ward. There was a weak relationship between the PaO_2 on arrival at hospital and the presence of acidosis, suggesting that in at least some patients, respiratory acidosis had been precipitated by high flow oxygen therapy administered in the ambulance on the way to hospital.

Long-term effects of NIV for acute exacerbations

The avoidance of intubation may have beneficial effects in the longer term. Confalonieri et al.[36] looked at the outcome up to 1 year in 24 patients who received NIV during their acute exacerbation of COPD and compared this with that in 24 well-matched historical controls. Mean admission pH was 7.29 and all were hypoxic and hypercapnic. The survival at 1 year was 71% in the NIV group compared with 50% in the controls. Further days in hospital during that year with exacerbations were also significantly lower in the NIV group (7 + 10 vs. 25 + 22 days, $P = 0.003$). These findings were confirmed in another retrospective study[37] comparing face mask ventilation with ETI and intermittent mandatory ventilation. Although no differences were seen in in-hospital survival there was a marked difference at 3 (23 vs. 48% mortality) and 12 (30 vs. 63% mortality) months favoring the non-invasive approach. In addition the number of new ICU admissions during the follow-up at 1 year was reduced in those ventilated non-invasively (0.12 vs. 0.30, $p < 0.05$). Within each group 1-year mortality was greater ($p < 0.01$) in patients with pneumonia. Imperfect matching is one possible explanation but patients who are intubated and mechanically ventilated may lose a considerable amount of muscle bulk[38] rendering them susceptible to further episodes of ventilatory failure. The observation of a better long-term outcome with NIV needs to be confirmed in further prospective trials. Longer-term follow-up from the YONIV study[39] failed to show any statistically significant benefit from NIV compared with conventional therapy, though importantly the study showed a median survival in both groups of over a year indicating that the patients salvaged by NIV were not just those who had a very poor prognosis. It may be significant that few patients in either group were intubated and ventilated and this is an important difference when compared with the studies mentioned above.

WEANING AND THE TREATMENT OF POST-EXTUBATION RESPIRATORY FAILURE

Some patients require ETI and intermittent mandatory ventilation from the outset or after a failed trial of NIV, and in this situation NIV may have a role. Nava et al.[40] performed a prospective multicenter randomized controlled trial of the use of NIV as a means of weaning patients with COPD, who had failed a T-piece weaning trial after 48 hours of ETI, controlled mechanical ventilation and aggressive suctioning to clear secretions. Fifty-six per cent of the patients had required ETI on presentation and 44% after a failed trial of NIV (mean pH at presentation = 7.18). If patients failed the weaning trial they were randomized to further intubation and mechanical ventilation or NIV. NIV was associated with a shorter duration of ventilatory support (10.2 days vs. 16.6 days), a shorter ITU stay (15.1 days vs. 24 days), less nosocomial pneumonia (0/25 vs. 7/25) and an improved 60-day survival (92% vs. 72%). Girault et al.[41] in a further randomized controlled trial involving 33 patients showed a reduction in the duration of invasive mechanical ventilation (4.6 + 1.9 vs. 7.7 + 3.8 days) and a reduced mean daily ventilatory support, but an increased total duration (11.5 + 5.2 vs. 3.5 + 1.4 days) of ventilatory support when the non-invasive approach was used. There was no difference in percentage of patients successfully weaned or in complication rates.

A proportion of patients weaned from invasive ventilation subsequently deteriorate and require further ventilatory support. Hilbert et al.[42] reported 30 patients with COPD who developed hypercapnic respiratory distress within 72 hours of extubation. They were treated with mask bilevel pressure support ventilation. Only six of these 30 patients as compared to 20 of 30 historical controls required reintubation. Although in hospital mortality was not significantly different, the mean duration of ventilatory assistance and length of intensive care stay related to the event were significantly shortened by NIV.

The use of NIV opens up new opportunities in the management of patients with ventilatory failure, particularly with regard to location and the timing of intervention. With NIV paralysis and sedation are not needed and ventilation outside the ICU is an option; given the considerable pressure on ICU beds in some countries, the high costs and that for some patients admission to ICU is a distressing experience[43] this is an attractive option. The largest study[31] suggests that early intervention is advantageous, certainly before ETI would normally be considered necessary. In patients not suitable for NIV from the outset or those who fail, ETI for 24–48 hours to gain control and then early extubation onto NIV has significant advantages over prolonged endotracheal intubation.

LIMITATIONS OF NIV AND PREDICTION OF OUTCOME (Table 27.2)

A number of contraindications to NIV have been suggested.[44] Some of these are self evident such as severe facial deformity or trauma, which prevent effective mask application. Others are primarily for theoretical reasons and because patients with these features have been excluded from previous studies and not because there is any evidence that intermittent mandatory ventilation is superior in these situations; they include coma or confusion, upper gastrointestinal bleeding, high risk of aspiration, excessive secretions, hemodynamic instability or uncontrolled arrhythmia. The issue of whether patients should receive a trial of NIV in these circumstances will depend upon the individual situation; for instance if intubation has been refused or is considered inappropriate there is little to be lost by a trial of NIV.

Attempts to predict which patients can be managed successfully with NIV yield conflicting results. Acidosis is an indicator of the severity of decompensation in acute on chronic ventilatory failure and has been shown to predict death in a number of studies of acute exacerbations of COPD.[13,33,45,46] It is therefore a logical starting point for identifying patients who might benefit from NIV. In a retrospective review aimed at identifying patients with COPD who could be successfully treated with NIV, Ambrosino et al.[47] found that patients with COPD failing NIV were significantly more acidotic at baseline compared with those successfully treated (pH 7.22 (SD 0.08) vs. 7.28 (SD 0.04), $p < 0.005$). Although using a discriminant analysis a number of variables had a predictive value of more than 0.80 for successful NIV, when tested together using logistic regression analysis, only baseline pH maintained a significant predictive effect with a sensitivity of 97% and specificity of 71%. Brochard et al.,[20] using a priori criteria for the need for intubation, found that success was less likely the lower the starting pH. In the study of Plant et al.[39] $[H^+]$ (OR 1.22 per nmol/L 95% CI 1.09–1.37, $p < 0.01$) and $PaCO_2$ (OR 1.14 per kPa 95% CI 1.14–1.81, $p < 0.01$) at enrollment were associated with treatment failure. Analysis of subgroups stratified according to admission pH showed a worse outcome with NIV delivered according to a simple protocol and not individually adjusted to the patients' requirements if the pH was < 7.3 (Figure 27.2). Allocation to NIV was still protective (OR 0.39, 95% CI 0.19–0.80). A number of studies have failed to show any

Table 27.2 Limitations of NIV and prediction of outcome

Relative contraindications to NIV	NIV less likely to be successful if:
Severe facial deformity or trauma	Severe acidosis
Coma or confusion	Reduced level of conciousness
Upper gastrointestinal bleeding	Presence of comorbidity
High risk of aspiration	Poor tolerance
Excessive secretions	Large mask leak
Hemodynamic instability	Edentulous patient
Uncontrolled arrhythmia	No improvement in blood gas tensions after a period of NIV
	No fall in respiratory rate with NIV
	Low activities of daily living score

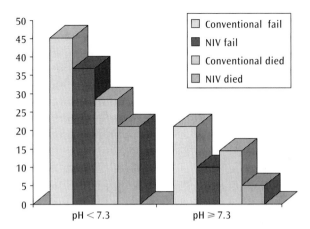

Figure 27.2 *Outcome with simple protocol delivered NIV on a general ward. (Reproduced from ref. 31 with permission.)*

relationship between baseline arterial blood gas tensions and the response to NIV.[48–53]

The severity of the illness at presentation, as judged by the APACHE II scores, has been shown to be greater in patients who failed NIV compared with those who were successfully treated in two studies (21 ± 4 vs. 15 ± 4 p = 0.02[50], 29 ± 4 vs. 18 ± 4 p < 0.0001[47]). However these results are not supported by other studies.[48,52,53] Using the Simplified Acute Physiology Score (SAPS) Benhamou *et al.*[49] also found no difference between successful and unsuccessful NIV in their study of elderly patients with acute respiratory failure (ARF) and a number of different underlying lung pathologies. It has been suggested that an altered level of consciousness is a contraindication to NIV,[54] though this is largely for theoretical reasons and because such patients have usually been excluded from clinical trials. However a better level of consciousness at baseline[47,53] and after 1 hour of NIV[53] has been shown to correlate with success. Brochard *et al.*[20] noted that the encephalopathy score dropped significantly in patients successfully treated with NIV during the course of their treatment. However three other studies have shown no such relationship.[49,52,55]

A number of other factors such as age, severity of airways obstruction, body weight and the presence of comorbid disease might be expected to have an influence upon outcome. Age however is not a bar to NIV, which has been used successfully in the elderly.[49] Ambrosino *et al.*[47] found that underweight patients did less well with NIV and that the FVC was significantly lower in patients failing with NIV. However surprisingly in another study Anton *et al.*[53] found that a successful outcome with NIV was more likely with a lower FEV$_1$ (27% predicted ± 11 vs. 38 ± 11 p < 0.01). The cause of the acute exacerbation is also not a reliable predictor of outcome from NIV.[47–50,53] In two studies[47,50] radiological consolidation was more common in the group failing NIV, but in a

prospective randomized controlled trial evaluating NIV against conventional treatment in patients with pneumonia, Confalonieri *et al.*[56] found that in the subgroup of patients who also had COPD the 2-month survival was better in the NIV group.

Once NIV has been started progress with treatment may indicate the likely outcome. Not surprisingly the ability of the patients to tolerate NIV is a factor. Benhamou *et al.*[49] found that 'tolerance' of NIV was the only factor of prognostic value. Ambrosino *et al.*[47] also found that better compliance was associated with a greater likelihood of success with NIV and in their prospective case series of 12 patients with hypercapnic ARF Soo Hoo *et al.*[50] noted that successfully treated patients were able to tolerate NIV for longer than the patients who could not be successfully treated with NIV. Larger volumes of air leak were noted in patients who failed with NIV[50] and these patients also tended to be edentulous and to breathe through pursed lips.

A number of studies have shown that the change in arterial blood gas tensions, particularly pH, after a short period of NIV predicts a successful outcome.[13,20,39,47,48,50,51] An improvement in pH and/or PaCO_2 at 30 minutes,[52] 1 hour[51] or after a longer period[50,51] predict successful NIV. In the YONIV study improvement in acidosis (OR 0.89 per nmol/L 95% CI 0.82–0.97, p < 0.01) and fall in respiratory rate (OR 0.92 per breath/min 95% CI 0.84–0.99, P = 0.04) after 4 hours of therapy were associated with success.[39]

Patients who have been intubated and are likely to fail a weaning attempt adopt a pattern of rapid shallow breathing when disconnected from the ventilator,[57] indicating that they are breathing against an unsustainable load. A reduction in respiratory rate with NIV has been variably shown in a number of studies, with larger falls generally being associated with a successful outcome from NIV,[20,50,51] though this is not always seen.[53] In the absence of a priori criteria for endotracheal intubation it is not surprising that a failure of commonly measured physiologic variables to improve prompts an escalation of therapy, which in this case is a switch to invasive ventilation.

Patients failing NIV do not exclusively fail shortly after initiation of NIV. Late failure (after 48 hours of successful NIV) is recognized, with rates reported at 0–20% and has been associated with poor outcomes. In a study of 137 patients admitted with COPD and acute hypercapnic respiratory failure initially successfully treated with NIV, 23% deteriorated after 48 hours of NIV.[58] These so-called 'late failures' were then assigned to either an increased number of hours of NIV (the mean number of hours/day of NIV at the time of late failure was 9.2) or intubation and mechanical ventilation depending on the patients'/relatives' wishes. Importantly it should be noted that patients assigned to increased NIV did significantly worse with a mortality of 92% compared with 53% in those invasively ventilated. At the time of relapse those patients treated with increased NIV were more acidotic than those who were intubated (pH 7.1 vs. pH 7.29). Although this difference was not statistically significant and may just reflect the small number of patients, this suggests that the patients who were treated with increased NIV were sicker than those who were intubated. There is also the possibility that patients who were not intubated were self selected as a group with more advanced disease, since they were not offered or declined ETI. The 3-month survival after hospital discharge between the initial successes and late failures were similar, indicating that the acute event itself did not signify a worse long-term outcome.

At the time of admission 'late failures' had significantly lower activities of daily living (ADL) scores and blood pressure, were more tachycardic and more likely to have associated complications, in particular hyperglycemia. pH was not different between the groups at admission, at 1 hour or 24 hours. Using logistic regression analysis a low pH, a low ADL score and the presence of associated complications at admission were more likely in patients who failed after 48 hours or longer of NIV. Neither the APACHE II score nor age were predictive of failure.

CHOICE OF VENTILATOR AND INTERFACE

Ventilators usually used for NIV are either volume or pressure targeted. There are theoretical advantages to each mode, but broadly speaking they are comparable in efficacy. Volume-targeted ventilators have been shown to produce more complete offloading of the respiratory muscles, but at the expense of comfort.[59] In intubated patients however assist pressure controlled ventilation has been shown to be more effective than assist control volume ventilation at reducing various parameters of respiratory muscle effort, though this difference was only seen at moderate tidal volumes and low flow rates.[60] In stable patients little difference in gas exchange was seen with different types of ventilator.[11,61] In terms of outcome Vitacca et al.[62] found that there was no difference whether volume-targeted or pressure-targeted machines were used, but pressure-targeted machines were better tolerated by patients.

A new mode of proportional assist ventilation (PAV) improves gas exchange and dyspnea in stable COPD[63] and has been used successfully in the treatment of acute respiratory failure of various etiologies.[64] PAV delivers ventilation according to patient demand, which should theoretically be more comfortable, but makes the assumption that the patient with respiratory failure knows best what he/she needs in terms of ventilatory support. PAV using flow assistance and PEEP achieved greatest improvement in minute ventilation, dyspnea and reduction in pressure time product per breath of the respiratory muscles and diaphragm in patients of COPD with acute respiratory failure.[65] It has been shown to decrease patient effort and work of breathing and neuromuscular drive ($P_{0.1}$) in patients with COPD being weaned off invasive mechanical ventilation.[66,67] Further data are needed comparing PAV with conventional modes of ventilation to establish whether these physiological advantages translate into improved outcomes. Pressure-cycled machines are usually cheaper than volume-cycled flow generators and this together with the fact that they tend to be better tolerated makes them the machines of first choice. In addition most of the randomized controlled trials have used pressure-cycled machines.

The ideal machine for non-invasively ventilating patients with COPD should be able to compensate well for leaks,[68] have a sensitive and responsive trigger (usually flow triggered[69]), be used in assist control mode and have the facility to add extrinsic PEEP, for the reasons outlined above. In-built monitoring is advantageous and is a feature of the new generation of portable ventilators available for use in the acute situation.

The choice of interface is critical to the success of NIV. A wide variety are now available and there are little data to base recommendations upon. Nasal and full-face masks from a variety of manufacturers or customized to the individual have been used in published studies. Mouth pieces have also been described when NIV is initiated as a means of acclimatizing the patient to the sensation of positive pressure.[64] Only one study[70] has compared the physiological effects of different masks in patients with chronic respiratory failure. A nasal mask was better tolerated than nasal plugs or full-face mask and $PaCO_2$ was significantly lower with a full-face mask or nasal plugs than with a nasal mask. Minute ventilation was significantly higher with a full-face mask than with a nasal mask because of an increase in tidal volume. The most important factor will be patient preference and physiogonomy. In the acute situation a full-face mask is often necessary at the outset because of the tendency of patients with an acute exacerbation of COPD to mouth breathe.

LONG-TERM NIV IN CHRONIC VENTILATORY FAILURE DUE TO COPD

A number of studies have shown that NIV is feasible at home during sleep in patients with COPD[71–77] and bronchiectasis[78] and that abnormal physiology can be corrected using NIV; gas exchange during sleep can be improved,[72] excessive respiratory muscle activation reduced[9,10] and exercise capacity and diurnal arterial blood gas tensions can be improved.[72,76] Use of healthcare resources is also reduced.[77]

However there have been few controlled trials and most of these had small numbers of patients followed over a short period of time. Strumpf et al.[79] performed a randomized controlled crossover study in 19 patients with COPD and found that seven were unable to tolerate the nasal mask and a further five withdrew because of intercurrent illness. In the seven who did complete the study, there were significant differences only in the neuropsychologic testing. Acclimatization was performed as an outpatient, but with regular visits from a respiratory therapists and ventilation was assessed during wakefulness by measurement of end tidal CO_2 tensions, though this measure is unreliable in patients with severe COPD. No measurements were made during sleep and it is therefore difficult to come to any definite conclusions since adequate ventilation was not confirmed. In addition the patients were not particularly hypercapnic (mean $PaCO_2$ 46 mmHg).

Meecham Jones et al.[80] performed a similarly designed crossover study of the use of nasal pressure support ventilation and oxygen with oxygen alone and showed statistically significant improvements in daytime arterial blood gas tensions, sleep quality and quality of life during the pressure support limb of the study. The improvement in daytime $PaCO_2$ correlated with a reduction in overnight transcutaneous CO_2. Lin[81] studied 12 patients in a prospective randomized crossover study of oxygen alone, NIV alone and oxygen plus NIV each for 2 weeks. There were no differences in tidal volume, minute volume, spirometry, diurnal arterial blood gas tensions, mouth pressures or ventilatory drive. Sleep efficiency was worse during NIV than with oxygen alone. However the maximum tolerated inspiratory pressure ranged from only 8 cmH_2O to a maximum of 15 cmH_2O. No data were given about the effect of NIV on blood gas tensions during ventilation and there was no statistically significant improvement in sleep hypoventilation with NIV. Given this it is perhaps not surprising that no effect on daytime function was seen. Gay et al.[82] randomized 13 clinically stable patients with severe COPD and daytime hypercapnia ($PaCO_2 > 45$ mmHg) to NIV ($n = 7$) or sham ($n = 6$) treatment, consisting of nightly use of a bilevel positive airway pressure device set to deliver an inspiratory positive airway pressure (IPAP) either 10 or 20 cmH_2O. The device was used in the spontaneous or timed mode and set to an EPAP of 2 cmH_2O. Patients underwent extensive physiologic testing including polysomnography and were introduced to the bilevel PAP system during a 2.5-day hospital stay. However only four patients in the NIV group were still using it at the completion of the 3-month trial, as opposed to all six patients in

the sham group. Only one patient had a significant reduction in diurnal $PaCO_2$. Compared with the positive study[80] in which the mean level of IPAP was 18 cmH_2O the level of IPAP in this study was very modest and may explain the absence of benefit; during overnight polysomnography transcutaneous PCO_2 was not measured and there was no change in mean or nadir SaO_2 which lends support to this hypothesis. Importantly two patients in the sham group reported that their breathing considerably improved despite unchanged results of the objective measures suggesting a significant placebo effect.

Case series of patients with COPD[74,75] suggest survival comparable to that seen in the oxygen-treated patients in the MRC and NOTT studies.[83–85] Although direct comparison cannot be made with historical controls from 20 years ago, it is important to note that the patients with COPD selected for home ventilation were often those who had 'failed' (not rigorously defined) on oxygen therapy and were usually hypercapnic. A number of studies suggest that hypercapnia is a poor prognostic sign.[83,86,87] The MRC study suggested that the presence of hypercapnia was a marker for a lack of benefit from oxygen therapy.[83] On the other hand a study from Japan of 4552 patients with obstructive lung disease did not show any difference in outcome between patients with hypercapnia and those who were normocapnic;[88] indeed hypercapnic patients who had had a thoracoplasty had a better prognosis than those who were normocapnic. It is therefore possible that the patients with a better prognosis are being selected out for home NIV.

The exact place of NIV in chronic ventilatory failure secondary to COPD remains unclear and needs to be evaluated by further large randomized controlled trials with clearly defined end-points. Long-term oxygen therapy (LTOT) is one of only two interventions which have been shown to prolong life in patients with COPD and remains the gold standard for the treatment of ventilatory failure due to COPD. Preliminary results from two multicenter European trials comparing NIV with LTOT in COPD suggest that NIV does not improve survival, but may reduce the need for hospitalization.[89,90]

Until further data are available a trial of NIV can only at present be justified in patients who have symptoms of nocturnal hypoventilation (morning headaches, daytime sleepiness, etc.) despite maximal bronchodilator therapy or cannot tolerate LTOT, even with careful administration using Venturi masks or a low flowmeter. It should also be considered in patients with intractable peripheral edema, because of possible beneficial effects of reducing $PaCO_2$ upon renal blood flow,[91] or repeated episodes of hospitalization with hypercapnic ventilatory failure. Most studies suggest that it is the patients with more severe hypercapnia who are likely to benefit and there is no place for nocturnal NIV, at present, in those without sustained daytime hypercapnia. Adequate control of nocturnal hypoventilation should be confirmed since this has been a feature of the studies in which benefit has been seen.[72,80]

CONCLUSIONS AND RECOMMENDATIONS
(Table 27.3)

There is now a robust evidence base for the use of NIV in acute exacerbations of COPD. Benefit has been shown when NIV is started when the pH is less than 7.35 after initial therapy has had a chance to work. It should be appreciated however that most patients with a pH between 7.30 and 7.35 will get better without the addition of NIV. However only 10 patients need to be treated to prevent one intubation and the advantages of starting NIV before the patient is severely acidotic outweigh any disadvantages.[31] Once the pH drops below 7.30 the prognosis is much worse.[20,31] It is reasonable therefore not to push NIV too hard on the patient who finds it difficult to tolerate if the pH is between 7.30 and 7.35. However once the pH drops below 7.30 the need for NIV becomes more pressing and it should be strongly encouraged, even if the patient does not like it very much, since the alternative is the need for intubation and possible death. The more acidotic the patient is from the outset the less likely a successful outcome and late failure is more likely in those with poor functional status and significant comorbidities. The response to an initial trial of NIV is a reasonably good predictor of subsequent outcome and will help to determine when NIV should be abandoned in favor of ETI and invasive ventilation. If the patient requires intubation, either from the outset or after a failed trial of NIV, early extubation onto NIV should be considered. The best location for an acute NIV service is dependent upon local factors, but staff expertise and training are critical. The place of home NIV in patients with COPD requires further evaluation.

Table 27.3 *Recommendations for non-invasive ventilation (NIV) in acute exacerbations of COPD*

NIV not attempted or failed and invasive ventilation commenced
> **Consider early extubation onto NIV**

pH < 7.3 after initial treatment – high incidence of need for IMV and risk of death
> **NIV strongly advocated, even if tolerance poor**

pH 7.30–7.35 after initial treatment – reduced need for intubation, improved survival and more rapid relief of breathlessness has been demonstrated. However majority of patients will get better without NIV
> **NIV recommended, but not mandatory if poorly tolerated**

REFERENCES

1. Macklem PT. Hyperinflation. *Am Rev Respir Dis* 1984; **129**:1–2.
2. Ionescu AA, Chatham K, Davies CA, Nixon LS, Enright S, Shale DJ. Inspiratory muscle function and body composition in cystic fibrosis. *Am J Respir Crit Care Med* 1998;**158**:1271–6.
3. Decramer M, Stas KJ. Corticosteroid-induced myopathy involving respiratory muscles in patients with chronic obstructive pulmonary disease or asthma. *Am Rev Respir Dis* 1992;**146**:800–2.
4. Douglas NJ, Calverley PMA, Leggett RJE, Brash HM, Flenley DC, Brezinova V. Transient hypoxaemia during sleep in chronic bronchitis and emphysema. *Lancet* 1979;**i**:1–4.
5. Douglas NJ. Sleep in patients with chronic obstructive pulmonary disease. *Clin Chest Med* 1998;**19**:115–25.
6. Westlake EK, Simpson T, Kaye M. Carbon dioxide narcosis in emphysema. *Q J Med* 1955;**94**:155–73.
7. Moxham J. Respiratory muscle fatigue: mechanisms, evaluation and therapy. *Br J Anaesth* 1990;**65**:43–53.
8. Juan G, Calverley P, Talamo C, Schnader J, Roussos C. Effect of carbon dioxide on diaphragmatic function in human beings. *N Engl J Med* 1984;**310**:874–9.
9. Elliott MW, Mulvey DA, Moxham J, Green M, Branthwaite MA. Inspiratory muscle effort during nasal intermittent positive pressure ventilation in patients with chronic obstructive airways disease. *Anaesthesia* 1993;**48**:8–13.
10. Carrey Z, Gottfried SB, Levy RD. Ventilatory muscle support in respiratory failure with nasal positive pressure ventilation. *Chest* 1990;**97**:150–8.
11. Elliott MW, Aquilina R, Green M, Moxham J, Simonds AK. A comparison of different modes of noninvasive ventilatory support: effects on ventilation and inspiratory muscle effort. *Anaesthesia* 1994;**49**:279–83.
12. Girault C, Richard J, Chevron V, *et al.* Comparative physiological effects of noninvasive assist-control and pressure support ventilation in acute hypercapnic respiratory failure. *Chest* 1997;**111**:1639–48.
13. Bott J, Carroll MP, Conway JH, *et al.* Randomized controlled trial of nasal ventilation in acute ventilatory failure due to chronic obstructive airways disease. *Lancet* 1993;**341**:1555–7.
14. Brochard L, Isabey D, Piquet J, *et al.* Reversal of acute exacerbations of chronic obstructive lung disease by inspiratory assistance with a face mask. *N Engl J Med* 1990;**323**:1523–30.
15. Diaz O, Iglesia R, Ferrer M, *et al.* Effects of noninvasive ventilation on pulmonary gas exchange and hemodynamics during acute hypercapnic exacerbations of chronic obstructive pulmonary disease. *Am J Respir Crit Care Med* 1997;**156**:1840–5.
16. Nava S, Bruschi C, Fracchia C, Braschi A, Rubini F. Patient–ventilator interaction and inspiratory effort during pressure support ventilation in patients with different pathologies. *Eur Respir J* 1997;**10**:177–83.
17. Appendini L, Patessio A, Zanaboni S, *et al.* Physiologic effects of positive end-expiratory pressure and mask pressure support during exacerbations of chronic obstructive pulmonary disease. *Am J Respir Crit Care Med* 1994;**149**:1069–76.
18. Ferguson GT, Gilmartin M. CO_2 rebreathing during BiPAP ventilatory assistance. *Am J Respir Crit Care Med* 1995; **151**:1126–35.
19. Ambrosino N, Nava S, Torbicki A, *et al.* Haemodynamic effects of pressure support and PEEP ventilation by nasal

route in patients with stable chronic obstructive pulmonary disease. *Thorax* 1993;**48**:523–8.

20. Brochard L, Mancebo J, Wysocki M, *et al*. Noninvasive ventilation for acute exacerbations of chronic obstructive pulmonary disease. *N Engl J Med* 1995;**333**:817–22.

21. Kramer N, Meyer TJ, Meharg J, Cece RD, Hill NS. Randomized, prospective trial of noninvasive positive pressure ventilation in acute respiratory failure. *Am J Respir Crit Care Med* 1995;**151**:1799–806.

22. Celikel T, Sungur M, Ceyhan B, Karakurt S. Comparison of noninvasive positive pressure ventilation with standard medical therapy in hypercapnic acute respiratory failure. *Chest* 1998;**114**:1636–42.

23. Martin TJ, Hovis JD, Costantino JP, *et al*. A randomized, prospective evaluation of noninvasive ventilation for acute respiratory failure. *Am J Respir Crit Care Med* 2000; **161**:807–13.

24. Nourdine K, Combes P, Carton M-J, Beuret P, Cannamela A, Ducreux J-C. Does noninvasive ventilation reduce the ICU nosocomial infection risk? A prospective clinical survey. *Intens Care Med* 1999;**25**:567–73.

25. Girou E, Schortgen F, Delclaux C, *et al*. Association of noninvasive ventilation with nosocomial infections and survival in critically ill patients. *JAMA* 2000;**284**:2361–7.

26. Fagon JY, Chastre J, Hance A, Montravers P, Novara A, Gibert C. Nosocomial pneumonia in ventilated patients: a cohort study evaluating attributable mortality and hospital stay. *Am J Med* 1993;**94**:281–7.

27. Torres A, Aznar R, Gatell JM. Incidence, risk and prognosis factors of nosocomial pneumonia in mechanically ventilated patients. *Am Rev Respir Dis* 1990;**142**:523–8.

28. Baldwin DR, Allen MB. Non-invasive ventilation for acute exacerbations of chronic obstructive pulmonary disease. *Br Med J* 1997;**314**:163–4.

29. Angus RM, Ahmed AA, Fenwick LJ, Peacock AJ. Comparison of the acute effects on gas exchange of nasal ventilation and doxapram in exacerbations of chronic obstructive pulmonary disease. *Thorax* 1996;**51**:1048–50.

30. Bardi G, Pierotello R, Desideri M, Valdisseri L, Bottai M, Palla A. Nasal ventilation in COPD exacerbations: early and late results of a prospective, controlled study. *Eur Respir J* 2000;**15**:98–104.

31. Plant PK, Owen JL, Elliott MW. Early use of non-invasive ventilation for acute exacerbations of chronic obstructive pulmonary disease on general respiratory wards: a multicentre randomized controlled trial. *Lancet* 2000;**355**: 1931–5.

32. Barbe F, Togores B, Rubi M, Pons S, Maimo A, Agusti AGN. Noninvasive ventilatory support does not facilitate recovery from acute respiratory failure in chronic obstructive pulmonary disease. *Eur Respir J* 1996;**9**:1240–5.

33. Jeffrey AA, Warren PM, Flenley DC. Acute hypercapnic respiratory failure in patients with chronic obstructive lung disease: risk factors and use of guidelines for management. *Thorax* 1992;**47**:34–40.

34. Wood KA, Lewis L, Von Harz B, Kollef MH. The use of noninvasive positive pressure ventilation in the emergency department. *Chest* 1998;**113**:1339–46.

35. Plant PK, Owen J, Elliott MW. One year period prevalance study of respiratory acidosis in acute exacerbation of COPD; implications for the provision of non-invasive ventilation and oxygen administration. *Thorax* 2000;**55**:550–4.

36. Confalonieri M, Parigi P, Scartabellati A, *et al*. Noninvasive mechanical ventilation improves the immediate and long-term outcome of COPD patients with acute respiratory failure. *Eur Respir J* 1996;**9**:422–30.

37. Vitacca M, Clini E, Rubini F, Nava S, Foglio K, Ambrosino N. Non-invasive mechanical ventilation in severe chronic obstructive lung disease and acute respiratory failure: short- and long-term prognosis. *Intens Care Med* 1996; **22**:94–100.

38. Coakley JH, Nagendran K, Ormerod IE, Ferguson CN, Hinds CJ. Prolonged neurogenic weakness in patients requiring mechanical ventilation for acute airflow limitation. *Chest* 1992;**101**:1413–16.

39. Plant PK, Owen JL, Elliott MW. Non-invasive ventilation in acute exacerbations of chronic obstructive pulmonary disease: long term survival and predictors of in-hospital outcome. *Thorax* 2001;**56**:708–12.

40. Nava S, Ambrosino N, Clini E, *et al*. Noninvasive mechanical ventilation in the weaning of patients with respiratory failure due to chronic obstructive pulmonary disease. A randomized, controlled trial. *Ann Intern Med* 1998;**128**: 721–8.

41. Girault C, Daudenthun I, Chevron V, Tamion F, Leroy J, Bonmarchand G. Noninvasive ventilation as a systematic extubation and weaning technique in acute-on-chronic respiratory failure. A prospective, randomized controlled study. *Am J Respir Crit Care Med* 1999;**160**:86–92.

42. Hilbert G, Gruson D, Porel L, Gbikpi-Benissan G, Cardinaud JP. Noninvasive pressure support ventilation in COPD patients with post extubation hypercapnic respiratory insufficiency. *Eur Respir J* 1998;**11**:1349–53.

43. Easton C, MacKenzie F. Sensory-perceptual alterations: delirium in the intensive care unit. *Heart Lung* 1988; **17**:229–37.

44. Ambrosino N. Noninvasive mechanical ventilation in acute respiratory failure. *Eur Respir J* 1996;**9**:795–807.

45. Soo Hoo GW, Hakimian N, Santiago SM. Hypercapnic respiratory failure in COPD patients. *Chest* 2000;**117**:169–77.

46. Warren PM, Flenley DC, Millar JS, Avery A. Respiratory failure revisited: acute exacerbation of chronic bronchitis between 1961–68 and 1970–76. *Lancet* 1980;**i**:467–70.

47. Ambrosino N, Foglio K, Rubini F, Clini E, Nava S, Vitacca M. Non-invasive mechanical ventilation in acute respiratory failure due to chronic obstructive airways disease: correlates for success. *Thorax* 1995;**50**:755–7.

48. Meduri GU, Turner RE, Abou-Shala N, Wunderink R, Tolley E. Noninvasive postive pressure ventilation via face mask – first line intervention in patients with acute hypercapnic and hypoxemic respiratory failure. *Chest* 1996; **109**:179–93.

49. Benhamou D, Girault C, Faure C, Portier F, Muir JF. Nasal mask ventilation in acute respiratory failure. *Chest* 1992; **102**:912–17.

50. Soo Hoo GW, Santiago S, Williams AJ. Nasal mechanical ventilation for hypercapnic respiratory failure in chronic obstructive pulmonary disease: determinants of success and failure. *Crit Care Med* 1994;**22**:1253–61.

51. Meduri GU, Abou-Shala N, Fox RC, Jones CB, Leeper KV, Wunderink RG. Noninvasive face mask mechanical ventilation in patients with acute hypercapneic respiratory failure. *Chest* 1991;**100**:445–54.

52. Poponick JM, Renston JP, Bennett RP, Emerman CL. Use of a ventilatory support system (BiPAP) for acute respiratory failure in the emergency department. *Chest* 1999;**116**:166–71.

53. Anton A, Guell R, Gomez J, *et al*. Predicting the result of noninvasive ventilation in severe acute exacerbations of patients with chronic airflow limitation. *Chest* 2000;**117**: 828–33.

54. Ambrosino N. Noninvasive mechanical ventilation in acute respiratory failure. *Eur Respir J* 1996;**9**:795–807.

55. Wysocki M, Tric L, Wolff MA, Gertner J, Millet H, Herman B. Noninvasive pressure support ventilation in patients with acute respiratory failure. *Chest* 1993;**103**:907–13.

56. Confalonieri M, Potena A, Carbone G, Porta RD, Tolley EA, Meduri UG. Acute respiratory failure in patients with severe community-acquired pneumonia. A prospective randomized evaluation of noninvasive ventilation. *Am J Respir Crit Care Med* 1999;**160**:1585–91.

57. Yang KL, Tobin MJ. A prospective study of indexes predicting the outcome of trials of weaning from mechanical ventilation. *N Engl J Med* 1991;**324**:1445–50.

58. Moretti M, Cilione C, Tampieri A, Fracchia C, Marchioni A, Nava S. Incidence and causes of non-invasive mechanical ventilation failure after initial success. *Thorax* 2000;**55**:819–25.

59. Girault C, Richard JC, Chevron V, *et al.* Comparative physiologic effects of noninvasive assist-control and pressure support ventilation in acute hypercapnic respiratory failure. *Chest* 1998;**111**:1639–48.

60. Cinnella G, Conti G, Lofaso F, *et al.* Effects of assisted ventilation on the work of breathing: volume-controlled versus pressure-controlled ventilation. *Am J Respir Crit Care Med* 1996;**153**:1025–33.

61. Meecham Jones DJ, Wedzicha JA. Comparison of pressure and volume preset nasal ventilator systems in stable chronic respiratory failure. *Eur Respir J* 1993;**6**:1060–4.

62. Vitacca M, Rubini F, Foglio K, Scalvini S, Nava S, Ambrosino N. Non-invasive modalities of positive pressure ventilation improve the outcome of acute exacerbations in COLD patients. *Intens Care Med* 1993;**19**:450–5.

63. Ambrosino N, Vitacca M, Polese G, Pagani M, Foglio K, Rossi A. Short-term effects of nasal proportional assist ventilation in patients with chronic hypercapnic respiratory insufficiency. *Eur Respir J* 1997;**10**:2829–34.

64. Patrick W, Webster K, Ludwig L, Roberts D, Wiebe P, Younes M. Non-invasive positive-pressure ventilation in acute respiratory distress without prior respiratory failure. *Am J Respir Crit Care Med* 1996;**153**:1005–11.

65. Ranieri VM, Grasso S, Mascia L, *et al.* Effects of proportional assist ventilation on inspiratory muscle effort in patients with chronic obstructive pulmonary disease and acute respiratory failure. *Anaesthesiology* 1997;**86**:79–91.

66. Wrigge H, Golisch W, Zinserling J, Sydow M, Almeling G, Burchardi H. Proportional assist versus pressure support ventilation: effects on breathing pattern and respiratory work of patients with chronic obstructive pulmonary disease. *Intens Care Med* 1999;**25**:790–8.

67. Appendini L, Purro A, Gudjonsdottir M, *et al.* Physiological response of ventilator-dependent patients with chronic obstructive pulmonary disease to proportional assist ventilation and continuous positive airway pressure. *Am J Respir Crit Care Med* 1999;**159**:1510–17.

68. Bunburaphong T, Nishimura M, Kacmarek RM. Performance characteristics of bilevel pressure ventilators – a lung model study. *Chest* 1997;**111**:1050–60.

69. Nava S, Ambrosino N, Bruschi C, Confalonieri M, Rampulla C. Physiological effects of flow and pressure triggering during non-invasive mechanical ventilation in patients with chronic obstructive pulmonary disease. *Thorax* 1997;**52**:249–54.

70. Navalesi P, Fanfulla F, Frigerio P, Gregoretti C, Nava S. Physiologic evaluation of noninvasive mechanical ventilation delivered with three types of masks in patients with chronic hypercapnic respiratory failure. *Crit Care Med* 2000;**28**: 1785–90.

71. Carroll N, Branthwaite MA. Control of nocturnal hypoventilation by nasal intermittent positive pressure ventilation. *Thorax* 1988;**43**:349–53.

72. Elliott MW, Simonds AK, Carroll MP, Wedzicha JA, Branthwaite MA. Domiciliary nocturnal nasal intermittent positive pressure ventilation in hypercapnic respiratory failure due to chronic obstructive lung disease: effects on sleep and quality of life. *Thorax* 1992;**47**:342–8.

73. Marino W. Intermittent volume cycled mechanical ventilation via nasal mask in patients with respiratory failure due to COPD. *Chest* 1991;**99**:681–4.

74. Leger P, Bedicam JM, Cornette A, *et al.* Nasal intermittent positive pressure ventilation. Long-term follow-up in patients with severe chronic respiratory insufficiency. *Chest* 1994;**105**:100–5.

75. Simonds AK, Elliott MW. Outcome of domiciliary nasal intermittent positive pressure ventilation in restrictive and obstructive disorders. *Thorax* 1995;**50**:604–9.

76. Sivasothy P, Smith IE, Shneerson JM. Mask intermittent positive pressure ventilation in chronic hypercapnic respiratory failure due to chronic obstructive pulmonary disease. *Eur Respir J* 1998;**11**:34–40.

77. Jones SE, Packham S, Hebden M, Smith AP. Domiciliary nocturnal intermittent positive pressure ventilation in patients with respiratory failure due to severe COPD; long term follow up and effect on survival. *Thorax* 1998;**53**:495–8.

78. Benhamou D, Muir JF, Raspaud C, *et al.* Long-term efficiency of home nasal mask ventilation in patients with diffuse bronchiectasis and severe chronic respiratory failure: a case-control study. *Chest* 1997;**112**:1259–66.

79. Strumpf DA, Millman RP, Carlisle CC, *et al.* Nocturnal positive-pressure ventilation via nasal mask in patients with severe chronic obstructive pulmonary disease. *Am Rev Respir Dis* 1991;**144**:1234–9.

80. Meecham Jones DJ, Paul EA, Jones PW, Wedzicha JA. Nasal pressure support ventilation plus oxygen compared with oxygen therapy alone in hypercapnic COPD. *Am J Respir Crit Care Med* 1995;**152**:538–44.

81. Lin CC. Comparison between nocturnal nasal positive pressure ventilation combined with oxygen therapy and oxygen monotherapy in patients with severe COPD. *Am J Respir Crit Care Med* 1996;**154**:353–8.

82. Gay PC, Hubmayr RD, Stroetz RW. Efficacy of nocturnal nasal ventilation in stable, severe chronic obstructive pulmonary disease during a 3-month controlled trial. *Mayo Clin Proc* 1996;**71**:533–42.

83. Medical Research Council Working Party Report. Long term domiciliary oxygen therapy in chronic hypoxic cor pulmonale complicating chronic bronchitis and emphysema. *Lancet* 1981;**i**:681–5.

84. Nocturnal Oxygen Therapy Trial Group. Continuous or nocturnal oxygen therapy in hypoxaemic chronic obstructive lung disease, a clinical trial. *Ann Intern Med* 1980;**93**:391–8.

85. Hamnegard CH, Wragg SD, Mills GH, *et al.* Clinical assessment of diaphragm strength by cervical magnetic stimulation of the phrenic nerves. *Thorax* 1996;**51**:1239–42.

86. Cooper CB, Waterhouse J, Howard P. Twelve year clinical study of patients with hypoxic cor pulmonale given long term domiciliary oxygen therapy. *Thorax* 1987;**42**: 105–10.

87. Connors AF Jr, Dawson NV, Thomas C, *et al.* Outcomes following acute exacerbation of severe chronic obstructive lung disease. The SUPPORT investigators. *Am J Respir Crit Care Med* 1996;**154**:959–67.

88. Aida A, Miyamoto K, Nishimura M, *et al.* Prognostic value of hypercapnia in patients with chronic respiratory failure during long term oxygen therapy. *Am J Respir Crit Care Med* 1998;**158**:188–93.

89. Muir J F, de la Salmoniere P, Cuvelier A, Chevret S, Tengang B, Chastang C, and on behalf of the NIPPV Study Group. Survival of severe hypercapnic COPD under long term home mechanical ventilation with NIPPV + oxygen versus oxygen therapy alone: preliminary results of a European multicentre study. *Am J Respir Crit Care Med* 1999;**159**:A295.

90. Clini E, Sturani C, and on behalf of AIPO. The Italian multicentric study of non-invasive nocturnal pressure support ventilation (NPSV) in COPD patients. *Am J Respir Crit Care Med* 1999;**159**:A295.

91. Sharkey RA, Mulloy EM, O'Neill SJ. The acute effects of oxygen and carbon dioxide on renal vascular resistance in patients with an acute exacerbation of COPD. *Chest* 1999;**115**:1588–92.

28

Invasive ventilation and the intensive care unit

M JEFFERY MADOR AND WILLIAM J GIBBONS

INDICATIONS FOR INVASIVE VENTILATION

As outlined in Chapter 27, non-invasive ventilation is an important component of the care of patients with COPD and acute respiratory failure. Non-invasive ventilation is associated with fewer complications than invasive ventilation.[1] In particular, the incidence of nosocomial pneumonia is reduced during non-invasive ventilation.[2] However, a percentage of patients with COPD and acute respiratory failure are too sick on arrival for a trial of non-invasive positive-pressure ventilation. These patients require endotracheal intubation. The recommended criteria for bypassing a trial of non-invasive ventilation and going immediately to endotracheal intubation are: (i) respiratory arrest or near respiratory arrest; (ii) cardiovascular instability – hypotension, serious dysrhythmia, myocardial ischemia; (iii) inability to protect the airway; and (iv) uncooperative patient.[3] Patients with a depressed level of consciousness due to CO_2 retention will require endotracheal intubation if they are unable to protect their airway or cooperate with therapy. Non-invasive ventilation is less likely to be successful if the patient has copious secretions or severe anxiety.

In patients in whom non-invasive ventilation is tried, it will not always be successful. Between 20 and 25% of patients sick enough to require ICU admission will fail a trial of non-invasive ventilation and require invasive ventilation.[4,5] Because there are no validated criteria to determine when endotracheal intubation should take place, failure is defined somewhat arbitrarily as a lack of improvement in arterial blood gases and/or clinical status. Most patients who fail non-invasive ventilation will do so early on. However, 15–25% of patients who do well initially with non-invasive ventilation will subsequently fail.[6] Late failures are more likely to occur in patients with more severe disease, with significant comorbidities or who develop complications during their hospital stay (particularly nosocomial pneumonia). These patients do poorly particularly if intensification of non-invasive ventilation is tried rather than endotracheal intubation and invasive ventilation.

MECHANICAL VENTILATION: SUPPORT PHASE

When considering how mechanical ventilation can be used optimally, two pathophysiological events are of particular relevance in patients with COPD and acute respiratory failure: (i) inspiratory muscle fatigue and (ii) dynamic hyperinflation. Inspiratory muscle fatigue occurs when the demands imposed on the inspiratory muscles exceed their capacity (see Chapter 15). In patients with COPD and acute respiratory failure, the load faced by the inspiratory muscles is high while their capacity is reduced by hyperinflation. However, the diaphragm in patients with COPD undergoes several structural adaptations, an increased proportion of type 1 fibers, an increase in mitochondrial content and a reduction in sarcomere length, all of which will increase its fatigue resistance.[7–9] Whether overt contractile fatigue of the inspiratory muscles occurs in patients with COPD and acute respiratory failure is still unknown. Teleologically, when faced with an unsustainable load, patients can let $PaCO_2$ rise and keep inspiratory muscle work at a non-fatiguing level (central fatigue) or choose to try and maintain CO_2 homostasis at the cost of progressive contractile fatigue of the inspiratory muscles which must eventually result in failure of the inspiratory muscles with resultant progressive hypercapnia. When anesthetized animals are faced with an unsustainable load, progressive hypercapnia occurs prior to the development of diaphragmatic fatigue.[10] However anesthesia impairs the response to loading. Performing similar experiments in unanesthetized animals would be unethical. To unambiguously document contractile fatigue of the diaphragm and/or the inspiratory muscles is difficult in humans, and to obtain these measurements in patients in acute respiratory failure is virtually impossible. However, it is possible to obtain such measurements in patients before and after an unsuccessful 'weaning trial'. Since fatigue is long lasting, it is possible to obtain measurements during a period of controlled mechanical ventilation before and after the weaning trial. In a recent study, Laghi and colleagues measured twitch transdiaphragmatic pressure (TwPdi), a measure of diaphragmatic fatigue, before and after an unsuccessful weaning trial.[11] In the vast majority of patients, TwPdi was unchanged after the weaning trial indicating that diaphragmatic fatigue did not occur. Of course, a weaning trial is stopped before patients develop the severity of respiratory failure that is often seen when patients initially present to the emergency room. Thus, it remains possible that contractile fatigue of the inspiratory muscles could occur in some patients with COPD and acute respiratory failure. Because of this possibility, one of the goals of mechanical ventilation should be to reduce the patient's work of breathing. However, the work of breathing does not need to be totally eliminated. Prolonged muscle inactivity can result in muscle deconditioning and atrophy. In an anesthetized rat preparation, controlled mechanical ventilation for just 48 hours resulted in a reduction in both diaphragmatic mass and *in vitro* diaphragmatic force production.[12]

DYNAMIC HYPERINFLATION

Patients with COPD and acute respiratory failure have severe airway obstruction and decreased pulmonary elastic recoil. Maximal expiratory flow is markedly reduced

and a prolonged expiratory time is required to permit complete exhalation of inspired gas volume. These patients commonly are tachypneic and have increased ventilatory requirements. These factors result in a shortened expiratory time so that the next inspiration starts before expiration has been completed resulting in dynamic hyperinflation and an alveolar pressure that remains positive at endexpiration (auto- or intrinsic-PEEP). The resulting increase in lung volume forces the patient to breathe in the upper less compliant portion of the pressure–volume curve, thereby increasing the elastic load to breathe. Hyperinflation forces the respiratory muscles to operate at an unfavorable position on their length–tension curve. Finally, the inspiratory muscles must generate sufficient pressure to counterbalance the positive alveolar pressure at end expiration before inspiratory flow can begin.[13] Thus, auto-PEEP behaves like an inspiratory threshold load. The effect of dynamic hyperinflation can seriously compromise inspiratory muscle function and significantly increase the patient's work of breathing. Thus, a goal of mechanical ventilation should be to try and reduce dynamic hyperinflation as much as possible and in particular not to inadvertently worsen dynamic hyperinflation by an injudicious choice of settings for the ventilator.

VENTILATOR MODES

Controversy exists as to the optimal mode of ventilation. Physiologic studies have increased our understanding of patient–ventilator interaction during the different modes of ventilation. However, no study has demonstrated that the mode of ventilation used in the support phase alters patient outcome. It is our opinion that the choice of ventilator mode is of relatively minor consequence provided that the chosen mode is used in an optimal fashion.

Assist-control ventilation

During assist-control ventilation, the ventilator delivers a positive-pressure breath at a preset tidal volume when triggered by a patient's inspiratory effort (assisted ventilation). The ventilator will also deliver breaths at a preset rate (backup rate) if no patient effort occurs within a preselected time period (controlled ventilation). With this ventilator mode patients are able to set their own respiratory rate. If the patient's spontaneous rate drops below the preset backup rate, controlled ventilation will be provided until the patient's spontaneous rate exceeds the backup rate.

Despite the fact that the ventilator inflates the lung, patients still perform substantial amounts of work during assisted ventilation.[14,15] In the assist mode, the patient

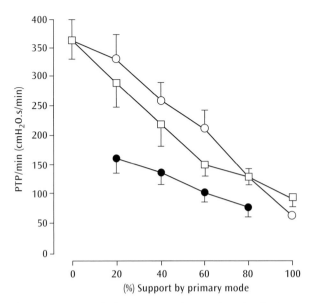

Figure 28.1 *Cumulative pressure–time product (PTP) of both triggering and non-triggering efforts (PTP/min) increased as the level of pressure support (PS) alone was decreased, or intermittent mandatory ventilation (IMV) alone was decreased, and as IMV was decreased in the presence of PS 10 cmH$_2$O (P < 0.0005 in each instance). At proportional levels of ventilator assistance, PTP/min was not different during IMV alone (open circles) and PS alone (open square) , but both were higher than that of combined IMV and PS 10 cmH$_2$O (filled circle). (Reproduced from ref. 17 with permission.)*

must generate a set negative pressure to trigger the ventilator to deliver gas into the inspiratory circuit. Measurement of the diaphragmatic electromyogram shows that patients are unable to stop their inspiratory effort once the ventilator is triggered, rather effort continues throughout inspiration.[16] In one study, in which the majority of patients had COPD, patient effort estimated by the pressure–time product averaged approximately 25% of that observed during spontaneous breathing (Figure 28.1).[17] Thus, the work of breathing was substantially reduced (thereby allowing any inspiratory muscle fatigue if it ever occurs to resolve) but not eliminated (hopefully preventing or diminishing muscle atrophy and deconditioning). Patient work of breathing will substantially increase if the peak flow is set too low to meet the patient's ventilatory demands.[18] The work of breathing will also increase if respiratory drive is heightened, the trigger setting is not sufficiently sensitive, or with dynamic hyperinflation.

Synchronized intermittent mandatory ventilation (SIMV)

During SIMV, the patient receives a preset number of positive-pressure breaths at a preset volume. The machine

breaths are patient triggered similar to assist-control ventilation. Between mandatory machine breaths, the patient is allowed to breathe spontaneously. When SIMV was originally described, it was thought that patient effort would decrease in proportion to the degree of ventilatory support provided to the patient, i.e. if the ventilator provided 50% of the patient's minute ventilation, the work of breathing would be 50% of that observed during spontaneous breathing. Subsequent studies have clearly shown that this does not happen (Figure 28.1). As ventilatory support is reduced from full ventilatory assistance (assist-control) by decreasing the SIMV rate, the work of breathing increases for both the spontaneous and machine-assisted breaths, i.e. patients are not able to regulate inspiratory muscle output on a breath-by-breath basis.[19,20] When the level of ventilatory support is low (less than 40% of the patient's minute ventilation), the work of breathing can be very high, often exceeding 80% of the work performed during spontaneous breathing.[19] This level of work will be too high for many patients leading to considerable patient distress. At higher levels of ventilatory support, the work of breathing will be less but may still be too high for some patients.

Pressure support ventilation

During pressure support ventilation, the physician sets a level of positive pressure (rather than volume) that augments each inspiratory effort. Each breath is triggered by the patient, airway pressure is then raised to the preset level. When inspiratory flow falls below a machine-specific threshold value, the ventilator cycles to the expiratory phase. Tidal volume is determined by the set level of pressure, the patient's effort and pulmonary mechanics. Because all breaths are triggered by the patient, as a safety feature, most ventilators have the capability to provide controlled mechanical ventilation if the patient becomes apneic.

Pressure support ventilation can be used successfully as the primary mode of ventilation in patients with COPD and acute respiratory failure. Pressure support is titrated by increasing the level of pressure support until the respiratory rate falls below 27–30 breaths/min. When the respiratory rate is below 27–30 breaths/min, inspiratory effort is usually within an acceptable range.[21,22] By contrast, measurement of exhaled tidal volume is less useful at predicting inspiratory muscle effort.[22] At high levels of pressure support, some patients develop expiratory muscle activity before inspiration is terminated.[22] In these patients machine inspiratory time exceeds the patient's neural inspiratory time leading to patient–ventilator asynchrony.

Proportional assist ventilation

Proportional assist ventilation is an experimental method of partial ventilatory support in which the ventilator generates flow and volume, in proportion to patient effort, to reduce the resistive and elastic load.[23] The patient must have an intact respiratory drive. The patient's elastance and resistance must be measured accurately usually during a period of controlled mechanical ventilation and these measurements need to be repeated continuously as patient mechanics change. If flow or volume assist is set too high, higher than the patient's resistance and elastance, inspiration will not stop at the end of the patient's inspiratory effort but will continue into neural expiration. This phenomenon has been termed 'runaway'. The patient will only be able to initiate expiration by abdominal muscle recruitment. Uncompensated dynamic hyperinflation causes problems with all ventilator modes but particularly with proportional assist ventilation. Addition of external PEEP at levels below the auto-PEEP level can successfully address this problem. In a small study of patients with COPD and acute respiratory failure, addition of external PEEP to counterbalance auto-PEEP plus flow assist (to reduce the resistive load) reduced the pressure generated by the inspiratory muscles per breath by 44%.[24] Addition of volume assist (to reduce elastic load) further reduced patient effort but 'runaway' was observed in some patients (because patient elastance was reduced during proportional assist ventilation compared with that observed during controlled mechanical ventilation) and the degree of volume assist was determined during controlled mechanical ventilation. Proportional assist ventilation is not commercially available at the present time. Its utility in the clinical setting compared with other modes of ventilation remains to be determined.

In summary, regardless of the ventilator mode employed, the level of ventilatory support should be high to ensure sufficient ventilatory muscle unloading.

VENTILATOR SETTINGS

Fractional inspired oxygen fraction (FIO2)

FIO_2 should be adjusted to achieve an arterial oxygen tension (PaO_2) of 60–70 mmHg. Higher levels will not substantially increase tissue oxygenation. If oxygenation is estimated by pulse oximetry, it must be remembered that oximeter accuracy is only to within 2–4%. Pulse oximetry is less accurate in darkly pigmented patients. In one study, if the oximeter reading was greater than 92% in white patients, the PaO_2 was always 60 mmHg or higher.[25] By contrast, in black patients the oximeter reading had to

be 95% or higher to ensure that the PaO_2 was always 60 mmHg or greater.

Tidal volume

In the past it had been customary to use a tidal volume of 10–15 ml/kg during volume-assisted ventilation. More recently, the hazards of alveolar overdistension have become appreciated. Low tidal volumes (6 ml/kg) have been definitively shown to be beneficial in patients with adult respiratory distress syndrome.[26] In patients with COPD, low tidal volumes may reduce the risk of dynamic hyperinflation and barotrauma. We use a tidal volume of 5–8 ml/kg in these patients. With pressure support and proportional assist ventilation, tidal volume is not set.

Ventilator rate

During assist-control ventilation, the machine backup rate should be set close to the patient's actual spontaneous rate. This will ensure that patients remain adequately ventilated if they suddenly become apneic (due to oversedation for example). The backup rate also determines machine inspiratory time. If the patient's spontaneous rate increases dramatically and the backup rate is not appropriately increased, expiratory time can be dramatically shortened leading to inverse-ratio ventilation and progressive dynamic hyperinflation.

During SIMV it had been suggested that the ventilator rate should be gradually reduced as long as blood gases remain acceptable. However, the work of breathing during SIMV can be very high at low levels of support.[19] Respiratory muscle unloading may be particularly important in patients with COPD and acute respiratory failure. We recommend that the ventilator rate be set at $\geq$80% of the rate during assist-control ventilation. With pressure support and proportional assist the rate is not set.

Pressure level

As mentioned previously, the pressure level should be titrated upward until the respiratory rate is below 27–30 breaths/min. If the respiratory rate is below this threshold, inspiratory muscle effort should be reduced to an acceptable level.

Inspiratory flow rate

Inspiratory flow can be an important determinant of the patient's work of breathing.[18] If the ventilator flow rate chosen is less than the patient's flow demands, the patient will increase his or her inspiratory efforts in an attempt to increase gas delivery. To minimize the work of breathing, the ventilator flow rate should be set above the patient's peak flow demands. Constant flow rates of 60–65 L/min are usually well tolerated in ventilator-dependent patients without dynamic hyperinflation, excessively high minute ventilations or heightened respiratory drive.

In patients with COPD and acute respiratory failure, high flow rates will shorten inspiratory time allowing for a longer expiratory time, thus potentially reducing the degree of dynamic hyperinflation.[27] In patients with COPD and acute respiratory failure, an increase in flow from 40 to 100 L/min increased PaO_2, decreased the dead space/tidal volume ratio and increased static compliance.[28] The improvement in gas exchange was believed to be due to better ventilation of poorly ventilated alveoli due to the prolongation of expiratory time. The increase in static compliance likely reflects a decrease in dynamic hyperinflation. Thus, in patients with COPD and dynamic hyperinflation, high flow rates are recommended.

Assisted breaths are usually delivered with a square wave flow wave form (constant flow). Sine wave, accelerating and decelerating waveforms are available on some ventilators. Decelerating flow has become popular among many respiratory care practitioners. However, unless peak flow is increased sufficiently, mean flow will be lower during decelerating flow prolonging inspiratory time. In patients with COPD and acute respiratory failure, we recommend using constant flow.

During pressure support ventilation, the speed of pressurization is usually fixed but varies between different ventilator brands. The speed of pressurization primarily depends on the initial flow rate. With some newer ventilators, the speed of pressurization can be adjusted. In patients with COPD and acute respiratory failure, faster speeds of pressurization (i.e. a high initial flow rate) will lead to a lower patient work of breathing.[29]

Trigger sensitivity

During assisted ventilation, a set negative pressure must be generated by the patient to trigger the ventilator to deliver a positive pressure breath. The negative pressure required to trigger the ventilator can be adjusted by the clinician from a minimum value of 0.5–1.0 cmH$_2$O to greater than 5 cmH$_2$O. As trigger sensitivity is reduced (greater pressure required to trigger the ventilator), the work of breathing increases.[18] At maximum sensitivity, the ventilator will often autocycle. The trigger should be set at the minimum pressure that does not cause autocycling, usually 1–2 cmH$_2$O.

In any demand flow system, there is a delay from the time a patient initiates an inspiratory effort until the time the machine starts to deliver a positive pressure breath.

The delay time is a function of the speed at which airway pressure falls with the patient's inspiratory effort (primarily determined by the patient's inspiratory muscle strength and respiratory drive), trigger sensitivity level (the more sensitive the shorter the time delay) and machine factors.[30] In older ventilators, the demand valve system was poorly responsive resulting in a considerable increase in the patient's work of breathing. In newer microprocessor ventilators, the demand valve system is better resulting in a reduction in the work of breathing during the trigger phase. Some newer ventilators also offer the option of flow triggering in which the demand valve is triggered by flow not pressure. Flow triggering can substantially reduce the work of breathing compared to pressure triggering.[31]

Dynamic hyperinflation is often present in patients with COPD and acute respiratory failure (see Chapters 13 and 15). With dynamic hyperinflation, alveolar pressure will be positive at end expiration. This phenomenon has been called auto-PEEP. When auto-PEEP is present, the patient must decrease airway pressure by an amount equivalent to the auto-PEEP level plus the sensitivity setting before triggering can occur (Figure 28.2). Auto-PEEP effectively decreases trigger sensitivity increasing patient work of breathing. If auto-PEEP is present, efforts should be made to decrease the patient's minute ventilation and ventilator settings should be adjusted if possible to reduce inspiratory time and prolong expiratory time. If these measures are unsuccessful, extrinsic PEEP can be cautiously added, always to a level below the auto-PEEP level. When extrinsic PEEP is added, triggering will occur

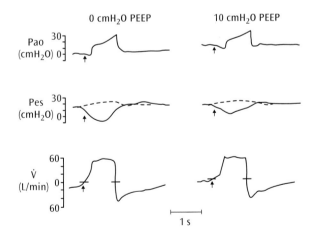

Figure 28.2 *Effect of adding external PEEP on the effective triggering threshold pressure in one patient. At a PEEP of zero, a 9 cmH$_2$O drop in esophageal pressure (Pes) is required to lower pressure at airway opening (Pao) and trigger flow. When 10 cmH$_2$O of PEEP is added, inspiratory threshold pressure imposed by auto-PEEP is overcome and less subject effort is required to trigger ventilation. (Reproduced from ref. 32 with permission.)*

when airway pressure falls below the extrinsic PEEP level rather than below zero.[32] Thus, extrinsic PEEP will improve the effective trigger sensitivity reducing the patient's inspiratory effort (Figure 28.2).

Positive end-expiratory pressure (PEEP)

In the past PEEP was avoided in patients with COPD because of the fear that hyperinflation would be aggravated. However, as mentioned above, it is now recognized that addition of external PEEP will improve the effective trigger sensitivity during assisted breaths reducing the patient's work of breathing. Auto-PEEP accounts for a substantial proportion of the patient's work of breathing.[33] Therefore, efforts to reduce this work component can be quite beneficial. Addition of external PEEP will not worsen hyperinflation because addition of a small amount of pressure downstream from the flow-limiting segment will have no effect on expiratory flow or end-expiratory lung volume provided the applied pressure is less than the critical closing pressure.[34]

As described in the monitoring section, measurement of auto-PEEP is relatively simple during controlled mechanical ventilation since the patient is not making any breathing efforts. However, during assisted ventilation, measurement of auto-PEEP in the clinical setting (i.e. without measurement of esophageal and gastric pressure) is difficult. Monitoring airway pressure during the addition of extrinsic PEEP is helpful. If there is little change in peak and plateau pressure following the addition of extrinsic PEEP; extrinsic PEEP is likely to be helpful. By contrast, if peak and plateau pressures rise in parallel to the level of extrinsic PEEP, this suggests additional hyperinflation and extrinsic PEEP is likely to be detrimental.

DISCONTINUATION OF MECHANICAL VENTILATION

Recent studies have clearly shown that the majority of patients undergoing mechanical ventilation do not require gradual withdrawal of ventilatory support. In these studies if the patient met certain clinical and physiologic criteria, they underwent a 2-hour trial of spontaneous breathing. If the patient tolerated this trial of spontaneous breathing, they were extubated. Approximately 75% of patients passed the spontaneous breathing trial in both studies.[35,36] The reintubation rate in these patients was 15.6–17.2%.[35,36] Thus, in most patients mechanical ventilation can be abruptly discontinued and gradual withdrawal of ventilatory support will only unnecessarily prolong the duration of mechanical ventilation. These studies were performed in a heterogeneous

population of patients with diverse causes of respiratory failure. The question arises as to whether the conclusions from these studies can be applied to patients with COPD and acute respiratory failure. Fortunately, several studies have applied a similar approach to extubation in patients with COPD. The percentage of patients who passed the 2-hour spontaneous breathing trial was lower in patients with COPD; 39 and 65%, respectively.[37,38] However, the reintubation rate was also lower; 0 and 4%, respectively. Thus, we believe that this approach can and should be applied to patients with COPD and acute respiratory failure.

When is a patient ready for a spontaneous breathing trial? While there are no firm guidelines but a number of clinical criteria have been employed in several studies and seem intuitively logical. These include: (i) the underlying cause for respiratory failure should have improved or resolved; (ii) PaO_2 should be greater than 60 mmHg with an FiO_2 less than or equal to 40%; (iii) PEEP should be less than or equal to 5 cmH$_2$O; (iv) the patient should be afebrile; (v) gross metabolic disturbances should be corrected; (vi) the patient should be hemodynamically stable off vasoactive drugs; and (vii) the patient's level of consciousness should be adequate to tolerate extubation.[35,36] There is evidence to suggest that physicians may be overly conservative in their estimation of when a patient can tolerate discontinuation of mechanical ventilation. A simple screening protocol employed in a university teaching hospital in the United States reduced the duration of mechanical ventilation by 25%.[39] In this study, if the patient met clinical criteria not dissimilar to those outlined above and had a rapid shallow breathing index (breathing frequency (f)/tidal volume (V_T)) (a predictor of weaning outcome)[40] of less than or equal to 105 breaths/min/L, they underwent a 2-hour trial of spontaneous breathing. If the patient passed the 2-hour trial of spontaneous breathing, a sticker was placed in the chart stating that the patient had an 85% chance of successfully staying off mechanical ventilation for 48 hours. Fifty-five per cent (48/88) of such patients were extubated that day. If all of the patients who passed the spontaneous breathing trial had been immediately extubated, the reduction in the duration of mechanical ventilation compared to standard physician-directed therapy might have been even greater. We believe that every patient undergoing mechanical ventilation should be assessed every day for his or her readiness to extubate. If the clinical criteria outlined above are not met, the patient remains on mechanical ventilation. If the clinical criteria are met, we have the patient undergo a spontaneous breathing trial.

A number of physiologic parameters have been examined as predictors of the outcome of a spontaneous breathing trial. In a heterogeneous population of patients, the f/V_T (rapid shallow breathing index) was found to be the best predictor of the outcome of a spontaneous breathing trial.[40] The f/VT is measured by connecting a portable spirometer to the endotracheal tube and measuring minute ventilation (VE) and respiratory rate (f). Tidal volume (VT) is calculated by dividing VE by f. The threshold value for the rapid shallow breathing index was 100–105 breaths/min/L. Those patients with a rapid shallow breathing index greater than 100 breaths/min/L had a 95% chance of failing a spontaneous breathing trial while those patients with an index less than 100 breaths/min/L had an 80% chance of being successfully extubated. However, the diagnostic accuracy of the rapid shallow breathing index may not be as good in patients with COPD and acute respiratory failure.[38,41] Furthermore, this parameter was prospectively validated as a predictor of the initial spontaneous breathing trial. It does not appear to be as accurate and may have a different threshold value when it is used serially in patients with COPD and acute respiratory failure to determine when a spontaneous breathing trial will be successful.[38]

A recent study in patients with COPD and acute respiratory failure suggested that two additional indices might be better predictors. These indices were the swing in inspiratory pressure at the airway opening (ΔPI) during occluded spontaneous inspiration divided by the maximal inspiratory pressure (MIP)[38] and an integrative index, CROP (compliance, rate, oxygenation, pressure), which equals effective dynamic compliance $\times$ 1/f (respiratory rate) $\times$ PaO$_2$/ PAO$_2$ (alveolar PO$_2$) $\times$ MIP.[40] Effective dynamic compliance of the respiratory system (effective Crs) is obtained from the ventilator dials by dividing VT by the difference between peak airway pressure and the value of applied or intrinsic PEEP. A correction for compliance of the ventilator tubing should be made. However neither index was prospectively validated after the threshold value was determined. Thus, at the present time we do not use any index to predict the outcome of a spontaneous breathing trial.

What physiologic criteria determine whether a patient passes or fails a spontaneous breathing trial? If the patient develops progressive hypercapnia or hypoxemia, it is clear that they have failed. A pH less than 7.32 or PaO$_2$ less than 55 mmHg generally indicates the need for reinstitution of mechanical ventilation. However, even if blood gases remain within acceptable limits, signs of respiratory distress are sufficient to indicate failure of the spontaneous breathing trial. These include an f greater than 35 breaths/min, an increase in heart rate or systolic blood pressure of 20% or more, agitation, diaphoresis, severe anxiety or depressed mental status.

How should the spontaneous breathing trial be performed? The clinician should anticipate the possibility of a spontaneous breathing trial and adjust sedation so that the patient is sufficiently alert in the morning to tolerate extubation should they pass the spontaneous breathing trial and to prevent depression of respiratory drive during the spontaneous breathing trial. The spontaneous breathing trial can be performed with a T-piece in which the patient is disconnected from the mechanical ventilator, through the continuous positive airway pressure (CPAP) circuit of the ventilator or with a small amount of pressure support. When the patient breathes on a CPAP circuit, demand valves need to be opened within the ventilator that will increase the work of breathing. However, when the patient is connected to the ventilator, all the ventilator alarms are operative which in the USA markedly increases the comfort of the nursing staff who are usually responsible for assessing the patient after the initial few minutes of the trial.

The endotracheal tube imposes a resistive load on the respiratory muscles. Pressure support ventilation has been advocated to counteract the extra work imposed by the endotracheal tube and ventilator. The amount of pressure support required to compensate for the extra work imposed by the endotracheal tube and ventilator averaged 7 cmH$_2$O but ranged from 3 to 14 cmH$_2$O in one study.[42] If pressure support overcompensates for this extra work patients may pass the spontaneous breathing trial but then subsequently require reintubation for respiratory failure. Alternatively, no compensation for this extra work could cause patients to fail a spontaneous breathing trial who might tolerate extubation. To further complicate the issue, some investigators have found that the work of breathing immediately post-extubation is often larger than expected possibly due to upper airway narrowing.[43] A recent large study has directly compared extubation outcome following a spontaneous breathing trial with a T-tube or pressure support ventilation arbitrarily set at 7 cmH$_2$O.[44] Reintubation rates were the same with both approaches. The percentage of patients passing the spontaneous breathing trial was significantly higher with pressure support ventilation (86%) than with T-tube (78%) but the magnitude of this difference was small. The authors concluded that spontaneous breathing trials could be performed with either approach. Because pressure support ventilation at 7 cmH$_2$O was marginally better, we favor this approach.

How long should the spontaneous breathing trial last? In the initial studies, a 2-hour trial of spontaneous breathing was employed. Recently, spontaneous breathing trials of 30 minutes and 120 minutes were compared.[45] There were no differences in the reintubation rate or in the percentage of patients passing the spontaneous breathing trial. Patients were only studied during the initial spontaneous breathing trial. Thus, for the initial assessment of a patient's ability to discontinue mechanical ventilation, 30 minutes appears sufficient. Whether 30 minutes is sufficient for patients who have previously failed a spontaneous breathing trial has not been evaluated. Therefore, in patients who have previously failed a spontaneous breathing trial, we use the standard duration of 2 hours.

What is the approach to the patient who fails a spontaneous breathing trial? The clinician should carefully evaluate the patient to look for any potentially reversible contributors to weaning failure. It should also be appreciated that the transition from positive-pressure ventilation to spontaneous breathing will increase left ventricular preload and afterload which can precipitate cardiogenic pulmonary edema in patients with left ventricular dysfunction or who are fluid overloaded.[46]

Two recent large studies have compared different 'weaning' strategies in patients who failed their initial spontaneous breathing trial.[35,36] In one study, weaning with pressure support ventilation, SIMV and progressive T-tube trials were compared. In the other study, the aforementioned three techniques were also compared to once-daily spontaneous breathing trials. For standardization purposes, withdrawal of ventilatory support with each weaning technique was relatively constrained. In the first study, pressure support ventilation resulted in a shorter weaning period than T-piece or SIMV. In the second study, once-daily trials of spontaneous breathing or T-tube trials resulted in a shorter weaning period than either pressure support or SIMV (Figure 28.3). The conflicting results of the two studies likely reflect differences in the implementation of the different weaning strategies. From these studies we can conclude that: (i) no method of gradual withdrawal of ventilatory support has been definitely proven to be better than once-daily spontaneous breathing trials; (ii) SIMV led to the longest weaning periods in both studies and probably should not be used to wean patients from mechanical ventilation; and (iii) the way a weaning strategy is implemented may be more important than what strategy is chosen. In a recent survey of intensivists from Spain, Portugal, North and South America, pressure support (22%), SIMV plus pressure support (an unstudied weaning mode) (29%) and intermittent spontaneous breathing trials (34%) were the most popular weaning methods.[47] Daily spontaneous breathing trials were preferred by only 7.2% of intensivists.

Non-invasive positive pressure ventilation has been shown to be useful in the treatment of patients with COPD and acute respiratory failure (see Chapter 27). As mentioned previously, many patients who arrive in the emergency room are too sick to be started on non-invasive ventilation and require immediate endotracheal intubation. Many of these patients can be stabilized relatively quickly and two studies have explored the possibility of converting these patients to non-invasive ventilation at 48 hours.[48,49] The rationale for this approach is that non-invasive ventilation is potentially associated with fewer complications, particularly nosocomial pneumonia,

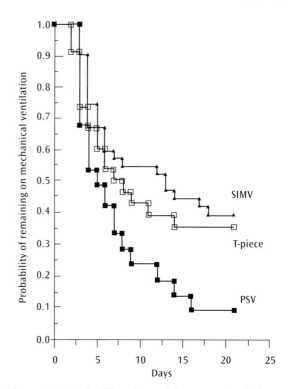

Figure 28.3 *Probability of remaining on mechanical ventilation in patients with prolonged difficulties in tolerating spontaneous breathing. This probability was significantly lower for pressured support ventilation (PSV) than for T-piece or synchronized intermittent ventilation (SIMV) (cumulative probability for old, p < 0.03 with the log-rank test) (From ref. 35 ©200 × Massachusetts Medical Society. All rights reserved.)*

compared with invasive ventilation. At 48 hours, patients who met clinical criteria for a spontaneous breathing trial underwent a 2-hour spontaneous breathing trial. If they passed the spontaneous breathing trial, they were extubated. If they failed the trial, they were randomly assigned to either continue with invasive ventilation or to be extubated and receive mechanical ventilation non-invasively. In the first study, the non-invasive group had a significantly lower mortality, a shorter duration of mechanical ventilation, a shorter ICU stay and a higher percentage of patients successfully liberated from mechanical ventilation. In the second study, which included patients with restrictive causes of hypercapnic respiratory failure, there were no significant differences in the percentage of patients successfully liberated from mechanical ventilation, ICU stay or mortality. Further study is required before this approach can be recommended. However, these studies do give the clinician confidence in pursuing an aggressive approach to extubation. If a borderline patient is extubated and subsequently fails, these studies suggest that non-invasive ventilation can be tried with a reasonable chance of successfully avoiding reintubation.

ADMINISTRATION OF BRONCHODILATOR MEDICATION TO INTUBATED PATIENTS

Bronchodilators are obviously an important component of therapy in patients with COPD and acute respiratory failure. The administration of bronchodilators in patients intubated and mechanically ventilated is potentially more complicated than in ambulatory patients because of the potential for medication to deposit on the ventilator circuit tubing and the endotracheal tube.[50] Bronchodilators can be administered by nebulizer or by metered dose inhaler with a spacer. In stable mechanically ventilated patients with COPD, near maximal bronchodilation can be achieved by administration of four puffs of albuterol salbutamol from a metered dose inhaler and spacer or with 2.5 mg of albuterol via nebulizer.[51,52] Anticholinergic agents have also been shown to be effective bronchodilators in mechanically ventilated patients.[53,54] Whether the combination of beta-agonist and anticholinergic agents can achieve greater bronchodilation in mechanically ventilated patients then either agent alone has not been determined. One study has compared the combination of anticholinergic and beta-agonist therapy to anticholinergic therapy alone in mechanically ventilated patients with COPD.[55] However, in this study the dose of ipratropium (2 puffs – dose 40 μg) was lower than the currently recommended dosage of four puffs for mechanically ventilated patients. Thus, it is not surprising that under these circumstances, combination therapy was more effective than the use of a single agent. Because anticholinergic agents have a good safety profile, combination therapy can be considered while we await future studies that will address this issue. The recommended dose of ipratropium is 4 puffs from a metered dose inhaler and spacer or 0.5 mg from a nebulizer. The details of delivery are exceedingly important. A technique for using a metered dose inhaler with spacer is shown in Table 28.1. A technique for using a nebulizer is shown in Table 28.2. If a metered dose inhaler is used, it must be used with a spacer. Attachment of a metered dose inhaler without a spacer, leads to a four- to six-fold reduction in overall delivery and the possibility of completely ineffective therapy.[56–58] In ambulatory patients a breathhold at end inspiration is recommended but in mechanically ventilated patients with COPD an end-inspiratory pause had no effect on bronchodilator effectiveness.[59] A collapsible chamber is the easiest spacer to use because it can remain in the ventilator circuit while

Table 28.1 *Technique for using metered dose inhalers (MDIs) in mechanically ventilated patients*

1 Assure tidal volume >500 ml (in adults) during assisted ventilation
2 Aim for an inspiratory time >0.3 of total breath duration
3 Ensure that the ventilator breath is synchronized with the patient's inspiration
4 Shake the MDI vigorously
5 Place canister in actuator of a cylindrical spacer situated in inspiratory limb of a ventilator circuit
6 Actuate MDI to synchronize with precise onset of inspiration by the ventilator
7 Allow passive exhalation
8 Repeat actuations after 20–30 s until total dose is delivered

Table 28.2 *Technique for using nebulizers in mechanically ventilated patients*

1 Place drug solution in nebulizer to optimal fill volume (2–6 ml depending on nebulizer)
2 Place nebulizer in inspiratory line at least 30 cm from the patient
3 Ensure airflow of 6–8 L/min through the nebulizer
4 Ensure adequate tidal volume (≥500 ml in adults). Attempt to use duty cycle >0.3 if possible
5 Adjust minute ventilation, sensitivity trigger, and alarms to compensate for additional airflow through the nebulizer, if required. Turn off flow-by or continuous flow mode on ventilator, remove heat and moisture exchanger from between nebulizer and patient
6 Observe nebulizer for adequate aerosol generation throughout use
7 Disconnect nebulizer when all medication is nebulized or when no more aerosol is being produced. Store nebulizer under aseptic conditions
8 Reconnect ventilator circuit and return to original ventilator and alarm settings

a non-collapsible spacer chamber needs to be removed between treatments. It is important to synchronize actuation of the metered dose inhaler with the onset of inspiration by the ventilator which requires some skill on the part of the practitioner. With the use of a nebulizer, the nebulizer should be placed in the inspiratory line at least 30 cm from the patient because this allows the ventilator tubing to act as a spacer for the aerosol to accumulate between inspirations.[50] The rate of aerosol production by commercial jet nebulizers can be highly variable even within a single brand.[60] Furthermore, particle size can vary greatly with different nebulizer brands.[60] The efficiency of a nebulizer changes with the pressure of the driving gas. The gas pressure supplied by the ventilator to drive the nebulizer during inspiration is lower than that supplied by a piped system which can significantly decrease nebulizer efficiency. Therefore, it is important to determine the effectiveness in a ventilator circuit of the particular brand of nebulizer in use at your hospital before it is used in ventilator-supported patients.

How frequently should aerosolized bronchodilators be administered? A recent study suggests that the bronchodilator response to albuterol salbutamol lasts up to 4 hours in mechanically ventilated patients, suggesting that the common practice of administering aerosolized bronchodilators every 4 hours is reasonable in mechanically ventilated patients with COPD.[49] Some practitioners administer bronchodilators more frequently up to every 2 hours particularly during the first day of therapy but data to support this practice are not available.

SEDATION AND ANALGESIA

Intubated patients with COPD frequently experience discomfort, anxiety and agitation during the process of mechanical ventilation for acute-on-chronic respiratory failure. For example, in one survey up to one-third of patients in intensive care units remember moderate-to-severe pain.[61] These agents are prescribed with the intent to provide comfort, promote synchronous breathing with the mechanical ventilator and provide amnesia. These agents are also used as a kind of 'chemical restraint' to reduce the risk of inadvertent removal of endotracheal and other tubes by the patient, and to reduce oxygen consumption. Thus, intravenous (IV) sedative and analgesic agents are common elements of the contemporary approach to care of mechanically ventilated patients with COPD. One survey reported a wide variety of sedative agents, i.e. 18 in use in the USA.[62] They may be administered by intermittent IV boluses or continuous IV drip. A partial list of commonly available IV sedative and analgesic agents used for these purposes in the USA is shown in Table 28.3.

Several important general limitations regarding the use of these agents in critically ill patients should be acknowledged before discussing these agents and their clinical use. Pharmacokinetic studies have been obtained only in healthy subjects and not in critical care unit patient populations.[63] Scales used for rating the effectiveness of sedation, such as the Ramsay scale (Table 28.4), have not been validated in these patient populations.[64] These limitations have an important implication for the prescription of these agents for mechanically ventilated patients with COPD: unanticipated responses may occur in some patients despite using recommended prescription guidelines, and accordingly, careful regular monitoring by the patient's physician is required.

Several general types of complications may occur as a result of usage of intravenous sedative and analgesic agents during mechanical ventilation of patients with COPD.[63] Hypotension due to a reduction in systemic

Table 28.3 *Selected sedative agents for mechanically ventilated patients with COPD*

Sedative category	Commonly used agents	Duration of usage	Bolus dosing as needed	Continuous infusion dosing
Benzodiazepines	Midazolam	• Short term only	• 0.03 mg/kg	• Initially 0.03 mg/kg/h and then titrated to desired effect
	Lorazepam	• Short term only	• 0.044 mg/kg every 2–4 h	
Opiates	Morphine	• Short or long term	• 0.05 mg/kg over 5–15 min every 1–2 h	• 4–6 mg/h
	Hydromorphone	• Short or long term	• Initiate with 0.5 mg; later 1–2 mg every 1–2 h may be needed	
	Fentanyl	• Short or long term	• 1–2 µg/kg	• 1–2 µg/kg/h
Anesthetics	Propofol	• Short term only		• Initially 0.5 mg/kg/h and titrated upwards by 0.5 mg/kg every 5 min; 'maintenance' infusion rates are typically 0.5–3.0 mg/kg/h
Selective alpha$_2$-adrenergic agonist	Dexmedetomidine	• Short term only		• Initiate with 1.0 µg/kg over 10 min, then 0.2–0.7 µg/kg/h
Neuroleptics	Haloperidol	• Short term only	• 2–10 mg intravenously every 2–4 h	

Table 28.4 *The Ramsay Scale for assessment of adequacy of sedation*

Score	Level of sedation achieved
1	Patient anxious, agitated or restless
2	Patient cooperative, oriented and tranquil
3	Patient responds to commands
4	Asleep, but with brisk response to light glabellar tap or loud auditory stimulus
5	Asleep, sluggish response to light glabellar tap or loud auditory stimulus
6	Asleep, no response

vascular resistance may occur. Psychologic distress may arise from the inability to remember experiences during critical illness.[65] Lack of physiologic sleep with prolonged usage of intravenous sedative agents during mechanical ventilation is another potential complication. Their usage represents an independent risk factor for ventilator-associated pneumonia[66] and prolonged duration of mechanical ventilation.[67] Regarding the latter potential complication, some recent evidence exists to support the practice of daily interruptions of continuous IV infusions of sedatives in order to shorten the duration of mechanical ventilation.[68] However, this study failed to track several important safety outcomes of daily awakenings, such as patients' perceptions of distress, cardiovascular effects and precipitation of drug-withdrawal syndromes.[63]

Short-acting benzodiazepines, such as midazolam and lorazepam, are probably the most commonly used class of sedative agents (Table 28.3). Benzodiazepines act by binding with γ-aminobutyric acid receptors in central nervous system neuron. This complex acts to hyperpolarize these neurons through increasing intracellular chloride flow.[69] Although their use consistently results in anterograde amnesia, it should be remembered they have no analgesic effects to address discomfort from endotracheal and other tubes. Midazolam has a relatively short onset of action, i.e. within 2–3 minutes when injected into the blood, due to its lipophilic properties.[69] Its relatively short duration of action is related to rapid redistribution after intravenous administration by bolus. Lorazepam, by contrast, is less lipophilic than midazolam, resulting in a slower onset of action and longer duration of action.[69] On the other hand, lorazepam is less expensive and is less likely to cause hypotension than midazolam.

Opiates such as morphine, a phenanthrene-derivative opiate agonist, and fentanyl, are commonly-used analgesic agents with sedative effects.[70,71] Opiates provide pain relief, especially from the discomfort of endotracheal and other invasive tubes by acting at several sites within the CNS; however, the precise mechanism of action has not been fully elucidated. Opiate agonists act principally on the CNS at certain receptors including the μ-receptor, localized in pain modulating regions, and the κ-receptor, localized in the cerebral cortex. Opiate antagonist activity at the μ-receptor can result in precipitation of withdrawal. Opiates cause respiratory depression with a diminished CO_2 ventilatory response which may be mediated more by μ_2-receptors than μ_1-receptors, the latter being more involved in analgesia effects. Kappa and other agonist receptors may also be contributory to respiratory depression. Plasma morphine concentrations are greater than the corresponding CNS concentration because of the blood–brain barrier. Morphine is metabolized principally in the liver by conjugation with glucuronic acid to form the pharmacologically inactive morphine-3-glucuronide metabolite and the pharmacologically active morphine-6-glucuronide metabolite. Plasma concentrations of these metabolites are greater than those of the parent compound. Of note, accumulation of morphine-6-glucuronide occurs in patients with COPD and coexistent renal impairment, resulting in prolonged and intensified pharmacological effects. Myoclonic spasms of skeletal muscle may occur with parent compound and active metabolite accumulation.

Fentanyl, an alternative to morphine, is a synthetic phenylpiperidine-derivative opiate agonist.[72] It has the advantages of greater potency and faster onset of action than morphine due to its relatively greater lipophilic properties. Possible histamine release with potential risks of bronchoconstriction and hypotension during morphine use is not as great a concern with fentanyl, suggesting a potential advantage for patients with chronic airways diseases such as asthma or COPD. In addition, fentanyl has a short half-life after a single dose due to rapid redistribution into peripheral tissues, and no active metabolites to raise concern about accumulation. However, relative disadvantages of fentanyl include lengthening of fentanyl half-life sometimes during prolonged continuous IV infusion due to tissue accumulation, chest wall rigidity and greater cost compared to morphine.

Short-acting anesthetic agents, such as propofol offer an additional approach to achieving and removing sedation more rapidly than with many other sedatives. The onset of action of propofol is very rapid, within 1–2 minutes, and duration of action short, 10–15 minutes, necessitating use by continuous infusion only. These features represent a potential advantage for rapid removal of sedation for assessment of neurological status, with relatively rapid re-establishment of adequate sedation afterwards. Similarly, these features of propofol may potentially assist the mechanical ventilator 'weaning' process of some patients with COPD whose degree of anxiety while intubated is felt to be a significant obstacle to successful extubation which precludes a gradual reduction in sedative infusion dosage. With prolonged administration of propofol over days, hyperlipidemia may result, an important consideration for patients simultaneously receiving total parenteral nutrition which includes intralipids. Hypotension with myocardial depression is another significant potential side effect with prolonged administration. Lastly, the cost of propofol should be considered, especially with prolonged infusions over days.

Dexmedetomidine is a relatively new short-acting anesthetic agent with alpha$_2$-adrenoceptor agonist properties which holds some promise for short-term sedation usage in critical care settings.[73,74] Like propofol, it has a relatively rapid onset and brief duration of action. Dexmedetomidine is metabolized almost completely by direct N-glucuronidation to inactive metabolites, as well as by the cytochrome P450 system. A principal advantage of dexmedetomidine, especially for patients with COPD, is absence of respiratory depression when administered at doses between 0.2 and 0.7 µg/kg by IV infusion. Other attractive features of dexmedetomidine are that its pharmacokinetics are not significantly altered by age, gender or severe renal impairment, its plasma protein binding is unaffected by simultaneous fentanyl use, and it does not significantly alter protein binding of warfarin, theophylline and certain other drugs. The most common side effects of dexmedetomidine include hypotension, nausea and bradycardia. Co-administration of midazolam can enhance the sedative effects of dexmedetomidine. Dexmedetomidine clearance may be prolonged, with less parent compound bound to plasma proteins, in patients with hepatic impairment. Dexmedetomidine is not indicated for infusions lasting longer than 24 hours.

Despite widespread clinical use, available information evaluating the comparative efficacy of different long-term (i.e. greater than 24 hours) IV sedative infusions is scanty. Furthermore, only a minority of commonly used sedative agents (i.e. midazolam and propofol) have been studied extensively in determining comparative efficacy of sedation lasting longer than 24 hours.[64] Inconsistent results regarding the superiority of sedation with propofol versus midazolam have been reported across published comparative studies; however, time to extubation seems shorter and hypotension more frequent with propofol versus midazolam.[64] No superiority of midazolam over lorazepam in terms of quality of sedation has been demonstrated thus far,[64] but more studies are needed to settle this question. Lastly, a deficiency exists in available data regarding an important outcome of use of long-term IV sedative infusions, i.e. the relative financial costs of different sedative agents.

The use of combined sedative and/or analgesic IV infusions can be entertained under certain circumstances for mechanically ventilated patients with COPD.[75] Combination infusions would be rational to consider in individual patients where sedative infusions for anxiety, such as a benzodiazepine, are not addressing coexistent acute pain, for example pain from the presence of an endotracheal tube. Other situations where it may be reasonable to consider the simultaneous use of two IV agents would be when there is an expected delayed onset of effect of a single agent, concern about cumulative and prolonged effects from use of a single agent, toxicity occuring from use of a single agent at high dosage and high financial costs resulting from the use of some single agents at high dosage.[75] However, certain potential risks of combined infusions must be acknowledged, including unpredictable synergistic actions and pharmacokinetics alterations in an individual patient, as well as additive toxicities of using two agents. Potential disadvantages include difficulty sorting out which agent is responsible for any occurrence of oversedation, high financial costs resulting from use of two agents simultaneously, and absence of guidelines for reducing dosages of the two respective agents.[75]

When patients with COPD are judged near ready for mechanical ventilator liberation and extubation, reduction or removal of sedative and analgesic infusions is indicated. Unfortunately, prolonged effects of sedative and analgesic infusions are not infrequently encountered for various reasons, and the process of mechanical ventilator liberation and extubation is delayed.[67] The role of daily interruptions of sedative infusions in mechanically ventilated patients for this purpose is controversial.[63] Evidence from a recent randomized controlled trial suggests that this strategy may significantly reduce duration of mechanical ventilation and length of stay in an intensive care unit.[68] However, the safety of this strategy in terms of precipitating acute sedative and analgesic withdrawal syndromes and possibly aggravating myocardial ischemia remains to be determined.[63,76]

Occasionally, benzodiazepine and opiate antagonists can be employed to rapidly reverse the effects of sedative or analgesic infusions to facilitate mechanical ventilator liberation and extubation or to assess underlying neurological status in a mechanically ventilated patient. Flumazenil is the preferred Federal Drug Agency (FDA)-approved agent to reverse the sedative effects of benzodiazepines.[69] However, at high doses flumazenil reverses the anticonvulsant effects of benzodiazepines, an obvious disadvantage in patients with prior history of seizure disorder. Flumazenil's effects on respiratory depression appear to be variable and brief.[77] Nonetheless, it may facilitate successful ventilator weaning and extubation in certain patients who have received only short-term (less than 24 hours) mechanical ventilation.[78] Incremental dosing of flumazenil can be accomplished with 0.2 mg IV boluses every 2 minutes up to a maximum of 1.0 mg. Continuous IV infusions of lower dose flumazenil can also be utilized at a rate of 0.5–1.0 µg/kg/min.[69] For opiates, naloxone is the FDA-approved parenteral agent used to reverse their effects.[69] Bolus administration of naloxone 0.4 mg IV every 5 minutes can be employed to desired effect, but this approach must be done with caution to avoid inducement of acute pain and agitation.

Neuroleptics, such as haloperidol, a butyrophenone, are indicated for and commonly used in mechanically ventilated patients with delirium manifested by agitation and confusion.[79] Intravenous administration produces effects within 1 hour, and duration of effect may be up to 8 hours. Some caution should be observed with neuroleptic administration in the mechanically ventilated patient: alternative etiologies of agitation and confusion (e.g. worsening hypoxemia) should be sought and excluded before the administration of neuroleptics. These agents do not provide any anxiolysis or sedation so sedatives are still needed. Concomitant use of medications which can prolong the electrocardiographic QT interval should be avoided since neuroleptics can produce QT interval prolongation. Hyperpyrexia from neuroleptic malignant syndrome is a rare complication of use.

Because of a prior lack of consensus among critical care physicians, the Society of Critical Care Medicine decided to publish recommendations in 1995 for the prescription of analgesic and sedative agents.[79] In their view, morphine sulfate is the preferred analgesic agent in the critically ill patient; hydromorphone is an acceptable alternative. Fentanyl is recommended for those with hemodynamic instability. Midazolam or propofol are the preferred anxiolytics for use over less than 24 hours, while lorazepam is recommended if anxiolytics are deemed required for more than 24 hours. Haloperidol is recommended for treatment of delirium.

Certain drugs are not advisable for use (e.g. meperidine and diazepam) in the setting of mechanical ventilation of the patient with COPD.[79] The disadvantage of use of meperidine is its metabolite, normeperidine, which can accumulate leading to CNS excitation. This can be especially problematical for mechanically ventilated patients with COPD and concomitant renal disease and/or pre-existent seizure disorder wherein risk for seizures is increased. Diazepam has a longer duration of action than other shorter-acting benzodiazepines such as lorazepam and midazolam.

Neuromuscular blocking agents have little role to play in facilitating adequate mechanical ventilation in most intubated patients with COPD because sedative and analgesic agents can usually facilitate patient–ventilator synchrony adequately. If selected for use, non-depolarizing neuromuscular blocking agents, such as pancuronium, vecuronium and atracurium, are preferred over depolarizing agents, such as succinylcholine, because of a longer duration of action.[80] Regardless of which non-depolarizing neuromuscular blocking agent is chosen, adequate sedation must be provided simultaneously to avoid a severe anxiety and terror reaction to complete paralysis. Adequacy of paralysis is best assessed by serial use of a peripheral nerve stimulator. Among the non-depolarizing

neuromuscular blocking agents, pancuronium is the least expensive with the longest activity. However, tachycardia and hypotension are potential complications of use; prologation of effect can be encountered in patients with advanced age, liver disease or renal disease. Vecuronium has an intermediate duration of action, with less potential for an adverse effect on blood pressure than pancuronium. Unfortunately, its effects can also be prolonged in patients with advanced age or liver disease. Atracurium undergoes plasma degradation only, so it is relatively unaffected by advanced age, liver disease or renal disease, making it an ideal choice for those patients. It also has less potential for an adverse effect on blood pressure compared with pancuronium.

A note of caution, however, about use of atracurium in patients with COPD is potential risk of histamine release with resulting bronchoconstriction. Prolongation or potentiation of effects of these nondepolarizing neuromuscular blocking agents can be encountered in several clinical settings: edema states where accumulation of medication occurs in edema fluid, certain electrolyte disturbances (hypokalemia, hypermagnesemia, hypocalcemia, hyponatremia), concomittant use of certain medications (e.g. calcium channel blockers, clindamycin, aminoglycosides) and certain acid – base disturbances (e.g. respiratory acidosis, metabolic alkalosis). Of particular concern to patients with COPD is the risk of acute myopathy when these agents and systemic corticosteroids are used simultaneously.[81] Diffuse flaccid weakness with failure to wean from mechanical ventilation and selective loss of thick filaments in muscle biopsy specimens are common features of acute myopathy of intensive care.[81] Lastly, avoidable potential complications of use of paralyzing agents include development of decubitus ulcers, corneal abrasions and nerve compression syndromes.

MONITORING OF MECHANICALLY VENTILATED PATIENTS

In patients with COPD receiving mechanical ventilation for acute-on-chronic respiratory failure, monitoring is essential for patient safety and a rational prescription strategy.

Respiratory system mechanics

Several non-invasive variables are available for assessment and have received considerable attention in the medical literature (see also Chapter 13). Probably the most important measurable non-invasive parameter for a mechanically ventilated patient with COPD is intrinsic

PEEP or 'auto-PEEP', which reflects the degree of dynamic hyperinflation present.[82,83] Unrecognized dynamic hyperinflation can have dire consequences, including reduced venous return resulting in a decreased cardiac output and hypotension, pneumothorax, misinterpretation of hemodynamic data and additional inspiratory elastic work to overcome before inflation begins.[83] During conventional volume-cycled ventilation, intrinsic PEEP (PEEPi) is defined as the difference between airway opening pressure (e.g. at the proximal end of an endotracheal tube) and alveolar pressure at end expiration in the absence of residual respiratory muscle activity. Although PEEPi is often related to expiratory flow limitation (EFL) in patients with COPD,[84] PEEPi is sometimes iatrogenically induced by clinicians who prescribe suboptimal ventilator settings which induce dynamic hyperinflation. Expiratory flow limitation can be suspected from inspection of the expiratory flow–time curve while the expiratory line resistance of the ventilator is removed.[85,86] Alternatively, failure to augment expiratory flow during application of a low level ($\sim$5 cmH$_2$O) of negative pressure at the airway opening during tidal breathing ('NEP' technique) can indicate presence of EFL.[86]

Intrinsic PEEP can increase whenever minute ventilation, tidal volume, inspiratory time, respiratory rate, or expiratory resistance increase and/or whenever expiratory time or static compliance of the lungs decrease. Bedside clues to the presence of increased PEEPi include abrupt termination of expiratory airflow at the onset of inflation, recognized at the bedside by inspection of a flow–time curve provided by the mechanical ventilator. Another potential clue to increased PEEPi is a large discrepancy between the frequency of a patient's spontaneous inspiratory efforts and the set machine breath rate.[32] The presence of increased PEEPi can also be inferred from the observation of unexplained rising 'plateau' pressures (Pplat) (measured during an automated end-inspiratory pause) over time, suggesting worsening compliance due to worsening dynamic hyperinflation. In passive patients without spontaneous respiratory muscle activity (e.g. well-sedated and/or paralyzed), simple automated end-expiratory line occlusions or using a Braschi valve in the inspiratory tubing, combined with simultaneous inspection of in-line pressure gauge can provide an estimate of average PEEPi.[87]

Another relatively simple approach to obtaining a non-invasive estimate of PEEPi is comparing the difference in Pplat before and after a prolonged expiration.[88] In the actively breathing patient esophageal balloon manometry coupled with inspection of the simultaneous airway flow curve is one approach to obtaining an estimate of dynamic hyperinflation.[89,90] The change in esophageal pressure generated prior to the onset of inspiratory flow is measured to yield 'dynamic PEEPi' (PEEPi,dyn). This PEEPi,dyn can underestimate the true magnitude of dynamic hyperinflation by up to 90% due to non-homogeneous mechanical properties within the lungs.[89]

Other relatively easily measured and derived non-invasive variables applied to assess the state of respiratory mechanics in patients with COPD during volume-cycled ventilation are peak airway pressure (peak Pao), effective dynamic compliance of the respiratory system (effective Crs)[91] and static compliance of the respiratory system (Crs).[82,92] Both peak Pao and effective Crs provide information about inspiratory airflow resistance. Peak airway pressure represents the sum of pressures used to overcome resistive and elastic forces opposing inflation of the respiratory system, i.e. endotracheal tube, lungs and chest wall. Serial comparison of peak Pao can provide information about trends in the severity of airflow obstruction during machine inflation. These trends could, in turn, be used to assess the effectiveness of bronchodilating regimens. By partitioning peak Pao into its inspiratory resistive and elastic components through measurement of Pplat, inspiratory resistive pressure can be compared serially to yield similar trend information, provided machine tidal volume, machine rate and inspiratory flow rate settings remain unchanged between peak Pao measurement time points. The effective Crs is calculated by dividing machine tidal volume by peak Pao minus any applied PEEP or PEEPi. Compressible volume of tubing must also be accounted for and subtracted from machine tidal volume in this calculation.[93] The dynamic characteristic can also be compared serially to assess the severity of airflow obstruction during machine inflation.[91] It should be noted that serial comparison of effective Crs provides the same information as serial comparison of peak Pao when machine tidal volume is held constant. For the proper interpretation of both peak Pao and effective Crs by the clinician, the confounding effect of any patient inspiratory muscle activity on these two variables has to be acknowledged; accordingly, these variables are best obtained in well-sedated and/or paralyzed patients. Reduction in static Crs from baseline values can be a clue to worsening dynamic hyperinflation.[92] Calculation of static Crs requires knowledge of machine tidal volume corrected for tubing compressible volume, as well as Pplat minus any applied PEEP or PEEPi.

Another more technically challenging but meaningful respiratory mechanics variable in a patient with COPD during volume-cycled ventilation is expiratory airflow resistance.[85,94] Expiratory resistance assessed in this situation represents the sum of resistance contributions from the endotracheal tube, expiratory valve as well as the degree of airways obstruction (lung and chest wall expiratory resistances are neglected). Expiratory resistance can be estimated by several techniques, including the 'flow interruption'[85] and 'passive exhalation time constant'[94] methods. Because of the requirement for additional equipment and expertise with these methods, their routine application in the daily clinical care of mechanically ventilated patients with COPD is relatively impractical.

External work of breathing and other indices of spontaneous patient effort

When using ventilator modes that provide partial support for patients with COPD in acute respiratory failure, external inspiratory work of breathing can be monitored to avoid excessive imposed workloads,[18] to improve patient–ventilator interactions[22] and to help minimize additional resistive work due to endotracheal tubes.[95] External inspiratory work of breathing is the product of mean inspiratory pressure at the airway opening and tidal volume for any machine breath. It is expressed in joules, which is the energy required to move 1 liter of air through a pressure gradient of about $10 \, cmH_2O$. If Crs and total resistance of the respiratory system are known and relatively constant in a passive patient while using machine settings of constant inspiratory flow during volume-cycled ventilation, then mean inspiratory pressure at the airway opening can be calculated using the equation of motion.[96] This yields an estimate of inspiratory work per liter of minute ventilation provided by the mechanical ventilator. If this value is then compared with values obtained while the patient is actively using inspiratory muscles, such as with assisted ventilation mode, an estimate of inspiratory work of breathing performed by the patient can be obtained.[18] A better estimate of energy consumed by the inspiratory muscles under conditions of variable ventilatory support, for example SIMV mode, can be obtained with an invasive parameter, the inspiratory pressure–time product (mean inspiratory pressure multiplied by inspiratory time).[19] Esophageal or transdiaphragmatic pressures can be used with this calculation. In a passive patient, additional resistive work of breathing imposed by an endotracheal tube can be estimated if one subtracts pressure at the distal tip of the endotracheal tube from airway opening pressure.[95]

Monitoring of gas exchange during mechanical ventilation

Arterial blood gas analysis (ABGs) is the most common and conventional method of monitoring gas exchange in the mechanically ventilated patient. Arterial blood samples for repeated ABGs can be obtained by repeated punctures or by indwelling arterial catheter. When changes in FIO_2 are made, the clinician need only wait approximately 10 minutes to repeat ABGs rather than the common practice of at least 30 minutes.[97] It is important in the patient with COPD to adjust mechanical ventilator settings (e.g. FIO_2, $\dot{V}E$) to obtain PaO_2 and $PaCO_2$ that

mimic the patient's usual baseline PaO_2 and $PaCO_2$ (if these are known). This avoids the problem of over-ventilation and consequent alkalemia with its attendant risk for inducing arrhythmias and seizures. An unexpected rise in $PaCO_2$ without concomitant adjustments in ventilator settings, i.e. $\dot{V}e$ is stable, should suggest acute pulmonary embolism (increased 'deadspace' ventilation) or initiation of nutritional supplementation (increased CO_2 production) in the absence of ventilator tubing leakage.

Pulse oximetry is another commonly used means of monitoring oxygenation in mechanically ventilated patients.[98] This spectrophotometric technique exploits the fact that oxyhemoglobin has different absorption spectra using red and infrared light wavelengths compared to reduced hemoglobin. This information in a given patient can be compared to a calibration algorithm obtained from normal subjects to yield an estimate of the patient's oxyhemoglobin saturation (SpO_2). When true oxyhemoglobin saturation (SaO_2) falls below 80%, accuracy of SpO_2 falls.[98] In mechanically ventilated patients, accuracy of SpO_2 may be off by an average of 5% when true oxyhemoglobin saturation is 90% or less.[99] In view of the fact that SpO_2 provides no information about acid–base status or ventilatory level, as well as in view of its inherent biases, SpO_2 should not be considered a replacement for ABGs. On the other hand, trends in SpO_2 changes track changes in true oxyhemoglobin values reasonably well.[99] Besides its biases, clinicians should be aware of underestimation of true SaO_2 by SpO_2 in the setting of dark-colored nail polish, motion artefact, low cardiac output states, drug-induced vasoconstriction (e.g. dopamine infusions), hypothermia, peripheral vascular disease, infusions of intravenous dyes (e.g. methylene blue).[98] Cardiac arrhythmias can interfere with the quality of the pulse tracing, potentially resulting in inaccurate SpO_2. Oxyhemoglobin saturation has been found spuriously low more frequently in critically ill African-Americans than critically ill Caucasians.[25] True SaO_2 is overestimated in the setting of significant methaemoglobinaemia,[98] an inadvertent complication that may develop after administration of large amounts of local anesthetic agents (e.g. lidocaine (lignocaine)), or with significant carboxyhemoglobinemia.

Capnography involves the continuous non-invasive monitoring of end-tidal CO_2 concentration as a first approximation of arterial blood PCO_2.[98] This capnographic approximation of $PaCO_2$ is only acceptable if the alveolar deadspace is minimal. When alveolar deadspace is increased, the difference between $PaCO_2$ and end-tidal PCO_2 widens. In patients with COPD, alveolar deadspace is increased and distribution of ventilation uneven; accordingly, the capnograph displays a rising concentration line in contrast to the relatively flat concentration line seen in normals. Unfortunately, trend changes in capnographic end-tidal CO_2 concentration in mechanically ventilated patients track changes in $PaCO_2$ only modestly well.[100] Sudden decreases in end-tidal CO_2 concentration can signal ventilator disconnection or circuit leak, acute pulmonary embolism, air embolism and esophageal intubation, among other complications.[98] The complication of inadvertent rebreathing can be heralded by an unexpected sudden rise in end-tidal CO_2 concentration.[98]

COMPLICATIONS OF MECHANICAL VENTILATION

Unfortunately, a number of different complications can plague the mechanically ventilated patient with COPD.

Pulmonary barotrauma

Pulmonary barotrauma is a feared complication of mechanical ventilation which likely results from alveolar rupture. Clinical forms vary and include pneumothorax, tension pneumothorax, subcutaneous emphysema, pneumomediastinum, pneumoperitoneum, among others. Pulmonary barotrauma occurs more frequently in mechanically ventilated patients with adult respiratory distress syndrome (ARDS) than in those with COPD.[101] Development of pulmonary barotrauma seems to be more closely associated with the presence of ARDS than with maximal airway pressures or other variables (minute ventilation, tidal volume, respiratory rate, applied positive end-expiratory pressure, patient age or gender).[102] Radiographic recognition of pulmonary barotrauma such as pneumothorax is dependent on patient positioning and underlying pulmonary disease.[103] Treatment of pneumothorax in a mechanically ventilated patient typically involves urgent placement of a chest tube. Although pulmonary barotrauma from significant intrinsic PEEP (PEEPi) is a concern, currently there is little published data establishing a direct link between them in clinical practice.

Endotracheal intubation to facilitate mechanical ventilation and secure the patient's airway can lead to subsequent complications. Endotracheal tube cuff leaks, obstruction and displacement are reported in approximately 6% of cases.[104] Delayed stenoses of the larynx and/or trachea can occur from mucosal injuries.[104] When the stenosis leaves an effective luminal diameter of 1 cm or less, exertional dyspnea occurs.[105] Stridor is present when luminal diameter is 0.5 cm or less.[106] Inadvertent self-extubation may result in additional traumatic injury. Tracheostomy is used in mechanically ventilated patients with the intention to help avoid significant injury from translaryngeal intubation, as well as improve patient comfort and airway protection, and facilitate the liberation (weaning) process from mechanical ventilation.

There are no available consensus guidelines about when exactly is best to perform a tracheostomy. Expert opinion suggests that after about 1 week of translaryngeal intubation and mechanical ventilation, an estimation should be made as to whether the patient is likely to be successfully extubated within another week; if not, then early tracheostomy should be considered.[107]

Arrhythmias

Asymptomatic arrhythmias are very prevalent in the stable COPD population; 76% may have episodic supraventricular tachycardia.[108] Atrial and ventricular extrasystoles and arrythmias also occur frequently in mechanically ventilated patients with COPD.[109] Multifocal atrial tachycardia (MAT) is particularly associated with COPD.[110,111] The type of arrhythmia that occurs in patients with COPD is influenced by the presence of coexisting coronary heart disease, cor pulmonale, severe blood gas abnormalities, electrolyte disturbances and certain medications. For example, elevated theophylline blood levels may precipitate cardiac rhythm disturbances.[111] The addition of theophylline to salbutamol generally increases heart rate and supraventricular extrasystoles, but there is usually no significant increase in ventricular arrhythmias in stable patients with COPD.[108] The presence of sustained ventricular arrhythmias in mechanically ventilated patients with COPD is believed to be associated with a poor prognosis.[112] Therapy of significant atrial or ventricular arrhythmias in mechanically ventilated patients with COPD must include correction of hypoxemia, acidosis and electrolyte disturbances (e.g. hypokalemia, hypomagnesemia); potentially arrythmogenic medications like theophylline should be held. Correction of these factors is particularly important in treating MAT where the role of acute administration of intravenous medications such as digoxin, adenosine and diltiazem is unclear; intravenous magnesium, metoprolol and verapamil may hold some promise for acute treatment of MAT.[113]

Stress ulcer prophylaxis

Critically ill patients requiring mechanical ventilation have a significantly elevated risk for a stress ulcer with upper gastrointestinal (GI) bleeding.[114] In mechanically ventilated patients with COPD, there is up to a 20% incidence of upper GI bleeding without prophylaxis.[115] Continuous enteral feeding seems to decrease the incidence of upper GI bleeding in mechanically ventilated patients.[116] In addition, keeping gastric pH above 4.0 seems to reduce the incidence of significant upper GI bleeding in mechanically ventilated patients.[117] This latter observation has led many clinicians to empirically employ H_2-blockers, such as ranitidine for upper GI bleed prophylaxis. Mucosal cytoprotective agents such as sulcralfate which do not affect gastric pH have also been used for upper GI bleed prophylaxis. However, there is some controversy about the efficacy of ranitidine compared with sulcralfate for upper GI bleed prophylaxis, as well as controversy over its effects on the incidence of ventilator-related pneumonias and mortality.[118] For example, in one of the better performed recent randomized controlled trials, clinically important GI hemorrhage occurred less frequently in ranitidine-prophylaxed patients than in those treated with sulcralfate (1.7% versus 3.8%, respectively).[119] It was estimated that one significant bleeding episode would be prevented for about every 50 patients given ranitidine.[119] However, in this study use of ranitidine was not associated with any difference in ventilator-related pneumonia or reduced mortality rates.[119]

Prophylaxis for thromboembolism

Since mechanically ventilated patients with COPD are immobile, may have peripheral edema from cor pulmonale and are often elderly, venous thromboembolism (VTE) is a significant risk.[120] Deep venous thrombosis (DVT) can occur in up to almost one-third of mechanically ventilated patients with COPD who receive no prophylaxis.[121] In the mechanically ventilated patient with COPD, acute pulmonary embolism may present with non-specific findings such as new tachypnea, tachycardia, hypoxemia or signs of bronchospasm; acute elevation of internal jugular venous pressures and otherwise unexplained hypotension may signal acute cor pulmonale from a VTE. An abrupt and otherwise unexplained rise in arterial CO_2 tension without a change in total minute ventilation may herald an acute VTE. Confirmation of the diagnosis of pulmonary embolism is often problematical because lung ventilation-perfusion scans can be difficult to interpret in the patient with COPD.[122] Since the majority of pulmonary emboli originate in the lower extremities, non-invasive techniques to diagnose DVT can potentially add useful information in this situation. For example, non-invasive ultrasonography at the bedside can detect DVT accurately in greater than 95% or so of patients.[123] However, pulmonary arteriography may ultimately be needed. A popular recent alternative to pulmonary arteriograms is the 'spiral' or helical chest CT scan:[124] it is less invasive and often more readily available than conventional pulmonary arteriography. Current enthusiasm for its use should be tempered by recognition of its limitations;[125] an NIH-sponsored trial in 2001 of contrast-enhanced helical CTs will examine its sensitivity and specificity in diagnosing VTE.[126] Certain modifications to the helical CT

technique hold promise for a diagnostic yield comparable to that of pulmonary arteriography.[127] According to the 6th American College of Chest Physicians Consensus Conference on Antithrombotic Therapy, treatment of acute uncomplicated VTE can be started with low-molecular-weight heparin or unfractionated intravenous heparin using an activated PTT that corresponds to a plasma heparin level of 0.2–0.4 IU/ml by protamine sulfate as a target for adequacy of dosage.[128] Oral anticoagulation should be overlapped with this heparinoid therapy for about 5 days.[128] Low-dose-unfractionated heparin (e.g. 5000 units subcutaneously every 12 hours) or low-molecular-weight heparin (e.g. enoxaparin 0.5 mg per kg subcutaneously every 12 hours) are current suggested regimens to provide DVT prophylaxis in patients with COPD at bedrest.[129]

Ventilator-associated pneumonia

Ventilator-associated pneumonia (VAP) has a tremendous cost for any mechanically ventilated patient: crude mortality from VAP is estimated at around 30%,[130] and a US hospital can potentially absorb a net loss of approximately $5800 US dollars (in 1991) per Medicare patient treated with nosocomial pneumonia.[131] Ventilator-associated pneumonia is defined as pneumonia acquired at least 48 hours after intubation and initiation of mechanical ventilation; 'early-onset' VAP are those that occur between 48 and 72 hours after intubation and 'late-onset' VAP are those that occur after 72 hours.[130] Microorganisms involved in 'early-onset' VAP tend to be antibiotic-sensitive, such as *Haemophilus influenzae*, methicillin-sensitive *Staphylococcus aureus* and pneumococcus, whereas bacteria involved in 'late-onset' VAP are often antibiotic-resistant, such as *Pseudomonas aeruginosa*, *Acinetobacter* species and methicillin-resistant *Staphylococcus aureus*.[132] A clinical diagnosis of VAP using the presence of fever, leukocytosis, purulent secretions and radiographic infiltrates for diagnostic criteria is often not accurate when compared to a combination of histological evidence of pneumonia and post-mortem cultures as a 'gold standard' for VAP: these clinical criteria have a sensitivity of 69% and specificity of 75%.[133] From a practical standpoint, positive blood cultures represent another convenient 'gold standard'.

Examples of alternatives to VAP in the differential diagnosis include chemical aspiration, pulmonary hemorrhage and atelectasis among others. Sampling of respiratory secretions for quantitative culture can be done with bronchoscopic techniques (bronchoalveolar lavage, protected brush specimen) that provide reasonable correlation with histological specimens, but these are necessarily invasive, require local expertise, are costly and have not been clearly shown to improve patient outcome.[134]

More recently, 'blind' non-bronchoscopic sampling (blind bronchial suctioning, 'mini' bronchoalveolar lavage or even simple endotracheal aspirates) for quantitative cultures has been introduced, with reasonably comparable yields to the invasive bronchoscopic methods.[135] Furthermore, 'blind' sampling methods can be performed safely by respiratory therapists.[136]

Ventilator-associated pneumonia most likely occurs as a result of prior bacterial colonization of the aerodigestive tract and aspiration of contaminated secretions into the lower airway.[130] Invasive tubing (nasogastric tubes, endotracheal tubes) and the ventilator circuit are important contributors to the development of VAP.[130] Appropriate systemic antibiotics are the key to treatment of VAP; indeed, the adequacy of initial empirical antibiotics is more critical to mortality from VAP than whether invasive bronchoscopic procedures for culture are performed.[137] The incidence of VAP can be reduced by use of proven successful preventative measures, for example with rigorous hand-washing, avoidance of unnecessary antibiotics, limitation of stress-ulcer prophylaxis, anti-pneumococcal and anti-influenzal vaccinations and with continuous aspiration of subglottic secretions.[130,138] Short-course empirical antibiotics for suspected VAP[139] and regular timed rotation of empirical antibiotics for VAP[140] are two newer strategies that hold promise for the future in reducing antibiotic-resistant gram-negative bacteria-related VAP.

Nosocomial sinusitis

Nosocomial sinusitis (NS) often accompanies VAP in mechanically ventilated patients.[141,142] Micro-organisms causing NS tend to be the same as those cultured from invasive procedures (e.g. protected specimen brush) performed for VAP, and is, accordingly, considered a risk factor for VAP.[143,144] Polymicrobial infections are common with infectious NS; gram-negative rods such as *Pseudomonas*, along with *Staphylococcus aureus* are frequently encountered in maxillary sinus cultures from puncture drainage procedures.[141–144] The putative pathogenesis of NS is thought to be narrowing and/or occlusion of sinus ostia preventing normal drainage of sinus secretions which, in turn, leads to overgrowth of commensal and colonizing micro-organisms in the affected sinuses.[141] Increases in systemic venous pressure from the supine body position and use of positive-pressure ventilation are believed to lead to sinus mucosal edema and ostial narrowing.[141] Mechanical blockage of sinus ostia by nasotracheal and nasogastric tubes are postulated to be important factors in the pathogenesis of NS,[141,142] but not all investigators have found an increased risk of NS in transnasally intubated patients.[145] Nosocomial infectious sinusitis should be suspected in febrile, intubated patients who have been mechanically ventilated for more than 3 days. Purulent nasal discharge or aspirated tracheal secretions in an intubated, mechanically ventilated patient without pulmonary infiltrates can suggest the diagnosis of NS. Sinus CT scanning may show sinus mucosal thickening, sinus opacification and air–fluid levels in patients with NS, but does not by itself confirm infectious NS. Confirmation of infectious NS is made through transnasal puncture of maxillary sinuses, with positive cultures defined as growth of micro-organisms in numbers greater than 10^3 cfu/ml.[141,142] Treatment with systemic antibiotics alone appears to be insufficient;[146] removal of all transnasal tubes, elevation of the patient's head, application of topical decongestants are strongly recommended. Potential complications of untreated infectious NS include meningitis, brain abcess, osteomyelitis and cavernous sinus thrombosis.[141]

PROGNOSIS

Determination of prognosis in patients with COPD after an episode of respiratory failure requiring mechanical ventilation is more difficult than in clinically stable outpatients with COPD. In the latter group, a better estimate of prognosis in a given patient with clinically stable COPD can be generated due to the availability of a number of well-designed longitudinal studies that included relatively large number of patients with a wide range of severity of COPD.[147–149] In clinically stable patients with severe COPD (i.e. $FEV_1 < 42.5\%$ predicted), estimated 3-year survival rate is approximately 75% in patients younger than 65 years and approximately 60% in patients older than 65 years.[147] Well-accepted mortality predictors in these patients include post-bronchodilator FEV_1 and age.[147] On the other hand, estimation of prognosis in patients with COPD after mechanical ventilation is more problematical due to a relative paucity of data, use of retrospective analysis in many published series, differing co-morbidity in patients across and within published series, and undefined (and potentially different) selection criteria for mechanical ventilation treatment across published series.[150] In addition, some variability in reported survival rates may be related to the wide range of time over which studies were published; changes in approach to medical treatment and mechanical ventilator usage strategies have occurred over the same time period.[150]

With these limitations in mind, the available data suggest that prognosis after mechanical ventilation for COPD is not encouraging. For example, in 13 patients with COPD mechanically ventilated for at least 10 days, survival was only 15% at 1 year in a small study from 1987.[151] In a later retrospective study, Menzies *et al.* reported a 1-year survival rate after mechanical ventilation of 38% in 95 patients with predominantly severe

COPD; the 1-year survival rate was associated with pre-ventilation levels of activity at home, FEV_1, serum albumin (used as an index of nutritional status) and severity of dyspnea.[152] In this study, pre-ventilation presence of cor pulmonale, chronic hypercarbia and left ventricular dysfunction were more common in patients who died in hospital. A roughly comparable 1-year survival rate after mechanical ventilation, i.e. 25%, was reported by Anon et al. in a more recent study of patients with severe COPD manifested by pre-ventilation need for long-term home oxygen therapy;[153] 1-year survival in that study was associated with pre-ventilation FEV_1. Data from a diagnostically-heterogeneous group of 1008 patients with acute respiratory failure culled from 11 years at a US university medical center found that 2-year survival among the subgroup of 94 patients with COPD was only 42%.[154]

Some data from large, more recent prospective studies is also available. Connors et al. performed a prospective multicenter study of the relationship between patient characteristics and length of survival in 1016 patients admitted to hospital with an exacerbation of COPD and a $PaCO_2$ of at least 50 mmHg.[155] Survival time was independently related to severity of illness, body mass index, patient age, prior functional status, PaO_2/FIO_2 ratio, congestive heart failure, serum albumin and the presence of cor pulmonale; the 1-year and 2-year survival rates in this prospective study were low at 57% and 51%, respectively, but modestly better than that reported in the older retrospective studies.[155] In another prospective multicenter cohort study, 362 admissions were analyzed to identify variables associated with hospital and 1-year survival for patients admitted to an intensive care unit with an acute exacerbation of COPD; a significant hospital mortality was reported, i.e. 24%, with development of non-respiratory organ system dysfunction being the major predictor of hospital mortality.[156] For patients aged 65 years or older, 1-year survival was only 41%.[156]

Financial costs for an episode of mechanical ventilation in patients with COPD are substantial. In the study by Connors et al., median cost of the index hospitalization (median length of stay = 9 days) was expensive at US$7100.[155] In another recent US study, median intensive care unit respiratory care costs for patients with COPD were US$2422 versus US$1580 for other patients without COPD, despite similar lengths of ICU stay and mechanical ventilation.[157] Most of the differential in financial costs in this study was accounted for by cost of nebulizers, metered dose inhalers and pulse oximetry in the patients with COPD. Cost per quality-adjusted life year was estimated at between US$26 000 and US$45 000 in a cost-utility analysis of patients with severe COPD after an episode of mechanical ventilation.[153]

In summary, it appears from the available published data that prognosis after an episode of mechanical ventilation in patients with COPD is limited and is related to factors such as pre-ventilation severity of COPD (degree of airflow obstruction, need for supplementary oxygen, hypercarbia, cor pulmonale), patient age, pre-ventilation level of activity and nutritional status. Costs to subsidize this treatment in patients with COPD are significant and greater than that for other mechanically ventilated patients.

ADVANCE DIRECTIVES

During the course of COPD, episodes of severe acute respiratory failure requiring invasive mechanical ventilatory support occur unpredictably in many patients. Unfortunately, certain patients with COPD and acute respiratory failure will not be able to be liberated from mechanical ventilatory support. To address this possible outcome of mechanical ventilation, written or verbal 'advance directives' by patients with COPD has become a part of their medical care in recent years.[158] Advance directives are a means to maintain patient autonomy at a time when the patient may be unable for various reasons to clearly express their personal preferences for provision of or limitations to critical care, especially mechanical ventilatory support.[159] An important advantage of advance directives is that they can provide an effective means to help resolve personal and emotional difficulties that physicians, nurses and families may have in dealing with decision-making once mechanical ventilation has already been initiated.

Unfortunately, only a small fraction of patients with COPD actually have advance directives in force.[159,160] In one survey of 40 patients with COPD who attended a general medical or pulmonary outpatient clinic, only 14% stated they had had prior discussions about their preferences regarding mechanical ventilation with their personal physicians.[160] In another survey, only 14.3% of patients believed their personal physician understood their end-of-life wishes.[159] These findings contrast with the observation that this patient population is generally receptive to advance care planning.[161] For example, most patients with COPD enroled in pulmonary rehabilitation programs will state they are interested in more information about advance directives and mechanical ventilation if asked.[159]

The pulmonary rehabilitation program setting represents a special opportunity to provide further information and education about advance directives since patients are clinically stable and return to the same point of care several times a week for several weeks. Indeed, more stable outpatients with COPD enroled in pulmonary rehabilitation programs have opinions about mechanical ventilation than those surveyed outside of participation in pulmonary rehabilitation.[159,160] However, still less than half of patients with COPD enroled in US pulmonary rehabilitation programs have advance directives in force.[159,162] In a recent survey, only one-third of responding pulmonary rehabilitation programs asked patients if they had advance directives and less than half (42%) distributed educational materials regarding advance directives.[163] In the USA, men and minority racial groups participating in pulmonary rehabilitation seem to have advance directives in force less frequently than their gender and racial counterparts.[162] Another study found that patient willingness to receive future mechanical ventilation appears to vary according to baseline health, survival likelihood and anticipated health following extubation.[159]

Information and advice from a patient's physician can significantly influence development of advance directives. In one US survey, patients with COPD who have had discussions with their physicians about advanced directives were more likely to have made a choice about future mechanical ventilation than those who had not.[160] In a survey of 279 of 401 eligible Canadian respirologists, physicians most often initiated discussions about future mechanical ventilation when patients had advanced COPD manifested by severe dyspnea and/or $FEV_1 < 30\%$ predicted.[164] Interestingly, only about 30% of Canadian respirologists reported that their patients made a decision about future mechanical ventilation after considering the physician's opinion; over half (53%) of these 279 respirologists admitted modifying information provided at least occasionally in order to influence their patient's decision about future mechanical ventilation.[164]

Other interventions can also potentially help patients with COPD decide about advanced directives.[161,165] In one randomized controlled trial of formal advanced directives education for patients with COPD enroled in a pulmonary rehabilitation program, the effect strength was greater in the educational intervention group compared to controls for durable powers of attorney for health care, advance directives discussions with physicians, initiation of life-support discussions and development of patient assurance that their physician understood their preferences.[161] In a Canadian pilot study of an instrument designed to help patients with mechanical ventilation decisions, all 20 patients with COPD reached a decision about future mechanical ventilation; of note, all 10 women with COPD declined future mechanical ventilation.[165]

REFERENCES

1. Brochard L, Mancebo J, Wysocki M, *et al*. Non-invasive ventilation for acute exacerbations of chronic obstructive pulmonary disease. *N Engl J Med* 1995;**333**:817–22.

2. Nourdine K, Combes P, Carton MJ, Beuret P, Cannamela J, Ducreux JC. Does non-invasive ventilation reduce the ICU nosocomial infection risk? A prospective clinical survey. *Intensive Care Med* 1999;**25**:567–73.

3. Bach JR, Brougher P, Hess DR, *et al*. Consensus statement: non-invasive positive pressure ventilation. *Respir Care* 1997;**42**:365–9.

4. Ambrosino N, Foglio K, Rubini F, Clini E, Nava S, Vitacca M. Non-invasive mechanical ventilation in acute respiratory failure due to chronic obstructive pulmonary disease: correlates for success. *Thorax* 1995;**50**:755–7.

5. Anton A, Guell R, Gomez J, Serrano J, *et al*. Predicting the result of non-invasive ventilation in severe acute exacerbations of patients with chronic airflow limitation. *Chest* 2000;**117**:828–33.

6. Moretti M, Cilione C, Tampieri A, Fracchia C, Marchioni A, Nava S. Incidence and causes of non-invasive mechanical ventilation failure after initial success. *Thorax* 2000;**55**:819–25.

7. Levine S, Kaiser L, Leferovich J, Tikunov B. Cellular adaptations in the diaphragm in chronic obstructive pulmonary disease. *N Engl J Med* 1997;**33**:1799–806.

8. Mercadier JJ, Schwartz K, Schiaffino S, *et al*. Myosin heavy chain gene expression changes in the diaphragm in chronic obstructive pulmonary disease. *Am J Physiol* 1998;**274**:L527–34.

9. Orosco-Levi M, Gea J, Lloreta JL, *et al*. Subcellular adaptation of the human diaphragm in chronic obstructive pulmonary disease. *Eur Respir J* 1999;**13**:371–8.

10. Sassoon CS, Greur SE, Sieck GC. Temporal relationships of ventilatory failure, pump failure and diaphragm fatigue. *J Appl Physiol* 1996;**81**:238–45.

11. Laghi F, Cattapon SE, Jubran A, Parthasarathy S, Warshawsky P, Choi YS, Tobin MJ. Is wearing failure caused by low-frequency fatigue of the diaphragm? *Am J Respir Crit Care Med* 2003;**1067**:120–7.

12. LeBourdeiller G, Viirer N, Boczkowski J, Seta N, Pavlovic D, Aubier M. Effect of mechanical ventilation on diaphragmatic contractile properties in rats. *Am J Respir Crit Care Med* 1994;**149**:1539–44.

13. Fleury B, Murciano D, Talamo C, Aubier M, Pariete R, Milic-Emili J. Work of breathing in patients with chronic obstructive pulmonary disease in acute respiratory failure. *Am Rev Respir Dis* 1985;**131**:822–82.

14. Marini JJ, Rodriguez RM, Lamb V. The inspiratory workload of patient-initiated mechanical ventilation. *Am Rev Respir Dis* 1986;**134**:902–9.

15. Ward ME, Corbeil C, Gibbons W, Newman S, Macklem PT. Optimization of respiratory muscle relaxation during mechanical ventilation. *Anesthesiology* 1988;**69**:29–35.

16. Flick GR, Bellamy PE, Simmons DH. Diaphragmatic contraction during assisted mechanical ventilation. *Chest* 1989;**96**:130–5.

17. Leung P, Jubran A, Tobin MJ. Comparison of assisted ventilator modes on triggering, patient effort and dyspnea. *Am J Respir Crit Care Med* 1997;**155**:1940–8.

18. Marini JJ, Capps JS, Culver BH. The inspiratory work of breathing during assisted mechanical ventilation. *Chest* 1985;**87**:612–18.

19. Marini JJ, Smith TC, Lamb VJ. External work output and force generation during synchronized intermittent mechanical ventilation: effect of machine assistance on breathing effort. *Am Rev Respir Dis* 1988;**138**:1169–79.

20. Imsand C, Feihl F, Perret C, Fitting JW. Regulation of inspiratory neuromuscular output during synchronized

intermittent mechanical ventilation. *Anesthesiology* 1994;**80**:13–22.

21. Brochard L, Harf A, Lorino H, Lemaire F. Inspiratory pressure support prevents diaphragmatic fatigue during weaning from mechanical ventilation. *Am Rev Respir Dis* 1989;**139**:531–21.

22. Jubran A, Van de Graaff WB, Tobin MJ. Variability of patient–ventilator interaction with pressure support ventilation in patients with chronic obstructive pulmonary disease. *Am J Respir Crit Care Med* 1995;**152**:129–36.

23. Younes M. Proportional assist ventilation. In: MJ Tobin, ed. *Principles and Practice of Mechanical Ventilation.* McGraw-Hill, New York, 1994, pp 349–69.

24. Ranieri VM, Grasso S, Mascia L, *et al.* Effects of proportional assist ventilation on inspiratory muscle effort in patients with chronic obstructive pulmonary disease and acute respiratory failure. *Anesthesiology* 1997;**86**:79–91.

25. Jubran A, Tobin MJ. Reliability of pulse oximetry in titrating supplemental oxygen therapy in ventilator dependent patients. *Chest* 1990;**97**:1420–5.

26. The Acute Respiratory Distress Syndrome Network. Ventilation with lower tidal volumes as compared with traditional tidal volumes for acute lung injury and the acute respiratory distress syndrome. *N Engl J Med* 2000;**342**: 1301–8.

27. Tuxen DV, Lane S. The effects of ventilatory pattern on hyperinflation, airway pressures, and circulation in mechanical ventilation of patients with severe airflow obstruction. *Am Rev Respir Dis* 1987;**136**:872–9.

28. Connors AF, McCaffree DR, Gray BA. Effect of inspiratory flow rate on gas exchange during mechanical ventilation. *Am Rev Respir Dis* 1981;**124**:537–43.

29. Bonmarchand G, Chevron V, Chopin C, *et al.* Increased initial flow rate reduces inspiratory work of breathing during pressure support ventilation in patients with exacerbation of chronic obstructive pulmonary disease. *Intensive Care Med* 1996;**22**:1147–54.

30. Sassoon CSH. Mechanical ventilator design and function:the trigger variable. *Respir Care* 1992;**37**:1056–9.

31. Giulioni R, Mascia L, Recchia F, Caracciolo A, Fiore T, Ranieri VM. Patient–ventilator interaction during synchronized intermittent mandatory ventilation. Effects of flow triggering. *Am J Respir Crit Care Med* 1995;**151**:1–9.

32. Smith TC, Marini JJ. Impact of PEEP on lung mechanics and work of breathing in severe airflow obstruction. *J Appl Physiol* 1988;**65**:1488–99.

33. Coussa ML, Guerin C, Eissa NT, *et al.* Partitioning of work of breathing in mechanically ventilated COPD patients. *J Appl Physiol* 1993;**75**:1711–19.

34. Tobin MJ, Lodato RF. PEEP, auto PEEP, and waterfalls. *Chest* 1989;**96**:449–51.

35. Brochard L, Rauss A, Benito S, *et al.* Comparison of three methods of gradual withdrawal from ventilatory support during weaning from mechanical ventilation. *Am J Respir Crit Care Med* 1994;**150**:896–903.

36. Esteban A, Frutos F, Tobin MJ, *et al.* A comparison of four methods of weaning patients from mechanical ventilation. *N Engl J Med* 1995;**332**:345–50.

37. Vallverdu L, Calaf N, Subirana M, Net A, Benito S, Mancebo J. Clinical characteristics, respiratory functional parameters, and outcome of a two-hour T-piece trial in patients weaning from mechanical ventilation. *Am J Respir Crit Care Med* 1998;**158**:1855–62.

38. Alvisi R, Volta CA, Righini ER, *et al.* Predictors of weaning outcome in chronic obstructive pulmonary disease patients. *Eur Respir J* 2000;**15**:656–62.

39. Ely EW, Baker AM, Dunagan DP, *et al.* Effect on the duration of mechanical ventilation of identifying patients capable of breathing spontaneously. *N Engl J Med* 1996;**335**:1864–9.

40. Yang KL, Tobin MJ. A prospective study of indexes predicting the outcome of trials of weaning from mechanical ventilation. *N Engl J Med* 1991;**324**:1445–50.

41. Vassilakopoulos T, Zakynthinos S, Roussos C. The tension–time index and the frequency/tidal volume ratio are the major pathophysiologic determinants of weaning failure and success. *Am J Respir Crit Care Med* 1998;**158**: 378–85.

42. Esteban A, Alia I, Gordo F, *et al.* Extubation outcome after spontaneous breathing trials with T-tube or pressure support ventilation. *Am J Respir Crit Care Med* 1997;**156**:459–65.

43. Brochard L, Rua F, Lorino H, Lemaire F, Harf A. Inspiratory pressure support compensates for the additional work of breathing caused by the endotracheal tube. *Anesthesiology* 1991;**75**:739–45.

44. Ishaaya AM, Nathan SD, Belman MJ. Work of breathing after extubation. *Chest* 1995;**107**:204–9.

45. Esteban A, Alia I, Tobin MJ, Gil A, Gordo F, Vallverdu I. Effect of spontaneous breathing trial duration on outcome of attempts to discontinue mechanical ventilation. *Am J Respir Crit Care Med* 1999;**159**:512–18.

46. Lemaire F, Teboul J, Cinotti L, *et al.* Acute left ventricular dysfunction during unsuccessful weaning from mechanical ventilation. *Anesthesiology* 1988;**69**:171–9.

47. Esteban A, Anzueto A, Immaculada A, *et al.* How is mechanical ventilation employed in the intensive care unit? An international utilization review. *Am J Respir Crit Care Med* 2000;**161**:1450–8.

48. Nava S, Ambrosino N, Clini E, *et al.* Non-invasive mechanical ventilation in the weaning of patients with respiratory failure due to chronic obstructive pulmonary disease. A randomized controlled trial. *Ann Intern Med* 1998;**128**:721–8.

49. Girault C, Daudenthun I, Chevron V, Tamion F, Leroy J, Bonmarchand G. Non-invasive ventilation as a systematic extubation and weaning technique in acute-on-chronic respiratory failure. A prospective randomized controlled study. *Am J Respir Crit Care Med* 1999;**160**:86–92.

50. Fink JB, Tobin MJ, Dhand R. Bronchodilator therapy in mechanically ventilated patients. *Respir Care* 1999;**44**:53–69.

51. Duarte AG, Momii K, Bidani A. Bronchodilator therapy with metered-dose inhaler and spacer versus nebulizer in mechanically ventilated patients: comparison of magnitude and duration of response. *Respir Care* 2000;**45**:817–23.

52. Dhand R, Duarte AG, Jubran A, *et al.* Dose–response to bronchodilator delivered by metered-dose inhaler in ventilator-supported patients. *Am J Respir Crit Care Med* 1996;**154**:388–93.

53. Fernandez A, Lazaro A, Garcia A, Aragon C, Cerda E. Bronchodilators in patients with chronic obstructive pulmonary disease on mechanical ventilation. Utilization of metered-dose inhalers. *Am Rev Respir Dis* 1990;**141**:164–8.

54. Yang SC, Yang SP, Lee TS. Nebulized ipratropium bromide in ventilator-assisted patients with chronic bronchitis. *Chest* 1994;**105**:1511–15.

55. Fernandez A, Munoz J, de la Calle B, *et al.* Comparison of one versus two bronchodilators in ventilated COPD patients. *Intensive Care Med* 1994;**20**:199–202.

56. Manthous CA, Hall JB, Schmidt GA, Wood LDH. Metered-dose inhaler versus nebulized albuterol in mechanically ventilated patients. *Am Rev Respir Dis* 1993;**148**:1567–70.

57. Rau JL, Harwood RJ, Groff JL. Evaluation of a reservoir device for metered-dose bronchodilator delivery to intubated adults: an *in vitro* study. *Chest* 1992;**102**:924–30.

58. Fuller HD, Dolovich MB, Turpie FH, Newhouse MT. Efficiency of bronchodilator aerosol delivery to the lungs from the metered dose inhaler in mechanically ventilated patients: a study comparing four different actuator devices. *Chest* 1994;**105**:214–18.

59. Mouloudi E, Katsanoulas K, Anastasaki M, Askitopoulou E, Georgopoulos D. Bronchodilator delivery by metered-dose inhaler in mechanically ventilated COPD patients:influence of end-inspiratory pause. *Eur Respir J* 1998;**12**:165–9.

60. Alvine GF, Rodgers P, Fitzsimmons KM, Ahrens RC. Disposable jet nebulizers: how reliable are they. *Chest* 1992;**101**:316–19.

61. Puntillo KA. Pain experiences of intensive care unit patients. *Heart Lung* 1990;**19**:526–33.

62. Hansen-Flaschen JH, Brazinsky S, Basile C, Lanken, PN. Use of sedating agents and neuromuscular blocking agents in patients requiring mechanical ventilation for respiratory failure. *JAMA* 1991;**266**:2870–5.

63. Heffner JE. A wake-up call in the intensive care unit. *N Engl J Med* 2000;**342**:1520–2.

64. Ostermann ME, Keenan SP, Seiferling RA, Sibbald WJ. Sedation in the Intensive Care Unit: a systematic review. *JAMA* 2000 **283**:1451–9.

65. Griffiths RD, Jones C, Macmillan RR. Where is the harm in not knowing? Care after intensive care. *Clin Intensive Care* 1996;**7**:144–5.

66. Rello J, Diaz E, Roque M, Valles J. Factors for developing pneumonia within 48 hours of intubation. *Am J Respir Crit Care Med* 1999;**159**:1742–6.

67. Kollef MH, Levy NT, Ahrens TS, Schaiff R, Prentice D, Sherman G. The use of continuous i.v. sedation is associated with prolongation of mechanical ventilation. *Chest* 1998; **114**:541–8.

68. Kress JP, Pohlman AS, O'Connor MF, Hall JB. Daily interruption of sedative infusions in critically ill patients undergoing mechanical ventilation. *N Engl J Med* 2000; **342**:1471–7.

69. Murray MJ, DeRuyter ML, Harrison BA. Opioids and benzodiazepines. *Crit Care Clin* 1995;**11**:849–73.

70. McEvoy GK, ed. *AHFS Drug Information.* American Society of Health-System Pharmacists, Bethesda, MD, 2000, pp 1886–7.

71. McEvoy GK, ed. *AHFS Drug Information.* American Society of Health-System Pharmacists, Bethesda, MD, 2000, pp 1907–12.

72. McEvoy GK, ed. *AHFS Drug Information.* American Society of Health-System Pharmacists, Bethesda, MD, 2000, pp 1891–7.

73. Schrefer J, ed. *Mosby's GENRx,* 10th edn. Mosby, St Louis, MO.

74. Khan ZP, Ferguson CN, Jones RM. Alpha-2 and imidazoline receptor agonists:their pharmacology and therapeutic role. *Anaesthesia* 1999;**54**:146–65.

75. Stoltzfus DP. Advantages and disadvantages of combining sedative agents. *Crit Care Clin* 1995;**11**:903–12.

76. Srivastava S, Chatila W, Amoateng-Adjepong Y, *et al.* Myocardial ischemia and weaning failure in patients with coronary artery disease: an update. *Crit Care Med* 1999; **27**:2109–12.

77. Shalansky SJ, Naummann TL, Englander FA. Effect of flumazenil on benzodiazepine-induced respiratory depression. *Clin Pharmacol* 1993;**12**:483–7.

78. Pepperman MI. Double-blind study of the reversal of midazolam-induced sedation in the intensive care unit with flumazenil (Ro 15–1788): effect on weaning from ventilation. *Anaesth Intensive Care* 1990;**18**:38–44.

79. Shapiro BA, Warren J, Egol AB, *et al.* Practice parameters for intravenous analgesia and sedation for adult patients in the intensive care unit: an executive summary. *Crit Care Med* 1995;**23**:1596–600.

80. Wheeler AP. Sedation, analgesia, and paralysis in the intensive care unit. *Chest* 1993;**104**:566–77.

81. Lacomis D, Giuliani MJ, Van Cott A, Kramer DJ. Acute myopathy of intensive care: clinical, electromyographic, and pathological aspects. *Ann Neurol* 1996;**40**:645–54.

82. Rossi A, Gottfried SB, Zocchi L, *et al.* Measurement of static compliance of the total respiratory system in patients with acute respiratory failure during mechanical ventilation: the effect of 'intrinsic' PEEP. *Am Rev Respir Dis* 1985;**131**: 672–7.

83. Rossi A, Ploese G, Brandi G, Conti G. Intrinsic positive end-expiratory pressure. *Intensive Care Med* 1995;**21**:522–36.

84. Rossi A, Polese G. Auto-positive end-expiratory pressure: its clinical significance. In: C Roussos, ed. *Mechanical Ventilation from Intensive Care to Home Care.* European Respiratory Society Journals, Sheffield, UK, 1998, p 419.

85. Gottfried SB, Rossi A, Higgs BD, *et al.* Non-invasive determination of respiratory system mechanics during mechanical ventilation for acute respiratory failure. *Am Rev Respir Dis* 1985;**131**:414–20.

86. Valta P, Corbeil C, Lavoie A, *et al.* Detection of expiratory flow limitation during mechanical ventilation. *Am J Respir Crit Care Med* 1994;**150**:1311–17.

87. Gottfried SB, Reissman H, Ranieri VM. A simple method for measuring intrinsic positive end-expiratory pressure during controlled and assisted modes of mechanical ventilation. *Crit Care Med* 1992;**20**:621–9.

88. Shapiro RS, Kacmarek RM. Monitoring of the mechanically ventilated patient. In: Marini JJ, Slutsky AS, eds. *Physiologic Basis of Ventilatory Support.* Marcel Dekker, New York, 1998, p 743.

89. Maltais F, Reissman H, Navalesi P, *et al.* Comparison of static and dynamic measurements of intrinsic PEEP in mechanically ventilated patients. *Am J Respir Crit Care Med* 1994;**150**: 1318–24.

90. Gluck EH, Barkoviak MJ, Balk RA, Casey LC, Silver MR, Bone RC. Medical effectiveness of esophageal balloon pressure manometry in weaning patients from mechanical ventilation. *Crit Care Med* 1995;**23**:504–10.

91. Gay PC, Rodarte JR, Tayyab M, Hubmayr RD. Evaluation of bronchodilator responsiveness in mechanically ventilated patients. *Am Rev Respir Dis* 1987;**136**:880–5.

92. Leatherman JW, Ravenscraft SA. Low measured intrinsic positive end-expiratory pressure in mechanically ventilated patients with asthma: hidden auto-PEEP. *Crit Care Med* 1996;**24**:541–6.

93. Hess D. Monitoring during mechanical ventilation. *Can Respir J* 1996;**3**:386–93.

94. Truwit JD, Marini JJ. Evaluation of thoracic mechanics in the ventilated patient. Part II: applied mechanics. *J Crit Care* 1988;**3**:199–213.

95. Banner MJ, Kirby RR, Blanch PB, Layton AJ. Decreasing the imposed work of the breathing apparatus to zero using pressure-support ventilation. *Crit Care Med* 1993;**21**:1333–8.

96. Marini JJ. Strategies to minimize breathing effort during mechanical ventilation. In: Tobin MJ, ed. *Mechanical Ventilation.* WB Saunders, Philadelphia, 1990.

97. Sasse SA, Jaffe MB, Chen PA, Voelker KG, Mahutte CK. Arterial oxygenation time after an F_{IO_2} increase in mechanically ventilated patients. *Am J Respir Crit Care Med* 1995;**152**: 148–52.

98. Jubran A, Tobin MJ. Monitoring during mechanical ventilation. *Clin Chest Med* 1996;**17**:453–73.

99. Severinghaus JW, Naifeh KH. Accuracy of response of six pulse oximeters to profound hypoxia. *Anesthesiology* 1987;**67**:551–8.

100. Hoffman R.A, Krieger BP, Kramer MR, *et al*. End-tidal carbon dioxide in critically ill patients during changes in mechanical ventilation. *Am Rev Respir Dis* 1989;**140**:1265–8.

101. Gammon RB, Shin MS, Buchalter SE. Pulmonary barotrauma in mechanical ventilation. Patterns and risk factors. *Chest* 1992;**102**:568–72.

102. Gammon RB, Shin MS, Groves RH, *et al*. Clinical risk factors for pulmonary barotrauma: a multivariate analysis. *Am J Respir Crit Care Med* 1995;**152**:1235–40.

103. Tocino IM, Miller MH, Fairfax WR. Distribution of pneumothorax in the supine and semi-recumbent critically ill adult. *AJR* 1985;**144**:901–5.

104. Stauffer JL, Olson DE, Petty TL. Complications and consequences of endotracheal intubation and tracheotomy. *Am J Med* 1981;**70**:65–75.

105. Streitz JM, Shapshay SM. Airway injury after tracheotomy and endotracheal intubation. *Surg Clin N Am* 1991;**71**: 1211–30.

106. Pingleton SK. Complications of critical illness: nosocomial pneumonia, pulmonary barotrauma and complications of endotracheal intubation. In: C Roussos, ed. *Mechanical Ventilation from Intensive Care to Home Care*. European Respiratory Society Journals, Sheffield, UK, 1998, pp 430–57.

107. Heffner JE. Timing of tracheotomy in mechanically ventilated patients. *Am Rev Respir Dis* 1993;**147**:968–71.

108. Eidelman DH, Sami MH, McGregor M, Cosio MG. Combination of theophylline and salbutamol for arrhythmias in severe COPD. *Chest* 1987;**91**:808–12.

109. Holford FD, Mithoefer JC. Cardiac arrythmias in hospitalized patients with chronic obstructive pulmonary disease. *Am Rev Respir Dis* 1973;**108**:879–85.

110. Shine KI, Kastor JA, Yurchak PM. Multifocal atrial tachycardia. Clinical and electrocardiographic features in 32 patients. *N Engl J Med* 1968;**15**:344–9.

111. Levine JH, Michael JR, Guarnieri T. Multifocal atrial tachycardia: a toxic effect of theophylline. *Lancet* 1985;**i**:12–14.

112. Gorecka D. Cardiac arrhythmias in chronic obstructive pulmonary disease. *Monaldi Arch Chest Dis* 1997;**52**:278–81.

113. McCord J, Borzak S. Multifocal atrial tachycardia. *Chest* 1998;**113**:203–9.

114. Cook DJ, Fuller HD, Guyatt GH, *et al*. Risk factors for gastrointestinal bleeding in critically ill patients. *N Engl J Med* 1994;**330**:377–81.

115. Harris (Pingleton) SK, Bone RC, Ruth WE. Gastrointestinal hemorrhage in patients in a respiratory intensive care unit. *Chest* 1977;**72**:301–4.

116. Pingleton SK, Hadzima SK. Enteral alimentation and gastrointestinal bleeding in mechanically ventilated patients. *Crit Care Med* 1983;**11**:13–16.

117. Hastings PR, Skillman JJ, Bushness LS, Silen W. Antacid titration in the prevention of acute gastrointestinal bleeding. *N Engl J Med* 1978;**298**:1041–5.

118. Messori A, Trippoli S, Vaiani M, *et al*. Bleeding and pneumonia in intensive care patients given ranitidine and sucralfate for prevention of stress ulcer: meta-analysis of randomised controlled trials. *Br Med J* 2000;**321**:1103–6.

119. Cook D, Guyatt G, Marshall J, *et al*. A comparison of sucralfate and ranitidine for the prevention of upper gastrointestinal bleeding in patients requiring mechanical ventilation. Canadian Critical Care Trials Group. *N Engl J Med* 1998;**338**:791–7.

120. Jain M, Schmidt GA. VTE:prevention and prophylaxis. *Semin Respir Crit Care Med* 1997;**18**:79–90.

121. Fraisse F, Holzapfel L, Couland J-M, *et al*. Nadroparin in the prevention of deep venous thrombosis in acute decompensated COPD. *Am J Respir Crit Care Med* 2000;**161**:1109–14.

122. Lesser BA, Leeper KV, Stein PD, *et al*. The diagnosis of pulmonary embolism in patients with chronic obstructive pulmonary disease. *Chest* 1992;**102**:17–22.

123. Grant BJ. Non-invasive tests for acute venous thromboembolism. *Am J Respir Crit Care Med* 1994;**149**;1044–7.

124. Mayo JR, Baile EM, Pare PD. Helical computed tomography for diagnosing pulmonary embolism. *Ann Intern Med* 2000;**133**:483–4.

125. Gotway MB, Patel RA, Webb WR. Helical CT for the evaluation of suspected acute pulmonary embolism:diagnostic pitfalls. *J Comput Assist Tomogr* 2000;**24**:267–73.

126. Stein PD. Observations in venous thromboembolism. *Am J Med* 2001;**110**:69–70.

127. Qanadli SD, Hajjam ME, Mesurolle B, *et al*. Pulmonary embolism detection:prospective evaluation of dual-section helical CT versus selective pulmonary arteriography in 157 patients. *Radiology* 2000;**217**:447–55.

128. Hyers TM, Agnelli G, Hull RD, *et al*. Antithrombotic therapy for venous thromboembolic disease. *Chest* 2001;**119**: 176S–93S.

129. Geerts WH, Heit JA, Clagett GP, *et al*. Prevention of venous thromboembolism. *Chest* 2001;**119**:132S–75S.

130. Kollef M. Current concepts: the prevention of ventilator-associated pneumonia. *N Engl J Med* 1999;**340**:627–34.

131. Boyce JM, Potter-Bynoe G, Dziobek L, Solomon SL. Nosocomial pneumonia in Medicare patients. Hospital costs and reimbursement patterns under the prospective payment system. *Arch Intern Med* 1991;**151**:1109–14.

132. Bauer TT, Ferrer R, Angrill J, *et al*. Ventilator-associated pneumonia: incidence, risk factors, and microbiology. *Semin Respir Infect* 2000;**15**:272–9.

133. Fabregas N, Ewig S, Torres A, *et al*. Clinical diagnosis of ventilator associated pneumonia revisited: comparative validation using immediate post-mortem lung biopsies. *Thorax* 1999;**54**:867–73.

134. Fagan JY, Chastre J, Wolff M, *et al*. Invasive and non-invasive strategies for management of suspected ventilator-associated pneumonia. A randomized trial. *Ann Intern Med* 2000;**132**:621–30.

135. Papazian L, Thomas P, Garbe L, *et al*. Bronchoscopic or blind sampling techniques for the diagnosis of ventilator-associated pneumonia. *Am J Respir Crit Care Med* 1995;**152**:1982–91.

136. Kollef MH, Bock KR, Richards RD, Hearns MI. The safety and diagnostic accuracy of minibronchoalveolar lavage in patients with suspected ventilator-associated pneumonia. *Ann Intern Med* 1995;**122**:743–8.

137. Luna CM, Vujacich P, Niederman MS, *et al*. Impact of BAL data on the therapy and outcome of ventilator-associated pneumonia. *Chest* 1997;**111**:676–85.

138. Kollef MH, Skubas NJ, Sundt TM. A randomized clinical trial of continuous aspiration of subglottic secretions in cardiac surgery patients. *Chest* 1999;**116**:1339–46.

139. Singh N, Rogers P, Atwood CW, *et al*. Short-course empiric antibiotic therapy for patients with pulmonary infiltrates in the intensive care unit: a proposed solution for indiscriminate antibiotic prescription. *Am J Respir Crit Care Med* 2000;**162**:505–11.

140. Gruson D, Hilbert G, Vargas F, *et al*. Rotation and restricted use of antibiotics in a medical intensive care unit: impact on the incidence of ventilator-associated pneumonia caused by

antibiotic-resistant gram-negative bacteria. *Am J Respir Crit Care Med* 2000;**162**:837–43.

141. Torres A, el-Ebiary M, Rano A. Respiratory infectious complications in the intensive care unit. *Clin Chest Med* 1999;**20**:287–301.

142. Bert F, Lambert-Zechovsky N. Sinusitis in mechanically ventilated patients and its role in the pathogenesis of nosocomial pneumonia. *Eur J Clin Microbiol Infect Dis* 1996;**15**:533–44.

143. Holzapfel L, Chastang C, Demingeon G, Bohe J, Piralla B, Coupry A. A randomized study assessing the systematic search for maxillary sinusitis in nasotracheally mechanically ventilated patients. Influence of nosocomial maxillary sinusitis on the occurrence of ventilator-associated pneumonia. *Am J Respir Crit Care Med* 1999;**159**:695–701.

144. Rouby JJ, Laurent P, Gosnach M, *et al.* Risk factors and clinical relevance of nosocomial maxillary sinusitis in the critically ill. *Am J Respir Crit Care Med* 1994;**150**:776–83.

145. Holzapfel L, Chevret S, Madinier G, *et al.* Influence of long-term oro- or nasotracheal intubation on nosocomial maxillary sinusitis and pneumonia: results of a prospective, randomized, clinical trial. *Crit Care Med* 1993;**21**:1132–8.

146. Souweine B, Mom T, Traore O, *et al.* Ventilator-associated sinusitis: microbiological results of sinus aspirates in patients on antibiotics. *Anesthesiology* 2000;**93**:1255–60.

147. Anthonisen NR, Wright EC, Hodgkin JE. Prognosis in chronic obstructive pulmonary disease. *Am Rev Respir Dis* 1986;**133**:14–20.

148. Traver GA, Cline MG, Burrows B. Predictors of mortality in COPD. *Am Rev Respir Dis* 1979;**119**:895–902.

149. Burrows B, Bloom JW, Traver GA, Cline MG. The course and prognosis of different forms of chronic airways obstruction in a sample from the general population. *N Engl J Med* 1987;**317**:1309–14.

150. Weiss SM, Hudson LD. Outcome from respiratory failure. *Crit Care Clin* 1994;**10**:197–215.

151. Spicher JE, White DP. Outcome and function following prolonged mechanical ventilation. *Arch Intern Med* 1987;**147**:421–5.

152. Menzies R, Gibbons W, Goldberg P. Determinants of weaning and survival among patients with COPD who require mechanical ventilation for acute respiratory failure. *Chest* 1989;**95**:398–405.

153. Anon JM, Garcia de Lorenzo A, Zarazaga A, Gomez-Tello V, Garrido G. Mechanical ventilation of patients on long-term oxygen therapy with acute exacerbations of chronic obstructive pulmonary disease: prognosis and cost-utility analysis. *Intensive Care Med* 1999;**25**:452–7.

154. Ludwigs UG, Baehrendtz S, Wanecek M, Matell G. Mechanical ventilation in medical and neurological diseases:11 years experience. *J Intern Med* 1991;**229**:117–24.

155. Connors AF Jr, Dawson NV, Thomas C, *et al.* Outcomes following acute exacerbation of severe chronic obstructive lung disease: The SUPPORT investigators (Study to Understand Prognoses and Preferences for Outcomes and Risks of Treatments). *Am J Respir Crit Care Med* 1996; **154**:959–67.

156. Seneff MG, Wagner DP, Wagner RP, Zimmerman JE, Knaus WA. Hospital and 1-year survival of patients admitted to intensive care units with acute exacerbation of chronic obstructive pulmonary disease. *JAMA* 1996;**274**:1852–7.

157. Ely EW, Baker AM, Evans GW, Haponik EF. The distribution of costs of care in mechanically ventilated patients with chronic obstructive pulmonary disease. *Crit Care Med* 2000;**28**:408–13.

158. Heffner JE. End-of-life ethical issues. *Respir Care Clin N Am* 1998;**4**:541–59.

159. Heffner JE, Fahy B, Hilling L, Barbieri C. Attitudes regarding advance directives among patients in pulmonary rehabilitation. *Am J Respir Crit Care Med* 1996;**154**:1735–40.

160. Travaline JM, Silverman HJ. Discussions with outpatients with chronic obstructive pulmonary disease regarding mechanical ventilation as life-sustaining therapy. *South Med J* 1995;**88**:1034–8.

161. Heffner JE, Fahy B, Hilling L, Barbieri C. Outcomes of advance directive education of pulmonary rehabilitation patients. *Am J Respir Crit Care Med* 1997;**155**:1055–9.

162. Gerald LB, Sanderson B, Fish L, Li Y, Bittner V. Advance directives in cardiac and pulmonary rehabilitation patients. *J Cardiopulm Rehabil* 2000;**20**:340–5.

163. Heffner JE, Fahy B, Barbieri C. Advance directive education during pulmonary rehabilitation. *Chest* 1996;**109**:373–9.

164. McNeely PD, Hebert PC, Dales RE, *et al.* Deciding about mechanical ventilation in end-stage chronic obstructive pulmonary disease: how respirologists perceive their role. *CMAJ* 1997;**156**:177–83.

165. Dales RE, O'Connor A, Hebert P, Sullivan K, McKim D, Llewellyn-Thomas H. Intubation and mechanical ventilation for COPD: development of an instrument to elicit patient preferences. *Chest* 1999;**116**:792–800.

29

Domiciliary oxygen therapy

JAN ZIELINSKI

INTRODUCTION

Oxygen was discovered independently by three scientists: Joseph Priestley, Wilhelm Scheele and Antoine Lavoisier.[1,2]

Priestley, in his experiment performed on 1 August 1774, was the first person to breathe this pure 'dephlogisticated air' and subsequently remarked 'Who can tell but that in time this pure air may become a fashionable article of luxury'.[1] Shortly after Lavoisiere named the gas, *oxygène*. Two hundred years later, thanks to technologic progress, oxygen has become a widely used lifesaving drug.

John Cotes and Alvan Barach were among the first to administer oxygen to patients with COPD to relieve dyspnea and improve exercise capacity.[3,4] Those two fields of oxygen application developed largely. They are discussed separately in the chapter on breathlessness (see Chapter 16) and the chapter on exercise (see Chapter 18).

Campbell introduced the concept of controlled oxygen therapy which allowed safe continuous oxygen treatment for COPD patients admitted to hospital with severe respiratory failure and edema due to cor pulmonale.[5]

The clinical effects of oxygen were spectacular. An objective proof of the beneficial effects of oxygen was seen in a rapid reduction of hypoxic pulmonary hypertension after a few days of treatment.[6] At that time, cor pulmonale was a common ultimate cause of death in COPD patients.[7] Oxygen appeared to be a miraculous drug.

The realization that oxygen may be an important, if not the most important, drug in the treatment of chronic respiratory failure occurred independently, on opposite sides of the Atlantic. Two teams of investigators, one led by Thomas Petty in Denver, Colorado, and the other by John Bishop in Birmingham, England, studied the effects of continuous oxygen therapy in patients with severe COPD.[8,9] They reported that 1 month of continuous oxygen treatment resulted, not only in the reduction of pulmonary arterial pressure (PAP), but also in the reduction of red cell mass and hematocrit.

Both of these studies were performed using stationary methods of oxygen delivery that restricted mobility. Petty and Finigan reported the effects of from 6 to 18 months of continuous ambulatory oxygen therapy using portable liquid oxygen.[10] They found an improvement in right heart function, reduction in hematocrit and an increase in dry body weight for most patients, with the ambulatory oxygen therapy.

The question of how many hours of oxygen therapy per day were required to achieve improvement in pulmonary hemodynamics was addressed by a series of clinical investigations. Stark *et al.* observed a fall in mean PAP after 8 months of oxygen therapy given for 15 or 18 hours daily.[11] However, 12 hours of oxygen per day did not appear to improve pulmonary hemodynamics.[12] The studies described above were observational in nature and based on small numbers of patients.

Table 29.1 *Baseline characteristics in MRC study*

	Oxygen	Controls
Number of subjects	42	45
M/F	33/29	33/12
Age (yr)	59	57
FEV_1 (L)	0.7	0.7
FVC (L)	1.8	1.8
Pao_2 (mmHg)	50	52
$Paco_2$ (mmHg)	55	54
PAP (mmHg)	34	34
PCV (%)	51	53

PAP: mean pulmonary arterial pressure; PCV: packed cell volume.

Table 29.2 *Baseline characteristics of COT and NOT groups*

Characteristics	COT	NOT
Oxygen (h/day)	18	12
Number of subjects (males, %)	101 (77)	102 (80)
Age (yr)	65	66
FEV_1 (%n)	30	30
FVC (%n)	53	54
Pao_2 (mmHg)	51	51
$Paco_2$ (mmHg)	43	44
PAP (mmHg)	30	29
PCV (%)	48	47

Definition of abbreviations: see Table 29.1.

CONTROLLED CLINICAL TRIALS

Two randomized controlled long-term clinical trials of domiciliary oxygen therapy in COPD were performed in the second half of the 1970s. These landmark studies were the Medical Research Council (MRC) trial performed in the United Kingdom, and Nocturnal Oxygen Therapy Trial (NOTT) performed in the USA.[13,14]

Eighty-seven stable COPD patients were enroled in the MRC study.[13] The main inclusion criteria were: an arterial oxygen pressure (Pao_2) from 40 to 60 mmHg and a past history of at least one episode of right heart failure. Baseline characteristics of the MRC patients are given in Table 29.1. The patients were randomized to receive oxygen therapy for 15 hours per day ($n = 42$) or no oxygen therapy (controls, $n = 45$). The period of follow-up was 5 years.

In the NOTT, 203 stable COPD patients with Pao_2 below 60 mmHg were selected from 1043 COPD patients screened for the study.[14] They were randomly assigned to continuous oxygen therapy (COT), ($n = 101$) or nocturnal oxygen therapy (NOT), ($n = 103$). Continuous oxygen therapy patients were to receive oxygen continuously but, in fact, breathed oxygen for a mean of 17.7 hours per day. Nocturnal oxygen therapy patients breathed oxygen for 12 hours per day including the period during sleep. The study continued for 3 years. Baseline characteristics of the NOTT patients are given in Table 29.2.

The main end-point for both studies was overall survival. In the MRC trial there was an improvement in survival from 25% to 41% (Figure 29.1) over 5 years for the group receiving oxygen therapy. However, there was no difference in mortality for male patients up to 500 days from the start of the study. In female patients, survival was improved for the oxygen-treated group from the commencement of treatment. However, the number of female patients in the study was small (9 treated and 12 controls).

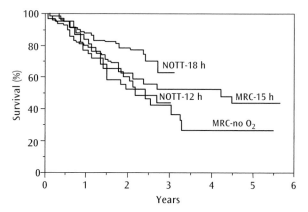

Figure 29.1 *Survival curves of patients in MRC and NOTT studies.*

In the NOTT survival at 6 months was similar for both COT and NOT groups. At 12, 24 and 36 months there was a significant improvement in survival for the COT over the NOT group ($P < 0.01$) (Figure 29.1). The NOTT study also reported that long-term oxygen therapy (LTOT) reduced secondary polycythemia, improved pulmonary hemodynamics and neuropsychologic function.

It is worth mentioning that COT patients were provided with ambulatory oxygen therapy contrary to the NOT patients and to the majority of the MRC patients who used a stationary source of oxygen. Petty recently suggested that the opportunity to exercise may have had a positive effect on survival in the COT patients.[15] Evidence for LTOT in COPD patients was recently reviewed by Crockett *et al.*[16,17]

INDICATIONS FOR DOMICILIARY OXYGEN THERAPY

The effects of hypoxemia on tissue oxygenation are closely related to the dissociation of oxyhemoglobin.

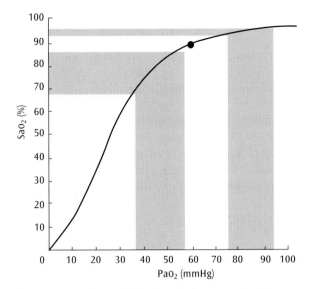

Figure 29.2 *Oxyhemoglobin dissociation curve. Relations between Pao_2 and Sao_2. For explanations see text.*

Oxygen pressure in the arterial blood represents only a small fraction of oxygen transported to the tissues. The amount of oxygen dissolved in plasma is negligible at sea level barometric pressure conditions. The oxygen content in arterial blood depends on the level of oxyhemoglobin saturation (Sao_2).

Relationships between Pao_2 and Sao_2 are shown in Figure 29.2. The rationale behind the indications for LTOT in COPD patients is based on those relationships. Because of the sigmoid shape of the oxyhemoglobin dissociation curve large changes in Pao_2, in the range from 100 to 60 mmHg, have little effect on Sao_2 and oxygen transport, assuming a normal hemoglobin concentration and a normal cardiac output. For pressures below Pao_2 of 60 mmHg (the steep area of the oxyhemoglobin curve), a small decrease in Pao_2 results in a significant reduction in Sao_2.

Since the publication of the MRC and NOTT studies domiciliary long-term oxygen therapy (LTOT) has become a routine method of treatment for COPD patients at an advanced stage of their disease. The NOTT inclusion criteria were adopted for clinical practice in the USA. In 1989, the European Society of Pneumonology (SEP) Task Group published recommendations for LTOT.[18] This group suggested that patients were eligible for LTOT if they had a Pao_2 less than or equal to 55 mmHg. They also suggested that patients with a Pao_2 ranging from 56 to 65 mmHg and signs of pulmonary hypertension might also benefit from domiciliary oxygen. Shortly after, the Rehabilitation Working Group of the European Society of Respiratory Physiology (SEPCR) recommended a Pao_2 less than or equal to 55 mmHg as a main inclusion criterion for LTOT.[19] Many pneumonologic societies have now

issued their own guidelines for LTOT,[20–23] which have recently been reviewed (Table 29.3).[24]

Worldwide, the indications for LTOT are very similar. The main inclusion criterion for LTOT is severe hypoxemia, with a Pao_2 less than or equal to 55 mmHg. In all countries, patients with moderate hypoxemia, Pao_2 from 56 to 59 (or 60) mmHg, are also eligible for LTOT. In these patients, LTOT is warranted if they present with an elevated hematocrit and signs of cor pulmonale, (pulmonary hypertension, peripheral edema). In some countries, nocturnal supplemental oxygen or oxygen during exercise is prescribed for patients desaturating in either of these situations. These indications are discussed later in this chapter (see 'Nocturnal oxygen therapy' and 'Oxygen during exercise' below).

EVALUATION AND FOLLOW-UP

The stability of the degree of hypoxemia should be confirmed by monitoring the patient for a period of 4 weeks under optimal medical therapy. During this period, Pao_2 should not increase by more than 5 mmHg and remain below 55 mmHg. Patients with an initial Pao_2 of between 56 and 60 mmHg should be reassessed after a period of 3 months.

Often LTOT is proposed for a patient on hospital discharge after being admitted for an exacerbation of COPD and treated with oxygen therapy. These patients should be re-evaluated after 1–3 months[25] as it has been shown that in COPD, a recovery in pulmonary function after an exacerbation can take up to 3 months.[26] At this time, around one-third of the patients provisionally accepted for LTOT will not meet inclusion criteria.[27,28]

Patients with a Pao_2 of between 56 and 59 mmHg prescribed LTOT should be re-evaluated after a 12-month period.[29] Around 11% COPD patients with such a level of hypoxemia, included in a Polish study, were found to improve and no longer qualify for oxygen therapy after 1 year. In Sweden, 18% of patients selected for LTOT did not fulfil the inclusion criteria for domiciliary oxygen therapy after 12 months of treatment.[30,31]

Arterial oxygen pressure should be assessed by direct arterial blood sampling or by taking arterialized blood from a hyperperfused ear lobe. Some studies reported good agreement between arterialized capillary and arterial Po_2.[32,33] However, Sauty *et al.* reported a significant underestimation (4 mmHg) of Pao_2 in the capillary blood.[34]

Non-invasive measurement of arterial blood saturation (Sao_2) with the use of pulse oximetry is not recommended. However, if required a Sao_2 less than or equal to 88% approximates a Pao_2 less than or equal to 55 mmHg and a Sao_2 less than or equal to 89% a Pao_2 less than or equal to 59 mmHg.

Table 29.3 *National guidelines or recommendations for long-term oxygen therapy (LTOT)** (Reproduced from ref. 24 with permission)*

Country	Primary indication	Secondary indication	Tertiary indication	Smoking policy
Austria NG	$Pao_2 < 7.3$ kPa (55 mmHg)	$Pao_2 < 7.3$ kPa (55 mmHg) on exercise at 0.5 W/kg	Nocturnal desaturation (Sao_2 drops below 75%), exclusion of OSAS requested	Smoking no contraindication
Belgium NG	$Pao_2 \leqq 7.3$ kPa (55 mmHg)	$Pao_2 = 7.4$–8.0 kPa (56–60 mmHg) accompanied by Ht > 55% and/or signs of cor pulmonale	Nocturnal hypoxemia (Sao_2 <88% for at least 1 hour of sleep), exercise hypoxemia in patients with Pao_2 55–60 mmHg desaturating on exercise (Sao_2 <88%)	Cessation of smoking requested
France SR	$Pao_2 \leqq 7.3$ kPa (55 mmHg)	$Pao_2 = 7.4$–7.8 kPa (56–59 mmHg) accompanied by one or more of the following signs Ht > 55%, clinical signs of cor pulmonale or pulmonary hypertension, ($PAP \geqq 20$ mmHg)	Nocturnal desaturation documented by pulse oximetry	Patients urged to stop smoking
Greece SR	$Pao_2 \leqq 7.3$ kPa (55 mmHg)	$Pao_2 = 7.4$–7.8 kPa (56–59 mmHg) accompanied by elevated Ht, cor pulmonale, edema		Patients urged to stop smoking. (not an exclusion criterion)
Netherlands CP	$Pao_2 \leqq 7.3$ kPa (55 mmHg)	$Pao_2 = 7.4$–7.8 kPa (56–59 mmHg) accompanied by cor pulmonale	Nocturnal hypoxemia (Sao_2 <90% for >2 h) or exercise hypoxemia	Not a contraindication
Poland NG	$Pao_2 \leqq 7.3$ kPa (55 mmHg)	$Pao_2 = 7.4$–7.8 kPa (56–59 mmHg) accompanied by Ht ≥ 55%, signs of pulmonary hypertension and right ventricle hypertrophy		Complete cessation of smoking requested
Portugal SG	$Pao_2 < 7.3$ kPa (55 mmHg)	$Pao_2 = 7.3$–8.6 kPa (55–65 mmHg) accompanied by polycythemia or cor pulmonale	Nocturnal hypoxemia (Sao_2 <90% for >30% of night) or exercise desaturation	Smoking an exclusion criterion
Slovakia NG	$Pao_2 < 7.3$ kPa (55 mmHg)	$Pao_2 = 7.3$–8.0 kPa (55–60 mmHg) plus at least one of following: signs of pulmonary hypertension on chest radiogram, ECG or echocardiogram; clinical signs of cardiac decompensation; Ht > 55% or $Paco_2 > 46$ mmHg; VC < 2 L or $FEV_1 < 1.5$ L	$Pao_2 > 60$ mmHg if pulmonary hypertension present verified by catheterization of pulmonary artery	Smoking an absolute contraindication
Spain SR	$Pao_2 < 7.3$ kPa (55 mmHg)	$Pao_2 = 7.3$–8.0 kPa (55–60 mmHg) accompanied by pulmonary hypertension, cor pulmonale, heart failure, cardiac arrhythmias; Ht > 55%	Nocturnal hypoxemia, exercise hypoxemia	Smoking discouraged

Sweden NG	$Pa_{O_2} < 7.3$ kPa (55 mmHg)	$Pa_{O_2} = 7.3–8.0$ kPa (55–60 mmHg) accompanied by polycythemia, peripherial edema, pulmonary hypertension, intellectual reduction	Nocturnal hypoxemia or exercise hypoxemia if on oxygen, dyspnea reduced or exercise capacity improved by 50% or by two steps on Borg's scale	Smoking discouraged
Switzerland SG	$Pa_{O_2} < 7.3$ kPa (55 mmHg)	$Pa_{O_2} = 7.3$ kPa (55 mmHg) accompanied by polycythemia and cor pulmonale		Cessation of smoking requested
UK NG	$Pa_{O_2} < 7.3$ kPa (55 mmHg)	$Pa_{O_2} = 7.3–8.0$ kPa (55–60 mmHg) accompanied by secondary polycythemia or nocturnal hypoxemia ($Sa_{O_2} < 90\%$ for at least a third of night) or evidence of pulmonary hypertension		LTOT should not be prescribed to smokers unwilling to stop the habit
USA NG	$Pa_{O_2} < 7.3$ kPa (55 mmHg) $Sa_{O_2} \leq 89\%$	$Pa_{O_2} < 7.3–7.8$ kPa (56–59 mmHg) $Sa_{O_2} = 89\%$ Accompanied by (a) dependent edema owing to congestive heart failure, or (b) cor pulmonale or pulmonary hypertension by ECG, gated pool scan, or pulmonary artery measurement, or (c) hematocrit greater than 56%	Nocturnal oxygen for: nocturnal $Pa_{O_2} \leq 55$ mmHg or $Sa_{O_2} \leq 88\%$, during sleep or a drop in Pa_{O_2} of more than 10 mmHg or in Sa_{O_2} of more than 5% with signs of or symptoms of hypoxemia (e.g. cognitive process, restlessness or insomnia). Oxygen with exercise for: $Pa_{O_2} \leq 55$ mmHg or $Sa_{O_2} \leq 88\%$ on exercise	
Japan SG	$Pa_{O_2} \leq 7.3$ kPa (55 mmHg)	$Pa_{O_2} < 7.4–7.8$ kPa (56–60 mmHg) Accompanied by pulmonary hypertension or severe hypoxemia during sleep or on exercise		

* Applicable as for June 1997.
NG: national guidelines; SG: society guidelines; CP: current practice; PAP: mean pulmonary arterial pressure; OSAS: obstructive sleep apnea syndrome.

Patients prescribed domiciliary oxygen should be encouraged to breathe oxygen continuously, at least 18 hours per day, and always overnight. Oxygen flow should be adjusted to increase PaO_2 above 60 mmHg (SaO_2 greater than 89%). Usually this is achieved with an oxygen flow of 1–2 liters per minute. It has been suggested that oxygen flow should be increased by 1 liter per minute during sleep and exercise.[21,22] In patients with severe hypercapnia, it may be difficult to increase PaO_2 to 60 mmHg because of high carbon dioxide tension in the alveoli. Higher oxygen flows may induce further increase in arterial carbon dioxide tension ($PaCO_2$) resulting in respiratory acidosis.[35] Transtracheal oxygen delivery may then be an option. (see 'Transtracheal catheter' below). The application of non-invasive positive-pressure ventilation overnight may also be appropriate (see Chapter 27).

Ideally, the prescription of domiciliary oxygen therapy should be made by a pulmonary physician. However, in many countries, oxygen therapy may be prescribed by general practitioners or respiratory therapists.[22,23] Studies performed in countries with developed home oxygen programmes have shown that prescriptions of LTOT by general practitioners may result in up to 60% of the patients receiving oxygen therapy not fulfilling inclusion criteria.[36–39] However, Guyatt et al. reported that there was no difference between the accuracy of LTOT prescription by a pulmonary specialist or a primary care physician in Ontario, Canada.[40] Recently, Oba et al. have suggested that by re-evaluating a patient on LTOT and discontinuing unnecessary oxygen therapy, up to $150 million per year might be saved in the USA.[41]

Monitoring of patients using domiciliary oxygen should be mandatory. In the USA a five-state survey found that more than 30% of patients prescribed LTOT because of abnormal blood gas measurements during hospitalization were using home oxygen either sporadically or not at all.[42] Six monthly follow-up and reassessment is recommended in the UK.[23] More frequent, every 2 months, visits have not been shown to improve outcomes such as the number of emergency department visits, the number of hospitalizations, the number of days hospitalized or mortality.[43]

Improved oxygenation in a patient who was originally severely hypoxic, PaO_2 less than or equal to 55 mmHg, may be temporary and does not necessarily justify cessation of oxygen therapy. [29,44]

SMOKING POLICY

Continued smoking by a person using LTOT largely negates its benefits.[45] A high carboxyhemoglobin level in smokers reduces oxygen transport to the tissues. Smoking also increases the risk of physical hazards such as burns and fire (see 'Non-medical hazards' below). However, policy concerning the prescription of LTOT for patients who continue to smoke varies between countries (Table 29.3). Chemical analysis of filters of oxygen concentrators has found cigarette smoke particles in 50% of the units tested suggesting that at least one-half of the patients or their families were smoking cigarettes.[46]

TELEMETRIC MONITORING

Telemetry systems that enable monitoring of some physiologic parameters and instrument performance by the home care company or physician are currently under development. Information regarding the operation of oxygen therapy equipment, compliance with hours of prescribed oxygen and flow, and the need for preventive maintenance can be obtained through these systems. In addition, daily monitoring of the patient's clinical status is possible. Pulse oximetry (to assess oxygenation of the patient), heart rate, respiratory rate and breath sounds may be periodically assessed via telemetry.[47] In Japan, a remote monitoring system for oxygen concentrators has been developed.[48] Concentration of produced oxygen, oxygen flow rate and usage time are continuously stored and periodically transmitted via a telephone line to a monitoring center. Another telemetric system allows remote monitoring of SaO_2 and heart rate. This system has been found to be of value in the early detection of acute exacerbations.[49]

COMPLIANCE WITH TREATMENT

Compliance with LTOT is a major issue. Results of controlled studies have clearly demonstrated that beneficial effects on survival and organ function are related to the minimum of 15 hours of oxygen breathing per day. Numerous reports based on large numbers of subjects using LTOT in the community, suggest that this requirement is difficult to achieve.

Pépin et al. reported the compliance with LTOT of a sample of 930 COPD patients from 14 regional centers in France.[50] The mean duration of oxygen use was 14.5 ± 5 hours per day, but only 45% of the patients breathed oxygen for more than 15 hours per day. Greater compliance with oxygen therapy was found in patients with more severe disease and more frequent hospitalizations.

Compliance to oxygen from an oxygen concentrator in 1000 patients on LTOT was assessed in Poland.[51] Mean oxygen breathing time was 13.9 hours per day. Thirty-two per cent of the patients used oxygen for more than 15 hours per day. Morrison et al. reported that 44% of LTOT patients in Scotland used less than 15 hours of oxygen therapy daily.[52] Recently Otis et al. reported that only 28% of 1100 patients receiving domiciliary oxygen used oxygen for more than 15 hours daily.[53] The authors believe that the lack of education and of follow-up were responsible for insufficient oxygen use.

In other studies, based on limited numbers of subjects, from 17 to 70% of the patients used oxygen for more than 15 hours per day.[54–58] It was found that patients increased their daily oxygen use when their condition deteriorated.[57] Kampelmacher et al. reported that the most common complaint contributing to oxygen treatment non-compliance was restricted autonomy.[58]

Treatment compliance may be improved by several measures. Patient education is of prime importance. Emphasis should be placed on the expected benefits of oxygen therapy such as improved survival, prevention of edema, and pulmonary emboli, better cardiac function, improved cognitive function, sexual relations and mood.[50] Education should be repeated as often as possible in non-compliant patients. Pepin et al. reported that patients who received education at the time of commencement of oxygen therapy and had follow-up educational sessions at home used a longer daily duration of oxygen therapy.[50]

Supplementary education by a nurse, technician or physiotherapist can be of great value.[50,59] Compliance also appears to be improved if the prescription of oxygen therapy is made by a pulmonary physician.[52,60] Provision of ambulatory oxygen has been shown to improve compliance in some studies[61–64] but not in others.[65]

EFFICACY OF OXYGEN SUPPLEMENTATION

Prescription of LTOT is based on resting PaO_2. Oxygen flow rate is also titrated at rest. To achieve maximum benefit from LTOT it is important that SaO_2 remains above 90% while the patient is breathing oxygen during activities of daily living. Recently formal protocols for resting and exercise oxygen prescription were proposed.[66]

A 24-hour assessment of SaO_2 is possible using pulse oximetry recording. It has been found that SaO_2 may fall on exercise or during sleep.[67]

Śliwiński et al. studied 34 COPD patients undergoing LTOT.[68] Patients breathed oxygen for 19.3 hours daily. The mean SaO_2 in patients at rest, breathing oxygen at a flow rate of 2 L/min was 94%. However, oxygen breathing did not protect 85% of the patients studied from significant falls in SaO_2 during daily activities and sleep. Desaturations were related to eating, washing, housework, naps and sleep. For 2.2 hours per day SaO_2 was below 90% despite breathing oxygen.

Similar results were obtained by Abdulla et al.[69] They reported a very satisfactory mean SaO_2 of 94% during 24-hour pulse oximetry recordings in 26 COPD patients on LTOT. The patients breathed supplementary oxygen for a mean of 19.5 hours per day. However, despite breathing oxygen, the patients were hypoxemic for 2.5 hours per day. Hypoxemia accompanied certain daily activities such as walking, washing and eating. During sleep, SaO_2 averaged 94%. Morrison et al. reported that three of 11 COPD patients receiving supplemental oxygen desaturated to below 90% during a large part of the night.[70]

CLINICAL EFFECTS OF DOMICILIARY OXYGEN TREATMENT

Oxygen breathing seems to improve the function of all hypoxia-sensitive cells. However, in many instances such improvement cannot be clinically assessed. The effects of oxygen on survival, neuropsychologic function, quality of life, pulmonary circulation and the erythropietic system have been most extensively studied.

Survival

Chronic alveolar and tissue hypoxia lead to remodeling of the pulmonary vascular bed and of the heart. Both develop in a clinical picture of cor pulmonale, a major complication of COPD, generally resulting in a poor prognosis. Before the era of LTOT mean survival after the first episode of right heart failure ranged from 1[71] to 4 or 5 years.[72–76] Patients with signs of cor pulmonale and a PaO_2 below 40 mmHg did not survive for more than 4 years.[77] Mean PAP was found to be an important prognostic factor. Seventy per cent of patients with PAP above 30 mmHg survived less than 5 years.[78,79]

Hypoxemia and pulmonary hypertension are closely related to the degree of airflow limitation, the most sensitive prognostic factor in COPD patients.[76,80] However, Anthonisen, using data from the NOTT study[14] and the IPPB trial,[80] was able to demonstrate an independent effect of hypoxemia on survival for a given degree of airflow obstruction.[81]

The effects of long-term oxygen treatment on survival had already been studied by the end of the 1960s. Neff and Petty reported in 1970 that LTOT prolonged life in patients with severe COPD.[82] The survival rate of patients treated with continuous ambulatory oxygen for 2 years was compared with that of a historical group of similarly severe patients who did not receive oxygen therapy.[83] The mortality of patients with severe hypoxemia treated with oxygen therapy was 31% compared with a 71% mortality in the historical group. The reduction in mortality rate was most clearly seen in patients with clinical signs of cor pulmonale. Recent data confirm that

Table 29.4 *Cause of death in 215 COPD patients undergoing LTOT (Reproduced from ref. 84 with permission)*

Cause of death	Patients n	%
Respiratory failure	82	38
Cor pulmonale with edema	28	13
Pulmonary infection	24	11
Pulmonary embolism	21	10
Fatal arrhythmia	18	8
Lung cancer	16	7
Myocardial infarction	12	6
Others	14	7
Total	215	100

Others comprised: carcinoma of organs other than the lungs (4); gastrointestinal bleeding (4); pneumothorax (2); cerebrovascular accident (1); multiorgan failure (1); peritonitis (1); suicide (1).

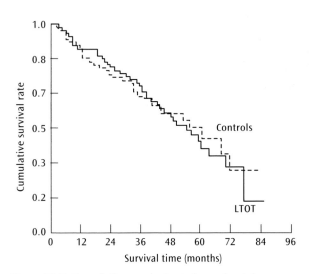

Figure 29.3 *Cumulative survival rate in moderately hypoxemic patients receiving oxygen and controls. Difference between groups is not statistically significant (P = 0.892). (From ref. 94.)*

right heart failure is now an infrequent cause of death in COPD patients treated with domiciliary oxygen. In a multicenter European study, circumstances of death were retrospectively assessed in 215 COPD patients undergoing domiciliary oxygen therapy. Causes of death are shown in Table 29.4.[84]

The effects of oxygen treatment on survival in controlled studies (MRC, NOTT) have been presented earlier in this chapter (see 'Controlled clinical trials'). Apart from oxygen breathing hours survival depended on some physiologic variables at the beginning of treatment. Severity of pulmonary hypertension,[85,86] low PaO_2 and FEV_1,[87] and low CO transfer factor[88] were found to unfavorably affect survival on LTOT. Women survived better on LTOT[13,89] then men except those women who were on long-term systemic steroid medication.[89]

It has been suggested that the prognosis of COPD patients undergoing LTOT is related to the acute effects of oxygen breathing on mean PAP.[90,91] Patients with a fall in PAP of more than 5 mmHg (responders) were found to have better survival than those in whom the fall in PAP after short-term oxygen administration was less than 5 mmHg (non-responders). This phenomenon has not been confirmed by other authors.[92] The discrepancy in results obtained by the various groups may be explained by the fact that 'responders' may have been investigated soon after exacerbation of their disease when the vaso-constrictive component of pulmonary hypertension was still important.[6,93]

Survival on LTOT in patients with moderate hypoxemia

Although the upper limit of PaO_2 for inclusion into the NOTT and MRC studies was 60 mmHg, both of these controlled studies on LTOT recruited severely hypoxemic patients. The mean PaO_2 was 51 mmHg in the MRC study

and 51.5 mmHg in the NOTT study with very few patients with PaO_2 above 55 mmHg at entry. The results of these studies appear to apply only to COPD patients with severe hypoxemia.

Recently, Górecka *et al.* performed a controlled study of the effects of LTOT on survival in COPD patients with moderate hypoxemia, (PaO_2 greater than 55 mmHg).[94] One hundred and thirty-five consecutive COPD patients with severe airways obstruction, mean FEV_1 0.83 ± 0.28 L, referred for LTOT were studied. The patients were randomly allocated to control – no oxygen ($n = 67$), and LTOT ($n = 68$) groups and were followed-up for at least 3 years. Seventy patients died during the observation period, 32 in the control and 38 in the LTOT group. No significant differences were found in survival rates between patients treated with LTOT or controls (Figure 29.3). Younger age, better VC and FEV_1 and greater body mass index predicted longer survival. Further analysis showed that patients who used oxygen for more than 15 hours per day did not have improved survival over patients who used less oxygen.

The results of the Górecka *et al.* study were recently confirmed by an ANTADIR group from France. Veale *et al.* followed a group of 7700 COPD patients prescribed LTOT of which 1425 (18.5%) had a PaO_2 equal to or greater than 60 mmHg at entry into the study.[95] Over 11 years of follow-up, no difference in survival was found between patients with $PaO_2 \geqslant 60$ mmHg and patients with PaO_2 between 50 and 59 mmHg. The results of both of these studies suggest that LTOT in COPD patients with PaO_2 above 55 mmHg does not prolong life. Neff and Petty previously reported this phenomenon in 1970.[82]

Why does LTOT not prolong life in patients with moderate hypoxemia? One may speculate that most probably, this is because this degree of hypoxemia does not influence the natural course of the disease. The majority of ANTADIR patients with moderate hypoxemia presented with a clinical picture of emphysema. The lungs of such patients are severely hyperinflated with intrinsic positive end-expiratory pressure.[96,97] The work of breathing in these patients is increased.[98,99] One may speculate that during an acute exacerbation of the disease, which seems to be the most frequent cause of death in COPD,[84] some of these patients may die due to respiratory muscle fatigue.[100] Modern techniques of evaluation of the diaphragmatic and respiratory muscle function may provide data to address such a hypothesis.[101]

Neuropsychologic function

The brain is the most oxygen-sensitive vital organ. To ensure that its needs are met, the brain, representing only 2% of the adult body mass, receives 20% of the cardiac output.

Chronic hypoxia leads to a variety of disorders of neuropsychologic functions. Hypoxemic COPD patients suffer from cognitive impairment[102–104] and emotional disorders.[105–107] A progressive worsening of neuropsychologic function with increasing severity of hypoxaemia has also been observed.[103,104] Perceptual learning, problem-solving, and simple motor skills were found to be the most affected. However, other authors have not confirmed these associations.[108] Cognitive function decline in severe COPD patients was recently studied by Incalzi et al.[109] Forty-nine per cent of the patients with COPD had a specific pattern of cognitive deterioration. The most disturbed functions were verbal and verbal memory tasks, visual memory and copying skills.

The emotional status of hypoxemic COPD patients is characterized by a high level of anxiety, stress and depression. Somatic preoccupation, and withdrawal are common in patients with severe COPD. The effects of low PaO_2 on emotional status are difficult to separate from the effects of dyspnea, a common feature of COPD.[110,111] In many studies dyspnea has been shown to increase depression, anxiety and psychologic tension. Patients with hypercapnia are known to experience less dyspnea than normocapnic subjects, as well as showing less anxiety and psychological tension.[112,113] This raises the possibility that permissive hypercapnia may be a useful breathing strategy.

The neurological effects of a short period (1 month) of oxygen therapy have been evaluated by Krop et al.[103] They studied 22 patients with advanced COPD; 10 with severe hypoxemia (PaO_2 less than 56 mmHg) and 12 with a similar reduction of FEV_1, but with PaO_2 greater than 56 mmHg. Patients with severe hypoxemia were treated with continuous oxygen, the remainder served as controls. At baseline, severely hypoxemic patients were found to be worse than controls in neuropsychologic tests. Treated patients improved significantly after oxygen treatment with respect to cognitive function and emotional status.

Cognitive function and emotional status in COPD patients undergoing LTOT was extensively studied in the NOTT.[104] At entry patients demonstrated lowered mood and deficits in cognitive function. After 6 months of oxygen treatment 42% of patients showed evidence of improved cognitive function, with greatest improvement in sequencing efficiency, flexibility of thinking and motor speed, but little change in emotional status. No difference between continuous oxygen (COT) and nocturnal oxygen (NOT) patients was seen. In a smaller group of patients neuropsychologic testing was repeated after a further 6 months of oxygen treatment. The improvement in cognitive function was maintained in the COT group but not in the NOT group.

The largest prospective study on changes in cognitive function and psychologic status variables after LTOT was recently published by Borak et al.[114] One hundred and twenty-four COPD patients were studied. Assessments included: IQ, ability to concentrate, memory recall of spatial, visual and verbal stimuli; levels of anxiety, depression and emotional tension; self-evaluation and attitude towards therapy. Ninety patients who survived 1 year of LTOT were reevaluated. The mean oxygen breathing time was calculated to be 15 hours per day. Recent memory and speed of work improved. There was no significant change in the IQ score, and visual and spatial memory. Contrary to the results of the NOTT study there was also a significant improvement in emotional status. There was a decrease in the depression and anxiety score and an improvement in the psychologic tension, general mood, self-esteem and attitude towards life and therapy. It is worth noting that improvement in neuropsychologic status was attained despite deterioration in lung function. The beneficial effects of LTOT on neuropsychologic function may have resulted from better oxygenation of the nervous system. However, the non-specific effects of improved mobility, reduced breathlessness and the sense of security resulting from the frequent follow-up visits may have also played a role.

Quality of life

The quality of life (QoL) of COPD patients has been studied using both general and disease-specific questionnaires. General questionnaires such as the Sickness Impact Profile questionnaire or the Quality of Well-Being questionnaire have been shown not to be sensitive to changes in COPD interventions.[115–118] More recently, the St George's Respiratory Questionnaire (SGRQ), a fully standardized, self-administered, sensitive to changes and reproducible, disease-specific questionnaire has been developed.[119] This questionnaire contains 76 items that are weighted to produce three component scores: symptoms, activities and impacts. A 100-point scale has been adopted with 100 points equivalent to maximum disability.

In general, COPD patients, particularly those with FEV_1 below 50% of predicted, have significant impairment of QoL.[120] High QoL scores have been found to be related to the severity of dyspnea rather than severity of hypoxemia. Correlation between severity of hypoxemia and QoL scores have been found to be poor.[105,116] In one study in patients qualified to receive LTOT no correlation was found between hypoxemia and impaired health as measured by a general health questionnaire.[121] However, a relationship has been reported between hypoxemia and SGRQ with lower PaO_2 associated with higher QoL scores. The effect of PaO_2 on QoL was independent of mood state characterized by depression and anxiety. Interestingly, no correlation between FEV_1 and SGRQ was found. Health status of COPD patients seems to depend not only on the severity of the disease but also on the number of exacerbations per year.[122]

Effects of LTOT on health status may be equivocal. LTOT improves organ function but imposes certain restrictions especially on patients provided only with a stationary oxygen source.

In the NOTT study a small but significant improvement in QoL was found after 6 months of oxygen treatment.[104] In an uncontrolled study LTOT had no effect on general activity and independence or coping skills over 6 months of treatment.[123] In another uncontrolled study 83% of patients receiving LTOT via oxygen concentrator felt that their general well-being had improved because of treatment.[124]

Okubadejo et al. studied COPD patients on LTOT and found that during 6 months of treatment there was a slight but not significant improvement in QoL score.[125] The authors concluded that LTOT does not impair health status.

The mode of delivery of oxygen used for home therapy affects QoL. In a crossover study comparing liquid and gaseous oxygen for ambulatory use it was found that liquid oxygen was used for a longer period per day than oxygen cylinders and that the majority of subjects preferred liquid oxygen.[126] However, there were no differences between the study groups in the mean scores of any of the four domains of the Chronic Respiratory Questionnaire.

In another study comparing the liquid ambulatory system with an oxygen concentrator, QoL in patients on the ambulatory system was better than that measured for patients using a stationary oxygen source.[127] Abdulla et al. found similarly high SGRQ scores in groups of COPD patients on LTOT from either a stationary or an ambulatory source.[69] Recently Okubadejo et al. studied a group of COPD patients on LTOT and a control group with severe COPD (comparable FEV_1) but no hypoxemia.[128] They found similar scores between the groups in QoL. However, activities of daily living scores were lower in the LTOT group.

Janssens et al.[129] studied 79 patients (63% COPD) who were treated with LTOT by an oxygen concentrator. In this community-based study QoL was measured using SGRQ. Quality of life in these patients was poor. High QoL scores were most strongly correlated with the distance walked during the day ($r = -0.55$) and the number of days spent in hospital during 1 year ($r = 0.5$).

Perrin et al.[130] evaluated the effects of LTOT combined with nasal intermittent positive-pressure ventilation (NIPPV), applied during night hours, on QoL in COPD hypercapnic patients. Quality of life was assessed using the SGRQ and the Nottingham Health Profile (NHP) before and after 6 months of treatment. Scores in both questionnaires improved only slightly.

Monso et al.[131] found a significantly reduced QoL in COPD patients undergoing LTOT. They studied 47 patients, with severe airways obstruction, $FEV_1 = 0.91 \pm 0.34$ L. Quality of life was measured using the NHP and the activities of daily living questionnaire. All dimensions characterizing QoL – energy, emotional reactions, sleep, social life and physical mobility – were affected. The impairment in QoL correlated with the impairment in the lung function. Lung function explained 39–45% of the variation in the QoL dimensions.

Recently Crockett et al. reported improvement in QoL in women undergoing LTOT. They studied 114 patients with COPD before and after 1 year of treatment. Female patients experienced significant improvements in the energy, emotional reactions, sleep, physical mobility and mental health. In males improvements were less pronounced.[132]

Pulmonary circulation

Acute alveolar hypoxia leads to pulmonary vasoconstriction and functional, reversible, pulmonary hypertension. This phenomenon was described by Von Euler and Liljestrand more than half a century ago.[133] Chronic alveolar hypoxia results in remodeling of the distal part of the pulmonary arterial bed. Hypertrophy of smooth muscles in the muscular pulmonary arteries, muscularization of pulmonary arterioles which normally have no muscular layer, intimal fibrosis and hypertrophy reduce vascular lumen and compliance of the vascular wall.[134] This leads to structural 'irreversible' pulmonary hypertension.[135]

The pathophysiology of pulmonary hypertension in COPD has been revisited more recently in comprehensive reviews by MacNee.[136,137] Long-term pulmonary hypertension leads to right ventricle hypertrophy known as cor pulmonale.[138]

In mild to moderate COPD, pulmonary hypertension is moderate in the range of 21–30 mmHg. In the largest published series of COPD patients ($n = 587$) with pulmonary hemodynamic assessment by direct measurements of pulmonary arterial pressure, mean PAP was 24 ± 11 mmHg.[139]

Exacerbation of COPD leads to an acute increase in PAP mainly due to aggravation of alveolar hypoxia. Hypoxic pulmonary vasoconstriction is much greater than in normal subjects. In patients with advanced COPD admitted to hospital due to exacerbation of the disease mean PAP may rise to 80 mmHg.[6] The reaction of the pulmonary vascular bed to acute hypoxia in COPD patients is markedly variable. Weitzenblum et al. were able to discriminate 'responders' in whom acute hypoxia induced a pronounced increase in pulmonary vascular resistance (PVR) and 'poor responders' in whom an increase in PVR was small or even absent.[140]

Such a severe afterload imposed on the right ventricle, working in the unfavorable conditions of hypoxia and acidosis, results in right ventricle dilatation and failure. Raised jugular venous pressure, hepatomegaly and dependent edema are typical signs of decompensated cor pulmonale.[141,142] Mechanisms of fluid retention in cor pulmonale are complex and discussed in Chapter 17.

Uncontrolled studies have invariably shown a reduction in PAP after LTOT.[143,144] In the MRC study pulmonary arterial hypertension (PH) was stabilized in patients receiving oxygen therapy whereas a calculated annual increase in a mean PAP by 2.8 mmHg was found in controls.[13] In the NOTT trial, PAP did not change over 6 months in patients receiving oxygen for 12 hours per day. A reduction in PAP by 3 mmHg was found for patients receiving oxygen for 18 hours a day during the 6-month period.[14]

Weitzenblum et al. studied pulmonary hemodynamics three times: before LTOT, at the commencement of LTOT, and after 31 months of oxygen treatment for 15–18 hours per day.[145] They found an increase in PAP by 2.9 mmHg per year before oxygen treatment and a decrease in PAP by 2.3 mmHg per year after the commencement of LTOT.

In one recent study pulmonary hemodynamics were prospectively investigated for 6 years in 95 COPD patients undergoing LTOT.[146] Oxygen treatment resulted in a reduction of PAP over the first 2 years of treatment with a slow return to baseline values over the next 4 years. There was also a significant long-term increase in the cardiac output. The stabilization of pulmonary hemodynamics was observed despite progression of COPD – decrease in FEV_1, PaO_2 and increase in $PaCO_2$. The study

confirmed that there is a long-lasting stabilization of hypoxic PH in COPD patients treated with oxygen on average from 13 to 15 hours per day. Although LTOT did not stop the natural course of COPD, it did prevent progression of hypoxic pH.

Why does PAP not normalize, even after many years of breathing oxygen? One of the reasons may be an insufficient number of hours of oxygen use. The MRC and NOTT studies showed improved effects on pulmonary hemodynamics of 18 versus 15 hours of oxygen breathing.[13,14] Animal experiments showed that as little as 4 hours of hypoxia per day results in PH and right ventricular hypertrophy after a certain number of exposures.[147] Selinger et al. demonstrated that removal of oxygen from patients with COPD who had been receiving LTOT caused immediate increases in PAP and PVR.[148] Śliwiński et al. showed that COPD patients breathing supplemental oxygen at 2 L/min may experience significant arterial blood desaturations.[68] This may result in episodes of increased PAP. Histopathologic studies of the pulmonary arteries of patients who died after being treated with domiciliary oxygen have shown persistent structural changes, especially in the intima of small pulmonary arteries and arterioles.[149,150] There is no evidence so far that LTOT is able to reverse the noncellular intimal fibroelastosis resulting from the activity of myofibroblasts in the walls of pulmonary vessels.[151,152] Apart from insufficient oxygen-breathing hours, the inability to raise arterial oxygen above 60 mmHg in some patients, and abnormal distribution of inspired air leaving a certain number of alveoli deprived of supplemental oxygen, may contribute to the persistence of the structural changes in pulmonary arteries.

Sleep

Oxygen supplementation during sleep has beneficial effects on sleep in COPD patients with hypoxemia. This topic is discussed in detail in Chapter 19.

Polycythemia

Chronic hypoxia triggers a compensatory erythropietic reaction. Hypoxia-sensitive cells in the juxtaglomerular parts of the kidneys increase erythropietin release resulting in an increase in the red cell mass and blood volume. Hypoxemia needs to last continuously for more than 2 hours with a PaO_2 less than 60 mmHg to trigger erythropietin release.[153,154]

This compensatory mechanism increases oxygen transport to the tissue by increasing the number of hemoglobin molecules ready to accept available oxygen from the lung. However, this compensatory mechanism has undesirable consequences. Increased packed cell volume leads to hyperviscosity of the blood. Acutely induced changes in blood viscosity and volume increase pulmonary vascular resistance and pressure.[155-157] Hematocrit above 55% is associated with significantly increased PVR.[158,159]

Domiciliary oxygen treatment has resulted in a decrease in polycythemia of variable intensity. A significant decrease in the red cell mass was found in early studies on the effects of continued oxygen treatment.[8-10] Similar results were observed in the NOTT and MRC studies.[13,14] In the NOTT study, hematocrit fell by 9.2% in the continuous oxygen therapy group, but not in patients receiving nocturnal oxygen therapy.[14] In the MRC study, red cell mass decreased in oxygen-treated patients.[13]

In other studies based on large groups of patients undergoing routine domiciliary oxygen treatment, a reduction in hematocrit was less pronounced.[51,95] Insufficient oxygen breathing hours may explain this phenomenon.

ADVERSE EFFECTS OF OXYGEN

The adverse effects of oxygen include both medical and non-medical hazards. Medical hazards include both direct oxygen toxicity on the lung tissue and hypercapnia. Explosion and fire are the main non-medical hazards related to the use of LTOT.

Pulmonary oxygen toxicity

A high inspired concentration of oxygen (FIO_2), greater than 0.5, may cause acute tracheobronchitis.[160] Inhalation of 100% oxygen results in regional atelectasis in units with low $\dot{V}/\dot{Q}$ ratios.[161] In animal models, breathing gas mixtures containing more than 60% oxygen leads to acute changes – edema, cellular damage and hyaline membrane formation.[162] The prolonged exposure to high oxygen concentrations results in a proliferative process leading to fibrosis.[163] Similar changes have been reported in humans after prolonged mechanical ventilation with high FIO_2 applied prior to death.[164] High oxygen concentrations are not used in domiciliary oxygen therapy. Oxygen toxicity has recently been reviewed.[165]

Petty et al. described histologic changes consistent with chronic oxygen toxicity in 6 out of 12 patients who died after being treated with domiciliary oxygen for between 7 and 61 months.[166] In no case did oxygen therapy appear to contribute to the cause of death, and six patients with histologic changes attributed to oxygen therapy had the same survival curve as patients without such changes. Similar pathologic changes were described in one out of five autopsies by Stewart et al.[167] There were no other reports of histopathologic changes from oxygen toxicity in subjects using low-flow oxygen.

Hypercapnia

In the early years of oxygen use in COPD patients an increase in $PaCO_2$ was an important clinical problem[168] usually attributed to suppression of the hypoxic ventilatory drive.[169,170]

In patients with severe hypoxemia the drive to breathe comes from peripheral receptors in the carotid body and the aortic arch, sensitive to hypoxia. Reaction of the respiratory center to carbon dioxide is blunted due to longstanding hypercapnia. Oxygen breathing suppresses hypoxic drive leading to a reduction in minute ventilation and a further increase in $PaCO_2$.

Another mechanism by which $PaCO_2$ may increase in COPD patients receiving oxygen during acute exacerbations was proposed by Aubier et al.[171,172] According to these authors, oxygen breathing leads to pulmonary arterial vasodilatation in low $\dot{V}/\dot{Q}$ regions leading to increased carbon dioxide in arterial blood. More recently Robinson et al. suggested that both hypoventilation and $\dot{V}/\dot{Q}$ redistribution are responsible for oxygen-induced hypercapnia during acute exacerbations of COPD.[173] Oxygen breathing may also increase $PaCO_2$ by shifting the CO_2 dissociation curve (Haldane effects)[174] and increasing the $\dot{V}/\dot{Q}$ imbalance.[175]

A computer model of the changes of CO_2 in response to oxygen breathing in COPD patients indicates that the change of $PaCO_2$ can be explained by the effects of changes in $\dot{V}/\dot{Q}$ ratio and the Haldane effect without changes in respiratory drive.[176]

The increase in $PaCO_2$ under oxygen administration is frequently observed in patients with acute respiratory failure. In stable COPD patients CO_2 retention is rather modest and not much influenced by oxygen treatment. High CO_2 levels are well tolerated by COPD patients.[177] Carbon dioxide tensions of up to 80 mmHg may be balanced by bicarbonate retention keeping pH at the normal range. Respiratory acidosis, rather than the high $PaCO_2$ by itself, seems to be responsible for the deleterious effects on body homostasis.[178]

On the other hand higher alveolar CO_2 concentration means better CO_2 elimination for a given level of minute ventilation. More efficient CO_2 elimination has been suggested as an adaptive mechanism in some patients with severe respiratory failure.[179]

Non-medical hazards

Oxygen supports combustion and may become explosive when delivered in pressurized cylinders. During domiciliary oxygen use major fire risks or burns can be associated with: ignition of the nasal cannula, caused by a patient smoking while breathing oxygen, and flammability of nearby objects (bedclothes, curtains, rugs) due to oxygen leakage from nearby oxygen delivery systems.[180] The incidence of burns injuries caused by cigarette ignition of the oxygen delivery system is not known. One burns unit admitted 21 LTOT patients with face, ear and neck burns over a 7-year period.[181]

Despite the large numbers of patients on home oxygen therapy and obvious hazards related to oxygen use, reports of fire or explosion unrelated to cigarette smoking are very rare.[46,47,182]

SPECIAL ISSUES

Nocturnal oxygen therapy

Radwan and Dufmats and Koo *et al.* were among the first investigators to perform serial measurements of arterial blood gases during sleep in COPD patients.[183,184] They reported a fall in PaO_2 and an increase in $PaCO_2$.

The introduction of non-invasive monitoring of arterial blood saturation has enabled more precise measurements.[185,186] Nocturnal desaturations were found to be rather common occurring mainly during REM sleep[187] and caused by alveolar hypoventilation.[188]

Recently Plywaczewski *et al.* found that all COPD patients eligible for LTOT experienced episodes of desaturation during sleep.[189] About half of the studied patients spent more than 30% of the night with SaO_2 less than 90% despite breathing oxygen at an airflow ensuring good oxygenation at rest and while awake.

Levi-Valensi *et al.*[190] defined nocturnal oxygen desaturation (NOD) as spending 30% of total sleep time with SaO_2 less than or equal to 90%. Fletcher *et al.*[191] diagnosed NOD if SaO_2 remained less than 90% for at least 5 minutes with a nadir SaO_2 of 85% or less during REM sleep. Using these definitions both groups reported that 25–45% of COPD patients who are not hypoxemic during the day (resting PaO_2 greater than 60 mmHg) experience NOD during sleep. Nocturnal oxygen administration abolished desaturation during REM sleep.[191]

Pulmonary artery catheterization measurements of these patients found mild pulmonary hypertension (PAP > 20 mmHg) in the majority of studied subjects.[190–193] Over 3 years of follow-up NOD patients treated with nocturnal oxygen showed a slight but steady reduction in mean PAP averaging 3.7 mmHg. Nocturnal oxygen desaturating patients given compressed air (sham group) had an increase in PAP by 3.9 mmHg over the same time period. No change in PAP was observed in non-desaturators.[194]

In a 3-year retrospective multicenter study, untreated patients with nocturnal hypoxemia appeared to have an increased risk of death.[195] Interestingly, 26% of patients without evidence of NOD at initial evaluation, subsequently developed this when re-studied 42 months later.[196]

Alveolar hypoxia is the main pathogenic mechanism of hypoxic pulmonary hypertension. Fletcher's observations supported hypotheses put forward by Flenley[197] and Block *et al.*[198] that nocturnal desaturation in COPD patients may be an important factor in the development of pulmonary hypertension and of clinical signs of cor pulmonale.

Thus nocturnal desaturation is a criterion for oxygen supplementation during sleep in patients satisfactorily oxygenated during the day. It is included in national guidelines for domiciliary oxygen therapy in Europe and in Japan, although the eligibility criteria varies from one country to another.

In the USA, to qualify for nocturnal oxygen supplementation, overnight pulse oximetry should demonstrate SaO_2 equal to or below 88% regardless of the duration of desaturation. Nocturnal oxygen is also indicated if there is a decrease in PaO_2 during sleep of more than 10 mmHg or in SaO_2 of more than 5% with signs or symptoms of hypoxemia (disorders of cognitive process, restlessness or insomnia).

Apart from pulmonary hypertension and reduced survival, the suspected deleterious effects of worsening hypoxemia during sleep include increased mortality during sleep[199] and poor sleep quality as reported by Cormick in COPD patients with marked daytime hypoxemia (PaO_2 less than 55 mmHg).[200] This may not necessarily apply to COPD patients with less severe daytime hypoxemia.[201]

Recently, the rationale for nocturnal oxygen treatment was challenged by the European working group.[202] The group investigated the effects of nocturnal desaturations on pulmonary hemodynamics in COPD patients with moderate hypoxemia during the day. Contrary to Fletcher's results, who found a significantly higher mean PAP in desaturators (23.3 ± 4.8 mmHg versus 20.4 ± 4.2 mmHg),[193] there was no difference in PAP between desaturators and non-desaturators in the Weitzenblum group at rest (19.4 ± 5.3 versus 18.7 ± 4.4 mmHg) and during steady-state exercise of 40 watts (37.4 ± 8.7 versus 36.5 ± 8.8 mmHg). These results seem to suggest that nocturnal desaturations do not induce clinically significant pulmonary hypertension in COPD patients without or with only moderate daytime hypoxemia.

After the initial investigation, patients who desaturated during sleep were randomly allocated to two groups. Forty-one patients commenced nocturnal oxygen supplementation, and 31 patients served as controls. End-points of the study were pulmonary hemodynamics and survival.[203] Nocturnal oxygen therapy did not modify the evolution of pulmonary hemodynamics. In both groups the increase in PAP after 2 years was negligible. Over a 3-year follow-up period, nine patients from the treated group and seven patients from the control group died (NS). The authors concluded that the prescription of nocturnal oxygen therapy is probably not justified in COPD patients with isolated NOD. In the most recent study the group confirmed that isolated nocturnal hypoxemia or sleep-related worsening of moderate daytime hypoxemia do not appear to favor the development of pulmonary hypertension.[204]

All COPD patients with NOD should have an obstructive sleep apnea syndrome (OSAS) excluded.[205] A crude assessment may be done by assessing the graphical output of overnight SaO_2 recorded with a pulse oximeter. Nocturnal desaturation episodes in COPD usually last approximately 20–30 minutes.[189] Desaturations in OSAS are short, lasting around 20–30 seconds. In patients with an overlap syndrome the combination of both features may be observed.[206]

The treatment of all COPD patients who desaturate during sleep with nocturnal oxygen would result in a large number of subjects treated at an enormous cost. The rationale for the treatment of isolated NOD needs further studies.

Oxygen during exercise

Exercise capacity in COPD patients without concomitant disease depends on the severity of airflow limitation, dynamic hyperinflation and the development of an inefficient ventilatory pattern with exercise.[207,208] Schenkel et al. studied a group of COPD patients without resting hypoxemia[209] but who desaturated during walking, washing and eating. Fewer hypoxemic episodes were observed during the night hours although mean SaO_2 was lower at night than during the day.

Arterial oxygen desaturation seems not to be an important limiting exercise factor. However, supplemental oxygen may improve exercise capacity in a number of ways. Oxygen can reverse exercise-induced hypoxemia.[210] Increase in alveolar oxygen pressure can reduce pulmonary arterial pressure rise and reduce the right ventricle afterload.[211] Oxygen may reduce dyspnea and increase the exercise endurance.[212,213] Numerous studies have found an increase in exercise performance with supplemental oxygen[214–216] also in patients who did not desaturate on exercise[215] perhaps by reducing the level of ventilation at a given level of exercise.[210] Reduction of dyspnea by supplemental oxygen in patients not hypoxemic at exercise may also result from reduced dynamic hyperinflation.[216–218]

McDonald et al. studied effects of 6 weeks of oxygen supplementation in COPD patients with exercise hypoxemia.[219] Six weeks of oxygen use resulted in a small but significant increase in 6-minute walking distance (6MWD) and quality of life score. However, there was no difference in level of improvement between treated and control group. Kramer et al. studied effects of the rehabilitation program in COPD patients performed at the depression of the Dead Sea (−402 m).[220] The sojourn there was equal to oxygen supplementation. Improvement in exercise performance was preserved for 2 weeks after return to Jerusalem (800 m). By contrast, Royackers et al. in a carefully controlled study did not find better effects of rehabilitation in patients trained with supplemental oxygen compared to patients breathing air, suggesting a placebo effect.[221]

Air travel with oxygen

Commercial aircraft fly at altitudes between 9 and 11 thousand meters (27–33 000 feet). The pressure inside the cabin is maintained at the equivalent of 2500 meters (8000 feet). At this altitude atmospheric oxygen pressure falls to 109 mmHg. Short laboratory exposure of COPD patients to this pressure has been found to be well tolerated.[222] However, if PaO_2 of the potential traveler falls during flight to below 50 mmHg, supplemental oxygen is recommended. The expected fall in PaO_2 during flight may be calculated from preflight assessment of PaO_2 and FEV_1.[222–226]

Patients on domiciliary oxygen therapy cannot use their equipment on board commercial airlines. Thus, passengers on LTOT should contact the airline in advance informing of their need to use oxygen during flight. It is suggested that 2 L/min increase in oxygen flow rate above flow rate at sea level would ensure adequate PaO_2 during flight. Problems of air travel with oxygen were recently reviewed by Stoller.[227]

SOURCES OF OXYGEN

Three oxygen delivery systems are currently available for home use: gaseous cylinders, liquid oxygen systems and oxygen concentrators. Compressed gaseous oxygen was introduced before the end of the 19th century. Liquid oxygen, although available for hospital use in the early 1900s, was adapted for home use in the mid 1960s.[8] The oxygen concentrator was introduced for the delivery of home oxygen therapy in 1973[228] and soon, after technical improvements, became the primary method of delivery of domiciliary oxygen therapy.

Oxygen concentrator

The oxygen concentrator (OC) (Figure 29.4) is the most commonly used home oxygen delivery system.[229] Oxygen

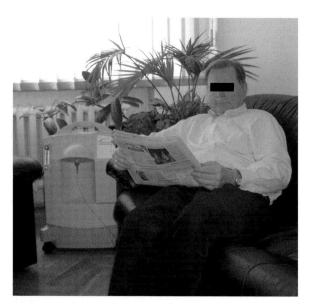

Figure 29.4 *Patient breathing oxygen from an oxygen concentrator.*

concentrators in current use are able to function continuously for approximately 10 000 hours with little maintenance. A concentration of approximately 95% oxygen at flow rates of up to 5 L/min is possible. They are the most economic method of providing LTOT and are easy to install and service. The major drawback of the OC system is that it is a stationary apparatus activated by electric power.

The principle on which the OC works is rather simple. Room air is drawn into the unit through a series of particle filters, into a compressor and heat exchanger. Gas is then directed to one of two cylinders containing molecular sieve materials. Within the molecular sieve nitrogen is adsorbed on very fine granular crystal zeolite. Smaller molecules like oxygen and trace gases pass through the sieve to a storage cylinder connected to a flow-meter and outlet. The apparatus operates in 10–12-second cycles. During one cycle, room air passes through one cylinder to produce oxygen. During the second cycle, oxygen is concentrated in the other cylinder while nitrogen is exhausted from the first cylinder. In the majority of models flow-meters are calibrated at 1–5 L of oxygen per minute. A lower flow rate results in a higher concentration of delivered oxygen.[230]

Modern OC produce relatively low noise levels, below 50 dB. The concentrator should be installed in a well-aerated space, away from heat and fire sources. The majority of models weigh around 20–25 kg (40–50 lb) and have two to four wheels allowing the patient to move the unit around. Up to 15 meters of oxygen tubing is provided to allow the patient freedom to use oxygen at a distance from the unit. Power consumption varies from 200 to 440 watts. Concentrators are equipped with a water

humidifier. However, due to the low effectiveness of the bubble humidifier,[231] at flow rates up to 4 L/min with nasal cannulae use of a humidifier can be eliminated. If used, the humidifier should be washed daily to prevent bacterial and fungal colonization. If the humidifier is not used a patient is only required to clean an external filter. This procedure is important to preserve adequate functioning of the unit, especially if OC is installed in dusty surroundings.

Oxygen concentrators are equipped with visual and sound alarms. They alert the user of power or pressure failure. The majority of models are supplied with an oxygen-sensing device triggering an alarm if the oxygen concentration falls below 80%. This alarm is very important as the patient may be unaware of a reduction in oxygen concentration which can be a major health risk.[232] OC are a low pressure system and cannot be used to operate pressure-driven nebulizers. To allow the patient to use the OC outside the home, smaller, lighter units that can be powered from a DC source (car battery) are also available. At least one OC model is capable of transfilling oxygen to a small high pressure portable cylinder[47] to allow a patient to use oxygen outdoors. However, such a unit is considerably more expensive than an ordinary OC. An oxygen concentrator that transfills portable liquid oxygen unit is currently being developed.

Current LTOT reimbursement policy in the USA recommends a combination of OC for stationary oxygen use plus small lightweight gaseous oxygen cylinders with an oxygen-conserving device for ambulation. As OC function depends on uninterrupted electric power a backup cylinder of pressurized oxygen is recommended to assure an uninterrupted oxygen supply. During the first decade of large OC use, there were several reports of malfunctions and reduced performance.[232–234] More recent models have achieved satisfactory reliability.

Liquid oxygen

At very low temperature gaseous oxygen may be converted to the liquid phase. This allows a large quantity of gas to be stored in a very small place. One liter of liquid oxygen equals 840 liters of gaseous oxygen. Liquid oxygen for home use is stored in large reservoirs containing from 20 to 40 liters of oxygen. Forty liters of liquid oxygen equals 33 600 liters of gaseous oxygen. At a flow rate of 2 L/min this system provides sufficient oxygen to last 11 days.

The oxygen container is designed like a thermos keeping the liquid at a temperature of $-165°C$ ($-297.3°F$). The insulation is not perfect. There is a small continuing loss of gaseous oxygen, estimated to be about 40–50 L/h, by evaporation. By opening the valve and closing the container, liquid oxygen passes through a warming coil and is converted into a gaseous form. The large storage tank is equipped with a quick-connect valve allowing a small portable liquid oxygen unit to be filled.

Oxygen flow rate from the container may be set at up to 8 L/min which exceeds the usual requirements of COPD patients. The portable units contain 1.0–2 liters of liquid oxygen weighing, when full, from 2.0 to 3.5 kg (4–7 lb). Oxygen flow rates of from 1 to 5 L/min are achievable. At a flow rate of 2 L/min a portable unit will last from 6 to 8 hours allowing the treated patient to perform out-of-doors activities, exercise and travel. Oxygen-conserving devices (see 'Oxygen-conserving systems' below) may double the time of use of a portable unit.

Liquid oxygen systems are more expensive than OC. The total cost includes the cost of equipment, oxygen and delivery. The logistics of liquid oxygen delivery to the patient's home may be a crucial part of total costs. A large number of patients living close to the delivery station can reduce the cost considerably.

Liquid oxygen systems are ideal for domiciliary oxygen therapy, providing the patient with 100% oxygen at a flow rate of up to 6 L/min. Liquid oxygen therapy does not require a power source and allows the patient to work, travel and participate in social activities.[235]

Oxygen cylinders

The first source of domiciliary oxygen was a large, heavy, pressurized gas cylinder. In the last two decades the OC and the liquid oxygen system have largely reduced their use. In developed countries, gaseous oxygen is now mainly used to backup the OC system. Small, lightweight, oxygen bottles are also used for ambulation. There are numerous different oxygen cylinder sizes available for home use. The range of sizes is designated by letters, from the A cylinder weighing 1.2 kg (2.5 lb) to the H cylinder, weighing (full) 70 kg (140 lb). Recently, aluminum cylinders specifically for home use have been developed that are less than 50% of the weight of a comparable size steel cylinder. The main problem associated with oxygen cylinders is their limited gas volume. The largest H cylinder can provide a continuous oxygen flow of 2 L/min for less than 3 days.

For decades, an additional problem occurring with cylinder use was the changing of the regulator from an empty cylinder to a full one. However, this problem has now been overcome and, in most cases, it can be easily changed by the patient or a family member. Special care is required when handling the cylinder to avoid injury from the weight of the cylinder, the use of oils and grease near the cylinder and to protect the cylinder from fire hazard.[236–239] For a backup oxygen supply E cylinders are most convenient. They contain 600 liters of oxygen allowing the patient to breathe oxygen at 2 L/min for 5 hours or up to 10 hours with an oxygen-conserving device. Small B and A cylinders contain 150 and 76 liters

of oxygen respectively and last for little over 1 hour and 30 minutes respectively at a standard flow of 2 L/min.

OXYGEN DELIVERY SYSTEMS

Conventional nasal cannulae are the most commonly used method of oxygen delivery. They are relatively unobtrusive allowing the user to communicate, eat, cough and sleep without encumbrance. When used at a low oxygen flow they rarely cause nasal mucosa dryness and irritation. Oxygen delivery is assured even in patients who mouth breathe,[240] although a considerable variability of inspired oxygen concentration may be observed.[241]

Some patients using nasal oxygen may experience nasal congestion, irritation of the nasal mucosa and epistaxis related to mucosal drying. Allergic reactions to the plastic materials used in some nasal cannulae have been reported.[242]

Transtracheal catheter

Continuous oxygen delivery by a small transtracheal catheter was developed and reported by Heimlich in 1982.[243] Delivery of oxygen directly to the trachea reduced deadspace, improved oxygenation, and the patient did not require a nasal cannula. Christopher et al. after long-term observation of 100 patients with transtracheal cannula reported that the catheter provided improved oxygenation at a lower oxygen flow than required for nasal cannula.[244] Compliance was very good (96%) and complications rare. Several systems of cannulation were developed in the USA[245,246] and Europe.[247–249]

The procedure is performed on an ambulatory basis under local anesthesia. A large catheter is introduced by the Seldinger technique between the second and third tracheal cartilage. This catheter serves to establish a small mini-tracheostomy tract that is epithelialized during 4–6 weeks. Through the orifice a small flexible oxygen catheter is introduced. Patients are taught to remove, clean and change such catheters twice daily. In some systems a large catheter is left in place permanently and changed every month.

Transtracheal oxygen delivery (TTO) reduces resting oxygen flow by up to 50%[244,247] and improves PaO_2 which is sometimes difficult to achieve with nasal cannula. Transtracheal oxygen therapy has been found to increase patient compliance, decrease the number of days of hospitalization[250] and increase exercise tolerance.[251] In some patients TTO improves self-image.[248]

The most frequent complication of TTO is formation of a mucous ball on the catheter that may cause serious airflow obstruction.[252] Less frequent complications include infections, subcutaneous emphysema, hemoptysis, catheter dislodgement and cough.[253]

The number of patients using TTO is difficult to estimate. One recent review estimated less than 1% of all patients receiving domiciliary oxygen in the USA were receiving TTO.[253] In Europe the use of TTO seems to be rare.[254,255]

OXYGEN-CONSERVING SYSTEMS

In COPD patients, expiration lasts more than a half of the breathing cycle. With a constant oxygen flow more than a half of oxygen is wasted. Although such a waste is not important when oxygen is provided by an OC, considerable cost and restriction of activity occur when a patient is using gaseous or liquid oxygen. Oxygen-conserving devices have been developed to reduce the cost and improve the efficiency and effectiveness of oxygen therapy.

The first simple devices, were based on the principle of attaching a small (20 ml) reservoir to a nasal cannula. Such reservoirs were placed below the nose (moustache type) or on the upper part of the chest (pendant-type).[256,257] During expiration oxygen filled the reservoir for subsequent delivery during early inspiration. This allowed the patient to achieve satisfactory oxygenation with reduced oxygen usage.

Reservoir cannulas, although effective,[258–260] are now rarely used. They have been replaced by electronically controlled intermittent flow devices.[261] The oxygen-conserving device (OCD) senses the patient's inspiratory effort and delivers oxygen during early inspiration assuring delivered oxygen reaches the alveoli.

Several models of OCD are commercially available. They are of three types: pulse, demand and hybrid.[261–263] In the pulse system, a short bolus of oxygen is delivered at the onset of inspiration. The demand system delivers oxygen during inspiration at a flow rate prescribed for continuous flow. A hybrid system is a mixture of pulse and demand system. Oxygen-conserving devices are either pressure or time cycled and are powered by batteries.

Although installation of OCD adds an additional cost to oxygen therapy, cuts on reimbursement of LTOT in the USA increased their use considerably. In 1998 approximately 80 000 OCDs were sold in the USA. When introducing such a device in the oxygen delivery system in an individual patient its clinical efficacy should be tested by pulse oximetry measurements.[264–266] Especially during exercise changeable breathing pattern, breathing frequency and tidal volume may reduce the amount of oxygen reaching a gas exchange zone in the lung and may cause hypoxemia.[267,268] It was also suggested that inspiratory signal sensitivity should be set for each individual patient during sleep.[269]

The OCD and techniques were recently reviewed by McCoy.[269]

FUTURE DIRECTIONS

The MRC and NOTT studies showed that increased oxygen breathing hours per day give better survival and improvement in many bodily functions. It may be assumed that really continuous oxygen treatment may give even better results. It may be achieved only by ambulatory oxygen, giving patients opportunities to enjoy work and family and social life. Advantages of ambulatory oxygen are related not only to increased oxygen breathing hours but also to opportunity of regular exercise. It seems that physical exercise, a key part of rehabilitation programs, may contribute to prolonged survival.[15,270]

Another field that should be explored further is ensuring a patient is normoxemic while breathing oxygen. Earlier in this chapter numerous papers were cited showing that patients on LTOT experience prolonged periods of hypoxemia during exercise and during sleep while breathing oxygen. Empirically recommended increase in oxygen flow by 0.5–1 liters during exercise and sleep should be objectively studied, assessing its efficacy and safety.[271]

The value of supplemental oxygen for nocturnal and exercise hypoxemia requires further study. The quality of life seems to be a better end-point to be evaluated in this respect than physiologic variables.

Ambulatory oxygen seems to add years to the life of patients on domiciliary oxygen. However it happens too often that domiciliary oxygen only adds years to life of a home-bound COPD patient.[272] A portable oxygen concentrator would be a great breakthrough in this direction.

REFERENCES

1. Priestley J. Observations on different kinds of air. *Phil Trans Lond* 1772;**62**:147–55.
2. *The New Encyclopaedia Britannica*, vol 9, 15th edn. Joseph Priestley, Chicago, 1991, pp 696–7.
3. Cotes J, Gilson JC. Effect of oxygen on exercise ability in chronic respiratory insufficiency: use of a portable apparatus. *Lancet* 1956;**i**:1084–5.
4. Barach AL. Ambulatory oxygen therapy: oxygen inhalation at home and out-of-doors. *Dis Chest* 1959;**35**:229–41.
5. Campbell EJM. A method of controlled oxygen administration which reduces the risk of carbon-dioxide retention. *Lancet* 1960;**ii**:12–14.
6. Abraham AS, Cole RB, Green ID, Hedworth-Whitty RB, Clarke SW, Bishop JM. Factors contributing to the reversible pulmonary hypertension of patients with acute respiratory failure studied by serial observations during recovery. *Circ Res* 1969;**24**:51–60.

7. Stuart-Harris C. A hospital study of congestive heart failure, with special reference to cor pulmonale. *Br Med J* 1959;**2**:201–8.
8. Levine BE, Bigelow DB, Hamstra RD, *et al.* The role of long-term continuous oxygen administration in patients with chronic airway obstruction with hypoxemia. *Ann Intern Med* 1967;**66**:639–50.
9. Abraham AS, Cole RB, Bishop JM. Reversal of pulmonary hypertension by prolonged oxygen administration to patients with chronic bronchitis. *Circ Res* 1968;**23**:147–57.
10. Petty TL, Finigan MM. Clinical evaluation of prolonged ambulatory oxygen therapy in chronic airway obstruction. *Am J Med* 1968;**45**:242–52.
11. Stark RD, Finnegan P, Bishop JM. Daily requirement of oxygen to reverse pulmonary hypertension in patients with chronic bronchitis. *Br Med J* 1972;**3**:724–8.
12. Stark RD, Finnegan P, Bishop JM. Long-term domiciliary oxygen in chronic bronchitis with pulmonary hypertension. *Br Med J* 1973;**3**:467–70.
13. Medical Research Council Working Party. Long term domiciliary oxygen therapy in chronic hypoxic cor pulmonale complicating chronic bronchitis and emphysema. *Lancet* 1981;**i**:681–5.
14. Nocturnal Oxygen Therapy Trial Group. Continuous or nocturnal oxygen therapy in hypoxemic chronic obstructive lung disease: a clinical trial. *Ann Intern Med* 1980; **93**:391–8.
15. Petty TL, Bliss PL. Ambulatory oxygen therapy, exercise, and survival with advanced chronic obstructive pulmonary disease (the nocturnal oxygen therapy trial revisited). *Respir Care* 2000;**45**:204–11.
16. Crockett AJ, Moss JR, Cranston JM, Alpers JH. Domiciliary oxygen in chronic obstructive pulmonary disease (Cochrane Review) In: *The Cochrane Library*, issue 3. Update Software, Oxford, 1999.
17. Crockett AJ, Cranston JM, Moss JR, Alpers JH. A review of long-term oxygen therapy for chronic obstructive pulmonary disease. *Respir Med*, 2001;**95**:437–43.
18. Levi Valensi P, Aubry P, Donner CF, Robert B, Ruhle KH, Weitzenblum E. Recommendations for long term oxygen therapy. *Eur Respir J* 1989;**2**:160–4.
19. Zieliński J, Śliwiński P. Indications for and methods of long-term oxygen therapy (LTOT). *Eur Respir Rev* 1991; **1**:536–40.
20. Pulmonary Physiology Committee affiliated with Japan Society of Chest Diseases. Guidelines for home oxygen therapy. *Jpn J Thorac Dis* 1988;**26**:923–5.
21. Siafakas NM,Vermeire P, Pride NB, *et al.* Optimal assessment and management of chronic obstructive pulmonary disease (COPD). *Eur Respir J* 1995;**8**:1398–420.
22. Standards for the diagnosis and care of patients with chronic obstructive pulmonary disease. *Am J Respir Crit Care Med* 1995;**152**(5/2): S77–120.
23. BTS guidelines for the management of chronic obstructive pulmonary disease. *Thorax* 1997;**52**(suppl 5):S1–28.
24. Zieliński J. Indications for long-term oxygen therapy: a reappraisal. *Monaldi Arch Chest Dis* 1999;**54**:178–82.
25. Conference report: new problems in supply, reimbursement and certification of medical necessity for long-term oxygen therapy. *Am Rev Respir Dis* 1990;**142**:721–4.
26. Seemungal TAR, Donaldson GC, Bhowmik A, Jeffries DJ, Wedzicha JA. Time course and recovery of exacerbations in patients with chronic obstructive pulmonary disease. *Am J Respir Crit Care Med* 2000;**161**:1608–13.
27. Levi-Valensi P, Weitzenblum E, Pedinielli JL, Racineux JL, Duwoos H. Three-month follow-up of arterial blood gas determinations in candidates for long-term oxygen therapy. *Am Rev Respir Dis* 1986;**133**:547–51.
28. Eaton TE, Grey C, Garrett JE. An evaluation of short-term oxygen therapy: the prescription of oxygen to patients with chronic lung disease hypoxic at discharge from hospital. *Respir Med* 2001;**95**:582–7.
29. Górecka D, Śliwiński P, Zieliński J. Adherence to entry criteria and one year experience of long-term oxygen therapy in Poland. *Eur Respir J* 1992;**5**:848–52.
30. Ström K, Boe J. A national register for long-term oxygen therapy in chronic hypoxia: preliminary results. *Eur Respir J* 1988;**1**:952–8.
31. Ström K, Boe J. Quality assessment and predictors of survival in long-term domiciliary oxygen therapy. *Eur Respir J* 1991;**4**:50–8.
32. Pitkin AD, Roberts CM, Wedzicha JA. Arterialised earlobe blood gas analysis: an underused technique. *Thorax* 1994;**49**:364–6.
33. Dar K, Williams T, Aitken R, Woods KL, Fletcher S. Arterial versus capillary sampling for analysing blood gas pressures. *Br Med J* 1995;**310**:24–5.
34. Sauty A, Uldry C, Debetaz LF, Leuenberger P, Fitting JW. Differences in Po_2 and Pco_2 between arterial and arterialized earlobe samples. *Eur Respir J* 1996;**9**:186–9.
35. Goldstein RS, Ramcharan V, Bowes G, McNicholas WT, Bradley D, Phillipson EA. Effect of supplemental nocturnal oxygen on gas exchange in patients with severe obstructive lung disease. *N Engl J Med* 1984;**310**:425–9.
36. Walshaw MJ, Lim R, Evans CC, Hind CRK. Prescription of oxygen concentrators for long-term oxygen treatment: reassessment in one district. *Br Med J* 1988;**297**:1030–2.
37. Bongard JP, De Haller R. Oxygenotherapie au long cours en Suisse. *Schweiz Med Wochenschr* 1989;**119**:110–15.
38. Dilworth JP, Higgs CMB, Jones PA, White RJ. Prescription of oxygen concentrators: adherence to published guidelines. *Thorax* 1989;**44**:576–8.
39. Baudouin SV, Waterhouse JC, Tahtamouni T, Smith JA, Baxter J, Howard P. Long-term domiciliary oxygen treatment for chronic respiratory failure reviewed. *Thorax* 1990;**45**: 195–8.
40. Guyatt GH, McKim DA, Austin P, *et al.* Appropriateness of domiciliary oxygen delivery. *Chest* 2000;**118**:1303–8.
41. Oba Y, Salzman GA, Willsie SK. Reevaluation of continuous oxygen therapy after initial prescription in patients with chronic obstructive pulmonary disease. *Respir Care* 2000;**45**:401–6.
42. US Department of Health and Human Services, Office of Inspector General. *Office of Audit. National Review of Medical Necessity for Oxygen Concentrators.* Audit Control No A-04-88-02055. 1990.
43. Cottrell JJ, Openbrier D, Lave JR, Paul C, Garland JL. Home oxygen therapy. A comparison of 2 vs 6 month patient reevaluation. *Chest* 1995;**107**:358–61.
44. O'Donohue WJ Jr. Oxygen therapy in pulmonary rehabilitation. In: JE Hodgkin, BR Celli, GL Connors, eds. *Pulmonary Rehabilitation. Guidelines to Success*, 3rd edn. Lippincott/Williams & Wilkins, Philadelphia, 2000, pp 135–46.
45. Calverley PMA, Leggett RJ, McElderry L, Flenley DC. Cigarette smoking and secondary polycythemia in hypoxic cor pulmonale. *Am Rev Respir Dis* 1982;**125**:507–10.
46. Benditt JO. Adverse effects of low-flow oxygen therapy. *Respir Care* 2000;**45**:54–61.
47. Kacmarek RM. Delivery systems for long-term oxygen therapy. *Respir Care* 2000;**45**:84–94.

48. Sano M. Quality assurance of oxygen concentrators in the home setting. In: S Kira, TL Petty, eds. *Progress in Domiciliary Respiratory Care. Current Status and Perspective*. Elsevier Science BV, Amsterdam, 1994, pp 269–75.

49. Miwa T, Furui H, Kishi F, Machida K, Takagi H, Kimura K. A supporting system for home oxygen therapy: transmission of patient's Sao_2 data by telephone line. In: S Kira, TL Petty, eds. *Progress in Domiciliary Respiratory Care. Current Status and Perspective*. Elsevier Science BV, Amsterdam, 1994, pp 259–68.

50. Pépin JL, Barjhoux CE, Deschaux Ch, Brambilla Ch. Long-term oxygen therapy at home. Compliance with medical prescription and effective use of therapy. *Chest* 1996;**109**: 1144–50.

51. Zieliński J, Śliwiński P, Tobiasz M, Górecka D. Long-term oxygen therapy in Poland. *Monaldi Arch Chest Dis* 1993;**48**:479–80.

52. Morrison D, Skwarski K, MacNee W. Review of the prescription of domiciliary long term oxygen therapy in Scotland. *Thorax* 1995;**50**:1103–5.

53. Atiş St, Tutloğlu B, Buğdayci R. Characteristics and compliance of patients receiving long-term oxygen therapy (LTOT) in Turkey. *Monaldi Arch Chest Dis* 2001;**56**:105–9.

54. Vergeret J, Tunon de Lara M, *et al.* Compliance of COPD patients with long-term oxygen therapy. *Eur J Respir Dis* 1986;**69**(suppl 146):421–5.

55. Walshaw MJ, Lim R, Evans CC, Hind CRK. Factors influencing the compliance in patients using oxygen concentrators for long-term home oxygen therapy. *Respir Med* 1990;**84**:331–3.

56. Restrick LJ, Paul EA, Braid GM, Cullinan P, Moore-Gillon J, Wedzicha JA. Assessment and follow-up of patients prescribed long-term oxygen treatment. *Thorax* 1993;**48**:708–13.

57. Howard P, Waterhouse JC, Billings CG. Compliance with long-term oxygen therapy by concentrator. *Eur Respir J* 1992;**5**:128–9.

58. Kampelmacher MJ, van Kesteren RG, Alsbach GPJ, *et al.* Characteristics and complaints of patients prescribed long-term oxygen therapy in the Netherlands. *Respir Med* 1998;**92**:70–5.

59. Peckham DG, McGibbon K, Tonkinson J, Plimbley G, Pantin C. Improvement in patients compliance with long-term oxygen therapy following formal assessment with training. *Respir Med* 1998;**92**:1203–6.

60. Ringbaek TJ, Lange P, Viskum K. Geographic variation in long-term oxygen therapy in Denmark. Factors related to adherence to guidelines for long-term oxygen therapy. *Chest* 2001;**119**:1711–16.

61. Vergeret J, Brambilla C, Mounier L. Portable oxygen therapy: use and benefit in hypoxaemic COPD patients on long-term oxygen therapy. *Eur Respir J* 1989;**2**:20–5.

62. Lock SH, Paul EA, Rudd RM, Wedzicha JA. Portable oxygen therapy: assessment and usage. *Respir Med* 1991;**85**:407–12.

63. Leach RM, Davidson AC, Chinn S, Twort CHC, Cameron IR, Bateman NT. Portable liquid oxygen and exercise ability in severe respiratory disability. *Thorax* 1992;**47**:781–9.

64. Ringbaek T, Lange P, Viskum K. Compliance with LTOT and consumption of mobile oxygen. *Respir Med* 1999;**93**:333–7.

65. Howard P, De Haller R. Domiciliary oxygen by liquid or concentrator? *Eur Respir J* 1991;**4**:1284–7.

66. Guyatt GH, McKim DA, Weaver B, *et al.* Development and testing of formal protocols for oxygen prescribing. *Am J Respir Crit Care Med* 2001;**163**:942–6.

67. Estopa RM, Monasterio C, Escarrabill J. Daily life desaturations in COPD patients on LTOT: International Oxygen Club Multicentre European Study. *Monaldi Arch Chest Dis* 1993;**48**:426–8.

68. Śliwiński P, Lagosz M, Górecka D, Zieliński J. The adequacy of oxygenation in COPD patients undergoing long-term oxygen therapy assessed by pulse oximetry at home. *Eur Respir J* 1994;**7**:274–8.

69. Abdulla J, Godtfredsen N, Pisinger C, Wennike P, Tonnesen P. Adequacy of oxygenation in a group of Danish patients with COPD on long-term oxygen therapy. *Monaldi Arch Chest Dis* 2000;**55**:279–82.

70. Morrison D, Skwarski KM, MacNee W. The adequacy of oxygenation in patients with hypoxic chronic obstructive pulmonary disease treated with long-term domiciliary oxygen. *Respir Med* 1997;**91**:287–91.

71. Vandenbergh E, Clement J, Van de Woestijne KP. Course and prognosis of patients with advanced chronic obstructive pulmonary disease. *Am J Med* 1973;**55**:736–46.

72. Ude AC, Howard P. Controlled oxygen therapy and pulmonary heart failure. *Thorax* 1971;**26**:572–8.

73. Weitzenblum E, Rasaholinjanahary J, Meyer PD, Hirth C, Oudet P. Evolution clinique, fonctionnelle et hemodynamique de bronchiteux chroniques au stade du coeur pulmonaire chronique. *Poumon Coeur* 1976;**32**: 299–304.

74. Weitzenblum E, Hirth C, Ducolone A, Mirhom R, Rasaholinjanahary J, Ehrhart M. Prognostic value of pulmonary artery pressure in chronic obstructive pulmonary disease. *Thorax* 1981;**36**:752–8.

75. Bishop JM, Cross KW. Physiological variables and mortality in patients with various categories of chronic respiratory diseases. *Bull Europ Physiopathol Resp* 1984;**20**:495–500.

76. Burrows B, Earle RH. Course and prognosis of chronic obstructive lung disease. A prospective study of 200 patients. *N Engl J Med* 1969;**280**:397–404.

77. Bishop JM. Hypoxia and pulmonary hypertension in chronic bronchitis. *Progr Resp Res* 1975;**9**:10–16.

78. Ourednik A, Susa Z. How long does the pulmonary hypertension last in chronic obstructive bronchopulmonary disease? *Progr Resp Res* 1975;**9**:24–8.

79. Schrijen F, Uffholtz H, Polu JM, Poincelot E. Pulmonary and systemic hemodynamic evolution in chronic bronchitis. *Am Rev Respir Dis* 1978;**117**:25–31.

80. Intermittent positive pressure breathing therapy of chronic obstructive pulmonary disease: a clinical trial. *Ann Intern Med* 1983;**99**:612–20.

81. Anthonisen NR. Prognosis in chronic obstructive pulmonary disease: results from multicenter clinical trials. *Am Rev Respir Dis* 1989;**140**:S95–9.

82. Neff TA, Petty TL. Long-term continuous oxygen therapy in chronic airway obstruction: mortality in relationship to cor pulmonale, hypoxia and hypercapnia. *Ann Intern Med* 1970;**72**:621–6.

83. Boushy SF, Coates EO Jr. Prognostic value of pulmonary function tests in emphysema: with special reference to arterial blood studies. *Am Rev Respir Dis* 1964;**90**:553–63.

84. Zieliński J, MacNee W, Wedzicha J, *et al.* Causes of death in patients with COPD and chronic respiratory failure. *Monaldi Arch Chest Dis* 1997;**52**:43–7.

85. MacNee W. Predictors of survival in patients treated with long-term oxygen therapy. *Respiration* 1992;**59**(suppl 2):5–7.

86. Dallari R, Barozzi G, Pinelli G, Marazotti M, Tartoni PL. Predictors of survival in subjects with chronic obstructive pulmonary disease treated with long-term oxygen therapy. *Respiration* 1994;**61**:8–13.

87. Skwarski K, MacNee W, Wraith PK, Śliwiński P, Zieliński J. Predictors of survival in patients with chronic obstructive pulmonary disease treated with long-term oxygen therapy. *Chest* 1991;**100**:1522–7.

88. Dubois P, Jamart J, Machiels J, Smeets F, Lulling J. Prognosis of severely hypoxemic patients receiving long-term oxygen therapy. *Chest* 1994;**105**:469–74.

89. Ström K. Survival of patients with chronic obstructive pulmonary disease receiving long-term domiciliary oxygen therapy. *Am Rev Respir Dis* 1993;**147**:585–91.

90. Ashutosh K, Mead G, Dunsky M. Early effects of oxygen administration and prognosis in chronic obstructive pulmonary disease and cor pulmonale. *Am Rev Respir Dis* 1983;**127**:399–404.

91. Ashutosh K, Dunsky M. Noninvasive tests for responsiveness of pulmonary hypertension to oxygen. Prediction of survival in patients with chronic obstructive lung disease and cor pulmonale. *Chest* 1987;**92**:393–9.

92. Śliwiński P, Hawryłkiewicz I, Górecka D, Zieliński J. Acute effect of oxygen on pulmonary arterial pressure does not predict survival on long-term oxygen therapy in patients with chronic obstructive pulmonary disease. *Am Rev Respir Dis* 1992;**146**:665–9.

93. Głuskowski J, Jędrzejewska-Mąkowska M, Hawryłkiewicz I, Vertun B, Zieliński J. Effects of prolonged oxygen therapy on pulmonary hypertension and blood viscosity in patients with advanced cor pulmonale. *Respiration* 1983;**44**:177–83.

94. Górecka D, Gorzelak K, Śliwiński P, Tobiasz M, Zieliński J. Effects of long term oxygen therapy on survival in patients with chronic obstructive pulmonary disease with moderate hypoxaemia. *Thorax* 1997;**52**:674–9.

95. Veale D, Chailleux F, Taytard A, Cardinaud JP. Characteristics and survival of patients prescribed long term oxygen therapy outside prescription guidelines. *Eur Respir J* 1998;**12**:780–4.

96. Haluszka J, Chartrand DA, Grassino AE, Milic-Emili J. Intrinsic PEEP and arterial Pco_2 in stable patients with chronic obstructive pulmonary disease. *Am Rev Respir Dis* 1990;**141**:1194–7.

97. Yan S, Kayser B, Tobiasz M, Śliwiński P. Comparison of static and dynamic intrinsic positive end-expiratory pressure using the Campbell diagram. *Am J Respir Crit Care Med* 1996;**154**:938–44.

98. Coussa ML, Guerin C, Eissa NT, et al. Partitioning of work of breathing in mechanically ventilated COPD patients. *J Appl Physiol* 1993;**75**:1711–19.

99. Śliwiński P, Kamiński D, Zieliński J, Yan S. Partitioning of the elastic work of inspiration in COPD patients during incremental exercise. *Eur Respir J* 1998;**11**:416–21.

100. Śliwiński P, Macklem PT. Inspiratory muscle dysfunction as a cause of death in COPD patients. *Monaldi Arch Chest Dis* 1997;**52**:380–3.

101. Sinderby C, Lindstrom L, Grassino AE. Automatic assessment of electromyogram quality. *J Appl Physiol* 1995;**79**:1803–15.

102. Wilson DK, Kaplan RM, Timms RM, Dawson A. Acute effects of oxygen treatment upon information processing in hypoxemic COPD patients. *Chest* 1985;**88**:239–43.

103. Krop HD, Block AJ, Cohen E. Neuropsychiatric effects of continuous oxygen therapy in obstructive pulmonary disease. *Chest* 1973;**64**:317–22.

104. Heaton RK, Grant I, McSweeny AJ, Adams KM, Petty TL. Psychologic effects of continuous and nocturnal oxygen therapy in hypoxemic chronic obstructive pulmonary disease. *Arch Intern Med* 1983;**143**:1941–7.

105. McSweeny AJ, Grant I, Heaton RK, Adams KM, Timms RM. Life quality of patients with chronic obstructive pulmonary disease. *Arch Intern Med* 1982;**142**:473–8.

106. Grant I, Heaton RK, McSweeny AJ, Adams KM, Timms RM. Neuropsychologic findings in hypoxemic chronic obstructive pulmonary disease. *Arch Intern Med* 1982;**142**:1470–6.

107. Borak J, Śliwiński P, Piasecki Z, Zieliński J. Psychological status of COPD patients on long-term oxygen therapy. *Eur Respir J* 1991;**4**:59–62.

108. Pedinielli JL, Bertagne P, Campoli C, Levi-Valensi P. Depression, alexithymie et handicap chez les insuffisants respiratoires chroniques. *Psychol Med* 1991;**2**:178–82.

109. Incalzi RA, Gemma A, Marra C, Muzzolon R, Capparella O, Carbonn P. Chronic obstructive pulmonary disease: an original model of cognitive decline. *Am Rev Respir Dis* 1993;**148**:418–22.

110. Gift AG, Plaut SM, Jacox A. Psychologic and physiologic factors related to dyspnoea in subjects with chronic obstructive pulmonary disease. *Heart Lung* 1986;**15**:595–601.

111. Gift AG, Cahill CA. Psychophysiologic aspects of dyspnoea in chronic obstructive pulmonary disease: a pilot study. *Heart Lung* 1990;**19**:252–7.

112. Burrows B, Fletcher CM, Heard BE, Jones NL, Wootliff JS. The emphysematous and bronchial types of chronic airways obstruction. *Lancet* 1966;**i**:830–5.

113. Sweer L, Zwillich CW. Dyspnoea in the patient with chronic obstructive pulmonary disease. *Clin Chest Med* 1990;**11**:417–45.

114. Borak J, Śliwiński P, Tobiasz M, Górecka D, Zieliński J. Psychological status of COPD patients before and after one year of long-term oxygen therapy. *Monaldi Arch Chest Dis* 1996;**51**:7–11.

115. Kaplan RM, Atkins CJ, Timms R. Validity of a quality of well-being scale as an outcome measure in chronic obstructive pulmonary disease. *J Chronic Dis* 1984;**37**:85–95.

116. Prigatano GP, Wright EC, Levin D. Quality of life and its predictors in patients with mild hypoxemia and chronic obstructive pulmonary disease. *Arch Intern Med* 1984;**144**:1613–19.

117. Jones PW. Quality of life measurement for patients with diseases of the airways. *Thorax* 1991;**46**:676–82.

118. Ries AL, Kaplan RM, Limberg TM, Prewitt LM. Effects of pulmonary rehabilitation on physiologic and psychosocial outcomes in patients with chronic obstructive pulmonary disease. *Ann Intern Med* 1995;**122**:823–32.

119. Jones PW, Quirk FH, Baveystock CM, Littlejohns P. A self-complete measure of health status for chronic airflow limitation. The St George's Respiratory Questionnaire. *Am Rev Respir Dis* 1992;**145**:1321–7.

120. Ferrer M, Alonso J, Morera J, et al. Chronic obstructive pulmonary disease stage and health-related quality of life. *Ann Intern Med* 1997;**127**:1072–9.

121. Okubadejo AA, Jones PW, Wedzicha JA. Quality of life in patients with chronic obstructive pulmonary disease and severe hypoxaemia. *Thorax* 1996;**51**:44–7.

122. Seemungal TAR, Donaldson GC, Paul EA, Bestall JC, Jeffries DJ, Wedzicha JA. Effect of exacerbation on quality of life in patients with chronic obstructive pulmonary disease. *Am J Respir Crit Care Med* 1998;**157**:1418–22.

123. Lahdensuo A, Ojanen M, Ahonen A, et al. Psychosocial effects of continuous oxygen therapy in hypoxaemic chronic obstructive pulmonary disease patients. *Eur Respir J* 1989;**2**:977–80.

124. Dilworth JP, Higgs CMB, Jones PA, White RJ. Acceptability of oxygen concentrators: the patient's view. *Br J Gen Pract* 1990;**40**:415–17.

125. Okubadejo AA, Paul EA, Jones PW, Wedzicha JA. Does long-term oxygen therapy affect quality of life in patients with chronic obstructive pulmonary disease and severe hypoxaemia? *Eur Respir J* 1996;**9**:2335–9.

126. Lock SH, Blower G, Prynne M, Wedzicha JA. Comparison of liquid and gaseous oxygen for domiciliary portable use. *Thorax* 1992;**47**:98–100.

127. Andersson A, Ström K, Brodin H, *et al.* Domiciliary liquid oxygen versus concentrator treatment in chronic hypoxaemia: a cost – utility analysis. *Eur Respir J* 1998;**12**:1284–9.

128. Okubadejo AA, O'Shea L, Jones PW, Wedzicha JA. Home assessment of activities of daily living in patients with severe chronic obstructive pulmonary disease on long-term oxygen therapy. *Eur Respir J* 1997;**10**:1572–5.

129. Janssens JP, Rochat T, Frey JG, Dousse N, Pichard C, Tschopp JM. Health-related quality of life in patients under long-term oxygen therapy: a home-based descriptive study. *Respir Med* 1997;**91**:592–602.

130. Perrin C, El Far Y, Vandenbos F, *et al.* Domiciliary nasal intermittent positive pressure ventilation in severe COPD: effects on lung function and quality of life. *Eur Respir J* 1997;**10**:2835–9.

131. Monso E, Fiz JM, Izquierdo J, *et al.* Quality of life in severe chronic obstructive pulmonary disease: correlation with lung and muscle function. *Respir Med* 1998;**92**:221–7.

132. Crockett AJ, Moss JR, Cranston JM, Alpers JH. Effects of long-term oxygen therapy on quality of life and survival in chronic airflow limitation. *Monaldi Arch Chest Dis* 1999;**54**:193–6.

133. Euler US, von, Liljestrand G. Observations on the pulmonary arterial blood pressure in the cat. *Acta Physiol Scand* 1946;**12**:301–20.

134. Hasleton PS, Heath D, Brewer DB. Hypertensive pulmonary vascular disease in states of chronic hypoxia. *J Pathol Bacteriol* 1968;**95**:431–40.

135. Fishman AP. State of the art: chronic cor pulmonale. *Am Rev Respir Dis* 1976;**114**:775–94.

136. MacNee W. Pathophysiology of cor pulmonale in chronic obstructive pulmonary disease. Part one. *Am J Respir Crit Care Med* 1994;**150**:833–52.

137. MacNee W. Pathophysiology of cor pulmonale in chronic obstructive pulmonary disease. Part two. *Am J Respir Crit Care Med* 1994;**150**:1158–68.

138. World Health Organization. Chronic cor pulmonale: report of an expert committee. *Circulation* 1963;**27**:594–615.

139. Bishop JM, Cross KW. Use of other physiological variables to predict pulmonary arterial pressure in patients with chronic respiratory disease. Multicentre study. *Eur Heart J* 1981;**2**:509–17.

140. Weitzenblum E, Schrijen F, Mohan-Kumar T, Colas-des Francs V, Lockhart A. Variability of the pulmonary vascular response to acute hypoxia in chronic bronchitis patients. *Chest* 1988;**94**:772–8.

141. Anand IS, Chandrashekhar Y, Ferrari R, *et al.* Pathogenesis of congestive state in chronic obstructive pulmonary disease. Studies of body water and sodium, renal function, hemodynamics, and plasma hormones during edema and after recovery. *Circulation* 1992;**86**:12–21.

142. Weitzenblum E, Apprill M, Oswald M, Chaouat A, Imbs JL. Pulmonary hemodynamics in patients with chronic obstructive pulmonary disease before and during an episode of peripheral edema. *Chest* 1994;**105**:1377–82.

143. Leggett RJ, Cooke NL, Clancy L, Leitch AG, Kirby BJ, Flenley DC. Long-term domiciliary oxygen therapy in cor pulmonale complicating chronic bronchitis and emphysema. *Thorax* 1976;**31**:414–18.

144. Cooper CB, Waterhouse J, Howard P. Twelve year clinical study of patients with hypoxic cor pulmonale given long-term domiciliary oxygen therapy. *Thorax* 1987;**42**:105–10.

145. Weitzenblum E, Oswald M, Apprill M, Ratomaharo J, Kessler R. Evolution of physiologic variables in patients with chronic obstructive pulmonary disease before and during long-term oxygen therapy. *Respiration* 1991;**58**:126–31.

146. Zieliński J, Tobiasz M, Hawryłkiewicz I, Śliwiński P, Paasiewicz G. Effects of long-term oxygen therapy on pulmonary hemodynamics in COPD patients. *Chest* 1998;**113**:65–70.

147. Widimský J, Urbanová D, Ressl J, Ostadal B, Pelouch V, Prochazka J. Effect of intermittent altitude hypoxia on the myocardium and lesser circulation in the rat. *Cardiovasc Res* 1973;**7**:798–808.

148. Selinger SR, Kennedy TP, Buescher P, *et al.* Effect of removing oxygen from patients with chronic obstructive pulmonary disease. *Am Rev Respir Dis* 1987;**136**:85–91.

149. Magee F, Wright JL, Wiggs BR, Pare PD, Hogg JC. Pulmonary vascular structure and function in chronic obstructive pulmonary disease. *Thorax* 1988;**43**:183–9.

150. Wilkinson M, Langhorne CA, Heath D, Barer GR, Howard P. A pathophysiological study of 10 cases of hypoxic cor pulmonale. *Q J Med* 1988;**66**:65–85.

151. Scott KWM, Barer GR, Leach E, Mungall IPF. Pulmonary ultrastructural changes in hypoxic rats. *J Pathol* 1978;**27**:126–31.

152. Meyrick B, Reid L. Endothelial and subintimal changes in rat hilar pulmonary artery during recovery from hypoxia: a quantitative and ultrastructural study. *Lab Invest* 1980;**42**:603–15.

153. Fitzpatrick MF, Mackay T, Whyte KF, Allen M, Tam RC, Dore CJ. Nocturnal desaturation and serum erythropoietin: a study in patients with chronic obstructive pulmonary disease and in normal subjects. *Clin Sci* 1993;**84**:319–24.

154. Eckardt KU, Boutellier U, Kurtz A, Schopen M, Koller EA, Bauer C. Rate of erythropoietin formation in humans in response to acute hypobaric hypoxia. *J Appl Physiol* 1989;**66**:1785–8.

155. Segel N, Bishop JM. The circulation in patients with chronic bronchitis and emphysema at rest and during exercise with special reference to the influence of changes in blood viscosity and blood volume on the pulmonary circulation. *J Clin Invest* 1966;**45**:1555–68.

156. Enson Y, Schmidt DH, Ferrer MI, Harvey RM. The effect of acutely induced hypervolemia on resistance to pulmonary blood flow and pulmonary arterial compliance in patients with chronic obstructive lung disease. *Am J Med* 1974;**57**:395–401.

157. Giuntini C, Mariani M. Capacitance of pulmonary vasculature in chronic pulmonary disease. *Scand J Respir Dis* 1971;**77**(suppl):66–71.

158. Lockhart A, Benis AM. Influence of rheology of perfusate on pressure–flow curves in isolated lung lobe of the dog. *Progr Resp Res* 1970;**5**:61–75.

159. Weisse AB, Moschos CB, Frank MJ, Levison GE, Cannilla JE, Regan TJ. Hemodynamic effects of staged hematocrit reduction in patients with stable cor pulmonale and severely elevated hematocrit levels. *Am J Med* 1975;**58**:92–8.

160. Sackner MA, Hirsch JA, Epstein S, Rywlin AM. Effect of oxygen in graded concentrations upon tracheal mucous velocity: a study in anesthetized dogs. *Chest* 1976;**69**:164–7.

161. Wagner PD, Laravuso RB, Uhl RR, West JB. Continuous distributions of ventilation-perfusion ratios in normal subjects breathing air and 100 per cent O_2. *J Clin Invest* 1974;**54**:54–68.

162. Fracica PJ, Knapp MJ, Crapo JD. Patterns of progression and markers of lung injury in rodents and subhuman primates exposed to hyperoxia. *Exp Lung Res* 1988;**14**(suppl): 869–85.

163. Crapo JD. Morphologic changes in pulmonary oxygen toxicity. *Annu Rev Physiol* 1986;**48**:721–31.

164. Barber RE, Hamilton WK. Oxygen toxicity in man: a prospective study in patients with irreversible brain damage. *N Engl J Med* 1970;**283**:1478–84.

165. Corraway MS, Piantadosi CA. Oxygen toxicity. *Respir Care Clin North Am* 1999;**5**:265–95.

166. Petty TL, Stanford RE, Neff TA. Continuous oxygen therapy in chronic airway obstruction: observations on possible oxygen toxicity and survival. *Ann Intern Med* 1971; **75**:361–7.

167. Stewart BN, Hood CI, Block JA. Long-term results of continuous oxygen therapy at sea level. *Chest* 1975; **68**:486–92.

168. Donald K. Neurological effects of oxygen. *Lancet* 1949;**ii**:1056–7.

169. Nunn J. *Nunn's Applied Respiratory Physiology*. Oxford University Press, Oxford, 1993, pp 421–8.

170. Dunn WF, Nelson SB, Hubmayr RD. Oxygen-induced hypercarbia in obstructive pulmonary disease. *Am Rev Respir Dis* 1991;**144**:526–30.

171. Aubier M, Murciano D, Fourrier M, Milic-Emili J, Pariente R, Derenne JP. Central respiratory drive in acute respiratory failure of patients with chronic obstructive pulmonary disease. *Am Rev Respir Dis* 1980;**122**:191–9.

172. Aubier M, Murciano D, Milic-Emili J, *et al.* Effects of the administration of O_2 on ventilation and blood gases in patients with chronic obstructive pulmonary disease during acute respiratory failure. *Am Rev Respir Dis* 1980;**122**: 747–54.

173. Robinson TD, Freiberg DB, Regnis JA, Young IH. The role of hypoventilation and ventilation-perfusion redistribution in oxygen-induced hypercapnia during acute exacerbations of chronic obstructive pulmonary disease. *Am J Respir Crit Care Med* 2000;**161**:1524–9.

174. Lenfant C. Arterial-alveolar difference in PCO_2 during air and oxygen breathing. *J Appl Physiol* 1966;**21**:1356–62.

175. West JB. Causes of carbon dioxide retention in lung disease. *N Engl J Med* 1971;**284**:1232–6.

176. Hanson CW 3rd, Marshall BE, Frasch HF, Marschall C. Causes of hypercarbia with oxygen therapy in patients with chronic obstructive pulmonary disease. *Crit Care Med* 1996;**24**:23–8.

177. Neff TA, Petty TL. Tolerance and survival in severe chronic hypercapnia. *Arch Intern Med* 1972;**129**:591–6.

178. Jeffrey AA, Warren PM, Flenley DC. Acute hypercapnic respiratory failure in patients with chronic obstructive lung disease: risk factors and use of guidelines for management. *Thorax* 1992;**47**:34–40.

179. Barach AL. Hypercapnia in chronic obstructive lung disease – an adaptive response to low-flow oxygen therapy. *Chest* 1974;**66**:112–13.

180. West GA, Primeau P. Nonmedical hazards of long-term oxygen therapy. *Respir Care* 1983;**28**:906–12.

181. Muchlberger T, Smith MA, Wong L. Domiciliary oxygen and smoking: an explosive combination. *Burns* 1998;**24**:658–60.

182. Lampton L. Home and out-patient oxygen therapy. In: R Brashear, M Rhodes, eds. *Chronic Obstructive Lung Disease: Clinical Treatment and Management*. CV Mosby, St Louis, 1978, pp 122–51.

183. Radwan L, Dufmats H. Variations of arterial oxygen and carbon dioxide tension during 24 hours in chronic respiratory insufficiency. *Scand J Respir Dis* 1974;**55**:99–104.

184. Koo KW, Sax DS, Snider GL. Arterial blood gases and pH during sleep in chronic obstructive pulmonary disease. *Am J Med* 1975;**58**:663–70.

185. Flick MR, Block AJ. Continuous in vivo monitoring of arterial oxygenation in chronic obstructive lung disease. *Ann Intern Med* 1977;**86**:725–30.

186. Douglas NJ, Calverley PMA, Leggett RJE, Brash HM, Flenley DC, Brezinova V. Transient hypoxaemia during sleep in chronic bronchitis and emphysema. *Lancet* 1979;**i**:1–4.

187. Wynne JW, Block AJ, Hemenway J, Hunt LA, Flick MR. Disordered breathing and oxygen desaturation during sleep in patients with chronic obstructive lung disease (COLD). *Am J Med* 1979;**66**:573–9.

188. Hudgel DW, Martin RJ, Capehart M, Johnson B, Hill P. Contribution of hypoventilation to sleep oxygen desaturation in chronic obstructive pulmonary disease. *J Appl Physiol* 1983;**55**:669–77.

189. Pływaczewski R, Śliwiński P, Nowinski A, Kaminski D, Zieliński J. Incidence of nocturnal desaturation while breathing oxygen in COPD patients undergoing long-term oxygen therapy. *Chest* 2000;**117**:679–83.

190. Levi-Valensi P, Aubry P, Rida Z. Nocturnal hypoxemia and long-term therapy in COPD patients with daytime Pao_2 60–70 mmHg. *Lung* 1990;**168**(suppl):770–5.

191. Fletcher EC, Miller J, Divine GW, Fletcher JG, Miller T. Nocturnal oxyhemoglobin desaturation in COPD patients with arterial oxygen tension above 60 mmHg. *Chest* 1987;**92**:604–8.

192. Fletcher EC, Levin DC. Cardiopulmonary hemodynamics during sleep in subjects with chronic obstructive pulmonary disease: the effect of short- and long-term oxygen. *Chest* 1984;**85**:6–14.

193. Fletcher EC, Luckett RA, Miller T, Fletcher JG. Exercise hemodynamics and gas exchange in patients with chronic obstruction pulmonary disease, sleep desaturation and a daytime Pao_2 above 60 mmHg. *Am Rev Respir Dis* 1989; **140**:1237–45.

194. Fletcher EC, Luckett RA, Goodnight-White S, Miller CC, Qian W, Costarangos-Galarza C. A double blind trial of nocturnal supplemental oxygen for sleep desaturation in patients with chronic obstructive pulmonary disease and a daytime Pao_2 above 60 mmHg. *Am Rev Respir Dis* 1992: **145**:1070–6.

195. Fletcher EC, Donner CF, Midgren B, *et al.* Survival in COPD patients with a daytime $Pao_2 > 60$ mmHg with and without nocturnal oxyhemoglobin desaturation. *Chest* 1992;**101**:649–55.

196. Fletcher EC, Scott D, Qian W, Luckett RA, Miller CC, Goodnight-White S. Evolution of nocturnal oxyhemoglobin desaturation in patients with chronic obstructive pulmonary disease and a daytime Pao_2 above 60 mmHg. *Am Rev Respir Dis* 1991;**144**:401–5.

197. Flenley DC. Clinical hypoxia: causes, consequences and correction. *Lancet* 1978;**i**:542–6.

198. Block AJ, Boysen PG, Wynne JW. The origins of cor pulmonale: a hypothesis. *Chest* 1979;**75**:109–10.

199. McNicholas WT, Fitzgerald MX. Nocturnal deaths among patients with chronic bronchitis and emphysema. *Br Med J* 1984;**289**:878.

200. Cormick W, Olson LG, Hensley MJ, Saunders NA. Nocturnal hypoxemia and quality of sleep in patients with chronic obstructive lung disease. *Thorax* 1986;**41**:846–54.

201. Fleetham J, West P, Mezon B, Conway W, Roth T, Kryger M. Sleep arousals and oxygen desaturation in chronic obstructive pulmonary disease: the effect of oxygen therapy. *Am Rev Respir Dis* 1982;**126**:429–33.

202. Chaouat A, Weitzenblum E, Kessler R, *et al*. Sleep-related O_2 desaturation and daytime pulmonary haemodynamics in COPD patients with mild hypoxaemia. *Eur Respir J* 1997;**10**:1730–5.
203. Chaouat A, Weitzenblum E, Kessler R, *et al*. A randomised trial of nocturnal oxygen therapy in chronic obstructive pulmonary disease patients. *Eur Respir J* 1999;**14**:1002–8.
204. Chaouat A, Weitzenblum E, Kessler R, *et al*. Outcome of COPD patients with daytime hypoxaemia with or without sleep-related oxygen desaturation. *Eur Respir J* 2001;**17**:848–55.
205. Bassiri AG, Guilleminault Ch. Clinical features and evaluation of obstructive sleep apnea-hypopnea syndrome. In: MH Kryger, T Roth, WC Dement, eds. *Principles and Practice of Sleep Medicine*, 3rd edn. WB Saunders, Philadelphia, 2000, pp 869–78.
206. Flenley DC. Sleep in chronic lung disease. *Clin Chest Med* 1985;**6**:651–61.
207. Killian KJ, Leblanc P, Martin DH, Summers E, Jones NL, Campbell EJM. Exercise capacity and ventilatory, circulatory, and symptom limitation in patients with chronic airflow limitation. *Am Rev Respir Dis* 1992;**146**:935–40.
208. Bye PTP, Esau SA, Levy RD, *et al*. Ventilatory muscle function during exercise in air and oxygen in patients with chronic air-flow limitation. *Am Rev Respir Dis* 1985;**132**:236–40.
209. Schenkel NS, Burdet L, de Muralt B, Fitting JW. Oxygen saturation during daily activities in chronic obstructive pulmonary disease. *Eur Respir J* 1996;**9**:2584–9.
210. Jolly EC, Di Boscio V, Aguirre L, Luna CM, Berensztein S, Gene RJ. Effects of supplemental oxygen during activity in patients with advanced COPD without severe resting hypoxemia. *Chest* 2001;**120**:437–43.
211. Olvey SK, Reduto LA, Stevens PM, Deaton WJ, Miller RR. First pass radionuclide assessment of right and left ventricular ejection fraction in chronic pulmonary disease: effect of oxygen upon exercise response. *Chest* 1980;**78**:4–9.
212. Cuvelier A, Nuir JF, Chakroun N, Aboab J, Onega G, Benhamou D. Refillable oxygen cylinders may be an alternative for ambulatory oxygen therapy in COPD. *Chest* 2002;**122**:451–6.
213. Dean NC, Brown JK, Himelman RB, Doherty JJ, Gold WM, Stulbarg MS. Oxygen may improve dyspnoea and endurance in patients with chronic obstructive pulmonary disease and only mild hypoxemia. *Am Rev Respir Dis* 1992;**146**:941–5.
214. King AJ, Cooke NJ, Leitch AG, Flenley DC. The effects of 30% oxygen on the respiratory response to treadmill exercise in chronic respiratory failure. *Clin Sci* 1973;**44**:151–62.
215. Woodcock AA, Gross ER, Geddes DM. Oxygen relieves breathlessness in 'pink puffers'. *Lancet* 1981;**1**:907–9.
216. O'Donnell DE, Bain DJ, Webb KA. Factors contributing to relief of exertional breathlessness during hypoxia in chronic airflow limitation. *Am J Respir Crit Care Med* 1997;**155**:530–5.
217. O'Donnell DE, D'Arsigny C, Webb KA. Effects of hyperoxia on ventilatory limitation during exercise in advanced chronic obstructive pulmonary disease. *Am J Respir Crit Care Med* 2001;**163**:892–8.
218. Somfay A, Porszasz J, Lee SM, Casaburi R. Dose-response effect of oxygen on hyperinflation and exercise endurance in nonhypoxaemic COPD patients. *Eur Respir J* 2001;**8**:77–84.
219. McDonald CF, Blyth CM, Lazarus MD, Marschner I, Barter CE. Exertional oxygen of limited benefit in patients with chronic obstructive pulmonary disease and mild hypoxemia. *Am J Respir Crit Care Med* 1995;**152**:1616–19.
220. Kramer MR, Springer C, Berkman N, *et al*. Rehabilitation of hypoxemic patients with COPD at low altitude at the Dead Sea, the lowest place on earth. *Chest* 1998;**113**:571–5.
221. Rooyackers JM, Dekhuijzen PN, Van Herwaarden CL, Folgering HT. Training with supplemental oxygen in patients with COPD and hypoxaemia at peak exercise. *Eur Respir J* 1997;**10**:1278–84.
222. Wadell K, Henriksson–Larsen K, Lundgren R. Physical training with and without oxygen in patients with chronic obstructive pulmonary disease and exercise-induced hypoxemia. *J Rehabil Med* 2001;**33**:200–5.
223. Berg BW, Dillard TA, Derderian SS, Rajagopal KR. Hemodynamic effects of altitude exposure and oxygen administration in chronic obstructive pulmonary disease. *Am J Med* 1993;**94**:407–12.
224. Dillard TA, Berg BW, Rajagopal KR, Dooley JW, Mehm WJ. Hypoxemia during air travel in patients with chronic obstructive pulmonary disease. *Ann Intern Med* 1989;**111**:362–7.
225. Dillard TA, Rosenberg AP, Berg BW. Hypoxemia during altitude exposure: a meta-analysis of chronic obstructive pulmonary disease. *Chest* 1993;**103**:422–5.
226. Cramer D, Ward S, Geddes A. Assessment of oxygen supplementation during air travel. *Thorax* 1996;**51**:202–3.
227. Stoller JK. Oxygen and air travel. *Resp Care* 2000;**45**:214–21.
228. Stark RD, Bishop JM. New method for oxygen therapy in the home using an oxygen concentrator. *Br Med J* 1973;**2**:105–6.
229. Fauroux B, Howard P, Muir JF. Home treatment for chronic respiratory insufficiency: the situation in Europe in 1992. *Eur Respir J* 1994;**7**:1721–6.
230. Johns DP, Rochford PD, Streeton JA. Evaluation of six oxygen concentrators. *Thorax* 1985;**40**:806–10.
231. Campbell EJ, Baker D, Crites-Silver P. Subjective effects of humidification of oxygen for delivery by nasal cannula: a prospective study. *Chest* 1988;**93**:289–93.
232. Bongard JP, Pahud C, De Haller R. Insufficient oxygen concentration obtained at domiciliary controls of eighteen concentrators. *Eur Respir J* 1989;**2**:280–2.
233. Gould GA, Scott W, Hayhurst MD, Flenley DC. Technical and clinical assessment of oxygen concentrators. *Thorax* 1985;**40**:811–13.
234. Evans TW, Waterhouse J, Howard P. Clinical experience with the oxygen concentrator. *Br Med J* 1983;**287**:459–61.
235. Burns M. Traveling with oxygen. In: BL Tiep, ed. *Portable Oxygen Therapy: Including Oxygen Conserving Methodology*. Futura, Mount Kisco, NY, 1991, pp 421–36.
236. Langenderfer R, Branson RD. Compressed gases: manufacture, storage, and piping systems. In: RD Branson, D Hess, RL Chatbum, eds. *Respiratory Care Equipment*, 2nd edn. Lippincott, Philadelphia, 1998, pp 21–54.
237. Thalken R. Production, storage and delivery of medical gases. In: CG Scanlan, CB Spearman, RL Sheldon, eds. *Egan's Fundamentals of Respiratory Care*, 6th edn. Mosby, St Louis, 1995, pp 633–55.
238. Kacmarek RM. Oxygen delivery systems for long-term oxygen therapy. In: WJ O'Donohue, ed. *Long-term Oxygen Therapy. Scientific Basis and Clinical Application*. Marcel Dekker, New York, 1995, pp 219–34.
239. Ward J. Medical gas therapy. In: GG Burton, JE Hodgkin, JJ Ward, eds. *Respiratory Care: A Guide to Clinical Practice*. Lippincott, Philadelphia, 1997, pp 335–404.
240. Gould GA, Forsyth IS, Flenley DC. Comparison of two oxygen conserving nasal prongs systems and the effects of nose and mouth breathing. *Thorax* 1986;**41**:808–9.

241. Bazuaye EA, Stone TN, Corris PA, Gibson GJ. Variability of inspired oxygen concentration with nasal cannulas. *Thorax* 1992;**47**:609–11.

242. Mc Laughlin AL Jr. Allergic contact dermatitis from oxygen cannulas. *Respir Care* 1980;**25**:1024–6.

243. Heimlich HJ. Respiratory rehabilitation with transtracheal oxygen system. *Ann Otol Rhinol Laryngol* 1982;**91**:643–7.

244. Christopher KL, Spofford BT, Petrun MD, McCarty DC, Goodman JR, Petty TL. A program for transtracheal oxygen delivery. Assessment of safety and efficacy. *Ann Intern Med* 1987;**107**:802–8.

245. Christopher KL, Spofford BT, Brannin PK, Petty TL. Transtracheal oxygen therapy for refractory hypoxemia. *JAMA* 1986;**256**:494–7.

246. Heimlich HJ, Carr GC. The Micro-trach: a seven year experience with transtracheal oxygen therapy. *Chest* 1989, **95**:1008–12.

247. Banner NR, Govan JR. Long term transtracheal oxygen delivery through microcatheter in patients with hypoxemia due to chronic obstructive airways disease. *Br Med J* 1986;**293**:111–14.

248. Leger P, Gerard M, Robert D. Simultaneous use of a pulsed dose demand valve with a transtracheal catheter TTC: an optimal O$_2$ saving for long term O$_2$ therapy. *Am Rev Respir Dis* 1986;**133**:A350.

249. Shneerson J. Transtracheal oxygen catheters. *Br J Hosp Med* 1992;**48**:24–6.

250. Hoffman LA, Denber JH, Wesmiller SW, Ferson PF, Johnson ST, Zullo TG. Nasal cannula and transtracheal oxygen: a comparison of patient response following six months use each technique. *Am Rev Respir Dis* 1988; **137**:153–6.

251. Wesmiller SW, Hoffman LA, Sciurga FC, Ferson PF, Johson JT, Dauber JH. Exercise tolerance during nasal cannula and transtracheal oxygen delivery. *Am Rev Respir Dis* 1990; **141**:789–91.

252. Fletcher EC, Nickeson D, Costarangos-Galarza C. Endotracheal mass resulting from a transtrachel oxygen catheter. *Chest* 1988;**93**:438–9.

253. Huber GL, Carter R, Makajan VK. *Transtracheal Oxygen Therapy. Scientific Basis and Clinical Application.* Marcel Dekker, New York, 1995, pp 257–309.

254. Sampablo I, Escarrabill J, Rosell A, Manresa F, Estopa R. Transtracheal catheter acceptance and adverse events in long-term home oxygen therapy. *Monaldi Arch Chest Dis* 1998;**53**:123–6.

255. Kampelmacher MJ, Deenstra M, Kesteren van RG, Melissant CF, Douze JMC, Lammers J-WJ. Transtracheal oxygen therapy: an effective and safe alternative to nasal oxygen administration. *Eur Respir J* 1997; **10**:828–33.

256. Tiep BL, Nicotra B, Belman MJ, Mittman C. Evaluation of a low-flow oxygen conserving nasal cannula. *Am Rev Respir Dis* 1984;**130**:500–2.

257. Soffer M, Tashkin DP, Shapiro BJ, Littner M, Harvey E, Farr S. Conservation of oxygen supply using a reservoir nasal cannula in hypoxemic patients at rest and during exercise. *Chest* 1985;**88**:663–8.

258. Tiep BL, Nicotra B, Carter R, Philips R, Otsap B. Evaluation of an oxygen conserving nasal cannula. *Respir Care* 1985;**30**:19–25.

259. Block AJ. Intermittent flow oxygen devices – technically feasible, but rarely used. *Chest* 1984;**86**:657–8.

260. Tiep BL. *Portable Oxygen Therapy: Including Oxygen Conserving Methodology.* Futura, New York, 1991, pp 221–375.

261. Bliss PL, McCoy RW, Adams AB. A bench study comparison of demand oxygen delivery systems and continuous flow oxygen. *Respir Care* 1999;**44**:925–31.

262. Carter R, Tashkin D, Djahed B, Hathaway E, Nicotra MB, Tiep BL. Demand oxygen delivery for patients with restrictive lung disease. *Chest* 1989;**96**:1307–11.

263. Yuan LC, Jun Z, Min LP. Clinical evaluation of pulse-dose and continuous-flow oxygen delivery. *Respir Care* 1995;**40**:811–14.

264. Garrod R, Bestall JC, Paul E, Wedzicha JA. Evaluation of pulsed dose oxygen delivery during exercise in patients with severe chronic obstructive pulmonary disease. *Thorax* 1999;**54**:242–4.

265. Hagarty EM, Skorodin MS, Langbein WE, Hultman CI, Jessen JA, Maki KC. Comparison of three oxygen delivery systems during exercise in hypoxemic patients with chronic obstructive pulmonary disease. *Am J Respir Crit Care Med* 1997;**155**:893–8.

266. Roberts CM, Bell J, Wedzicha JA. Comparison of the efficacy of a demand oxygen delivery system with continuous low flow oxygen in subjects with stable COPD and severe oxygen desaturation on walking. *Thorax* 1996;**51**:831–4.

267. Braun SR, Spratt G, Scott GC, Ellersieck M. Comparison of six oxygen delivery systems for COPD patients at rest and during exercise. *Chest* 1992;**102**:694–8.

268. Yaeger ES, Goodman S, Hoddes E, Christopher KL. Oxygen therapy using pulse and continuous flow with a transtracheal catheter and nasal cannula. *Chest* 1994; **106**:854–60.

269. McCoy R. Oxygen-conserving techniques and devices. *Respir Care* 2000;**45**:95–103.

270. MacNee W, Zieliński J. Survival. In: CF Donner, M Decramer, eds. *Pulmonary Rehabilitation*, vol 5. European Respiratory Society, Sheffield, 2000, pp 7–15.

271. Cutaia M. New insights into the temporal pattern of hypoxemia in COPD. *Chest* 2000;**118**:1521–2.

272. Zieliński J. Long-term oxygen therapy in COPD patients with moderate hypoxaemia: does it add years to life? *Eur Respir J* 1998;**12**:756–8.

30

Pulmonary rehabilitation

EFM WOUTERS

INTRODUCTION

Chronic obstructive pulmonary disease is a devastating disorder that accounts for exorbitant human suffering. Impaired exercise tolerance and breathlessness are important features of the patient suffering from COPD. Despite the definition of COPD as a disease state characterized by the presence of a generally progressive and irreversible airflow limitation, the primary treatment was directed during many years on pharmacologic modulation of the airflow limitation by bronchodilating and anti-inflammatory agents. Despite the symptomatic relief after administration of bronchodilating agents, in most COPD patients a functional deficit persists after optimal pharmacologic treatment. Based on generally accepted treatment goals in COPD, pharmacologic treatment can therefore no longer be considered as sufficient in the state of the art management of patients with symptomatic COPD. Indeed, besides lessening of airflow limitation, reduction of symptoms and improvement in health status as well as prevention of secondary complications are also widely accepted management goals for COPD.[1,2]

The concept of rehabilitation, involving holistic efforts to restore patients with debilitating and disabling disease to an optimally functioning state, is a relatively recent practice in pulmonary medicine. In 1974 a committee of the American College of Chest Physicians defined pulmonary rehabilitation as 'an art of medical practice wherein an individually tailored, multidisciplinary program is formulated which through accurate diagnosis, therapy, emotional support and education stabilises or reverses both physio-pathologic and psycho-pathologic manifestations of pulmonary diseases and attempts to return the patient to the highest possible functional capacity allowed by his handicap and overall life situation'.[3]

More recent definitions were formulated by the National Institute of Health (NIH) and by a task force of the European Respiratory Society (ERS). The NIH defined pulmonary rehabilitation as a multidimensional continuum of services directed to persons with pulmonary disease and their families, usually by an interdisciplinary team of specialists, with the goal of achieving and maintaining the individual's maximum level of independence and functioning in the community.[4] According to the ERS task force, pulmonary rehabilitation must be considered as 'a process which systematically uses scientifically based diagnostic management and treatment options in order to achieve the optimal daily functioning and health related quality of life of individual patients suffering from impairment and disability due to chronic respiratory diseases as measured by clinically and/or physiologically relevant outcome measures'.[5] The statement of the American Thoracic Society (ATS) on pulmonary rehabilitation supports previous definitions by defining pulmonary rehabilitation as a multidisciplinary program of care for patients with chronic respiratory impairment which is individually tailored and designed to optimize physical and social performance and autonomy of the patient.[6]

These definitions refer to the philosophic concept of rehabilitation as a process to restore an individual to the fullest medical, mental, emotional, social and vocational potential of which a person is capable. This holistic approach of rehabilitation is based on the definition of health by the World Health Organization (WHO) as a state of complete physical, mental and social well-being. Present definitions are also based on the widely applied international classification model for impairments, disabilities and handicaps (ICIDH).[7] Impairment in this concept is used in terms of organ system impairment. Disability is generally used to describe the loss in exercise capacity caused by the particular organ system impairment, while the total effect of the disability on the ability of the person to function in society is called handicap: handicap is similar to the term disability according to the American usage. Based on the generally accepted concept of irreversible organ impairment in COPD as a consequence of airway abnormalities and lung parenchymal changes and the limited outcome of modulation of organ impairment on symptomatology and level of disability, the whole continuum of multidisciplinary services was considered part of the 'rehabilitation' process, directed to manage the consequences of impairment and disability on patient's life.

Present knowledge about pathophysiologic factors, intrinsically linked to the process of COPD and contributing to the level of disability, allows a more precise definition of rehabilitation in the management of patients with chronic respiratory diseases as COPD. Rehabilitation in this more strict definition refers to the continuum of multidisciplinary services, directed to modulate the impact of the disease process on a patient's life. Intervention strategies directed to modulate impairment or the level of disability, based on scientifically based insights, have to be considered as non-pharmacologic treatment of the disease process in order to obtain presently accepted treatment goals. These non-pharmacologic treatment modalities have to be integrated in the COPD management process, based on careful and systematic diagnostic work-up of the patient with COPD. This approach fits with the view of ICIDH-2 that healthy functioning and disability form a continuum as outcomes of an interaction between a person's physical or mental condition and the physical and social environment in which they live.[8]

SELECTION OF CANDIDATES FOR NON-PHARMACOLOGIC TREATMENT AND REHABILITATION

Although pulmonary rehabilitation programs have been widely applied in COPD patients, there is poor evidence about which patients benefit most. The ATS statement considers pulmonary rehabilitation to be indicated for patients with chronic impairment who despite optimal medical management are dyspneic, have reduced exercise tolerance or experience a restriction in activities.[6] In fact, these criteria can no longer be considered as indications

for pulmonary rehabilitation alone, being internationally defined treatment goals for COPD. Present medical management, usually limited to pharmacologic interventions with bronchodilating agents or anti-inflammatory medication, can no longer be considered as a sufficient disease intervention strategy: indeed, the limited outcome of these intervention strategies is widely accepted, at least with respect to the symptoms experienced by the patient.[9,10] Furthermore, the present limited focus of COPD management on the modulation of airflow limitation is not supported by studies trying to predict different independent factors in the disease process. Thus, Ries et al. reported by factor analysis that besides FEV_1 as measure of disease severity, maximal oxygen uptake, lung volumes and expiratory flow independently contribute to fully describe the process of COPD.[11] Others have identified exercise capacity, dyspnea and quality of life ratings as well as pulmonary hyperinflation as determining components, while in the study reported by Mahler et al. maximal respiratory pressures contribute to the severity of the COPD.[12,13]

Furthermore, in rehabilitation programs improvements in dyspnea and exercise tolerance are considered as attainable targets of the intervention without consideration of the complexity of pathogenetic conditions contributing to these disabling symptoms.

Therefore, pulmonary rehabilitation refers to the whole spectrum of non-pharmacologic treatment interventions, directed to attenuate the persistent impaired health status after present pharmacologic treatment. As dyspnea and impaired functional status are now considered as part of the disease process of COPD, these interventions have to be considered as management options in every COPD patient, independent of the degree of airflow limitation.[14] Similar gains in physical performance and health status were reported in COPD patients with severe, moderate and mild disease based on spirometric criteria (ATS).

DIMENSIONS OF PULMONARY REHABILITATION PROGRAMS

Based on the historically defined approach of pulmonary rehabilitation, each patient enroled in a rehabilitation program has to be considered as a unique individual with specific physiologic and psychopathologic impairment caused by the underlying disease. Therefore, pulmonary rehabilitation incorporated many different therapeutic modalities applied as a comprehensive, multidisciplinary care program including pharmacologic treatment. Specific components in this non-pharmacologic approach to patients with COPD are supported by scientific data supporting the efficacy and effectiveness of the applied

Table 30.1 *Dimensions of pulmonary rehabilitation*

Aim of the intervention	Level of focusing of the intervention	Directness of the intervention
Reduction and control of respiratory symptoms	Individual	Direct
Improvement in physical functioning	Group	Indirect
Improvement in quality of life	Environment	Supported by educational material
Reduction of the number of acute exacerbations		
Promotion of self-management behavior		
Improvement of cognition and behavior		
Reduction of psychologic impact of physical impairment and disability		
Improvement of survival		

intervention procedure. In order to improve quality of life or to promote self-management behavior of chronically ill patients with COPD, it is also important to consider the different dimensions of the rehabilitation program. In general, a distinction has to be made between (i) the aim of the intervention, (ii) the level at which the intervention is focused and (iii) the directness of the intervention.[15] For pulmonary rehabilitation in general, these dimensions are described in Table 30.1.

Based on this approach, interventions directed at improvement of, for example, quality of life, have to be focused on improvement of general psychologic, social, practical and physical well-being of the patient. Dependent upon the aim and the phase the patient is in, the interventions can involve physical exercise programs as well as stress-management programs, social skills training or different kinds of counseling and support. The level of focusing of the intervention has to be decided depending on the aim of the intervention and the expected efficiency. Group training is much appreciated by patients; psychologic group interventions directed at patients and partners can increase efficiency in order to obtain management goals. Furthermore, interventions can be directed at changing or adaptation of the environment of the COPD patient. These interventions are often specified by the term 'social engineering', because they are directed at modification of living-, work-, or leisure-time situations and healthy lifestyles of the patient from a social or patient perspective.[16] Finally, the directness of the intervention has to be considered. As part of a comprehensive intervention, indirect interventions can be considered in order to improve social support for the patient or to train other professionals in intervention skills.

This theoretical approach of intervention programs is still largely unattainable in most rehabilitation programs, based on the limited resources currently spent on non-pharmacologic intervention strategies in COPD. In this approach, components of a rehabilitation program are individualized based on a careful assessment of the patient, not limited to lung function testing, but addressing physical and emotional deficits, know-ledge of the disease, cognitive and psychosocial functioning as well as nutritional assessment. Furthermore, this assessment must be an ongoing process during the whole rehabilitation process.

COMPREHENSIVE REHABILITATION PROGRAMS IN COPD

The outcome of comprehensive pulmonary rehabilitation programs is at present well documented based on different reports analyzing the short-term as well as the long-term outcome parameters. Ries *et al.* compared the effects of a comprehensive pulmonary rehabilitation program including exercise reconditioning with those of education alone on physiologic and psychosocial outcomes in COPD.[17] Pulmonary rehabilitation consisted of twelve 4-hour sessions that included education, physical and respiratory care instruction, psychosocial support and supervised exercise training, followed by monthly reinforcement sessions for 1 year. The education group received 2-hour sessions that included videotapes, lectures and discussions. This comprehensive rehabilitation program produced a significant increase in maximal exercise tolerance, maximal oxygen uptake, exercise endurance and self-efficacy for walking, and these effects were associated with a marked reduction of perceived breathlessness, muscle fatigue and shortness of breath. Most of these effects persisted for 18–24 months although benefits tended to diminish after 1 year.

These positive effects of rehabilitation on dyspnea were confirmed by the results of O'Donnell et al., who demonstrated that supervised multimodality endurance exercise training relieved both chronic and acute activity-related breathlessness and that this relief of breathlessness was related to a fall in ventilatory demand during exercise as a result of enhanced mechanical efficiency. This improvement in breathlessness was translated into important increases in exercise capacity and into the ability to participate to a greater extent in activities of daily living.[18]

Similar results were reported by Goldstein et al.[19] They performed a prospective randomized controlled trial of respiratory rehabilitation in 89 subjects. Exercise activities included interval training, treadmill, upper-extremity training and leisure walking as part of an 8-week inpatient rehabilitation program. Significant improvements in exercise tolerance, measured by submaximal cycle time and walking distance, were demonstrated and sustained for 6 months in the rehabilitation group. There were also significant differences in questionnaire assessment of dyspnea and dyspnea index.

Studies demonstrated that beneficial effects are even achieved after home-based pulmonary rehabilitation programs: improvements in maximal workload, symptom-limited oxygen uptake and maximal inspiratory pressure together with a decrease in lactate, inspiratory muscle load and dyspnea during maximal exercise were reported and these effects were maintained over 18 months.[20,21] Wedzicha et al.[22] tested the hypothesis that severity of respiratory disability affected the outcome of pulmonary rehabilitation: in a randomized, controlled study, patients with COPD were stratified for dyspnea using the Medical Research Council (MRC) dyspnea score and the patients were randomly assigned to an 8-week program of either exercise plus education or education alone. Improvements in exercise performance and health status were higher in patients with moderate levels of dyspnea.

Others have confirmed these positive effects in the short term and long term even by inexpensive, comprehensive outpatient programs,[23–25] although continuation of supervised training is generally recommended in order to stabilize obtained training effects. A meta-analysis of respiratory rehabilitation demonstrated that pulmonary rehabilitation relieves dyspnea and improves the control over COPD and these improvements were con-sidered clinically important. The value of the improvement in exercise capacity was not so convincing.[26]

More recent studies further evaluated the outcome of pulmonary rehabilitation, including aspects of cost-effectiveness in the outcome assessment. Goldstein et al.[27] reported an economic analysis of 2 months of inpatient rehabilitation followed by 4 months of outpatient supervision (Figure 30.1). The incremental cost of achieving improvements beyond the minimal clinically important difference in dyspnea, emotional function and mastery

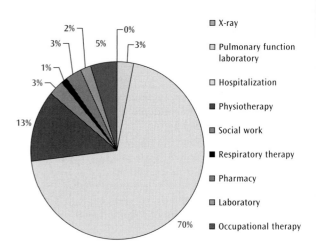

Figure 30.1 *Cost of 2-month inpatient respiratory rehabilitation by hospital service. (Reproduced from ref. 27 with permission.)*

was $11.597 (Canadian). More than 90% of this cost was attributable to the inpatient phase of the program. Of the non-physician healthcare professionals, nursing was identified as the largest cost center, followed by physical therapy and occupational therapy.

Troosters et al. reported that a 6-month outpatient rehabilitation program that involved moderate-to-high training intensity did not alter pulmonary function, but did improve functional and maximal exercise performance, peripheral and respiratory muscle strength, and quality of life when compared with usual care in patients with severe COPD.[28] These improvements in functional and maximal exercise performance were clinically relevant and were maintained 18 months after the onset of training (Figure 30.2).

This outpatient program had a mean cost per patient of approximately $2600 to achieve a mean improvement of 52 meters in 6-minute walking distance at 6 months. Griffiths et al.[29] analyzed the effects of outpatient pulmonary rehabilitation on use of health care and patients' well being over 1 year. They reported that there was no difference between the rehabilitation and control groups in the numbers of patients admitted to the hospital but the number of days these patients spent in hospital differed significantly (Figure 30.3).

Furthermore, they demonstrated that the rehabilitation group had more primary-care consultations at the general practitioners' premises than did the control group but fewer primary-care home visits. The rehabilitation group showed greater improvements in walking ability and in general as well as in disease-specific health status. Benefits in heath status as well as in hospitalizations that persist for a period of 2 years after an outpatient rehabilitation program are confirmed in literature.[30] In conclusion, there is now a lot of evidence in literature demonstrating the efficacy and effectiveness of comprehensive pulmonary rehabilitation programs.

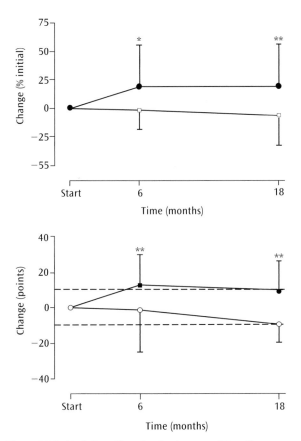

Figure 30.2 *Training effect for 6-minute walking distance (upper panel) and dyspnea (lower panel). (Reproduced from ref. 28 with permission.)*

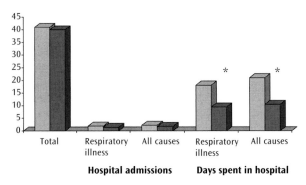

Figure 30.3 *Outcome of pulmonary rehabilitation: use of secondary care. Pale bars: control group; dark bars: rehabilitation group. *P < 0.05. (From ref. 29.)*

COMPONENTS OF REHABILITATION PROGRAMS

Exercise training

Impaired exercise tolerance is a prominent feature especially in patients suffering from COPD. Exercise limitation, particularly in patients with COPD, is the result of

complex changes including a wide spectrum of variables: reduced expiratory airflow as a consequence of poor elastic recoil; increased airways resistance leading to increased work of breathing and increased ventilatory drive; reduced pulmonary vascular bed and increased pulmonary vascular resistance contributing to exercise-induced hypoxemia; impaired cardiac output by impediment of right heart filling and left ventricular systolic function and skeletal muscle dysfunction. In addition leg fatigue attributable to peripheral muscle weakness has now been generally recognized as a common limiting symptom during exercise in COPD[31] reflecting in part skeletal muscle dysfunction. Several factors have been suggested to explain the occurrence of skeletal muscle dysfunction in COPD: chronic inactivity and deconditioning, systemic inflammation, systemic corticosteroid administration, hypoxemia, electrolyte disturbances and muscle depletion as a consequence of chronic tissue wasting. A variety of COPD-related changes in structure and metabolism of the skeletal muscles have been reported: decreased oxidative capacity,[32] a greater proportion of fatigue-susceptible fibers as a consequence of shifts from type 1 fibers to type 2 fibers[33] as well as changes in energy rich phosphagen metabolism.[34] Lower capacity for muscle aerobic metabolism is related to an increased lactic acidosis for a given exercise work rate and enhances ventilatory demand by increasing non-aerobic carbon dioxide production. This requirement imposes an additional burden on the respiratory muscles already facing an increased impedance to breathing. Exercise in COPD also induces an early onset of muscle intracellular acidosis.[35]

Remarkably, opposite changes in diaphragmatic fiber composition are now reported especially in more severe COPD patients with a shift towards a higher proportion of fatigue-resistant fibers.[36] Inspiratory muscle weakness has been shown to be related to dyspnea, fatigue and exercise limitation in COPD patients. Besides these changes in intrinsic diaphragmatic muscle structure, mechanical disadvantages and altered muscle fiber length mainly as a consequence of static and dynamic hyperinflation as well as an altered muscle environment contribute to a dysfunction of inspiratory muscles and especially of the diaphragm in COPD. A possible imbalance between inspiratory muscle function and increased muscle load related to the increased resistive and elastic load is an important determinant of dyspnea, susceptibility to inspiratory muscle fatigue, drive on the respiratory muscles and hypercapnia.[37]

The outcome of exercise training as part of a rehabilitation program has to be interpreted in the light of these complex interacting processes. Pulmonary rehabilitation programs always include a measure of exercise training which is generally based on transfer of standard recommendations for exercise training from healthy subjects to these disabled pulmonary patients. Unfortunately this usually ignores the complexity of bodily changes

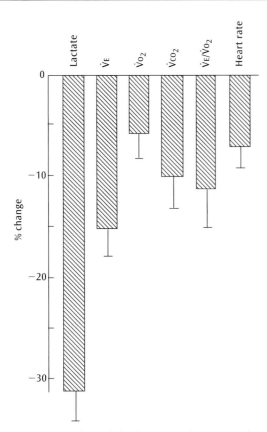

Figure 30.4 *Exercise training in COPD: change occuring from baseline after high work rate training. (Reproduced from ref. 38 with permission.)*

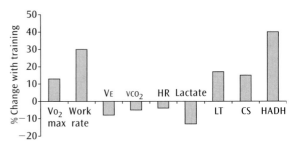

Figure 30.5 *Physiologic training effect and COPD. (Reproduced from ref. 32 with permission.) LT = Lactate threshold; CS = citrate synthase; HADH = hydroxyacyl-CoA dehydrogenase.*

related to or that are a consequence of the disease state. It is sensible to determine the nature of exercise limitation, for example cardiocirculatory, ventilatory, diffusion limitation, limitation in the pulmonary circulation or peripheral muscle limitation in the indivual patient, before deciding on the individual exercise regime to be used.

Physiological outcome of training in COPD

Although exercise training is now considered as the cornerstone of every rehabilitation program, it was unclear until the 1990s if there were physiologic reasons for improvement in exercise tolerance. It was generally thought that these patients are unable to achieve a training intensity sufficiently high to train exercising muscles. Casaburi *et al.*[38] clearly showed evidence that physiologic training responses could be observed in COPD patients (Figure 30.4). At a given level of exercise, significant reductions in blood lactate, CO_2 production, minute ventilation, O_2 consumption and heart rate were observed.

The ventilatory requirement for exercise fell after an effective training program in proportion to the drop in blood lactate at a given exercise stress level. Based on these data and the results of other studies,[39] it can be concluded that physiological adaptation to training develops

in these COPD patients. A reduction in lactic acid production by the contracting muscles is probably the main mechanism in the process of adaptation. Early lactic acid production during exercise is reported in COPD patients. A number of factors can contribute to this. Maltais *et al.* demonstrated by muscle biopsy studies that the oxidative capacity of the vastus lateralis muscle is reduced in COPD and that this reduction in oxidative capacity is significantly related to the decreased exercise capacity.[32] Others have demonstrated a relationship between this early lactic acid production and changes in intermediary amino acid metabolism, especially the glutamate concentrations in muscle biopsies.[40] The physiologic response to endurance training in patients with COPD was therefore evaluated by analyzing changes in skeletal muscle aerobic enzyme activities. Maltais and his group[39] clearly demonstrated an increase in aerobic enzyme activity after an endurance training program and that this improvement in skeletal muscle oxidative capacity was related to the reduction in exercise-induced lactic acidosis in these patients (Figure 30.5).

Beneficial effects of training in patients with COPD are also seen in skeletal muscle bioenergetics: the half-time of phosphocreatine (PCr) recovery fell significantly after an 8-week endurance training program and at a given submaximal work rate, improved bioenergetics were reflected in a decreased inorganic phosphate to phosphocreatine ratio and an increased intracellular pH. These data indicate that the physiologic changes provoked by endurance training essentially took place at the level of the skeletal muscle during submaximal exercise.[41]

These results clearly indicated that skeletal muscle adaptations related to physiologic parameters can occur after training even in severe patients with COPD.

EXERCISE PRESCRIPTION

Although exercise training is recognized as an important component of the treatment of patients with COPD, the optimal method of exercise training still remains a matter of debate. In general, exercise training can be divided into two types: aerobic or endurance training and strength training. The majority of the studies of exercise training in COPD have focused on endurance training. However, no clear recommendations for COPD are yet available. However, in normal subjects clear recommendations are available about duration, intensity and frequency for aerobic training.[42,43] According to these recommendations, aerobic training calls for rhythmical, dynamic activity of large muscles, performed three to four times a week for 20–30 minutes per session at an intensity of at least 50% of maximal oxygen consumption. Such a program of aerobic training is capable of inducing structural and physiologic adaptations that provide the trained individual with improved endurance for the performance of high-intensity activity. Most of the rehabilitation programs include exercise sessions of at least 30 minutes, three to four times a week. Although no ideal duration has been established, duration in many programs is around 8 weeks. In one randomized controlled trial, patients were randomized to either a standard 7-week twice-weekly outpatient-based program or a comparable but shortened 4-week course in order to assess the optimal duration of a pulmonary rehabilitation program. A 7-week course of pulmonary rehabilitation provides greater benefits to patients than a 4-week course in terms of improvement in health status.[44]

Limited information is also available regarding the physiological outcome of different types of exercise testing. Most studies have investigated the physiologic response of continuous training at a given workload in order to stress the oxidative pathways. Otherwise, interval training, alternating high and lower training load, resembles more closely the daily life activity pattern especially in severe COPD patients and this form of training stresses in addition the glycolytic pathways. Continuous training seemed to be related to physiological improvement while interval training had more marked effects on leg pain in COPD patients.[45] Indeed, continuous training results in a significant increase in oxygen consumption, and a decrease in minute ventilation and ventilatory equivalent for carbon dioxide at peak exercise capacity, while no changes in these measures were observed after interval training. A significant reduction in lactic acid production was observed after both training modalities but was most pronounced in the continuous training group. Remarkably, in the interval training group a decrease in leg pain was reported as well as a significant increase in peak workload. Therefore, it seems that different physiologic training response patterns can be obtained after interval or continuous training in COPD, possibly related to specific training effects in either oxidative or glycolytic muscle metabolic pathways (Figure 30.6).

Limited data are available comparing concentric exercise (positive work) with eccentric exercise (negative work) as part of the rehabilitation program. In patients with COPD the ventilatory requirements of eccentric exercise are considerably lower than those of concentric exercise at similar workloads resulting in a greater ventilatory

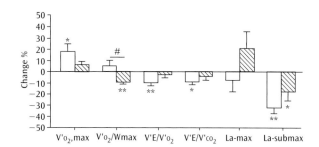

Figure 30.6 *Physiologic outcomes with continuous (white bars) versus interval (hatched bars) training. (From ref. 45.)*

reserve and less disturbed gas exchange.[46] Therefore, eccentric work might be a suitable type of exercise and training in patients with limited ventilatory reserves. In one randomized trial, the effects of eccentric exercise training in addition to general exercise training on exercise performance and quality of life were compared. It was reported that pulmonary rehabilitation improved exercise performance and quality of life similarly in both training groups but that physiologic training effects were observed only in the group which had trained eccentrically.[47]

It remains questionable how optimal training intensity should be modulated in COPD patients. In healthy subjects training is normally targeted by means of percentage of maximal heart rate (60–90% of predicted) or the percentage of maximal oxygen uptake (50–80% predicted) achieved.[42] However, the principles of exercise training intensity derived from normal subjects are often not applicable to pulmonary patients who are limited by breathing capacity and dyspnea. Some investigators have reported that high-intensity training can be tolerated by patients with COPD and that they can be trained at an intensity which represents a higher percentage of maximum exercise tolerance than recommended for normals because these patients can sustain ventilation at high percentages of their maximum breathing capacity.[48–50] In some studies, it was even concluded that high-intensity training might be superior to low-intensity training.[38] Indeed, Casaburi *et al.* compared high work rate training versus low work rate training and concluded that physiologic training effects were much less marked in patients who trained at low work rate even though the total amount of work involved in the training regimen was the same irrespective of the training group to which the patient was assigned. Others concluded that most patients with COPD were unable to achieve high-intensity training, defined as a training intensity of 80% of baseline maximal power output.[51] Furthermore, these authors demonstrated that the intensity of training achieved, in percentage of baseline maximal power output, is not influenced by the initial baseline maximal oxygen consumption, age or the degree of airflow limitation. Despite the impossibility to maintain high-intensity training, significant improvement in exercise capacity was obtained and physiological adaptation to endurance training occurred.

An interesting study was reported by Clark *et al.*:[52] they investigated the physiologic benefits of an exercise program designed for rehabilitation of COPD patients and concentrated on isolated conditioning of peripheral skeletal muscles rather than whole-body aerobic training on the premise that a cumulative set of individual limb exercises should be better tolerated by the patients than whole-body exercise. The training group showed significant improvement in a variety of measures of upper and lower peripheral muscle performance, with no additional breathlessness. Furthermore, the training group showed a reduction in ventilatory equivalents for oxygen and carbon dioxide, both at peak exercise and at equivalent work rate. An increase in efficiency of peripheral oxygen extraction by the skeletal muscle was hypothesized to explain these physiologic responses.

The intensity of training depends on the chosen setting of training. Although patients can tolerate high-intensity training in a monitored setting, low intensity may be tolerated and maintained better over the long term. Additional research is needed to identify optimal exercise strategies for subgroups of patients with pulmonary disease.

Vallet *et al.*[53] tested the effect of two methods of training, one individualized at the heart rate corresponding to the gas exchange threshold and the other at the heart rate corresponding to 50% of maximal heart reserve. They reported a significant increase in symptom-limited oxygen uptake and maximal oxygen pulse after an individualized protocol, whereas standardized training exhibited no significant changes. Individualized training also exhibited a concomitant and gradual decrease in minute ventilation, carbon dioxide production and venous lactate concentration. These results clearly indicate that despite an apparently similar target training level, individualized training clearly optimized the physiologic training effects in patients with chronic airflow limitation and, more particularly, decreased their ventilatory requirement.

Only limited data are available on the effects of strength training in patients with pulmonary disease. Strength training involves the performance of explosive tasks such as weightlifting over a short period of time. Simpson *et al.* reported a 73% increase in cycling endurance time at 80% of maximal power output following 8 weeks of weightlifting training of the upper and lower extremity muscles.[54] Otherwise, no significant changes in maximal cycling exercise capacity or walking distance were observed. Others confirmed that weight training can improve treadmill walking endurance of patients with mild COPD and that this improvement in treadmill endurance correlated with improvements in upper and lower limb isokinetic sustained muscle strength following training.[55] The outcome of combination of strength training and endurance training also needs further evaluation. In one study

combination of aerobic endurance training and strength training resulted in increases in quadriceps strength, thigh muscle cross-sectional area and pectoralis major muscle strength without influence on peak work rate, walking distance or health status.[56]

Upper extremity training

Patients with COPD frequently report disabling dyspnea for daily activities involving the upper extremities such as combing their hair, brushing their teeth or shaving. It is known that even in healthy persons arm exercise is relatively more demanding than leg exercise. Some studies have demonstrated that arm elevation is related to a disproportionate increase in the diaphragmatic contribution to the generation of ventilatory pressures[57] and that arm elevation is a fatiguing task for the muscles involved as assessed by electromyographic data. In COPD patients, studies have reported that arm exercise has effects on breathing pattern, recruitment of expiratory muscles as well as on the pattern of metabolic and ventilatory response.[58–62] Therefore, exercise training of the upper extremities may be beneficial for these patients, since exercise training is specific to the muscles and tasks involved in the training. However, relatively few data exist assessing the results of upper extremity (UE) training compared with those available for lower extremity training. Studies have demonstrated that UE training leads to improved arm muscle endurance during isotonic arm ergometry[63] and that arm training conducted during a pulmonary rehabilitation program led to a reduced metabolic demand associated with arm exercise.[57] Based on present findings, it can be concluded that strength and endurance training of the UE improves arm function and that these exercises are safe and should be included in rehabilitation programs for patients with pulmonary diseases. Further studies are needed to explore the effects of arm training on functional outcomes, to evaluate different forms of arm exercise training programs and to determine the effect of arm exercise training on respiratory muscle function.

Ventilatory muscle training

There is accumulating evidence for the occurrence of respiratory muscle dysfunction, especially in COPD patients. Four main factors may explain especially inspiratory muscle dysfunction in COPD: (i) mechanical disadvantage associated with hyperinflation; (ii) altered muscle fiber length as an important determinant of the force-generating capacity; (iii) alterations in the intrinsic muscle structure, manifested by changes in fiber type composition and muscle mass; and finally (iv) changes in muscle environment manifested by a variety of electrolyte disturbances, changes in oxygen and carbon dioxide tension or levels of inflammatory mediators.[64] This imbalance between the function of the inspiratory muscles and the load they are facing plays an important role in the sensation of dyspnea, the level of hypercapnia and could even be an important determinant of survival in COPD. Interventions directed to improve respiratory muscle performance have to affect two possible variables – the force developed during contraction as a fraction of the maximal force (measured by the ratio Pbreath/Pmax) and the duty cycle, represented by the ratio T_I/T_{TOT} for the inspiratory muscles. Changes in duty cycle are difficult to obtain. Therefore, interventions directed to improve respiratory muscle performance focus on lowering the ratio Pbreath/Pmax by reducing the load on the respiratory muscles or by improving their force-generating capacity. Ventilatory muscle training is generally practised in order to increase respiratory muscle strength.

Two types of training are commonly applied in ventilatory muscle training: normocapnic sustained hyperpnea and inspiratory resistance breathing. During normocapnic hyperpnea, a supernormal target ventilation is required for 15–20 minutes, during which carbon dioxide tension is kept constant. This form of training requires complicated equipment to monitor the patients and a medical facility to train them. Inspiratory resistance training uses small hand-held devices based on a resistance, flow-dependent system or by applying a threshold valve as a flow-independent device.

In a meta-analysis on ventilatory muscle training the effects of inspiratory resistive training have been reviewed.[65] The effects of 17 reviewed studies were rather disappointing: non-significant changes in Pmax were reported in the 11 studies in which it was evaluated and in respiratory muscle endurance in the nine studies where this was measured. These findings demonstrate that control of the training stimulus may be exceedingly important if the expected physiologic training response is to be produced. Other studies have now demonstrated that respiratory muscle training, if properly applied, results in improved respiratory muscle strength or endurance.[66] This improvement in respiratory muscle function is associated with a decreased sensation of dyspnea. In patients with ventilatory limitation of exercise capacity, the association of target-flow inspiratory muscle training and peripheral muscle exercise training allows for an additional improvement of walking distance and maximal exercise capacity compared with exercise training alone.[67,68] However, the role of ventilatory muscle training in improvement of exercise capacity remains controversial because the positive outcome of this form of training on exercise capacity could not be reproduced in patients with better preserved inspiratory muscle function.[69,70]

Future studies on ventilatory muscle training should taken into account the striking differences in muscle structural alterations in lower limb and respiratory muscles

in COPD patients, reflecting the degree of activity of these muscles and the load they face: fiber shifts in the diaphragm are already parallel to those observed in endurance training making the diaphragm more resistant to muscle fatigue, a beneficial adaptation of a muscle chronically facing an increase workload.[36] Selection of good candidates for muscle training and of training modalities based on pathological and physiological insights in muscle function adaptations can contribute to provide further scientific evidence for this intervention modality.[71]

Education

Patient education is generally used as an 'umbrella term for various forms of goal-directed and systematically applied communication processes, directed at the improvement of cognition, understanding and motivation, and the improvement of action- and decision-making possibilities of a patient to improve the coping with and recovery of the disease'.[72] Ideally, patient education is more than provision of information to the patient but is a 'planned learning experience using a combination of methods such as teaching, counseling and behavior modification techniques which influence patient knowledge and health behavior'.[73] Promotion of self-management behavior in COPD can be directed to improve adherence to medical advice with respect to medication and healthy lifestyle, directed at the stabilization or retardation of the progression of the clinical picture or at the avoidance of undesirable consequences and complications. Medical advice to chronically ill patients can also be directed at various aspects of cognition and behavior.[16]

Studies concerning patient education in COPD patients are limited.[74–78] Most of the reported studies are directed at the improvement of self-management, decrease of medical consumption, decrease of life stress, increase of social support and improvement of quality of life. Most educational programs are conducted by a range of professionals, the environment of the patient is generally not involved and most of the studies do not pay attention to the problems of partners. The overall impression in most studies is that programs do have effects on various aspects of COPD. Characteristics like depression, anxiety and optimism, well being, the number and length of hospital admissions and use of health services can be influenced positively by patient education programs.

Most of these studies have only short-term effects. Van den Broek reported the effects of a patient education group intervention program as part of a pulmonary rehabilitation program.[16] Patients were randomly assigned to an experimental group and a control group. Partners participated in the study. Patients in the control group received medical advice and standard clinical care. The experimental group followed a structured educational program consisting of two components: an informative part and an educational part. The total program was directed at teaching self-management skills. Patients were followed for 12 months after the end of the rehabilitation program. Limited or no effects could be demonstrated on variables for psychologic functioning, physical functioning or for social and practical functioning.

The characteristics of an optimal educational program for patients with COPD have been formulated:[16]

1 The program should be conducted by experts specially trained in techniques to change behavioral or irrational cognitions.
2 Information should be provided in a structured way.
3 A group program is preferable from a health economical perspective, but a combination of an individualized program and a group program may be most effective.
4 Both participation in the social environment and attention to the problems of the partners should have a high priority to maintain newly acquired skills and cognitions in the home situation.
5 Both medical and psychosocial parameters have to be emphasized.
6 The responsibility of the patient for his/her own health must be emphasized.
7 In order to promote the patient's self-activity and to support the maintenance of behavioral changes in the home situation, additional materials should be made available to the patient to be used at home.
8 Follow-up sessions are necessary to support the patient and his or her partner in the home situation.
9 Specific patient education interventions should be implemented in a multidisciplinary program in addition to standard care to improve physical and psychological functioning.
10 Short- and long-term effects have to be evaluated by valid measurements.

Stabilization or reversal of disease-related psychopathology was one of the initially defined goals of pulmonary rehabilitation. Personality traits and intrapsychic conflicts as well as acute psychologic states such as panic, anxiety or depression are widely recognized problem categories in patients with COPD. Specific psychosocial intervention strategies are usually required in order to modify these problems. Kaptein and Dekker recently reviewed the nature of psychosocial support in different rehabilitation programs. They concluded that relaxation techniques as a predominantly passive form of intervention were the most frequently applied type of psychosocial support, aimed at more controlled and efficient breathing.[79] The authors concluded that future research is needed to assess the outcome of more specific psychosocial intervention strategies as well as to delineate the contribution of

psychosocial intervention itself over and above pulmonary rehabilitation programs.

Nutritional support

Although the importance of nutrition in health and disease is intuitively acknowledged, the role of nutrition in the management of COPD has only gained interest during the last decades. Traditionally, weight loss was considered to be an inevitable and irreversible terminal event related to the severity of the disease process. An adequate analysis of the underlying mechanisms or related functional consequences was completely lacking and weight loss was even considered as an adaptive mechanism in COPD in order to decrease oxygen consumption. From this viewpoint, it could be argued that nutritional support might actually influence the disease adversely by inducing additional metabolic and ventilatory stress on the respiratory system. Studies demonstrating the disturbed energy balance during weight loss in COPD have, however, challenged this approach. Modifying body composition should be considered as an essential component in every rehabilitation program. Indeed, in normal subjects the body cell mass (BCM) or fat-free mass is the determining factor of functional capacity, while exercise training can be considered as a metabolic stress test, increasing the activity-related energy expenditure. Insights into body compositional changes, energy expenditure as well as on intervention strategies are necessary to explain the results of pulmonary rehabilitation programs.

BODY COMPOSITION IN COPD PATIENTS

Patients suffering from a chronic wasting condition like COPD are generally characterized by their body weight. Patients are considered underweight if they have a body weight less than 90% of their ideal weight; indices of relative weight as body mass index (BMI) or Quetelet index (body weight/height^2) are also widely used. The assessment of body composition has gained importance, as new indirect techniques have become available to estimate the various body compartments accurately with no discomfort for the investigated subjects. The best known body composition model is a two-compartment model, which divides the body into a fat compartment (FM, fat mass) and the fat-free mass (FFM). The FFM can be further subdivided into two compartments: the intracellular compartment or body cell mass (BCM), which represents the energy exchanging part, and the extracellular compartment, which represents substance outside the cells and mainly functions as support and transport tissue. BCM reflects the quantity of actively metabolizing (liver, gut, immune system) and contracting (muscle) tissue. Approximately 60% of BCM is composed of muscle tissue.

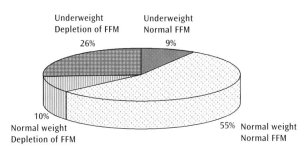

Figure 30.7 *Body composition in stable COPD. (Reproduced from ref. 81 with permission.)*

Independently of the underlying disease state or condition, a loss of BCM of up to 40% is inevitably associated with death. The importance of body composition analysis was demonstrated in studies characterizing large groups of clinically stable COPD patients. It was found that COPD patients can be stratified into four groups based on a two-compartment model: (i) COPD with normal weight and normal FFM; (ii) underweight patients and depletion of FFM; (iii) underweight patients with preservation of FFM; and (iv) normal weight patients but with depletion of FFM (Figure 30.7).

In clinically stable patients with moderate to severe COPD, depletion of FFM has been reported in 20% of COPD outpatients and in 35% of those eligible for pulmonary rehabilitation.[80,81]

Especially from a functional point of view, depletion of FFM is very important to consider in COPD patients. Indeed, FFM is a significant determinant of muscle strength,[82] exercise capacity and exercise response in patients with COPD.[83–85] Patients with a depleted FFM are also characterized by lower peak oxygen consumption and peak work rate and early onset of exercise-induced lactic acidosis compared with non-depleted patients.[83] These functional consequences of being underweight and particularly of FFM depletion as quantified in exercise tests have also been reflected as a decreased health status as measured by the St George's Respiratory Questionnaire (SGRQ).[86] In another study, patients with depleted FFM irrespective of body weight showed greater impairment in the impact and activity scores of the SGRQ and the domain invalidity of the Medical Psychological Questionnaire for Lung Diseases, in comparison with depleted patients with relative preservation of FFM.[87] The effects of FFM depletion on activity and impact of the SGRQ were mediated by a decreased exercise performance, but independent of exercise capacity a relationship was found between FFM depletion and the experienced invalidity of the patients.

ENERGY METABOLISM IN COPD

Weight loss, and particularly loss of fat mass, occurs if energy expenditure exceeds dietary intake. More specifically, muscle wasting is a consequence of an imbalance between protein synthesis and protein breakdown. These impairments in total energy balance and protein metabolism may occur simultaneously, but these processes can also be dissociated. Based on the concept that in most rehabilitation programs exercise training is considered as a key element in order to improve the functional and health status of the patient suffering from COPD, insights in the pattern and components of daily energy expenditure are important in order to give adequate advice to the patient.

Total daily energy expenditure (EE) is usually divided into three components: (i) resting energy expenditure (REE), comprising sleeping metabolic rate and the energy cost of arousal; (ii) diet-induced thermogenesis; and (iii) physical activity-induced thermogenesis. Several studies have measured REE in COPD, based on the assumption that REE is the major component of total daily EE in sedentary persons. In COPD patients, an increased REE has been reported in different studies. REE was found to be elevated in 25% of patients with COPD after adjustment for the metabolically active FFM.[93] Drug therapy, especially use of beta-agonists, increased work of breathing as well as systemic inflammation has been related to this increase in REE. There is increasing evidence that hypermetabolism in COPD is related to the level of systemic inflammation.[94,95] Despite the high prevalence of hypermetabolism in COPD patients, the contribution of hypermetabolism to depletion of FFM is very limited: similar percentages of depleted COPD patients could be found in normometabolic as well as in hypermetabolic patients.[93]

In normal subjects, the most important determinant of total EE is the amount of voluntary or obligatory physical activity once the maintenance requirements of basal metabolic rate, DIT and the minimal essential amount of movement necessary to maintain life are accounted for. In general, the intensity and duration of physical activity determines this level of daily EE. Presumably as a consequence of the lower load of activities in COPD, EE for activities is generally considered to be low in these patients. However, despite the methodologic difficulties in measuring TDE, recent studies have focused attention on activity-related energy expenditure in patients with COPD. They found that patients with COPD not only had a significantly higher TDE than healthy subjects, but that the activity-related component of TDE was significantly higher in patients with COPD than in the healthy subjects.[96] No differences in TDE were reported between hypermetabolic and normo-metabolic patients with COPD; furthermore, REE adjusted for FFM did not correlate significantly with TDE, indicating that different mechanisms may underlie metabolic alterations in subgroups of patients with COPD.[97]

Several processes may account for the increased activity-related energy expenditure in patients with COPD. The mechanical efficiency of leg exercise is decreased in patients with COPD.[96] Clearly, part of the increased oxygen consumption during exercise can also be related to inefficient ventilation in the presence of increased ventilatory demand, especially under conditions of dynamic hyperinflation.[98] Furthermore, inefficient muscle metabolism may contribute to an increased TDE. Several studies indeed showed severely impaired oxidative phosphorylation during exercise in COPD, accompanied by an increased and highly anerobic metabolism involving both the energy release of high-energy phosphate compounds as well as enhanced glycolysis. It is generally known that anerobic metabolism is less efficient than aerobic metabolism.[99]

The habitual level of physical activity seems also to be very important in order to maintain the energy balance in ambulatory COPD patients. Goris et al.[100] reported that patients with a lower physical activity level, as measured by a simultaneous 7-day assessment of physical activity with a tri-axial accelerometer for movement basal metabolic rate, were able to eat sufficient for their energy needs and remained in energy balance. However, patients with a high physical activity level were unable to maintain energy balance and lost weight.

OUTCOME OF NUTRITIONAL INTERVENTION IN PATIENTS WITH COPD

The first clinical trials investigating the efficacy of nutritional intervention consisted of nutritional supplementation by means of oral liquid supplements or enteral nutrition. These short-term studies showed that 2–3 weeks of nutritional supplementation lead to a significant increase in body weight and respiratory muscle function.[101,102] The short-term effects noted in these studies are probably partly attributable to repletion of muscle water, electrolytes and cellular energy state rather than to constitution of muscle protein nitrogen. Significant improvements in respiratory and peripheral skeletal muscle function, exercise capacity and health-related quality of life were observed in one inpatient and one outpatient study following 3 months' oral supplementation of about 1000 kcal daily.[103,104] These data are not reproduced in other intervention studies: besides non-compliance and biological characteristics, a poor treatment response may be attributed to inadequate baseline assessment of energy requirements and to the observation that patients take supplements instead of their regular meals. A recent meta-analysis of nine randomized, controlled trials of caloric supplementation given for more than 2 weeks failed to demonstrate any significant improvement in anthropometric measures, lung function or exercise capacity.[105]

The limited therapeutic outcome in some of these studies could be related in part to the failure to include a comprehensive rehabilitation program in the treatment regime. The authors advocate combining nutritional support with an anabolic stimulus such as exercise to

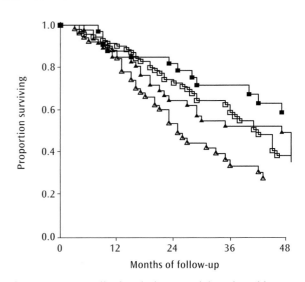

Figure 30.8 *Mortality in relation to weight gain. White square: non-depleted non responder; black square: non-depleted responder; white triangle: depleted non-responder; black triangle: depleted responder. (Reproduced from ref. 107 with permission.)*

optimize function. Indeed, in a large clinical trial a daily nutritional supplement given as an integrated part of a comprehensive pulmonary rehabilitation program resulted in a significant weight gain despite a daily supplementation that was much less than that used in most other outpatient studies.[106] Combining nutritional support and exercise not only increased body weight but also resulted in a significant improvement of FFM and respiratory muscle strength. The clinical relevance of this treatment response was further shown in a post hoc survival analysis of the study material that demonstrated that weight gain and increase in respiratory muscle strength were associated with significantly increased survival rates[107] (Figure 30.8).

Non-response to nutritional supplementation may also be related to biological characteristics underlying the disease process of COPD. In one study, non-response to nutritional therapy was associated with aging, relative anorexia and an elevated systemic inflammatory response.[108] New insights in the mechanisms of altered metabolism and substrate handling in COPD can contribute to further improvement of nutritional intervention strategies in these patients. A flow chart for nutritional screening and therapy is provided in Figure 30.9.

Simple screening can be based on measurement of the BMI and the weight course. Based on the BMI, patients are divided into underweight (BMI $< 21 \text{ kg/m}^2$; age > 50 years), normal weight $(21 < \text{BMI} < 25 \text{ kg/m}^2)$ and overweight patients $(25 < \text{BMI} < 30 \text{ kg/m}^2)$. Criteria used to define weight loss are: weight loss greater than 10% in the past 6 months or greater than 5% in the past month. Nutritional supplementation in indicated subgroups should initially consist of adaptations of the patients'

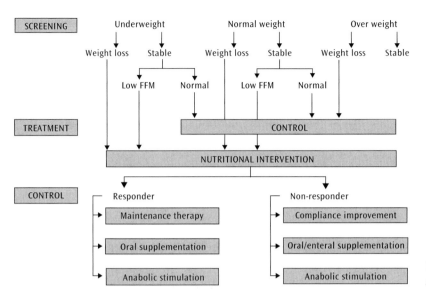

Figure 30.9 *Flow chart for nutritional screening and therapy.*

dietary habits (food choice, meal pattern). Nutritional support should be given as energy-dense supplements in quantities well divided during the day to avoid loss of appetite and adverse metabolic and ventilatory efforts resulting from a high caloric load.

It was long believed that because of their ventilatory limitation, patients with respiratory disease should consume a fat-rich diet to decrease carbon dioxide load. Scientific evidence supporting this theory is scarce and not convincing. More recent data show that patients experience less dyspnea after a liquid carbohydrate-rich supplement than after an equicaloric fat-rich supplement. These data are in line with a more rapid gastric emptying after a carbohydrate supplement than after a fat-rich supplement.[109] Based on data in other chronic wasting conditions, daily protein intake should be at least 1.5 g/kg/body weight to allow optimal protein synthesis. When feasible, patients should participate in an exercise program to stimulate an anabolic response and increase in FFM rather than fat storage. If weight gain and functional improvement occur, therapy is continued or moved to a maintenance regimen. If the desired response is not noted, it may be necessary to identify compliance issues. If compliance is not the problem, more calories may be needed by oral supplements or by enteral routes. Nevertheless, one should recognize that despite these interventions some patients may still not reach the intended effect because of underlying mechanisms of weight loss that are as yet not reversible.

In case of non-response adjuvant therapy with anabolics can be considered as an alternative intervention. Indeed, anabolic steroids given as adjuvant therapy to nutritional supplementation in COPD had a more favorable distribution of the body weight gain toward a larger increase in FFM and a larger improvement in respiratory muscle strength.[106] Further studies are indicated to investigate whether an anabolic response may be

enhanced by modulation of cellular metabolism of the muscle by bioactive nutrients involved in muscle energy and substrate metabolism such as creatine, carnitine, antioxidants and amino acids.

The exciting new area of research in nutraceuticals may result in the future to a shifting of nutritional therapy as a form of supportive care to a direct metabolic intervention strategy in order to modulate metabolism and functional capacity.

SUMMARY

Pulmonary rehabilitation refers to the whole spectrum of non-pharmacological intervention strategies, directed at improving the health and functional status of patients with chronic respiratory diseases. It is now clearly established that these multidisciplinary programs improve exercise capacity, reduce symptoms, improve quality of life and reduce medical consumption in COPD patients.[110] Exercise training, peripheral muscle training and nutritional support are evidence-based important components in the management approach of the COPD patient. Additional non-pharmacological treatment has therefore to be considered an integrated part of the disease management of every COPD patient.

REFERENCES

1. Siafakas NM, Vermeire P, Pride NB, *et al.* Optimal assessment and management of chronic obstructive pulmonary disease. ERS consensus statement. *Eur Respir J* 1995;**8**:1398–420.
2. ATS statement. Standards for the diagnosis and care of patients with chronic obstructive pulmonary disease. *Am J Respir Crit Care Med* 1995;**152**:S77–120.

3. Petty TL. Pulmonary rehabilitation. In: Basic of RD. American Thoracic Society, New York, 1975.

4. Pulmonary Rehabilitation Research NIH Workshop Summary. *Am Rev Respir Dis* 1994;**49**:828.

5. Selection criteria and programmes for pulmonary rehabilitation in COPD patients: ERS Task Force Position Paper. *Eur Respir J* 1997;**10**:744–57.

6. Pulmonary rehabilitation: official statement of the American Thoracic Society. *Am J Respir Crit Care Med* 1999;**159**:1666–82.

7. World Health Organisation. *International Classification of Impairments, Disabilities and Handicaps.* WHO, Geneva, 1980.

8. Towards a Common Language for Functioning and Disablement: ICIDH-2. http://www.who.ch/icidh. World Health Organization, Geneva, 1999.

9. Pauwels RA, Lofdahl CG, Laitinen LA, *et al.* Long-term treatment with inhaled budesonide in persons with mild chronic obstructive pulmonary disease who continue smoking. European Respiratory Society Study on Chronic Obstructive Pulmonary Disease. *N Engl J Med* 1999;**340**:1948–53.

10. Burge PS, Calverley PM, Jones PW, Spencer S, Anderson JA, Maslen TK. Randomised, double blind, placebo controlled study of fluticasone propionate in patients with moderate to severe chronic obstructive pulmonary disease: the ISOLDE trial. *Br Med J* 2000;**320**:1297–303.

11. Ries AL, Kaplan RM, Blumberg E. Use of factor analysis to consolidate multiple outcome measures in chronic obstructive pulmonary disease. *J Clin Epidemiol* 1991;**44**:497–503.

12. Wegner RE, Jorres RA, Kirsten DK, *et al.* Factor analysis of exercise capacity, dyspnoea ratings and lung function in patients with severe COPD. *Eur Respir J* 1994;**7**:725–9.

13. Mahler DA, Faryniarz K, Tomlinson D, *et al.* Impact of dyspnea and physiologic function on general health status in patients with chronic obstructive pulmonary disease. *Chest* 1992;**102**:395–401.

14. Berry MJ, Rejeski WJ, Adair NE, Zaccaro D. Exercise rehabilitation and chronic obstructive pulmonary disease stage. *Am J Respir Crit Care Med* 1999;**160**:1248–53.

15. Maes S. Chronische ziekten. [Chronic illnesses.] In: *Handboek Klinische Psychologie* 1993.

16. Van den Broek AHS. Patient Education and Chronic Obstructive Pulmonary Disease. Thesis, University of Leiden, 1995.

17. Ries AL, Kaplan RM, Limberg TM, Prewitt LM. Effects of pulmonary rehabilitation on physiologic and psychosocial outcomes in patients with chronic obstructive pulmonary disease. *Ann Intern Med* 1995;**122**:823–32.

18. O'Donnell DE, McGuire M, Samis L, Webb KA. The impact of exercise reconditioning on breathlessness in severe chronic airflow limitation. *Am J Respir Crit Care Med* 1995;**152**:2005–13.

19. Goldstein RS, Gort EH, Stubbing D, Avendano MA, Guyatt GH. Randomised controlled trial of respiratory rehabilitation. *Lancet* 1994;**344**:1394–7.

20. Strijbos JH, Postma DS, van Altena R, Gimeno F, Koeter GH. A comparison between an outpatient hospital-based pulmonary rehabilitation program and a home-care pulmonary rehabilitation program in patients with COPD. A follow-up of 18 months. *Chest* 1996;**109**:366–72.

21. Wijkstra PJ, van der Mark TW, Kraan J, van Altena R, Koeter GH, Postma DS. Effects of home rehabilitation on physical performance in patients with chronic obstructive pulmonary disease (COPD). *Eur Respir J* 1996;**9**:104–10.

22. Wedzicha JA, Bestall JC, Garrod R, Garnham R, Paul EA, Jones PW. Randomized controlled trial of pulmonary rehabilitation in severe chronic obstructive pulmonary

disease patients, stratified with the MRC dyspnoea scale. *Eur Respir J* 1998;**12**:363–9.

23. Swerts PM, Kretzers LM, Terpstra Lindeman E, Verstappen FT, Wouters EF. Exercise reconditioning in the rehabilitation of patients with chronic obstructive pulmonary disease: a short-and long-term analysis. *Arch Phys Med Rehabil* 1990;**71**:570–3.

24. Cambach W, Chadwick-Straver RVM, Wagenaar RC, *et al.* The effects of a community-based pulmonary rehabilitation programme on exercise tolerance and quality of life: a randomized controlled trial. *Eur Respir J* 1997;**10**:104–13.

25. Bendstrup KE, Ingemann Jensen J, Holm S, Bengtsson B. Out-patient rehabilitation improves activities of daily living, quality of life and exercise tolerance in chronic obstructive pulmonary disease. *Eur Respir J* 1997;**10**:2801–6.

26. Lacasse Y, Wong E, Guyatt GH, King D, Cook DJ, Goldstein RS. Meta-analysis of respiratory rehabilitation in chronic obstructive pulmonary disease. *Lancet* 1996;**348**:1115–19.

27. Goldstein RS, Gort EH, Guyatt GH, Feeny D. Economic analysis of respiratory rehabilitation. *Chest* 1997;**112**:370–9.

28. Troosters T, Gosselink R, Decramer M. Short- and long-term effects of outpatient rehabilitation in patients with chronic obstructive pulmonary disease: a randomized trial. *Am J Med* 2000;**109**:207–12.

29. Griffiths TL, Burr ML, Campbell IA, *et al.* Results at 1 year of outpatient multidisciplinary pulmonary rehabilitation: a randomised controlled trial. *Lancet* 2000;**355**:362–8.

30. Foglio K, Bianchi L, Ambrosino N. Is it really useful to repeat outpatient pulmonary rehabilitation programs in patients with chronic airway obstruction?: a 2-year controlled study. *Chest* 2001;**119**:1696–704.

31. Killian KJ, Leblanc P, Martin DH, *et al.* Exercise capacity and ventilatory, circulatory, and symptom limitation in patients with airflow limitation. *Am Rev Respir Dis* 1992;**146**:935.

32. Maltais F, Simard AA, Simard C, *et al.* Oxidative capacity of the skeletal muscle and lactic acid kinetics during exercise in normal subjects and in patients with COPD. *Am J Respir Crit Care Med* 1996;**153**:288.

33. Satta A, Migliori GB, Spanevello A, *et al.* Fibre types in skeletal muscles of chronic obstructive pulmonary disease patients related to respiratory function and exercise tolerance. *Eur Respir J* 1997;**10**:2853.

34. Pouw EM, Schols AMWJ, Van der Vusse GJ, *et al.* Elevated inosine monophosphate levels in resting muscle of patients with stable chronic obstructive pulmonary disease. *Am J Respir Crit Care Med* 1998;**157**:453.

35. Wuyam B, Payen JF, Levy P, *et al.* Metabolism and aerobic capacity of skeletal muscle in chronic respiratory failure related to chronic obstructive pulmonary disease. *Eur Respir J* 1992;**5**:157.

36. Levine S, Kaiser L, Leferovich J, *et al.* Cellular adaptation in the diaphragm in chronic obstructive pulmonary disease. *N Engl J Med* 1997;**337**:1799.

37. O'Donnell DE, Webb KA. Exertional breathlessness in patients with chronic airflow limitation. The role of lung hyperinflation. *Am Rev Respir Dis* 1993;**148**:1351–7.

38. Casaburi R, Patessio A, Ioli F, *et al.* Reductions in exercise lactic acidosis and ventilation as a result of exercise training in patients with obstructive lung disease. *Am Rev Respir Dis* 1991;**143**:9.

39. Maltais F, Leblanc P, Simard C, *et al.* Skeletal muscle adaptation to endurance training in patients with chronic obstructive pulmonary disease. *Am J Respir Crit Care Med* 1996;**154**:442.

40. Engelen M, Schols A, Does J, *et al.* Altered glutamate metabolism is associated with reduced muscle glutathione

levels in patients with emphysema. *Am J Respir Crit Care Med* 2000;**161**:98–103.

41. Sala E, Roca J, Marrades R, *et al.* Effects of endurance training on skeletal muscle bioenergetics in chronic obstructive pulmonary disease. *Am J Respir Crit Care Med* 1999;**159**:1726–34.

42. American College of Sports Medicine. The recommended quantity and quality of exercise for developing and maintaining cardiorespiratory and muscular fitness in healthy adults. *Med Sci Sports Exerc* 1990;**23**:265–74.

43. Casaburi R. Exercise training in chronic obstructive lung disease. In: R Casaburi, TL Petty, eds. *Principles and Practice of Pulmonary Rehabilitation.* WB Saunders, Philadelphia, 1993, pp 204–24.

44. Green R, Singh S, Williams J, Morgan M. A randomised controlled trial of four weeks versus seven weeks of pulmonary rehabilitation in chronic obstructive pulmonary disease. *Thorax* 2001;**56**:143–5.

45. Coppoolse R, Schols A, Baarends E, *et al.* Interval versus continuous training in patients with severe COPD. *Eur Respir J* 1999;**14**:258–63.

46. Rooyackers J, Dekhuijzen P, van Herwaarden C, Folgering H. Ventilatory response to positive and negative work in patients with chronic obstructive pulmonary disease. *Respir Med* 1997;**91**:143–9.

47. Rooyackers J. Pulmonary Rehabilitation in Patients with Severe Chronic Obstructive Pulmonary Disease. Thesis Katholieke Universiteit Nijmegen, the Netherlands.

48. Ries AL, Kaplan RM, Limberg TM, *et al.* Effects of pulmonary rehabilitation on physiologic and psychosocial outcomes in patients with chronic obstructive pulmonary disease. *Ann Intern Med* 1995;**122**:823–32.

49. Punzal PA, Ries AL, Kaplan RM, *et al.* Maximum intensity exercise training in patients with chronic obstructive pulmonary disease. *Chest* 1991;**100**:618–23.

50. Ries AL, Archibald CJ. Endurance exercise training at maximal targets in patients with chronic obstructive pulmonary disease. *J Cardiopulm Rehab* 1987;**7**:594–601.

51. Maltais F, LeBlanc P, Jobin J, *et al.* Intensity of training and physiologic adaptation in patients with chronic obstructive pulmonary disease. *Am J Respir Crit Care Med* 1997;**155**:555–61.

52. Clark C, Cochrane L, Mackay E. Low intensity peripheral muscle conditioning improves exercise tolerance and breathlessness in COPD. *Eur Respir J* 1996;**9**:2590–6.

53. Vallet G. Ahmaïdi S, Serres I, *et al.* Comparison of two training programmes in chronic airway limitation patients: standardized versus individualized protocols. *Eur Respir J* 1997;**10**:114–22.

54. Simpson K, Killian K, McCartney N, *et al.* Randomised controlled trial of weightlifting exercise in patients with chronic airflow obstruction. *Thorax* 1992;**47**:70–5.

55. Clark CJ, Cochrane LM, MacKay E, *et al.* Skeletal muscle strength and endurance in patients with mild COPD and the effects of weight training. *Eur Respir J* 2000; **15**:92–7.

56. Bernard S, Whittom F, LeBlanc P, *et al.* Aerobic and strength training in patients with chronic obstructive pulmonary disease. *Am J Respir Crit Care Med* 1999;**159**:896–901.

57. Couser JI, Maryinez FJ, Celli BR. Respiratory response and ventilatory muscle recruitment during arm elevation in normal subjects. *Chest* 1992;**101**:336–40.

58. Celli BR, Rassulo J, Make BJ. Dyssynchroneous breathing during arm but not leg exercise in patients with chronic airflow obstruction. *N Engl J Med* 1986;**314**: 1485–90.

59. Criner GJ, Celli BR. Effect of unsupported arm exercise on ventilatory muscle recruitment in patients with severe airflow obstruction. *Am Rev Respir Dis* 1988;**138**:856–61.

60. Dolmage TE, Maestro L, Avendano MA, Goldstein RS. The ventilatory response to arm elevation of patients with chronic obstructive pulmonary disease. *Chest* 1993; **104**:1097–100.

61. Martinez FJ, Couser JL, Celli BR. Respiratory response to arm elevation in patients with chronic airflow obstruction. *Am Rev Respir Dis* 1991;**143**:476–80.

62. Baarends E, Schols A, Slebos D, *et al.* Metabolic and ventilatory response pattern to arm elevation in patients with COPD and healthy age-matched subjects. *Eur Respir J* 1995;**8**:1345–51.

63. Ries AL, Ellis B, Hawkins R. Upper extremity exercise training in chronic obstructive pulmonary disease. *Chest* 1988;**93**: 688–92.

64. Marchand E, Decramer M. Respiratory muscle function and drive in chronic obstructive pulmonary disease. *Clin Chest Med* 2000;**21**:679–92.

65. Smith K, Cook D, Guyatt GH, *et al.* Respiratory muscle training in chronic airflow limitation: a meta-analysis. *Am J Respir Crit Care Med* 1995;**145**:533–9.

66. Harver A, Mahler DA, Daubenspeck JA. Targeted inspiratory muscle training improves respiratory muscle function and reduces dyspnea in patients with chronic obstructive pulmonary disease. *Ann Intern Med* 1989;**111**:117.

67. Dekhuijzen PNR, Folgering THM, Van Herwaarden CLA. Target-flow inspiratory muscle training during pulmonary rehabilitation in patients with COPD. *Chest* 1991;**99**:128.

68. Wanke T, Formanek D, Lahrmann H, *et al.* Effects of combined inspiratory muscle and cycle ergometer training on exercise performance in patients with COPD. *Eur Respir J* 1994;**7**:2205.

69. Benditt JO, Wood DE, McCool FD, *et al.* Changes in breathing and ventilatory muscle recruitment patterns induced by lung volume reduction surgery. *Am J Respir Crit Care Med* 1997; **155**:279.

70. Larson JL, Covey MK, Wirtz SE, *et al.* Cycle ergometer and inspiratory muscle training in chronic obstructive pulmonary disease. *Am J Respir Crit Care Med* 1999;**160**:500.

71. Pulmonary Rehabilitation. Joint ACCP/AACVPR Evidence-based Guidelines. *Chest* 1997;**112**:1363–96.

72. Damoiseaux V. Patiëntenvoorlichting: een terreinverkenning. [Patient education: an exploration.] Symposiumbundel patiëntenvoorlichting 1984. GVO cahiers, University of Maastricht.

73. Jones K, Tilford S, Robinson Y. *Health Education. Effectiveness and Efficiency.* Chapman and Hall, India, 1990.

74. Jensen PS. Risk, protective factors, and supportive interventions in chronic airway obstruction. *Arch Gen Psychiatry* 1983;**40**:1203–7.

75. Atkins CJ, Kaplan RM, Timms RM, *et al.* Behavioural exercise programs in the management of chronic obstructive pulmonary disease. *J Couns Clin Psychol* 1984;**52**:591–603.

76. Howland J, Nelson EC, Barlow PB, *et al.* Chronic obstructive airway disease. Impact of health education. *Chest* 1986; **90**:233–8.

77. Tougaard L, Krone T, Sorkanaes A, *et al.* Economic benefits of teaching patients with chronic obstructive pulmonary disease about their illness. The *Lancet* 1992;**339**:1517–20.

78. Toshima MT, Kaplan RM, Ries AL. Experimental evaluation of rehabilitation in chronic obstructive pulmonary disease: short-term effects on exercise endurance and health status. *Health Psychol* 1990;**9**:237–52.

79. Kaptein AA, Dekker FW. Psychosocial support. *Eur Respir Mon* 2000;**5**:58–69.

80. Engelen MP, Schols AM, Baken WC, Wesseling GJ, Wouters EF. Nutritional depletion in relation to respiratory and peripheral skeletal muscle function in out-patients with COPD. *Eur Respir J* 1994;**7**:1793–7.

81. Schols AM, Soeters PB, Dingemans AM, Mostert R, Frantzen PJ, Wouters EF. Prevalence and characteristics of nutritional depletion in patients with stable COPD eligible for pulmonary rehabilitation. *Am Rev Respir Dis* 1993;**147**:1151–6.

82. Engelen MP, Schols AM, Does JD, Wouters EF. Skeletal muscle weakness is associated with wasting of extremity fat-free mass but not with airflow obstruction in patients with chronic obstructive pulmonary disease. *Am J Clin Nutr* 2000;**71**:733–8.

83. Baarends EM, Schols AM, Mostert R, Wouters EF. Peak exercise response in relation to tissue depletion in patients with chronic obstructive pulmonary disease. *Eur Respir J* 1997;**10**:2807–13.

84. Palange P, Forte S, Felli A, Galassetti P, Serra P, Carlone S. Nutritional state and exercise tolerance in patients with COPD. *Chest* 1995;**107**:1206–12.

85. Palange P, Forte S, Onorati P, *et al*. Effect of reduced body weight on muscle aerobic capacity in patients with COPD. *Chest* 1998;**114**:12–18.

86. Shoup R, Dalsky G, Warner S, *et al*. Body composition and health-related quality of life in patients with obstructive airways disease. *Eur Respir J* 1997;**10**:1576–80.

87. Mostert RM, Goris A, Weling-Scheepers C, *et al*. Tissue depletion and health related quality of life in patients with chronic obstructive pulmonary disease. *Respir Med* 2000;**94**:859–67.

88. Braun SR, Keim NL, Dixon RM, Clagnaz P, Anderegg A, Shrago ES. The prevalence and determinants of nutritional changes in chronic obstructive pulmonary disease. *Chest* 1984;**86**:558–63.

89. Goldstein S, Askanazi J, Weissman C, Thomashow B, Kinney JM. Energy expenditure in patients with chronic obstructive pulmonary disease. *Chest* 1987;**91**:222–4.

90. Fitting JW, Frascarolo P, Jequier E, Leuenberger P. Energy expenditure and rib cage-abdominal motion in chronic obstructive pulmonary disease. *Eur Respir J* 1989;**2**:840–5.

91. Wilson DO, Donahoe M, Rogers RM, Pennock BE. Metabolic rate and weight loss in chronic obstructive lung disease. *J Parenter Enteral Nutr* 1990;**14**:7–11.

92. Schols AM, Mostert R, Soeters PB, Wouters EF. Body composition and exercise performance in patients with chronic obstructive pulmonary disease. *Thorax* 1991;**46**:695–9.

93. Creutzberg EC, Schols AM, Bothmer Quaedvlieg FC, Wouters EF. Prevalence of an elevated resting energy expenditure in patients with chronic obstructive pulmonary disease in relation to body composition and lung function. *Eur J Clin Nutr* 1998;**52**:396–401.

94. Nguyen LT, Bedu M, Caillaud D, *et al*. Increased resting energy expenditure is related to plasma TNF-alpha concentration in stable COPD patients. *Clin Nutr* 1999;**18**:269–74.

95. Schols AM, Buurman WA, Staal van den Brekel AJ, Dentener MA, Wouters EF. Evidence for a relation between metabolic derangements and increased levels of inflammatory mediators in a subgroup of patients with chronic obstructive pulmonary disease. *Thorax* 1996;**51**:819–24.

96. Baarends EM, Schols AM, Pannemans DL, Westerterp KR, Wouters EF. Total free living energy expenditure in patients with severe chronic obstructive pulmonary disease. *Am J Respir Crit Care Med* 1997;**155**:549–54.

97. Baarends EM, Schols AM, Westerterp KR, Wouters EF. Total daily energy expenditure relative to resting energy expenditure in clinically stable patients with COPD. *Thorax* 1997;**52**:780–5.

98. O'Donnell DE, Lam M, Webb, KA. Measurement of symptoms, lung hyperinflation, and endurance during exercise in chronic obstructive pulmonary disease. *Am J Respir Crit Care Med* 1998;**158**:1557–65.

99. Kutsuzawa T, Shioya S, Kurita D, Haida M, Ohta Y, Yamabayashi H. ^{31}P-NMR study of skeletal muscle metabolism in patients with chronic respiratory impairment. *Am Rev Respir Dis* 1992;**146**:1019–24.

100. Goris A. Validation of the Assessment of Food Intake in Humans. Thesis, 2001.

101. Whittaker JS, Ryan CF, Buckley PA, Road JD. The effects of refeeding on peripheral and respiratory muscle function in malnourished chronic obstructive pulmonary disease patients. *Am Rev Respir Dis* 1990;**142**:283–8.

102. Wilson DO, Rogers RM, Sanders MH, Pennock BE, Reilly JJ. Nutritional intervention in malnourished patients with emphysema. *Am Rev Respir Dis* 1986;**134**:672–7.

103. Rogers RM, Donahoe M, Costantino J. Physiologic effects of oral supplemental feeding in malnourished patients with chronic obstructive pulmonary disease. A randomized control study. *Am Rev Respir Dis* 1992;**146**:1511–17.

104. Efthimiou J, Fleming J, Gomes C, Spiro SG. The effect of supplementary oral nutrition in poorly nourished patients with chronic obstructive pulmonary disease. *Am Rev Respir Dis* 1988;**137**:1075–82.

105. Ferreira IM, Brooks D, Lacasse Y, Goldstein RS. Nutritional support for individuals with COPD: a meta-analysis. *Chest* 2000;**117**:672–8.

106. Schols AM, Soeters PB, Mostert R, Pluymers RJ, Wouters EF. Physiologic effects of nutritional support and anabolic steroids in patients with chronic obstructive pulmonary disease. A placebo-controlled randomized trial. *Am J Respir Crit Care Med* 1995;**152**:1268–74.

107. Schols AM, Slangen J, Volovics L, Wouters EF. Weight loss is a reversible factor in the prognosis of chronic obstructive pulmonary disease. *Am J Respir Crit Care Med* 1998;**157**:1791–7.

108. Creutzberg EC, Schols AM, Weling Scheepers CA, Buurman WA, Wouters EF. Characterization of nonresponse to high caloric oral nutritional therapy in depleted patients with chronic obstructive pulmonary disease. *Am J Respir Crit Care Med* 2000;**161**:745–52.

109. Vermeeren M, Baarends E, Nelissen L, *et al*. Immediate postprandial effects of a nutritional supplement on symptoms and exercise capacity in patients with chronic obstructive pulmonary disease (COPD). *Eur Respir J* 1997;**10**:2264–9.

110. Global initiative for chronic Obstructive Lung Disease (GOLD), a collaborative project of the US National Heart, Lung and Blood Institute (NHLBI) and the World Health Organization (WHO).

Health status

PAUL W JONES

INTRODUCTION

The primary effects of COPD occur in the lungs but, as with many chronic diseases, it has secondary effects on other organs and systems. These include the skeletal muscle, in which wasting can occur through disuse atrophy and the effects of cachexia (see Chapter 30). Cardiovascular disturbances include pulmonary hypertension and effects on myocardial function and skeletal muscle due to lack of physical exercise (see Chapter 18). Fatigue is a common, complex and ill-understood process in COPD,[1] but for reasons that are not well understood, patients do not readily volunteer that it is a problem until they are asked directly.[2] Higher brain function is disturbed with sleep disruption (see Chapter 19), cognitive dysfunction[3] and the development of mood impairment.

The development of ill health due to chronic disease does not follow a simple linear path (Figure 31.1) and within each pathway there may be multiple mechanisms. For example breathlessness may be due to expiratory airflow limitation, an increase in static lung volume, dynamic hyperinflation and hypoxia-induced stimulation of breathing. Furthermore, some of these paths are circular. Perhaps, the simplest to understand is the effect of exercise limitation. This causes muscle wasting due to disuse atrophy, which itself will induce exercise limitation. The existence of such feedback loops leads to 'local autonomy' with the induction of secondary self-maintaining disease processes that are entirely unrelated

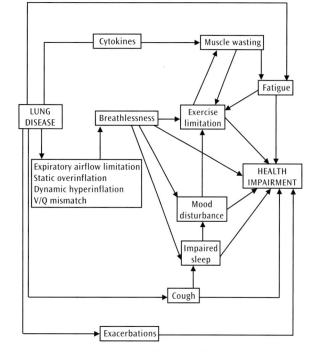

Figure 31.1 *Links between disease in the lungs and resulting breathlessness.*

to the original disease trigger. It is clearly inappropriate to consider COPD just as a condition of the lungs; it is a multisystem disease and so its assessment should reflect this.

Table 31.1 *Frequency of self-reported activity limitations in 2500 COPD patients. (Data from British Lung Foundation survey)*

Activity	Frequency reported (%)
Sleep disturbance	52
Washing/bathing	55
Making the bed	59
Housework	65
Walking outside the house	68
Gardening	75
Climbing stairs	79

SYMPTOMS AND THEIR EFFECTS IN COPD

Symptoms may have both direct and indirect effects. Breathlessness and fatigue both cause exercise limitation, but the experience of breathlessness may also induce anxiety, which, if severe, becomes panic. Exercise limitation may induce depression. Fatigue may be a feature of both chronic disease and depression and have a complex relationship with impaired mood. Many secondary effects of COPD symptoms are due to their effects on mobility and limitation of activity. The latter may be divided into those that are essential to normal daily life such as washing and dressing and those that restrict social functioning and recreation. The frequency of these disturbances may be very high (Table 31.1). The data presented in this table were provided by patients' self-report and could have been highly influenced by responder bias. Nevertheless this was a large sample of patients and does show that many have daily limitation of their activity due to their symptoms.

Finally, it should be recognized that whilst breathlessness and fatigue can cause the well-recognized specific consequences of COPD through their effects on activity, it should also be recognized that malaise and a general sense of impaired well being also occur, especially during and after exacerbations. These are more difficult to define and quantify but they undoubtedly contribute to the distress that results from this disease.

ASSESSING THE OVERALL EFFECT OF COPD

Since COPD is such a complex disease with multiple effects on the patient's health produced by many different pathophysiologic pathways, it is clear that assessments confined to one specific aspect of the disease will fail to address other important effects. There is a need for an overall integrative measure that aggregates the discrete effects of the disease into a simple summary score. Bearing in mind the fact that several important aspects of

COPD lie outside the lungs, this summary measure should bring together effects due primarily to disturbances of lung function and those resulting from effects on other organs. Only two types of measure can currently provide this integrative function in COPD: cardiopulmonary exercise testing and questionnaires.

In many respects exercise tests are very attractive as an overall measure of COPD because they are objective and can be standardized. Their main disadvantage is that they do not address factors such as sleep disturbance, effects of cough and sputum production, impact of exacerbations and feelings of malaise and impaired well being. To tackle these areas of impaired health, it is necessary to question the patient. This is the basis of clinical history taking, which is still the first clinical skill taught to medical students. Modern medicine is now greatly reliant upon laboratory-based measurements and pulmonary medicine led the way with the early adoption of laboratory methods for measuring pulmonary function routinely. But this has not invalidated the process of questioning patients to detail and quantify their symptoms. It is worth noting that the specificity of patients' descriptions of the quality of their dyspnea can help elucidate the cause of breathlessness in those in whom laboratory investigations have not been helpful.[4]

Clinical histories vs. questionnaires

In routine practice, a clinical history is taken to make a diagnosis and formulate an overall assessment of the manner and degree to which the disease is affecting the patient. The outcome of this assessment is a summary or description that will be unique to each patient. A well-taken and comprehensive clinical history can provide a clear and detailed picture of the effect of COPD on the patient's health and well being. If this is documented and sufficiently well-taken, it will be relatively easy for the clinician to establish what changes had occurred over the intervening period when the patient is next reviewed.

These qualitative assessments are entirely appropriate to the purpose to which they are put. By contrast, the requirements of clinical trials are quite different. Such studies are performed in groups of patients and their results averaged across all the individuals within the study. This means that all patients must be measured in the same way. To achieve this, the assessments are standardized so that each patient's symptoms and the effect of the disease on their life is assessed in exactly the same way as for all the others in the study. Then, to calculate an average and summarize the results of the study, it is necessary to convert the patients' descriptions of their disease into numbers. For these reasons, the patient's history must be obtained in a standardized manner using a questionnaire.

Quality of life vs. health status measurement

The term 'quality of life' is used very widely and often there is a failure to distinguish between quality of life that covers all aspects of an individual's life and 'health-related quality of life' which is limited to those areas of life disturbed specifically by disease. The distinction is important, because health is only a minor factor in determining quality of life, even in patients with serious disease. The more restricted concept of 'health-related quality of life' still has disadvantages and incautious use may lead to confusion as to what is being assessed. People's lives are very varied, so life quality will be affected by disease in many different ways. A simple example may illustrate this. COPD patients are middle aged or older, so may have grandchildren. Playing with grandchildren can be very important to some people, but it is not a feature of the lives of all older people. Not all patients have grandchildren or, if they do, they may live too far away or be grown up. Even if there are grandchildren of a suitable age, other factors that are external to the patient may determine whether COPD affects this potentially important area of life. For example, the energy cost of playing football with an energetic 7-year-old is very different from that needed to play chess with a 10-year-old. One activity may be severely disturbed by COPD, the other not at all. Thus it is the interests of the child rather than the patient that will determine their health-related quality of life. It is useful, therefore, to think of health-related quality of life as being unique to each patient.

Questionnaires that are designed to measure the effect of COPD on symptoms, daily activities and sense of well being in groups of patients must be standardized, so that all patients are assessed in exactly the same way. This means that all of the items in the questionnaire must be relevant (at least potentially) to every patient to whom it will be administered. Items that may not apply universally should not be included – for example those about grandchildren. Methods have been developed for identifying the items that are most important and frequent in COPD patients, but they result inevitably in a questionnaire that is composed of items that are universal to all patients, in other words individuality is selectively omitted. For this reason, I now suggest that it may be better to use the term 'health status measurement' to distinguish this process from 'health-related quality of life' assessment. The latter is best reserved for the assessment of individuals, is assessed during an interview and is summarized in words. 'Health status measurement' is carried out in groups of patients using standardized questionnaires and is summarized using numbers.

Health status questionnaires treat each patient as if they were a 'typical' or 'average' patient, so the score for an individual should be interpreted in that light. Results from a clinical trial give the average result from that group of patients. Benefit to an individual's health-related quality of life will depend on their circumstances and will vary between patients. In part it will be conditioned by those unique aspects of the patient's life that can only be assessed through a clinical interview. In other words, 'health-related quality of life' applies in clinical practice, 'health status measurement' to clinical studies. Most of the remaining portions of this chapter concern health status measurement and what it can tell us about COPD and its treatment.

HEALTH STATUS QUESTIONNAIRES

Health status questionnaires fall into two broad types: disease specific and general health. The major differences between them lie in terms of their content. As implied by the name, general health questionnaires are designed to assess the impact of any disease, whereas the content of disease-specific questionnaires is chosen for the disease in question.

General health questionnaires

General questionnaires were the first instruments used to measure health status in patients with respiratory disease. A number have been used.

MEDICAL OUTCOMES STUDY SF-36

The Medical Outcomes Study Short-form 36-item (SF-36) questionnaire covers eight dimensions of health: physical functioning, physical role limitation, social functioning, emotional role limitation, general health, vitality, mental health and bodily pain.[5,6] Each dimension is scored separately and transformed to a 0–100-point scale. Two global scores are obtained for a Physical Component Summary and a Mental Component Summary. This instrument can be completed by patients in 5–10 minutes. It has been validated in COPD and is used quite widely in COPD studies.[7] Generic health instruments tend to be less sensitive than disease-specific questionnaires in clinical trials, although the SF-36 has shown responsiveness to change with treatment, both with rehabilitation[8] and inhaled corticosteroids.[9] The disadvantage with the SF-36, as a general health measure, is that its scoring range does not include death, which limits its usefulness for health economic analyses.

QUALITY OF WELLBEING SCALE

The Quality of Wellbeing (QWB) scale is a general health scale with utility properties – its scores range from perfect health (1) to death (zero) so it can be used in cost–utility analyses. It contains 50 items with three components: mobility, physical activity and social activity. It is quite complex to use and takes approximately 10–15 minutes to be completed through an interview. It has been validated for use in obstructive airways disease,[10] although in one long-term study of pulmonary rehabilitation it failed to show any significant change even though there were improvements in exercise endurance and reductions in breathlessness and leg fatigue during exercise.[11]

EQ-5D (or EuroQol)

The EQ-5D is a utility scale that provides a simple and brief method for individuals to rate health status using a visual analog scale for five dimensions (mobility, self-care, usual activities, pain/discomfort and anxiety/depression).[12] It is probable that this will be used increasingly in clinical trials, especially those sponsored by pharmaceutical companies.

OTHER GENERAL QUESTIONNAIRES

The Sickness Impact Profile was one of the first general health instruments that was developed and was used in the Nocturnal Oxygen Therapy Trial.[13] It appears to be insensitive in patients with mild to moderate lung impairment[14] and is now little used in COPD. The Nottingham Health Profile includes 38 items covering six dimensions: energy, pain, emotional reaction, sleep, social isolation and physical mobility. It is self-administered and takes 5–10 minutes to complete. It has some validity in COPD, but as with most general health questionnaires, its validity is not as strong as that of disease-specific instruments.[15,16]

Disease-specific questionnaires

There are a number of questionnaires developed specifically for COPD.

CHRONIC RESPIRATORY DISEASE QUESTIONNAIRE

The Chronic Respiratory Disease Questionnaire (CRQ) was designed as an evaluative instrument to quantify changes in health.[2,17] It consists of four components: dyspnea (five items); fatigue (four items); mastery (four items); and emotion (seven items). Each item is graded by the patient using a 7-point Likert scale. For the dyspnea component, the subject is asked to describe the five most common activities that caused dyspnea over the past 2 weeks by recall and then by reading a list of 26 different activities. It takes 15–20 minutes for the first assessment. An interviewer is required to assist the patient in making these selections, but a standardized self-complete version will be available soon.

ST GEORGE'S RESPIRATORY QUESTIONNAIRE

The St George's Respiratory Questionnaire (SGRQ) was developed for patients with asthma or COPD.[18,19] Its three components are symptoms (distress attributable to cough, wheeze, and acute exacerbations), activity (disturbance of physical activity and mobility caused by dyspnea), and impacts (psychosocial effects of the disease). It takes 10–20 minutes to complete. It was designed for supervised self-administration, but has also been validated for use by telephone administration. The method of scoring differs from other disease-specific instruments because each item has its own empirically derived weight that is independent of age, gender, disease severity and duration[20] and largely independent of country.[21]

OTHER DISEASE-SPECIFIC QUESTIONNAIRES

A number of other disease-specific questionnaires have been produced in recent years. Among them are the Breathing Problems Questionnaire (BPQ)[22,23] and the QOL-RIQ – a questionnaire developed originally in Dutch but also available in English.[24] Similar questionnaires developed in the USA include the Seattle Obstructive Lung Disease Questionnaire[25] and two questionnaires that concentrate two function-limitation questionnaires that are similar in many respects to health status instruments: the Modified Pulmonary Functional Status and Dyspnea Questionnaire (PFSDQ-M)[26] and the Pulmonary Functional Status Scale (PFSS).[27] The latter questionnaires are in wide use in pulmonary rehabilitation programmes in the USA. All health status questionnaires tend to be rather long, which makes them largely unsuitable for use in the clinic. For this reason a short questionnaire, the AQ20, was developed for routine use in asthma and COPD.[28,29] It requires 2–3 minutes to complete and score.

QUESTIONNAIRES FOR SEVERE DISEASE

Most of the disease-specific questionnaires were developed for patients who have at least some degree of mobility, but some patients particularly those with respiratory failure may have severe restriction of daily activity and be largely housebound. This may place them at one end of the scoring range of a questionnaire, with the risk of so-called 'floor-effects', so that many patients produce the worst possible score. Furthermore, a questionnaire designed for patients who are less severely restricted may not have enough items to discriminate well between different levels of very severe disease. The general health questionnaires, especially those that include death at one end of the scaling range, may be more suitable for such patients, although this has not been proven. To meet the need for a disease-specific instrument suitable for such patients, two different types of instrument have been developed. One, the London Chest Activity of Daily Living Scale (LCADL), was designed specifically to assess limitations of activities of daily living in COPD patients.[30] The other is a comprehensive measure of health status impairment for patients with respiratory failure irrespective of cause.[31] There is evidence for the validity of these two questionnaires, although it is not yet clear whether either offers any distinct advantages over the existing instruments.

DISEASE-SPECIFIC QUESTIONNAIRES: SUMMARY

The content of disease-specific questionnaires varies between those with a relatively high psychologic content (e.g. CRQ and QOL-RIQ) and those with a higher proportion of physical items (e.g. PFSDQ-M and PFSS), although the differences overall are not very great. The chief distinction between them lies in the format of the responses that are required. Most use Likert scales with response categories such as: 'a little', 'somewhat' etc, as exemplified by the CRQ. A few employ dichotomous responses with simple answers to each item such as: 'yes'/'no', 'true'/'false', as used in the SGRQ and AQ20. In theory, Likert scales may permit better short-term responsiveness to change than dichotomous response formats. On the other hand, Likert scales may be susceptible to a phenomenon known as 'response-shift' in which patients may, over time, change the way in which they scale severity. For example, what is judged to be 'moderate' when they first become ill may be assessed as being 'a little' when they have experienced the symptoms for some time. In theory, dichotomous responses may be more suitable for long-term studies.

VALIDATION OF HEALTH STATUS QUESTIONNAIRES

This is a complex topic, filled with arcane terminology, but basically it is concerned with two questions:

1 Does the questionnaire do what it claims to do, i.e. measure impaired health?
2 Does it have the properties that make it a reliable measurement instrument?

One complication is that questionnaires are often required to have two different purposes:

1 To detect differences in health between patients – discriminative properties.
2 To detect longitudinal changes within patients – evaluative properties.

Not all questionnaires used in COPD have both, although it is an advantage if they do. There is no single step that can be used to test whether a questionnaire measures

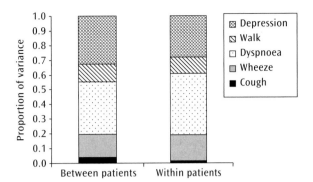

Figure 31.2 *Left-hand bar: proportion of variance in SGRQ total score attributable to frequency of cough, frequency of wheeze, dyspnea (MRC Dyspnea Scale), 6-minute walking distance and depression (Hospital Anxiety and Depression Scale). Right-hand bar: proportional variance in change in SGRQ score attributable to changes in these five covariates over 1 year. The variances have been normalized to 100% to permit comparison between the between-patient and within-patient analyses.*

impaired health. Rather, it is a process of testing whether it behaves in the way that we would expect it to do, if it did measure health. Thus we would expect it to detect differences between patients in terms of their level of symptoms, physiological impairment, mood state, hospital admissions, etc. This topic has been reviewed in depth elsewhere and there are now many studies that, taken together, show that the questionnaires used most widely in COPD are valid measures of health impairment.[32]

One of the major objectives of these questionnaires is to integrate a range of different effects of the disease into an overall score. The success of this can be tested by using multivariate analysis and regressing the questionnaire score against other measures of disease activity that are important in COPD. With the SGRQ it can be shown that the determinants, or partial correlates, of the health status score are very similar, whether tested in terms of a cross-sectional analysis (across patients) or longitudinal (within patients).[19] This is an important point since it shows that the questionnaire behaves in the same way, whether used to distinguish between patients or detect changes within patients (Figure 31.2).

PHYSIOLOGIC CORRELATES OF HEALTH STATUS

COPD is a disease that is characterized by expiratory airflow limitation, so a correlation with the FEV_1 should be expected.[33] There is a clear relationship between FEV_1 and health status across patient groups, as shown in Figure 31.3. The worse the degree of airway obstruction,

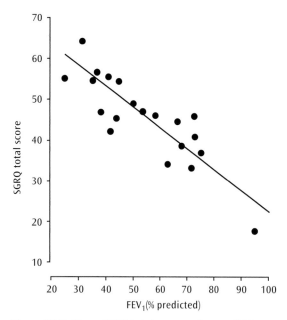

Figure 31.3 *Mean SGRQ total score and mean FEV$_1$ from 20 studies in asthma and COPD. A higher score indicates worse health.*

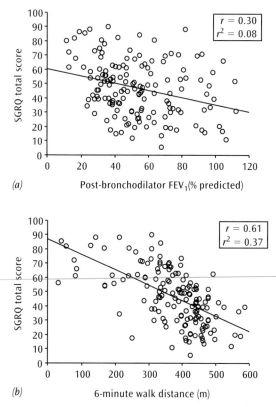

Figure 31.4 *(a) Relationship between SGRQ total score and post-bronchodilator FEV$_1$. (b) Relationship between SGRQ total score and 6-minute walking distance. Exercise performance is a better correlate of impaired health status than the FEV$_1$.*

the worse is the health status. A graph of this type provides a useful method by which a validation check can be carried out, to test whether results from a particular study fit the overall pattern obtained with this particular questionnaire. This plot is misleading in one important way, however, since averaged data such as this do not reflect the true nature of the relationship between health status and FEV$_1$. This is illustrated better in Figure 31.4(a), in which SGRQ and FEV$_1$ data from individual patients are plotted. The most immediate feature of this figure is that the correlation is weak. At first sight, this may call into question the validity of the health status questionnaires (or this one in particular), but it should not be surprising in view of the complexity of the pathways linking lung disease and health status (Figure 31.1). In fact there are other stronger physiologic correlates of health status than the FEV$_1$, as illustrated in Figure 31.4(b). This uses data from the same patients as Figure 31.4(a), but shows SGRQ scores plotted against exercise performance. It is quite clear that exercise is a stronger determinant of impaired health than expiratory airflow limitation.[19] It is worth noting also that arterial PaO$_2$ appears to be a consistently better correlate of impaired health than the FEV$_1$.[19,31]

BASELINE ASSESSMENT OF HEALTH STATUS

The weak correlation with spirometric measurements shows that the evaluation of patients with COPD requires more than just the FEV$_1$, if we wish to get a picture of the overall effect of the disease. Figure 31.4(a) shows that there are many patients who have relatively mild limitation of expiratory airflow, yet exhibit quite severely impaired health due to other COPD-related factors. It is very important to recognize those patients because treatment for COPD is directed largely towards symptom reduction and they are clearly highly symptomatic. For this reason therapeutic decisions should be based on the level of symptoms, not just on the FEV$_1$.

There is no agreed method of assessing the health or disability of COPD patients in routine practice, but questionnaires such as the CRQ and SGRQ do not appear to be the solution because they are too complex and time consuming for routine use. On the other hand, the simple 5-point MRC Dyspnea Questionnaire can be used routinely and it has been shown to distinguish quite well between different levels of severity of COPD and correlates well with health status measured using the SGRQ.[19,34] However, even the MRC scale may be more complex than is actually needed to identify patients with the greatest likelihood of impaired health. Perhaps only one or two screening questions may be all that are required, although they have yet to be identified.

THRESHOLDS FOR CLINICAL SIGNIFICANCE

One of the most useful aspects of health status measurement is the identification of a score that is described variously as a: 'threshold for clinical significance', 'minimum important difference', 'minimum clinically important difference', etc. These terms are used to convey the concept that there is a particular health status score or change in score that indicates a clinically significant boundary. The establishment of these thresholds is a complex process and the different methods of assessing such thresholds are discussed in depth elsewhere.[35] However, it appears that, for any given questionnaire, the threshold value appears to be consistent across the different methods of estimation. With the CRQ, the minimum clinically important difference appears to be 0.5 for all four components of that instrument.[36] With the SGRQ, the corresponding value is 4 units for both the total and impacts scores.[18] No estimate has been calculated for the symptoms and activity components.

An important and frequently overlooked aspect of these thresholds is the fact that they are average values that have been estimated in populations of patients. As a result, they can be applied only to groups of patients. In the same way that health status questionnaires treat each patient as if they were an average patient, the clinically significant threshold or minimum important difference applies only to the 'average' or 'typical' patient. It is inappropriate to use a 4-point change in SGRQ score or 0.5-unit change in CRQ score to indicate whether an individual patient had a worthwhile response to therapy.

HEALTH STATUS RESULTS FROM CLINICAL TRIALS

An increasing number of clinical trials are using health status measurement as an outcome measure. These questionnaires were adopted first in rehabilitation trials. This may be due in part to the multidisciplinary approach that is needed for pulmonary rehabilitation dictating the need for a less specific, more overall, measure of clinical efficacy. There is now good evidence from a meta-analysis of rehabilitation trials using the CRQ that pulmonary rehabilitation produces an improvement in health that is significantly greater than the minimum clinically important difference.[37] In particular it will be noted that the lower confidence interval for two of the domains either just touches or does not even cross the threshold of significance (Figure 31.5). This finding has now been confirmed in a single large study using the CRQ, SRGQ and SF-36.[8] All three questionnaires showed a large improvement immediately after the end of the rehabilitation period, but this wore off over the following year

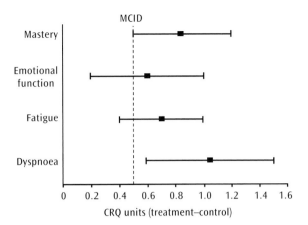

Figure 31.5 *Meta-analysis of CRQ scores from randomized controlled trials of pulmonary rehabilitation. The bars indicate the 95% confidence intervals. The dotted line at 0.5 is the threshold for a minimum clinically significant difference between the two treatment groups.*

and only the SGRQ score was found to remain clinically significant at the end of this period. Some of this apparent fall off in effect seen with the CRQ may have been due in part to 'response shift' – i.e. patients resetting their judgement as to the severity of the effect of their symptoms on their daily life and well being.

The contribution of health status measurements to pharmacologic studies was first most clearly illustrated by a 16-week study that compared two doses (standard and high dose) of the long-acting bronchodilator beta$_2$-agonist Salbutamol in a three-armed randomized placebo-controlled study.[38] The most important observation from this study was that, whilst the two doses produced the same increase in FEV$_1$ (approx 115 ml), only the standard dose produced a statistically and clinically significant improvement in health. The higher dose did not. Data obtained using the generic SF-36 questionnaire suggested that this was because the higher dose produced more side effects. This dose-dependent effect on health gain has been confirmed in another study that used two different doses of formoterol – another long-acting beta$_2$-agonist.[39] This is an important observation, because it shows that dose of the drug may influence the size of the symptomatic gain, even though it may not alter spirometric benefit.

A recent study with tiotropium, a long-acting anticholinergic bronchodilator, has shown that the time course of the spirometric and health status changes may be very different.[40] The improvement in lung function was seen within the first day of therapy, but the health status gain took many weeks to develop fully (Figure 31.6). Reasons for this delayed improvement may be multifactorial. First, it may take time for patients to become aware of their improvement and so translate it into improved daily activities. Second, some of the health benefits may develop slowly. For example, improved sleep quality may take some while to become fully apparent and for the patient to become aware of a sustained change. Another area of improvement that would take time to develop is a reduction in the number of exacerbations. It is known that frequent exacerbations are associated with poor health status[41] and there is evidence that bronchodilators may reduce exacerbations.[39,42] Since exacerbations occur on average only one or two times a year, any health status benefit from a reduction in their frequency will take time to accrue.

The studies discussed here show why it is relevant to measure health status in COPD. Neither the size, nor the time course of the symptomatic or health status response to therapy were predictable from the changes in FEV_1. Clearly formal measurements provide information about COPD that is complementary to that from spirometry.

LONGITUDINAL CHANGES IN HEALTH STATUS

COPD is known to be a progressive disease, as shown by the characteristic worsening of FEV_1, so it should be no surprise that health status declines at a measurable rate. This has been demonstrated only recently however. Whilst the concept of deterioration in health status score is quite easy to understand, attaching meaning to the estimated rates of decline is more difficult. In part this will come with experience and as more studies are published (as was the case with estimates for the rate of decline of FEV_1). However, health status measurement has one advantage in this respect because the threshold for clinical significance forms a useful reference point that permits rates of deterioration to be translated into something that is more clinically meaningful – the time to reach a clinically significant change.

Rates of decline in lung function have been calculated using sophisticated statistical techniques that allow calculation of a 'weighted regression'. A similar approach has now been used for health status assessed using the SGRQ and SF-36.[9] The rate of deterioration for COPD patients treated either with bronchodilators alone or with high-dose inhaled corticosteroid in the form of fluticasone 1000 μg/day is shown in Figure 31.7. Note that with this questionnaire, deterioration is shown as a rise in score. The rate of deterioration in the bronchodilator-alone patients was 3.4 units per year. Thus on average the patients decline by a clinically significant amount every 15 months. This is very much faster than would be expected in healthy subjects. No longitudinal studies have

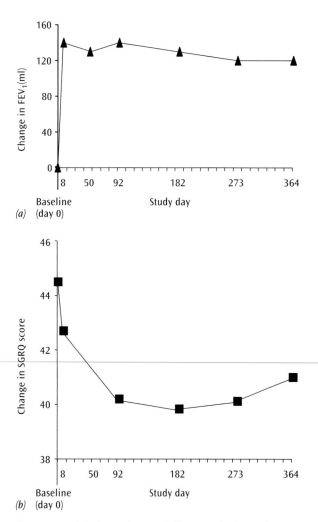

Figure 31.6 (a) Change in trough (i.e. morning) FEV_1 in patients given tiotropium over 1 year. (b) SGRQ score in the same patients. A fall in score indicates improved health.

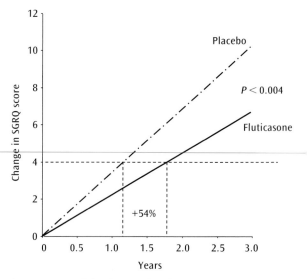

Figure 31.7 Weighted regression for change in SGRQ total score over 3 years from the ISOLDE study of fluticasone vs. placebo. Note that the higher the slope, the faster the rate of decline in health. The dotted line at 4 units is the threshold for a clinically significant change.

yet been performed in healthy people, but our own cross-sectional data suggest that the deterioration will be less than 0.5 units per year. As shown in Figure 31.7, addition of fluticasone reduced the rate of decline so that a clinically significant degree of deterioration occurred every 20 months.[43] Whilst this would appear to be a worthwhile treatment effect, perhaps the most important feature of the data in Figure 31.7 is that the SGRQ scores in the two treatment groups moved further apart over time – i.e. benefit from the drug increased progressively, at least up to the end of this 3-year study. This constitutes evidence for a disease-modifying effect of inhaled corticosteroid, at least if COPD is recognized as being a multisystem disease whose severity is not reflected entirely by the FEV_1.

In the context of a study such as this, the principal strength of health status measurement – its ability to aggregate multiple treatment effects into a single overall measure – is also its weakness because it does not identify any mechanism for the progressive improvement with treatment. Similarly it does not explain why there is such a big variation in the rate of change in health status between patients (Figure 31.8). Some patients treated with bronchodilators alone showed a small improvement over the course of 3 years, whilst some deteriorated at a rate that would produce a clinically significant level of deterioration every 6 months. Multivariate analysis of these results has shown that both the FEV_1 and the frequency of exacerbations are independent predictors of the decline in SGRQ score. The FEV_1 effect is predictable from the cross-sectional analysis shown in Figure 31.2, but the effect of exacerbations may be more complex. It is known that exacerbation frequency has an impact on health status, although its effect on rate of decline is unexplained. One plausible hypothesis is that exacerbations

have a direct impact on health, perhaps through the release of circulating cytokines,[44] but they may also have an effect through the period of enforced inactivity that they produce. This can lead to physical detraining and muscle wasting, which may lead secondarily to reduced exercise tolerance. In support of this hypothesis is the observation that fluticasone reduced the exacerbation frequency, and also had its greatest effect on the Activity component of the SGRQ and the physical aspects of the SF-36.[43]

ASSESSING THERAPEUTIC RESPONSE IN PRACTICE

It is appropriate to start any consideration of the assessment of treatment response in routine clinical practice by first considering the criteria against which the response may be judged. As argued throughout this chapter, COPD is a multisystem disease with many different effects, so improvement with treatment may potentially take many forms. This presents a major challenge to any attempt to formalize a method of routine assessment.

What is a clinically significant improvement?

To get an idea of what a clinically significant improvement might mean for an individual patient, it is possible to 'back calculate' from a notional improvement in score that corresponds to a clinically significant change to identify combinations of responses to questionnaire items that would produce a change of that magnitude. This has been done for the SGRQ.[35] For example, to achieve a 4-unit improvement a patient would have to report that: they no longer took a long time to wash or dress and could now walk up stairs without stopping and could now leave the house for shopping or recreation. It is important to note that the patient would have to have reported all of these improvements to achieve a 4-unit improvement. Whilst some of these improvements may tend to occur together, their combination still constitutes quite a striking improvement. This suggests that the threshold is conservative, since major changes in activity must occur for the improvement to register as being clinically significant. Indeed, it may be argued that the threshold is too conservative for the assessment of individual patients, since each of these limitations is so severe that an improvement in any one may be judged clinically worthwhile.

The example of a clinically significant improvement in health status given above is derived from a population-based estimate of the threshold for clinical significance for a population-based questionnaire. There are, however,

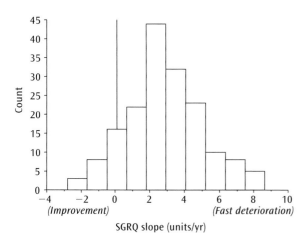

Figure 31.8 *Frequency distribution for the slope of deterioration in SGRQ score in patients given only bronchodilators for 3 years. A high positive slope indicates a high rate of decline. Approximately 6% of patients improved slightly over this period.*

many more factors that determine the health-related quality of life of an individual. These tend to be social or recreational rather than the typical health status questionnaire items that concentrate more on essential activities of daily living. There are many examples of activities undertaken by older people that cannot appear in standardized questionnaires. For example: playing with grandchildren; walking the dog; being able to pick up the newspaper from the local shop (every day regardless of weather); camping holidays; dancing; sailing; home decorating; visiting shopping malls, etc. Whilst none of these may be important to all patients, each may be very important to the patient who undertakes the activity.

Assessing responses in individuals

Health status questionnaires are valid measures in groups of patients although they may not be suitable for an individual patient. Clinicians treat individuals, however. As illustrated above, many activities that are important to patients would never find their way into health status questionnaires. For this reason, assessment must be individualized. One approach is to agree some therapeutic objectives with the patient. This principle was used for the dyspnea component of the CRQ,[17] but in practice that approach proved quite difficult to apply since it is time consuming and patients cannot always identify even a small number of areas of physical activity that are important to them. Clinical experience has also shown that therapeutic benefits may be unexpected. Furthermore, patients may not expect some benefits because they have had their symptoms so long that they expect no improvement. In practice, there seems little alternative to asking the patients whether they noticed any change, and if they do notice a benefit what was it and was it worthwhile?

The approach that I have just advocated may seem at first sight to take clinical pulmonary medicine back 40 years before the advent of routine spirometry. However, it should be recalled that therapies for COPD can have effects that are not reflected in the FEV_1. As a result, the correlation between FEV_1 and health status is weak and this applies also to changes with therapy. Furthermore, the response in terms of FEV_1 is also small (typically 100–150 ml) which lies within the repeatability of the measurement. Most treatments for COPD are symptomatic, so treatment response should be judged in terms of symptomatic gain. For these reasons, whilst spirometric measurements are important, treatment decisions about symptomatic therapy should be based upon evidence of symptomatic response. This suggestion is supported by scientific evidence. Patients in a double-blind randomized study who reported, in response to the question 'How effective was your treatment?' that the treatment

was 'Effective', had a 4-unit improvement in SGRQ score.[38] Those who said the treatment was 'Satisfactory' had negligible improvement. Similar results were obtained using the physicians' estimate of treatment efficacy. Thus even the simplest possible approach to assessing efficacy appears to be valid and reliable.

SUMMARY

Health status measurement is perhaps the only truly integrative method of assessing COPD patients and their response to treatment. It is providing new insights into COPD and its natural history. It is important to distinguish between health status measurements made in groups of patients and health-related quality of life assessments in individuals. The chief limitation of health status measurement is that any practicable questionnaire must treat each patient as being an 'average' or 'typical' patient. This becomes particularly important when addressing an individual's response to therapy. Treatment-associated symptomatic quality of life improvements in individual patients can only be assessed by asking the patient whether they noticed a change and whether any improvement was worthwhile.

REFERENCES

1. Breslin E, van der Schans C, Breukink S, et al. Perception of fatigue and quality of life in patients with COPD. Chest 1998;114:958–64.
2. Guyatt GH, Townsend M, Berman LB, Pugsley SO. Quality of life in patients with chronic airflow limitation. Br J Dis Chest 1987;81:45–54.
3. Grant I, Prigatano GP, Heaton RK, McSweeny AJ, Wright EC, Adams KM. Progressive neuropsychologic impairment and hypoxemia. Relationship in chronic obstructive pulmonary disease. Arch Gen Psychiatry 1987;44:999–1006.
4. Schwartzstein RM. The language of dyspnea. In: DA Mahler, ed. Dyspnea. Marcel Dekker, New York, 1998, pp 35–62.
5. Stewart AL, Hays R, Ware JE. The MOS short-form general health survey. Reliability and validity in a patient population. Med Care 1988;26:724–32.
6. Ware JE, Gandeck B. Overview of the SF-36 health survey and the International Quality of Life Assessment (IQOLA) Project. J Clin Epidemiol 1998;51:903–12.
7. Mahler DA, Mackowiak JI. Evaluation of the short-form 36-item questionnaire to measure health-related quality of life in patients with COPD. Chest 1995;107:1585–9.
8. Griffiths TL, Ionescu A, Mullins J, Turner-Lawlor P, Thomas J, Burr M. Use of the SF-36 questionnaire as an outcome measure in a randomised controlled trial of pulmonary rehabilitation. Am J Respir Crit Care Med 1998;157:A257.
9. Spencer S, Calverley PMA, Burge PS, Jones PW. Health status deterioration in patients with chronic obstructive pulmonary disease. Am J Respir Crit Care Med 2001; 163:122–8.

10. Kaplan RM, Atkins CJ, Timms R. Validity of a quality of well-being scale as an outcome measure in chronic obstructive pulmonary disease. *J Chron Dis* 1984; **37**:85–95.

11. Ries AL, Kaplan RM, Limberg TM, Prewitt LM. Effects of pulmonary rehabilitation on physiologic and psychosocial outcomes in patients with chronic obstructive pulmonary disease. *Ann Intern Med* 1995;**122**:823–32.

12. EuroQol Group. EuroQol – a new facility for the measurement of health-related quality of life. *Health Policy* 1990;**20**:329–32.

13. Nocturnal oxygen therapy trial (NOTT) group. Continuous or nocturnal oxygen therapy in hypoxemic chronic obstructive lung disease. *Ann Intern Med* 1980;**93**:391–8.

14. Jones PW. Quality of life measurement for patients with diseases of the airways. *Thorax* 1991;**46**:676–82.

15. Tsukino M, Nishimura K, Ikeda A, Koyama H, Mishima M, Izumi T. Physiologic factors that determine the health-related quality of life in patients with COPD. *Chest* 1996;**110**:896–903.

16. Prieto L, Alonso J, Ferrer M, *et al.* Are results of the SF-36 health survey and the Nottingham Health Profile similar?: a comparison in COPD patients. *J Clin Epidemiol* 1997;**50**: 463–73.

17. Guyatt GH, Berman LB, Townsend M, Pugsley SO, Chambers LW. A measure of quality of life for clinical trials in chronic lung disease. *Thorax* 1987;**42**:773–8.

18. Jones PW, Quirk FH, Baveystock CM. The St George's Respiratory Questionnaire. *Respir Med* 1991;**85**:25–31.

19. Jones PW, Quirk FH, Baveystock CM, Littlejohns P. A self-complete measure for chronic airflow limitation – the St George's Respiratory Questionnaire. *Am Rev Respir Dis* 1992;**145**:1321–7.

20. Quirk FH, Jones PW. Patients' perception of distress due to symptoms and effects of asthma on daily living and an investigation of possible influential factors. *Clin Sci* 1990;**79**:17–21.

21. Quirk FH, Baveystock CM, Wilson RC, Jones PW. Influence of demographic and disease related factors on the degree of distress associated with symptoms and restrictions on daily living due to asthma in six countries. *Eur Respir J* 1991;**4**: 167–71.

22. Hyland ME, Bott J, Singh S, Kenyon CA. Domains, constructs and the development of the breathing problems questionnaire. *Qual Life Res* 1994;**3**:245–56.

23. Hyland ME, Singh SJ, Sodergren SC, Morgan MP. Development of a shortened version of the Breathing Problems Questionnaire suitable for use in a pulmonary rehabilitation clinic: a purpose-specific, disease-specific questionnaire. *Qual Life Res* 1998;**7**:227–33.

24. Maille AR, Koning CJ, Zwinderman AH, Willems LN, Dijkman JH, Kaptein AA. The development of the 'Quality-of-life for Respiratory Illness Questionnaire (QOL-RIQ)': a disease-specific quality-of-life questionnaire for patients with mild to moderate chronic non-specific lung disease. *Respir Med* 1997;**91**:297–309.

25. Tu SP, MB M, Spertus JA, Steele BG, Fihns SD. A new self-administered questionnaire to monitor health-related quality of life in patients with COPD. *Chest* 1997;**112**:614–22.

26. Lareau SC, Breslin EH, Meek PM. Functional status instruments: outcome measure in the evaluation of patients with chronic obstructive pulmonary disease. *Heart Lung* 1996;**25**:212–24.

27. Weaver TE, Narsavage GL, Guilfoyle MJ. The development and psychometric evaluation of the Pulmonary Functional Status Scale: an instrument to assess functional status in pulmonary disease. *J Cardiopulmon Rehabil* 1998;**18**:105–11.

28. Barley EA, Quirk FH, Jones PW. Asthma health status in clinical practice: validity of a new short and simple instrument. *Respir Med* 1998;**92**:1207–14.

29. Hajiro T, Nishimura K, Jones PW, *et al.* A novel, short and simple questionnaire to measure health-related quality of life in patients with chronic obstructive pulmonary disease. *Am J Respir Crit Care Med* 1999;**159**:1874–8.

30. Garrod JC, Bestall EA, Paul EA, Wedzicha JA, Jones PW. Development and validation of a standardized measure of activity of daily living in patients with severe COPD: the London Chest Activity of Daily Living Scale (LCADL). *Respir Med* 2000;**2000**:589–96.

31. Carone M, Bertolotti G, Anchisi F, Zotti AM, Donner CF, Jones PW. Analysis of factors that chrraracterize health impairment in patients with chronic respiratory failure. *Eur Respir J* 1999;**13**:1293–300.

32. Jones PW. Health status measurement in chronic obstructive pulmonary disease. *Thorax* 2001;**56**:880–7.

33. Ferrer M, Alonso J, Morera J, *et al.* Chronic obstructive pulmonary disease stage and health-related quality of life. *Ann Intern Med* 1997;**127**:1072–9.

34. Bestall JC, Paul EA, Garrod R, Garnham R, Jones PW, Wedzicha JA. Usefulness of the Medical Research Council (MRC) dyspnoea scale as a measure of disability in patients with chronic obstructive pulmonary disease. *Thorax* 1999;**54**:581–6.

35. Jones PW. Interpreting thresholds for a clinically significant changes in health status in asthma and COPD. *Eur Respir J* 2002;**19**:398–404.

36. Jaeschke R, Singer J, Guyatt GH. Measurement of health status. Ascertaining the minimal clinically important difference. *Controlled Clin Trials* 1989;**10**:407–15.

37. Lacasse Y, Wong E, Guyatt GH, King D, Cook DJ, Goldstein RS. Meta-analysis of respiratory rehabilitation in chronic obstructive pulmonary disease. *Lancet* 1996;**348**:1115–19.

38. Jones PW, Bosh TK. Changes in quality of life in COPD patients treated with salmeterol. *Am J Resp Crit Care Med* 1997;**155**: 1283–9.

39. Dahl R, Greefhorst LAPM, Nowak D, *et al.* Inhaled formoterol dry powder versus ipratropium bromide in chronic obstructive pulmonary disease. *Am J Respir Crit Care Med* 2001;**164**:778–84.

40. Vincken W, van Noord JA, Greeforst APM, *et al.* Improved health outcomes in patients with COPD during 1 year's treatment with tiotropium. *Eur Respir J* 2002;**19**:217–26.

41. Seemungal TAR, Donaldson GC, Paul EA, Bestall JC, Jefferies DJ, Wedzicha JA. Effect of exacerbation on quality of life in patients with chronic obstructive pulmonary disease. *Am J Respir Crit Care Med* 1998;**157**:1418–22.

42. Casaburi R, Mahler DA, Jones PW, *et al.* A long-term evaluation of once daily inhaled tiotropium in chronic obstructive pulmonary disease. *Eur Respir J* 2002;**19**: 209–16.

43. Burge PS, Calverley PM, Jones PW, Spencer S, Anderson JA, Maslen TK. Randomised, double blind, placebo controlled study of fluticasone propionate in patients with moderate to severe chronic obstructive pulmonary disease: the ISOLDE trial. *Br Med J* 2000;**320**:1297–303.

44. Schols A, Buurman WA, Staal-van den Brekel AJ, Dentener MA, Wouters EFM. Evidence for a relation between metabolic derangements and increased levels of inflammatory mediators in a subgroup of patients with chronic obstructive pulmonary disease. *Thorax* 1996;**51**:819–24.

Surgery for emphysema

BARTOLOME R CELLI

The past few decades have witnessed the rise of COPD as an important cause of morbidity and mortality, not only in the developed world but also in the rest of the world. Indeed, COPD is predicted to be the third highest cause of death and is estimated to be fifth in overall morbidity in the world by the year 2020.[1] Over the same time period, treatment for the disease has also improved, with great advances in the treatment of smoking addiction, oxygen therapy, pharmacotherapy and pulmonary rehabilitation. Despite or perhaps due to these advances, more patients reach more severe stages of the disease and continue to complain of dyspnea and exercise limitation that impairs even the activities of daily living. This has paved the way for the exploration of several surgical alternatives, of which the one that has found acceptance is lung transplantation (see Chapter 33). However, the difficulties associated with the selection, preparation and treatment of patients who are transplanted and, more important, the limited number of donors, has restricted this option to relatively few patients (compared to the number of candidates) and few centers worldwide.

Other options have been tried and abandoned because of poor results.[2,3] Surgical attempts to improve chest mobility such as costochondrectomy and transverse sternotomy failed when it was realized that thoracic enlargement was the result and not the cause of emphysema. Subsequently, attempts were made to decrease the size of the thoracic cage through thoracoplasty and phrenicectomy. A similar but less radical approach was the introduction of air into the abdominal cavity or pneumoperitoneum with the objective of re-shaping the flattened diaphragm. Needless to say, the passage of time proved many of these approaches to be not only impractical but also by and large ineffective and they were never really popular. Efforts were also made to alleviate the airway obstructive component using procedures such as denervation, which attempted to relieve the airway tone and the placement of intratracheal and bronchial stents. All of these approaches once again proved to be temporizing solutions without any real proof of their value and for practical purposes remain historical anecdotes.

In the late 1950s, Brantigan and colleagues proposed a new and unique approach.[4,5] They hypothesized that by removing wedges of the most affected portion of the lungs unevenly affected by emphysema, reduction surgery would restore the outward elastic pull on the small airways and reduce expiratory airway obstruction. The procedure by definition would also decrease lung volume and by allowing the diaphragm to adopt a more physiologically normal position, would also improve diaphragmatic function. The original report noted significant symptomatic improvement in most of the patients, but unfortunately, six of the 33 patients died and this relatively high operative mortality (18%) prevented wide application of the operation.

The idea remained as a solid one and the development of new operative techniques and resources allowed its re-birth. Using targeted laser resection, Wakabayashi et al. reported symptomatic improvement associated with modest physiologic changes.[6,7] But it really was the group of Cooper and colleagues who pushed the concept of lung volume reduction surgery (LVRS) to its present state.[8] The group already had vast experience in unilateral and bilateral lung transplantation and using median sternotomy to resect areas of inhomogeneous emphysema targeted preoperatively using modern radiological techniques previously unavailable to Brantigan and colleagues. In addition, better anesthesiology support and the use of pericardial strips to prevent dreaded air leaks led to the first publications, which reported dramatic improvements not only in airflow obstruction but also in dyspnea and quality of life.[9] These results literally shook the world and prompted a rush to perform the surgery in many instances without adequate preparation and patient selection. The unfortunate consequence was the accumulation of poor results in many centers. Two reviews[10,11] sponsored by the Health Care Financial Administration (HCFA) analyzed the crude outcomes of 772 patients who underwent LVRS as defined by the agency using the *International Classification of Diseases*, 9th edition. The procedures performed between October 1995 and January 1996 were associated with a 14% mortality at 3 months and a 17% mortality at 6 months. The agency used these results as an argument to stop payment for this procedure for the elderly patients covered by MEDICARE in the USA. The debate about the benefit of lack thereof of this decision still lingers on, and awaits the result of several large randomized trials comparing LVRS with medical treatment before it can be resolved. The subsequent report to Congress in 1998 described a 23% mortality at 12 months and a 28% mortality at 18 months. Interestingly, LVRS has served to bring to the medical community the unanswered question of whether new surgical procedures should be submitted to the same strict research testing that has become the gold standard for the introduction of new medical therapies, namely, the randomized controlled trial. Arguments for both positions are heated[13,14] and their resolution will weigh heavily on the ways that new surgical procedures will be evaluated in the future.

The objective of this chapter is to review the large volume of published data without attempting to resolve the debate created around the procedure. Many peer-reviewed publications prove the interest and the need to decide the true value, if any, of LVRS. As we go to print, the final results of the larger trials are still pending.

PATIENT SELECTION

The selection of patients that could benefit from LVRS is not entirely clear. As originally proposed by Brantigan and coworkers[5] then expanded upon by Cooper *et al.*[8] the patients should have severe airflow obstruction, important hyperinflation as demonstrated by body plethysmographic TLC higher than 120% of predicted and even higher values for RV (>150% predicted). The presence of non-communicating areas of air trapping can be determined by evaluating the difference between plethysmographic and helium or nitrogen washout determined FRC. As we will discuss below, in most studies[14,15] the presence of inhomogeneous distribution of emphysema is also a favorable characteristic, especially if the emphysema is preferentially located in the upper lobes. The original authors also warned that important hypercapnia, presence of pulmonary hypertension, associated asthma, treatment with high doses of corticosteroids and poor functional performance made candidates too risky to undergo surgery. Many of these empirically suggested inclusion and exclusion criteria have gradually been proven true. Szekley and coworkers[16] were the first to confirm that patients with elevated $Paco_2$ (>45 mmHg) and unable to walk more than 150 meters were significantly more likely to develop postoperative morbidity and mortality (18%).

Data from a group of patients ($n = 140$) from the NETT trial that had a high mortality (20%) and confirmed that patients with very low FEV_1 (<20% predicted), very low diffusion capacity for carbon monoxide (DL_{CO}, <20% predicted) and homogeneous emphysema manifested a mortality that was significantly higher than that of the patients in the control group.[17] Indeed, the findings of this study confirm that the suggested criteria proposed by Cooper *et al.* were not only logical but also valid. Furthermore, the difference in mortality between the operated (36%) and non-operated patients (3%) was so large that the NETT investigators chose to stop recruiting patients presenting with those radiological and physiologic characteristics.

Most authors have also suggested that the patients should have no significant co-morbidity, stable psychologic and social status and be able to undergo rehabilitation.[5,6,18,19] Indeed, many programs will not include anyone unable to complete a rehabilitation plan or who remains functionally severely limited after rehabilitation.[8] The inclusion in a rehabilitation program is very important, not only as a prognostic factor but also because occasional patients may benefit so much from rehabilitation that after completion of the program they may cease to be candidates for LVRS.[8] Indeed, some of the groups that have completed a large number of patients believe that the inability to perform some minimum of exercise is an important criterion to select for surgery.[20]

The criteria that can help evaluate patients with COPD being considered for LVRS are shown in Table 32.1.

SURGICAL METHODS

As is true for patient selection, there is no absolute agreement as to the best surgical methods. Two schools using different procedures have produced what appear to be similar results. The procedure originally described by

Table 32.1 *Proposed criteria to select patients with COPD who may be considered for lung volume reduction surgery*

Hyperinflation: total lung capacity > 120% predicted and residual volume > 150% predicted

Severe obstruction: $FEV_1 < 40\%$ but higher than 20% predicted

Inhomogeneous emphysema by CT and by scintillographic scan

Able to complete pulmonary rehabilitation and walk >200 meters in 6 minutes

$Paco_2 < 55\,mmHg$

No pulmonary hypertension and no clinically important bronchiectasis

No more than 10 mg daily of corticosteroids

No alpha-1-antitrypsin deficiency

Table 32.2 *Post-LVRS change in FEV_1 in selected observational studies. Data presented as per cent improvement from baseline*

Author	3–6 months (%)	1 year (%)	2 years (%)	3 years (%)	4 years (%)
Cooper et al.[9]	76	62		35	24
Gelb et al.[39]	42		20		15
Roue et al.[36]	30		20		0
Brenner et al.[49]	40	38	32		

Cooper *et al.* includes median sternotomy with resection,[8,9] whereas other centers have promoted the resection using video-assisted thoracoscopy in either one side[21] or bilateral operations in one or two sittings.[22,23] The use of laser resection[24] has been largely abandoned because the results of trials comparing it with stapled resection have been shown significant improvement in the latter not only in FEV_1 but also a lower rate of complications.[25] The use of a procedure that reduces lung volume without cutting has been proposed but not received widespread evaluation.[26]

A more difficult task is to define advantages for either the median sternotomy or video assisted thoracoscopy (VAT) resection.[27] There are a few comparative studies and all have confirmed that bilateral procedures are better than unilateral, but no decisive advantage of either technique over the other.[28,29] With the currently available data, it seems as if both procedures produce similar results and complication rates. Based on this, it has been suggested that the selection of a technique depends on the surgeon's preference and experience.[30] The current National Emphysema Surgical Trial (NETT) is comparing outcome in centers using both techniques.[19] The results from this and other similar trials will help clarify if there is any real advantage of one technique over the other.

OUTCOME OF LVRS

The number of studies evaluating the results of LVRS on multiple outcomes is impressive.[5,8–10,16–49] Unfortunately, most series have been small, with relatively short follow-up time and using different selection and operative criteria. On the other hand the recent publication of some larger randomized trials begin to allow the emergence of some form of consensus.[17,18,20,40] Overall, the 30-day mortality ranges from 0 to 18%. Most recognized centers with large number of patients report 3 to 6% mortality,

which is acceptable for procedures of this magnitude. The original wider range probably reflected differences in inclusion and exclusion criteria, in surgical technique and experience and, equally important, in the overall perioperative management.

Physiologic outcomes

PULMONARY FUNCTION

These have been the most frequently reported outcome data. The original report by Cooper *et al.* described a close to 80% improvement over the preoperative FEV_1, 6 months after LVRS.[8] This dramatic improvement has not been duplicated by any other group. However it is fair to say that the 15–60% improvement reported in multiple studies between 3 and 6 months after surgery have been the most significant changes reported by any medical or non-medical therapy excluding lung transplant. Indeed, Table 32.2 shows the improvements in FEV_1 that have been reported in several selected large series. It is important to note that all authors comment on the marked variability in individual patient's responses. Thus, some patients have improvements that can be a high as 150% whereas a sizable minority manifest either no improvement or worse, a decrease in the postoperative FEV_1. Improvement in FEV_1 is usually accompanied by a similar or bigger improvement in VC with an increase in lung recoil pressure at TLC[31] following the reduction in mismatch between lung and chest wall size. Attempts to determine which factors predict a good FEV_1 response have met with limited success (see Chapter 13 for a more detailed account of potential mechanisms). Ingenito *et al.*[50] have shown that responders had a lower inspiratory lung resistance preoperatively than non-responders, but this method is not easy to compute and, more important, only has a modest capacity to actually predict FEV_1 response. Furthermore other outcomes such as exercise endurance, quality of life and dyspnea may improve independent of FEV_1[44,46] and thus determinations of predictors for FEV_1 response may need to be tested as predictors of other outcomes before they can be widely recommended.

A more uniform response is the description of decrease in lung volumes.[5,8,24–29,35–48] This makes sense since the procedure is designed to resect areas that tend to retain trapped air and in essence contribute to lung volume but not gas exchange. A review of the data demonstrates that TLC decreases anywhere from 4 to 25% whereas the FRC and RV fall is in the range of 3–40%. The change in the FRC and resting lung volume may be important because it determines the operating length of the diaphragm. This re-shaping places the diaphragm in a better contractile position and may be the reason why several small studies have documented a small but significant improvement in diaphragmatic strength and endurance.[34,44,45]

Very few studies have reported that changes in diffusion capacity (DLcosb). The few that have done so have documented no major change compared to the preoperative value.[9] However, a very low DLcosb (<20% predicted) was one of the strongest predictors of poor outcome in the subset of patients of the NETT trial with the highest postoperative mortality.[17] In general, most centers have avoided operating patients with such DLco and that may be the explanation why those centers have not reported similar findings. It is interesting that LVRS does not seem to affect DLco. One would have thought that resection of lung in patients with an already low value could induce an extreme reduction of DLco that could signify important loss of vascular bed. The data are very interesting, because if confirmed in the larger trials they may indicate that the vascular reserve is larger than previously thought.

The results of changes in arterial blood gases have been more frequently reported. Indeed, one of the dominating features of the initial report by Cooper and colleagues was the significant increase in PaO$_2$ that led to the discontinuation of oxygen in close to 50% of the patients needing it preoperatively.[8,9] By contrast, there are no major changes in postoperative PaCO$_2$. Once more, specific breakdown of the blood gas changes suggest the heterogeneity of response, with some patients manifesting significant improvement in oxygenation and some actually being worse after the pro-cedure. Albert et al. observed no correlation between arterial blood gas change and change in spirometry, lung volume or DLco.[51] Therefore, they concluded that the change in gases was mainly due to changes in alterations in ventilation-perfusion heterogeneity and not really in improvement in ventilation. The clinical consequence of the improved oxygenation is the possible discontinuation of oxygen in close to 25% of operated patients and a decrease in oxygen needs in close to 50%. Unfortunately, the improvement in oxygenation in most of the patients is transitory and the majority require reintroduction of oxygen often within 2 years after the procedure.

RESPIRATORY MUSCLE FUNCTION AND CENTRAL DRIVE

Although the procedure was primarily conceived to improve airflow limitation, Brantigan and coworkers already hypothesized that decreasing lung volume and placing the diaphragm closer to its physiologic position should result in improvement in respiratory muscle function.[5] Indeed, several groups[44,45,52,53] have documented not only increases in the volitionally dependent maximal inspiratory pressure that range from 5 to 40% but also improvement in diaphragmatic contractility, as shown by the determination of maximal transdiaphragmatic pressure, and twitch Pdi during involuntary electrical stimulation.[45] There have been no systematic evaluations of the effect of LVRS on accessory muscle use, but it is appealing to think that a decrease in lung volume results in lengthening of the accessory muscles also and this should facilitate force generation.

Two studies[44,54] have evaluated the effect of LVRS on central respiratory drive, one used diaphragmatic EMG and reported a decrease in electrical activity of the diaphragm after surgery. We have also reported that using mouth occlusion pressure (P$_{0.1}$), LVRS resulted in a significant decrease in its resting value and more important a decrease in the slope of response to CO$_2$ administered by the closed circuit method. Thus the data can be interpreted as showing that the mechanical changes produced by LVRS result in a decrease in the need of the central controller to maintain high levels of central output, a proven characteristic of the breathing pattern of patients with severe COPD.

Exercise performance

Together with pulmonary function, this has been the most evaluated form of outcome after LVRS. However, the tools used to document the changes have varied. The most frequently used tool has been the timed walk, usually the 6-minute walk distance (6MWD). Most if not all of the studies that have used this tool show an improvement that ranges from 5 to 120%.[8,16–18,20,24,34–36,40,42] In addition, many reports fail to provide information as to whether the baseline value is the one obtained before preoperative rehabilitation or the value after rehabilitation or right before surgery. In support of the changes noted above are the better characterized changes reported in few randomized trials reported. Indeed, the 60 meters improvement reported by Geddes et al.[20] using the shuttle walk distance is within the value reported by those using the 6MWD. Further, even the most recent NETT study[17] that reported important negative consequences of LVRS in patients with homogeneous emphysema and very low FEV$_1$ or DLco, did show an improvement in the 6MWD that was significant when compared to baseline and to patients randomized to medical treatment.

That the improvement report in the walked distance is real is further supported by the results of the fewer studies that have evaluated the patients using formal cardiopulmonary exercise testing.[34,37,41,42] Most if not all have documented an improvement in maximal workload (Watts), modest but significant increase in peak oxygen uptake ($\dot{V}O_2$) and in achieved maximal ventilation ($\dot{V}E$). Several of these studies have analyzed the changes in breathing pattern and muscle function that are observed after surgery.[34,44,55] The most evident and important ones are: a decrease in respiratory rate associated with an increase in tidal volume at the same level of mechanical work and a decrease in the work of breathing under similar circumstances. In addition, Martinez et al.[44] have shown that there is a decrease in dynamic hyperinflation, the magnitude of which seems to be the main factor responsible for the development of dyspnea during exercise. Other observations that have been reported include a decrease in the V_D/V_T with decrease in $PaCO_2$ during exercise.

Very important are the observations related to the changes in pulmonary vascular pressure after LVRS. That the procedure could result in a significant and clinically relevant increase in overall pulmonary vascular pressure was a real concern. Furthermore, pulmonary circulatory hypertension could reach undesirable levels during exercise, when the increase in metabolic demand can only be met with increase in cardiac output. Although the number of studies is limited,[56,57] the results indicate that there may be a small but perhaps not clinically significant increase in the vast majority of patients. The findings probably represent the careful evaluation criteria of the groups reporting the results where patients with resting increased mean pulmonary artery pressure (45 mmHg) were excluded from the trials. Interestingly, most centers do not require cardiac catheterization to document the pressure in the pulmonary circulation. Right side catheterization is limited to those patients whose clinical examination reveal signs of right heart strain such as loud pulmonic sound, increased jugular vein distention, leg edema or a pattern of right ventricular strain in the electrocardiogram. In most centers a cardiac echogram precedes the right side catheterization.

In summary, improvement in exercise performance has been documented in the vast majority of patients who have undergone successful LVRS. It is important to note that the changes may occur independent of the changes in resting pulmonary function, indicating that the mechanism for improvement may not be the same. Whereas FEV_1 improvement is most likely related to improvement in lung elastic recoil as documented by Sciurba et al.[31] the benefits observed in exercise may be influenced by the deflation produced by the procedure

and its effect on dynamic hyperinflation and respiratory muscle function.

Dyspnea and health status

Dyspnea is the dominant symptom and the most frequent reason why patients request the procedure. Indeed, all of the programs require that a significant degree of dyspnea be documented for patients to be considered for LVRS. Again, the majority of the studies have documented a decrease in the perceived perception of breathlessness independent of the tool used to evaluate the symptom.[9,18,20,24,27,28,34–36,41,47–49,58] Several authors have used the Medical Research Council scale and have shown decreases that range from 50 to 70% improvement with the mean values decreasing from around 3.8 to 1.2. Other groups have used the Baseline and Transitional Dyspnea Index scale with improvements that are higher than the 1 unit that has been deemed clinically significant. Again, very few studies have evaluated individual responses and have attempted to correlate those responses to physiologic changes, which may help explain the results. Brenner et al. studied the effect of LVRS on MRC dyspnea grades.[59] They observed that the improvement in MRC dyspnea correlated poorly with the change in FEV_1 (r = -0.3), whereas the change correlated better with the degree of hyperexpansion. Interestingly, although 28% of the patients had minimal or no improvement in FEV_1, 10 of 37 patients noted an improvement of 2 or more in the MRC scale, a value that is very significant when one considers the range of the scale which goes from 0 to 4. The dissociation between change in FEV_1 and dyspnea has been described for the dyspnea measured during exercise. Indeed, using the Visual Analog or the Borg scale, Martinez et al.[44] showed that 16 of 17 patients manifested improvement in the symptom during exercise, independent of the change obtained in the FEV_1. Furthermore, the improvement in exercise dyspnea correlated better with the decrease in dynamic hyperinflation than with the change in FEV_1.

The systematic evaluation of health status was less consistent in the initial reports and comparison of studies is plagued by the lack of uniformity in the timing of the evaluations and the tools utilized. Several groups have reported significant improvement in health status using the generic tool SF-36.[9,18–20,47] The improvements were significant and included the domains of vitality, social functioning, physical functioning and general status. The findings are supported by those observed in the randomized trials that have evaluated this outcome. Indeed, the study by Geddes et al.[20] documented a 1-year improvement in health status that was significantly higher than the progressive decrease reported by the control group and still higher at that point than at baseline.

Table 32.3 *Change in FEV$_1$ and mortality in four published randomized trials. FEV$_1$ values expressed as percent change from baseline*

	3–6 months		1 year		Mortality (%)	
Author	LVRS (%)	Medicine (%)	LVRS (%)	Medicine (%)	LVRS (%)	Medicine (%)
Criner et al.[18]	15	0				
Geddes et al.[20]			20	−5	16	2
Pompeo et al.[40]						
NETT[19]	5	−4			33	2

Somewhat surprisingly there are less data where disease-specific instruments have been utilized. In the study reported by Bagley and colleagues[49] improvements were noted in all domains of the Chronic Respiratory Disease Questionnaire (CRDQ), the dyspnea, fatigue, emotional function and mastery. Similarly, Norman and coworkers documented large improvements in the overall St George's Respiratory Questionnaire score.[60] The improvement of 31 units is extremely significant for a test where the clinically significant difference has been reported to be a change in 4 units.

From the data so far published, LVRS results in significant short-term improvement in functional and exercise dyspnea and in health status, the duration of which we still do not totally know. Indeed, the most important question, which has plagued the procedure, is the duration of the beneficial effects. For a procedure that has certain mortality and considerable cost, the final description of the duration of its effect may help clarify its true role as an option in the treatment of patients with severe lung emphysema. Table 32.3 provides a summary of the information available regarding outcomes and mortality in the few published randomized trials.

DURATION OF THE EFFECTS

There is a general consensus that LVRS is more a palliative procedure than one that prolongs life. One study[61] compared 3-year survival in 65 patients operated with LVRS who were covered by Medicate versus a group of 22 similar patients that could not be operated because of the stop payment order issued by Medicare. No differences were observed in baseline age, clinical characteristics or pulmonary function. During the time available for follow-up, 17% of the surgical patients died compared with 36% that could not be operated. The difference in mortality was not significant statistically. Interestingly, there was an increase of 60% in the FEV$_1$ in the operated group whereas there was minimal deterioration in the medical survivors.

The long-term changes in pulmonary function have only been reported in the uncontrolled trials.[36,38,39] It is

unlikely that this procedure should be associated with a change in the natural rate of decline of lung function that occurs as a function of age. The big question is whether the rate of decline is higher than that reported for patients with COPD. The question remains open and will only be answered when the long-term analysis of the randomized trials become available.

In a very small report including 12 patients, Roue and coworkers[36] noted that four of six patients evaluated at 2 years manifested a 20% improvement in FEV$_1$. This improvement had disappeared at 2 years in the two patients who had reached that point. The group at Washington University[62] has reported FEV$_1$ changes in patients followed for up to 3 years. In those survivors, the mean FEV$_1$ is still 20% higher than the preoperative value, although there was a continuous decline compared with the close to 60% improvement noted at 6 months. The most detailed long-term studies have been reported by Gelb and coworkers[63] who have not only evaluated FEV$_1$ but also lung elastic recoil, compliance and upstream resistance. This group had data spanning 1–5 years before the procedure and was therefore able to compare the postoperative rate of decline in FEV$_1$ with that observed preoperatively. In this small group of patients, the rate of decline of FEV$_1$ was similar to that observed before LVRS. The findings are in contrast with the results reported by Fessler and Wise,[64] who compared the rate of decline in FEV$_1$ reported in seven LVRS trials with the historical rate of decline in smoking and non-smoking COPD. In that report, the rate of FEV$_1$ loss was greater in all of the trials than in the non-operated historical and not well-matched controls. The largest available study is the retrospective analysis of Brenner et al. which reported 376 patients who underwent LVRS in one single institution.[59] The report included patients who underwent unilateral thoracoscopic surgery, unilateral thoracoscopic staple resection and bilateral thoracoscopic staple surgery. Overall, peak improvements occurred at 6 months and although there was a progressive decline after that point, the values for the unilateral and, most impressively, the bilateral staple were still observed 20 months after the procedure.

PROBLEMS WITH LVRS

If, as the majority of the published trials suggest, LVRS is such a good procedure why is there still skepticism? Several reasons should lead us to be cautious. First and foremost is the obligation to do no harm. There is a significant mortality associated with this procedure. The widespread performance of LVRS without a deep understanding of the possible good candidates for the procedure could lead to unfavorable results that could hamper its true value. Some reports[16,17] documented a 19% mortality which affected primarily patients with high $PaCO_2$, those that could not walk more than 200 meters in a 6-minute walking test, those with FEV_1 lower than 20% predicted or $DLCO$ of that same magnitude and patients with homogeneous emphysema. Those reports very strongly support the role of pulmonary rehabilitation as not only a therapeutic tool but also as a screening test to select patients more likely to be fit and to be able to withstand the stress associated with surgery.

The second problem is the difficulty in selecting the patient who may benefit from the surgery and who would have the least chance of dying or getting worse from the operation.[65–68] Based on the model described above, the current concept is that patients with the more severe hyperinflation and inhomogeneous emphysema, and those with poor but not extremely severe lung function and those with a preserved systemic function, appear to be the best candidates for the procedure. Table 32.4 summarizes the current available information about factors that may help predict outcome in the published series that have addressed this question.

There is the issue of cost, and the issue of importance in an era that is driven by healthcare cost containment. Society as a whole will have to deal with this problem if the operation does prove to be useful for a selected group of patients with COPD. In this regard, LVRS is less expensive than lung transplantation, and may be an alternative for patients who while on a transplant waiting list may benefit from a temporary solution.

Finally, it must be remembered that patients who successfully survive LVRS only accrue partial gains. In all published series, the gain is significant, but patients continue to have severe COPD. If the natural history of the operated patients parallels that of patients without surgery, the natural decline of lung function will continue and at some point their function will be back to where it was before surgery. LVRS is a palliative and not curative procedure. Therefore, the final decision will be determined by the 'time' of improved function that the operation may buy and the relative value of that time compared with the cost and risk of the operation. This balance, moreover, will undoubtedly change so both issues of patient selection and surgical techniques are resolved. Bronchoscopic lung volume reduction techniques currently being investigated[69] may reduce mortality and cost.

Nevertheless, LVRS has provided a fresh revival to the lessons learned from applied physiology. In addition, from the lessons learned in performing this procedure and the determination of its successfulness in a selected group of patients, LVRS will offer a new avenue for many patients with few other alternatives.[70] Finally, as an indirect result, LVRS may help alleviate the current 'bottleneck' in the transplantation waiting process by allowing many patients with COPD to opt for LVRS and thus shorten the waiting time for patients who have no such option.

EDITORIAL NOTE

As we go to press, the intention to treat analysis of the NETT study has been published.[71] Even excluding the 140 high-risk patients described previously[17], there was no overall survival advantage with surgery although significant improvements in exercise capacity, health status and dyspnea were seen. Post hoc analysis identified a subgroup of patients with a combination of predominant upper lobe disease and a low exercise capacity as having lower mortality as well as the greatest symptomatic benefit when treated surgically compared to similar patients randomized to medical therapy. A parallel cost-effectiveness analysis suggests that in this subgroup, surgery costs $98,000 per quality year of life-year (QALY) gained.[72] Overall costs were a formidable $190,000 per QALY, much higher than other surgical interventions in cardiology but still cheaper than lung transplantation. Further analysis of these data are planned although an empirical decision restricting funding for surgery to those with upper lobe predominant disease and possibly those with a limited exercise capacity post-rehabilitation seems likely.

Another important development has been the publication of a pilot study describing successful lung volume reduction by the bronchoscopic placement of one-way

Table 32.4 *Factors that predict outcome after LVRS*

	Favorable factor	Detrimental factor
Mortality and morbidity	Younger (<75 years) No co-morbidity	FEV_1 < 20% predicted DLCOsb < 20% predicted Non-homogeneous emphysema 6-minute walk distance <150 m Hypercapnia
Physiology	Inhomogeneous emphysema Small increase in inspiratory resistance	Alpha-1-antitrypsin deficiency Extreme hyperinflation Pulmonary hypertension

valves in the upper lobes of patients medically unfit for LVRS. The procedure was well tolerated with no major morbidity.[73] Other groups are developing endobronchial occlusion using biologic glue or opening collateral channels to the upper lobes by implanting spiracles in the airway wall. If such techniques result in sustained benefit they could have major implications for patient selection and costs.

REFERENCES

1. Murray CJ, Lopez AD. Mortality by cause for eight regions of the world: Global Burden of Disease Study. *Lancet* 1997; **349**:1269–76.
2. Gaensler E, Cugell D, Knudson R, *et al.* Surgical management of emphysema. *Clin Chest Med* 1983;**4**:443–63.
3. Deslauriers J. History of surgery for emphysema. *Sem Thorac Cardiovasc Surg* 1996;**8**:43–51.
4. Brantigan OC, Mueller EA, Kress MB. A surgical approach to pulmonary emphysema. *Am Surgeon* 1957;**23**:789–804.
5. Brantigan OC, Kress M, Mueller EA. A surgical approach to pulmonary emphysema. *Am Rev Respir Dis* 1959;**39**:194–202.
6. Wakabayasi A, Brenner M, Kayaleh RA, *et al.* Thoracoscopic carbon dioxide laser treatment of bullous emphysema. *Lancet* 1991;**337**:881–3.
7. Wakabayashi A. Thoracoscopic laser pneumoplasty in the treatment of diffuse bullous emphysema. *Ann Thorac Surg* 1995;**60**:936–42.
8. Cooper JD, Trulock KP, Traintafillou AN, *et al.* Bilateral pneumectomy (volume reduction) for chronic obstructive pulmonary disease. *J Thorac Cardiovasc Surg* 1995;**109**: 106–19.
9. Cooper JD, Patterson GA, Sundaresan RS, *et al.* Results of 150 consecutive bilateral lung volume reduction procedures in patients with severe emphysema. *J Thorac Cardiovasc Surg* 1996;**112**:1319–30.
10. Holohan T, Handelsman H. *Lung Volume Reduction Surgery for End-Stage Chronic Obstructive Pulmonary Disease.* Agency for Health Care Policy Research, Rockville, MD, 1996.
11. *Report to Congress: Lung Volume Reduction Surgery and Medicare Coverage Policy: Implications of Recently Published Evidence.* Department of Health and Human Services, Washington DC, 1998.
12. Lung Volume Reduction Surgery. Statement of the American Thoracic Society. *Am J Respir Crit Care Med* 1996;**154**:1151–2.
13. Berger R, Celli B, Meneghetti A, *et al.* Limitations of randomized clinical trials for evaluating emerging operations. The case of lung volume reduction surgery. *Ann Thorac Surg* 2001;**72**:649–57.
14. Gierada DS, Sloan RM, Bae KT, Yusen RD, Lefrak SS, Cooper JD. Pulmonary emphysema: comparison of preoperative quantitive CT and physiologic index values with clinical outcome after lung-volume reduction surgery. *Radiology* 1997;**205**:235–42.
15. Weder W, Thurnheer R, Stammberger U, Burge M, Russi EW, Bloch KE. Radiologic emphysema morphology is associated with outcome after lung volume reduction. *Ann Thorac Surg* 1997;**64**:313–19.
16. Szekely LA, Oelberg DA, Wright C, *et al.* Preoperative predicators of operative morbidity and morality in COPD patients undergoing bilateral lung volume reduction surgery. *Chest* 1997;**111**:550–8.
17. National Emphysema Treatment Trial Group. Patients at high risk of death after lung volume reduction surgery. *N Engl J Med* 2001;**345**:1075–83.
18. Criner GJ, Cordova FC, Furukawa S, *et al.* Prospective randomized trial comparing bilateral lung volume reduction surgery to pulmonary rehabilitation in severe chronic obstructive pulmonary disease. *Am J Respir Crit Care Med* 1999;**160**:2018–27.
19. National Emphysema Treatment Trial Research Group. Rationale and design of the National Emphysema Treatment Trial (NETT): a prospective randomised trial of lung volume reduction surgery. *J Thorac Cardiovasc Surg* 1999;**118**:518–28.
20. Geddes D, Davis M, Koyama H, *et al.* Effect of lung volume reduction surgery in patients with severe emphysema. *N Engl J Med* 2000;**343**:239–45.
21. Keenan RJ, Landrenau RJ, Sciurba FC, *et al.* Unilateral thoracoscopic surgical approach for diffuse emphysema. *J Thorac Cardiovasc Surg* 1996;**111**:308–15.
22. Brenner M, Yusen R, McKenna R, *et al.* Lung volume reduction surgery for emphysema. *Chest* 1996;**110**:206–18.
23. Iwa T, Watanabe Y, Fukatani G. Simultaneous bilateral operations for bullous emphysema by median strenotomy. *J Thorac Cardiovasc Surg* 1981;**81**:732–7.
24. Hazelrigg S, Boley T, Henkle J, *et al.* Thoracoscopic laser bullectomy: a prospective study with three-month results. *J Thorac Cardiovasc Surg* 1996;**112**:319–26.
25. McKenna R, Brenner M, Gelb A, *et al.* A randomized, prospective trial of stapled lung reduction versus laser bullectomy for diffuse emphysema. *J Thorac Cardiovasc Surg* 1996;**111**:317–22.
26. Swanson S, Mentzer S, DeCamp M, *et al.* Non-cut thoracoscopic lung placation: a new technique for lung volume reduction surgery. *J Am Coll Surg* 1997;**185**:25–32.
27. McKenna R, Brenner M, Fischel R, *et al.* Should lung volume reduction surgery for emphysema be unilateral or bilateral? *J Thorac Cardiovasc Surg* 1996;**112**:1331–8.
28. Kotloff RM, Tino G, Bavaria JE, *et al.* Bilateral lung volume reduction surgery for advanced emphysema – a comparison of median sternotomy and thoracoscopic approaches. *Chest* 1996;**110**:1399–406.
29. Wisser W, Tschernko E, Senbaklavaci O, *et al.* Functional improvement after volume reduction sternotomy versus videoendoscopic approach. *Ann Thorac Surg* 1997;**63**:822–8.
30. Naunbeim K, Ferguson M. The current status of lung volume reduction operations for emphysema. *Ann Thorac Surg* 1996;**61**:601–12.
31. Sciurba FC, Rogers RM, Keenan RJ, *et al.* Improvement in pulmonary function and elastic recoil after lung volume reduction surgery for diffuse emphysema. *N Engl J Med* 1996;**334**:1095–9.
32. Fujita RA, Barnes GB. Morbidity and morality after thoracoscopic pneumoplasty. *Ann Thorac Surg* 1996;**62**:251–7.
33. McKenna RJ, Brenner M, Fischel RJ, *et al.* Patient selection criteria for lung volume reduction surgery. *J Thorac Cardiovasc Surg* 1997;**114**:957–64.
34. Benditt JO, Lewis S, Wood DE, Klima L, Albert RK. Lung volume reduction surgery improves maximal O_2 consumption, maximal minute ventilation, O_2 pulse, and dead space to tidal ratio during leg cycle ergometry. *Am J Respir Crit Care Med* 1997;**156**:561–6.
35. Bringisser R, Zollinger A, Hauser M, *et al.* Bilateral volume reduction surgery for diffuse pulmonary emphysema by video-assisted thoracoscopy. *J Thorac Cardiovasc Surg* 1996;**112**:875–82.
36. Roue C, Mal H, Sleiman C, *et al.* Lung volume reduction in patients with severe diffuse emphysema. A retrospective study. *Chest* 1996;**110**:28–34.
37. Keller CA, Ruppel G, Hibbett A, *et al.* Thoracoscopic lung volume reduction surgery reduces dyspnea and improves

exercise capacity in patients with emphysema. *Am J Respir Crit Care Med* 1997;**156**:60–7.

38. Flaherty KR, Kazerooni EA, Curtis JL, *et al*. Short-term and long-term outcomes after bilateral lung volume reduction surgery: prediction by quantitative CT. *Chest* 2000;**119**: 1337–46.

39. Gelb AF, McKenna RJ, Brenner M, Shein MJ, Samel NN, Fischel R. Lung function 4 years after lung volume reduction surgery for emphysema. *Chest* 1999;**116**:1608–15.

40. Pompeo E, Marino M, Nofroni I, Matteucci G, Mineo TC. Reduction pneumoplasty versus respiratory rehabilitation in severe emphysema: a randomised study. *Ann Thorac Surg* 2000;**70**:948–53.

41. Sugi K, Kaneda Y, Esato K. Subjective symptoms and prognosis after lung volume reduction surgery in patients with severe pulmonary emphysema. *Jpn J Thorac Cardiovasc Surg* 1999;**47**:489–94.

42. Gelb AF, McKenna RJ, Brenner M. Expanding knowledge of lung volume reduction. *Chest* 2001;**119**:1300–2.

43. Butler CW, Snyder M, Wood DE, Curtis JR, Albert RK, Benditt JO. Underestimation of mortality following lung volume reduction surgery resulting from incomplete follow up. *Chest* 2001;**119**:1056–60.

44. Celli BR, Montes de Oca M, Mendez R, *et al*. Lung reduction surgery in severe COPD decreases central drive and ventilatory response to CO_2. *Chest* 1997;**112**:902–6.

45. Laghi F, Jubran A, Topeli A, *et al*. Effect of lung volume reduction surgery on neuromechanical coupling of the diaphragm. *Am J Respir Crit Care Med* 1998;**157**:475–83.

46. Ferguson GT, Fernandez E, Zamora M, *et al*. Improved exercise performance following lung volume reduction surgery for emphysema. *Am J Respir Crit Care Med* 1998; **157**:1195–203.

47. Cordova F, O'Brien G, Furukawa S, *et al*. Stability of improvements in exercise performance and quality of life following bilateral lung volume reduction surgery in severe COPD. *Chest* 1997;**112**:907–15.

48. Brenner M, McKenna R, Gelb A, *et al*. Rate of FEV_1 change following lung volume reduction surgery. *Chest* 1998;**113**: 652–9.

49. Bagley P, Davis S, O'Shea M, *et al*. Lung volume reduction surgery at a community hospital: programme development and outcomes. *Chest* 1997;**111**:1552–9.

50. Ingenito E, Evans R, Loring S, *et al*. Relation between preoperative inspiratory lung resistance and the outcome of lung volume reduction surgery. *N Engl J Med* 1998;**338**: 1181–5.

51. Albert R, Benditt J, Hildebrandt J, *et al*. Lung volume reduction surgery has variable effects on blood gases in patients with emphysema. *Am J Respir Crit Care Med* 1998;158–71.

52. Tschernko E, Gruber E, Jacksch P, *et al*. Ventilatory mechanics and gas exchange during exercise before and after lung volume reduction surgery. *Am J Respir Crit Care Med* 1998;**158**:1424–31.

53. Benditt J, Wood D, McCool D, *et al*. Changes in breathing and ventilatory muscle recruitment pattern induced by lung volume reduction surgery. *Am J Respir Crit Care Med* 1997;**155**:279–84.

54. Teschler H, Starmatis G, El-Raouf F, *et al*. Effect of surgical lung volume reduction on respiratory muscle function in pulmonary emphysema. *Eur Respir J* 1996;**9**:1179–84.

55. O'Donnell D, Webb K, Bertley J, *et al*. Mechanism of relief of exertional dyspnoea following unilateral bullectomy and lung volume reduction surgery in emphysema. *Chest* 1996;**110**: 18–27.

56. Web IL, Rossof L, McKeon K, Graver LM, Scharf SM. Development of pulmonary hypertension after lung volume reduction surgery. *Am J Respir Crit Care Med* 1999;**159**:552–6.

57. Oswald-Mammoser M, Kessler R, Massard G, *et al*. Effect of lung volume reduction surgery on gas exchange and pulmonary hemodynamics at rest and during exercise. *Am J Respir Crit Care Med* 1999;**158**:1020–5.

58. Holbert J, Brown M, Sciurba F, *et al*. Changes in lung volume and volume of emphysema after unilateral lung reduction surgery: analysis with CT and densitometry. *Radiology* 1996;**201**:793–7.

59. Brenner M, McKenna R, Gelb A, *et al*. Dyspnoea response following bilateral thoracoscopic staple lung volume reduction surgery. *Chest* 1997;**112**:916–23.

60. Norman M, Hillerdal G, Orre L, *et al*. Improved lung function and quality of life following increase in elastic recoil after lung volume reduction surgery in emphysema. *Respir Med* 1998;**92**:653–8.

61. Meyers B, Yusen R, Lefrak S, *et al*. Outcome of Medicare patients with emphysema selected for, but denied, a lung volume reduction operation. *Ann Thorac Surg* 1998;**6**: 331–6.

62. Yusen R, Pohl M, Richardson V, *et al*. 3 year results after lung volume reduction surgery. *Am J Respir Crit Care Med* 1998;**157**:A335.

63. Gelb A, McKenna R, Brenner M, *et al*. Lung function 5 years after lung volume reduction surgery for emphysema. *Am J Respir Crit Care Med* 2001;**163**:1562–6.

64. Fessler H, Wise R. Lung volume reduction surgery; is less really more? *Am J Respir Crit Care Med* 1999;**159**:1031–5.

65. Glaspole IN, Gabbay E, Smith JA, Rabinov M, Snell GI. Predictors of perioperative morbidity and mortality in lung volume reduction surgery. *Ann Thorac Surg* 2000;**69**: 1711–16.

66. Pompeo E, Sergiacomi G, Nofroni I, Roscetti W, Simonetti G, Mineo TC. Morphologic grading of emphysema is useful in the selection of candidates for unilateral or bilateral reduction pneumoplasty. *Eur J Cardiothorac Surg* 2000;**17**:680–6.

67. Ingenito EP, Loring SG, Moy ML, *et al*. Comparison of physiological and radiological screening for lung volume reduction surgery. *Am J Respir Crit Care Med* 2001;**163**: 1068–73.

68. Tschernko EM, Kritzinger M, Gruber EM, *et al*. Lung volume reduction surgery: preoperative functional predictors for postoperative outcome. *Anesth Analg* 1999;**88**:28–33.

69. Toma TP, Hopkinson NS, Hillier J, Hansell DM, Morgan C, Goldstraw PG, Polkey MI, Geddes DM. Bronchoscopic volume reduction with valve implants in patients with severe emphysema. *Lancet* 2003;**361**:931–933.

70. Keller CA, Naunheim K, Osterloch J, *et al*. Histopathologic diagnosis made in lung tissue resected from patients with severe emphysema undergoing lung volume reduction surgery. *Chest* 1997;**111**:941–7.

71. National Emphysema Treatment Trial Research Group. A randomized trial comparing lung-volume reduction surgery with medical therapy for severe emphysema. *N Engl J Med* 2003;**348**:2059–73.

72. National Emphysema Treatment Trial Research Group. Cost effectiveness of lung-volume reduction surgery for patients with severe emphysema. *N Engl J Med* 2003;**348**:2092–102.

73. Toma TP, Hopkinson NS, Hillier J, Hansell DM, Morgan C, Goldstraw PG *et al*. Bronchoscopic volume reduction with valve implants in patients with severe emphysema. *Lancet* 2003;**361**:931–3.

33

Lung transplantation

PAUL A CORRIS

INTRODUCTION

The modern era for lung transplantation began in 1981 when Bruce Reitz and colleagues from Stanford University introduced heart–lung transplantation for patients with pulmonary vascular disease.[1] Indications for combined heart and lung transplants (HLT) were subsequently widened to include various pulmonary conditions.[2] Survival rates were good and in marked contrast with results obtained for single lung transplantation over the preceding 25 years.[3] The success of HLT was based on reliable healing of the tracheal anastomosis compared with the bronchial anastomotic breakdown seen frequently following single lung transplantation (SLT). This reliable healing reflected a good blood supply to the proximal donor trachea via donor coronary artery/bronchial artery anastomoses, in contrast to the lack of blood supplied to the proximal donor bronchus following transplantation of a single lung. The lack of success with SLT was also based on both poor selection of potential recipients, some of whom were septic and had multiorgan failure, and the apparently insuperable problems of rejection and infections.

It was realized that many patients undergoing HLT, however, received a new heart unnecessarily. After a period of research, the Toronto Group reported success with SLT in patients with fibrosing lung disease in 1986.[4]

Important potential factors were careful patient selection, restoration of a viable blood supply to the bronchial anastomosis by wrapping it with a pedicle of greater omentum and the introduction of ciclosporin A as the principal immunosuppressant. It has been shown subsequently that the bronchial anastomosis does not require a wrap of omentum for reliable healing and no centers now perform this procedure. Some centers experimented with direct revascularization of donor bronchial artery to ensure good blood supply to the donor bronchus but this practice has also been abandoned.

In 1988 the double lung transplant operation (DLT) using an en bloc transplantation of both lungs with a tracheal anastomosis was introduced by Patterson and colleagues.[5] However, this procedure was accompanied by much more frequent problems with airway healing than the HLT operation.[6] In addition, the operation was, if anything, more complex than HLT and the extensive mediastinal dissection frequently led to denervation of the recipient's native heart. Bleeding was at least as great a problem as that for HLT, and by 1989 the procedure as originally described had been largely abandoned. Noirclerc et al.[7] provided the solution to the problem of airway healing by performing two separate bronchial anastamoses, since as in SLT the donor bronchus is better vascularized initially if the anastomosis is close to the lung parenchyma. This concept was further developed by Pasque et al.[8] with the bilateral sequential lung transplant. As its name implies, two separated lungs are implanted with separate hilar anastomoses (each of bronchus, pulmonary artery and left atrial cuff). The heart and mediastinum are left largely undisturbed. The incision is a transverse bilateral thoracotomy, dividing the sternum horizontally. In contrast to HLT, SLT and bilateral sequential lung transplantation do not in general require cardiopulmonary bypass with associated anticoagulation. A final development comprises the use of living lobar transplantation involving the implantation of two lobes from two living donors. This procedure is only suitable for children or small adults and will not impact greatly on transplantation for COPD.

EVOLUTION OF LUNG TRANSPLANTATION IN COPD

It was originally believed that patients with end-stage COPD were not suitable for SLT. Objections to SLT for emphysema arose because of perceived problems with the native lung, which would be ventilated during a period of positive-pressure ventilation leading to air trapping, subsequent mediastinal shift and compression of the transplanted lung. Since perfusion would be directed towards the transplanted lung because of expected lower pulmonary vascular resistance, ventilation-perfusion ($\dot{V}A/\dot{Q}$) imbalance would result. These considerations proved to be more than theory and experience in the early 1970s demonstrated that severe ventilation-perfusion imbalance and hyperinflation of the native lung actually occurred.[9,10] Therefore patients with emphysema including those with inherited alpha-1-antitrypsin deficiency were initially treated with combined HLT. Moreover the successful results in patients with alpha-1-antitrypsin deficiency showed that such patients could undergo transplant procedures and retain normal lung function in the first 12–18 months without replacement therapy. The shortfall in donor heart lung blocks led to the introduction of the en bloc double lung transplant for emphysema, but as previously noted this operation was associated with tracheal anastomotic complications in 50% of patients and quickly lost favor. Successful introduction of single lung transplantation for patients with fibrosing lung disease led to re-examination of this procedure for patients with emphysema since techniques of donor lung preservation and surgical technique had improved dramatically from those methods used in the early 1970s.

After a preliminary report of successful SLT for emphysema by Mall and coworkers[11] in France in 1989, the Lung Transplant Group now at Washington University cautiously embarked on a program of SLT in patients with emphysema and demonstrated the utility and safety of this procedure in carefully selected patients.[8] Although the mechanics of the native lung remain the same, improvements in patient selection, lung preservation and anesthetic management have contributed to the success. Subsequent experience from other groups including our own has demonstrated the potential problem of residual infection in the native lung.[12] Moreover, most patients with large bilateral bullae may still show evidence of gross hyperinflation of the native lung in the early postoperative period after SLT and thus the bilateral sequential lung transplantation was successfully applied to patients with emphysema who were not suitable for SLT.

There is now reasonable agreement about technical approaches to transplantation for COPD, in particular emphysema where experience is greatest. Those patients with no evidence of large bilateral bullae are suitable for consideration of SLT. Those patients with frequent pulmonary sepsis or marked bullous disease may be considered for HLT[13] or bilateral sequential lung transplantation, with the latter procedure being increasingly used as the procedure of choice.[14]

INDICATIONS, CONSIDERATIONS AND CRITERIA FOR LUNG TRANSPLANTATION
(Table 33.1)

Age

The shortfall in suitable donor organs leads to an upper age limit of 55–60 years for transplantation of heart and lungs or both lungs alone, with an upper age limit of 65 for transplantation of single lung. The higher age limit for single lung reflects the increased availability of suitable single lungs.

Disease-specific guidelines

Transplantation is usually considered for a patient when estimated life expectancy is less than 18 months. It is inherently difficult to predict the survival in many patients with advanced obstructive disease however and it is now recognized that patients with COPD may experience improved functional capacity following transplantation but not necessarily improved survival. The International Society of Heart and Lung Transplantation Guidelines regarding referral of patients with chronic obstructive pulmonary disease are as follows:

- $FEV_1 < 25\%$ predicted without reversibility
- And/or $Pa_{CO_2} > 7.3$ kPa (55 mmHg)
- And/or pulmonary artery pressures elevated with progressive deterioration such as cor pulmonale

Table 33.1 *Guidelines for transplant referral*

$FEV_1 < 25\%$ predicted
Maximum medical treatment
Rehabilitation
Hypercapnea
Pulmonary hypertension
Unacceptable quality of life

- Preference should be given to those patients with elevated PaCO$_2$ with progressive deterioration who require long-term oxygen therapy as they have the poorest prognosis.[15,16]

Nutritional state

Many patients reaching the end stage of chronic pulmonary disease suffer from cachexia and malnutrition.[17] All recipients lose weight in the first week following transplantation and severe preoperative nutritional deficiency leads to an inability to withstand the rigors of the postoperative period, increasing susceptibility to infection and poor wound healing. Obesity, on the other hand, increases surgical risk, predisposing to atelectasis and impairing postoperative mobility which is essential following lung transplantation. Ideally recipients should weigh within 15 kg of their ideal body weight. There is an increased mortality in adult patients whose body weight is less than 40 kg. The early unsuccessful transplant recipients were all bed bound and the majority of transplant centers now require that recipients are capable of self-care and able to participate in gentle exercise rehabilitation to maintain muscle bulk and physical fitness.

Infection

Localized sepsis preoperatively may lead to severe systemic infection postoperatively because of the need for immunosuppressive therapy. Extrapulmonary sepsis therefore mitigates against successful transplantation. Patients with recurrent or persistent pulmonary infection are not suitable for SLT. Oral hygiene is important and all patients should have any dental sepsis eradicated preoperatively. The presence of subpleural aspergilloma is a contraindication to any form of lung transplantation. Removal of the lung containing an aspergilloma is likely to result in seeding of the pleural space with aspergillus leading to fungal empyema. Removal of the contralateral lung for single lung transplant leaves the aspergilloma in situ and subsequent immunosuppression inevitably will lead to disseminated aspergillus infection.

Previous surgery

There is a risk of life-threatening hemorrhage when the native lungs are removed if there are pleural scars or adhesions. Clearly there is a gradation of risk from scarring due to previous open lung biopsy via a limited thoracotomy to previous total pleurectomy and the latter is regarded as a contraindication for HLT. This has important consequences for the management of pneumothorax in potential recipients with emphysema.

If pleurodesis is required, surgeons should be advised to perform limited anterior pleurodesis. The use of the antifibrinolytic aprotinin during transplant surgery reduces bleeding in patients who have undergone previous thoracotomy,[18] and the recent development of bilateral sequential lung transplantation via a transverse bilateral thoracotomy allows the surgeon much better access to the pleural space than is afforded by a sternotomy. In this regard the bilateral sequential lung transplantation has advantages over the original HLT.

Systemic corticosteroids

Although early lung transplantation programs insisted on patients being weaned from corticosteroids, this proved very difficult to achieve in practice, particularly in patients with COPD. Data from Newcastle have shown that patients with bronchial anastomoses are at no greater risk when receiving up to 20 mg of prednisolone a day compared with those on no prednisolone[19] providing there is no evidence of steroid-induced thinning of the skin, osteoporosis or myopathy.

Osteoporosis

Patients with COPD who are being considered for transplantation may have already been treated with corticosteroids for many years and moreover their intrinsic disease leads to markedly decreased physical activity. These factors along with age and hormonal deficiencies frequently result in a substantial loss of bone mineral density. Immunosuppressive agents post-transplantation such as corticosteroids and cyclosporin accelerate loss of bone mineral. Accordingly patients who have severe osteoporosis or those with a history of compression fractures in the pre-transplantation period are at high risk for the development of the recurrence of fractures postoperatively. Symptomatic osteoporosis is now regarded as a contraindication for transplantation referral until therapy, usually with bisphosphonates, improves bone density.

Cardiac disease

Patients with COPD under consideration for SLT or bilateral sequential lung transplantation ideally should have sufficient preservation of right ventricular function to allow single lung anesthesia, obviating the need for cardiopulmonary bypass. The right ventricle has a very great capacity to show improved function after successful surgery when pulmonary vascular resistance falls to normal and the Toronto Group have successfully performed a single lung transplantation in a patient with a right ventricular ejection fraction of only 12%, although the mean right ventricular ejection fractions of a series of patients reported by this group were 31% and 38% for their SLT and DLT candidates respectively.[16] We have shown that following SLT for pulmonary fibrosis, pulmonary vascular resistance, pulmonary artery pressure and right ventricular performance returned to normal even when markedly abnormal preoperatively.[20] The presence of cor pulmonale complicating COPD is not a contraindication for successful SLT.

Psychologic factors

There is no procedure in medicine which provides more stress for recipients and family than lung transplantation. The process begins from the time of initial referral and lasts until postoperative rehabilitation is complete. Any potential recipient must be well motivated and want a lung transplant, be able to cope and have demonstrated a willingness to comply. A supportive family or circle of close friends is essential. Underlying psychiatric illness, abuse of alcohol or drugs including cigarettes constitutes contraindications.

Presence of other major organ dysfunction

Good renal and hepatic function is essential particularly in view of ciclosporin toxicity.[21] A creatinine clearance of over 50 ml/min is required. Only minor abnormalities of liver function are acceptable. This is clearly of importance in patients with alpha-1-antitrypsin deficiency who may have abnormalities of hepatic function as a result of their disease. The presence of portal hypertension would preclude consideration of lung transplantation alone. Type I diabetes mellitus if well controlled no longer rules out transplantation.

Volume reduction surgery

The successful introduction of volume reduction surgery may have appeared to have added an alternative surgical treatment option for patients under consideration for lung transplantation. In practice however, patients deemed suitable for lung volume reduction surgery represent a different subgroup of patients. The criteria for lung reduction surgery continue to evolve but it is clear that all patients should have ceased smoking and have a marked disability despite completing a comprehensive pulmonary rehabilitation program. All patients should have considerable airflow obstruction with an FEV_1 of less than 35% predicted and marked thoracic hyperinflation. Importantly the lungs should show sufficient heterogeneity in the distribution of emphysema to provide the surgeon with target areas of lung functioning volume occupying lung which is amenable to surgical resection. Patients with severe hypoxemia, hypercapnea or pulmonary hypertension are in general not suitable. Moreover patients with alpha-1-antitrypsin deficiency have been demonstrated to show a rapid decline following volume reduction surgery and this is now considered a contraindication in a majority of surgical units undertaking this procedure. Lung volume reduction surgery and lung transplantation need not however be considered as mutually exclusive procedures. There is now clear evidence that patients can undergo successful lung transplantation following volume reduction surgery in patients whose lung function and quality of life deteriorates after apparent benefit to the point where poor prognostic features develop.

Lung transplantation – an exercise in quality rather than quantity?

Two published studies have provided data suggesting that lung transplantation does not confer in general a survival benefit in patients with end-stage emphysema by 2 years of follow-up. The first study published by Hosenpud and colleagues[22] undertook analysis of data from the Joint United Network for Organ Sharing/International Society of Heart and Lung Transplantation Thoracic Registry. The aim was to clarify the actual survival benefit of lung transplantation in patients with cystic fibrosis, idiopathic pulmonary fibrosis and emphysema. Using a time-dependent non-proportional hazard analysis the risk of mortality after transplantation relative to that in patients on the waiting list was assessed. The data suggested a survival benefit following lung transplantation for patients with cystic fibrosis and idiopathic pulmonary fibrosis. By contrast, in patients with emphysema the mortality rate on the waiting list was low so survival following transplantation did not exceed waiting list survival during the 2-year follow-up.

Some caution is needed over the interpretation of these findings. Firstly, because the data was derived from many centers prior to publication of international guidelines, participating centers were unlikely to have a uniform listing policy for all patients. Moreover, some centers employed a policy of listing patients at an early stage in the development of severe lung dysfunction, giving a long waiting time for lung transplantation candidates. This practice clearly biases the analysis towards waiting list survival. The data presented selectively reported experience in the USA where waiting time is the most important determinant of organ allocation and this clearly encourages larger transplantation centers to list patients early. The Dutch Lung Transplant Group have also published data demonstrating no difference in survival in patients with emphysema who were transplanted compared with those remaining on the waiting list, although this study was underpowered to derive a clear conclusion. Moreover, it is important to note that the conclusions were based on group mean data and it is clear that individual patients with emphysema who were hypoxemic, hypercapnic, underweight, with pulmonary hypertension and a history of previous intubation for an episode of severe Type II respiratory failure have a very different prognosis compared with a disabled but stable patient.

Matching donor to recipient

Donor matching is based on ABO compatibility and size by calculating the predicted total lung capacity (TLC) of both donor and recipient using height, age and sex. There is no direct measurement of donor lung TLC. In patients with COPD who have much greater lung capacities than predicted, it is preferable to give larger lungs than predicted as above, particularly if carrying out SLT. The size discrepancy between the transplanted lung and hemithorax commonly prevents sealing of any parenchymal leak which if present may lead to pneumothoraces persisting for several days. The chest wall remains compliant, and in practice is observed to change shape in the first few days after transplantation. A screening lymphocytoxic cross-match using recipient serum and a banked pool of lymphocytes is carried out in all potential recipients accepted for transplantation to exclude the presence of pre-formed antibodies. Direct cross-match with lymphocytes from a potential donor is only carried out prospectively when this screening test is positive. Wherever possible donor and recipient are matched for cytomegalovirus (CMV) status. If a CMV-negative recipient receives a CMV-positive organ, serious CMV infection can ensue and most centers use prophylactic oral gancyclovir 1 g tds for the first 3 months. This approach prevents CMV disease when immunosuppression is highest and delays its onset until the host response aids recovery. Alternative strategies include the use of weekly testing for levels of antigenaemia by PCR and treating when levels rise.

Choice of operation (Table 33.2)

There are several reasons why unilateral lung transplantation is an attractive option in patients with emphysema. The procedure is technically straightforward and most recipients do not have pleural adhesions. Furthermore, the functional results of single lung transplantation are acceptable, most patients achieving an FEV_1 of 50%

Table 33.2 *Transplantation for COPD*

Single lung	Bilateral lung
Best use of resource	Better lung function but not exercise performance
Less extensive surgery	Better survival at 3 years and quality of life long term
Patients >50 years	Patients <50 years or with bilateral bullae

predicted. These improvements are not as dramatic as those achieved following bilateral lung transplantation. There are, however, no major differences in maximum exercise performance and in general a significant degree of limitation persists with maximum oxygen consumption ranging between 45 and 52% predicted for both procedures. Patients who remain free of obliterative bronchiolitis do, however, enjoy a normal lifestyle and a good quality of life. The obvious advantage of single lung transplantation over bilateral lung transplantation is that this procedure enables more transplantations to be conducted if both donor lungs were acceptable. Critics of the single lung transplantation option are concerned about hyperinflation of the native lung and potential compression of the contralateral graft. Although volume reduction on the opposite side can be considered, the use of single lung transplantation may be best limited to those patients without bullous disease and older patients who may be less able to tolerate the more major bilateral procedure. Furthermore, there is evidence that quality of life and long-term survival is slightly better in bilateral recipients than in their unilateral counterparts. The preference is therefore to offer bilateral lung transplantation to younger patients and those of large stature with significant bilateral bullous disease. One further consideration regarding choice of operation relates to the potential risk of native lung sepsis following single lung transplantation. As a consequence patients with a history of recurrent infective exacerbations associated with continued sputum production are usually offered bilateral lung transplantation. All patients considered for single lung transplantation undergo CT scanning to ensure there is no evidence of bilateral bronchiectasis which would again indicate the need for the bilateral lung procedure.

Finally, the choice as to whether one carries out left or right single lung transplantation is based on a preoperative perfusion scan. Where perfusion is equal then either right or left transplantation is carried out; however, where there is a difference in perfusion which is greater than 40% to the left and 60% to the right then the lung with the least functional contribution is transplanted out of preference.

POSTOPERATIVE COMPLICATIONS AND FOLLOW-UP

Immunosuppression and postoperative management

Most patients are extubated within 36 hours of surgery and then begin an active program of mobilization. Fluid intake is restricted in the early postoperative period with diuresis encouraged to avoid accumulation of fluid in the lungs. Prophylactic antibiotics in the form of flucloxacillin and metronidazole are given for the first 5 days and the donor lungs are lavaged with samples sent to microbiology, prior to implantation, so that appropriate antibiotics may be started early to cover 'donor acquired' pulmonary sepsis. At present patients receive azathioprine, antithymocyte globulin, methylprednisolone and ciclosporin during the immediate postoperative period. Alternative therapy by substituting azathioprine with mycophenolate mofetil or ciclosporin with tacrolimus is favored by some centers. Antithymocyte globulin is stopped after 3 days and methylprednisolone substituted by oral prednisolone at a rapidly tailing dose to a maintenance of 0.1 mg/kg. If patients have no evidence of lung rejection at 3 months, maintenance steroids may be withdrawn. Rejection episodes are treated with pulsed methylprednisolone 10 mg/kg i.v. for 3 days following by augmented oral prednisolone for 1 month. Patients with recurrent acute rejection episodes of steroid-resistant rejection are treated with antithymocyte globulin, photophoresis or methotrexate.

Assessment of graft function

Over the first few postoperative days analysis of blood gases and examination of chest radiographs are used to monitor graft function. Thereafter chest radiographs are performed daily for approximately 1 week and lung function is monitored by continuous oximetry, daily spirometry and regular measurement of lung volumes and diffusing capacity. Patients undergoing single lung transplantation for COPD undergo a ventilation perfusion scan in the first week to ensure good perfusion and ventilation to the newly transplanted lung. In patients with emphysema there is both early preferential ventilation and perfusion to the transplanted lung, unlike the situation following single lung transplantation for pulmonary fibrosis when preferential ventilation appears to lag being preferential perfusion by about 5 weeks.[23] The principal problem in the management of lung transplant recipients is that clinically it is impossible to separate opportunist infections of the lung from lung rejection. Both complications can present identical respiratory symptoms and identical respiratory physical signs. A chest radiograph is also unhelpful since pulmonary infiltrates may be common to both and in the early postoperative period may also occur as a result of reimplantation injury. Moreover the chest radiograph may be entirely normal in patients experiencing acute rejection. This is particularly true in the first month after transplantation. During most episodes of acute rejection and infection the FEV_1 and diffusing capacity show a sustained fall of greater than 10% and thus unlike other solid organ transplant patients graft function following lung transplantation can be monitored with ease. Many transplant units teach recipients to monitor their own FEV_1 using hand-held battery spirometers.

A diagnosis of rejection is currently based on transbronchial biopsy using alligator forceps under radiologic screening.[24] The principal morphologic changes found in acute rejection are perivascular infiltrates which may extend into alveolar septa at the later stages of rejection. Additionally bronchial tissue may also show evidence of lymphocytic infiltrate. It is our practice to carry out three or four biopsies from each lobe of one lung since rejection may be patchy and the use of multiple biopsies from multiple lobes affords greater chance of positive diagnosis. Moreover opportunist infection and rejection may coexist. In a series reported from Papworth Hospital just under 25% of the biopsies performed in the face of a deteriorating clinical condition or a reduction in lung function showed the presence of both infection and rejection. For this reason bronchoalveolar lavage is routinely combined with transbronchial biopsy and lavage submitted for both viral culture, monoclonal staining for pneumocystis and routine culture for bacteria and fungi. The practice of routine surveillance transbronchial lung biopsies on all patients at 1 week, 1 month, 3 months, 6 months, 12 months and thereafter on an annual basis is standard practice.

Results

Providing patients are appropriately selected the results of HLT, SLT and bilateral sequential single lung transplantation are good.[12–14,25] Approximately 10–15% of recipients will die in the first few weeks following transplantation, generally due to problems with poor lung preservation leading to diffuse alveolar damage, sepsis or both. The 1-year survival for centers in the UK lies between 70 and 80%, with a 3-year survival of 55–60%. The most important complications leading to death comprise opportunist infections and the development of obliterative bronchiolitis (OB). Current data suggest approximately 30% of patients surviving the perioperative period will subsequently develop OB within 5 years of their transplantation. This leads in the majority of cases to a progressive deterioration in lung function unresponsive to medical therapy and ultimate progression to respiratory failure, death or consideration of retransplantation after 6–12 months.

After SLT for COPD the transplanted lung receives approximately 80% of the total ventilation and perfusion over the first year. As one would predict the flow volume curve after SLT for emphysema shows a two-compartment pattern, the initial high flow originating from the transplanted lung and the subsequent 'tail' of low flow from the native lung. Lung function, CT scans and transbronchial lung biopsies have revealed normal results in patients up to 5 years after transplantation, indicating the potential for prolonged survival in patients who do not develop OB.

Long-term complications

OBLITERATIVE BRONCHIOLITIS

This process may be defined physiologically by the development of progressive irreversible airflow obstruction unresponsive to augmented steroids.[26] Pathology shows obliteration of bronchioles, the lumens of which are filled by organizing fibrin associated with fibroblasts and mononuclear cells. Immunohistology has revealed that the walls of the bronchioles are infiltrated by CD8 lymphocytes.[27] The small bronchioles are left as fibrous bands extending out to the pleura with associated dilatation and bronchiectasis of proximal airways. Vascular sclerosis affecting both pulmonary arteries and pulmonary veins may also be seen in conjunction with obliterative bronchiolitis. Current evidence suggests that the development of obliterative bronchiolitis is related to the trauma and severity of rejection occurring in the first 6–12 months following transplantation and it is the presence of persisting rejection after the first month which is probably most important. More recent evidence has demonstrated a clear relationship between the presence of both lymphocytic bronchiolitis which represents airway directed rejection and organizing pneumonia in the subsequent development of obliterative bronchiolitis.

The disease usually results in a progressive loss of function due to airflow obstruction over a 6–12-month period leading to respiratory failure and death. However, a few patients appear to 'stabilize' with evidence of inactive OB on biopsy and an attenuation of the loss in FEV_1. Some patients with OB have demonstrated a clinical response to increased immunosuppression.[28] In patients who are maintained on ciclosporin, a switch to tacrolimus or total lymphoid irradiation may stabilize lung function. Other approaches have included cyclophosphamide. Continued research aims to identify those patients at risk of this most important complication at an early stage when augmented immunosuppression may be successful in preventing irreversible bronchiolar obliteration.

LYMPHOPROLIFERATIVE DISORDERS

The association between immunosuppression and lymphoproliferative disorders has been well recognized and the most common form affects the B-cell lineage resulting in B-cell non-Hodgkin's lymphoma. These lymphomas are usually associated with the Epstein–Barr virus. Normal lymphatic tissue has been found within lung transplant parenchyma itself as well as in lymph nodes and spleen and the lymphoma usually responds to a reduction in the level of immunosuppression.

Disease recurrence

So far there is no evidence that patients with COPD including those with alpha-1-antitrypsin deficiency and emphysema, develop recurrence of their original disease. All transplantation centers regard the cessation of smoking as an absolute requirement for acceptance onto the active waiting list and thus providing that recipients do not take up smoking again it should reduce the potential risk of disease recurrence.

CONCLUSIONS

Lung transplantation now offers an effective therapy for patients with end-stage COPD. Debate remains as to which operation patients with COPD and particularly emphysema are most suited but in practice well-chosen recipients, without the presence of frequent pulmonary sepsis or bilateral bullae, appear to do well with single lung transplantation. Patients with these complications do as well with bilateral sequential single lung transplants as HLT. The major problems facing lung transplantation at this time is a shortfall in suitable donor organs compared to the number of potential recipients and for this reason we do not advocate that patients on the active waiting list should be intubated for chronic ventilation. In the early postoperative period opportunist infection and graft rejection remain the major problems and in the long term obliterative bronchiolitis will affect approximately 30% of patients leading to potential graft failure. There is much current research aimed at reducing this figure and certainly patients with COPD who have received lung transplants and remain free of this complication enjoy an excellent standard of life with normal or near normal restoration of activity and good prospects of prolonged survival.

REFERENCES

1. Reitz B, Wallwork J, Hunt SA, *et al*. Heart lung transplantation: a successful therapy for patients with pulmonary vascular disease. *N Engl J Med* 1982;**306**:557–63.

2. Penketh A, Higenbottam T, Hakim M, Wallwork J. Heart and lung transplantation in patients with end stage lung disease. *Br Med J* 1987;**295**:311–14.

3. Wildevuuer CRH, Benfield JR. A review of 23 lung transplantation by 20 surgeons. *Ann Thorac Surg* 1979; **9**:489–515.

4. Toronto Lung Transplant Group. Unilateral transplant for pulmonary fibrosis. *Journal* 1986;**314**:1140–5.

5. Patterson GA, Cooper JD, Goldman B, *et al*. Technique of successful clinical double lung transplantation. *Ann Thorac Surg* 1988;**45**:626–33.

6. Patterson GA, Todd TR, Cooper JD, *et al*. Airway complications following double lung transplantation. *J Thorac Cardiovasc Surg* 1990;**99**:14–21.

7. Noirclerc MJ, Metras D, Vaillant A, *et al*. Bilateral bronchial anastomosis in double lung and heart lung transplantations. *Eur J Cardiothorac Surg* 1990;**4**:314–17.

8. Pasque MK, Cooper JD, Kaiser LR, *et al*. Improved technique for bilateral lung transplantations: rationale and initial clinical experience. *Ann Thorac Surg* 1990;**46**:785–91.

9. Stevens PM, Johnson PC, Bell RL, *et al*. Regional ventilation and perfusion after lung transplantations in patients with emphysema. *N Engl J Med* 1970;**282**:245–9.

10. Vanderhoeft RJ, Roemans P, Nemry C, *et al*. Left lung transplantation in a patient with emphysema. *Arch Surg* 1974;**103**:505–9.

11. Mal H, Andreassin B, Fabrice P, *et al*. Unilateral lung transplantation in end stage pulmonary emphysema. *Am Rev Respir Dis* 1989;**26**:704–6.

12. Colquhoun IW, Gascoigne AD, Gould FK, *et al*. Native pulmonary sepsis following single lung transplantation. 1991;**52**:931–3.

13. Khagani A, Banner N, Ozdogan E, *et al*. Unilateral lung transplantation in end stage pulmonary emphysema. *J Heart Lung Transplant* 1991;**10**:15–21.

14. Kaiser LR, Pasque ML, Trulock EP, *et al*. Bilateral sequential lung transplantations: the procedure of choice for double lung replacement. *Ann Thorac Surg* 1991;**52**:438–46.

15. ISHLT International Guidelines for Selection of Lung Transplant Candidates. *J Heart Lung Transplant* 1998;**17**:703–9.

16. Morrison DL, Maurer JR, Grossman RF. Preoperative assessment for lung transplantation. *Clin Chest Med* 1990;**2**:207–15.

17. Hunter AMB, Carey MA, Larsh HE. The nutritional status of patients with chronic obstructive pulmonary disease. *Am Rev Respir Dis* 1981;**124**:376–81.

18. Bidstrup BP, Royston D, Supsford RW, Taylor KM. Reduction in blood loss and blood use after cardiopulmonary bypass with high dose aprotinin. *J Thorac Cardiovasc Surg* 1989; **93**:364–72.

19. Colquhoun IW, Gascoigne AD, Au J, *et al*. Airway complications following pulmonary transplantation. *Ann Thorac Surg* 1994;**57**:141–5.

20. Doig JC, Richens D, Corris PA, *et al*. Resolution of pulmonary hypertension after single lung transplantation. *Br Heart J* 1991;**66**:431–4.

21. Bennett WM, Pulliam JP. Ciclosporin nephrotoxicity. *Ann Intern Med* 1983;**99**:851–4.

22. Hosenpud JD, Bennett LE, Keck BM, Edwards EB, Novick EJ. Effect of diagnosis on survival benefit of lung transplantation for end stage lung disease. *Lancet* 1998;**351**:24–7.

23. McCleod AT, Stone TN, Hawkins T, *et al*. Ventilation perfusion relationships after single lung transplantation for pulmonary fibrosis. *Am Rev Respir Dis* 1989;**139**:A265.

24. Higenbottam T, Stuart S, Penketh A, Wallwork J. Transbronchial lung biopsy for the diagnosis of rejection in heart lung transplant recipients. *Transplantation* 1988;**46**:532–9.

25. Yacoub M, Khagani A, Theodoropoulos S, *et al*. Single lung transplantation for obstructive airways disease. *Transpl Proc* 1991;**23**:1213–14.

26. Scott JP, Higenbottam TW, Sharples C, *et al*. Risk factors for obliterative bronchiolitis in heart lung transplant recipients. *Transplantation* 1991;**51**:813–17.

27. Milne DS, Gascoigne AD, Wilkes J, *et al*. The immunohistological features of obliterative bronchiolitis following lung transplantation. *Transplantation* 1992; **54**:748–50.

28. Glanville AR, Baldwin JC, Bourke CM, *et al*. Obliterative bronchiolitis after heart lung transplantation: apparent arrest by augmented immunosuppression. *Ann Intern Med* 1987;**107**:300–4.

34

Guidelines for COPD management

PETER MA CALVERLEY AND WILLIAM MACNEE

There are now a large number of documents generated singularly and jointly by many national and international bodies, all of which offer recommendations about the diagnosis and management of COPD. Almost all of these have been produced since the first edition of this book was published and to date there is no sign that their number, either as new statements or in revised form, is diminishing. These documents are important as they act as benchmarks against which current practice in COPD care is judged. Despite attempts at careful wording in the titles of some documents,[1,2] they are used as guides to what should or should not be funded, at least in certain healthcare systems. Thus, it is important to be aware of their strengths and limitations and relate their contents to the individual physician's approach to COPD management.

It is a certainty that by the time this chapter is read new and somewhat different advice will be available in the revised versions of several of the international guidelines. Hence a detailed analysis of the similarities and differences of existing guidelines is not particularly fruitful since more detailed and authoritative information is available in the earlier chapters of this book, often written by the same people who formulate the international management guidance. Instead, we wish to examine several other features common to all the documents, consider areas where their recommendations may change in the next 5 years and, finally, suggest an approach to patient care based on current evidence.

GUIDELINES ON COPD – FORM AND CONTENTS

Although individual review articles have advocated approaches to COPD care for many years, the first guidelines about this topic supported by a national thoracic society were those of Canada, soon followed by the Australian and New Zealand Thoracic Society and their Swiss counterparts. These documents arose directly from the perceived success of the asthma management guidelines in the early 1990s which was seen as a valuable way of stimulating rational and effective therapy in patients who might not have received this previously. Although the capacity to produce dramatic improvements in individual patient well being is rather smaller in COPD than asthma, overall, substantial gains in health care should be possible by applying this approach. As with asthma the large international societies also formulated their views about management, the most important being those of the European Respiratory Society (ERS) and the American Thoracic Society (ATS), with the British Thoracic Society (BTS) also making a contribution somewhat later.[2–4] Finally, a group organized by the World Health Organization/National Heart Lung and Blood Institute (WHO/NHLBI) in the USA was founded with the acronym GOLD – The Global Initiative for Chronic Obstructive Lung Disease – and detailed recommendations were made available in early 2001 with a printed executive summary and additional information available on the internet.[5]

Until GOLD, all of the proceeding documents were expert consensus statements, reflecting knowledgeable but potentially selective reviews of the literature by the participants. The early statements arose only from thoracic physicians, although the BTS made specific efforts to include general physicians in both primary and secondary care, accident and emergency specialist nurses, and patient representatives, and also tried to offer relatively specific management advice. An earlier attempt by the ERS to develop a management flow chart to apply their

Table 34.1 *GOLD: objectives*

Increase awareness of COPD among health professionals,
 health authorities and the general public
Improve diagnosis, management and prevention
Stimulate research

recommendations proved to be too complex to use in routine practice.[3]

The GOLD program represents a further advance on the earlier approaches. Its aims and key features are summarized in Table 34.1. This is the first group to try and evaluate the strength of evidence for the statements made. The scaling adopted is a relatively simple one and may not meet the more rigorous approaches advocated by some enthusiasts for evidence-based medicine. Nonetheless, it does give a clear level of support for certain areas, for example mucolytic therapy, that had been dismissed in previous reviews. At present the BTS Guidelines have been subsumed within the UK National Institute for Clinical Excellence (NICE) guidelines program. The next revision is based on conducting multiple systematic reviews of all studies that have been reported as relevant to COPD. Whether the resulting recommendations will differ from those arrived at by using the simpler methodology developed by GOLD or indeed those arrived at by expert consensus is not at all clear. It may be that the literature published relevant to COPD will need to generate more controversy before the additional sophistication of the NICE approach is necessary.

A further novel feature of GOLD is the regular review of new scientific evidence and annual web-based updates in relation to the original recommendations. This process should overcome a major failing of all previous documents, that is the lengthy interval between revisions. Fortunately, a significant number of important studies have been reported in the last decade providing new evidence about the effects of existing therapy and evaluating new treatment approaches. Until now, a revision of the whole document was undertaken before this new information could be set into a clinical context. While this may not limit the therapeutic choices made by informed clinicians, it has delayed funding for treatment approaches that are clearly evidence based but not in the existing guidelines. The GOLD concept clearly permits a more timely inclusion of important information and the next revision of the now joint ERS/ATS guidelines will reflect this by being a web-based document.

Despite the advantages of existing documents it is still appropriate for some local modifications to take place and this again is encouraged as part of the GOLD plan. Clearly, resources will vary from country to country and the pattern of implementation is likely to be influenced by the existing methods of physician reimbursement and patient referral. The purpose of GOLD and future guidelines should be to ensure that treatment recommendations are based on evidence and the individual healthcare system will need to balance what has been recommended against what it perceives as appropriate to spend on COPD patients. It should no longer be acceptable to spend limited resources on treatments that are suboptimal or ineffective simply because that has always been the previous treatment norm.

DEFINING COPD

Several different definitions have been proposed by the various guidelines and several of these are shown in Table 34.2. No specific ATS definition is given here, as until recently this was based on the non-proportional Venn diagram developed by Snider to cope with the differential contributions of the underlying pathology to the individual COPD patient. The problems of defining COPD are dealt with in Chapter 1 but one further aspect should be stressed here. The definition selected by all guidelines leans towards terms that can be applied practically. Hence the emphasis on airflow obstruction (reduced FEV_1/FVC or, in the ERS version, slow forced emptying of the lungs) and lack of spontaneous variability (largely fixed in the BTS definition, not fully reversible in GOLD). Most definitions stress the progressive nature of the symptoms and physiological change and GOLD emphasizes the key role of inhaled insults as a pathogenic mechanism. Based on these approaches clinicians should be able to identify a patient with COPD and apply an appropriate management strategy. However, these definitions focus on the clinicophysiological outcomes of the processes that are occurring within the lower respiratory tract of the COPD patient. They are not the ideal way of identifying patients when a specific mechanism is to be studied, for example regulation of vascular endothelial growth factor (VEGF) in the pulmonary endothelium as a mechanism promoting apoptosis in emphysema.[6] They also do not account for the heterogeneity of the disease. Clearly, not all patients who meet the clinical definitions have a significant degree of emphysema. Thus studies of this mechanism or indeed of agents to promote alveolar regeneration would not necessarily be appropriate in a clinically defined COPD population. We are still ignorant of the role of individual pathologic phenotypes in the natural history of COPD, but the development of these mechanistic studies, together with the availability of quantitative CT scanning (see Chapter 21), may provide the necessary stimulus to initiate these longer-term investigations. Until such data are available, the definition of COPD will remain a compromise equivalent to that of 'cardiac failure' but without the specificity that allows us to subclassify cardiac dysfunction into systolic and diastolic or determine even more basic causes of

Table 34.2 *Definition of COPD*

European Respiratory Society 1995

Chronic obstructive pulmonary disease (COPD) is a disorder characterized by reduced maximum expiratory flow and slow forced emptying of the lungs; features which do not change markedly over several months. Most of the airflow limitation is slowly progressive and irreversible. The airflow limitation is due to varying combinations of airway disease and emphysema; the relative contribution of the two processes is difficult to define *in vivo*

British Thoracic Society 1997

Chronic obstructive pulmonary disease (COPD) is a chronic, slowly progressive disorder characterized by airflow obstruction (reduced FEV_1 and FEV_1/VC ratio) that does not change markedly over several months. Most of the lung function impairment is fixed, although some reversibility can be produced by bronchodilator (or other) therapy

GOLD 2001

Chronic obstructive pulmonary disease (COPD) is a disease state characterized by airflow limitation that is not fully reversible. The airflow limitation is usually both progressive and associated with an abnormal inflammatory response of the lungs to noxious particles or gases

Table 34.3 *Spirometric classification of COPD severity*

	FEV$_1$ (% predicted)		
	Mild/ stage I	Moderate/ stage II	Severe/ stage III
European Thoracic Society	>70	50–69	<50
American Thoracic Society	>50	35–49	<35
British Thoracic Society	60–79	40–59	<40
GOLD	>80	50–79 (A) 30–49 (B)	<30

the problem such as valvular abnormalities. Clearly, there is much work to be done in this area of COPD research.

CLASSIFYING DISEASE SEVERITY

Clinicians look to guidelines to offer a practical approach to grade the severity of disease and relate this to management decisions. In asthma, this has been indirectly related to the patient's symptoms and is usually based on the amount of rescue medication they use and the type of treatment employed to control symptoms. Although there is an approximate relationship of this empirical scheme to the diurnal variation to peak flow and/or the histamine responsiveness, these measures have never been incorporated as primary outcomes in the staging of asthma severity.[7]

A completely different approach has been used in COPD, which may not have always served the patients well. Until recently, most guidelines based their staging on the FEV_1, making the generally reasonable assumption that the lower is the FEV_1 as a percentage of predicted, then the greater would be the pathologic and symptomatic severity. Some of the different proposals about staging are shown in Table 34.3.

At least three problems limit this approach. The first is practical, as until recently spirometry has not been widely available, and this remains a problem especially in less developed countries and in primary care medicine.

Although there are still issues about how best to obtain technically satisfactory recordings (see Chapter 20), improvements in spirometer design and software are making this much easier. More important is the arbitrary nature of the boundaries selected for the severity classification (Table 34.3). Disease severity described spirometrically as a continuously distributed variable in any COPD population and FEV_1 itself will show modest day-to-day variability (see Chapter 20). Patients who lie close to the selected boundary may therefore be reclassified as more or less severe if seen on a different day.

Most important is the relatively poor relationship between health status and spirometry (see Chapter 31), which means that an individual patient with an FEV_1 of 60% predicted can be more symptomatic than one whose FEV_1 is 45% predicted, despite the fact that both are given the same treatment. Since the benefits of bronchodilator therapy and rehabilitation are based on symptomatic improvement (see Chapters 22 and 30) rather than altered lung mechanics, it is irrational to base management too precisely on a specified level of the FEV_1.

The authors of the GOLD guidelines were aware of this dilemma when they produced their severity scheme. They allowed a wide range of spirometric abnormality to encompass stage 2 (moderate) disease and have tried, less successfully than they originally anticipated, to stress that symptoms are the management driver in assessing which treatment should be selected. The most severe subgroup of COPD (<30% predicted in GOLD and <35% predicted in the ATS scheme) are chosen to highlight a population where persistent daytime hypoxemia is more likely to be found and hence where continuous domiciliary oxygen treatment is indicated (see Chapter 29). This clinical problem indicates the weakness of a purely symptom based method of classifying COPD as hypoxemic patients are not necessarily more or less symptomatic than those without this important clinical complication.

Thus, classifying COPD for clinical rather than epidemiologic purposes requires a hybrid approach. Several investigators are trying to develop scoring systems based on spirometry, assessment of dyspnea (such as the MRC dyspnea scale), arterial oxygen tension, body mass index (an important prognostic sign in more severe disease) with or without some measurement of exercise capacity. If successful this should provide a more robust and practical approach to classifying the severity of COPD and its impact on the individual.

GUIDELINES AND MANAGEMENT

Although they were produced at different times and for rather different audiences, there is a large measure of consensus between the different management guidelines about the most important goals of treatment in COPD and how to achieve these. The GOLD objectives for treatment are presented in Table 34.4 and provide a useful checklist, both of the desirable attributes of any new treatment and as a way of assessing how effective a particular treatment strategy has proven.

Often the evaluation of success is subjective, but as noted previously such changes can correspond to quite sophisticated functional improvements (see Chapter 18). Applying a list of this type to patient care does require that the physician be clear about what the intervention is or is not likely to achieve, something that the patient should be fully informed about.

Assessing the response to treatment

Since none of the existing medications for COPD have been shown to modify the long-term decline in lung function which is a hallmark of the disease, efforts in treatment have focused on the use of medications to control symptoms. A major shift in assessing the effects of treatment in COPD has been a move away from simply measuring changes in the degree of airflow limitation as assessed by the FEV_1 with the realization that by definition the FEV_1 in COPD will not change substantially in response to treatment. Recent guidelines have emphasized other end-points such as improvement in health status, exercise capacity and symptom scores, particularly breathlessness. Exercise

capacity and health status are sensitive indicators of the response to treatment and importantly the improvement experienced by the patient.[8,9] Reducing the frequency and severity of exacerbations is also now recognized as an important goal of treatment. The use of health status questionnaires, exercise tests or symptom scores have not reached daily practice as they are time consuming and difficult to apply to individual patients. However, use of simple, standardized questions may help the physician to assess the effect of treatment (Table 34.5).

Bronchodilators

All current guidelines recommend the use of bronchodilators for the relief of symptoms. More recent guidelines, particularly GOLD, recognize that the symptom benefit from the use of bronchodilators in COPD cannot be accurately predicted from the changes in the FEV_1 and relate more to reducing dynamic hyperinflation and hence improving symptoms and exercise tolerance. Considerable evidence has emerged since the publication of even the most recent guidelines, indicating a significant role for long-acting bronchodilators in the treatment of COPD, long-acting beta-agonists, such as salbutamol and formoterol,[10–13] and most recently the long-acting anticholinergic tiotropium.[14,15] The sustained relief of symptoms, convenience of use, improvements in health status and reduction in exacerbation rates in moderate to severe COPD will result in a change in the position of these drugs in future guidelines towards their use earlier in the course of COPD. All of the current guidelines recommend the use of combinations of bronchodilators in patients who remain symptomatic and it seems likely that the same will be applied to long-acting bronchodilators, although evidence is not available at present.

Theophyllines remain as a treatment option in most guidelines but as a second-line bronchodilator therapy because of their systemic administration, narrow therapeutic index and hence the potential for side effects. It remains to be seen whether recent evidence of the anti-inflammatory effect of low-dose theophylline[16] will be translated to clinical improvements in patients.

Table 34.4 *Objectives of COPD management*

Prevent disease progression
Relieve symptoms
Improve exercise tolerance
Improve health status
Prevent and treat exacerbations
Prevent and treat complications
Reduce mortality
Minimize side effects from treatment

Table 34.5 *Assessing the full impact of COPD on the patient's life: asking simple questions*

Has your treatment made a difference to you?
Is your breathing easier in any way?
Can you do some things now that you couldn't before, or do the same things but faster?
Can you do the same things as before, but are now less breathless when you do them?
Has your sleep improved?

Glucocorticosteroids

The role of inhaled glucocorticosteroids remains a controversial topic in the management of COPD, but is the therapeutic area for which considerable new information has recently become available. Many published guidelines have recommended their use only in COPD patients, with significant improvements in FEV_1 following a trial of glucocorticoids or in those with a large degree of reversibility. There is now considerable evidence that a short course of oral glucocorticoids is a poor predictor of the long-term response to inhaled glucocorticoids.[17] Thus, a therapeutic trial of inhaled glucocorticoids is no longer recommended in the most recent COPD guidelines (GOLD). There is still debate[18,19] over the use of inhaled corticosteroids in COPD. The unanimity of the lack of effect of inhaled corticosteroids on the decline in FEV_1 in the four trials which have been published provides sufficient evidence that at all stages of the disease inhaled glucocorticoids do not influence the decline in FEV_1. However, inhaled corticosteroids in moderate to severe COPD do appear to affect symptoms and improve health status, possibly by reducing exacerbation rates.[20,21] The most recent advice from the GOLD guidelines is to use inhaled corticosteroids in patients with documented spirometric response to inhaled glucocorticoids or based on the study showing a positive effect on exacerbations, in patients with an $FEV_1 < 50\%$ predicted (Stage IIB: moderate COPD and Stage III severe COPD) with repeated exacerbations requiring treatment, antibiotics and glucocorticoid steroids. The number of exacerbations that constitute repeated exacerbations is not defined but a figure of two or more exacerbations per year seems to be a consensus view.

The lack of a dramatic effect of inhaled corticosteroids is purported to reflect the lack of effect of corticosteroids on airspace inflammation in COPD.[22,23] However, the results of studies which have assessed airspace inflammation depends on the marker of airway inflammation which has been measured. The results are also likely to be influenced by the heterogeneity of the disease. The results of trials of inhaled corticosteroids do not accurately reflect the effects of inhaled corticosteroids in clinical practice and the possible variable effects in different clinical phenotypes of COPD, since in all inhaled corticosteroids studies considerable care is taken to exclude patients who show any signs of reversibility of their airways disease. It seem likely that in the future we may have biomarkers which may predict the response to corticosteroids and allow more rational application of this therapeutic intervention in patients with COPD.

Pulmonary rehabilitation

There is now consensus on the benefit of pulmonary rehabilitation in symptomatic patients with COPD, at all stages of the disease,[24] but still no consensus on whether repeated rehabilitation courses enable patients to sustain the benefits gained from the initial course of treatment. Guidelines have a role in advocating the use of pulmonary rehabilitation, since in many countries pulmonary rehabilitation is only available in a minority of respiratory centers, in spite of the fact that the evidence is overwhelming in support of a beneficial effect of pulmonary rehabilitation on health status. Indeed the improvement in health status and exercise tolerance following pulmonary rehabilitation outstrips any of the pharmacologic interventions in COPD.

Surgical interventions

Lung transplantation in COPD is now considered in COPD guidelines to have a limited role in improving quality of life and functional capacity in COPD, but its effect on survival is limited.[25] The results of large controlled trials of lung volume reduction surgery are still awaited to determine the benefit or otherwise of this form of treatment.[26]

EXACERBATIONS OF COPD

The importance of impact of exacerbations of COPD on healthcare utilization and the detrimental effects on the health status of patients is emphasized in all guidelines. Exacerbations are now an important target for therapeutic intervention.

The use of antibiotics in exacerbations of COPD remains somewhat controversial, although there is now increasing evidence which supports their use in exacerbations with clinical signs of airway infection (increased sputum volume, purulence, increased breathlessness).[27]

Recent studies have shown a small but significant benefit of oral glucocorticoids in the treatment of exacerbations of COPD (see Chapter 25). The exact dose and duration of treatment is still unknown. There is now a consensus for the use of non-invasive ventilation in COPD but the exact timing of this intervention is still unclear (see Chapter 27).

THE FUTURE OF GUIDELINES

Now that the initial flurry of local and national guidelines has begun to abate it is time to consider what future steps are required to make these documents more effective. The convergence of the different groups on specific recommendations is to be expected given the limited but generally consistent evidence available. Treatment is best considered as cumulative rather than stepping up and down as has been the recommendation in asthma. The obvious exception is the management of the acute exacerbation where persisting with high doses of oral corticosteroids can be both dangerous and damaging for the patient. This pattern is likely to continue until such time as disease modification allows for some of the lung damage that characterizes COPD to be reversed.

The major challenge is now one of implementing what is already known and developing 'user-friendly' clinical management plans that are easily understood by the trainee physician and patient alike. The focus on randomized controlled trial data sometimes detracts from the crucial role played by patients in their own care. If they have realistic expectations of what they can achieve with treatment and what their treatment is supposed to do for them, then disease management becomes substantially easier. If the guidelines drafted now can help achieve that goal as well then their authors should feel well rewarded.

REFERENCES

1. American Thoracic Society. Standards for the care of patients with chronic obstructive pulmonary disease (COPD) and Asthma. *Am Rev Respir Dis* 1987;**136**:225–44.
2. American Thoracic Society. Standards for the diagnosis and care of patients with chronic obstructive pulmonary disease. *Am J Respir Crit Care Med* 1995;**152**:S77–120.
3. Siafakas NM, Vermeire P, Pride NB, *et al.* Optimal assessment and management of chronic obstructive pulmonary disease (COPD). The European Respiratory Society Task Force. *Eur Respir J* 1995;**8**:1398–420.
4. Anonymous. BTS guidelines for the management of chronic obstructive pulmonary disease. The COPD Guidelines Group of the Standards of Care Committee of the BTS. *Thorax* 1997;**52**(suppl 5):S1–28.
5. Pauwels RA, Buist AS, Calverley PMA, Jenkins CR, Hurd SS. Global strategy for the diagnosis, management and prevention of chronic obstructive pulmonary disease. *Am J Respir Crit Care Med* 2001;**163**:1256–76.
6. Kasahara Y, Tuder RM, Cool CD, Lynch DA, Flores SC, Voelkel NF. Endothelial cell death and decreased expression of vascular endothelial growth factor and vascular endothelial growth factor receptor 2 in emphysema. *Am J Respir Crit Care Med* 2001;**163**:737–44.
7. Anonymous. The British guidelines on asthma management 1995 review and position statement. *Thorax* 1997;**52**(suppl 1):i–s21.
8. Hay JG, Stone P, Carter J, *et al.* Bronchodilator reversibility, exercise performance and breathlessness in stable chronic obstructive pulmonary disease. *Eur Respir J* 1992;**5**:659–64.
9. Griffiths TL, Burr ML, Campbell IA, *et al.* Results at 1 year of out-patient multidisciplinary pulmonary rehabilitation. *Lancet* 2000;**355**:362–8.
10. Rennard SI, Anderson W, Wallack R, *et al.* Use of a long-acting inhaled beta$_2$-adrenergic agonist, salmeterol xinafoate, in patients with chronic obstructive pulmonary disease. *Am J Respir Crit Care Med* 2001;**163**:1087–92.
11. Ramirez-Venegas A, Ward J, Lentine T, Mahler DA. Salmeterol reduces dyspnea and improves lung function in patients with COPD. *Chest* 1997;**112**:336–40.
12. Dahl R, Greefhorst LA, Nowak D, *et al.* Inhaled formoterol dry powder versus ipratropium bromide in chronic obstructive pulmonary disease. *Am J Respir Crit Care Med* 2001;**164**:778–84.
13. Rossi A, Kristufek P, Levine BE, *et al.* Comparison of the efficacy, tolerability, and safety of formoterol dry powder and oral, slow-release theophylline in the treatment of COPD. *Chest* 2002;**121**:1058–69.
14. Casaburi R, Mahler DA, Jones PW, *et al.* A long-term evaluation of once-daily inhaled tiotropium in chronic obstructive pulmonary disease. *Eur Respir J* 2002;**19**:217–24.
15. Vincken W, Van Noord JA, Greefhorst AP, *et al.* Improved health outcomes in patients with COPD during 1 year's treatment with tiotropium. *Eur Respir J* 2002;**19**:209–16.
16. Culpitt S, de Matos C, Russell RE, Donnelly LE, Rogers DF, Barnes PJ. Effect of theophylline on induced sputum inflammatory indices and neutrophil chemotaxis in chronic obstructive pulmonary disease. *Am J Respir Crit Care Med* 2002;**165**:1371–6.
17. Burge PS, Calverley PMA, Jones PW, Spencer S, Anderson JA. Prednisolone response in chronic obstructive pulmonary disease. *Thorax* 2003;(in press).
18. Calverley PMA. Inhaled corticosteroids are beneficial in chronic obstructive pulmonary disease. *Am J Respir Crit Care Med* 2000;**161**:341–2.
19. Barnes PJ. Inhaled corticosteroids are not beneficial in chronic obstructive pulmonary disease. *Am J Respir Crit Care Med* 2000;**161**:342–4.
20. Burge PS, Calverley PM, Jones PW, Spencer S, Anderson JA, Maslen TK. Randomised, double blind, placebo controlled study of fluticasone propionate in patients with moderate to severe chronic obstructive pulmonary disease: the ISOLDE trial. *Br Med J* 2000;**320**:1297–303.
21. Alsaeedi A, Sin DD, McAlister FA. The effects of inhaled corticosteroids in chronic obstructive pulmonary disease: a systematic review of randomized placebo-controlled trials. *Am J Med* 2002;**113**:59–65.
22. Keatings VM, Jatakanon A, Worsdell YM, Barnes PJ. Effects of inhaled and oral glucocorticoids on inflammatory indices in asthma and COPD. *Am J Respir Crit Care Med* 1997;**155**:542–8.
23. Culpitt SV, Maziak W, Loukidis S, *et al.* Effect of high dose inhaled steroid on cells, cytokines, and proteases in induced sputum in chronic obstructive pulmonary disease. *Am J Respir Crit Care Med* 1999;**160**:1635–9.
24. Ries AL, Carlin BW, Carlin V, *et al.* Pulmonary rehabilitation: Joint ACCP/AACVPR evidence-based guidelines. *J Cardiopulm Rehabil* 1997;**17**:371–405.
25. Hosenpud JD, Bennett LE, Keck BM, Edwards EB, Novick RJ. Effect of diagnosis on survival benefit of lung transplantation for end-stage lung disease. *Lancet* 1998;**351**:24–7 [see comments].
26. Anonymous. Rationale and design of the National Emphysema Treatment Trial (NETT): a prospective randomized trial of lung volume reduction surgery. *J Thorac Cardiovasc Surg* 1999;**118**:518–28.
27. Saint S, Bent S, Vittinghoff E, Grady D. Antibiotics in chronic obstructive pulmonary disease exacerbations. A meta-analysis. *JAMA* 1995;**273**:957–60.

Index